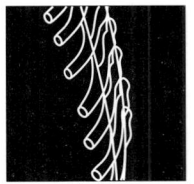

The Lumbar Spine

THE INTERNATIONAL SOCIETY FOR THE STUDY OF THE LUMBAR SPINE

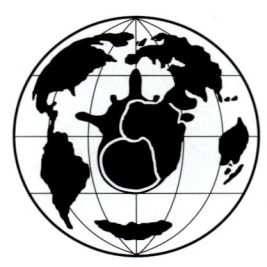

Editorial Committee

SAM W. WIESEL, M.D.
Professor and Chairman
Department of Orthopaedic Surgery
Georgetown University Medical Center
Washington, District of Columbia

JAMES N. WEINSTEIN, D.O.
Endowed Professor
University of Iowa College of Medicine
Iowa City, Iowa

HARRY N. HERKOWITZ, M.D.
Chairman, Department of Orthopaedic Surgery
William Beaumont Hospital
Royal Oak, Michigan

JIŘÍ DVOŘÁK, M.D.
Head, Department of Neurology, Spine Unit
W. Schulthess Hospital
Zurich, Switzerland

GORDON R. BELL, M.D.
Head, Section of Spinal Surgery
Department of Orthopaedic Surgery
Cleveland Clinic Foundation
Cleveland, Ohio

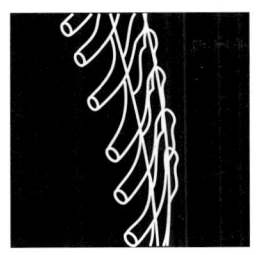

VOLUME 2

The Lumbar Spine

■

SECOND
EDITION

W.B. SAUNDERS COMPANY
A Division of Harcourt Brace & Company
PHILADELPHIA   LONDON   TORONTO   MONTREAL   SYDNEY   TOKYO

W.B. SAUNDERS COMPANY
A Division of Harcourt Brace & Company

The Curtis Center
Independence Square West
Philadelphia, Pennsylvania 19106

Library of Congress Cataloging-in-Publication Data

The Lumbar spine / the International Society for the Study of the Lumbar Spine; editorial committee, Sam W. Wiesel . . . [et al.].—2nd ed.

  p.   cm.

Includes bibliographical references and index.

ISBN 0–7216–4953–X (set)

1. Backache.   2. Lumbar vertebrae—Diseases.   I. Wiesel, Sam W.
II. The International Society for the Study of the Lumbar Spine.
[DNLM: 1. Lumbar Vertebrae.   2. Spinal Diseases. WE 750 L95665 1996]

RD771.B217L86   1996

617.5′6—dc20

DNLM/DLC   95–10052

The Lumbar Spine, 2nd edition

ISBN Volume 1   0–7216–6942–5
      Volume 2   0–7216–6943–3
      Two-Volume Set   0–7216–4953–X

Copyright © 1996, 1990 by W.B. Saunders Company.

All rights reserved. No part of this publication may be reproduced or transmitted in any form or by any means, electronic or mechanical, including photocopy, recording, or any information storage and retrieval system, without permission in writing from the publisher.

Printed in the United States of America.

Last digit is the print number: 9   8   7   6   5   4   3   2   1

*This text is dedicated to
Shirley Fitzgerald,
who has faithfully served as the Administrative Secretary
of the society for many years.
In large measure, our success is due
to her enthusiastic hard work.*

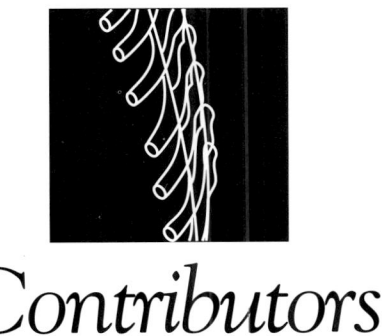

Contributors

TODD J. ALBERT, M.D.
Assistant Professor, Department of Orthopaedic Surgery, Thomas Jefferson University, Philadelphia, Pennsylvania. Attending Surgeon, Rothman Institute, Pennsylvania Hospital, Philadelphia, Pennsylvania

Chapter 21. Adult Scoliosis: Evaluation and Decision-Making

GUNNAR B. J. ANDERSSON, M.D., Ph.D.
Professor and Chairman, Department of Orthopedic Surgery, Rush Medical College, Chicago, Illinois. Chairman, Department of Orthopedic Surgery; Senior Attending, Rush-Presbyterian-St. Luke's Medical Center, Chicago, Illinois

Chapter 4. Biomechanics: Occupational Biomechanics; Chapter 18: Low Back Pain in Pregnancy

RICHARD A. BALDERSTON, M.D.
Professor, Chief of Scoliosis Service, Department of Orthopaedic Surgery, Thomas Jefferson University, Philadelphia, Pennsylvania

Chapter 8. Lumbar and Lumbosacral Spondylolisthesis: Surgical Treatment of Adult Degenerative Spondylolisthesis; Chapter 21. Adult Scoliosis: Evaluation and Decision-Making

MICHELE CRITES BATTIÉ, Ph.D.
Professor and Chair, Department of Physical Therapy, University of Alberta, Edmonton, Alberta, Canada

Chapter 1. Epidemiology: Epidemiology of Disc Disease; Chapter 17. Rehabilitation: Education and Training; Chapter 19. Industrial Low Back Pain: Risk Factors

GORDON R. BELL, M.D.
Head, Section of Spinal Surgery, Department of Orthopaedic Surgery, Cleveland Clinic Foundation, Cleveland, Ohio

Chapter 2. Anatomy of the Lumbar Spine: Developmental to Normal Adult Anatomy; Chapter 15. Complications of Lumbar Spine Surgery

MICHEL BENOIST, M.D.
Consultant Rheumatologist of Paris Hospitals, University of Paris VII, Paris, France

Chapter 7. Clinical Entities: Alternative Techniques for Disc Decompression: Percutaneous Discectomy and Chemonucleolysis; Chapter 11. Inflammatory Disorders: Inflammatory Spondyloarthropathies

CONTRIBUTORS

STANLEY J. BIGOS, M.D.
Professor in Orthopaedics, School of Medicine, University of Washington; Adjunct Professor of Environmental Health, School of Public Health, University of Washington, Seattle, Washington
Chapter 19. Industrial Low Back Pain: Risk Factors

SCOTT D. BODEN, M.D.
Associate Professor, Department of Orthopaedic Surgery, Emory University School of Medicine, Atlanta, Georgia. Director, Emory Spine Center, Emory University System of Health Care, Atlanta, Georgia
Chapter 7. Clinical Entities: Lumbar Spine Algorithm; Chapter 20. Multiply Operated Spine: Algorithmic Approach; Chapter 24. Fusion: Biology of Lumbar Spine Fusion and Bone Graft Materials

DAVID S. BRADFORD, M.D.
Professor and Chairman, Department of Orthopaedic Surgery, University of California, San Francisco, School of Medicine, San Francisco, California. Medical Staff, Moffitt/Long Hospital, San Francisco, California
Chapter 8. Lumbar and Lumbosacral Spondylolisthesis: Surgical Treatment of Isthmic and Dysplastic Spondylolisthesis in the Adult

PAUL BRINCKMANN, Prof. Dr. rer. nat.
Institute for Experimental Biomechanics, University of Münster, Münster, Germany
Chapter 4. Biomechanics: Effects of Repeated Loads and Vibration

CHARLES V. BURTON, M.D.
Medical Director, Institute for Low Back Care, Minneapolis, Minnesota
Chapter 26. The Ethics of Spine Care

JOHN M. CAVANAUGH, B.S., M.S., M.D.
Research Scientist, Bioengineering Center, Wayne State University, Detroit, Michigan
Chapter 3. Diagnosis and Neuromechanisms: Neurophysiologic Basis of Low Back Pain

RICK B. DELAMARTER, M.D.
Associate Clinical Professor, Department of Orthopaedic Surgery, UCLA School of Medicine, Los Angeles, California. Co-Director, UCLA Comprehensive Spine Center, Los Angeles, California
Chapter 7. Clinical Entities: Surgical Indications and Techniques; Chapter 20. Multiply Operated Lumbar Spine: Algorithmic Approach

RICHARD A. DEYO, M.D., M.P.H.
Professor, Departments of Medicine and Health Services, University of Washington, Seattle, Washington. Staff Physician, Veterans Affairs Medical Center, Seattle, Washington
Chapter 6. Radiology: Reproducibility and Accuracy of Lumbar Spine Imaging Studies

RONALD DONELSON, M.D.
Assistant Professor, Department of Orthopedic Surgery, State University of New York Health Science Center at Syracuse, Syracuse, New York. Medical Staff, State University Hospital, Syracuse, New York
Chapter 17. Rehabilitation: Mechanical Diagnosis and Therapy for Low Back Pain: Toward a Better Understanding

JOHN DOVE, F.R.C.S.
Stoke-on-Trent Spinal Service, Stoke-on-Trent, England
Chapter 20. Multiply Operated Lumbar Spine: Algorithmic Approach

JIŘÍ DVOŘÁK, M.D.
Head, Department of Neurology, Spine Unit, W. Schulthess Hospital, Zurich, Switzerland
Chapter 3. Diagnosis and Neuromechanisms: Clinical Neurophysiology and Electrodiagnostic Testing in Low Back Pain; Chapter 9. Lumbar Spinal Stenosis: Clinical, Radiologic, and Electrodiagnostic Diagnosis of Degenerative Lumbar Stenosis

ANTHONY P. DWYER, M.D.
Professor of Orthopaedics, University of Colorado Health Sciences Center, Denver, Colorado
Chapter 2. Anatomy of the Lumbar Spine: Clinically Relevant Anatomy

W. THOMAS EDWARDS, Ph.D.
Associate Professor, Orthopedic Research Laboratory, Department of Orthopedic Surgery, State University of New York Health Science Center at Syracuse, Syracuse, New York

Chapter 4. Biomechanics: Biomechanical Analyses of Loads on the Lumbar Spine

STEPHEN EISENSTEIN, Ph.D., F.R.C.S.
Director, Centre for Spinal Studies, The Robert Jones Agnes Hunt Orthopaedic Hospital, Oswestry, England. Senior Lecturer, Faculty of Postgraduate Medicine, Keele University, Staffordshire, England

Chapter 20. The Multiply Operated Lumbar Spine: Algorithmic Approach

FRANK EISMONT, M.D., F.A.C.S.
Professor of Orthopaedic Surgery, University of Miami School of Medicine, Miami, Florida

Chapter 12. Fractures of the Lumbar Spine: Evaluation, Classification, and Treatment

JOSEPH E. EPSTEIN, M.D.
Clinical Professor of Neurological Surgery, Albert Einstein College of Medicine, Bronx, New York. Honorary Attending, Department of Surgery, Division of Neurosurgery, The North Shore University Hospital, Manhasset, New York, and The Cornell University Medical College, New York, New York

Chapter 9. Lumbar Spinal Stenosis: Surgery for Spinal Stenosis

NANCY E. EPSTEIN, M.D.
Associate Clinical Professor of Surgery, Department of Surgery, Division of Neurosurgery, The North Shore University Hospital, Manhasset, New York, and The Cornell Medical College, New York, New York

Chapter 9. Lumbar Spinal Stenosis: Surgery for Spinal Stenosis

JEREMY C. T. FAIRBANK, M.D., F.R.C.S.
Honorary Clinical Lecturer in Orthopaedics, University of Oxford, Oxford, England. Consultant Orthopaedic Surgeon, Nuffield Orthopaedic Centre, Oxford, England

Chapter 3. Diagnosis and Neuromechanisms: History Taking and Physical Examination: Identification of Syndromes of Back Pain

YIZHAR FLOMAN, M.D.
Professor of Orthopedic Surgery, Hadassah-Hebrew University Medical School, Jerusalem, Israel. Head, Spine Surgery, Hadassah University Hospital, Jerusalem, Israel

Chapter 17. Rehabilitation: Psychologic Approaches to the Management and Treatment of Chronic Low Back Pain

ROBERT D. FRASER, M.B., B.S., M.D., F.R.A.C.S.
Clinical Professor, University of Adelaide, Adelaide, South Australia. Head of Spinal Unit, Department of Orthopaedics and Trauma, Royal Adelaide Hospital, Adelaide, South Australia

Chapter 13. Spinal Infections: Iatrogenic Discitis

BRUCE E. FREDRICKSON, M.D.
Professor of Orthopedic and Neurologic Surgery, State University of New York Health Science Center at Syracuse, Syracuse, New York

Chapter 22. Spinal Instrumentation: Internal Fixation: Indications, Technique, and Results

ANTHONY J. FREEMONT, B.Sc., M.B.B.S., M.D.
Professor of Osteoarticular Pathology, University of Manchester, Manchester, England

Chapter 11. Inflammatory Disorders: Fibrosis, Chronic Inflammation, and Vascular Damage in Mechanical Back Pain Syndromes

JOHN W. FRYMOYER, M.S., M.D.
Professor of Orthopaedic Surgery; Dean, College of Medicine, University of Vermont, Burlington, Vermont

Chapter 1. Epidemiology: Magnitude of the Problem; Chapter 10. Segmental Instability

CONTRIBUTORS

STEVEN R. GARFIN, M.D.
Professor of Orthopaedic Surgery, University of California, San Diego Medical Center, San Diego, California
Chapter 7. Clinical Entities: Lumbar Disc Degeneration: Normal Aging or a Disease Process? Chapter 12. Fractures of the Lumbar Spine: Evaluation, Classification, and Treatment

STANLEY GERTZBEIN, M.D., F.R.C.S.(C.)
Medical Director, The Spine Institute, Houston, Texas
Chapter 12. Fractures of the Lumbar Spine: Evaluation, Classification, and Treatment

C. J. M. GETTY, M.A., M.B., F.R.C.S.
Honorary Lecturer, Sheffield University Medical School, Sheffield, England. Consultant Orthopaedic Surgeon and Clinical Director in Orthopaedics, Northern General Hospital, Sheffield, England
Chapter 23. Surgical Approaches: Laminectomies

LARS G. GILBERTSON, Ph.D.
Post-doctoral Associate, Department of Biomedical Engineering, College of Engineering, University of Iowa, Iowa City, Iowa
Chapter 4. Biomechanics: Biomechanics of Thoracolumbar Spine Stabilization

KEVIN GILL, M.D.
Clinical Associate Professor, Orthopaedic Surgery, University of Texas Southwestern Medical Center, Dallas, Texas. Chief, Orthopaedic Surgery Department, St. Paul Medical Center, Dallas, Texas
Chapter 6. Radiology: Discography

VIJAY K. GOEL, Ph.D.
Professor and Chairman, Department of Biomedical Engineering, College of Engineering, University of Iowa, Iowa City, Iowa
Chapter 4. Biomechanics: Biomechanics of Thoracolumbar Spine Stabilization

SERGE A. GRACOVETSKY, Ph.D.
Associate Professor, Concordia University, Montréal, Québec, Canada
Chapter 4. Biomechanics: Function of the Spine from an Evolutionary Perspective

DIETER GROB, M.D.
Klinik Wihelm Schulthess, Zurich, Switzerland
Chapter 24. Fusion: Future of Spine Fusion

SCOTT HALDEMAN, M.D., Ph.D., F.R.C.P.(C.)
Associate Clinical Professor, Department of Neurology, University of California, Irvine, Irvine, California
Chapter 3. Diagnosis and Neuromechanisms: Clinical Neurophysiology and Electrodiagnostic Testing in Low Back Pain

HAMILTON HALL, M.D., F.R.C.S.C.
Professor, Department of Surgery, University of Toronto, Toronto, Ontario, Canada; Director, Spine Center, Orthopaedic and Arthritic Hospital, and Medical Director, Canadian Back Institute, Toronto, Ontario, Canada
Chapter 3. Diagnosis and Neuromechanisms: History Taking and Physical Examination: Identification of Syndromes of Back Pain

EDWARD N. HANLEY, JR., M.D.
Chairman and Program Director, Department of Orthopaedic Surgery, Carolinas Medical Center, Charlotte, North Carolina; Clinical Professor, Department of Surgery, University of North Carolina at Chapel Hill School of Medicine, Chapel Hill, North Carolina. Vice-President, Clinical Activities, Charlotte-Mecklenburg Hospital Authority, Carolinas Medical Center, Charlotte, North Carolina
Chapter 7. Clinical Entities: Surgical Indications and Techniques; Chapter 8. Lumbar and Lumbosacral Spondylolisthesis: Operative Treatment: Children and Adolescents

TOMMY HANSSON, M.D., Ph.D.
Division of Orthopaedics, Sahlgren University Hospital, Gothenburg, Sweden
Chapter 16. Osteoporosis of the Spine

MITSUO HASUE, M.D.
Chief, Department of Orthopaedic Surgery, Japanese Red Cross Medical Center, Tokyo, Japan

Chapter 3. Diagnosis and Neuromechanisms: Etiology of Sciatic Pain and Mechanisms of Nerve Root Compression

ROWLAND G. HAZARD, M.D.
Associate Professor of Orthopaedics and Rehabilitation, University of Vermont, Burlington, Vermont. Director of Rehabilitation, Spine Institute of New England, Williston, Vermont

Chapter 17. Rehabilitation: Functional Restoration for the Patient with Chronic Low Back Pain

KENNETH B. HEITHOFF, B.S., M.D.
Medical Director and Chairman, Center for Diagnostic Imaging, St. Louis Park, Minnesota

Chapter 6. Radiology: Myelography and Computed Tomography of the Lumbar Spine

HARRY N. HERKOWITZ, M.D.
Chairman, Department of Orthopaedic Surgery, William Beaumont Hospital, Royal Oak, Michigan

Chapter 7. Clinical Entities: Lumbar Disc Degeneration: Normal Aging or a Disease Process? Chapter 9. Lumbar Spinal Stenosis: Role of Arthrodesis; Chapter 24. Fusion: Present Role of Lumbar Spine Fusion

STEN H. HOLM, Ph.D.
Associate Professor, University of Gothenburg, Gothenburg, Sweden. Sahlgren University Hospital, Gothenburg, Sweden

Chapter 5. Biochemistry: Nutritional and Pathophysiologic Aspects of the Lumbar Intervertebral Disc

KEN HSU, M.D.
Clinical Instructor, Fellowship in Spine Surgery, St. Mary's Spine Center, San Francisco, California. Director of Orthopaedic Service, St. Mary's Spine Center, San Francisco, California

Chapter 22. Spinal Instrumentation: Complications of Transpedicle Spine Fixation

MALCOLM I. V. JAYSON, M.D., F.R.C.P.
Professor of Rheumatology, University of Manchester, Manchester, England. Consultant Rheumatologist, Rheumatic Diseases Centre, Hope Hospital; Director, Manchester and Salford Back Pain Centre, Salford, England

Chapter 11. Inflammatory Disorders: Fibrosis, Chronic Inflammation, and Vascular Damage in Mechanical Back Pain Syndromes

NEIL KAHANOVITZ, M.D.
Anderson Orthopaedic Institute, Arlington, Virginia

Chapter 7. Clinical Entities: Alternative Techniques for Disc Decompression: Percutaneous Discectomy and Chemonucleolysis

ALLISON M. KAIGLE, M.S.
Biomedical Engineer, Department of Occupational Orthopaedics, Sahlgren University Hospital, Gothenburg, Sweden

Chapter 4. Biomechanics: Degeneration, Injury, and Spinal Instability

TONY S. KELLER, Ph.D.
Associate Professor, Department of Mechanical Engineering; Associate Professor, Department of Orthopaedics and Rehabilitation, University of Vermont, Burlington, Vermont

Chapter 16. Osteoporosis of the Spine

ALBERT I. KING, B.S., M.S., Ph.D.
Distinguished Professor, Bioengineering Center, Wayne State University, Detroit, Michigan

Chapter 3. Diagnosis and Neuromechanisms: Neurophysiologic Basis of Low Back Pain

JOHN P. KOSTUIK, M.D.
Professor of Orthopaedics-Neurosurgery, Johns Hopkins University, Baltimore, Maryland. Chief, Division of Spinal Surgery, Department of Orthopaedic Surgery, Johns Hopkins Hospital, Baltimore, Maryland

Chapter 7. Clinical Entities: Controversies in Cauda Equina Syndrome and Lumbar Disc Herniation; Chapter 21. Adult Scoliosis: Assessment and Treatment

JUERGEN KRAEMER, M.D.
Professor of Orthopedics, University of Bochum, Bochum, Germany

Chapter 1. Epidemiology: Historical Perspective of Lumbar Spine Surgery

MARTIN KRAG, M.D.
Associate Professor, Department of Orthopaedics and Rehabilitation, McClure Musculoskeletal Research Center, University of Vermont, Burlington, Vermont. Director, Spine Institute of New England, Fletcher Allen Health Care, Williston, Vermont

Chapter 22. Spinal Instrumentation: Biomechanics of Transpedicle Spine Fixation; Complications of Transpedicle Spine Fixation

LAWRENCE T. KURZ, M.D.
Chapter 9. Lumbar Spinal Stenosis: Clinical, Radiologic, and Electrodiagnostic Diagnosis of Degenerative Lumbar Stenosis

NOSHIR A. LANGRANA, Ph.D.
Professor, Mechanical and Aerospace Engineering, Rutgers University College of Engineering, Piscataway, New Jersey. Adjunct Professor, Department of Orthopaedic Surgery, University of Medicine and Dentistry of New Jersey, Newark, New Jersey

Chapter 4. Biomechanics: Biomechanical Analyses of Loads on the Lumbar Spine

THOMAS LEHMANN, M.D.
Clinical Professor of Orthopaedic Surgery, University of Louisville, Louisville, Kentucky

Chapter 4. Biomechanics: Lumbosacral Orthosis

JOHN C. Y. LEONG, F.R.C.S., F.R.C.S.E., F.R.A.C.S., J.P.
Head of Department of Orthopaedic Surgery; Director of School of Postgraduate Medical Education and Training, Faculty of Medicine, University of Hong Kong, Hong Kong, China. Chief of Service, Department of Orthopaedics and Traumatology, Queen Mary Hospital, Pokfulam, Hong Kong, China

Chapter 13. Spinal Infections: Pyogenic and Tuberculous Infections

STEPHEN J. LIPSON, M.D.
Associate Professor of Orthopedic Surgery, Harvard Medical School, Boston, Massachusetts. Orthopedic Surgeon-in-Chief, Beth Israel Hospital, Boston, Massachusetts

Chapter 5. Biochemistry: Biochemistry and Cell Biology of the Intervertebral Disc: Aging Versus Degeneration

ANNE ELISABETH LJUNGGREN, Ph.D.
Professor, Faculty of Medicine, Department of Physical Therapy Science, University of Bergen, Bergen, Norway. Senior Scientist, Research Forum, Ullevål University Hospital, Oslo, Norway

Chapter 7. Clinical Entities: Natural History and Clinical Role of the Herniated Disc

MARK LORENZ, M.D.
Clinical Associate Professor of Orthopedic Surgery, Loyola University Medical School, Chicago, Illinois. Partner, Hinsdale Orthopedic Associates, Hinsdale, Illinois

Chapter 2. Anatomy of the Lumbar Spine: The Three-Joint Complex

KEITH D. K. LUK, M.Ch. (Orth.), F.R.C.S.E., F.R.C.S.G., F.R.A.C.S.
Reader of Department of Orthopaedic Surgery, Faculty of Medicine, University of Hong Kong, Hong Kong, China. Honorary Hospital Chief Executive, Duchess of Kent Children's Hospital, Hong Kong, China

Chapter 13. Spinal Infections: Pyogenic and Tuberculous Infections

WILLIAM S. MARRAS, B.S., M.S.I.E., Ph.D., C.P.E.
Professor, Department of Industrial Welding and Systems Engineering, Ohio State University, Columbus, Ohio. Director, Biodynamics Laboratory, Ohio State University, Columbus, Ohio

Chapter 4. Biomechanics: Occupational Biomechanics

TOM G. MAYER, M.D.
Clinical Professor, University of Texas Southwestern Medical Center, Dallas, Texas. Medical Director, Productive Rehabilitation Institute of Dallas for Ergonomics (PRIDE), Dallas, Texas

Chapter 17. Rehabilitation: Functional Restoration for the Patient with Chronic Low Back Pain

IAIN McCALL, F.R.C.R.
Department of Diagnostic Imaging, The Robert Jones and Agnes Hunt Orthopaedic Hospital, Oswestry, England

Chapter 6. Radiology: Plain Films of the Lumbar Spine; Magnetic Resonance Imaging of the Lumbar Spine

JOHN A. McCULLOCH, M.D., F.R.C.S.(C.)
Professor of Orthopedics, Northeastern Ohio University College of Medicine, Akron, Ohio. Summa Health Systems, St. Thomas Hospital, Akron, Ohio

Chapter 7. Clinical Entities: Surgical Indications and Techniques

ROBIN McKENZIE, P.T., Dip. M.T.
President; Spinal Consultant, McKenzie Institute International, Waikanae, New Zealand

Chapter 17. Rehabilitation: Mechanical Diagnosis and Therapy for Low Back Pain: Toward a Better Understanding

THOMAS W. McNEILL, M.D.
Associate Professor, Rush College of Medicine, Chicago, Illinois. Senior Attending Surgeon, Rush-Presbyterian-St. Luke's Medical Center, Chicago, Illinois

Chapter 7. Clinical Entities: Pelvic Visceral Dysfunction—Cauda Equina Syndrome

VERT MOONEY, M.D.
Professor of Orthopaedic Surgery, University of California, San Diego Medical Center, San Diego, California

Chapter 7. Clinical Entities: Facet Syndrome; Evaluation and Treatment of Sacroiliac Dysfunction

ROBERT J. MOORE, B.Sc., M.Sc., Ph.D.
Senior Hospital Scientist, Institute of Medical and Veterinary Science, Adelaide, South Australia

Chapter 5. Biochemistry: Biochemistry and Histology of the Intervertebral Disc: Animal Models of Disc Degeneration

ROBERT MULHOLLAND, F.R.C.S.
Special Professor in Orthopaedic and Accident Surgery, University of Nottingham, Nottingham, England

Chapter 6. Radiology: Magnetic Resonance Imaging of the Lumbar Spine

ALF NACHEMSON, M.D., Ph.D.
Professor and Chairman, Department of Orthopaedics, Institute of Surgical Sciences, University of Gothenburg; Sahlgren University Hospital, Gothenburg, Sweden

Chapter 1. Epidemiology: Future of Low Back Pain

KAORU NAKANO, M.D.
Vice-director, Nakano Orthopedic Hospital, Sapporo, Japan

Chapter 23. Surgical Approaches: Anterior Extraperitoneal Lumbar Discectomy Without Fusion

NOBORU NAKANO, M.D., Ph.D.
Instructor, Sapporo Medical University, Sapporo, Japan. Director, Nakano Orthopedic Hospital, Sapporo, Japan

Chapter 23. Surgical Approaches: Anterior Extraperitoneal Lumbar Discectomy Without Fusion

TOHRU NAKANO, M.D.
Vice-director, Nakano Orthopedic Hospital, Sapporo, Japan

Chapter 23. Surgical Approaches: Anterior Extraperitoneal Lumbar Discectomy Without Fusion

MARGARETA NORDIN, R.P.T., Dr. Sci.
Research Associate Professor, School of Medicine, New York University, New York, New York. Director, Occupational and Industrial Orthopaedic Center, Hospital for Joint Diseases, New York University Medical Center, New York, New York
Chapter 17. Rehabilitation: Education and Training

JOHN O'BRIEN, Ph.D., F.R.C.S.(Ed), F.A.C.S, F.R.A.C.S.
Consultant Surgeon in Spinal Disorders, England, United Kingdom
Chapter 6. Radiology: Plain Films of the Lumbar Spine

ORSO L. OSTI, M.D., Ph.D., F.R.A.C.S.
Lecturer, Department of Surgery, University of Adelaide, Adelaide, South Australia. Visiting Surgeon, Spinal Unit, Royal Adelaide Hospital; Orthopedic Department, Modbury Hospital, Adelaide, South Australia
Chapter 5. Biochemistry: Biochemistry and Histology of the Intervertebral Disc: Animal Models of Disc Degeneration; Chapter 7. Clinical Entities: Alternative Techniques for Disc Decompression: Percutaneous Discectomy and Chemonucleolysis; Chapter 13. Spinal Infections: Iatrogenic Discitis

MANOHAR M. PANJABI, Ph.D.
Professor and Director, Biomechanics Laboratory, Department of Orthopaedics and Rehabilitation, Yale University School of Medicine, New Haven, Connecticut
Chapter 4. Biomechanics: Degeneration, Injury, and Spinal Instability

STANLEY V. PARIS, Ph.D., P.T.
Professor, President, Institute of Physical Therapy, St. Augustine, Florida; Clinical Professor, Anatomy, P.T. Program, Medical College of Georgia, Augusta, Georgia. Director; Senior Clinician, Flagler Physical Therapy, St. Augustine, Florida
Chapter 17. Rehabilitation: Manipulation of the Lumbar Spine

MOHAMAD PARNIANPOUR, Ph.D.
Assistant Professor, Department of Industrial Welding and Systems Engineering; Assistant Professor, Biomedical Engineering, Ohio State University, Columbus, Ohio. Associate Director, Biodynamics Laboratory, Ohio State University, Columbus, Ohio
Chapter 19. Industrial Low Back Pain: Trunk Performance, Strength, and Endurance: Measurement Techniques and Applications

AVINASH G. PATWARDHAN, Ph.D.
Professor of Orthopedic Surgery; Director of Orthopedic Biomechanics Laboratory, Department of Orthopedic Surgery, Loyola University Medical School, Chicago, Illinois
Chapter 2. Anatomy of the Lumbar Spine: The Three-Joint Complex

MALCOLM H. POPE, Dr. Med. Sci., Ph.D.
Professor, Department of Biomedical Engineering, College of Engineering, University of Iowa, Iowa City, Iowa. Director, Iowa Spine Research Center, University of Iowa, Iowa City, Iowa
Chapter 4. Biomechanics: Effects of Repeated Loads and Vibration; Degeneration, Injury and Spinal Instability; Chapter 10. Segmental Instability

RICHARD W. PORTER, M.D., F.R.C.S., F.R.C.S.E.
Professor of Orthopaedic Surgery, University of Aberdeen, Aberdeen, Scotland
Chapter 9. Lumbar Spinal Stenosis: Development of the Vertebral Canal; Pathophysiology of Neurogenic Claudication

FRANCO POSTACCHINI, M.D.
Professor of Orthopaedic Surgery, University of Modena, Modena, Italy
Chapter 9. Lumbar Spinal Stenosis: Long-Term Results

WOLFGANG RAUSCHNING, M.D., Ph.D.
Professor in Clinical Anatomy, Department of Orthopaedic Surgery, Sahlgren University Hospital, Gothenburg, Sweden. Academic University Hospital, Uppsala, Sweden

Chapter 6. Radiology: Imaging Anatomy of the Lumbar Spine

STEPHEN L. G. ROTHMAN, M.D.
Consultant Radiologist, Spinal Injury Service, Rancho Los Amigos Hospital, Downey, California. Department of Radiology, San Pedro Peninsula Hospital, San Pedro, California

Chapter 8. Lumbar and Lumbosacral Spondylolisthesis: Classification, Diagnosis, and Natural History

BJÖRN RYDEVIK, M.D., Ph.D.
Associate Professor of Orthopaedics, University of Gothenburg, Gothenburg, Sweden. Associate Professor of Orthopaedics, Department of Orthopaedics, Sahlgren University Hospital, Gothenburg, Sweden

Chapter 3. Diagnosis and Neuromechanisms: Etiology of Sciatic Pain and Mechanisms of Nerve Root Compression

JEFFREY A. SAAL, M.D., F.A.C.P.
Associate Clinical Professor, Stanford University School of Medicine, Stanford, California

Chapter 8. Lumbar and Lumbosacral Spondylolisthesis: Comprehensive Nonoperative Care of Lytic Spondylolisthesis: Principles and Practice

JEFFREY H. SCHIMANDLE, M.D.
Department of Orthopaedic Surgery, Emory University School of Medicine, Atlanta, Georgia

Chapter 24. Fusion: Biology of Lumbar Spine Fusion and Bone Graft Materials

SHAUL SCHREIBER, M.D.
Instructor, Hadassah-Hebrew University Medical Center, Jerusalem, Israel. Senior Psychiatrist, Department of Psychiatry, Hadassah University Hospital, Jerusalem, Israel

Chapter 17. Rehabilitation: Psychologic Approaches to the Management and Treatment of Chronic Low Back Pain

DAVID SELBY, M.D.
Clinical Professor, University of Texas Southwestern Medical Center, Dallas, Texas. Spine Surgeon, Dallas Spine Group, Dallas, Texas

Chapter 7. Clinical Entities: Lumbar Spine Fusion: Different Types and Indications

MANOJ SHARMA, Ph.D.
Engineer III, Design and Analysis, Case Corporation, East Moline, Illinois

Chapter 4. Biomechanics: Biomechanical Analyses of Loads on the Lumbar Spine

DAN M. SPENGLER, M.D.
Professor and Chairman, Department of Orthopaedics and Rehabilitation, Vanderbilt University Medical Center, Nashville, Tennessee

Chapter 7. Clinical Entities: Lumbar Spine Algorithm

KEVIN F. SPRATT, Ph.D.
University of Iowa, Iowa City, Iowa

Chapter 25. Measuring Clinical Outcomes

DANIEL STEIN, M.D.
Head, Department of Child and Adolescent Psychiatry, Abrabanel Mental Health Center, Bat-Yam, Israel

Chapter 17. Rehabilitation: Psychologic Approaches to the Management and Treatment of Chronic Low Back Pain

MAREK SZPALSKI, M.D.
Stagemeester, Department of Experimental Anatomy/Manual Medicine, Vrij Universiteit, Brussel, Brussels, Belgium; Adjunct Assistant Professor in Orthopaedics and Rehabilitation, Vanderbilt University, Nashville, Tennessee. Senior Consultant, Department of Orthopaedics, Centre Hospitalier Moliere Longchamp, Brussels, Belgium; Senior Scientist, Department of Orthopaedic Surgery, Hospital for Joint Diseases, New York, New York

Chapter 19. Industrial Low Back Pain: Trunk Performance, Strength, and Endurance: Measurement Techniques and Applications

KAZUHISA TAKAHASHI, M.D.
Instructor, Department of Orthopaedic Surgery, School of Medicine, Chiba University, Chiba, Japan. Department of Orthopaedic Surgery, Chiba University Hospital, Chiba, Japan
Chapter 7. Clinical Entities: Surgical Indications and Techniques

JILL URBAN, Ph.D.
University Laboratory of Physiology, University of Oxford, Oxford, England
Chapter 5. Biochemistry: Disc Biochemistry in Relation to Function

ALEXANDER R. VACCARO, M.D.
Assistant Professor, Department of Orthopaedic Surgery, Thomas Jefferson University Hospital, Philadelphia, Pennsylvania
Chapter 8. Lumbar and Lumbosacral Spondylolisthesis: Surgical Treatment of Adult Degenerative Spondylolisthesis

PIETER F. VAN AKKERVEEKEN, M.D., Ph.D.
Orthopedic Surgeon and Managing Director, Rug Adviescentra, Utrecht, the Netherlands
Chapter 3. Diagnosis and Neuromechanisms: Pain Patterns and Diagnostic Blocks; Chapter 9. Lumbar Spinal Stenosis: History and Classification of Spinal Stenosis

EDWARD VAN HANSWYK, B.S.
Clinical Assistant Professor of Orthopedic Surgery, State University of New York Health Science Center at Syracuse, Syracuse, New York
Chapter 4. Biomechanics: Lumbosacral Orthosis

HEIKKI VANHARANTA, M.D.
Department of Physical Medicine, University of Oulu, Oulu, Finland
Chapter 17. Rehabilitation: Functional Restoration for the Patient with Chronic Low Back Pain

BARRIE VERNON-ROBERTS, M.B.B.S., M.D., Ph.D., F.R.C.P.A., F.R.C.Path.
Head of Department of Pathology; George Richard Marks Professor of Pathology, University of Adelaide, Adelaide, South Australia. Head of the Division of Tissue Pathology; Senior Visiting Pathologist, Royal Adelaide Hospital, Adelaide, South Australia
Chapter 13. Spinal Infections: Iatrogenic Discitis

TAPIO VIDEMAN, M.D., Dr. Med. Sci.
Professor in Sports Medicine, University of Jyväskylä, Jyväskylä, Finland
Chapter 1. Epidemiology: Epidemiology of Disc Disease

ROBERT G. WATKINS, M.D.
Associate Clinical Professor, Department of Orthopaedic Surgery, University of Southern California School of Medicine, Los Angeles, California; Orthopaedic Spine Surgeon, Kerlan-Jobe Orthopaedic Clinic, Los Angeles, California
Chapter 23. Surgical Approaches: Anterior Surgical Approach to the Thoracolumbar, Lumbar, and Lumbosacral Spine

PETER WEHLING, M.D.
Privat Dozent, Orthop. Universitatsuklinik, Düsseldorf, Germany. Leitender Arzt Orthopädie, Praxis u. Klinik Orthopädie, Düsseldorf, Germany
Chapter 3. Diagnosis and Neuromechanisms: Etiology of Sciatic Pain and Mechanisms of Nerve Root Compression

JAMES N. WEINSTEIN, D.O.
Endowed Professor, University of Iowa College of Medicine, Iowa City, Iowa
Chapter 4. Biomechanics: Biomechanics of Thoracolumbar Spine Stabilization; Chapter 14. Spinal Tumors; Chapter 25. Measuring Clinical Outcomes

THOMAS S. WHITECLOUD, III, M.D.
Professor and Chairman, Department of Orthopaedic Surgery, Tulane University Medical Center, School of Medicine, New Orleans, Louisiana
Chapter 23. Surgical Approaches: Laminectomies

SAM W. WIESEL, M.D.

Professor and Chairman, Department of Orthopaedic Surgery, Georgetown University Medical Center, Washington, District of Columbia

Chapter 7. Clinical Entities: Lumbar Spine Algorithm; Chapter 20. Multiply Operated Lumbar Spine: Algorithmic Approach

DAVID G. WILDER, Ph.D.

Visiting Associate Professor, Department of Biomedical Engineering, University of Iowa, Iowa City, Iowa. Senior Scientist, Iowa Spine Research Center, University of Iowa, Iowa City, Iowa

Chapter 4. Biomechanics: Effects of Repeated Loads and Vibration; Chapter 10. Segmental Instability

LEON L. WILTSE, M.D.

Clinical Professor of Orthopedic Surgery, University of California, Irvine, College of Medicine, Irvine, California. Staff, Long Beach Memorial Medical Center, Long Beach, California

Chapter 8. Lumbar and Lumbosacral Spondylolisthesis: Classification, Diagnosis, and Natural History

HANSEN YUAN, M.D.

Professor of Orthopedic and Neurological Surgery, State University of New York Health Science Center at Syracuse, Syracuse, New York. Chief, Division of Spine, Institute for Spine Care, SUNY Health Science Center at Syracuse, Syracuse, New York

Chapter 4. Biomechanics: Lumbosacral Orthosis; Chapter 22. Spinal Instrumentation: Internal Fixation: Indications, Technique, and Results

MICHAEL R. ZINDRICK, M.D.

Clinical Associate Professor of Orthopaedic Surgery, Department of Orthopaedic Surgery, Loyola University Medical School, Maywood, Illinois. Orthopedic Surgeon, Hinsdale Hospital, Hinsdale, Illinois; Good Samaritan Hospital, Downers Grove, Illinois; Loyola University Medical Center, Maywood, Illinois; Hines Veterans Administration Hospital, Hines, Illinois

Chapter 7. Clinical Entities: Lumbar Spine Fusion: Different Types and Indications

JAMES ZUCHERMAN, M.D.

Director of Spine Surgery Fellowship, St. Mary's Spine Center, San Francisco, California. Medical Director, St. Mary's Spine Center, San Francisco, California

Chapter 22. Spinal Instrumentation: Complications of Transpedicle Spine Fixation

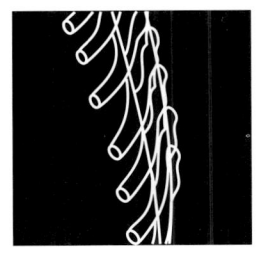

Preface

The goal of the second edition of *The Lumbar Spine* continues to be the presentation of an up-to-date review of the lumbar spine from both basic science and clinical perspectives. Emphasis has been placed on new information that has been generated since the first edition. Approximately 30 to 40% of the book contains new material and 95% of the book has been rewritten. This edition of *The Lumbar Spine* can serve as both a reference source for the study of low back disorders and a practical guide to the diagnosis and management of patients with specific problems.

The editorial committee has been expanded to bring new ideas into the second edition. It is hoped that we have identified the best authors for each topic. In updating each section, the authors have tried to eliminate those areas that are not current or are outdated and to focus on pertinent information that is relevant for both basic science and clinical care.

Finally and most importantly, it has again been a very exciting and stimulating experience to work with all the members of the International Society for the Study of the Lumbar Spine to complete this edition. Everyone has been enthusiastic. The editors are most appreciative of each contribution and are very proud of the final text.

SAM W. WIESEL, M.D.

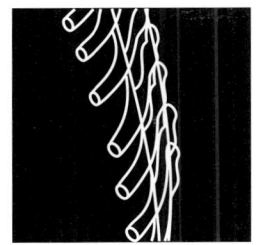

Contents

VOLUME 1

CHAPTER 1
Epidemiology 1

Historical Perspective of Lumbar Spine Surgery 1
JUERGEN KRAEMER

Magnitude of the Problem 8
JOHN W. FRYMOYER

Epidemiology of Disc Disease 16
TAPIO VIDEMAN
MICHELE CRITES BATTIÉ

Future of Low Back Pain 28
ALF NACHEMSON

CHAPTER 2
Anatomy of the Lumbar Spine 43

Developmental to Normal Adult Anatomy .. 43
GORDON R. BELL

The Three-Joint Complex 52
MARK LORENZ
AVINASH G. PATWARDHAN

Clinically Relevant Anatomy 57
ANTHONY P. DWYER

CHAPTER 3
Diagnosis and Neuromechanisms 74

Neurophysiologic Basis of Low Back Pain 74
ALBERT I. KING
JOHN M. CAVANAUGH

History Taking and Physical Examination Identification of Syndromes of Back Pain 85
JEREMY C. T. FAIRBANK
HAMILTON HALL

Pain Patterns and Diagnostic Blocks 105
PIETER F. VAN AKKERVEEKEN

Etiology of Sciatic Pain and Mechanisms of Nerve Root Compression 123
BJÖRN RYDEVIK
MITSUO HASUE
PETER WEHLING

Clinical Neurophysiology and Electrodiagnostic Testing in Low Back Pain . 141
SCOTT HALDEMAN
JIŘÍ DVOŘÁK

CHAPTER 4
Biomechanics 163

Biomechanical Analyses of Loads on the Lumbar Spine 163
NOSHIR A. LANGRANA
W. THOMAS EDWARDS
MANOJ SHARMA

Effects of Repeated Loads and Vibration 181
PAUL BRINCKMANN
DAVID G. WILDER
MALCOLM H. POPE

Degeneration, Injury, and Spinal
Instability 203
MANOHAR M. PANJABI
ALLISON M. KAIGLE
MALCOLM H. POPE

Biomechanics of Thoracolumbar Spine
Stabilization 212
VIJAY K. GOEL
JAMES N. WEINSTEIN
LARS G. GILBERTSON

Occupational Biomechanics 235
GUNNAR B. J. ANDERSSON
WILLIAM S. MARRAS

Lumbosacral Orthosis 251
HANSEN YUAN
EDWARD VAN HANSWYK
THOMAS LEHMAN

Function of the Spine from an Evolutionary
Perspective 259
SERGE A. GRACOVETSKY

CHAPTER 5

Biochemistry 271

Disc Biochemistry in Relation to
Function 271
JILL URBAN

Biochemistry and Histology of the
Intervertebral Disc: Animal Models of Disc
Degeneration 281
ORSO L. OSTI
ROBERT J. MOORE

Nutritional and Pathophysiologic Aspects
of the Lumbar Intervertebral Disc 285
STEN H. HOLM

Biochemistry and Cell Biology of the
Intervertebral Disc: Aging Versus
Degeneration 310
STEPHEN J. LIPSON

CHAPTER 6

Radiology 317

Imaging Anatomy of the Lumbar Spine 317
WOLFGANG RAUSCHNING

Plain Films of the Lumbar Spine 333
IAIN McCALL
JOHN O'BRIEN

Magnetic Resonance Imaging of the Lumbar
Spine 353
ROBERT MULHOLLAND
IAIN McCALL

Myelography and Computed Tomography
of the Lumbar Spine 376
KENNETH B. HEITHOFF

Discography 428
KEVIN GILL

Reproducibility and Accuracy of Lumbar
Spine Imaging Studies 434
RICHARD A. DEYO

CHAPTER 7

Clinical Entities 447

Lumbar Spine Algorithm 447
SCOTT D. BODEN
SAM W. WIESEL
DAN M. SPENGLER

Lumbar Disc Degeneration: Normal Aging
or a Disease Process? 458
STEVEN R. GARFIN
HARRY N. HERKOWITZ

Natural History and Clinical Role of the
Herniated Disc 473
ANNE ELISABETH LJUNGGREN

Surgical Indications and Techniques 492
EDWARD N. HANLEY, JR.
RICK B. DELAMARTER
JOHN A. McCULLOUCH
KAZUHISA TAKAHASHI

Alternative Techniques for Disc
Decompression: Percutaneous Discectomy
and Chemonucleolysis 524
NEIL KAHANOVITZ
MICHEL BENOIST
ORSO L. OSTI

Facet Syndrome 538
VERT MOONEY

Evaluation and Treatment of Sacroiliac
Dysfunction 559
VERT MOONEY

Pelvic Visceral Dysfunction—Cauda Equina
Syndrome 569
THOMAS W. McNEILL

Controversies in Cauda Equina Syndrome
and Lumbar Disc Herniation 582
JOHN P. KOSTUIK

Lumbar Spine Fusion: Different Types and
Indications 588
MICHAEL R. ZINDRICK
DAVID SELBY

VOLUME 2

CHAPTER 8

Lumbar and Lumbosacral Spondylolisthesis ... 621

Classification, Diagnosis, and Natural
History 621
LEON L. WILTSE
STEPHEN L. G. ROTHMAN

Comprehensive Nonoperative Care of Lytic
Spondylolisthesis: Principles and Practice 654
JEFFREY A. SAAL

Operative Treatment: Children and
Adolescents 669
EDWARD N. HANLEY, JR.

Surgical Treatment of Isthmic and
Dysplastic Spondylolisthesis in the Adult 684
DAVID S. BRADFORD

Surgical Treatment of Adult Degenerative
Spondylolisthesis 700
RICHARD A. BALDERSTON
ALEXANDER R. VACCARO

CHAPTER 9

Lumbar Spinal Stenosis ... 711

Development of the Vertebral Canal 711
RICHARD W. PORTER

Pathophysiology of Neurogenic
Claudication 717
RICHARD W. PORTER

Classification and Treatment of Spinal
Stenosis 724

History and Classification of Spinal
Stenosis 724
PIETER VAN AKKERVEEKEN

Clinical, Radiologic, and Electrodiagnostic
Diagnosis of Degenerative Lumbar
Stenosis 731
LAWRENCE T. KURZ
JIŘÍ DVOŘÁK

Surgery for Spinal Stenosis 737
NANCY E. EPSTEIN
JOSEPH E. EPSTEIN

Role of Arthrodesis 757
HARRY N. HERKOWITZ

Long-Term Results 766
FRANCO POSTACCHINI

CHAPTER 10

Segmental Instability ... 782
JOHN W. FRYMOYER
MALCOLM H. POPE
DAVID G. WILDER

CHAPTER 11

Inflammatory Disorders ... 797

Inflammatory Spondyloarthropathies 797
MICHEL BENOIST

Fibrosis, Chronic Inflammation, and
Vascular Damage in Mechanical Back Pain
Syndromes 812
MALCOLM I. V. JAYSON
ANTHONY J. FREEMONT

CHAPTER 12

Fractures of the Lumbar Spine: Evaluation, Classification, and Treatment 822
STEVEN GARFIN
STANLEY GERTZBEIN
FRANK EISMONT

CHAPTER 13

Spinal Infections 874

Pyogenic and Tuberculous Infections 874
JOHN C. Y. LEONG
KEITH D. K. LUK

Iatrogenic Discitis 899
ROBERT D. FRASER
BARRIE VERNON-ROBERTS
ORSO L. OSTI

CHAPTER 14

Spinal Tumors 917
JAMES N. WEINSTEIN

CHAPTER 15

Complications of Lumbar Spine Surgery 945
GORDON R. BELL

CHAPTER 16

Osteoporosis of the Spine 969
TOMMY HANSSON
TONY S. KELLER

CHAPTER 17

Rehabilitation 989

Education and Training 989
MICHELE CRITES BATTIÉ
MARGARETA NORDIN

Mechanical Diagnosis and Therapy for Low Back Pain: Toward a Better Understanding 998
ROBIN McKENZIE
RONALD DONELSON

Manipulation of the Lumbar Spine 1012
STANLEY V. PARIS

Psychologic Approaches to the Management and Treatment of Chronic Low Back Pain 1018
SHAUL SCHREIBER
DANIEL STEIN
YIZHAR FLOMAN

Functional Restoration for the Patient with Chronic Low Back Pain 1042
ROWLAND G. HAZARD
TOM G. MAYER
HEIKKI VANHARANTA

CHAPTER 18

Low Back Pain in Pregnancy 1057
GUNNAR B. J. ANDERSSON

CHAPTER 19

Industrial Low Back Pain 1065

Risk Factors 1065
STANLEY J. BIGOS
MICHELE CRITES BATTIÉ

Trunk Performance, Strength, and Endurance: Measurement Techniques and Applications 1074
MAREK SZPALSKI
MOHAMAD PARNIANPOUR

CHAPTER 20

Multiply Operated Lumbar Spine: Algorithmic Approach 1106
SAM W. WIESEL
STEPHEN EISENSTEIN
RICHARD DELAMARTER
JOHN DOVE
SCOTT BODEN

CHAPTER 21

Adult Scoliosis 1118

Evaluation and Decision-Making 1118
RICHARD A. BALDERSTON
TODD J. ALBERT

Assessment and Treatment 1130
JOHN KOSTUIK

CHAPTER 22

Spinal Instrumentation 1177

Biomechanics of Transpedicle Spine
Fixation 1177
MARTIN KRAG

Complications of Transpedicle Spine
Fixation 1203
KEN HSU
JAMES ZUCHERMAN
MARTIN KRAG

Internal Fixation: Indications, Technique,
and Results 1216
BRUCE FREDRICKSON
HANSEN YUAN

CHAPTER 23

Surgical Approaches 1230

Laminectomies 1230
C. J. M. GETTY
THOMAS S. WHITECLOUD, III

Anterior Surgical Approach to the
Thoracolumbar, Lumbar, and Lumbosacral
Spine 1252
ROBERT G. WATKINS

Anterior Extraperitoneal Lumbar
Discectomy Without Fusion 1271
TOHRU NAKANO
KAORU NAKANO
NOBORU NAKANO

CHAPTER 24

Fusion 1284

Biology of Lumbar Spine Fusion and Bone
Graft Materials 1284
SCOTT D. BODEN
JEFFREY H. SCHIMANDLE

Fusion: Its Current and Future Place in the
Degenerative Lumbar Spine 1307

Present Role of Lumbar Spine Fusion 1307
HARRY N. HERKOWITZ

Future of Spine Fusion 1309
DIETER GROB

CHAPTER 25

Measuring Clinical Outcomes 1313
KEVIN F. SPRATT
JAMES N. WEINSTEIN

CHAPTER 26

The Ethics of Spine Care 1339
CHARLES V. BURTON

Index i

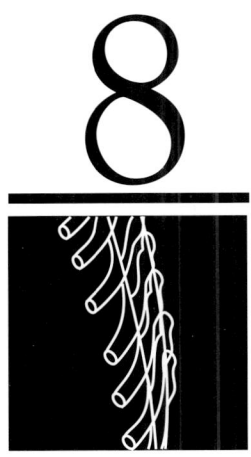

8

Lumbar and Lumbosacral Spondylolisthesis

Classification, Diagnosis, and Natural History

■

LEON L. WILTSE
STEPHEN L. G. ROTHMAN

Few conditions have fascinated orthopedic surgeons as has spondylolisthesis. Thousands of articles have been written on the subject, and scarcely a week goes by without a new one appearing in the world literature. A review of the world literature found that more than 300 articles have been published since 1990, when the first edition of this book was published.

In 1728, Herbinaux,[33] a Belgian obstetrician, noted that occasionally a bony prominence was present in front of the sacrum, and this was thought, perhaps, to cause problems in delivery. He is generally credited with having first described spondylolisthesis, probably the complete type, in which the body of L5 is actually lying in front of the sacrum (i.e., spondyloptosis).

Spondylolisthesis is the slippage of all or part of one vertebra onto another. The term, coined by Kilian[43] in 1854, is derived from the Greek *spondylos,* meaning "vertebra," and *olisthesis,* meaning "to slip or slide down a slippery incline." Kilian did not recognize the defect in the pars interarticularis but believed the lesion to be caused by a slow subluxation of the lumbosacral facets. One year later, Robert[77] of Koblenz established that the location of the fundamental lesion of the isthmic type is in the pars interarticularis, but he did not recognize the nature of the defect. In 1885, Lambl[47] demonstrated the lesion in the pars. Neugebauer,[56] in 1881, made an extensive study of anatomic specimens throughout Europe and was the first to recognize that anterior element slippage can occur by an elongation of the pars without its coming apart. He also noted that the entire vertebra can slip if the superior facets slide forward between the inferior facets. He did, however, confuse the degenerative type with the isthmic type of the disorder.

Newman,[58] in "The etiology of spondylolisthesis," published in 1963, coined the phrase degenerative spondylolisthesis. He was also the first to publish a satisfactory classification of the condition.[59] He separated congenital forms (or dysplastic forms as he called them) from isthmic forms. Macnab,[50] Rosenberg,[79] Gill and associates,[24] Taillard,[100] Wynne-Davies and Scott,[113] Saraste,[87] Grobler and coworkers,[27] and Osterman and associates,[66] to name a few, have been prominent in the development of the present knowledge of spondylolisthesis.

The types of spondylolisthesis are as varied as its causes. The type of greatest clinical importance in persons younger than 40 years is the isthmic type, in which the lesion is in the pars interarticularis. However, dysplasia and changes in facet orientation are prominent in its causation, and several other conditions permit slippage forward of one vertebra on another. This discussion is limited to the lumbar spine, although the disease occurs often in the cervical spine and a few reports of pars defects in the thoracic spine have been published. The classification of spondylolisthesis presented here is

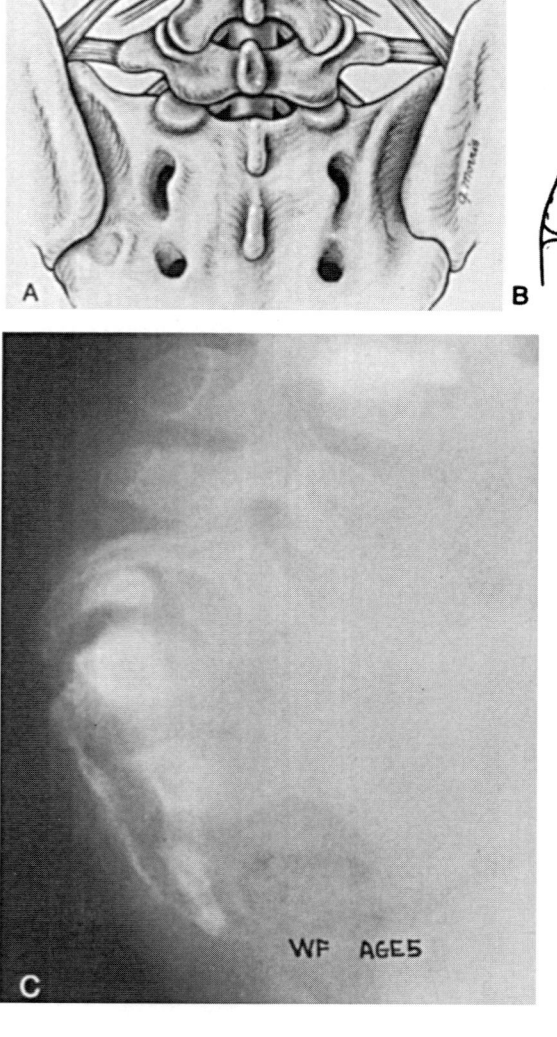
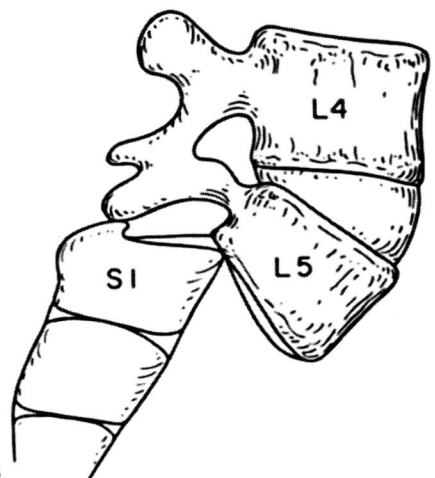

Figure 1. Congenital (dysplastic) spondylolisthesis in a 5-year-old girl. *A*, Note axially oriented facets. This is the hallmark of this type of spondylolisthesis. *B*, Lateral view. *C*, Lateral x-ray film of congenital type IA spondylolisthesis in a 5-year-old Caucasian girl. The partes are not elongated, but because of the flattening of the articular processes, one has the impression that they are. (From Wiltse, L.: Common problems of the lumbar spine: Spondylolisthesis and its treatment. J. Cont. Orthop. Educ. July 1979, p. 14.)

based on both anatomic and etiologic criteria.

CLASSIFICATION AND DIAGNOSIS OF SPONDYLOLISTHESIS

Anatomic Classification

The following classification of spondylolisthesis and spondylolysis has been derived from classifications previously published by various authors.[50, 58] This classification is anatomic and the basic congenital condition acting as the etiologic agent may be the same in more than one type or subtype.[57, 108]

I. Congenital
   A. This type has dysplastic articular processes at the level of olisthesis. They are axially oriented and are frequently associated with dysplasia of the superior vertebral end plate as well as with spina bifida.[59] This unstable condition permits the slippage to occur[69] (Fig. 1A to C).
   B. This type seen in the adult results from either sagittal (parallel) orientation of the articular processes or from anomalous, malformed articular processes that dislocate in adult life.
   C. Other congenital anomalies of the lumbar spine permit spondylolisthesis to occur. Congenital kyphosis is the principal one.[1]
II. Isthmic—The lesion is located in the pars interarticularis. Three types can be recognized.
   A. In the lytic type, there is a stress fracture of the pars[107] (Fig. 2).
   B. An elongated but intact pars is present secondary to healed stress fractures (Fig. 3A to D).
   C. Acute fracture of the pars results from major trauma.
III. Degenerative—This type results from long-standing intersegmental instability.
IV. Postsurgical
   A. A partial or complete loss of posterior bony and discogenic support occurs secondary to extensive decompressive facetectomy, often in patients with sagittally oriented facets.
   B. Postoperative stress fractures of the articular processes at their junction with the laminae produce this lesion.
V. Posttraumatic—This condition, always due to severe trauma, results from acute fractures in areas of the bony hook other than the pars (Fig. 4A to D).
VI. Pathologic—This lesion results from generalized or localized bone disease. Destruction of the posterior elements

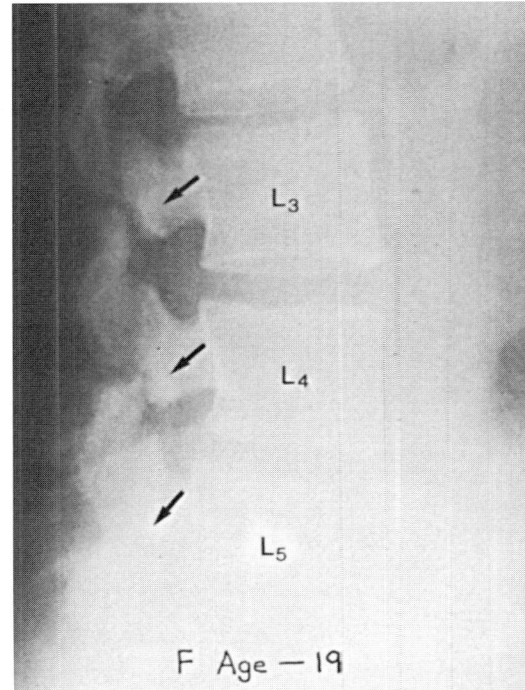

Figure 2. Typical stress fractures of the pars in a female equestrian, aged 19 years, competing for the Olympic games. The L3 lesion is older than the L4; L5 is intact.

Table 1

Forms of Spondylolisthesis
1. Developmental—due to { lysis / elongation
2. Acquired { traumatic—due to { acute fractures / stress fractures } / iatrogenic / pathologic / degenerative

From Marchetti, P. G., and Bartolozzi, P.: Spondylolisthesis. In Gaggi, A. (ed.): Spondylolisthesis. Bologna, Italy, A. Costa, 1986, p. 35.

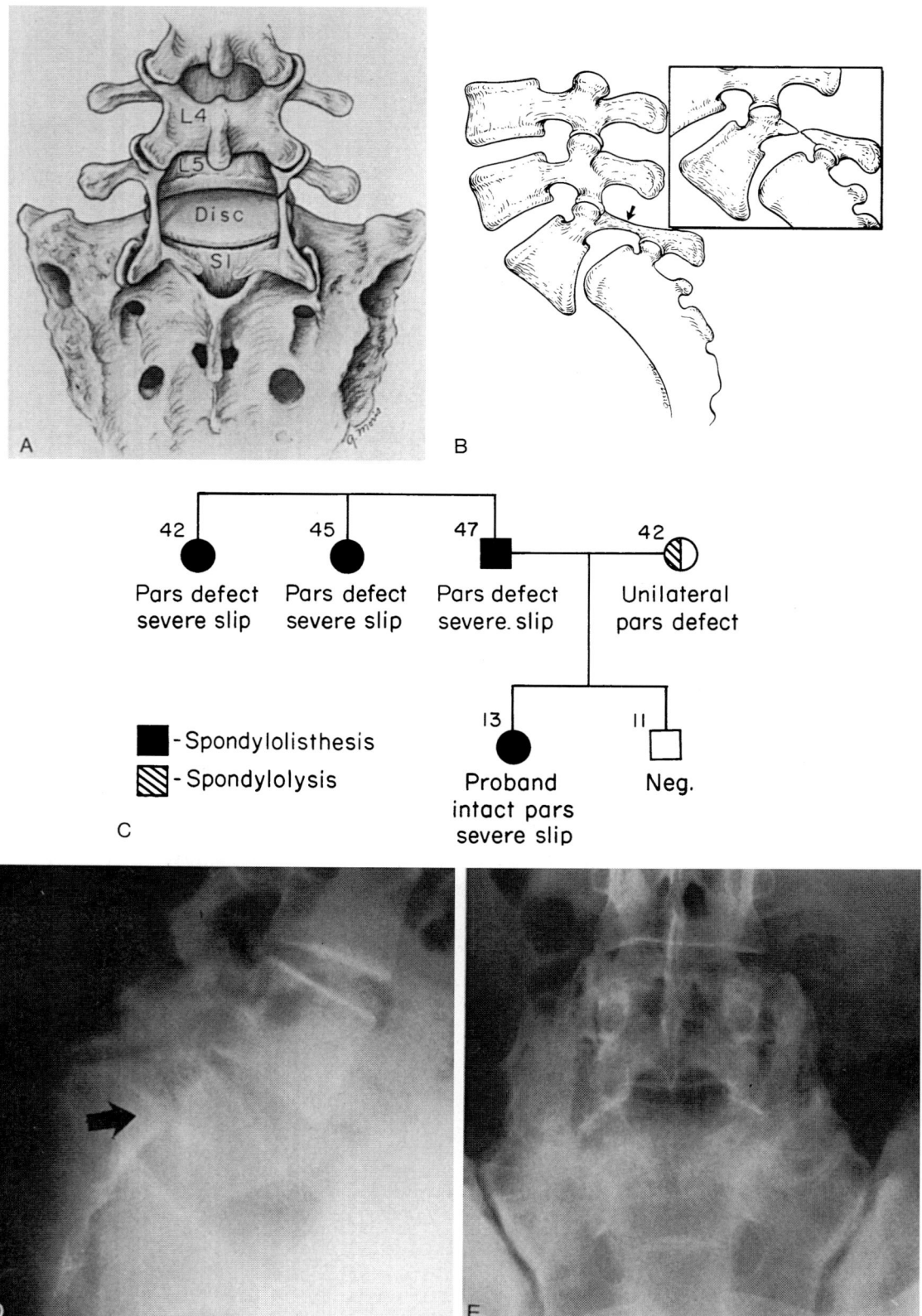

Figure 3 *See legend on opposite page*

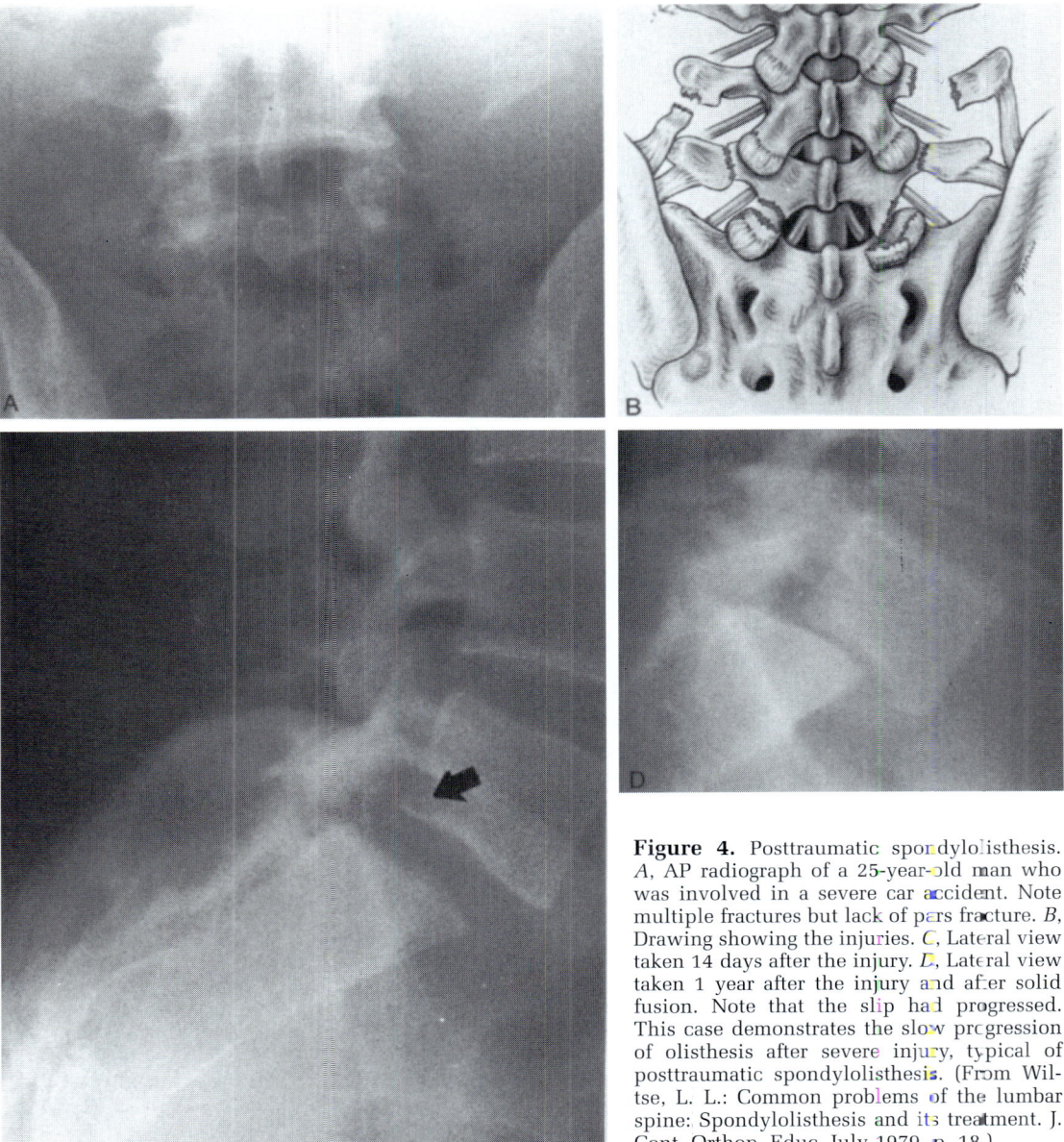

Figure 4. Posttraumatic spondylolisthesis. *A*, AP radiograph of a 25-year-old man who was involved in a severe car accident. Note multiple fractures but lack of pars fracture. *B*, Drawing showing the injuries. *C*, Lateral view taken 14 days after the injury. *D*, Lateral view taken 1 year after the injury and after solid fusion. Note that the slip had progressed. This case demonstrates the slow progression of olisthesis after severe injury, typical of posttraumatic spondylolisthesis. (From Wiltse, L. L.: Common problems of the lumbar spine: Spondylolisthesis and its treatment. J. Cont. Orthop. Educ. July 1979, p. 18.)

Figure 3. Elongated but intact pars (IIB classification). *A*, Drawing made at surgery of elongated but intact pars. On the right, the right pars has cracked through, and the left has elongated but remained intact. It might have healed even if the fusion had not been performed. *B*, Lateral drawing of type IIB. The pars may stretch for years and then crack and come apart. (From Ruge, D., and Wiltse, L. L.: Spondylolisthesis and its treatment: Conservative treatment, fusion with and without reduction. *In* Ruge, D., and Wiltse, L. L. (eds.): Spinal Disorders: Diagnosis and Treatment. Philadelphia, Lea & Febiger, 1977.) *C*, Family of one of the author's patients with elongated but intact pars. Only the proband had elongated, but intact, pars. All others had typical type IIA lesions in the pars. *D*, Preoperative lateral view of same patient as in *A*. Patient is a 16-year-old Caucasian woman. *E*, Anteroposterior (AP) radiograph, after fusion, of patient in *A*. (*C, E*, from Wiltse, L. L., Newman, P. M., Macnab, I: Classification of spondylolysis and spondylolisthesis. Clin. Orthop. 116:25, 1976.)

allows the cephalic vertebra to slip forward onto the one below it.
A. Generalized
B. Localized

Other Recent Classifications

Marchetti and Bartolozzi,[52] in their excellent monograph on spondylolisthesis published in 1986, presented a classification based exclusively on etiology. They divided all lesions into either developmental or acquired types (Table 1).

Variations in Classification Systems

There is actually little difference between the classification presented here and that of Marchetti and Bartolozzi.[52, 100]

The classification outlined previously is largely an anatomic one, yet each type has a clear-cut etiology. For example, the congenital type is markedly hereditary, yet upright posture causes the slipping (Rosenberg, N. J., personal communication, 1975). Although the isthmic type (acquired) has a strong hereditary component, every case is the result of stress fractures of the pars.

The degenerative type is largely acquired but has a significant congenital factor in its etiology, as noted in the sagittal orientation of the facets. The postsurgical type may even have a congenital component in a few cases. The pathologic type often has a hereditary element, as for example in osteoporosis[99] or Kuskokwim disease. The posttraumatic type is probably totally acquired.

The authors differ from Marchetti and Bartolozzi in strongly recommending that the term postsurgical be used instead of iatrogenic. The first meaning of the word iatrogenic in most English dictionaries is physician induced. In today's litigious atmosphere, the use of iatrogenic is probably unwise. Fortunately, because of the advent of the use of pedicle screws for fixation, the incidence of postsurgical spondylolisthesis will likely be reduced dramatically.

Types of Spondylolisthesis

Type I. Congenital

TYPE IA

In this subtype, anomalies of the lumbosacral area are frequently associated with spinal bifida occulta of the S1 or L5 segments (Fig. 5A,B). There is also dysplasia (underdevelopment) of the articular processes.[60] These dysplastic articular processes have an axial orientation, usually more on one side than on the other. The combination of dysplastic articular process, axial (horizontal) orientation of the facets, and spina bifida make the area unable to support superincumbent weight, and spondylolisthesis results. The pars interarticularis may remain unchanged. If it remains completely unchanged with subluxated facets and the ring is intact, the slip cannot exceed more than about 35% or there will be too much pressure on the cauda equina. Severe tightness of the hamstrings is likely to result. At least one case is on record in which a severe cauda equina compression syndrome resulted in paraplegia (Macnab, I., personal communication, June 1958). Usually, however, the pars interarticularis either elongates or comes apart. If it elongates, healing as it does, it is difficult to distinguish roentgenographically from type IIB, in which the pars cracks and heals, elongating as it does so. If the pars separates, the condition may be nearly impossible to distinguish from type IIA. If exposed at operation, the abnormal relationship and subluxation of the facets may still be difficult to identify. Careful study with computed tomographic (CT) scanning usually makes it possible to categorize this type accurately.

Occasionally, a wide-open upper sacrum exists and the L5 vertebra also shows wide spina bifida. The upper end of the superior surface of the body of S1 is often dysplastic (Fig. 6A to C). In a study by Wynne-Davies and Scott,[113] 11 of 12 patients with a dysplastic lesion had spinal bifida occulta in the lumbosacral area. No large series indicate the male/female ratio for the congenital type, but in the Wynne-Davies and Scott series, there were only seven male and five female patients (ratio of 1.4) in the dysplastic group. For the isthmic type with stress fracture, the male/female ratio was 25:10, with the male patients being more commonly affected.

There is a strong genetic element in both the dysplastic and the isthmic types of spondylolisthesis. In the study by Wynne-Davies and Scott,[113] a radiographic survey was carried out of the 147 first-degree relatives of 47 patients treated in Edinburgh for spondylolisthesis of L5; 12 patients had the congen-

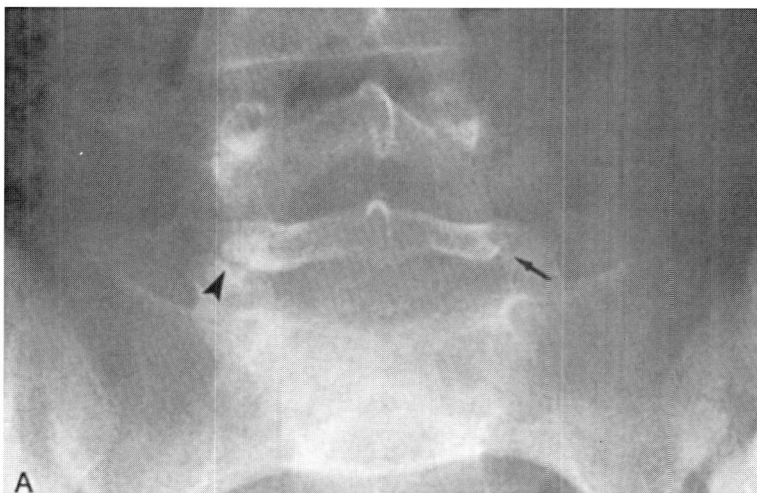
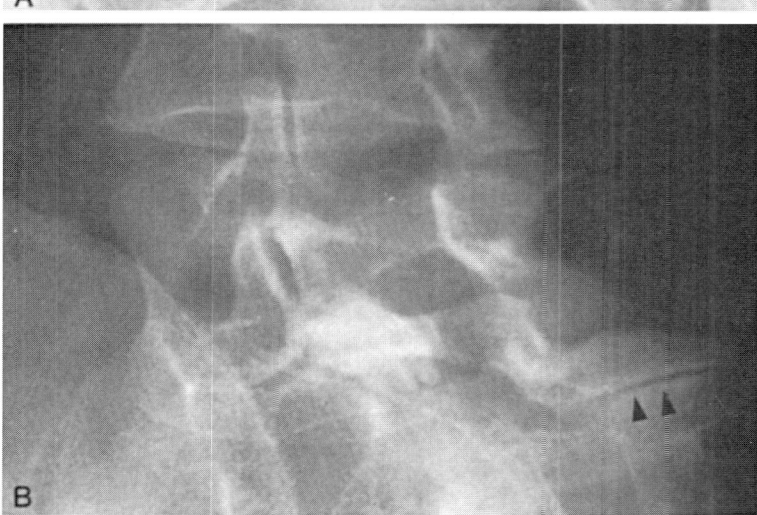

Figure 5. *A*, AP view of congenital type IA spondylolisthesis. This patient had 30% olisthesis. Note axial orientation of facets and tropism of facets. S1 spinous process is bifid, but L5 is not. *B*, Oblique view shows the markedly axial (horizontal) orientation of the left L5–S1 facet in the same case of congenital type IA as shown in *A*.

ital type, and 35 had an isthmic defect. The survey identified 19% of relatives with the opposite type from the patient. This suggests a close relationship between the causes of the congenital and isthmic types, which has prompted some researchers to postulate that the two are different manifestations of the same disease. Index patients with the congenital form had a higher proportion of affected relatives (33%) than did patients with the isthmic form.

Spina bifida occulta at L5 and/or S1 was more common among all persons with either congenital or isthmic types of spondylolysis than among their unaffected relatives (congenital form, 94%; isthmic type, 32%; and unaffected relatives, 7%). However, there was no single instance of a neural tube defect (e.g., anencephaly, spina bifida with or without meningocele, other generalized vertebral anomalies, and spinal dysraphism) among 826 first-, second-, or third-degree relatives. Wynne-Davies and Scott[113] concluded that the developmental defects of the vertebrae associated with spondylolysis are not etiologically related to neural tube defects.

Congenital spondylolisthesis of type IA can occur in newborn infants. Zembo and coworkers[115] reported a small series of this type in infants, two of whom had the condition at birth. Patients with this type appearing at birth usually have the lesion in the lower lumbar spine. Horizontal facets and a high grade of slip are nearly always present. This type is different from congenital kyphosis, which usually appears in the thoracolumbar area.

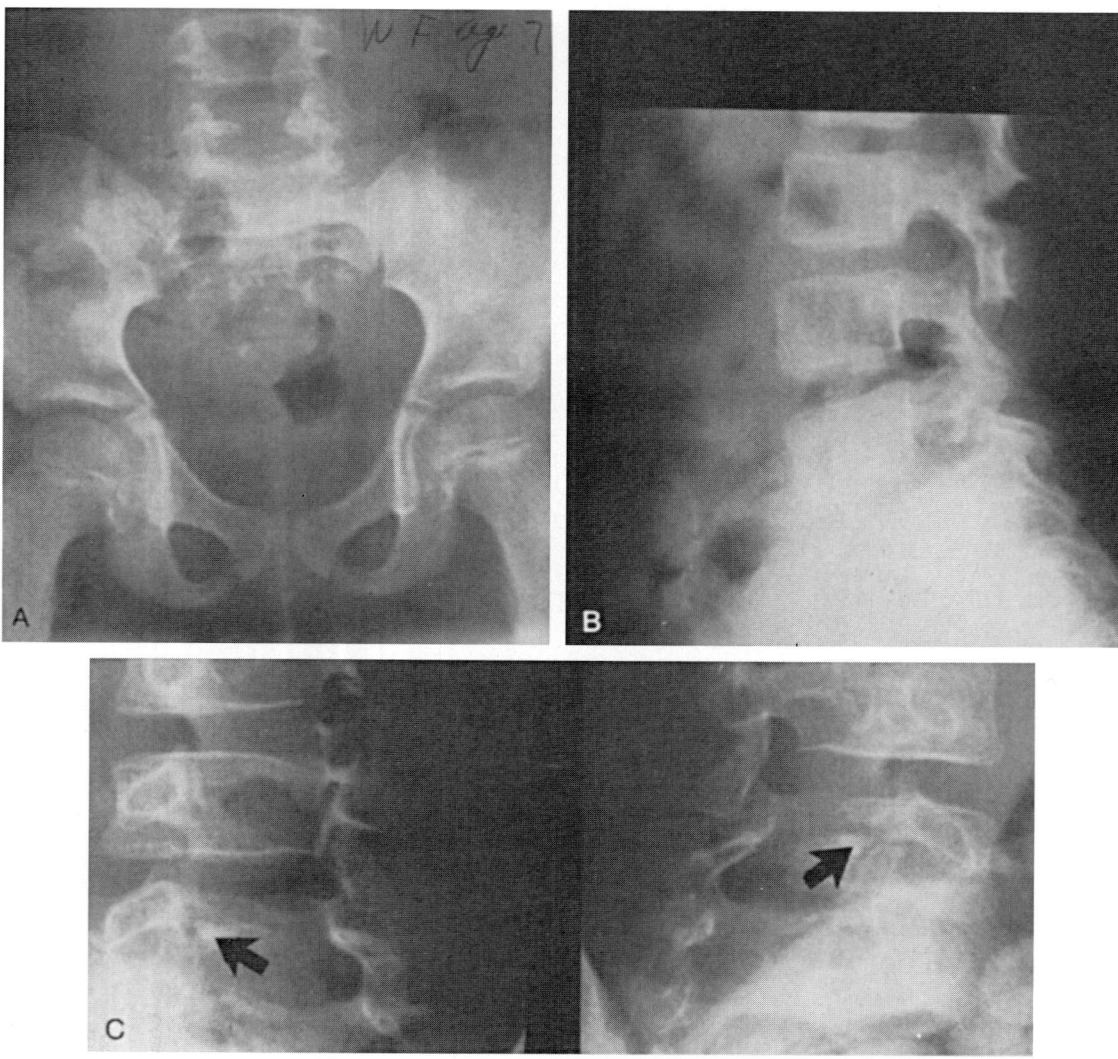

Figure 6. *A, B*, AP and lateral views spina bifida of L5 and a wide-open sacrum in a child. Note that in the lateral view, the pars fracture is also visualized. *C*, Oblique views of same patient, showing pars fractures.

TYPE IB

In this type of spondylolisthesis, there is congenital sagittal malorientation of the articular processes. As in type IA, the posterior elements are often poorly developed (Fig. 7*A* to *E*). The slip probably occurs because the facets have an unstable orientation of the facets and because the articular processes at the olisthetic level, besides being sagittally oriented, are rotated so that the posterior tip is more medial than the anterior tip on one side. This type seldom progresses to an extremely high degree of olisthesis because the neural ring is intact and severe neurologic change would develop before high-grade slip could occur.

TYPE IC. OTHER ABNORMALITIES OF THE LUMBAR SPINE

Other, often severe, congenital abnormalities of the lumbar spine permit partial or complete spondylolisthesis to occur. Most of these are of relatively little importance and are included here only because they have been reported in the literature.

Congenital kyphosis is probably the principal representative of this type.[115] Winter,[112] in a summary of his previous publications,

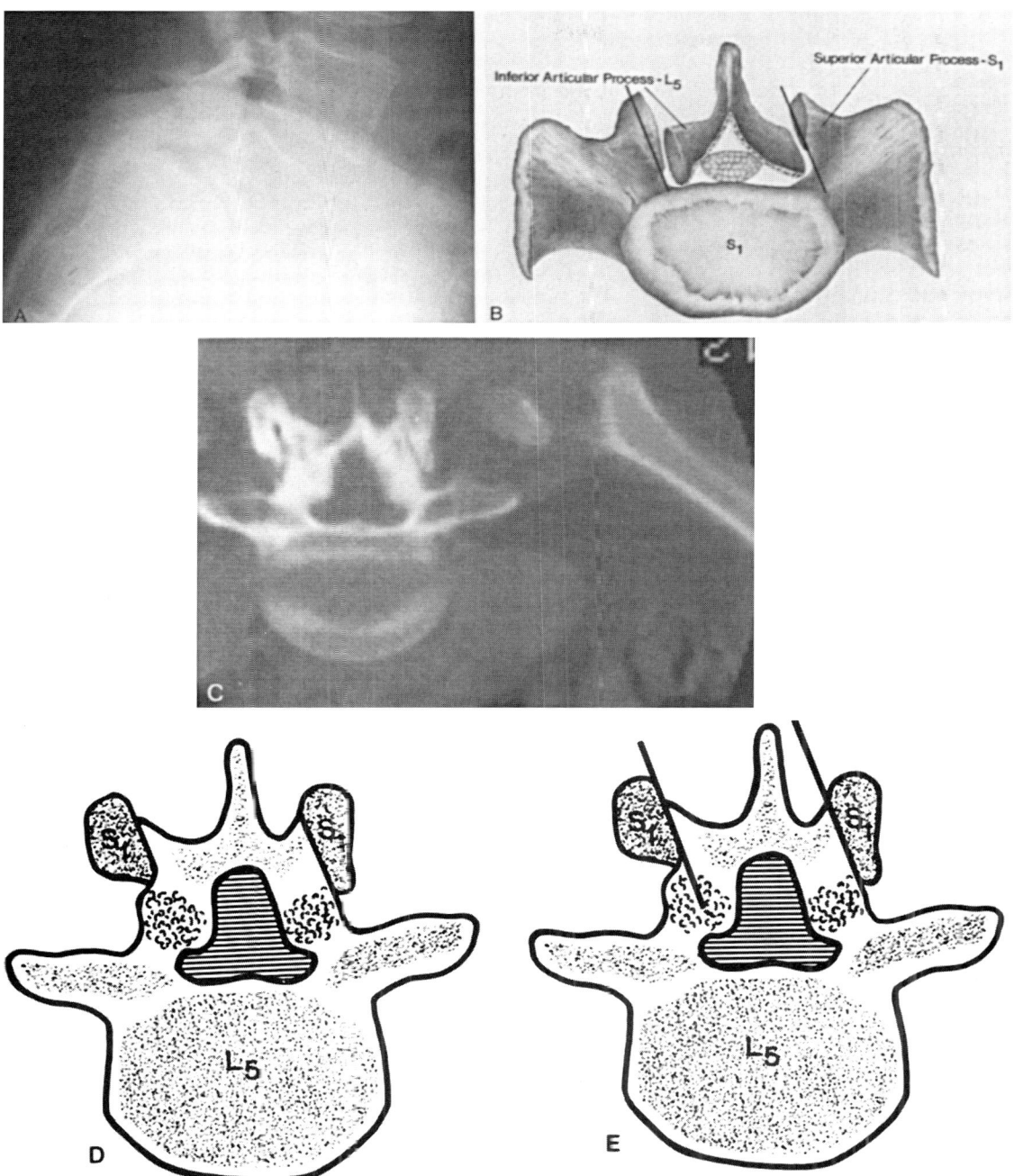

Figure 7. *A*, Lateral view of type IB. Note the intact pars and the relatively low degree of slip. The pars appears elongated, but what is actually seen is the side of the neural ring. *B* The cephalic end of the sacrum in type IB. This shows the sagittal orientation of the facets. Note that, on the left the facet is rotated in the direction opposite that of the facet on the right. This peculiar rotation effectively removes the stability normally supplied by the facets. *C*, Axial CT section through lower one fourth of the body of L5. Note the sagittal orientation of the facets. Also note how the facets on the right are rotated so that the posterior tip of the facet is more medial than the anterior tip. This peculiar rotation effectively removes the stability normally supplied by the facets. *D*, Drawing of axial CT section shown in *C*. Facets are sagittally oriented and are also in a state of tropism; the third peculiarity is that the posterior tips of the facets are more medial than the anterior tips. *E*, The lines show the direction of the facets in the axial plane. When both facets are in nearly the same plane, much of the stability normally supplied by the facets is lost.

recognized congenital failure of vertebral body formation, congenital failure of segmentation, and a mixed type of the disorder. Congenital failure of vertebral body formation is, by far, the most significant cause of complete spondylolisthesis in this type. This usually occurs at the thoracolumbar junction, rather than at L4 or L5.

Armstrong and Ye[5] described a congenital condition in which forward angulation of the upper sacrum permitted olisthesis. They described three types on the basis of the angles made by intersecting vertical lines; the first line is through the upper two sacral segments perpendicular to the end plate, and the second is through the remainder of the segments.

Type II. Isthmic

Isthmic spondylolisthesis always involves a fracture in the pars interarticularis. Secondary changes (e.g., alteration in the shape of the body of L5)[84] may occur, but these are not fundamental to its cause.

TYPE IIA. LYTIC (SPONDYLOLYTIC)

Lytic spondylolisthesis results from separation or dissolution of the pars after a stress fracture (Fig. 8). Statistically, it is seldom seen in patients younger than 5 years, but it occasionally occurs in this age group.[62] The authors' youngest patient with a confirmed lesion of the pars was only 8 months old when the lesion was first discovered.[105] This child's father also had the same lesion (West, F., personal communication). Borkow and Kleiger[9] reported on a patient in whom the lesion in the pars was first discovered when the child was only 4 months of age.

If a group of 100 children of 5 years of age were studied roentgenographically, probably none would have a pars defect.[81] However, if the same children were examined toward the end of the first grade (approaching 7 years of age), the incidence would be approximately 4.4%, which is just slightly below the United States national average. Baker and McHolick[6] and also Frederickson and associates[20, 21, 63] performed a study with this design. They were also able to examine roentgenographically the same group when they were approaching adulthood. They found that the incidence had increased 1.4% by the time the group reached age 18 years.[20] Most of this increase occurred between the ages of 11 and 16 years, the time of life when boys and girls are engaging in strenuous athletics that produce fatigue fractures.[21]

Why the lesion appears so frequently from 5½ to 7 years of age is not well known.[32] One might postulate either that it is because these children already have the anatomic predisposition for pars fractures, and this is the age when children start school and begin to push each other and tumble about, or that this is the first time when they sit for long periods with a lordotic posture. It is not known whether fracture in the pars is caused by flexion or extension stresses.[91] It probably results from both, as well as from torsional stresses.[17, 101, 102] There is considerable controversy concerning this point. It is known that the fracture never occurs in animals phylogenetically below humans and that only humans have true lordosis (Schultz, A. H., personal communication, 1962). This type also has a strong hereditary component.[105] Table 2 shows the proportions of first-degree relatives with spondylolysis or spondylolisthesis.

TYPE IIB

In this type of spondylolisthesis, there is elongation of the pars without separation.

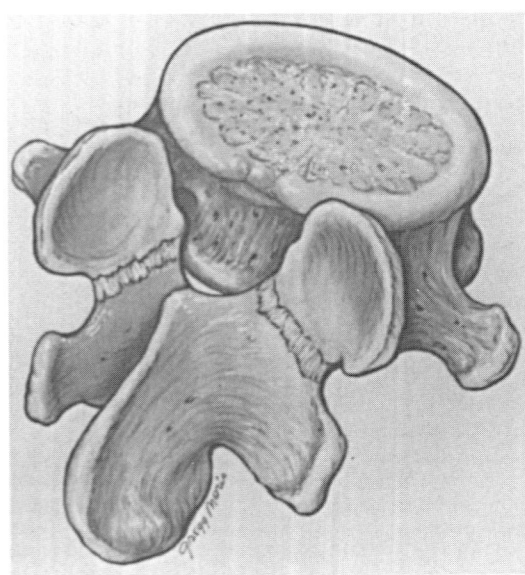

Figure 8. The defect in isthmic spondylolysis, classification IIA. (From Ruge, D., and Wiltse, L. L.: Spondylolisthesis and its treatment: Conservative treatment, fusion with and without reduction. *In* Ruge, D., and Wiltse, L. L. (eds.): Spinal Disorders: Diagnosis and Treatment. Philadelphia, Lea & Febiger, 1977.)

Table 2

Affected First-Degree Relatives of Patients with Spondylolysis or Spondylolisthesis

Patients	Parents	Siblings	Children	Total
Dysplastic (congenital) type	6 of 18	2 of 12	3 of 3	11 of 33 (33.0%)
Isthmic type	5 of 32	7 of 51	5 of 31	17 of 114 (14.9%)
Total	11 of 50 (22.0%)	9 of 63 (14.3%)	8 of 34 (23.5%)	28 of 147 (19.0%)

From Wynne-Davies, R., and Scott, J. H. S.: Inheritance and spondylolisthesis: A radiographic family survey. J. Bone Joint Surg. 61B:301–305, 1979.

This disease has the same cause as type IIA. It is secondary to repeated microfractures, which allow the pars to heal in a somewhat elongated position as the body of L5 slides forward, or to a single unilateral stress fracture, which causes the pars to heal in a displaced position.

One of the authors (L.L.W.) obtained x-ray studies of all available members of five families in whom the proband had an elongated but intact pars, whereas several other members of each of their immediate families had typical spondylolysis or spondylolisthesis with the classic pars defect, which is seen in type IIA. (As noted above, Wynne-Davies and Scott[113] found that patients with dysplastic pars had a high incidence of family members with fractures of the pars. Because their report preceded the CT scanning era, we can only presume that many of their dysplastic pars cases are actually healed pars fractures. In the authors' series of some 4000 imaging studies on patients with spondylolysis and spondylolisthesis, true congenital spondylolisthesis is considerably less common than in Wynne-Davies and Scott's studies.)

The pars may remain in continuity as it elongates, or it may thin out and finally separate, leaving stumps with a combined length much greater than that of a normal pars (Fig. 9A to D). If a separation finally occurs, the lesion is likely to be reclassified as type IIA, because it cannot be differentiated from that subtype. The fundamental disease is the same.

Since the advent of CT scanning, it has been possible to diagnose healed spondylolysis in many cases not previously recognized. Often, one can see a residual line representing the fracture site. There are two discernible patterns of healing. In some patients without slip, the pars becomes sclerotic and heals in situ. It is possible to identify subtle grooves in the inferior surface of the pars in some patients on lateral reformatted CT scans. Dense callus may form along the medial surface of the pars. This may successfully bridge the fracture. Ossification of the joint capsule also may occur as a further stabilizer of the motion segment. In many patients, only a "hockey stick" deformity of the pars can be identified. The presumption should be that this represents healed fractures and not a congenital anomaly.

TYPE IIC

Many investigators argue that acute pars fracture should logically not be included in the classification system because, at least in the adult, it virtually never occurs in isolation. There are almost always other injuries to the same vertebra, most commonly compression fracture, and the cause is always major trauma. The question then arises whether the pars defects were already present before the injury but were considered acute because they were discovered after a major trauma. Acute pars fractures probably do occur in children of 5 or 6 years of age.

Theory Supporting Common Etiologic Mechanism for Types I and II

It is likely that there is a common congenital component in all variations of both the congenital and isthmic types of spondylolisthesis.[1, 69] For this reason, the authors have formulated the following hypothesis of etiology.

It has been consistently observed that both congenital and isthmic types of spondylo-

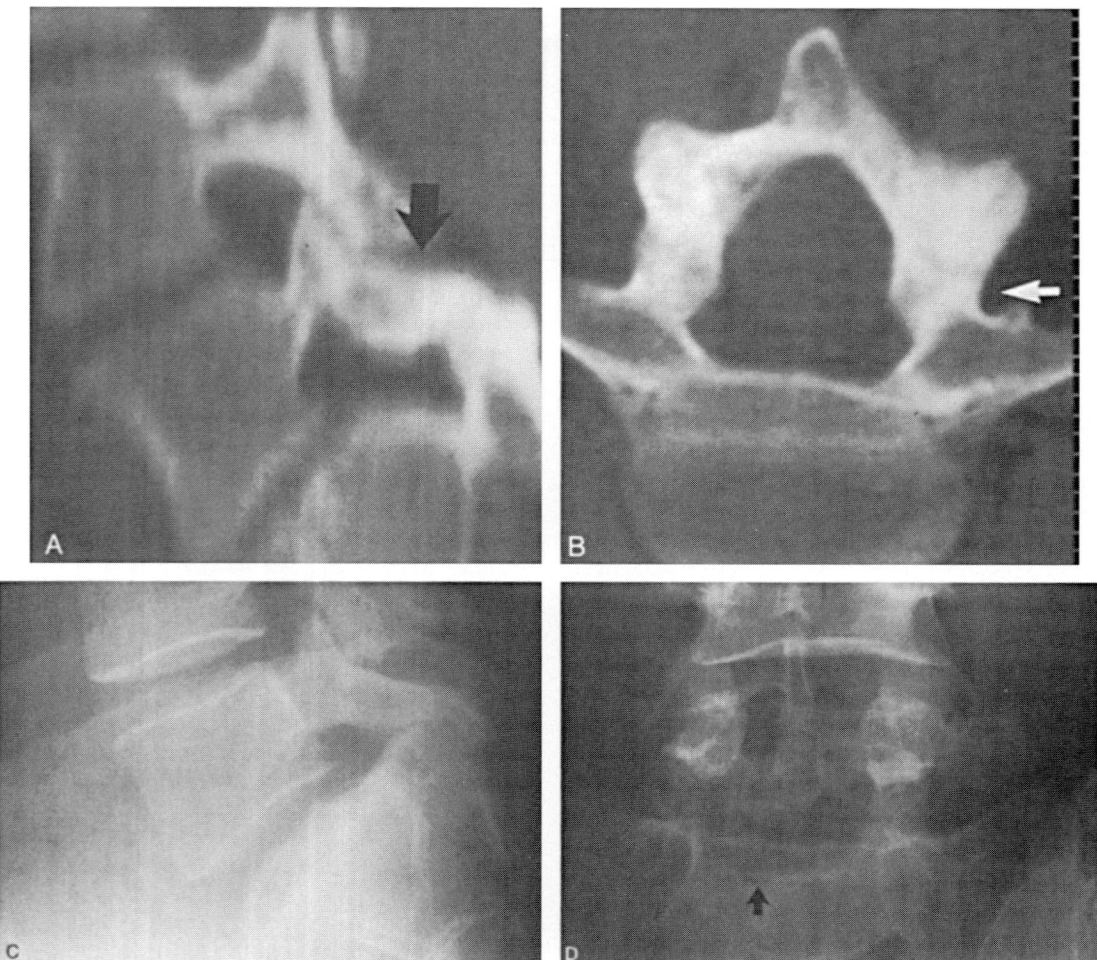

Figure 9. *A*, Reconstructed parasagittal view of a healed but elongated pars (type IIB classification). *B*, Axial view of healed bilateral pars fractures in the same patient as in *A*. Arrow points to healed area. Note elongated but healed pars. The radiologist reported, on the basis of the CT scan, "minor spina bifida occulta and hypoplasia of the lumbosacral facets." *C*, AP radiograph of the same patient as in *A*. Arrow points to a dysplastic area at the top of the body of S1. *D*, Lateral view of patient in *A*. Note dysplastic areas in cranial border of the body of S1. This patient had never been an athlete and stated that he was rather sedentary. Therefore, these fractures are not quite the same as those seen in the teenaged superathlete, who seldom has signs of dysplasia. This patient may have developed pars defects because he had abnormal growth of the upper sacrum and facets.

listhesis are often associated with spina bifida of the L5 or S1 segments. The spina bifida defect is much more common at S1 than at L5, but lesions at S1 and/or L5 occur considerably more often in patients with spondylolisthesis than in the normal population.[24] Since the advent of CT scanning, the ability to detect associated congenital anomalies has been immeasurably enhanced.[80] CT scans demonstrate hypoplasia of the superior articular process of S1 in most patients with either type of spondylolisthesis.

Except in the case of the young athlete (see below), there is a common congenital propensity for fracture at the pars, and also the slip in the dysplastic type is caused by hypoplasia of the posterior arches of L5 and/or S1, usually combined with an unstable orientation of the facets.[38]

In the presence of hypoplasia of the facets, because the area of contact is small, the L5 pars is predisposed to stress fracture because the fulcrum, which should be through the center of the pars, is displaced caudally. The increased length of the lever arm exerts greater stress on the pars, thus predisposing it to fracture.

Dysplasia of the L5–S1 joint area with abnormal orientation of the articular processes leads to congenital spondylolisthesis with the higher grades of slip. The facets may be sagittally or axially oriented but never coronally oriented. If they were coronally oriented, olisthesis would be impeded by direct bony contact of the facets. When facets are sagittally or axially oriented, especially when the facet on one side is more medial at its posterior tip than on its anterior tip, only the ligamentous structures check forward gliding. Because the spine is unstable at the articular processes, especially if there is a bifid spinous process, subluxation or luxation occurs.

Because, as is suggested here, the underlying processes are the same, both mechanisms may coexist. Therefore, patients can have both dysplastic facets and elongated pars. Usually, in the isthmic type, as the pars elongates or breaks, the laminae, including the spinous process and inferior articular processes, remain posterior as the anterior parts of the vertebrae slip forward; thus, the cauda equina is not compressed. This accounts for the frequently seen cases of an extremely high-grade slip with no neurologic changes and little dysfunction of any kind.

In some patients, after a certain amount of elongation, the pars finally fractures and does not heal. In other patients, the pars neither elongates nor fractures, but the superior facets glide forward on the inferior facets so that the entire neural ring subluxates forward, causing profound cauda equina compression, even with relatively low degrees of olisthesis. These probably account for the cases in which the severity of pain and hamstring spasm are out of proportion to the relatively low degree of slip (see Fig. 18A to F). The cases of cauda equina crisis are probably of this type.[75]

Inheritance Factor in Types I and II

To date, the pattern of inheritance for types I and II is not known with certainty. Haukipuro and colleagues[32] believe, as do Amusco and Mankin,[2] that the pattern definitely results from a dominant gene. Wynne-Davies and Scott[113] believe that it lies between autosomal dominant inheritance with reduced penetrance and multifactorial inheritance.[114]

On the basis of studies carried out in the 1950s,[105] the authors believed that the pattern of inheritance was attributable to a recessive gene with incomplete penetrance. However, in some families, the involved gene showed incomplete dominance, in that some affected individuals are carriers of the gene (heterozygous).

It is possible that the confusion encountered in determining the inheritance pattern arises because there are at least two distinct anatomic types, congenital and isthmic. Although these types each have subtypes with anatomic differences, they may have a common congenital cause. Much of the early work on the hereditary aspects of spondylolisthesis was done before the advent of CT scanning, when plain x-ray films were often of poor quality.

Stress Fracture of the Pars in the Young Athlete

Stress fracture of the pars is commonly seen in young athletes engaged in strenuous training.[30, 41] To the authors' knowledge, no genetic surveys have been conducted to determine whether there is an increased incidence among first-degree relatives of this group. In a study of 100 young female gymnasts,[33, 70, 90] 11 had pars defects. This is nearly four times the average for female adolescents. Of the 11, nine had spina bifida of the L5 and/or the S1 arch. This is higher than the average finding. One problem with studies of spinal bifida in children is that the posterior arch does not close until fairly late in adolescence or early adulthood, so the incidence is abnormally high even in children without pars defects.[53, 101, 102]

In a more recent study of six young athletes with fresh pars fractures, conducted by one of the authors (S.L.G.R.), all had normal bony anatomy. This leads to the surmise that, with regard to this one type of unquestionable stress fracture developing later (i.e., in adolescence), the cause is primarily the extreme stress placed on the pars, which is the most vulnerable point. Young athletes who have spina bifida may be slightly more likely to develop pars fractures than those with normal bony architecture.[67] This explains the increased incidence of spina bifida in the young athlete with fresh pars fractures.

Type III. Degenerative

The degenerative lesion is the result of long-standing intersegmental instability.[19, 34, 71, 74] Remodeling of the articular processes occurs at the level of involvement (Fig. 10A,B). Farfan (personal communication, 1988) believed that there are multiple small compression fractures of the inferior articular processes of the vertebra that slip forward. Because of this, the bone of the articular processes has a peculiar granular appearance on radiographs. As the slip progresses, the articular processes change direction and become more horizontal.[78]

Tropism of the facets is common.[80] When tropism is present, one side virtually always slips more than the other, and rotation of the vertebra at the level of olisthesis is an integral characteristic. The facets are sagittally oriented. The subluxation is more severe on the side of the more sagittally oriented facet. It is not possible to determine whether the more sagittal orientation occurs because one side has slipped further or whether the increased sagittal orientation is the cause of the increased slip on that side. However, there can be little doubt that rotary instability is part of degenerative spondylolisthesis.

According to Rosenberg,[79] degenerative spondylolisthesis occurs six times more frequently in women than in men, six to nine times more frequently at the L4 interspace than at adjoining levels, and four times more frequently when the L5 is sacralized than when it is not.[78, 79] When the lesion is at L4, the L5 vertebra is more stable and exhibits less lordosis than is average. A horizontal line drawn between the cephalic borders of the iliac crests (intercristal line) passes, on the average, through a more caudal level in the spine of patients in whom degenerative spondylolisthesis develops than in other patients. This arrangement increases stress on the joint between L4 and L5, leading to decompensation at the articular processes and multiple microfractures of the inferior articular processes of L4, thereby allowing forward slipping. Farfan (personal communication, 1988) stated that, when demonstrable degenerative spondylolisthesis is present, the olisthetic joint has lost 50% of its torsion and shear strength.

In previous years, the author (L.L.W.) had not seen this lesion in any patient younger

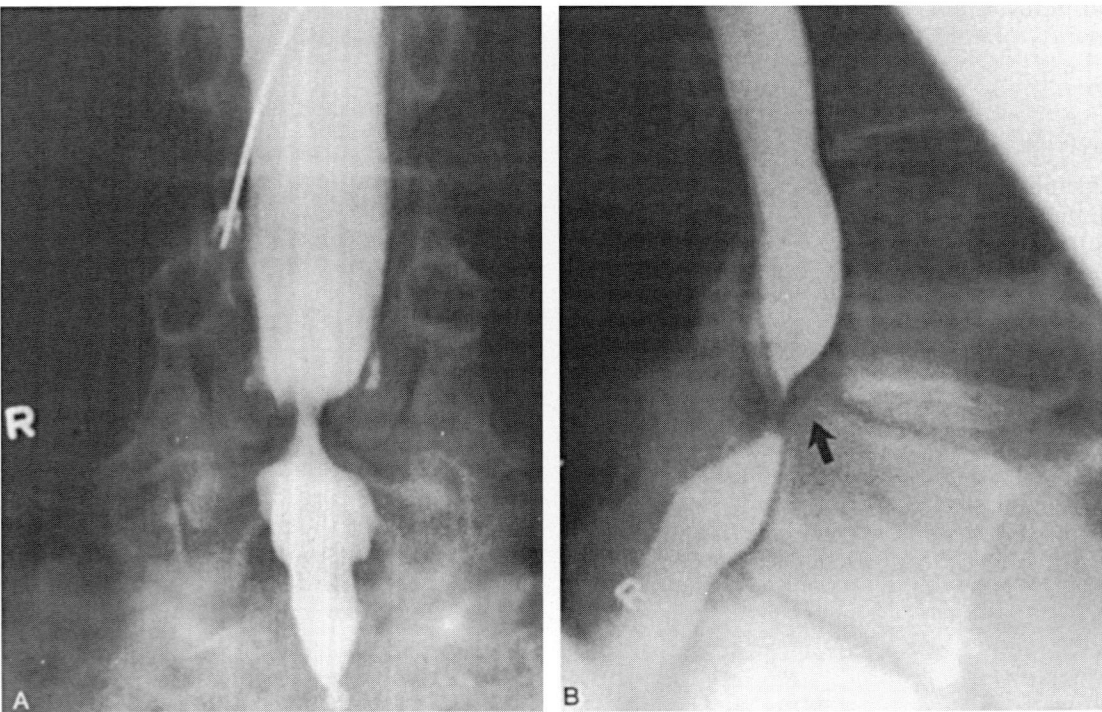

Figure 10. Typical AP (*A*) and lateral (*B*) myelograms of a patient with degenerative spondylolisthesis.

than 40 years, but as routine standing x-ray films of all patients are being taken, slippage is being seen in patients as young as in their late 30s. Knutsson[45] flexion and extension views also reveal dynamic instability, a frequent precursor of degenerative spondylolisthesis, at even earlier ages. At present, a condition is not called degenerative spondylolisthesis unless greater than 2 mm of slip is noted on the standing lateral view. Dynamic instability, on the other hand, is seen much more frequently and is the usual precursor of full-blown degenerative spondylolisthesis. For a condition to be classified as dynamic instability and not as degenerative spondylolisthesis, there should be anteriorposterior translation or intervertebral tilt on x-ray film beyond a normal extent, but the translation should be less than 2 mm.

Interestingly, the slip in spondylolisthesis seldom exceeds 30%, unless there has been surgical intervention.

Type IV. Postsurgical

TYPE IVA

This is a fairly frequent type of spondylolisthesis.[48, 104] The incidence varies in different reported series, but it was approximately 3% to 5% in the series reported by White and Wiltse.[104] The slip occurs because too much of the supporting structure has been removed in an effort to provide adequate decompression.[28] This group of patients includes those seen after extensive decompression for spinal stenosis, after laminectomy for disc removal, or after any other spine surgery in which it is necessary to destabilize the spine. Often, a minor degree of instability was present before surgery but could not be detected by ordinary x-ray examination. If a rather wide laminectomy is performed, as is often necessary to decompress the spine adequately, postoperative olisthesis is a common occurrence. Also, in the presence of osteoporosis and poor ligamentous support, unanticipated olisthesis may occur. Since the introduction and widespread use of pedicle screws, far fewer of these cases are being seen. Decompressive facetectomy done for spinal stenosis is the situation in which the use of pedicle screws is most clearly indicated.[26]

TYPE IVB

In a study of CT scans by one of the authors (S.L.G.R.) of patients who had undergone laminectomy, more than 10% were noted to have stress fractures of the pars where it joins the inferior articular process at the level of decompression. Mild postsurgical spondylolisthesis is common in these patients. This is somewhat different from instances in which too much bone has been removed. It is suggested that, in these cases, surgical weakening occurs at the base of the articular process, and fracture occurs during normal activity.

Type V. Posttraumatic

The posttraumatic type of spondylolisthesis is secondary to an acute injury that fractures parts of the supporting bone other than the pars and allows forward slip of the upper vertebra on the one below it as a secondary phenomenon. Fracture of one or both pedicles may also be present in this type.[51, 58]

This type of spondylolisthesis is always the result of severe trauma; the slip must occur gradually, over a period of weeks or longer. An acute fracture-dislocation should probably not be called spondylolisthesis, although the pathologic change may be virtually the same.

Type VI. Pathologic

In pathologic spondylolisthesis, either generalized or localized bone disease causes the bony mechanism (consisting of the pedicle, the pars, and the superior and inferior articular processes) to fail to hold the forward thrust of the superincumbent body weight, causing forward slip of the vertebra on the one below it. This type is rare.[73]

TYPE VIA. GENERALIZED

In this type of lesion, widespread generalized bony changes occur, as in the following examples.

Albers-Schönberg Disease (Osteoporosis). In this condition, fractures of the pars are frequent. These fractures sometimes heal and refracture. Spondylolysis often occurs[101] (Fig. 11A to C).

Arthrogryposis. In a type of arthro-

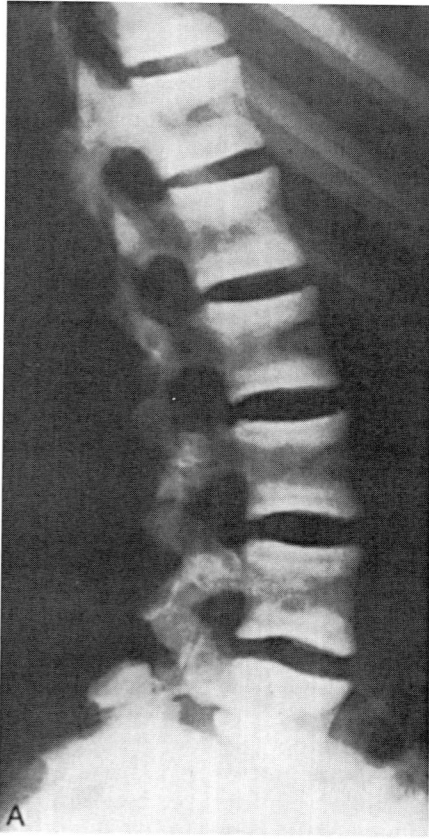

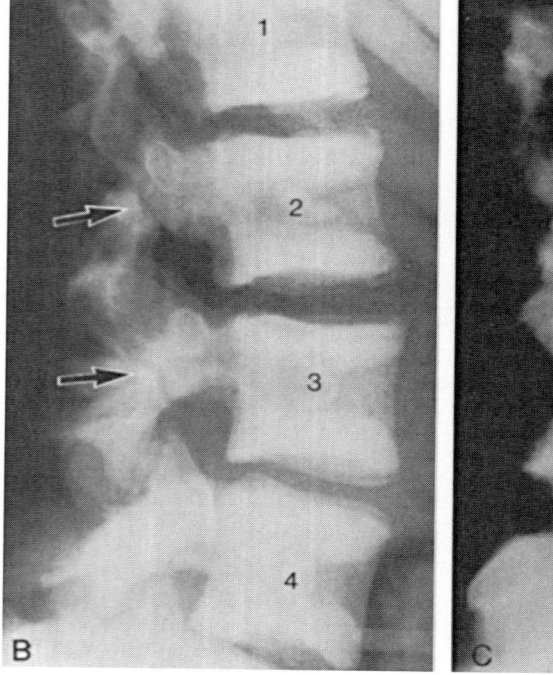

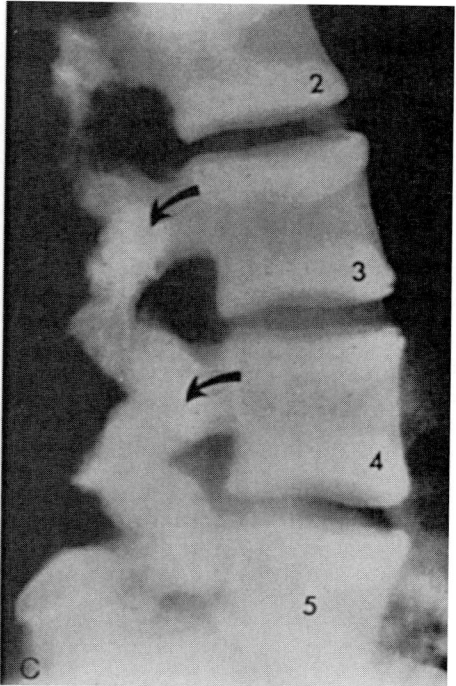

Figure 11. Pathologic spondylolisthesis secondary to osteopetrosis, showing cracking and healing of pars. *A*, A 12-year-old girl. Note pars fracture at L5. The partes of L2 and L3 are intact. *B*, Three months later, note spondylolysis of the L2 and the L3 partes. *C*, Seventeen months later, the partes of L2 and of L3 have healed. The pars of L5 shows an attempt at healing.

gryposis called Kuskokwim disease, several pedicles (but L5 in particular) may be elongated, producing spondylolisthesis of L5 on S1.

TYPE VIB. LOCALIZED

Localized bone infection, tumor, or some other localized destructive process may destroy the supporting structures sufficiently that the cranial vertebra slips forward on the vertebra that is more caudal.

Spondylolisthesis in the lumbar spine secondary to syphilitic gummas of the articular processes has been reported by Karaharjii and Hunnuksela.[42] It has been reported rarely in the United States in the past 30 years.

NATURAL HISTORY OF SPONDYLOLISTHESIS AND SPONDYLOLYSIS

This discussion of the natural history is limited to types IA, IB, IIA, IIB, and III. These are the congenital and isthmic types as well as degenerative spondylolisthesis.

Several studies have been made in an attempt to establish the natural history of types I (congenital) and II (isthmic),[70] but they have been only partially successful. It is essential that one be certain of the type of spondylolisthesis being studied. The slip that occurs in the isthmic type, in which the loose element remains in its normal position, behaves differently from the congenital type, in which there is neither a pars defect nor spina bifida. Most long-range studies also have the problem of poor x-ray films or no original x-ray films available at the time of the follow-up study, and one must depend on reports by radiologists who may not have been aware of these subdivisions.

Especially in children, if standing lateral films are not taken but only decubitus films, the physician may call a condition spondylolysis when, in actuality, some degree of slip would be seen if a standing film were taken. Also, when attempting to determine the incidence of a given type of spondylolisthesis in the general population, one must consider that most patients first come to the physician because of back pain. Because many people have slip, often severe, but have no back or leg pain, the statistics may be skewed.

It appears, on the basis of a review of several studies, that isthmic spondylolisthesis with olisthesis up to at least 10% carries about the same risk of low back trouble as that in the normal population without spondylolisthesis.[98] For slip of between 10% and 25%, there may be some increase in the incidence of back pain and sciatica.[37]

What about the higher grades (beyond 25%) of slip? Are these patients predisposed to have symptoms? The authors believe that they are, and there are some statistical studies to support this belief.[37,83,87] In large studies taken from preemployment x-ray films incidental to preemployment physical examinations, the incidence of high-grade slip is low and, in many studies, nonexistent. This suggests that people with high-grade slip do not apply for work in the general labor market. Unfortunately, no studies show the incidence of high-grade slip in the general population. Clinicians with large spine practices see a few cases of high-grade slip in the elderly as an incidental finding, suggesting that it is not frequent and also that, if slip is present in the elderly, it does not cause enough trouble for them to seek medical care.

Saraste[86] reported a 20-year observation of 255 spondylolysis and spondylolisthesis patients. She noted that progression of slip was small and not correlated with age at diagnosis or with the initial degree of olisthesis. Disc height reduction at the spondylolytic level occurred earlier and was more severe than in a control group. If the slip was greater than 25%, the patient was at an increased risk for symptoms compared with the normal population. Wedging of the L5 vertebral body and disc degeneration also increased the likelihood of back pain and sciatica, compared with those without spondylolysis or olisthesis. This finding was not confirmed in other studies.

Harris and Weinstein[32] compared the long-term clinical results (average of 18 years) in 11 patients with what appeared to be isthmic spondylolisthesis with olisthesis greater than 50%, who were treated nonoperatively, along with another group of 21 who had slip of a similar percentage treated by posterior fusion in situ. The two groups were compared as to degree of pain, residual neurologic change, bladder and bowel problems, and changes in lifestyle. At follow-up, the two groups had virtually equal clinical findings. Only one patient in each group had significant pain, and all were living normal, active lives. In two in the nonoperated group significant slip developed, and this progressive slip was an indication for in situ fusion.

Apel and coworkers[4] reported on a group of 12 patients with first-degree spondylolisthesis and an average follow-up period of 40 years. These patients were treated at Hines Veterans Administration Hospital in Chicago between 1944 and 1951. In each case, the slip had been classified as grade I and was at the L5–S1 level. Five patients had been treated conservatively, and seven were treated surgically with a Hibbs posterior fusion from L5 to S1. Of the conservatively managed patients, all functioned well during their working years, although one had chronic, nondisabling, low back pain. This same patient demonstrated radiographic evidence of progression to a grade II spondylolisthesis. Among those undergoing surgery, the poor results were confined to patients for whom attempts at fusion failed. The researchers concluded that the management of low-grade spondylolisthesis should be conservative whenever possible. They recommended that, when the low back pain is disabling and surgery is resorted to, failure to obtain fusion portends a poor clinical result. Interestingly, in this study, conservatively managed patients actually did somewhat better than those who were operated on.

It can be deduced from these studies that it is best to treat the patient who has either isthmic spondylolisthesis (types IIA or IIB) or congenital spondylolisthesis (types IA or IB) without resorting to surgery, if possible. If pain is severe and persistent to the degree that it alters the patient's lifestyle or if, in a young patient, the slip is increasing, fusion in situ is indicated.[84, 85] However, there is little danger in continuing conservative treatment indefinitely.

The natural history of the three most important types of spondylolisthesis (congenital, isthmic, and degenerative) can be summarized as follows.

Types IA and IB. Congenital

TYPE IA

If the posterior ring is intact, symptoms of cauda equina compression may occur with slip as low as 35%. It has been noted by many investigators that the olisthesis is seldom identified while it is developing, suggesting that it happens relatively slowly. If a wide-open spina bifida of L5 and/or S1 is present,[86] then

1. Olisthesis often appears earlier than in cases in which the posterior arch is present.[87]
2. Slip may be very severe.
3. These patients may have severe hamstring spasm but fare better neurologically than if the posterior elements are intact and still slip forward.
4. These patients probably need fusion more often than do other patients.

TYPE IB

This type shows altered facet orientation but often an intact posterior ring. The following are associated with the disorder:

1. High-grade slip is less common.
2. Leg pain, back spasm, hamstring spasm, and altered gait bring the patient to medical attention.
3. In L5 spondylolisthesis, the part of the cauda equina caudal to the L5 nerves is compressed.
4. If fusion in situ without decompression is performed on these patients, they are likely to have persistent tight hamstrings and altered gait, but they usually obtain a satisfactory result. If recovery is too slow, decompression can be done months or even years later with a good chance of improvement of symptoms.
5. This type is often seen in adults, usually in patients who have symptoms for the first time.

Types IIA and IIB. Isthmic

Patients with these lesions have either a separated fracture in the pars or a pars that has elongated as the vertebral body slips forward. This usually leaves the posterior elements in normal position.[39, 40]

1. Few cases are noted before age 5 years.
2. Most cases develop during the first year of school.[20, 81]

3. By 7 years of age, 4% of the cases have appeared.[5]

4. Another 1.4% appear before adulthood.

5. Most of the 1.4% appear between the ages of 11 and 15 years, and these represent stress fractures in the pars in athletic children.[14, 65, 107]

6. Children with spastic diplegia develop stress fractures in the pars four times as often as children in the general population.

7. In persons engaged in strenuous athletics, new cases appear even into early adulthood.[18]

8. Olisthesis develops any time after the pars fractures occur, but the majority of high-grade slips develop between 10 and 14 years of age (in girls, this occurs a year or so earlier than in boys).

9. High-grade slip is four times as likely in girls as in boys, yet pars defects are only half as frequent in girls as in boys.[14, 39]

10. Back and leg pain commonly bring the patient to the physician. Changes in body contour alone seldom bring patients to seek medical attention.[22, 92, 93]

11. Significant increases in olisthesis after adulthood are sufficiently uncommon that they are not considered a substantial problem.[15, 22, 23, 94]

12. Olisthesis up to 10%[33] appears not to increase the likelihood of back problems, even with heavy work.[2] With slip between 10% and 25%, there may be some question, and slip beyond 25%, clearly increases the likelihood of a patient's having low back symptoms, compared with what would be expected in a population without pars defects.[94, 95] Virta and associates[103] showed that a finding of pars defects at L5 in unselected middle-aged people is not associated with increased back symptoms or decreased function.[103]

13. Wedging of the body of L5 also increases the likelihood of symptoms, according to Saraste and associates.[82]

14. Increased sagittal rotation causes more change in body contour than does increased olisthesis.[40]

15. Spondylolisthesis, even high grade, causes no problem during pregnancy or delivery.[85]

16. Shelokov[96] showed that gait abnormalities associated with high-grade slip disappear when fusion has become solid.

17. As to what factors portend further olisthesis, only a few conditions can be incriminated. Degree of olisthesis,[23, 91, 94] wedging of the L5 vertebral body at an early age, and degenerative narrowing of the disc space have been incriminated but are not noted by every investigator.[20, 91, 94]

18. In a retrospective study involving several centers, Grobler and associates[27] concluded that L4–L5 isthmic spondylolisthesis occurs in about 9% of patients with isthmic spondylolisthesis. It usually becomes symptomatic in adulthood. It is more unstable than lesions at L5, and surgical treatment is required in a higher percentage of persons who present for treatment (approximately 37%) than if the lesion is not at L5.

Type III. Degenerative

Degenerative spondylolisthesis is characterized by the following:

1. It is seldom seen before age 40 years on ordinary x-ray films, but the incidence increases with age and it is common in the elderly.[19] Dynamic instability may be noted several years before age 40 years and often progresses to full-blown degenerative spondylolisthesis. Standing lateral x-ray films must show greater than 2 mm of slip before it is called degenerative spondylolisthesis.

2. Women are more commonly affected than men.[79]

3. Pain is of two types: (a) claudicant pain, characterized by pain in the calves brought on by walking,[75] and (b) the much more common sciatic type, in which pain extends down one leg, resembling the pain from a herniated disc.

4. Slip seldom progresses to more than 33% if no surgery is performed.

5. Severe paralysis is rare, but footdrop, unilateral or occasionally bilateral, occurs often.

6. Sciatic tension signs are often absent, even though the pain may be of the sciatic type.

7. Most patients can be treated nonoperatively. It has been reported that only one person in 10 with slip who goes to a physician needs surgery.[75]

8. The major instability is not flexion-extension instability (in other words, tilt) but axial-rotational and anterior-posterior transitional instability.[54]

SURGERY FOR SPONDYLOLISTHESIS

Types IIA and IIB. Isthmic

Because a complete discussion of the surgery for spondylolisthesis is beyond the scope of this paper, the discussion is limited to a few areas, especially areas of controversy. The opinions expressed and the type of surgery recommended are drawn from the senior author's (L.L.W.) experience, and no effort is made to discuss the many other types of surgery being performed by surgeons around the world.

In children with isthmic spondylolisthesis, fusion in situ is performed without decompression, no matter how high the degree of slip.[7, 66, 68, 75, 76, 111] This has been the authors' practice for the past 30 years. No child has had less than a good result. Complications have been negligible. A paraspinal approach[36] has been used since 1960[106] (Fig. 12). Most patients have been allowed to get up within a few days, and normally no corset or brace is used. There have been no failures of fusion[75] (Fig. 13A to G). To the authors' knowledge, in only one or two cases reported in the literature has a child with high-grade slip had a cauda equina syndrome present when first seen by a physician. The authors have never encountered this, but would perform a decompression immediately.

In a study of adults with high-grade isthmic spondylolisthesis and sciatica reported by Peek and coworkers,[68] eight consecutive patients were treated by fusion in situ without decompression.[24, 106] All patients had severe sciatica and neurologic deficits. Anterior displacement[44] ranged from 60% to complete spondylosis, with the average being 81%. Follow-up ranged from 2 to 14.1 years, with an average of 5 years. All eight cases had solid fusion with excellent relief of back pain and sciatica. Neurologic deficits resolved, with the exception of lost Achilles reflexes in two patients. There were no serious complications (Fig. 14A to C). Appearance was satisfactory in all cases. Osterman and Seitsalo[66] stated that pain and abnormal gait disappear after the fusion is solid.

When should the arthrodesis be limited to L5 and S1, and when should L4 be included? Considering the degree of sagittal rotation alone and ignoring, for the moment, such factors as ruptured disc at the L4 level or internal disc disruption[12] at that level, if the angle of the superior border of L5 to the horizontal (this is the new sacrohorizontal angle) is less than 55 degrees, the authors fuse only L5 to S1. If the angle is greater than 55 degrees, L4 is included in the fusion[109] (Fig. 15). If one is in doubt about including L4 in the fusion because of concerns about pain at that level, the discogram and the pain reproduction test may be used.[3] Anatomic degeneration alone is no reason to include the level above in the fusion.[16, 46, 72]

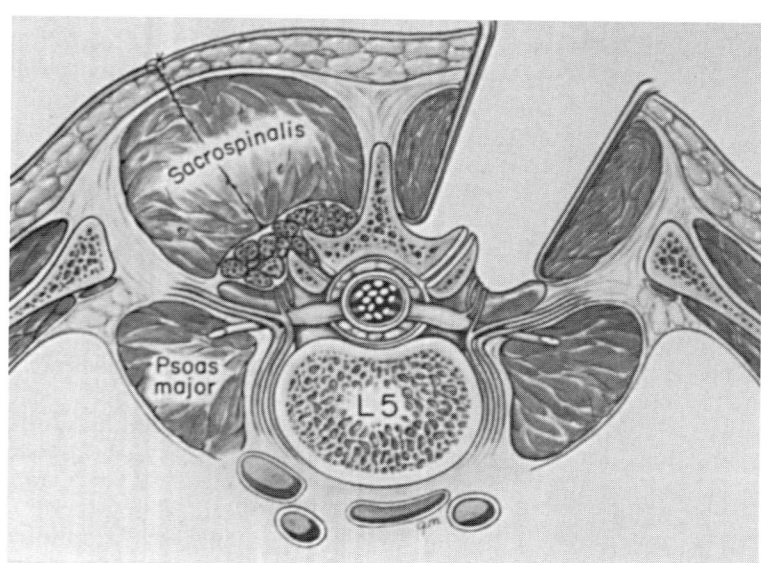

Figure 12. The paraspinal approach used in virtually all cases of spondylolisthesis type I and type II. (From Wiltse, L. L., Bateman, J. G., and Hutchenson, R. H.: The paraspinal sacrospinalis-splitting approach to the lumbar spine. J. Bone Joint Surg. 50A:919, 1968.)

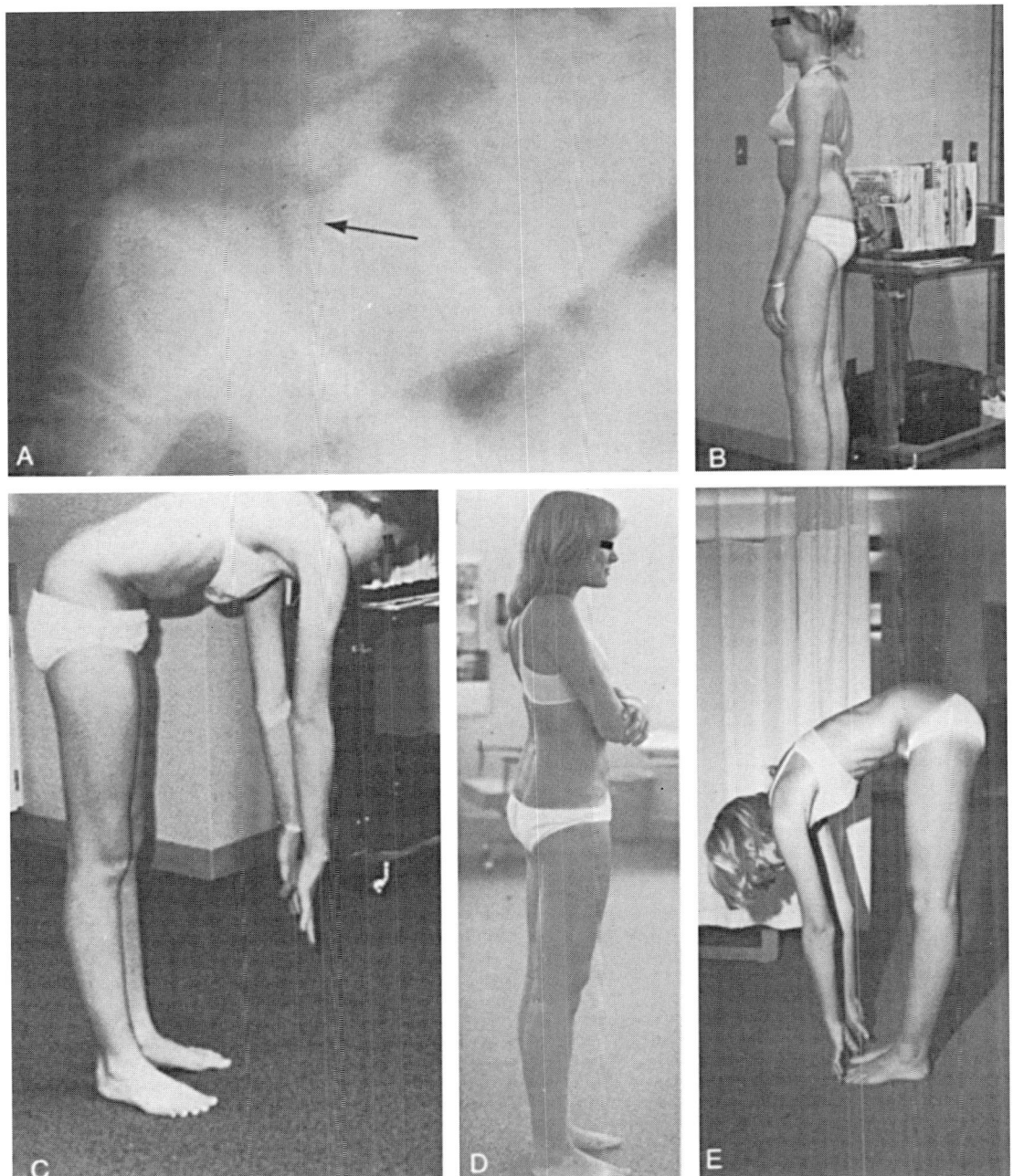

Figure 13. *A,* X-ray film of a typical 15-year-old female patient with high-grade slip and marked sagittal rotation of L5. The degree of sagittal rotation is much more important, in regard to the effect on bodily contour, than is the slip. Note that there has been an increase of a few degrees in sagittal rotation and a few degrees of decrease in sacral tilt, but none of olisthesis. This is characteristic. *B,* Note change in body contour. *C,* Note limitation in bending. *D,* One year after fusion. *E,* Bending 1 year after fusion.

Illustration continued on following page

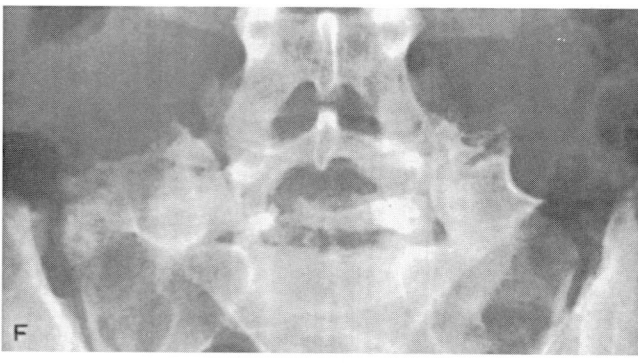
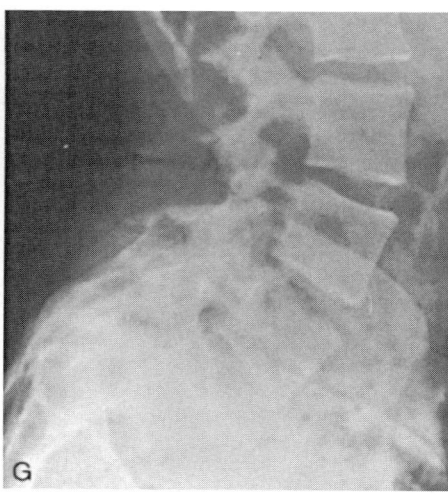

Figure 13. *Continued F,* AP x-ray film 11 years after fusion. *G,* Lateral x-ray film 11 years after fusion.

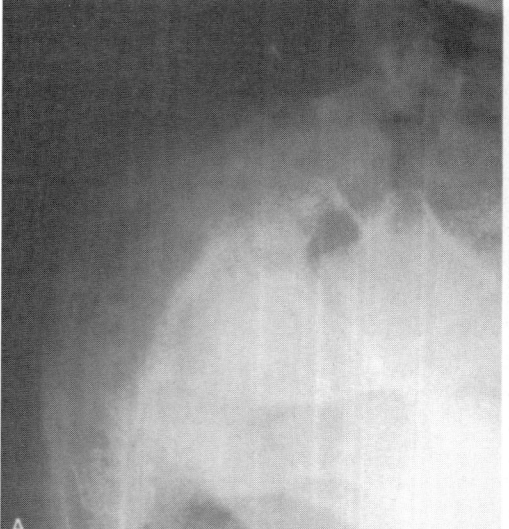
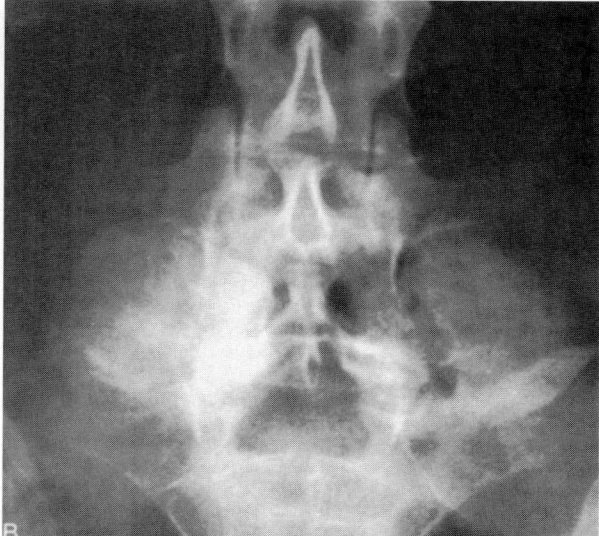
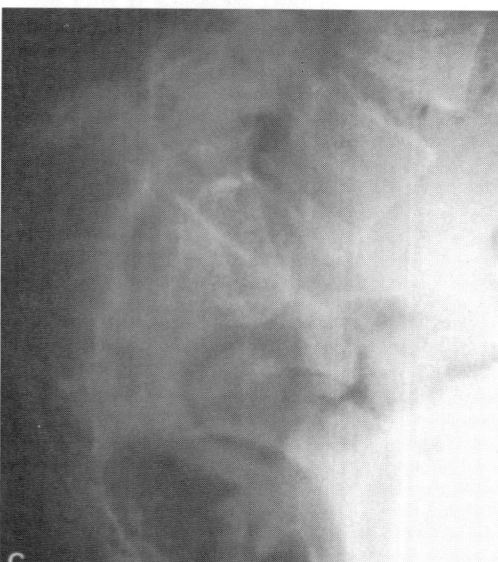

Figure 14. *A,* A 34-year-old Caucasian woman with high-grade slip, severe leg pain, and reflex and sensory change in painful leg. *B,* Three and a half years after fusion in situ, no decompression. She was allowed up immediately. No corset or brace was used. *C,* Lateral view. Note that no further olisthesis or sagittal rotation has occurred. She shows an excellent result.

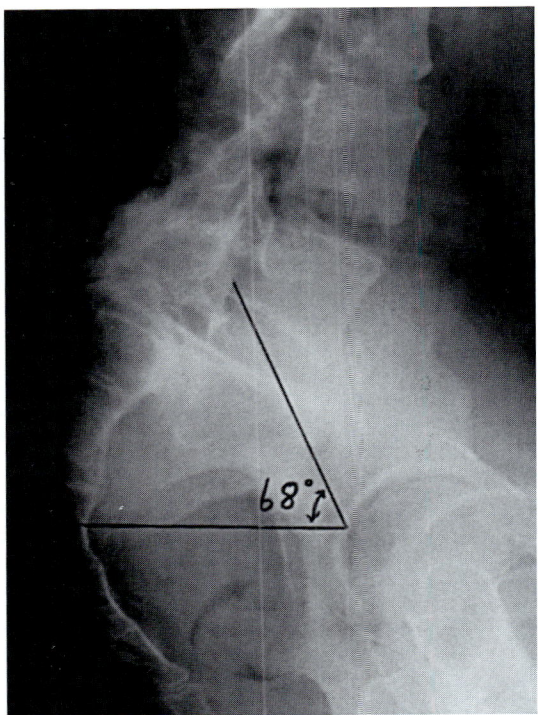

Figure 15. Sacrohorizontal angle (x-ray film must be taken with the patient standing). When a solid fusion of the lateral masses has been obtained from L5 to S1, it is as though there is a class IV transitional vertebra with the wings solidly fused to the alae. The top of L5 then becomes the new sacrohorizontal angle. The authors have arbitrarily chosen 55 degrees as the breakoff point for one-level fusions. For angles greater than 55 degrees, a two-level fusion is performed from L4 to S1.

Types IA and IB. Congenital

In the congenital type IA, surgery is identical to that done for the isthmic type, but in congenital type IB, in which the posterior arch is intact and there is no defect in the pars, the posterior ring slides forward and may compress the cauda equina. These patients may have more severe tightness of the hamstrings that is slower to resolve after surgery. In these cases, fusion in situ can be performed, but if the tight hamstrings and peculiar gait persist, a decompression procedure may be necessary and can be performed easily later. The authors have had to perform a late decompression in only one patient out of four with the congenital type of spondylolisthesis who had an intact ring.

After the fusion is solid, there is no danger of further olisthesis, and simple decompression at the L5–S1 level suffices. It appears that the nerves passing over the posterior superior rim of the body of S1 are compressed in these patients, but one is wise to decompress the L5 nerve as well. It is also important to get out far enough laterally on the L5 nerve to be sure that it is free. Thus, wide fusion should be performed in these patients, so that if decompression is required later, it can be done without compromising the solidity of the fusion. In the authors' experience, the tight hamstrings disappear rapidly after decompression. However, if the existing tightness is not too great and not too troublesome, the patient can be left undecompressed; the gait returns to normal and hamstring tightness disappears over a a few years. In either the isthmic or the congenital type, pain and hamstring tightness are likely to persist until the fusion is solid. A late decompression was necessary in only two cases in the authors' entire experience with the isthmic type of spondylolisthesis.

The question of whether discography should be carried out at the first unfused level above the proposed fusion is not dealt with here.

Postoperative Cauda Equina Syndrome

There have been a number of reports in the literature of postoperative cauda equina syndrome after fusion in situ without decompression.[89] The authors studied the reports carefully but have no ready explanation for this phenomenon. The following is a theoretic explanation.

As the parts of the vertebrae anterior to the pars slip forward, even though the pars is broken, there remain strong soft tissue structures attempting to pull the posterior elements forward. These soft tissue structures consist of the intraspinous ligaments, the ligamentum flavum, and also the scar tissue between the ends of the fractured pars (the "spondylolisthesis ligament"[16]). In many cases, the facets between L5 and S1 hold the loose element in its normal place, but in other cases, the superior articular processes slip between the inferior ones and the loose element follows the anterior parts forward, as they are pulled down against the posterior superior border of the body of S1.[11] Figure 16 shows such a situation.

This forward slip probably happens

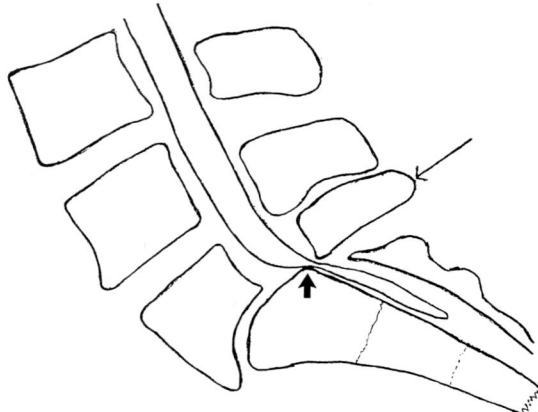

Figure 16. In some cases, the loose element of L5, instead of remaining back in its normal position, may be pulled forward by the various ligaments and thus partially follow the anterior elements as they slide forward. This happens in spite of the presence of pars fractures. By this mechanism, the caudal edge of the arch may compress the cauda equina between itself and the posterosuperior border of the body of S1. This may account for some cases of tight hamstrings. (Based on Buirski, G., McCall, I. W., and O'Brien, J. P.: Myelography in severe lumbosacral spondylolisthesis. Br. J. Radiol. 57:1067–1072, 1984.)

slowly enough that paralysis seldom occurs, but tight hamstrings do occur. Under general anesthesia, all muscle protection is lost. If this loose element is pressed on by the surgeon while the soft tissue is scraped off its posterior surface, it would seem that in rare cases damage could occur, causing an immediate cauda equina syndrome or a delayed one, owing to swelling of the nerves in a closed space.

It is difficult to know how much pressure is actually put on the pars during surgery, but based on testing with a mockup on a simple scale, using a Cobb elevator, it appears that 15 pounds (7 kg) can easily be exerted. Even pressing down with a Lecksell rongeur to remove soft tissue can easily exert considerable force. Obviously, one should ease the soft tissue off the loose element, decompress the L5 nerves out beyond the pars, and either reduce the slip or remove a generous amount of the posterior border of the sacrum, or probably both. This should be followed by the use of pedicle screws, if they are not contraindicated.

Pedicle Screws

In a further attempt to achieve fusion, pedicle screws are usually used in adult patients in whom there has been failure in previous surgery. The authors have not made a point of reducing the slip. In cases of alar transverse process impingement, decompression can be avoided by lifting L5 off the sacrum. Pedicle screws are essential in these cases.[110] With the use of pedicle screws, the L5 can be jacked cranially and posteriorly, which lifts the lateral masses off of the nerve. Only one level of vertebra need be fused. If the vertebrae are severely separated at surgery, the surgeon should add an interbody fusion to take the stress off the screws. Whenever reduction is performed by pulling on the screws, thus stressing them, an interbody fusion should be added. If the only reduction accomplished is the amount that occurs by positioning on the table, the screws are not severely stressed and an anterior support may be unnecessary.

If the surgeon prefers, the nerve can be decompressed by channeling far out laterally, then fixating the vertebrae with rods and pedicle screws and adding fusion (Fig. 17A to E).

If a Gill operation is performed on an adult, pedicle screws should always be used because the remaining fusion area is so small.[25] This is true even if an interbody fusion is added, because if most of the posterior support is removed by the Gill procedure followed by an interbody fusion, which removes much of the anterior ligamentous support, catastrophic instability is a real possibility.[44]

AREAS OF CONTROVERSY AND NEEDS FOR FURTHER RESEARCH

It is difficult to distinguish the congenital and isthmic types of spondylolisthesis. The distinction is important only in some instances in which the treatment is different. Both types involve a hereditary component in their etiology. Understanding the patterns of inheritance requires further research. The advent of CT scanning has made this type of study much more exact than in the past. Nevertheless, difficulties remain.

It is clear that if there is separation at the isthmus and the posterior element remains in the normal position, decompression by removal of the loose element is unnecessary and often harmful because it removes sup-

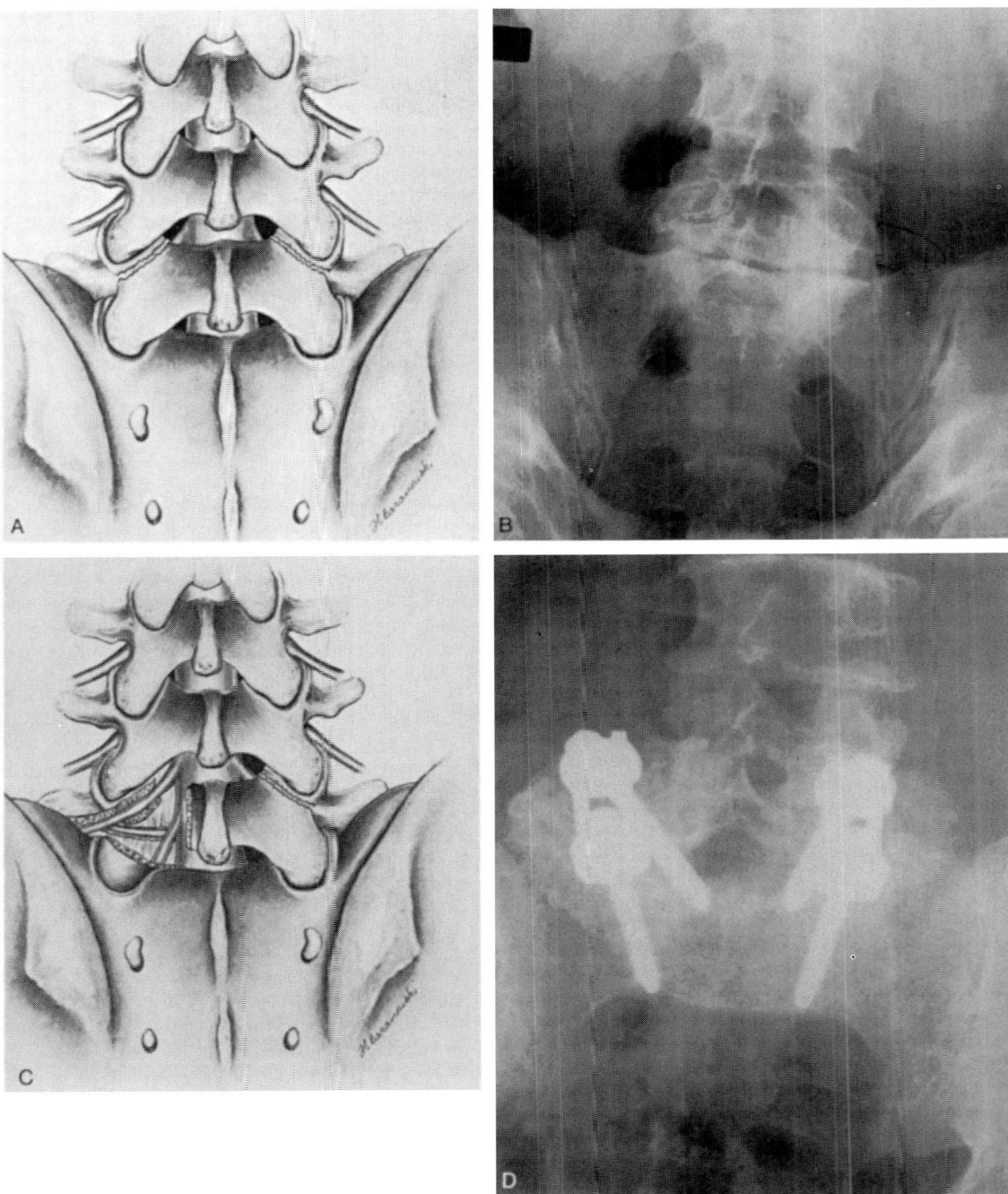

Figure 17. *A*, In spondylolisthesis, if the slip is as much as 20%, or perhaps even less, the lateral masses and transverse processes may drop down on the alae and compress the L5 nerve. The drawing attempts to demonstrate this. *B*, In this AP x-ray film of a patient with spondylolisthesis and 25% slip, there is also some tilt to the left. In this patient, the lateral mass was jammed down against the ala on the left. He had severe sciatica on the left. *C*, Traditionally, decompression is performed on the painful side, as in this drawing, and fusion on the other side only. In younger people, after wait of about 6 weeks, an anterior interbody fusion is performed. *D*, With the use of pedicle screws, decompression is possible, as in *C*, and pedicle screws and rods are added. An anterior interbody fusion is not necessary. Alternatively, the left side can be spread before tightening down the nuts and thus lift the lateal mass off the L5 nerve, in which case decompression is unnecessary.

Illustration continued on following page

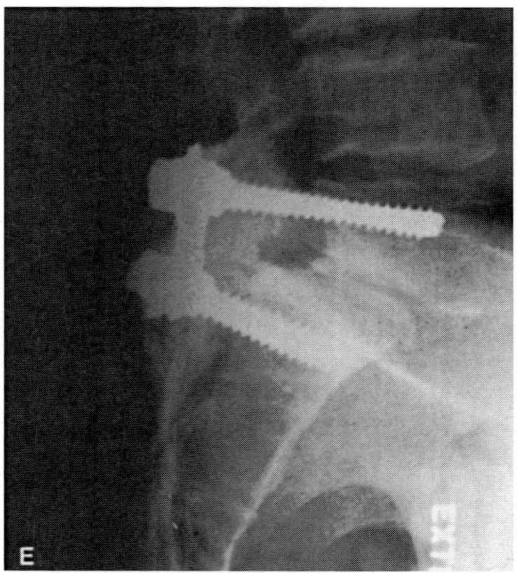

Figure 17. *Continued E,* Lateral view shows solid fusion with pedicle screws and rods in place.

port and also decreases the available fusion area. Not so clear is how to determine the circumstances under which decompression is necessary when the arch is intact and olisthesis exists. The CT scan, frontal and lateral axial and sagittal reformations, and physical examination should make this decision possible.

Buirski and coworkers[11] believed that in many cases, because of fibrous attachments between the tips of the broken pars and the ligamentum flavum, the loose element follows along as the body slips forward, thus presenting a clinical picture of cauda equina compression. These investigators reported that these patients have neurologic change with relatively small degrees of slip. This is an area needing further study by clinicians in collaboration with radiologists. With contrast enhancement and reformation of scans, it should be possible to confirm or refute the contention that, in some patients, symptoms occur because the loose element moves forward with the anterior elements as olisthesis progresses.

What causes tight hamstrings? Newman[59] theorized that this phenomenon is due to the body's attempt to hold the spine in the most comfortable position. Reflex spasm occurs, which ceases to be under voluntary control of the patient. At least in some cases, the cause is clearly nerve pressure, but is this always so? Perhaps traction on the nerves plays a part when there is a high-grade slip.

CASE ■ 1

The authors reported on a patient with congenital spondylolisthesis with about 40% slip (Fig. 18*A* to *F*). She had been fused from L5 to S1 and had a wide, solid arthrodesis. Her hamstrings before operation were extremely tight, so much so that she had to walk on tiptoe with her feet wide apart and her knees flexed. One year after fusion, her hamstring tightness remained unchanged. Her disability was such that she could not even attend school. A myelogram showed no tethering of the filum. Simple decompression of both L5 and S1 nerves was done, saving the wide fusion. The patient was walking normally within 3 weeks. This represents one case in which the tight hamstrings were caused by compression alone. After compression was removed, she resumed normal gait in a matter of weeks, after having been virtually unable to walk for longer than 2 years.

Marked disagreement still exists concerning when reduction should be performed.[26, 72] The results of simple fusion in situ, even in the most severe cases, have been good. Although a great deal of discussion has surrounded residual change in body contour, the patients themselves seem undisturbed about their build.[68] It seems likely that, as methods of reduction improve, reduction will gain favor in patients with high-grade olisthesis.

Will internal fixation be used frequently in the future? It appears that it will.

Treatment of stress fractures in young athletes remains controversial. The young athlete who is training to compete in the Olympics in gymnastics, for example, can frequently develop stress fractures of the pars or even the pedicles. This produces pain that sends him or her to the physician, who diagnoses an early stress reaction in the pars and rarely in the pedicle[41, 64] (Fig. 19). If there is an expectation that these fractures will heal, the patient must be taken off athletics and put into a brace or a corset (the authors use a heavy corset) for at least 8 months. The problem is that the healing rate is rather low (probably often because of noncompliance). If the patient is put into a cast from knees to nipples and kept in a horizontal position for at least 4 months, the early fractures always heal. This appears to

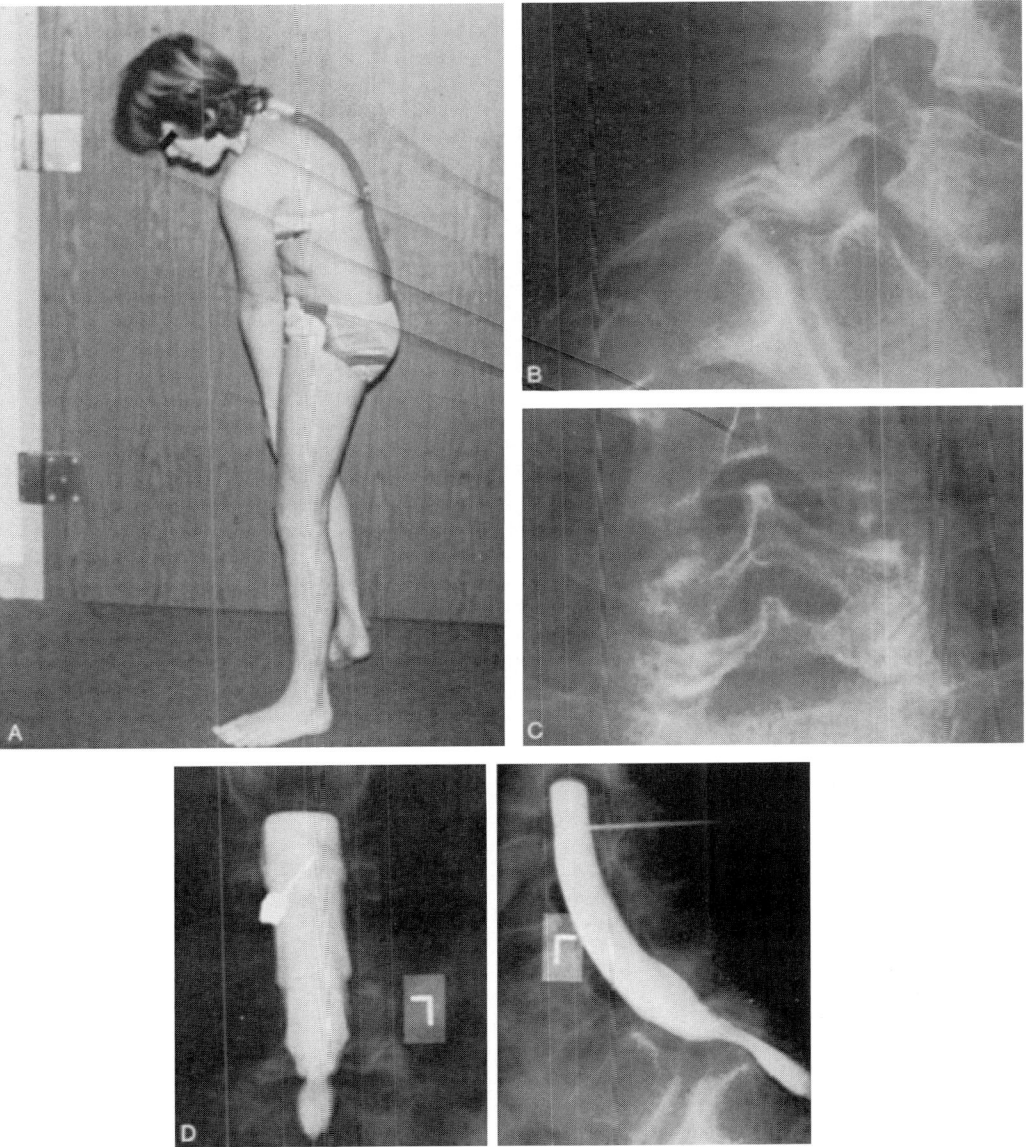

Figure 18. *A*, A 12-year-old child with a hamstring spasm so severe that she could not go to school. *B*, Standing lateral view shows a slip of about only 25%, but no pars defect. *C*, AP view shows typical axially oriented facets, and the facets show tropism. Most important, the posterior ring of L5 is intact. *D*, Myelogram shows near-block at L5–S1.

Illustration continued on following page

be far too severe a treatment, but the question remains, How vigorous should the surgeon be in trying to obtain healing of this relatively benign condition?

At the time of this writing, the authors are aware of no statistical studies indicating that pars fractures that occur in teenaged athletes have a hereditary element. However, some evidence suggesting a hereditary component exists, in that the incidence of spina bifida is increased in these adolescents.[39] Except for the increased incidence of spina bifida, the bony architecture appears normal on CT scans in the cases reviewed.

What is the place of pars interarticularis fusion?[29] At least three methods of fusing the fracture of the pars interarticularis are available.[60] The earliest was described by Buck,[10] who passed a screw down the pars interarticularis, drawing the fragments to-

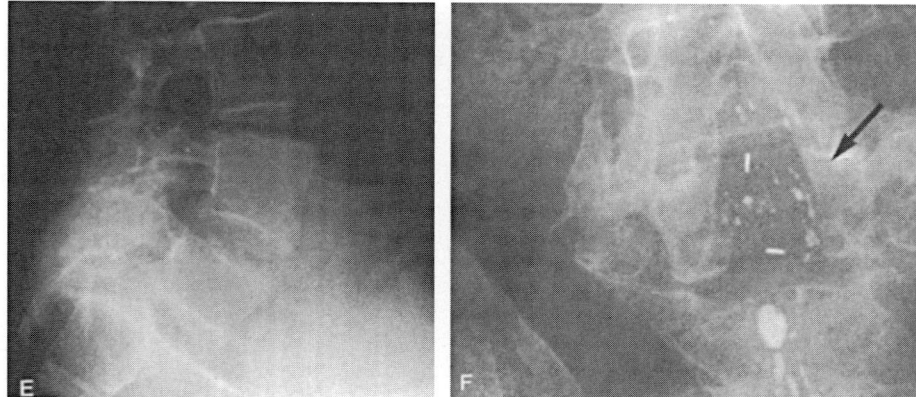

Figure 18. *Continued E*, Lateral view 6 months postoperatively shows solid fusion at L4 to S1 with no further slip. *F*, Because her hamstring spasm was unchanged, a decompression was performed. Within 3 weeks she could walk and bend normally. This case demonstrates that when the posterior arch is intact, a small amount of slip can be devastating. Also, simply removing the pressure cured the patient of all hamstring spasm in a matter of days. This case is important in that the cause of the hamstring spasm in such instances is still a matter of widespread discussion.

gether and then placing a graft. Nicol and associates[60, 61] advocated a method of passing wires around the base of the spinous process. Morscher and colleagues[55] in Switzerland developed another method using a tiny Harrington-type hook around the loose element and a screw into the lateral mass of L5. All of these methods work. All impose a fairly demanding surgical technique. The obvious problem is determining when it is

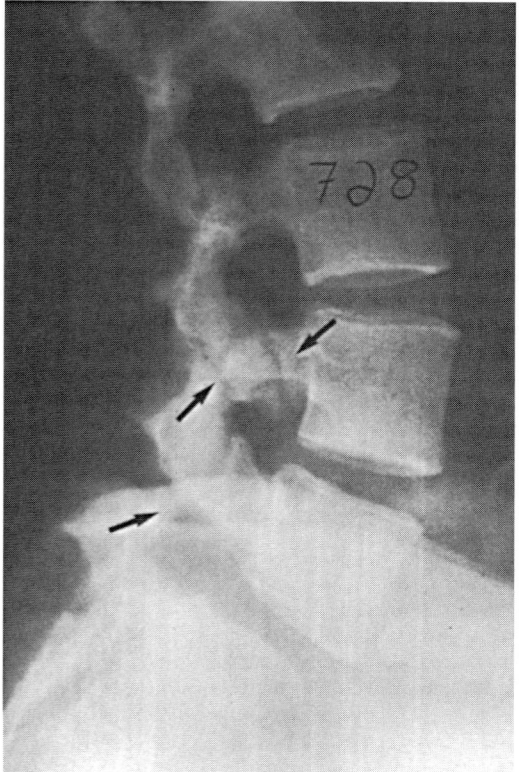

Figure 19. The radiograph shows a rare case, in which the pars is broken on one side and the pedicle on the other.

appropriate to perform this rather major operation for a condition from which the child will probably recover and live a nearly pain-free life.

Just where is the pain coming from in cases of spondylolysis? Does some of the pain come from the tissue between the broken ends of the pars? Eisenstein and his group[16] showed that this tissue between the ends of the pars, the spondylolysis ligament as he calls it, is innervated; thus, surgery for the condition should include removal of this ligament and replacement with bone graft.

Schlenzka and coworkers[88] in 1993 reported a comparison study of direct repair of the pars with a matched group having classic fusion. They found no statistical differences in the subjective clinical outcomes in the two groups.

In considering degenerative spondylolisthesis, should every case operated on be fused?[8, 13, 34, 35, 49, 97] The authors believe so. Differences of opinion exist, however, and Herron and Trippi[36] reported that patients with degenerative spondylolisthesis do just as well with decompression alone, without fusion. The authors reviewed the world literature of the past 6 years and found at least six articles recommending that fusion seldom be added and another eight or 10 recommending that fusion be performed only if the olisthetic level is clearly unstable.

What is the best way to fuse? The authors use an intertransverse process fusion at only the olisthetic level. Is internal fixation advisable? Because of the availability of pedicle screws and the ability to fuse short segments, internal fixation may be advisable. The question then arises, Is decompression necessary if one can pull the olisthetic vertebra back into place, spread it apart somewhat, and keep it in the proper degree of lordosis by internal fixation with pedicle screws? Perhaps decompression is not necessary if such a reduction can be accomplished. If the screws and rods are stressed severely, an interbody fusion should be added. Farfan (personal communication, 1988) has for years been an advocate of pulling the olisthetic vertebra backward, blocking it in place, and not performing decompression.

Should the L5–S1 level also be fused in cases of L4–L5 degenerative spondylolisthesis? In elderly patients, it is seldom necessary to perform a two-level fusion for L4–L5 olisthesis (Fig. 20A to D).

Should retrodisplacement be considered a form of spondylolisthesis and be included in the classification? The authors believe that it should not be included. Retrodisplacement does not meet the definition of spondylolisthesis, because olisthesis means to slip or slide down an incline. In retrodisplacement, the vertebra above slides posteriorly on the vertebra below it.

The word retrolisthesis is often used to describe this condition, but the authors prefer retrodisplacement. It is primarily a disease of the disc, and the posterior elements may be normal or nearly so. In fact, the authors have attached little importance to retrodisplacement when it is associated with spondylolisthesis and have seldom performed surgery for this condition alone.

DISCUSSION

Several reports in the literature state that the division between congenital and isthmic spondylolisthesis is an artificial one that should be abandoned in the classification. The authors have considered this statement but have continued to describe the division because the classification presented here is anatomic and only incidentally etiologic. It seems that continuing this separation is indicated because, for example, a patient with an intact posterior arch responds differently as olisthesis progresses from a patient with a pars fracture and a separated arch. Consider the child with an intact posterior ring at L5 and a wide-open sacrum, axially oriented facets between L5 and S1, a 30% slip, and severe hamstring tightness. Should such a case have the same classification as one involving a young athlete with fresh fractures of the pars but otherwise normal anatomy? The authors believe not. The major reason for separating the anatomic types is that their proper surgical treatment can be different.

An argument could be made for leaving the acute pars fracture resulting from major trauma out of this classification, because it is rare and, at least in the adult, virtually never occurs as an isolated lesion, but is seen as part of other severe bony injuries to the vertebra. It is included largely for completeness of the classification scheme.

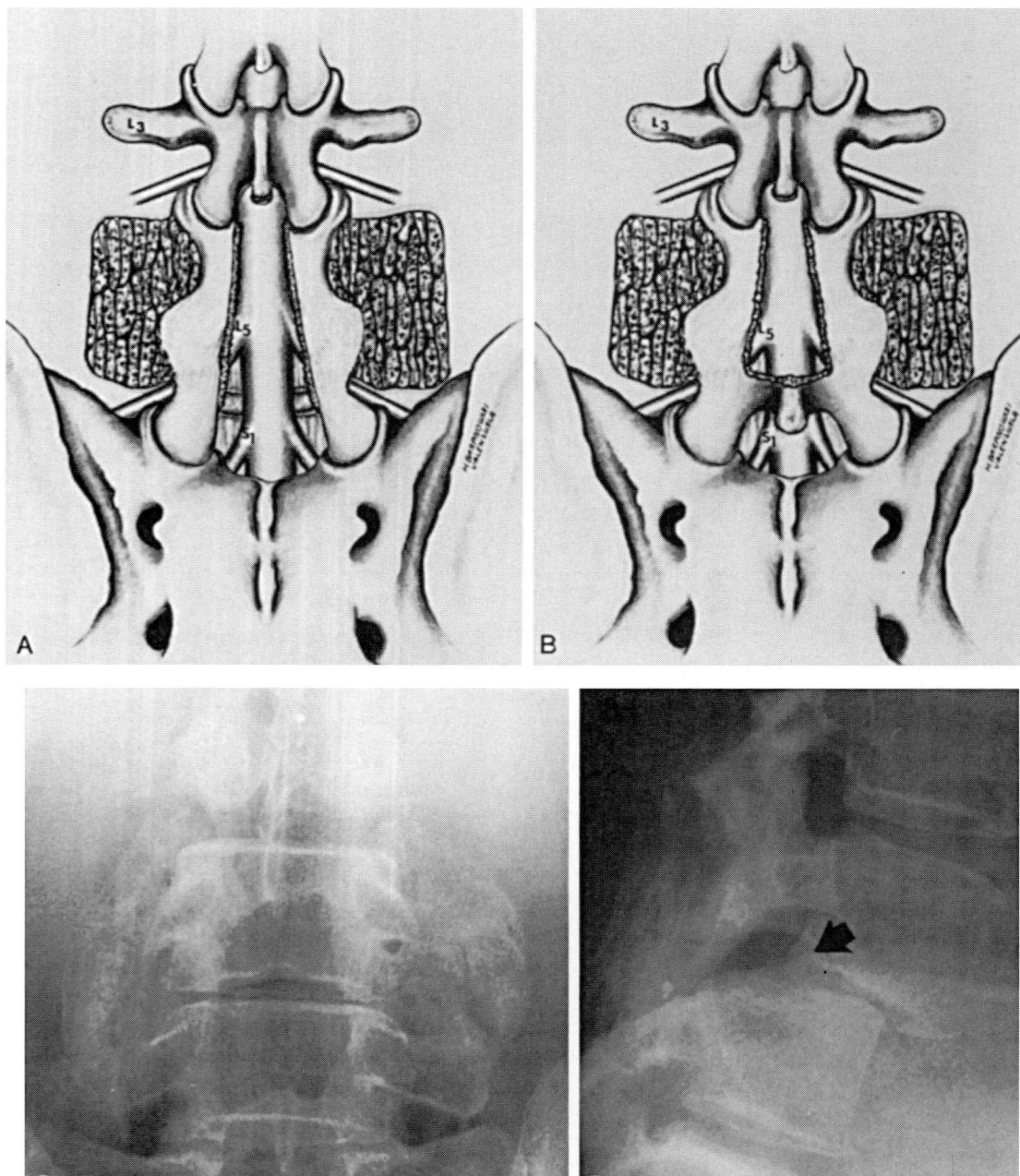

Figure 20. *A*, Type of decompression and fusion performed for degenerative spondylolisthesis. *B*, If the L5–S1 level is clearly uninvolved, the decompression is not extended all the way down to S1. *C*, AP x-ray film of a case in which the patient was treated in the above manner. *D*, Lateral x-ray film of a case treated in the above manner.

CONCLUSIONS

The classification presented recognizes great overlap in the fundamental causes of types I and II spondylolisthesis. For example, in consanguinity studies, both types have a strong hereditary component in their etiology. Both have dysplasia of the facets, and both have an increased incidence of spina bifida. Types IIA and IIB are actually the same disease, except that in type IIB the pars has healed.

However, important anatomic differences affect prognosis and treatment. For this reason, the authors have chosen to continue to separate the congenital (dysplastic) from the isthmic and have presented largely an anatomic classification. The authors believe that the division will help physicians in their surgical treatment of these patients. The term congenital is used instead of dysplastic, because both types have dysplastic articular processes. Admittedly, there are some problems with the word congenital, because both types have so many congenital etiologies.

The term postsurgical describes the type of olisthesis that occurs after too-extensive decompression. To call this type iatrogenic is to invite a malpractice suit.

The discussion of surgical treatment presents the methods that one of the authors (L.L.W.) has used to for many years with what he believes to be generally good results. In no way should this be construed as an attempt to encompass the whole field of surgery for spondylolisthesis.

The entire question of reduction and the several methods available to accomplish it are discussed by other authors in subsequent sections of this chapter.

REFERENCES

1. Albinase, M., and Pizzutillo, P. D.: Family study of spondylolysis and spondylolisthesis. J. Pediatr. Orthop. 2:496–499, 1982.
2. Amuso, S. J., and Mankin, H. J.: Hereditary spondylolisthesis and spina bifida. J. Bone Joint Surg. 49A:507–513, 1967.
3. Antti-Poika, I., Soini, J., Tallrota, K., et al.: Clinical relevance of discography combined with CT scanning in spondylolisthesis patients. J. Bone Joint Surg. 72B:480–485, 1990.
4. Apel, D., Lorenz, M., and Zindrick, M.: Symptomatic spondylolisthesis in adults: Four decades later. Spine 14:345–348, 1989.
5. Armstrong, G. W. D., and Ye, B. C.: Sacral configuration in dysplastic spondylolisthesis. J. Bone Joint Surg. 67B:335, 1985.
6. Baker, D. R., and McHolick, W.: Spondylolisthesis and spondylolysis in children. J. Bone Joint Surg. 38A:933, 1956.
7. Banta, C. J., Wiltse, L. L., Reynolds, J. B., et al.: Physical appearance and range of motion of high grade spondylolisthesis in patients with in situ arthrodesis—A video presentation. Presented at the Annual Meeting of the North American Spine Society, Monterey, CA, 1992.
8. Bolesta, M. J., and Bohlman, H. H.: Degenerative spondylolisthesis: The role of arthrodesis. Presented at the Annual Meeting of the American Academy of Orthopaedic Surgeons, Washington, DC, February 1992.
9. Borkow, S. E., and Kleiger, B.: Spondylolisthesis in the newborn, a case report. Clin. Orthop. 81:73–76, 1971.
10. Buck, J. E.: Direct repair of the defect in spondylolysis. J. Bone Joint Surg. 52B:432–437, 1970.
11. Buirski, G., McCall, I. W., and O'Brien, J. P.: Myelography in severe lumbosacral spondylolisthesis. Br. J. Radiol. 57:1067–1072, 1984.
12. Crock, H. V.: Observations on management of failed spinal operations. J. Bone Joint Surg. 58B:193, 1976.
13. Dall, B., and Gibbons, M.: Decompression and fusion for degenerative spondylolisthesis in the elderly. Presented at the Annual Meeting of the North American Spine Society, San Diego, CA, October 1993.
14. Dandy, D. J., and Shannon, M. J.: Lumbosacral subluxation. J. Bone Joint Surg. 53B 578–592, 1971.
15. Danielson, B. I., Frennered, A. K., and Irstam, L. K.: Radiologic progression of isthmic lumbar spondylolisthesis in young patients. Spine 16:422–425, 1991.
16. Eisenstein, S., Ashton, I., Roberts, S., and Darby, A.: The spondylolisthesis ligament. Presented at the of the International Society for the Study of the Lumbar Spine Meeting, Marseilles, France, June 1993.
17. Farfan, H. F.: Mechanical disorders of the low back. Philadelphia, Lea & Febiger, 1973.
18. Ferguson, R. J., McMarter, J. H., and Stanelski, C. L.: Low back pain in college football linemen. Am. J. Sports. Med. 2:63–69, 1974.
19. Fitzgerald, J., and Newman, P. H.: Degenerative spondylolisthesis. J. Bone Joint Surg. 58B:184, 1976.
20. Frederickson, B. E., Baker, D., McHolick, W. J., et al.: The natural history of spondylolysis and spondylolisthesis. J. Bone Joint Surg. 66A:699, 1984.
21. Frederickson, B. E., Baker, D., Murtland, A., et al.: Spondylolisthesis: The natural history age 5–40. Presented at the Annual Meeting of the International Intradiscal Therapy Society, Anaheim, CA, March 1991.
22. Frennered, A. K., Danielson B. I., and Nachemson, A. L.: Natural history of symptomatic low grade spondylolisthesis. J. Pediatr. Orthop. 11:209–213, 1991.
23. Frennered, A. K., Danielson, B. I., Nachemson, A. L., et al.: Midterm follow-up of young patients fused in situ for spondylolisthesis. Spine 16:409–416, 1991.
24. Gill, G. G., Manning, J. G., and White, H. L.: Surgical treatment of spondylolisthesis without spinal fusion. J. Bone Joint Surg. 33A:493, 1955.
25. Gill, G. G.: Long-term follow-up evaluation of a few patients with spondylolisthesis treated by excision of the loose lamina without spinal fusion. Clin. Orthop. 182:215–219, 1984.
26. Goutallier, D.: Results of treatment of spondylolisthesis by in situ interbody fusion. Presented at the Annual Meeting of the Societe Francaise de Chirurgie Orthopedique et Traumatologique, South Korea, Spring 1993.
27. Grobler, L. J., Haugh, L., Wiltse, L. L., et al.: L4/5

isthmic spondylolisthesis: Clinical and radiological review in 52 cases. Presented at the Annual Meeting of the American Orthopaedic Association, Coronado, CA, June 1993.
28. Grobler, L. J., et al.: Postoperative spondylolisthesis at L4–L5: The role of facet joint morphology. Presented at the Annual Meeting of the North American Spine Society, San Diego, CA, October 1993.
29. Hambly, M. F.: Tension band wiring with fusion for spondylolisthesis. Presented at the International Society for the Study of the Lumbar Spine Meeting, Miami, FL, April 1988.
30. Harada, T., Ebara, S., Anwar, M. M., et al.: The lumbar spine in spastic diplegia: A radiographic study. J. Bone Joint Surg. 75B:534–537, 1993.
31. Harris, I., and Weinstein, S.: Long-term follow-up of spondylolisthesis. J. Bone Joint Surg. 69A:960, 1987.
32. Haukipuro, K., Keranen, N., Koivisto, E., et al.: Familial occurrence of lumbar spondylolysis and spondylolisthesis. Clin. Genet. 13:471–476, 1978.
33. Herbinaux, G.: Traite sur divers accouchement laborieux et sur les polypes de la matrice. Bruxelles, De Boubers, 1792.
34. Herkowitz, H. N., and Kurtz, L. T.: Degenerative spondylolisthesis with spinal stenosis: A prospective study comparing decompression with decompression and intertransverse process arthrodesis. J. Bone Joint Surg. 73:802–808, 1991.
35. Herkowitz, H. N., and Kurtz, L. T.: Degenerative spondylolisthesis with spinal stenosis. J. Bone Joint Surg. 73:1104–1107, 1991.
36. Herron, L., and Trippi, A.: L4–L5 degenerative spondylolisthesis: The results of treatment by decompressive laminectomy without fusion. Spine 14:496–500, 1989.
37. Hult, L.: The Munkfors investigation. Acta Orthop. Scand. 16(suppl.), 1954.
38. Hutton, W. C., and Cyron, B. M.: Spondylolysis: The role of the posterior elements in resisting the intervertebral compressive force. Acta Orthop. Scand. 49:604–609, 1978.
39. Jackson, D. W., Wiltse, L. L., and Cirincione, R. J.: Spondylolisthesis in the female gymnast. Clin. Orthop. 117:68–73, 1976.
40. Johnson, J. R., Kerwin, E. O.: The long-term results of fusion in situ for severe spondylolisthesis. J. Bone Joint Surg. 65B:43, 1983.
41. Kaplansky, B., Lagallata, F., Heller, B., et al.: Single photo emission computed tomography for evaluation of lumbar spondylolisthesis. Presented at the Annual Meeting of the North American Spine Society, San Diego, CA, October, 1993.
42. Karaharjii, E., and Hunnuksela, M.: Possible syphilitic spondylitis. Acta Orthop. Scand. 44:289, 1973.
43. Kilian, H. F.: Schilderungen neuer Beckenformen und ihres Verhalten im leben Bassermann und Mathy (cit da Brocher). Mannheim, 1854.
44. Kirkham, B., Popp, C., and Transfeld, E.: Radiographic instability in spondylolisthesis. Presented at the Annual Meeting of the North American Spine Society, San Diego, CA, October 1993.
45. Knutsson, F.: Instability associated with disc degeneration. Acta Radiol. 15:593, 1944.
46. Lakatos, R., Handal, J., and Selby, D.: Lumbar disc degeneration associated with adult spondylolisthesis as assessed by discography. Presented at the Annual Meeting of the North American Spine Society, San Diego, CA, Oct., 1993.
47. Lambl, W.: Beitrage zur Geburtskunde und Gynackologue. Von F. W. Scanzoni, 1884.
48. Lee, C. K.: Lumbar instability (olisthesis) after extensive posterior spinal decompression. Spine 82:429–433, 1983.
49. Lombardi, J., Wiltse, L. L., Reynolds, J., et al: Treatment of degenerative spondylolisthesis. Spine 10:821, 1985.
50. Macnab, I.: Spondylolisthesis with an intact neural arch: The so-called pseudospondylolisthesis. J. Bone Joint Surg. 32:325, 1950.
51. Marchetti, P. G., Binazzi, R., Ponziana, L., et al.: Surgical technique of acute traumatic spondylolisthesis. Presented at the Annual Meeting of the Orthopaedic Trauma Association.
52. Marchetti, P. G., and Bartolozzi, P.: Spondylolisthesis. In Gaggi, A. (ed.): Spondylolisthesis. Bologna, Italy, A. Costa, 1986, p. 35.
53. McCarroll, J. R., Miller, J. M., and Ritter, M. A.: Lumbar spondylolysis and spondylolisthesis in college football players. Am. J. Sports Med. 14:404–406, 1986.
54. Mimura, M., Moriya, H., Takahashi, K., et al.: Rotational instability in degenerative spondylolisthesis.—A possible mechanical etiology of the disease. Presented at the International Society for the Study of the Lumbar Spine Meeting, Marseilles, France, June 1993.
55. Morscher, E., Gerber, B., and Fasel, J.: Surgical treatment of spondylolysis by bone grafting and direct stabilization of the spondylolysis by means of a hook screw. Arch. Orthop. Trauma Surg. 103:175–178, 1984.
56. Neugebauer, F. I.: Die entschung der spondylolisthesis. Zentrabl. Gynackol. 5:260–261, 1881.
57. Neuwirth, M.: Dysplastic and isthmic spondylolisthesis. Bull. Hosp. Joint Dis. Orthop. Inst. 41:95–104, 1981.
58. Newman, P. H.: The etiology of spondylolisthesis. J. Bone Joint Surg. 45B:39, 1963.
59. Newman, P. H.: A clinical syndrome associated with severe lumbosacral subluxation. J. Bone Joint Surg. 47B:472–481, 1965.
60. Nicol, R. O., and Scott, J.: Lytic spondylolysis repair by wiring. J. Bone Joint Surg. 67B:673, 1985.
61. Nicol, R. O., and Seall, J. H. S.: Lytic spondylolysis repair by wiring. Spine 11:117–130, 1987.
62. Oakley, R. H., and Carty, H.: Review of spondylolysis and spondylolisthesis in pediatric practice. Bone Joint Radiol. 57:877–885, 1984.
63. Ohata, H.: Spondylolysis: Familial occurrence and its genetic implication. J. Jpn. Orthop. Assn. 41:931–941, 1967.
64. Oland, C., Rineberg, B., Malberg, M., and Fried, S.: Fracture of the pedicle associated with contralateral spondylolysis. J. Bone Joint Surg. 68A:1454–1455, 1986.
65. O'Neill, D. B., and Micheli, L. J.: Postoperative radiographic evidence for fatigue fracture as the etiology in spondylolysis. Spine 14:1342–1355, 1989.
66. Osterman, K., and Seitsalo, S.: Fusion in situ in severe spondylolisthesis. Presented at the International Society for the Study of the Lumbar Spine Meeting, Miami, FL, April 1988.

67. Patwardhan, A., Lorenz, M., Orenstein, E., et al.: A biomechanical study of spina bifida occulta. Presented at the 13th Annual Meeting of the International Society for the Study of the Lumbar Spine, June 1986.
68. Peek, R. D., Wiltse, L. L., and Reynolds, J. B.: In situ arthrodesis without decompression in grade III or IV spondylolisthesis in adults who have severe sciatica. J. Bone Joint Surg. 71A:62–68, 1989.
69. Pfeil, J., Neithard, F., and Cotta, N.: Pathogenesis of pediatric spondylolisthesis. Z. Orthop. 125:526–533, 1987.
70. Porter, R. W., and Hibbert, C. S.: Symptoms associated with lysis of the pars interarticularis. Spine 9:755–785, 1984.
71. Postacchini, F., Cinotti, G., and Perugia, D.: Degenerative lumbar spondylolisthesis. II. Surgical treatment. Ital. J. Orthop. Traumatol. 17:467–477, 1991.
72. Poussa, M., Schlenzka, D., Seitsalo, S., et al.: Surgical treatment of severe isthmic spondylolisthesis in adolescents. Reduction vs. fusion in situ. Spine 18:894–901, 1993.
73. Rask, M. R.: Spondylolisthesis resulting from osteogenesis imperfecta. Clin. Orthop. 139:164–166, 1979.
74. Reynolds, J. B., and Wiltse, L. L.: Degenerative spondylolisthesis. Presented at the International Society for the Study of the Lumbar Spine Meeting, San Francisco, June 1978.
75. Reynolds, J. B., and Wiltse, L. L.: The surgical treatment of high-grade spondylolisthesis in children by in situ fusion. Presented at the International Society for the Study of the Lumbar Spine Meeting, Cambridge, Great Britain, Spring 1982.
76. Reynolds, J. B., and Banta, C. J.: High grade spondylolisthesis in children and adolescents in long term follow up in situ fusion. Presented at the Annual Meeting of the American Academy of Orthopedic Surgeons, Washington, DC, February 1992.
77. Robert (zu Koblenz): Eine eigentümliche angeborene Lordose wahrscheinlich bedingt eine Verschiebung des Korpers des letzten Lindenwirbels auf die vordere Flache des ersten Kreuzbeinwirbels (Spondylolisthesis, Kilian) nebst Bemerkungen über die Mechanik dieser Beckenformation. Monatsschr. Geburtskd. Frauenkrank 5:891–894, 1855.
78. Rosenberg, N. J.: Degenerative spondylolisthesis, surgical treatment. Clin. Orthop. 117:112, 1976.
79. Rosenberg, N. J.: Degenerative spondylolisthesis, predisposing factors. J. Bone Joint Surg. 57A:467, 1975.
80. Rothman, S. L. G., and Glenn, W. V.: CT multiplanar reconstruction in 253 cases of lumbar spondylolysis. AJNR 5:81–90, 1984.
81. Rowe, C. G., and Roche, M. B.: The etiology of separate neural arches. J. Bone Joint Surg. 35A:102, 1953.
82. Saraste, H., Bronström, L. A., and Aparisi, T.: Prognostic radiologic aspects of spondylolisthesis. Acta Radiol. [Diagn.] (Stockh.) 25 427–432, 1984.
83. Saraste, H.: Radiologic assessment of anatomic deviation in lumbar spondylolysis. Acta Radiol. [Diagn.] (Stockh.) 25:317–323, 1984.
84. Saraste, H.: The etiology of spondylolisthesis. Acta Orthop. Scand. 56:253–255, 1985.
85. Saraste, H.: Spondylolysis and pregnancy—a risk analysis. Acta Obstet. Gynecol. Scand. 65:727–729, 1986.
86. Saraste, H.: A radiologic follow up of spondylolysis and spondylolisthesis. J. Pediatr. Orthop. 7:631–638, 1987.
87. Saraste, H.: Long term clinical results: A radiological follow up of spondylolysis and spondylolisthesis. J. Pediatr. Orthop. 7:631–738, 1987.
88. Schlenzka, D., Seitsalo, S., Poussa, M., et al.: Operative treatment of symptomatic lumbar spondylolysis or mild isthmic spondylolisthesis in young patients: Direct repair of the defect or segmental spinal fusion? Presented at the International Society for the Study of the Lumbar Spine Meeting, Marseilles, France, 1993.
89. Schoenecker, P., Herring, J., Capello, A., et al.: Cauda equina syndrome following in situ fusion for spondylolisthesis. Presented at the Annual Meeting of the Pediatric Orthopaedic Society of North America, 1987.
90. Schreiber, A., et al.: Studies in the mechanical factors in the development of spondylolisthesis. Presented at the Annual Meeting of the Association of Bone and Joint Surgeons, 1984.
91. Schulitz, K. P., and Lethard, N.: Strain on the interarticular stress distribution. Arch. Orthop. Trauma Surg. 95:197–202, 1980.
92. Seitsalo, S.: Operative and conservative treatment of moderate spondylolisthesis in young patients. J. Bone Joint Surg. 72B:908–913, 1990.
93. Seitsalo, S., Osterman, K., Hyvarinen, H., et al.: Severe spondylolisthesis in children and adolescents—a long term follow up of fusion in situ. J. Bone Joint Surg. 72B:269–265, 1990.
94. Seitsalo, S., Osterman, K., Hyvarinen, H., et al.: Progression of spondylolisthesis in children and adolescents. A long-term follow-up of 272 patients. Spine 16:417–421, 1991.
95. Semon, R. L., and Spengler, D.: Significance of lumbar spondylolysis in college football players. Spine 6:172, 1981.
96. Shelokov, A. P.: Residual gait abnormalities in surgically treated spondylolisthesis. Presented at the Annual Meeting of the North American Spine Society, San Diego, CA, 1993.
97. Spencer, D.: Degenerative spondylolisthesis. Lecture presented at the 75th Annual Meeting of the Clinical Orthopaedics Society, Chicago, October 1987.
98. Splithoff, C. A.: The lumbosacral junction. JAMA 152:1610–1613, 1957.
99. Szappanos, L., Szepesi, K., and Thomazy, V.: Spondylolisthesis in osteoporosis J. Bone Joint Surg. [Br.] (in press).
100. Taillard, W.: Etiology of spondylolisthesis. Clin. Orthop. 117:30–39, 1976.
101. Troup, J. D. G.: The etiology of spondylolisthesis. Presented at the International Society for the Study of the Lumbar Spine Meeting, London, 1976.
102. Troup, J. D. G.: The etiology of spondylolisthesis. Orthop. Clin. North Am. 8:59–64, 1977.
103. Virta, L., Ronnemaa, T., and Osterman, K.: Low back pain in the middle-aged and elderly spondylolisthesis population. Rehabilitation Research Centre of the Social Insurance Institution, Turku, and the Orthopaedic Hospital of the Invalid Foundation, Helsinki, Finland.
104. White, A. H., and Wiltse, L. L.: Spondylolisthesis after extensive lumbar laminectomy (Proceedings). J. Bone Joint Surg. 57A:727, 1975.
105. Wiltse, L. L.: Etiology of spondylolisthesis. J. Bone Joint Surg. 44A:539–560, 1962.

106. Wiltse, L. L., Bateman, J. G., and Hutchinson, R. H.: The paraspinal sacrospinalis-splitting approach to the lumbar spine. J. Bone Joint Surg. 50A:919, 1968.
107. Wiltse, L. L.: Fatigue fracture: The basic lesion in isthmic spondylolisthesis. J. Bone Joint Surg. 57A:17–22, 1975.
108. Wiltse, L. L., Newman, P. H., and Macnab, I.: Classification of spondylolysis and spondylolisthesis. Clin. Orthop. 117:23–29, 1976.
109. Wiltse, L. L., and Winter, R. B.: Terminology and measurement in spondylolisthesis. J. Bone Joint Surg. 65A:768–772, 1983.
110. Wiltse, L. L., Guyer, R. D., Spencer, C. W., et al.: Alar transverse process impingement of the L5 spinal nerve: The far out syndrome. Spine 9:31–41, 1984.
111. Wiltse, L. L., Reynolds, J. B., and Banta, C. J.: High grade spondylolisthesis in children and adolescents in long term follow up in situ fusion. Presented at the Annual Meeting of the North American Spine Society, Monterey, CA, 1992.
112. Winter, R. B.: Congenital kyphosis. J. Bone Joint Surg. 55A:223–256, 1973.
113. Wynne-Davies, R., and Scott, J. H. S.: Inheritance and spondylolisthesis: A radiographic family survey. J. Bone Joint Surg. 61B:301–305, 1979.
114. Yano, T., Meyagi, S., and Ikari, T.: Studies of familial incidence of spondylolisthesis. Singapore Med. J. 8:203, 1967.
115. Zembo, M. M., Roberts, J. M., Burke, S. W., et al.: Congenital spondylolisthesis. Presented at the 21st Annual Meeting of the Scoliosis Research Society, Bermuda, September 1986.

Comprehensive Nonoperative Care of Lytic Spondylolisthesis: Principles and Practice

∎

JEFFREY A. SAAL

Rehabilitation of patients with low back pain is a comprehensive process that requires both accurate diagnosis and early intervention. The primary goal of rehabilitation should be to optimize function, although initially pain may be a patient's chief symptom. Patients may state that they are unable to participate in their normal activities because of pain and that their quality of life has diminished. They may no longer be able to work, take care of their household, or participate in recreational activities normally.

The focus of a rehabilitation program should be on improving function and quality of life instead of treating pain. The program should teach patients to assume control of their lumbar dysfunction instead of allowing their condition and pain to dictate their lives.

GOAL SETTING

One of the important tenets in rehabilitation medicine is goal setting. Short-term and long-term goals must be set for each individual case. The short-term goals require continual adjustment as the clinical progression is monitored during rehabilitation. Goal setting should take into consideration the following factors:

- Clinical subtype of spondylolisthesis
- Clinical symptom pattern
- Patient's activity level
- Structural pathologic processes
- Patient's perceived outcome
- Patient's age
- Patient's motivation to improve
- Patient's level of physical conditioning
- Psychosocial barriers to recovery

It is imperative that the patient be integrally involved in the goal-setting process. Patients should fully understand the realistic outcome of their clinical condition. Additionally, they must understand the time frame required and the methods to be used to achieve this outcome. If the physician and patient are not in accord on these issues, the outcome will be less than optimum.

REHABILITATION PRINCIPLES[71]

The goal of rehabilitation is to restore an optimum state of health and function. The physical rehabilitation process can be divided into phases, each of which is part of the overall plan to restore function[63] (Table 1).

The comprehensive nonoperative treatment program may include numerous elements (Table 2). The factors involved in goal setting determine whether and when to implement these treatment elements.

Specific Adaptation to Imposed Demands Principle

The principle of specific adaptation to imposed demands is an important concept in rehabilitation. It states that the body responds to a given demand with a specific, predictable adaptation.[2] If one can define the specific goals of the rehabilitation process, the program designed can be tailored to meet that need.

Team Approach

Rehabilitation is a multidisciplinary process. Therefore, a coordinated team is necessary to accomplish the goals. This entails a nonsurgical medical rehabilitation specialist as the team leader and the appropriate array of physical, occupational, and vocational therapists, psychologists, a psychiatrist, manual therapy experts, a radiology consultant, and a surgeon.

Table 2

Elements of Comprehensive Nonoperative Treatment Program

- Antiinflammatory medications
- Pain-modulating medications
- Physical modalities for pain control
- Detoxification from addictive and central nervous system–acting medications
- Therapeutic exercises to
  Control pain (flexion or extension stretching)
  Improve flexibility
  Improve range of motion
  Improve muscle strength
  Improve muscle endurance
  Improve balance
  Improve proprioception and coordination
  Improve cardiorespiratory aerobic and anaerobic capacity
  "Work harden"*
  Train for a particular sport, job, or activity
- Use of braces and orthoses
- Ergonomic evaluation and workplace modification
- Body mechanics instruction
- Psychosocial evaluation and intervention
- Psychiatric intervention (when necessary and appropriate)
- Family counseling
- Vocational counseling
- Nutritional counseling and weight reduction
- Smoking cessation
- Establishment of a successful physician-patient relationship

*Job-specific physical training programs to enhance fitness.

Treatment Timelines

The rehabilitation process should begin as soon as possible after disability onset and should be terminated only when the patient can successfully return to his or her maximum realistic level of active function. Careful outlining of the rehabilitation goals before rehabilitation as part of planning for function restoration can minimize the patient's frustration and discouragement. Early diagnostic intervention with the establishment of a precise diagnosis is the key to implementing the rehabilitation plan. An improper or imprecise diagnosis can lead to major pitfalls in the treatment regimen. Early intervention results in control of the

Table 1

Physical Rehabilitation Process

Phase I	Control of the inflammatory process
Phase II	Control of pain
Phase III	Restoration of joint range of motion and soft tissue extensibility
Phase IV	Improvement of muscle strength
Phase V	Improvement of muscle endurance
Phase VI	Development of specific biomechanical skill patterns (coordination retraining)
Phase VII	Improvement of general cardiovascular endurance
Phase VIII	Maintenance of exercise programs

inflammatory processes and speeds the recovery of normal articular and soft tissue range of motion. Early exercise also enhances the early improvement of muscle strength, which has been shown to correlate with the development of strong ligaments and tendons.[30, 55, 79, 80]

Patients should be advised that musculoskeletal maladaptations, including muscle and soft tissue contractures, muscle weakness, flexibility asymmetries, and segmental motion limitations, are developed over an extended period. Therefore, a rehabilitation plan must allow sufficient time to reverse these processes. Exercise physiologic principles dictate the time frames required to establish new length in shortened tissues, strengthen weakened muscle groups, improve flexibility, and improve segmental spinal motion. There are no quick remedies—the patient and the physician must understand this central issue. Successful rehabilitation requires sufficient time for the patient to optimize physical functioning and to control any outstanding psychosocial barriers to recovery.

The treatment program typically requires eight to 18 sessions of supervised active physical therapy followed by transition to an independent exercise program either at home or in a health club. The treatment plan requires the patient's participation in an exercise regimen three to four times weekly. The duration of symptoms (Table 3) and the type of functional deficits (Table 4), as well as the patient's improvement schedule, determine the exact time frames for treatment programs. Careful monitoring of the rehabilitation program is necessary to determine when alterations in the program are necessary or when an injection procedure (e.g., pain or inflammatory control procedure) may be fruitful. Additionally, careful monitoring avoids unnecessary treatment, overtreatment, or inappropriate resource allocation.

CLINICAL SUBTYPES OF SPONDYLOLISTHESIS

Patients with spondylolisthesis may be asymptomatic and never present for medical evaluation.[33, 72] Patients who seek medical evaluation do so with a variety of symptoms that yield clues to the underlying pathophysiologic mechanisms. The treating physician must understand the possible operant mechanisms and their variations to plan appropriate treatment strategies and options.

The clinical subtypes include

- Back pain (with no referral zone pain)
- Back pain with leg (and/or buttock) referral zone pain
- Paresthesia syndrome

Each of these clinical subtypes may have a distinct pattern of symptom presentation (e.g., back pain, back and leg pain, and lower extremity paresthesias). Recognition of the clinical subtypes and an understanding of their operant pathogenesis allow the clinician to plan appropriately the timing of treatment goals and resource allocation.

Back Pain

In discogenic syndromes, patients may report that back pain is worsened by activities that increase intradiscal pressure.[83] These activities include sitting, bending, and lifting. In cases of segmental instability, patients may note exacerbation of pain with position transition, such as changing posi-

Table 3

Clinical Patterns		
Pattern	Symptom Type	Duration
Acute onset	Persisting symptoms	<6 months
Chronic persistent	Persisting symptoms	>6 months
Chronic recurrent		
Type I	Frequent intermittent flare-ups with short pain-free intervals	Variable
Type II	Infrequent intermittent flare-ups with long pain-free intervals	Variable

Table 4

Activity Level		
Functional Level	Environment	Physical Limitations
Full, unrestricted	Home	Normal activity level
	Work	Normal activity level
	Recreation	Normal activity level
Partially restricted	Home	Limited heavy housecleaning
	Work	Full time
	Recreation	Decreased sport intensity
Restricted	Home	No housework
	Work	Part-time sedentary
	Recreation	Walk only
Severely restricted	Home	Sedentary existence
	Work	None
	Recreation	None

tion from sitting to standing. Patients with stenosis often report pain intensification when changing position and with walking.

The causes of back pain (with no referral zone pain) in patients with spondylolisthesis can be categorized into four pathophysiologic subsets:

1. Segmental instability of the spondylolisthetic segment.[24]
2. Disc degeneration at the level of or adjacent to the spondylolisthetic segment.[37, 53, 82]
3. Dorsal root ganglion compression (or mechanical perturbation) secondary to intervertebral nerve root canal compromise.[37] This compromise may be due to stenotic compression (i.e., fixed compression[37]) or due to segmental instability (i.e., dynamic compression[37]), or a combination of both processes.
4. Nonspinal causes: prostate disease, visceral pathologic change, neoplastic disease, infectious process, and so on.

The pathophysiology of back pain in patients with segmental instability is proposed to originate from a number of sources, either solely or in combination. The pain may be due to mechanical deformation of the annular collagen fibers, with nociception mediated through the dorsal primary ramus network.[59] Additionally, it may result from articular cartilage degeneration with compression and shear of the facet joint surfaces with activation of substance P–mediated free nerve endings.[59] Nociception may also emanate from the fibrocartilage within the lytic defect[3] or be caused by repetitive stretching of the capsular fibers of the facet joints.[52, 59] The common denominator in each of these syndromes is pain mediation through the dorsal primary ramus.

There may be an inflammatory focus within the facet joints[59] or within the lytic defect.[52] However, there is no compelling evidence to date that inflammation exists within the disc when segmental instability is the operant mechanism. Theoretically, the generation of soft tissue pain secondary to repeated mechanical deformation of ligaments or musculotendinous tissues may also be involved.[35, 61]

Disc degeneration at the level of the spondylolisthesis or at adjacent levels has been proposed as a potential pain source in this clinical subset. The pain mechanism associated with primary disc degeneration remains elusive.[48] However, it is clear that it involves more then structural factors alone. Biochemical and neurophysiologic evidence points toward a complex chemically mediated mechanism.[48] The mechanical and chemical factors associated with pain generation involve a variable combination of nociceptor excitation of the annulus fibrosus, the facet capsule, the subchondral bone of the articular pillars, the posterior longitudinal ligament, and the restraining soft tissues of the functional spinal segment.

Dorsal root ganglion compression or mechanical perturbation in the intervertebral nerve root canal may yield a clinical pattern of back pain with no referral zone pain. This can be considered a dorsal ramus syndrome with axial pain referral but no radiation to the extremities.[59] This is distinctly different from extremity referral zone pain mediated by the dorsal ramus network[62] or a ventral ramus syndrome and radicular referral zone pain with or without neurologic loss.

Back Pain with Leg (and/or Buttock) Referral Zone Pain

The second clinical subtype is back pain with leg (and/or buttock) referral zone pain. The referred pain may be mediated through the dorsal ramus network or via the ventral ramus. The dorsal ramus syndromes may cause nonspecific pain referral to the buttock, hip, or leg.[59] A dorsal ramus syndrome may never create a motor or reflex loss. Ventral ramus syndromes cause the more familiar radicular referral pain to the buttock, leg, calf, and foot.[62] The ventral ramus innervates the motor unit, and thus ventral ramus injuries may produce a neurologic deficit or a deep, aching pain.

The causes of back and leg pain syndromes include

1. Segmental instability, which causes repetitive mechanical deformation of the exiting nerve root.[24] The mechanical perturbation probably leads to repetitive neuronal discharges that can create a hyperalgesic state.[11]
2. Intervertebral nerve root canal stenosis or disc herniation at the listhetic level or at the adjacent level. Mechanical and inflammatory mechanisms appear to be operant in this clinical subset.[57, 58, 71] The mechanical aspect of the pathophysiologic mechanism may cause vascular alteration of the nerves and dorsal root ganglion nutritional pathways leading to neural dysfunction.[41] The inflammatory aspect of an intervertebral disc herniation can result in neural injury and hyperalgesia.[11]
3. Far-lateral compression secondary to an extraforaminal disc herniation[33, 84] or from the L5 transverse process.[67] This mechanism is similar to intervertebral nerve root canal pathologic changes.

The challenge for the clinician is that all of these patients have an identical primary symptom of leg pain. However, they all have distinctly different underlying pathologic processes that necessitate different treatment strategies.

Paresthesia Syndrome

The third clinical subtype is the leg or foot paresthesia syndrome. This syndrome typically occurs in elderly patients with severe intervertebral nerve root canal stenosis secondary to advanced disc space collapse at the level of the spondylolisthesis. Often, these patients do not have significant leg or back pain, but instead report constant paresthesias, primarily of the feet.

This syndrome is presumably secondary to compression of the sensory fibers of the mixed spinal nerve in the stenotic intervertebral canal. The symptoms of paresthesia may not be accompanied by a loss of sensibility. The degree and duration of compression determine the degree and reversibility of the findings.[46] This syndrome must be differentiated from peripheral neuropathic processes by electrodiagnostic studies.[64]

TREATMENT PROGRAM

The phases of rehabilitation have been described above. These phases are guideposts for the treatment algorithm. Additionally, a comprehensive treatment program includes the relevant elements described under Rehabilitation Principles (see Table 2).

Medications

The use of medications plays a minor role in the treatment of patients with pain from spondylolisthesis (see under Clinical Subtypes of Spondylolisthesis). However, the short-term use of nonsteroidal antiinflammatory drugs (NSAIDs) can be a valuable aspect of patient management. NSAIDs have both analgesic and antiinflammatory properties.[23] There is no credible evidence that one NSAID is any more potent at reducing inflammation than another.[23] The appropriate drug choice is based on the patient's tolerance, convenient dosing intervals, and the physician's preference. An adequate drug trial is 7 to 14 days.[23] If no effect or an adverse side effect occurs, another drug should be selected from one of the other chemical families. Blood studies to monitor for side effects should be undertaken after the first 6 weeks of continuing use. Thereafter, blood studies to monitor iron stores and hepatic and renal function should be undertaken every 3 to 6 months. Long-term administration of NSAIDs is occasionally necessary; however, the risks must be weighed against the treatment alternatives and the potential side effects.[23]

Opiate analgesics have no role in the long-term care of patients with low back pain. Short-term use may be indicated for severe flare-ups during the acute stage. However, the proper use of ice application, positioning exercises, and NSAIDs administration usually obviate the need for these medications. The use of muscle relaxant medications should also be avoided. These medications are central nervous system anxiolytics with only limited peripheral action.[23] They create mood alteration and depression and have significant addictive potential.[23] Similarly, sleep-inducing, or hypnotic, medications have no role in the treatment of patients with lumbar pain. Tricyclic antidepressant medication can be used to block serotonin pathways and to help modulate pain responses, and they can facilitate sleep without the central nervous system–depressing and addictive qualities of hypnotic medications.[81] It is much easier never to prescribe central nervous system–acting medications than it is to detoxify patients. The endorphin-suppressive action of these medications can present a substantial barrier to recovery and make it difficult for the patient to participate in active rehabilitation. Passive treatment modalities must be avoided if a treatment success is to be achieved.

Manipulation and Traction

Manipulation and traction do not have a well-established place in the treatment regimen of patients with painful spondylolisthesis. Time should not be wasted on these passive treatment modalities. Soft tissue mobilization techniques appear to be beneficial for some patients.[35, 61] These techniques should be used sparingly and only to facilitate participation in the active exercise regimen. In patients with significant soft tissue contractures, these passive techniques can be coupled with active stretching exercises to accomplish normal soft tissue extensibility. However, the long-term use of soft tissue mobilization techniques for pain relief performed in isolation creates a dependency on them that is contrary to the stated goals of rehabilitation.

Lumbar Braces and Corsets

Lumbar braces and corsets may have a limited role in management of the spondylolisthetic patient, although there are no published data to support their use. It is this author's contention that active improvement in trunk muscle strength and proper use of dynamic stabilization obviate the need for these appliances. In isolated circumstances, a manual laborer may require a lumbosacral corset to perform his or her job more comfortably. Additionally, elderly persons with segmental instability may derive benefit from a corset. However, most older patients with spondylolisthesis have stable lesions resulting from degeneration of the associated motion segment. The athlete with a pars fracture presents a special circumstance, and the interested reader is referred to an appropriate reference.[33]

Exercise Training

By definition, lumbar spondylolisthesis is an unstable lesion resulting in at least some degree of segmental instability. The core of the treatment regimen is an exercise program designed to teach the patient to use dynamic muscle control in order to maintain stabilization of the spine. This dynamic muscle stabilization program should allow the patient to reduce mechanical stress on the spine and thereby reduce the possibility of symptom production.[68] Arguably, the end effect of this training should not only ameliorate symptoms but also reduce the mechanical factors that accelerate the degenerative process. One can conceptualize this exercise training process as creating a muscle fusion that maintains spine stability. However, the goal is not to make the patient rigid and inflexible.[65, 66] On the contrary, the patient is taught to improve and maintain symmetric strength, flexibility, balance, proprioception, and trunk control.

To apply muscle fusion, adequate flexibility and spinal range of motion must be attained. Studies of the diurnal variations and stresses on the lumbar spine note changes in lumbar disc and ligament extensibility as the day progresses.[1] These changes are based on the creep of soft tissue structures that lead to increased range of motion. Adams and associates[1] noted that bending and lifting activities performed early in the morning, when undertaken by nonextensible ligamentous and annulus fibers, cause fatigue damage to the disc more easily than do similar activities performed later in the day. This finding suggests a need for flexibility of the structures to eliminate this repetitive fatigue stress on the intervertebral joint. The muscles that attach to the pelvis can be thought of as guy wires that effectively change the position and symmetry of the pelvis.

Given that the pelvis is the platform on which the lumbar spine rests, pelvic positioning is the key to postural control of the lumbar spine. Therefore, adequate flexibility of hamstring, quadriceps, iliopsoas, gastrocnemius-soleus, hip rotators, and iliotibial band muscles is important. There is also a need for flexible neural elements.

Training programs for the rehabilitation of the lumbar spine progress from floor exercises and manual resistance exercises to the use of resistance equipment. Training for strength and flexibility of the trunk and extremities is integral to the development of adequate postural control and stabilization skills. All patients must demonstrate a baseline level of skill in the floor exercise program before advancing to an unsupervised gymnasium–health spa type of training program. It is inadequate to simply tell a patient to "go to the gym and work out." Similarly, giving patients handout sheets with exercises to perform has been shown to yield unsatisfactory results.[56] A properly structured training program in a gymnasium can minimize the risk of injury through the use of weight-training equipment and maximize the gains from combined and coordinated muscle group activity. That type of training program should conceptually match the program of floor exercises, because both are based on the principles of dynamic muscular stabilization of the spine.

Every patient with spondylolisthesis does not need to commit to an extensive weight-training program. The overall rehabilitation program should be designed for an individual patient's needs, with realistic and functional goals. Patients who are avid recreational athletes usually require additional strength gains attainable only through a weight-training program. This is certainly true of professional and high-level competitive athletes. These same considerations exist for patients involved in manual labor or in activities that require performance of repetitive tasks with heavy loads.

The training goals of a gymnasium program are similar to those of a floor exercise program. Development of trunk strength is essential for functional stabilization of the spine.[1] Increasing the strength and endurance of extremity musculature limits the amount of stress placed on the spine and trunk during the performance of daily activities. Patients should be taught to use resistance equipment with safe techniques and in safe positions that are not harmful to the spine.

Extremity strength training techniques are targeted for the muscle groups that stabilize the trunk. These techniques are most commonly used during floor exercises and in safe lifting and bending techniques. However, the benefits of performing extremity strength exercises are greater than the targeting and training of specific sites of extremity strength. In addition, patients are instructed in cocontraction techniques that consist of active use of the trunk musculature to stabilize the spine while an extremity is working against resistance. Specific exercises are targeted for the prime trunk stabilizing muscles, including the abdominal obliques, the latissimus dorsi (including all of its segments), the spine extensors, and the interscapular (middle trapezius, serratus anterior, and rhomboids) muscles. A specific strengthening program is always tailored to an individual patient's needs.

The patient's physical capacity for occupational and recreational activities guides the program structure. The weight-training program is not geared solely toward strengthening the truncal musculature; taken a step further, it becomes a total fitness program. Incorporated in this total fitness program is aerobic and anaerobic training. Learning to stabilize the spine while riding a stationary bicycle, while running on the treadmill, or while swimming is an integral stage of the training program. Careful instruction that demonstrates proper spinal positioning during each of these activities is required. The injured worker is schooled in body mechanics and learns to transfer the newly found skills to the job site. Ergonomic evaluation and modification of the workplace may also be required.

The goal of exercise training is to develop an engram[28] of motor control to accomplish stabilization. An engram is a neurophysiologic phenomenon that describes the motor information necessary to perform a complex movement. All of the individual components of a complex motor act are stored together in the motor cortex as a unit, forming an engram. These data are retrievable without the need for conscious control. This phenomenon is identical to training for a specific athletic skill, such as a golf swing or a tennis stroke. During early training, conscious control is necessary. Later, the movement pattern becomes automatic and conscious control is no longer necessary.

Strength Training: Basic Physiologic Principles

The major principle to keep in mind is one of progressive resistance exercise.[20] This type of exercise must be performed on a regular basis at a minimum of three times per week. The initial programs involve progressive resistance exercise to the muscle groups designated as the prime movers in the injured area. Programs using frequent daily adjustable progressive resistive exercise (DAPRE) techniques appear to achieve maximum resistance. The DAPRE technique is based on the principle that strength can be redeveloped more quickly after injury than it was developed initially.[21] The key component of the program is performance of maximum repetitions during the third and fourth sets of exercises, with the number of repetitions performed used as a basis for adjusting the resistance applied during the fourth set and on the next day.[6, 9]

Maintenance strength programs are begun after the patient has achieved 90% to 95% of the expected strength gains. The limits of performance must be extended persistently to improve muscle strength. The rate of improvement appears to depend on the willingness of the subject to overload (to exercise the muscle to the absolute limit it can do, to fully exhaust the muscle by the end of the exercise).[14, 19]

To achieve maximum intensity of muscle contraction, the highest possible percentage of muscle mass should be involved at any given moment.[7, 9] To achieve this end, good form is of utmost importance. The resistance should be accelerated in a smooth fashion and briefly halted at the position of full muscle contraction. The speed used in raising and lowering the weight also trains the muscle to develop the appropriate speed of contraction for the types of sporting activity designated.[15, 50, 54]

Concentric exercise programs are used most frequently in rehabilitation. Eccentric training programs have been developed for the treatment of tendinitis.[75] Eccentric programs are believed to be beneficial in increasing load. The speed of the contraction is modified during the specialized eccentric program, which gradually increases the speed of movement while increasing the load on the tendon. This type of eccentric loading program parallels normal musculotendinous unit functions in movement patterns. It has been suggested that concentric programs may place greater stress on the musculotendinous unit and thus cannot increase the length of the soft tissues. Some researchers have reported that patients often report increased symptoms with concentric exercise programs and decreased symptoms with eccentric exercise programs.

The use of overload to attain muscle fatigue appears to be the most important factor in strengthening programs. Initial gains in muscle strength are related to improved levels of motor unit activity. After the first 2 weeks of training, additional force gains are made through muscle hypertrophy.[13, 19, 26]

The ability to synchronize the firing ratios of the motor units is a consequence of weight-training programs. Improvement in strength correlates with increased synchronization patterns. Therefore, carefully concentrated exercise performed at the proper skill level and speed allows synchronization of the motor units and improves the ability of the muscle to gain strength more rapidly.[4, 9, 10, 19] Overzealousness during the initial phases of the strengthening program can result in reactive inflammatory changes or joint synovitis. Careful progression of the strength training program is, therefore, imperative.

The strengthening program should begin with isometric exercises. The isometric phase can be carried out early, while joint motion is still protected. Manual resistance exercises can begin after the joint can be moved. In this situation, the therapist uses a program of progressive, carefully graded manual resistance. As the patient accomplishes this program with comfort, the therapist can note the range within which it is appropriate to work. It is important that the contractions be carried out in the patient's pain-free range.[47]

Strengthening programs advance from the isometric state and are used when range of motion is limited and when pain accompanies isotonic workouts. Muscle weakness and fatigability are pinpointed during the physical examination and efforts to reverse them are concentrated on in the rehabilitation process.

After the patient has carefully progressed through the manual resistance program and the isometric program, pain-free ranges can be carefully adjusted. Isometric contractions are optimally held for 5 to 6 seconds, with a rest period of 10 to 20 seconds. This ensures a proper muscle blood flow and removes the substrate of muscular contraction. The isometric contraction should be carried out frequently during the day, in sets of 10 to 12 repetitions.[2] The goal is to transfer this isometric strength development to an isotonic program. Persons who carry out isometric exercises with greater frequency develop greater endurance, which transfers to better performance of progressive resistive exercises.

The concept of specificity of exercise should constantly be kept in mind. Because most endeavors rely on dynamic muscle contraction, merely training the muscle with static contractions (i.e., isometric contractions) may not transfer to the dynamic activities,[2, 31, 38, 39] even though this method can increase absolute static strength.[60]

After the patient can successfully perform isometric and manual resistance exercises, progression to an isotonic program can begin. There is no evidence to support the use of isokinetic equipment for strength or endurance training. This type of equipment appears to be most beneficial as a measurement tool, not as a training tool.

Isotonic programs can use free weights, elastic bands, universal-type exercise machines, or cammed equipment such as Nautilus. The MedX equipment allows isolation patterns to be developed for training the erector spinae and the rectus abdominis muscles. Free weights are useful in isolation patterns, for example, the use of dumbbells for the upper extremity after a rotator cuff injury. Heavy free weights should be used only in a buddy system and by patients who are skilled lifters. For the novice, weight machines such as the Cybex, Universal machine, and Hydragym are especially useful. Isolation patterns are difficult to obtain, but the ease with which these machines can be used and their multiple stations make them extremely practical. The use of cammed equipment has many distinct advantages. This type of equipment is designed with a cam, which varies the resistance offered by a given load to try to match the average torque curves for each of a large number of muscle groups. This theoretically eliminates the dead areas noted in certain portions of the range of motion during training with free weights. Another advantage of cammed equipment is the individualized stations, which allow adjustment of foot rests and seat height.

The use of elastic bands is extremely practical, especially for home strengthening programs. Elastic bands can be used not only for resistance exercises but also for flexibility programs. Isolation patterns can be accomplished with the use of elastic bands. This type of exercise is extremely practical because the patient is able to travel with the exercise equipment. Maintenance programs using elastic bands can be helpful.

Occasionally, the buoyancy produced by water is useful during the initial phase of strengthening programs. A person can be placed in a pool and, with use of a life jacket, can begin to use the resistance of water against her or his body weight for strengthening. These water-based programs make it possible to maintain lower extremity strength and range of motion as well as aerobic endurance. This satisfies the patient's psychologic and physiologic goals. The use of a stationary bicycle with varying seat heights is also beneficial, in that it improves knee and ankle range of motion as well as progressive resistance.

Costill[13] demonstrated the necessity for

combining strength and endurance programs into the muscle rehabilitation portions of the program. Because there is a specific program response to the type of exercise performed, an exercise program must be tailored to meet the needs of each individual.[27] Steadman[76] employed a group of exercises that challenge the muscles in three different ways. High-repetition, moderate-weight sets are performed initially, followed by a rapid, low-resistance repetition until fatigue. The last step is maintenance of an isometric contraction for approximately 1 minute. This type of program improves not only absolute strength but also endurance. It also stresses the anaerobic pathway necessary for burst-type activities (rapid acceleration movements).[13] Gaining muscle endurance necessitates stressing the aerobic pathways and improving the oxidative enzyme capacity of slow-twitch muscle fibers,[19] which results in higher repetition work at lower weight levels.[7, 9] These muscle endurance sets are also useful as maintenance programs. Isolation of specific muscle contractions during endurance training is based on the person's specific activity requirements.

The threshold of change in the development of muscular endurance is unclear. Therefore, the degree of intensity placed on the muscle cannot be clearly defined. In one study, strength scores improved significantly when they were preceded by a program using high-repetition work. Therefore, it seems appropriate to start the patient on a high-repetition, low-weight program before embarking on a higher-resistance program.[21] This appears to allow time for cellular adaptation to occur and enhances the eventual strength gains of the program participant.

The use of the stationary bicycle with variable resistance is extremely beneficial in lower-extremity muscle endurance programs. Additionally, stair-steppers and stair-climbing machines are also beneficial. Swimming and other water exercises are useful in programs of upper-extremity muscle endurance. The maintenance of muscle endurance has been demonstrated to be a significant factor in the prevention of injury. This appears to be related to depletion of oxidative enzymes in slow-twitch fibers, leading to fatigue of the musculature and inability of the musculature to protect the joints.[22]

Flexibility Training

Training for flexibility is another essential component of a program of spine stabilization. For passive trunk flexion to occur at the hips rather than about the axis of the lumbar spine, adequate musculotendinous flexibility in the hip and leg extensors, hip abductors and external rotators, flexors, and knee extensors is important. The hamstrings, gluteus medius, short hip rotators, quadriceps, iliopsoas, and gastrocnemius-soleus complex are specific muscle sites that should be targeted for training. It is critical that stretching exercises be performed in a spine-safe manner (with positions that do not necessarily raise intradiscal pressure, torque the spinal segments, or excessively load the posterior elements).

Loaded trunk flexion and torsion are the primary areas of risk. Many of the flexibility techniques taught in school athletic programs and popular exercise videotapes are less than ideal for this reason, and they should be avoided. However, flexibility is important, including the flexibility of such structures as the abdominal oblique muscles, the facet joint capsules, and the thoracolumbar fascia. These stretches should be carried out passively in a spine-safe manner.

When prescribing flexibility exercises, clinicians need to keep in mind certain facts. Flexibility exercises increase the elasticity not only of loose connective tissue but also of the connective tissue of muscle and muscle contractile units.[70] Connective tissue behaves viscoelastically.[29] This means that it deforms in response to applied force, and if the force is large enough, it returns to a slightly longer length after the force stretching it is removed.[43] In addition, the viscoelasticity of tissue is enhanced in the presence of elevated temperature.[13, 45] Its increase in length is greater if force is applied slowly. Thus, one should apply a stretch slowly, for an adequate period of time, after warming the tissue.

Actual lengthening of the muscle contractile units is accomplished by slightly different physiologic principles, but the principles for tissue elasticity and for muscle contractile unit lengthening can be applied to good advantage together. The relationship of muscle fibers to one other is governed by neural factors as well as by physical principles. Relaxation of incoming neural input is essential to lengthen a contractile unit.[73] This is best accomplished by a stretch that occurs slowly and evenly and is accompanied by gentle contraction of the antagonist muscles. For example, gentle contraction of the ankle dorsiflexors with passive stretch of the gastrocnemius-soleus complex facilitates a better stretch.[40] Performance of stretching exercises both before and after an exercise period has been demonstrated to result in increased flexibility gains.[51] The ideal length of time for holding an isolated stretch is probably 15 to 30 seconds. Continuation of the stretch for a longer period does not generate any greater flexibility gains, except in the case of pathologic contracture.[42, 70]

For many years, flexibility training was an ignored aspect of injury rehabilitation and injury prevention.[63] However, the literature supporting flexibility training continues to grow, as it repeatedly demonstrates how to reduce sports injuries in various environments.[5, 8, 12] Flexibility programs with a sound scientific foundation should be incorporated into rehabilitation training programs.[17, 18] One such program, the proprioceptive neuromuscular facilitation procedure, is a proven, effective means of passive stretching.[78] This procedure involves an initial passive static flexibility maneuver of the agonist, followed by a 3-second maximum voluntary contraction and then static stretching. This type of flexibility program has been found to be more effective than the use of passive static flexibility methods alone.[78]

Flexibility programs can enhance the concentric contraction velocities of muscles. These programs can also reduce the subjective symptoms of muscle soreness after vigorous exercise.[32]

Aerobic Training

During the entire functional restoration program, the patient is not allowed to remain sedentary. As soon as possible, the patient should begin aerobic training with walking, which can be performed on a treadmill. Later, the stationary bicycle or stairstepper can be used for training. Depending on the patient's ability to stabilize the spine, many forms of aerobic conditioning are possible. Knee, hip, and foot problems are factors in determining the preferred type of aerobic conditioning. Exercises in a swimming pool are another way to keep the patient active without stressing the spine. The aerobic capacity of the patient should not be allowed to drop during the early phases of the program.

Aerobic conditioning can increase endorphin levels.[16] This improves the patient's sense of well-being and increases pain thresholds. This increase in pain threshold allows the patient to perform at higher levels of function before perceiving pain. However, one should not use aerobic conditioning as the sole form of exercise training for patients with low back pain. Aerobic conditioning can physiologically improve cardiorespiratory endurance but cannot enhance muscular strength, muscular endurance, balance, or body mechanics.

Contrary to popular opinion, there is neither direct nor inferential scientific evidence that running is injurious to the lumbar spine. Studies show that running did not adversely affect the articular cartilage of the hip and did not either create or progress arthritic degeneration.[44] If the hip appears to be unaffected, it seems reasonable to assume that the spine is uncompromised as well.

Program Prescription

It is important for the physician prescribing the exercise program to communicate certain key information to the physical therapist. At the time of the initial prescription, the medical report must contain detailed pathoanatomic diagnostic information that relates the pain generator and indicates whether an emphasis on flexion or on extension is preferred. Typically, a flexion-based exercise is most appropriate for patients with painful spondylolisthesis.[74] Precautions regarding peripheral joint pathologic processes that may interrupt active exercise training, for example, patellofemoral pain syndromes, must be adequately communicated. Additionally, specialized lower extremity or upper extremity rehabilitation programs should be incorporated in the lumbar exercise program. For example, the patient with rotator cuff tendinitis (i.e., an impingement syndrome) and lumbar disc herniation requires a combined program. If the shoulder pathologic change is not addressed, then the lumbar program will falter because of the patient's inability to carry out any exercises that involve the upper extremities.

Time goals must be given to the patient and the physical therapist. If these goals are not met, the program requires modification. For instance, in the case of a patient with an acute problem, the physical therapist should be informed that, if there is persistent leg pain after three sessions and the program cannot progress, the physical therapist should return the patient to the physician for an epidural injection of cortisone or other aggressive approaches to reduce radicular inflammatory response.[71]

The decision to discharge the patient from supervised exercise and to transfer the patient to a maintenance program must be made by the rehabilitation team overseeing the patient's care. Some patients, because of their athletic background and motivation, can learn the program quickly (in 6 to 8 visits) and thereby complete the supervised portion of the program. However, deconditioned, unathletic patients may need 18 sessions of supervised physical therapy to attain a level of training that allows the transitional program to begin.

Exercise training is not finished in the physical therapy gymnasium. All patients must be prepared for transition to home-based programs. Patients should receive detailed and clear information regarding the suggested maintenance program at the time of discharge from supervised physical therapy. This program should be updated again 4 to 6 weeks after discharge. In many circumstances, the exercise program continues in a neighborhood gymnasium. In this case, the physical therapist or trainer must accompany the patient to the gymnasium to instruct the patient about the program and proper weight training activities, using the specific equipment available. In some circumstances, the duration of supervised physical therapy can be shortened if a trained exercise instructor works with the patient. The exercise trainer can monitor the program progression and act as the patient's coach during the recovery process. The exercise trainer provides progress reports to the treating physician to allow smooth program progression.

Therapeutic Corticosteroid Regional Injections

The precise application of corticosteroids to an area of inflammation can either temporarily or permanently reduce pain associated with the inflammatory focus.[36] The clinical subtypes yield clues about whether and where an inflammatory focus may reside. Injection therapy should be used to facilitate participation in the active exercise regimen. The exercise regimen should be the mainstay and central aspect of the treatment program. The window of opportunity created by the corticosteroid effect must be used judiciously for advancement and progression of the active rehabilitation program.[67] Injections should be used only to facilitate program progression and not simply to provide short intervals of pain reduction.

Precise localization is imperative if corticosteroid injection therapy success is to be maximized. This can only be achieved by an x-ray film–guided technique.[3] For example, radicular leg pain produced by the inflammatory reaction associated with a posterolateral L5–S1 intervertebral herniated nucleus pulposus may be benefited by a translumbar or caudal cortisone epidural approach. A posterolateral herniated nucleus pulposus at L4–L5 or above is best approached with a targeted translumbar injection technique lateralized to the side correlated with the patient's pain symptom.

Lateral pathologic change may affect osseous or soft tissue and may involve the intervertebral nerve root canal or the extraforaminal nerve. The process may be static or dynamic compression. Lateral pathologic alterations may be best addressed with a transforaminal selective epidural injection to ensure adequate cortisone application to the spinal nerve root in the lateral canal or the extraforaminal zone. Combined central and lateral pathologic change may be best addressed by cortisone injection that combines the translumbar and transforaminal approaches. Posterior element inflammatory foci can be addressed with corticosteroid instillation in the intraarticular facet joint or the pars defect.

Nociception emanating from the posterior longitudinal ligament, possibly from a central contained protrusion, is probably best approached by one of the epidural techniques (caudal, translumbar, transforaminal, or a combination of these).

When a patient is unable to advance with an active exercise program, a decision must be made as to how to get beyond this plateau. Injection techniques should be considered as adjunctive treatment. Similarly, acupuncture can be used as adjunctive treatment, in selected cases, to control pain and thereby allow patients to participate in an active exercise regimen.[49] Typically, five sessions of acupuncture are required to create the desired effect. Acupuncture can be used to raise the patient's endorphin level,[77] thereby permitting discontinuance of analgesic medications and facilitating participation in an active exercise and recovery program. Additionally, the activation of endorphins supplements the endorphin generation associated with active exercise, creating a sense of well-being that invariably has a positive impact on the patient's recovery.

Pain must not be the limiting factor in program progression. As in athletic training, pain must be worked through for the patient to reach higher levels of physical fitness and training. However, sources of pain must be differentiated (e.g., nerve root pain versus the pain from stretching the hamstring muscles and tendons). Mechanical lumbar pain is not necessarily a signal to stop exercising; however, increased mechanical (axial) pain that does not resolve quickly after an exercise session, or that gradually increases in intensity in successive exercise sessions, should be a signal to reassess the patient.

Epidural injection of a corticosteroid is the author's treatment of choice for persistent radicular pain that does not permit the patient to advance with the rehabilitation program. Although a tapered course of oral corticosteroids may be prescribed, the reported side effects are probably more frequent and the results more variable.[25] Acupuncture is an alternative or additional therapy that can be used at this point.[49, 77] The results of injection therapy are assessed at 2 to 3 weeks. If disabling radicular pain persists, a second epidural corticosteroid injection may be administered. If the persistent back pain is consistent with posterior element pain, corticosteroid injections of the offending facet joint or the pars defect may be initiated. Injection therapy is used to facilitate progress in recovering function. Decisions to inject or reinject are based on the patient's progress with the active exercise program.

THE PHYSICIAN AS TRAINER

Patient motivation is the key to successful rehabilitation. It is the physician's responsibility and mandate to motivate the patient. The physician must explain to patients the reasons for their back pain. With diagrams and imaging tests such as magnetic resonance imaging and computed tomography, the patient can be shown a visual image of the problem. The patient can then be taught how the concept of dynamic muscle stabilization can be applied to treat the pain. The physician must elicit active cooperation from the patient for the program to be successful. As the program proceeds, the physician functions as a coach to motivate the patient to continue the program. At monthly and bimonthly intervals, the patient's progress is checked. The physical therapist should communicate the current stabilization level and the frequency and intensity of the patient's exercise program. At the time of checkups, the patient is reassessed and the level is tested. Standardized protocols for evaluation of fitness and stabilization level must be employed. It would be of enormous value if all physical therapy facilities used an identical system for monitoring patient progress. Additionally, new symptoms and previous symptoms should be noted.

During follow-up visits, patients should be asked to perform their exercises. If patients cannot perform these exercises in the office, they are not being done at home. It is helpful if the physician can demonstrate some exercises to the patient. This places the physician in the role of trainer. Physician-guided training can help solidify the stabilization program and ensure that the patients commit to a sustained, long-term rehabilitation process.

REFERRAL FOR SURGERY

The inability of the patient to advance with an aggressive active rehabilitation program is an indication to consider surgery. This does not guarantee surgical success, but it demonstrates that it is time for referral. Failure to improve function with passive, nonspecifically applied, unmonitored conservative care is not an appropriate indication for surgical referral.

Patients must be made aware of the likely natural history of their condition, and whether the surgical intervention being considered is likely to provide results superior to those with nonoperative care. Additionally, the patient must be apprised of the potential short-term and long-term risks and complications of the surgical alternatives available. The surgeon who elects to operate solely on the basis of the structure noted on an imaging study and a history of (relatively untreated) back and leg pain is, in the author's opinion, committing a grievous error.

One should not succumb to the pitfall of basing the treatment decisions on structural pathologic change alone. One must treat patients, not imaging test results. According to the basic laws of physiology, all patients can achieve a heightened level of fitness with an active exercise program. The question is whether the gains achieved in physical capability are sufficient without structural alteration of the spine (i.e., surgery) to improve their function. The key to successful treatment outcome, whether it be surgical or nonsurgical, is careful patient selection.

REFERENCES

1. Adams, M. A., Dolan, P., and Hutton, W. C.: Diurnal variations in the stresses on the lumbar spine. Spine, 12:130–137, 1987.
2. Allman, F. L.: Exercise in sports medicine. In Basmajian, J. V. (ed.): Therapeutic Exercise. Baltimore, Williams & Wilkins, 1984, pp. 485–509.
3. Aprill, C.: Diagnostic disc injection. In Frymoyer, J. W. (ed.): The Adult Spine. New York, Raven Press, 1991, pp. 403–442.
4. Basmajian, J. V., Harden, T. P., and Regenos, E. M.: Integrated actions of the four heads of quadriceps femoris: An EMG study. Anat. Rec. 172:15–20, 1972.
5. Beck, J. L., and Day, R. W.: Overuse injuries. Clin. Sports Med. 4:553, 1985.
6. Blackburn, T. A.: Rehabilitation of anterior cruciate ligament injuries. Orthop. Clin. North Am. 16:241–269, 1985.
7. Bonde-Petersen, F., Grandal, H., Hansen, J. W., et al.: The effect of varying the number of muscle contractions on dynamic muscle training. Eur. J. Appl. Physiol. 18:468–473, 1966.
8. Borms, J.: Importance of flexibility in overall physical fitness. Int. J. Phys. Ed. 21:15–26, 1984.
9. Burger, R. A.: Optimal repetitions for the development of strength. Res. Q. 33:334–333, 1962.
10. Chu, D. A.: Comparisons of Selected Electromyographic Data Under Isokinetic and Isotonic Stress Load. Menlo Park, CA, Stanford University, 1974.
11. Coderre, T. J., Katz, J., Vaccarino, A. L., and Melzack, R.: Contribution of central neuroplasticity to pathological pain: Review of clinical and experimental evidence. Pain 52:259–285, 1993.
12. Cornelius, W. L.: A flexibility method designed to establish suitable internal environment for strength. Int. Gymnast. Techn. 2(suppl.):33–34 1981.
13. Costill, D. L., Coyle, E. F., Fink, W. F. et al : Adaptations in skeletal muscle following strength training. J. Appl. Physiol. 46:149, 1976.
14. Costill, D. L., Fink, W. J., and Habansky, A. J.: Muscle rehabilitation after knee surgery. Phys. Sports Med. 5:71–74, 1977.
15. Coyle, E. F., Feiring, D. C., Rotkis T. C., et al.: Specificity of power improvements through slow and fast isokinetic training. J. Appl. Physiol. 51:1437–1442, 1981.
16. Davies, J. E., Gibson, T., and Tester, L.: The value of exercises in the treatment of low back pain. Rheumatol. Rehabil. 18:243, 1979.
17. de Vries, H. A.: Electromyographic observations of the effect of static stretching upon muscle distress. Res. Q. 32:468–480, 1961.
18. de Vries, H. A.: Evaluation of static stretching procedures for improvement flexibility. Res. Q. 33 222–230, 1962.
19. DeLateur, B. J.: Therapeutic Exercise. In Basmajian, J. V.: Exercise for Strength and Endurance. Baltimore, Williams & Wilkins, 1984.
20. DeLorme, T. L.: Restoration of muscle power by heavy-resistance exercises. J. Bone Joint Surg. 27A:645–667, 1945.
21. Dickinson, A. D., and Bennett, K. N.: Therapeutic exercise. Clin. Sports Med. 4:417–429, 1985.
22. Eriksson, E.: Anatomical, histological and physiological factors in experienced downhill skiers. Orthop. Clin. North Am. 7:159–165, 1975.
23. Farfan, H. F., Cossette, B., Robertson, G. H., et al.: The effects of torsion on the lumbar intervertebral joints: The role of torsion in the production of disc degeneration. J. Bone Joint Surg. 52A:468–497, 1970.
24. Farfan, H. F., Osteria, V., and Lamy, C.: The mechanical etiology of spondylosis and spondylolisthesis. Clin. Orthop. 117:40–55, 1976.
25. Fitzgerald, R. H., Jr.: Intrasynovial injection of steroids. Uses and abuses. Mayo Clin. Proc. 51:655, 1976.
26. Fug-sang-Fredriksen, A., and Sheel, U.: Transient decrease in number of motor units after immobilization in man. J. Neurol. Neurosurg Psychiatry 41:924–929, 1978.
27. Halling, A., and Dooley, J.: The importance of isokinetic power and its specificity to athletic conditions. Athletic Training 14:83–86, 1979.
28. Harris, F. A.: Facilitation techniques and technological adjuncts in therapeutic exercise. In Basmajian, J. V. (ed.): Therapeutic Exercise. Baltimore, Williams & Wilkins, 1984, pp. 110–178.
29. Haut, R., and Little, R.: A constitutive equation for collagen fibers. Biomechanics 5:423–430, 1972.
30. Hirsch, G.: Tensile properties during tendon healing. A comparative study of intact and sutured rabbit peroneus brevis tendons. Acta Orthop. Scand. [Suppl.] 153:1–145, 1974.
31. Holland, D. P.: Exercise prescription and therapeutic rehabilitation in sports medicine. Athletic Training, 17:283–286, 1982.
32. Hortobagyi, T., Faludi, J., Tihanyi, J., et al.: Effects of intense "stretching" flexibility training on the mechanical profile of the knee extensors and on the range of motion of the hip joint. Int. J. Sports Med. 6:317–321, 1985.
33. Jackson, R. P., and Glah, J. J.: Foraminal and extraforaminal lumbar disc herniation: Diagnosis and treatment. Spine, 12:577–585, 1987.

34. Kelemen, M. H., and Stewart, K. J.: Circuit weight training: A new direction for cardiac rehabilitation. Sports Med. 2:385–388, 1985.
35. Kellgren, J.: Observations on referred pain arising from muscle. Clin. Sci. 3:175–193, 1938.
36. Kennedy, J. C., and Baxter-Willis, R.: The effects of local steroid injections on tendons: A biochemical and microscopic correlative study. Am. J. Sports Med. 4:11–18, 1976.
37. Kikuchi, S., Sato, K., Konno, S., and Hasue, M.: Anatomic and radiographic study of dorsal root ganglia. Spine 19:6–11, 1994.
38. Knapik, J. J., Wright, J. E., Mawdlsley, R. H., et al.: Isometric, isotonic and isokinetic torque variations in four muscle groups through a range of joint motion. Phys. Ther. 63:939–947, 1983.
39. Knapik, J. J., Wright, J. E., Mawdlsley, R. H., et al.: Isokinetic, isometric and isotonic strength relationships. Arch. Phys. Med. Rehabil. 64:77–80, 1983.
40. Knott, M., and Voss, D. E.: Proprioceptive Neuromuscular Facilitation. New York, Harper & Row, 1956.
41. Kobayashi, S., Yoshizawa, H., Hachiya, Y., et al.: Vascogenic edema induced by compression injury to the spinal nerve root: Distribution of intravenously injected protein tracers and gadolinium enhanced MR imaging. Presented at the International Society for the Study of the Lumbar Spine Meeting, Marseilles, France, 1993.
42. Kottke, F., Pauley, D., and Ptak, R.: The rationale for prolonged stretching for correction of shortening of connective tissue. Arch. Phys. Med. Rehabil. 47:345–352, 1966.
43. LaBan, M.: Collagen tissue: Implications of its response to stress in vitro. Arch. Phys. Med. Rehabil. 43:461–466, 1962.
44. Lane, N. E., and Buckwalter, J. A.: Exercise: A cause of osteoarthritis. Rheum. Dis. Clin. North Am. 19:617–633, 1993.
45. Lehmann, J., Masock, S., Warren, C. G., et al.: Effect of therapeutic temperatures on tendon extensibility. Arch. Phys. Med. 51:481–487, 1970.
46. Lind, B., Massie, J. B., Lincoln, T., et al.: The effects of induced hypertension and acute graded compression on impulse propagation in the spinal nerve roots of the pig. Spine 18:1550–1555, 1993.
47. Lindh, M.: Increase of muscle strength from isometric quadriceps exercise at different knee angles. Scand. J. Rehabil. Med. 11:33–36, 1979.
48. Matsui, H., Olmarker, K., Cornefjord, M., et al.: Local electrophysiologic stimulation in experimental double level cauda equina compression. Spine 17:1075–1078, 1992.
49. Melzack, R., Stilwell, D. M., and Fox, E. J.: Trigger points and acupuncture points for pain: Correlations and implications. Pain 3:3–23, 1977.
50. Moffroid, M., and Whipple, R.: Specificity of speed of exercise. Phys. Ther. 50:1692–1700, 1970.
51. Moller, M., Oberg, B., and Gilquist, J.: Stretching exercise and soccer: Effect of stretching on range of motion in the low extremity in connection with soccer training. J. Sports Med. 6:50–52, 1985.
52. Mooney, J., and Robertson, J.: The facet syndrome. Clin. Orthop. 115:149–156, 1976.
53. Mooney, V.: Presidential Address. International Society for the Study of the Lumbar Spine: Where is the pain coming from? Spine 12:754–759, 1987.
54. Murray, M. P., Baldwin, J., Gardner, G., et al.: Maximum isometric knee flexor and extensor muscle contractions—normal patterns of torque versus time. Phys. Ther. 57:637–643, 1977.
55. Noyes, F. R.: Functional properties of knee ligaments and alterations induced by immobilization: A correlative biomechanical and histological study in primates. Clin. Orthop. 123:210–242, 1977.
56. Oldridge, N. B., and Steiner, D. L.: The health belief model: Predicting compliance and dropout in cardiac rehabilitation. Med. Sci. Sports Exerc. 22:678–683, 1990.
57. Olmarker, K., Rydevik, B., and Nordborg, C.: Autologous nucleus pulposus induces neurophysiologic and histologic changes in porcine cauda equina nerve roots. Spine 18:1425–1432, 1993.
58. Pedowitz, R. A., Garfin, S. R., Massie, J. B., et al.: Effects of magnitude and duration of compression on spinal nerve root conduction. Spine 17:194–199, 1992.
59. Pedrini-Mille, A., Weinstein, J. A., Found, E. M., and Chung, C. B.: Stimulation of dorsal root ganglion and degradation of rabbit anulus fibrosus. Spine 15:1252–1256, 1990.
60. Rasch, P. J., and Morehouse, L. E.: Effect of static and dynamic exercises on muscular strength and hypertrophy. J. Appl. Physiol. 11:29, 1957.
61. Reynolds, M.: Myofascial trigger point syndromes in the practice of rheumatology. Arch. Phys. Med. Rehabil. 62:111–113, 1981.
62. Rydevik, B., Brown, M., and Lundborg, G.: Pathoanatomy and pathophysiology of nerve root compression. Spine 9:7–15, 1984.
63. Saal, J. A.: General principles and guidelines for rehabilitation of the injured athlete. In Saal, J. A. (ed.): Physical Medicine and Rehabilitation: State of the Art Reviews, Vol. 1, Philadelphia, Hanley & Belfus, 1987, pp. 523–536.
64. Saal, J. A., and Saal, J. S.: Electrophysiologic evaluation of lumbar pain: Establishing the rationale for therapeutic management. In White, A. H., Rothman, R. H., and Ray, C. D. (eds.): Lumbar Spine Surgery: Techniques and Complications. St. Louis, C. V. Mosby, 1987, pp. 528–551.
65. Saal, J. A.: Rehabilitation of football players with lumbar spine injury (part 1). Phys. Sportsmed. 16:61–74, 1988.
66. Saal, J. A.: Rehabilitation of football players with lumbar spine injury (part 2). Phys. Sportsmed. 16:117–125, 1988.
67. Saal, J. A., and Saal, J. S.: Nonoperative treatment of herniated lumbar intervertebral disc with radiculopathy: An outcome study. Spine 14:431–437, 1989.
68. Saal, J. A.: Dynamic muscular stabilization in the nonoperative treatment of lumbar pain syndromes. Orthop. Rev. 19:691–700, 1990.
69. Saal, J. A.: Rehabilitation of the injured athlete. In DeLisa, J. A. (ed.): Principles and Practice of Rehabilitation Medicine. Philadelphia, J. B. Lippincott (in press).
70. Saal, J. S.: Flexibility training. In Saal, J. A. (ed.): Physical Medicine and Rehabilitation: State of the Art Reviews, Vol. 1. Philadelphia, Hanley & Belfus, 1987, pp. 537–554.
71. Saal, J. S., Franson, R. C., Dobrow, R., et al.: High levels of inflammatory phospholipase A2 activity in lumbar disc herniations. Spine 15:674–678, 1990.

72. Saraste, H.: Longterm clinical and radiological follow-up of spondylolysis and spondylolisthesis. J. Pediatr. Orthop. 7:631–638, 1987.
73. Sherrington, C. S.: The Integrative Action of the Nervous System. New Haven, CT, Yale University Press, 1961.
74. Sinaki, M., Lutness, M. P., Ilstrup, D. M., et al.: Lumbar spondylolisthesis: Retrospective comparison and three year follow up of two conservative treatment programs. Arch. Phys. Med. Rehabil. 70:594–598, 1989.
75. Stanish, W. D., Curwin, S., and Rubinovich, M.: Tendinitis analysis and treatment. Clin. Sports Med. 4:593–608, 1986.
76. Steadman, J. R.: Rehabilitation after knee ligament surgery. Am. J. Sports Med. 8:294–296, 1980.
77. Takagi, H.: Critical review of pain relieving procedures including acupuncture: Advances in pharmacology and therapeutics II CNS pharmacology. Neuropeptides 1:79–92 1982.
78. Tanigawa, M. C.: Comparison of the hold-relax procedure and passive mobilization on increasing muscle length. Phys. Ther. 52:725–735, 1972.
79. Tipton, C. M., James, S. I., and Mergner, W.: Influence of exercise in strength of medial collateral ligaments of dogs. Am. J. Physiol. 218:894–902, 1970.
80. Tipton, C. M., Schild, R. J., and Tomanek, R. J.: Influence of physical activity on the strength of knee ligaments in rats. Am. J. Physiol. 212:783–787, 1967.
81. Ward, N. G.: Tricyclic antidepressants for chronic low back pain. Spine 11:661–665, 1986.
82. Weinstein, J.: Mechanism of spinal pain: The dorsal root ganglion and its role as a mediator of low back pain. Spine 11:999–1001, 1986.
83. Weinstein, J., Claverie, W., and Gibson, S.: The pain of discography. Spine 13:1344–1348, 1988.
84. Wiltse, L. L., and Spencer, C. W.: New uses and refinements of the paraspinal approach to the lumbar spine. Spine 13:696–706, 1988.

Operative Treatment: Children and Adolescents

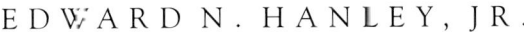

EDWARD N. HANLEY, JR.

Spondylolisthesis, the slippage of one vertebra on another, is the result of a loss of the mechanical integrity of the spinal column. Predominantly occurring at the lumbosacral articulation, it is thought to be accentuated by gravitational and postural forces acting on this area as a result of upright human posture. Although a variety of predisposing factors have been described for spondylolisthesis in children, two types of vertebral slippage predominate in childhood: dysplastic (I) and isthmic (II).[59, 88]

Spondylolisthesis is rarely seen in infancy, but its frequency appears to increase between the ages of 5 and 8 years and to stabilize before the third decade of life.[3, 9, 26, 84, 86] Heredity and activity patterns undoubtedly influence its occurrence.* Progression, when it occurs, appears to predominate in children with the dysplastic type; it is usually correlated with the adolescent growth spurt.[5, 22, 79] Increasing slippage is infrequently seen thereafter. Symptoms of pain and/or neurologic dysfunction, which are commonly the presenting symptoms in adults, are less frequently seen in children and adolescents.[11, 22, 35, 43, 51]

CONSIDERATION OF SURGERY

Although the majority of patients can be satisfactorily managed with nonoperative measures (i.e., rest, immobilization, exercises, and the administration of antiinflammatory medication),[33, 35, 36, 59, 77, 88] a subset of patients remain in whom symptoms or progression of deformity leads to consideration of surgical intervention. Knowledge of the natural history of the disease, risk factors for future problems, and the expected outcome of interventional treatment

---

*References 3, 9, 42–44, 46, 47, 75, 78, 83, 84, 86, and 88.

all play a role in therapeutic decision-making. Similarly, no one solution is appropriate for all patients.

When operative treatment is elected, one must judiciously select the most appropriate surgical and postsurgical treatment plan for a particular individual. Although arthrodesis in situ remains the standard for operative care, there are instances in which other procedures, such as isthmic defect repair or slip reduction, may be indicated. Appropriate selection of the procedure for the patient and meticulous attention to details of the operation minimize problems and complications while maximizing return of function.

When an individual presents for evaluation or is being followed with a diagnosis of spondylolysis or spondylolisthesis, certain factors should be considered so that an appropriate treatment or monitoring regimen can be instituted. Clinical and radiographic risk factors that may portend a poor result with nonoperative measures should be weighed each time the patient is assessed. Although no exact formula exists for determining when to advise surgery, the following factors should be considered.[36]

Clinical Risk Factors

Age. The progression of spondylolisthesis is most likely to occur in persons younger than age 15 years and is correlated with the adolescent growth spurt.[5, 22, 79] Significantly increased slippage after this period is unlikely.[11, 22, 30, 46, 71, 79]

Pain. Children with symptoms of back pain, particularly those that are unresponsive to nonoperative measures, are more likely to require surgery. Likewise, if radicular symptoms are present, the likelihood of the need for surgical treatment to control these symptoms is higher. In addition, patients with neural symptoms are likely to have a higher grade of slip (>50%). This condition alone may be an indication for surgery.[31, 79]

Sex. Female patients with spondylolisthesis are more likely than male patients to experience progression of displacement.[11, 22, 73, 87] This may be related to the generally more lax nature of their soft tissues.

Ligamentous Laxity. Generalized laxity of the soft tissues may be a predisposing factor for progressive slippage. Assessment of joint hyperextension, skin laxity, or a family history of related conditions may be beneficial.

Radiographic Risk Factors

Type of Slippage. In persons with incomplete or abnormal formation of the posterior elements at the lumbosacral articulation, spondylolisthesis of the dysplastic type (type I) is liable to occur and more likely to progress.[22, 35, 36, 42, 59, 86] Persons with the more common isthmic spondylolisthesis tend to acquire their disease later in childhood, and mechanical factors leading to profound progression are generally not present.[59, 86]

Mechanical Insufficiency. Persons with anatomic factors leading to mechanical insufficiency at the L5-to-sacrum level are more likely to exhibit progression. These factors include an eroded, rounded, or dome-shaped sacrum; a trapezoid shape of the L5 vertebral body; a seesaw (teeter-totter) type of alignment of L5 on S1, as described by Hensinger and coworkers[35, 36]; and an abnormally high slip angle (>40 to 50 degrees) indicative of localized kyphosis.* The slip angle normally ranges from 0 to 10 degrees. It should be measured in all patients with spondylolisthesis, as this is a reliable and reproducible sign that correlates well with propensity for further displacement.[11]

Degree of Slippage. Spondylolisthesis of greater than 30% is more likely to progress. In patients with 50% or greater olisthesis, the likelihood of progression is so great that many investigators advocate surgical treatment at this stage, regardless of whether symptoms are present.[3, 11, 35, 55, 79, 84]

Hypermobility. If the degree of slip increases when a standing lateral radiograph is compared with a supine view, a tendency to progression exists.[11, 56] Likewise, if on lateral flexion-extension radiographs, increased olisthesis or angular hypermobility with opening of the isthmic defect is present, the propensity to progression of slip is increased.[36]

---

*References 3, 11, 22, 35, 36, 46, and 79.

INDICATIONS FOR SURGERY

For children and adolescents, the indications for surgical intervention are different than those for adults. Likewise, the results of surgical treatment are generally more favorable in the younger population.[31] Children with spondylolysis or low-grade spondylolisthesis are likely to respond to nonoperative measures, and often surgery can be avoided in these patients without long-term sequelae.[*] This may be related to accelerated degeneration of the disc during adolescence, resulting in spontaneous stabilization of the spondylolisthetic segment.[71] On the other hand, it is generally in childhood that progression of slippage and initial presentation of higher-grade slips are seen. Some children with major grades of spondylolisthesis or even spondyloptosis have no symptoms.

During evaluation of spondylolysis or spondylolisthesis, many factors must be considered, and the indications for surgery may vary. However, on the basis of existing knowledge of the natural history of the disease, of individual risk factors, and of the outcome of surgical treatment for this condition, broad indications for surgical intervention may be determined. They are as follows:

1. Persistence of painful mechanical or neurologic symptoms, despite an appropriate course of nonoperative treatment[12, 13, 35]
2. Documentation of progressive slippage beyond 25% to 33%[12] (Fig. 1A,B)
3. Presentation with slip greater than 50%[12, 35, 47, 87]
4. Postural deformity and gait abnormality (relative indication)[35, 36] (Fig. 2A to D).

OPERATIVE OPTIONS

In Situ Fusion—One Level

In most instances, local one-level arthrodesis of the spine suffices, providing a stable fusion and symptomatic relief in the majority of patients.[11, 35, 66, 73, 79] This procedure is best performed through a bilateral approach with an intertransverse process—or a transverse process—sacral ala arthrodesis to stabilize flexion, extension, and rotational forces on the involved segment. For slip of less than 50% in children and adolescents, this is the procedure of choice. Further slippage postoperatively is less likely if bilateral muscle splitting, rather than a midline dissection, is used.[80]

In Situ Fusion—Two Levels

When the spondylolisthesis exceeds 50%, the anterior displacement of the vertebral body and thus the transverse processes to which the fusion is to be applied makes long-term stabilization with a one-level fusion less likely. In such instances, it is wise to extend the arthrodesis to L4.[12, 15] Despite the immobilization of the additional segment, mobility is remarkably well preserved when pain relief is achieved. The increased frequency of pseudarthrosis seen in adults with extension of the fusion is not observed in children.[31] However, even when the fusion does not appear radiographically solid, a good clinical result may be achieved.[48]

Schoenecker and coworkers[69] described the occurrence of cauda equina syndrome after in situ posterior arthrodesis for grade III or grade IV lumbosacral spondylolisthesis, even though no directed manipulation of the neural elements occurred. They postulated that this may result from relaxation of the stabilizing muscles under general anesthesia and with the dissection and exposure. When this occurs, they recommend acute decompression including sacral prominence excision.

Laminectomy or Laminectomy and Fusion

In adult patients with spondylolisthesis, radicular symptoms are encountered relatively frequently and are unrelieved without neural decompressive procedures. In contrast, radiculopathy due to spondylolisthesis is seen much less frequently in childhood. This is probably attributable to the relative lack of hypertrophic tissue about the pars interarticularis lesion, despite the magnitude of the slip. Even in relatively high-grade cases of olisthesis, laminectomy can be avoided because, with satisfactory arthrodesis and elimination of abnormal motion, nerve-related lower extremity symptoms usually resolve.[11, 30, 35, 39] In addition, removal of the pos-

---
*References 35, 36, 59, 71, 79, 84, 86, and 88.

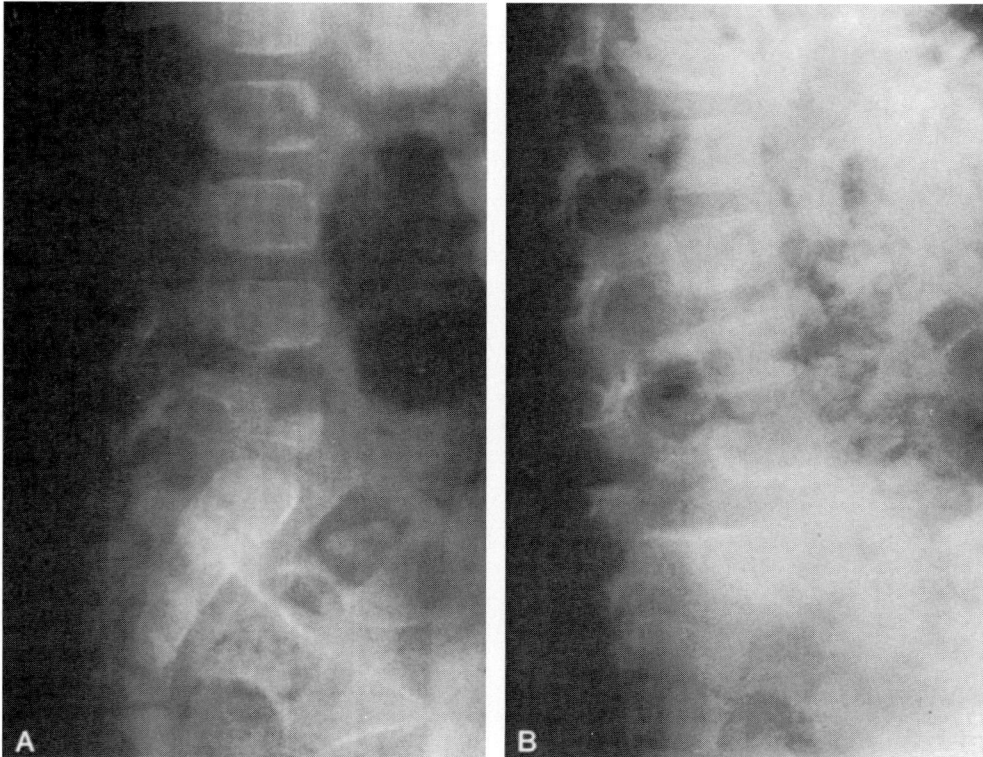

Figure 1. *A*, A 2-year-old child with back pain. Sclerosis of the pars interarticularis at L5 is present. *B*, At age 4, the pars defect is apparent and spondylolisthesis of 25% has occurred. Further progression is an indication for surgical stabilization.

terior ligamentous and osseous elements may add yet another destabilizing factor to an already unstable mechanical situation. This may result in predisposition to further slippage, even during the period of arthrodesis consolidation.[45, 87] Owing to these factors, laminectomy alone for spondylolisthesis is never indicated in children and should be performed along with fusion in certain circumstances. These situations include laminectomy performed in conjunction with the reduction of a high-grade spondylolisthesis and, occasionally, cases in which the preoperative symptoms are predominantly radicular and in which myelography, computed tomography, and/or magnetic resonance imaging shows a large, hypertrophic, fibrocartilaginous mass encroaching on the nerve roots at the level of the defect.

Anterior Fusion

The indications for anterior arthrodesis in childhood spondylolisthesis appear to be limited. Most patients, with the possible exception of those with high-grade (>75%) slips, achieve satisfactory results with posterior stabilization alone. Although, with experience, anterior lumbosacral interbody fusion is reported to be successful,[27, 72, 80, 82] the technical difficulties presented by the confluence of the great vessels at this level add risk to this operation. In addition, the possibility of inducing retrograde ejaculation, owing to violation of the presacral plexus in male patients, should be considered if this procedure is contemplated.[40] On occasion, however, when deformity is great and a posterior procedure is deemed insufficient, or in instances in which pseudarthrosis or plastic deformation of the fusion mass has occurred because of a high slip angle and/or a major translational displacement, a supplementary anterior fusion can be performed.[7, 17, 85] A few surgeons advocate a primary anterior approach with disc excision, thereby facilitating reduction.[50, 74, 76] Good results with interbody fusion through a posterior approach have been reported by Cloward.[21]

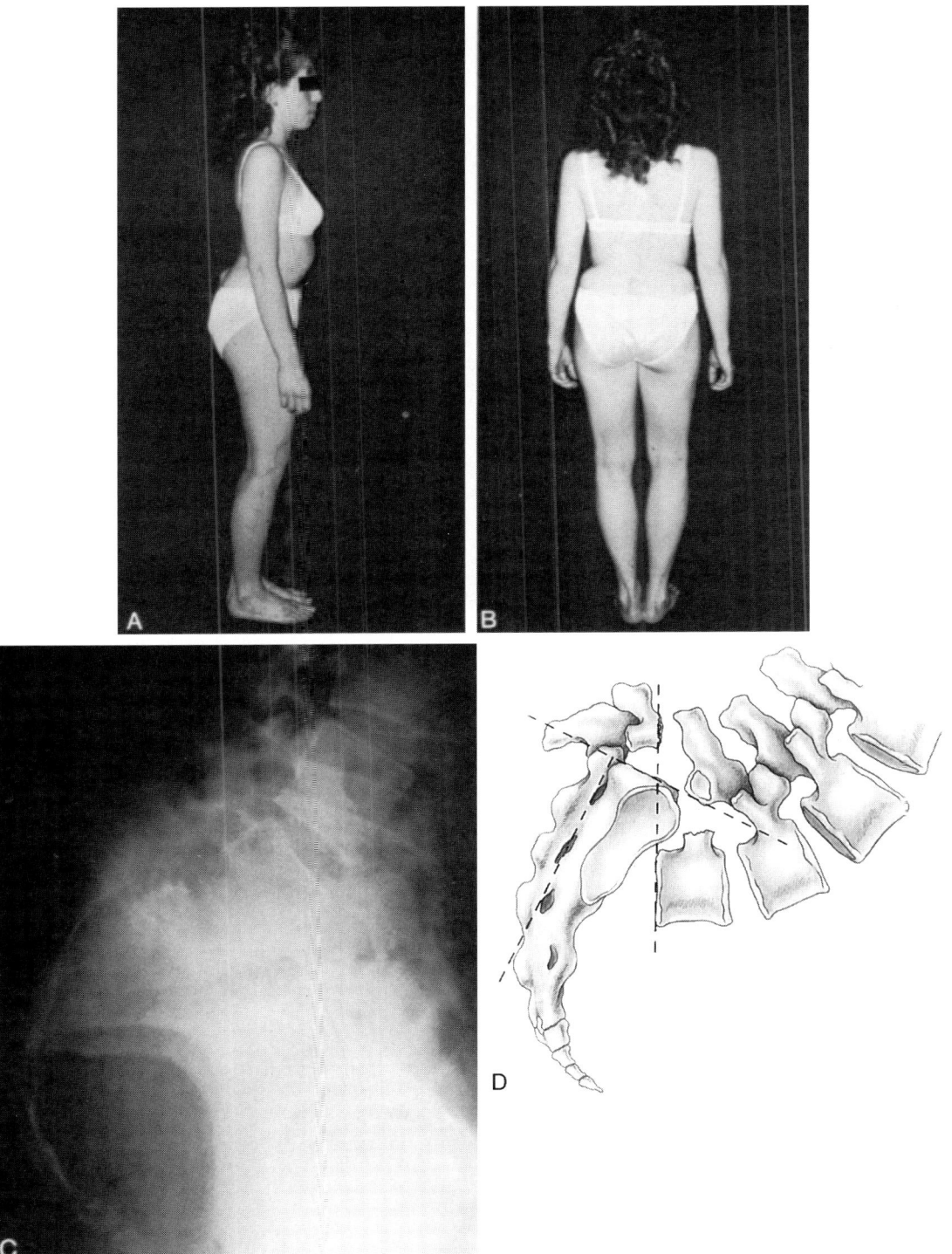

Figure 2. *A, B,* Teenaged girl with complete spondylolisthesis (spondyloptosis). Note the characteristic deformity. *C,* Standing lateral radiograph demonstrates complete slippage of the lumbar spine off the pelvis. *D,* Schematic drawing of this patient's radiograph. The slip angle measures 58 degrees and quantifies the localized kyphosis.

Isthmic Defect Repair

First popularized by Buck[19] in 1970, direct repair of isthmic defects can be performed for isolated spondylolysis or low-grade (<25%) spondylolisthesis.[14, 16, 60, 81] The appeal of this technique lies in the preservation of the involved motion segment, which minimizes abnormal stresses at adjacent levels. The repair may be performed by using a direct screw technique,[19, 65] plates,[50] or wires around the transverse processes and posterior elements, providing a tension band–like effect.[16, 38, 60] Repair can also be achieved by wiring the posterior elements to a pedicle screw[67] or by using a hook screw that facilitates compression across the grafted pars defect.[34, 57, 61, 89] The procedure is most easily performed, particularly when one is using the wire technique, at levels above the lumbosacral junction. Bone grafting of the pars defect to facilitate healing of the pars defect is mandatory. This procedure should not be attempted when the defect distance is substantial (>25% olisthesis) or when an abnormal slip angle is present. Nachemson[58] suggested direct defect repair in conjunction with lateral arthrodesis. Although seemingly attractive in most cases, this technique appears to add little to the already satisfactory results of lateral arthrodesis in situ.

Anterior and Posterior Fusion

Combined approaches for spondylolisthesis are advocated by some investigators for higher-grade and more unstable spondylolisthetic patterns.[13, 49, 82] As mentioned previously, this technique is most commonly used if a posterior procedure alone might be expected to fail or if a reduction technique is deemed to require a primary anterior release.[17] Possible vascular and neurologic complications should be considered if one elects this approach.

Reduction of Spondylolisthesis

Despite uncertainty as to the indications for reduction of partial or complete spondylolisthesis, a variety of techniques have been described.* These procedures include postoperative traction, with or without cast reduction, followed by posterior fusion (Lance[44] and Scaglietti and coworkers[68]); in situ fusion followed by postoperative reduction and casting (Burkus and colleagues[20]); posterior distraction techniques (DeWald and colleagues,[24] Harrington and Tullos,[32] and Kaneda and coworkers[41]); kyphosis reduction and sublaminar wiring (Schwend and colleague[70]); posterior element wiring with external traction reduction (Balderston and Bradford[4] and Snijder and colleagues[76]); spinal column shortening by L5 vertebrectomy (Gaines and Nichols[29] and Huizenga[37]); combined posterior and anterior procedures (Bradford and colleagues,[13, 17, 18] DeWald and colleagues,[24] and McPhee and O'Brien[52]); and pedicle screw techniques (Ani and associates,[1] Boos and coworkers,[8] Edwards,[25] Louis and Maresca,[49] McQueen and colleagues,[53] Matthiass and Heine,[54] and Sijbrandij[74]).

With all of these methods, a significant incidence (up to 30% in some series) of neural problems has been reported, most commonly involving postoperative dysfunction of the L5 and/or S1 nerve roots. Additionally, loss of reduction is not uncommon, owing to the tremendous mechanical forces that have caused the presenting deformity.[12] Regardless of the technique employed, meticulous attention to the bone grafting arthrodesis technique is necessary. Otherwise, deformity and recurrent symptoms ensue. To prevent tethering during the reduction maneuver, laminectomy and thorough clearing of the nerve roots at the deformity level are mandatory whenever reduction is undertaken. Nonetheless, neural pain or dysfunction may occur after such a procedure. The cause of this is unclear, but it is speculated that the pain or dysfunction may be related to unrecognized nerve root compression or tension or to vascular factors associated with repositioning of the roots and changes in spinal alignment.

Although pedicle screw techniques seem appealing at this time, the small size of the pedicle in children, particularly those with dysplastic variations of the disease, sometimes precludes appropriate placement of the screws. This may prevent the surgeon from obtaining an adequate mechanical grasp of the olisthetic vertebra for the reduction maneuver. Alternatively, the screw itself may impinge on neural structures.

---

*References 1, 4, 8, 13, 17, 18, 20, 23–25, 29, 32, 37, 41, 44, 49, 52–54, 68, 70, 74, and 76.

Regardless of the technique employed, postoperative immobilization of the pelvis, with either a cast or a brace incorporating one or both thighs, should be considered to decrease the patient's activity and to minimize the chances for loss of reduction.

Poussa and colleagues[64] compared adolescent patients who had severe spondylolisthesis (>50%) treated by pedicle screw instrumentation and reduction with those who were treated by fusion or arthrodesis in situ without instrumentation. Despite some improvement in slip degree and kyphosis in the patients who underwent reduction procedures, there were no differences in function or pain between the two groups. Operative time, complications, and reoperations were more common with reduction procedures.

Pseudarthrosis Repair

Pseudarthrosis of an attempted arthrodesis is relatively uncommon in children if appropriate surgical techniques are used.[11, 31] As with other arthrodesis procedures, the likelihood of pseudarthrosis is greater if procedures are extensive or when mechanical forces work against bone consolidation. In patients with high-grade slips or those with abnormal slip angles, the arthrodesis may be placed in tension, which increases the likelihood of pseudarthrosis This occurrence can be limited by using meticulous technique and adequate bone graft material and by minimizing stress on the fusion site during consolidation. This effect may be accomplished with casting, bracing, or internal fixation.

When failure of fusion occurs, it is generally accompanied by persistent pain, progression of slippage, or recurrence of deformity. Radiographs should be correlated with the clinical symptoms before a second procedure is considered. Often (at least in children), an additional few months of immobilization results in resolution of the problem. However, when symptoms persist or deformity progresses, with clear evidence of failure of fusion, repeated repair with clearing of all fibrous tissue at the defect and fresh bone grafting should be considered. Usually, this results in a satisfactory outcome. Secondary anterior arthrodesis or addition of instrumentation to the pseudarthrotic level is usually reserved for older patients, cases of higher-grade spondylolisthesis, or instances in which two or more posterior operations have failed. Postoperative immobilization for at least 3 months should be used after all pseudarthrosis repairs.

POSTOPERATIVE CARE

During childhood and adolescence, excellent success rates for fusion in spondylolisthesis have been reported, regardless of the form of immobilization employed. Good results in greater than 90% of patients have been reported by Wiltse and Jackson[36] and Rombold,[66] who did not use postoperative immobilization; by Bosworth and coworkers[10] and Nachemsen,[58] who used a corset; and by Turner and Bianco,[79] who used postoperative casting. Bradford[12, 14, 15] and Axelsson[2] stated that immobilization of the leg is usually unnecessary.

Despite these reports, there are situations in which gross activity restrictions imposed by immobilization of the lumbar spine and pelvis may play a role.[56] For patients with spondylolisthesis greater than 50% or for those in whom translational or slip angle reduction is attempted, the author employed a cast or brace incorporating the torso and one thigh. Likewise, when instrumentation is used for reduction purposes, this type of postoperative restriction may be beneficial in decreasing the incidence of instrument loosening and, hence, of reduction loss. Young people using such devices are always able to ambulate, albeit with some loss of speed, with minimum inconvenience.

A reduction of activity by whatever means for a period of 3 months postoperatively is generally sufficient for satisfactory fusion consolidation. Return to relatively normal activity is permitted after 6 months and is unlimited after 1 year if a good result has been achieved. The issue of whether these children should be allowed to return to high-stress endeavors, such as gymnastics and contact sports, after surgery for spondylolisthesis is controversial and should be resolved on an individual basis. For patients who have complete resolution of symptoms, a satisfactory radiographic appearance of the fusion, and normal spine motion, the author generally permits full return to athletic activities without restriction.

SPECIAL CONSIDERATIONS

Spondylolisthesis in Scoliosis

Most scoliosis associated with spondylolisthesis is antalgic and resolves with treatment of the symptomatic slippage. On occasion, however, a patient has spondylolisthesis in conjunction with a structural scoliosis. Each condition should be treated individually, on the basis of treatment criteria for that condition.[14] Thus, if the spondylolisthesis meets operative criteria and the scoliosis does not, the spondylolisthesis should be operated on and the scoliosis should be treated by whatever nonoperative measures are indicated. The opposite is also true. On rare occasions in which both conditions warrant surgery, it is best to avoid a contiguous fusion to the sacrum. At least a few open lumbar motion segments should be preserved between the two fused portions of the spine. A balanced, mobile spine with some deformity is preferable to a stiff one, regardless of the situation.

Spondylolisthesis Above a Previously Fused Level

In rare instances in children, a spondylolysis or spondylolisthesis develops above a previously fused segment.[6] This condition should be managed as if it were an isolated problem with whatever nonoperative or operative measures are indicated. If surgery is necessary, extension of the fusion should be limited to as few additional segments as possible, preferably to one segment only.

Iatrogenic Spondylolisthesis

Iatrogenic induction of spondylolisthesis in children generally occurs after laminectomy for tumorous conditions. Any child who has undergone such a procedure should be observed closely for the development of deformity. If this occurs, stabilization should be performed immediately. In patients, especially younger ones, who have had multiple-level laminectomies or in whom the pars interarticularis has been resected, a kyphotic and/or spondylolisthetic deformity predictably develops and a prophylactic stabilization procedure is indicated.

Operative Treatment of Spondylolisthesis

The author's approach to surgical treatment of spondylolisthesis varies, depending on the patient's symptoms and mechanical factors influencing the instability pattern. Factors that influence the outcome include the presence or absence of neural symptoms and the slip angle in relationship to the degree of olisthesis. Based on current knowledge of and experience with this disorder, the author has adopted relative guidelines to select the indicated procedure for each patient with spondylolisthesis (Table 1).

Patients with spondylolisthesis of less than 25% and no symptoms require observation only. It is most reasonable to follow them for 6 months. If unresponsive symptoms develop or progression to the next grade occurs, a direct repair or local one-level posterolateral arthrodesis is indicated. Similarly, a one-level stabilization procedure in situ is used for patients with grade 1 or grade 2 olisthesis whose symptoms have failed to show response. The slip angle is generally not a factor in such patients. Rarely, children and adolescents with slip of less than 50% have neural symptoms as a result of fibrocartilaginous hypertrophy about the pars interarticularis defect. When radiculopathy is encountered in this group of patients, back pain generally predominates and lower extremity symptoms usually resolve with a stabilization procedure and elimination of the abnormal motion causing the nerve root irritation. However, if radicular symptoms predominate (a situation commonly seen in adults) and appropriate studies reveal profound neural encroachment, laminectomy and removal of the hypertrophic tissue about the pedicle-pars region may be performed. It is important to do more than just remove the lamina, as failure to clear the roots of compressive tissue results in the continuation of symptoms. After such procedures, immobilization in a lumbar corset, a thoracolumbosacral orthosis, or a cast for 3 months facilitates fusion consolidation by generally reducing the patient's activity.

For patients with olisthesis of from 50%

Table 1

Guidelines for Treatment of Spondylolisthesis Based on Symptoms, Degree of Olisthesis, and Slip Angle

	Asymptomatic	Slip Angle <45 Degrees		Slip Angle >45 Degrees	
		Low Back Pain Only	Back and Neural Symptoms	Low Back Pain Only	Back and Neural Symptoms
I (<25%)	No treatment	One-level fusion*	One-level fusion* Rare neural decompression	One-level fusion*	One-level fusion* Rare neural decompression
II (25–50%)	No treatment versus one-level fusion* if progression is documented	One-level fusion*	One-level fusion* Selective neural decompression	One-level fusion*	One-level fusion* Selective neural decompression
III (50–75%)	Two-level fusion*	Two-level fusion*	Two-level fusion† Neural decompression	Two-level fusion‡ (selective reduction)	Two-level fusion‡ Selective neural decompression (selective reduction)
IV (75–100%)	Two-level fusion†	Two-level fusion† (selective reduction)	Two-level fusion Neural decompression† (selective reduction)	Two-level fusion‡	Two-level fusion‡ Neural decompression (selective reduction)
Complete spondylolisthesis	No treatment versus reduction for functionally cosmetic reasons†	Two-level fusion† (selective reduction)	Two-level fusion Neural decompression† (selective reduction)	Two-level fusion‡ (selective reduction)	Two-level fusion‡ Neural decompression (selective reduction)

*Corset, thoracolumbosacral orthosis, or cast
†Thoracolumbosacral orthosis, with thigh extension
‡Preoperative and postoperative extension cast

to 75% without abnormal kyphosis, extension of the arthrodesis to another level (e.g., L4 to sacrum for L5–S1 spondylolisthesis) usually results in a satisfactory outcome (Fig. 3A,B). Extension of the fusion is indicated in such instances, owing to the anterior positioning of the transverse processes, which permits an inadequate grasp of the translated vertebra by the fusion that is placed in tension. By extending the fusion, a more sagittally oriented arthrodesis in relative compression can be achieved. However, if a laminectomy is deemed necessary for relief of radicular disorders, another element of instability may be introduced. In such instances, it has been the author's practice to immobilize the torso and one thigh postoperatively to limit flexion at the fusion site.

When slip of greater than 50% is present and the slip angle exceeds 45 degrees, an attempt to reduce the local kyphotic deformity by extension casting followed by a two-level in situ fusion is employed. Continuation of this immobilization postoperatively facilitates fusion incorporation and limits postoperative progression, particularly in instances in which a midline approach and/or neural decompression has been performed.

In patients with spondylolisthesis of greater than 75% or complete spondylolisthesis, surgical decision-making becomes more difficult. In children and adolescents with higher-grade spondylolisthesis who are asymptomatic, it is probably best to perform a two-level in situ fusion to avoid the potential development of complete spondylolisthesis. In such instances, stabilization in situ accomplishes nothing and reduction of the deformity is difficult, possibly resulting in the development of neural dysfunction. It is probably best in these situations to do nothing unless a profound cosmetic abnormality and gait disturbance are present. If reduction is undertaken, the risk/benefit ratio must be weighed carefully and discussed with the patient and family before surgery.

The majority of patients with high-grade spondylolisthesis or complete spondylo-

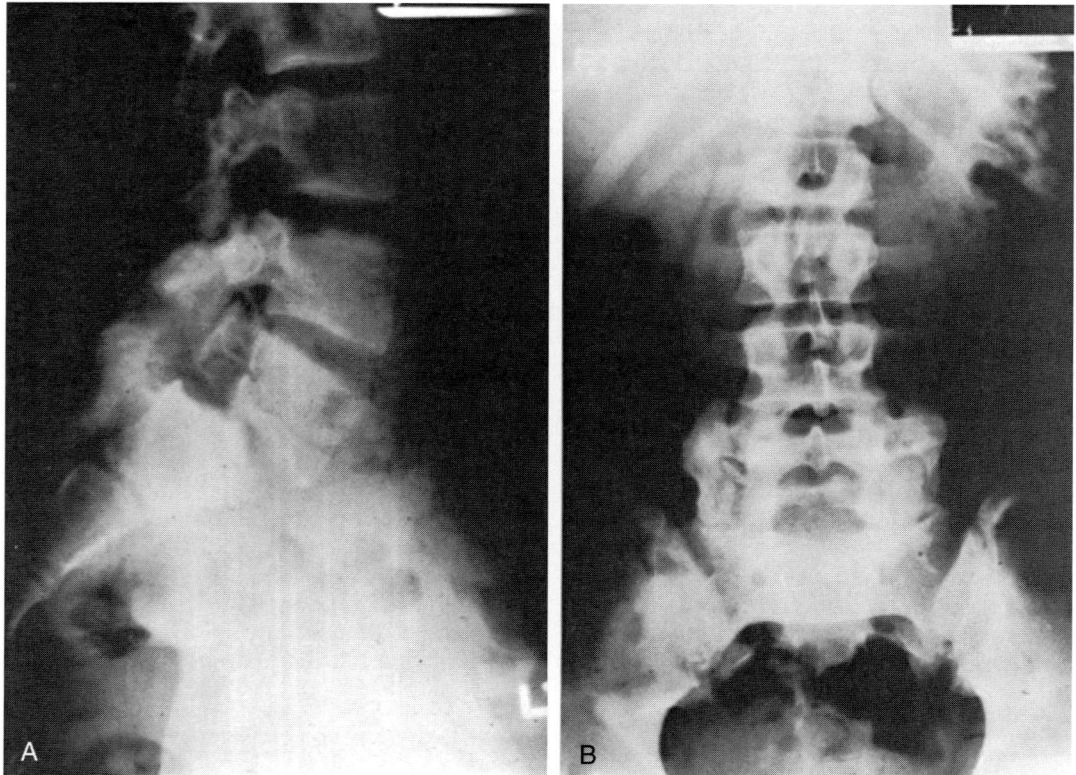

Figure 3. *A, B,* Posterolateral in situ arthrodesis for spondylolisthesis in a 14-year-old boy. At 1 year postoperatively, the fusion is consolidated and symptoms are resolved.

listhesis are symptomatic, and the deformity is of the dysplastic type. Almost always, an abnormally high slip angle is present. Frequently, radicular symptoms, motor symptoms, or sensory changes, or combinations of these problems, are present. In such situations, the minimum surgical intervention is a two-level arthrodesis in situ combined with neural decompression. Extension casting preoperatively and postoperatively is helpful in controlling the slip angle and thus in improving spinal balance while retarding pseudarthrosis and/or progression.

The question of whether to attempt reduction of a severe spondylolisthesis remains controversial, owing to the difficulty of accomplishing the reduction and the risk of causing or accentuating neurologic symptoms or deficits. For high-grade spondylolisthesis and complete spondylolisthesis, the author has attempted reduction in patients with preoperative neural symptoms and an abnormal slip angle. Previously, the author employed a distraction technique using Harrington rods. Although this usually resulted in an initial improvement of the translational abnormality, the slip angle was not decreased and was often accentuated by this technique. This resulted not only in instrumentation of an excessive portion of the lumbar spine, but also in gradual loss of reduction with time, regardless of whether a concomitant anterior fusion was performed.

In selected cases, the author's practice has been to perform a laminectomy and reduction using an isolated posterior approach, employing techniques and instrumentation devised by Charles Edwards of Baltimore[25] (Fig. 4*A,B*). Although the procedure is technically demanding and time-consuming, almost any degree of spondylolisthesis can be reduced with this technique. The procedure is based on the introduction of forces opposite those acting to produce the deformity, as well as on the principle of stress relaxation of soft tissues. A slow and gradual reduction, meticulous attention to preparation of a good fusion bed, and postoperative immobilization of the torso and pelvis are

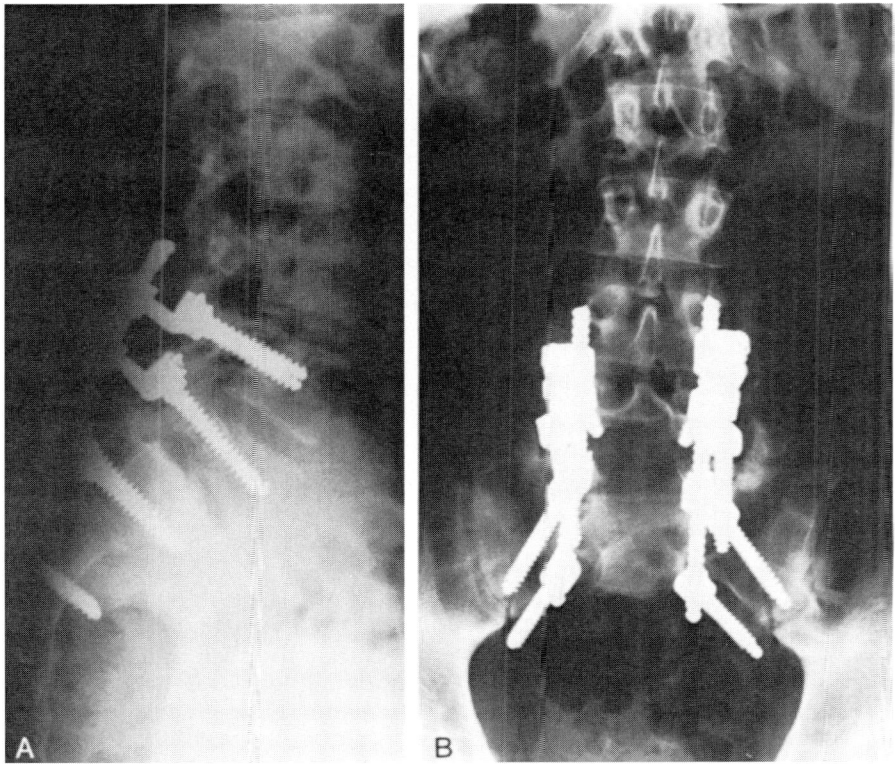

Figure 4. *A, B,* Radiographs following reduction and stabilization of spondylolisthesis utilizing a pedicle screw–rod technique. After distraction, posteriorly directed forces correct the translational malalignment. Two-level sacral fixation permits correction of the kyphotic deformity during the gradual reduction maneuver. Laminectomy of L5 has been performed.

mandatory to avoid instrumental or osseous failure and a resultant recurrence of the deformity. This procedure should not be performed without a thorough decompression of the L5 nerve roots before the reduction maneuver, nor should it be performed by persons unfamiliar with pedicle screw surgical techniques. In patients younger than age 12 years, the small size of the vertebral elements may preclude adequate screw placement. In these patients, other techniques of treatment, such as cast reduction, are advisable.

TECHNICAL SURGICAL CONSIDERATIONS

Posterolateral Spinal Arthrodesis

The procedure is similar for one- or two-level fusions (Fig. 5). When a laminectomy is unnecessary, the spine can be approached by muscle-splitting technique lateral to the midline, with exposure of the transverse processes, facet joints, and sacral ala. A single midline skin incision with subcutaneous dissection or a bilateral skin incision may be used. The transverse processes should be thoroughly denuded and decorticated, along with the lateral aspect of the facet joint and pedicle. It is not necessary to destroy the facet joint, and this should be avoided at the superior margin of the fusion so as to minimize damage to the adjacent motion segment. Exposure of the pars interarticularis defect is generally unnecessary. At the sacral ala, complete exposure is performed and a large drill hole (⅝ inch) placed into it from a superior-to-inferior direction. This establishes a good fusion bed of cancellous bone in the pelvis and permits the fusion mass to assume a more sagittal orientation, thus placing it in relative compression. A large volume of autologous cancellous bone graft is then obtained from the ilium and packed into the fusion bed.

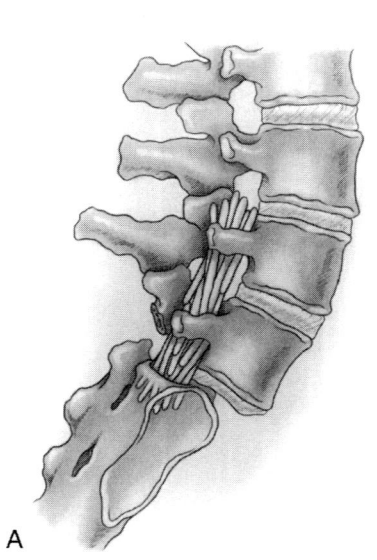 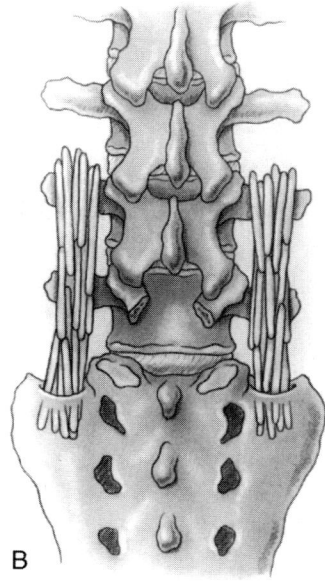

Figure 5. Posterolateral lumbosacral spinal arthrodesis. The bone graft extends into a drill hole placed in the sacral ala.

If nerve root decompression is performed in conjunction with arthrodesis, a midline approach is best. The hypermobile posterior elements are removed, either as a unit or in a piecemeal fashion. At this point, it is necessary to proceed superiorly in the epidural space and to identify the ventral area of the pars defect adjacent to the inferolateral aspect of the L4 lamina. Fibrocartilaginous tissue is noted to proliferate from the pedicle-pars region in a mushroomlike fashion, with the nerve root (L5) coursing under the cap of the mushroom as it exits through the foramen. Removal of this tissue is necessary to adequately relieve neural irritation and predictably to eliminate symptoms. The inferior roots (S1) at the laminectomy site are rarely the source of neural symptoms, and any irritative forces or stenotic factor will have been relieved by the laminectomy. After decompression, fusion is performed, as described previously. When a laminectomy has been performed, bleeding should be meticulously controlled and a drain inserted prior to closure to avoid the development of a symptomatic epidural hematoma.

Spondylolisthesis Reduction

This procedure is indicated in only carefully selected cases. The author's preferred technique for spondylolisthesis reduction is that developed by Edwards.[25] It is described for treatment of deformity at the L5-to-sacrum level. Through a posterior midline approach, the posterior and lateral elements of L4, L5, S1, and S2 are completely exposed. The loose posterior elements are then removed, and the L5 nerve roots are dissected free from the superior margin of the pedicle through the entire foramen. The L5 nerve roots must be completely free so as to permit their unobstructed migration superiorly and dorsally during the reduction maneuver.

With radiographic visualization, holes are drilled into the pedicles of L4 and L5 on either side. Pedicle screws of an appropriate length are inserted into these pedicles. At S1 and S2, screws are placed in a lateral orientation to take advantage of the more substantial bone present in this area of the sacrum. All screws are placed in a plane parallel with that of the adjacent vertebral end plate. At the L5 level, this often means an inferiorly directed angle of from 45 to 60 degrees.

After screw placement and radiographic confirmation of screw position, the lateral fusion sites are decorticated. Rods are then inserted, obtaining a stable two-segment base on the sacrum. This permits control of sacral rotation and therefore correction of the slip angle. Turnbucklelike pedicle connectors are then applied between the rods and L4 and L5. Moderate distraction force is instituted in stages, which permits gradual stretching of the soft tissue contractures. If necessary, supplementary distraction may be applied by the Harrington distraction rod (from L1 or L2 to the sacral ala), which can be removed after appropriate distraction has been accomplished. After initial distraction, the translational deformity is gradually corrected by sequential tightening of the threaded pedicle connectors. During this portion of the procedure, it is necessary to pause briefly each time that translational reduction forces are applied, to permit stress relaxation of the soft tissues and to avoid instrument pullout. Applying a combination of intermittent distraction and translation force permits one gradually to bring the malpositioned spine back into normal alignment. Throughout the procedure, the nerve roots should be observed for tethering and should be released where necessary. After reduction, all articulations are tightened, and bone graft is applied to the lateral masses. Postoperative immobilization of the torso and one thigh for at least 3 months is mandatory. After this period, gradual resumption of activity is permitted.

CONCLUSIONS

Spondylolysis and spondylolisthesis in childhood and adolescence are relatively common, but the majority of persons with these conditions are asymptomatic or can be effectively managed by nonoperative measures. Surgery may be indicated when symptoms are incapacitating and unresponsive to appropriate nonoperative measures, when documented progression of at least one grade has occurred, or when olisthesis at presentation is greater than 50%. In situ posterolateral arthrodesis of one or two segments is successful in most instances. Laminectomy in children with spondylolisthesis may predispose them to further deformity and should be avoided when unnecessary. On rare occasions, fusion or a combination of reduction and fusion can be considered for symptomatic high-grade spondylolisthesis or complete spondylolisthesis with neural symptoms, gait abnormalities, or significant cosmetic deformity. Experience with the techniques necessary to accomplish reduction and a stable arthrodesis, along with an awareness and acceptance of the possible complications of this maneuver, are prerequisites to its performance.

REFERENCES

1. Ani, N., Keppler, L., Biscup, R. S., and Steffee, A. D.: Reduction of high-grade slips (grade III–IV) with VSP instrumentation. Report of a series of 41 cases. Spine 16:S302–S310, 1991.
2. Axelsson, P., Johnsson, R., and Stromquist, B.: Lumbar orthosis with unilateral hip immobilization. Spine 18:876–879, 1993.
3. Baker, D. R., and McHolick, W.: Spondylolysis and spondylolisthesis in children. J. Bone Joint Surg. 38A:933–944, 1956.
4. Balderston, R. A., and Bradford, D. S.: Technique for achievement and maintenance of reduction for severe spondylolisthesis. Spine 10:376–382, 1985.
5. Blackburne, J. S., and Velikas, E. P.: Spondylolisthesis in children and adolescents. J. Bone Joint Surg. 59B:490–494, 1977.
6. Blasier, R. D., and Monson, R. C.: Acquired spondylolysis after posterolateral spinal fusion. J. Pediatr. Orthop. 7:215–217, 1987.
7. Bohlman, H. H., and Cook, S. S.: One-stage decompression and posterolateral and interbody fusion for lumbosacral spondyloptosis through a posterior approach. Report of two cases. J. Bone Joint Surg. 64A:415–418, 1982.
8. Bocs, N., Marchesi, D., Zuber, K., and Aebi, M.: Treatment of severe spondylolisthesis by reduction and pedicular fixation. A 4–6 year follow-up study. Spine 18:1655–1661, 1993.
9. Borkow, S. E., and Kleiger, B.: Spondylolisthesis in the newborn. Clin. Orthop. 81:73–76, 1971.
10. Bosworth, D. M., Fielding, W. J., Demarest, L., and Bonaquist, M.: Spondylolisthesis: A critical review of a consecutive series of cases treated by arthrodesis. J. Bone Joint Surg. 37A:767–786, 1955.
11. Boxall, D., Bradford, D. S., Winter, R. B., and Moe, J. H.: Management of severe spondylolisthesis in children and adolescents. J. Bone Joint Surg. 61A:479–495, 1979.
12. Bradford, D. S.: Spondylolysis and spondylolisthesis. In Chou, I. S. N., and Seljeskog, E. L. (eds.): Spinal Deformity and Neurological Dysfunction. New York, Raven Press, 1978.
13. Bradford, D. S.: Treatment of severe spondylolisthesis: A combined approach for reduction and stabilization. Spine 4:423–429, 1979.
14. Bradford, D. S.: Management of spondylolysis and spondylolisthesis. Instr. Course Lect. 32:151–162, 1983.
15. Bradford, D. S.: Spondylolysis and spondylolisthesis in children and adolescents. In Bradford, D. S., and Hensinger, R. W. (eds.): Pediatric Spine. New York, Thieme-Stratton, 1985.
16. Bradford, D. S., and Iza, J.: Repair of the defect in spondylolysis or minimal degrees of spondylolisthesis by segmental wire fixation and bone grafting. Spine 10:673–679, 1985.
17. Bradford, D. S., and Gotfried, Y.: Staged salvage reconstruction of grade IV and V spondylolisthesis. J. Bone Joint Surg. 69A:191–202, 1987.
18. Bradford, D. S., and Boachie-Adjei, O.: Treatment of severe spondylolisthesis by anterior and posterior reduction and stabilization. A long-term fol-

low-up study. J. Bone Joint Surg. 72A:1060–1066, 1990.
19. Buck, J. E.: Direct repair of the defect in spondylolisthesis. J. Bone Joint Surg. 52B:432–437, 1970.
20. Burkus, J. K., Lonstein, J. E., Winter, R. B., and Denis, F.: Long-term evaluation of adolescents treated operatively for spondylolisthesis. A comparison of in-situ arthrodesis only with in-situ arthrodesis and reduction followed by immobilization in a cast. J. Bone Joint Surg. 74A:693–704, 1992.
21. Cloward, R. B.: Spondylolisthesis: Treatment by laminectomy and posterior interbody fusion. Clin. Orthop. 154:74–82, 1981.
22. Dandy, D. J., and Shannon, M. J.: Lumbosacral subluxation. J. Bone Joint Surg. 53B:578–595, 1971.
23. Del Torto, U.: Surgical reduction and stabilization of spondylolisthesis. Clin. Orthop. 75:281–284, 1971.
24. DeWald, R. L., Faut, M. M., Taddonio, R. F., and Neuwirth, M. G.: Severe lumbosacral spondylolisthesis in adolescents and children: Reduction and staged circumferential fusion. J. Bone Joint Surg. 63A:619–626, 1981.
25. Edwards, C. C., and Bradford, D. S.: Controversies: Instrumented reduction of spondylolisthesis. Spine 19:1535–1537, 1994.
26. Frederickson, B. E., Baker, D., McHolick, W. J., et al.: The natural history of spondylolysis and spondylolisthesis. J. Bone Joint Surg. 66A:699–707, 1984.
27. Freebody, D., Bendall, R., and Taylor, R. D.: Anterior transperitoneal lumbar fusion. J. Bone Joint Surg. 53B:617–627, 1971.
28. Freeman, B. L., and Donati, H. L.: Spinal arthrodesis for severe spondylolisthesis on children and adolescents. A long-term follow-up study. J. Bone Joint Surg. 71A:594–598, 1989.
29. Gaines, R. W., and Nichols, W. K.: Treatment of spondyloptosis by two-stage L5 vertebrectomy and reduction of L4 onto S1. Spine 10:680–686, 1985.
30. Gill, G. G., Manning, J. G., and White, H. L.: Surgical treatment of spondylolisthesis without spine fusion. J. Bone Joint Surg. 37A:493–520, 1955.
31. Hanley, E. N., and Levy, J. A.: Surgical treatment of isthmic lumbosacral spondylolisthesis: Analysis of variables influencing results. Spine 14:48–50, 1989.
32. Harrington, P. R., and Tullos, H. S.: Spondylolisthesis in children; observations and surgical treatment. Clin. Orthop. 79:75–84, 1971.
33. Harris, I. E., and Weinstein, S. L.: Long-term follow-up of patients with grade III and IV spondylolisthesis. J. Bone Joint Surg. 69A:960–969, 1987.
34. Hefti, F., Seelig, W., and Morscher, E.: Repair of lumbar spondylosis with a hook-screw. Int. Orthop. 16:81–85, 1992.
35. Hensinger, R. N., Lang, J. R., and MacEwen, G. D.: Surgical management of spondylolisthesis in children and adolescents. Spine 1:207–216, 1976.
36. Hensinger, R. N.: Spondylolysis and spondylolisthesis in children. Instr. Course Lect. 32:132–151, 1983.
37. Huizenga, B. A.: Reduction of spondylolisthesis with two stage vertebrectomy. Orthop. Trans. 7:21, 1983.
38. Johnson, G. V., and Thompson, A. G.: The Scott wiring technique for direct repair of lumbar spondylolysis. J. Bone Joint Surg. 74B:426–430, 1992.
39. Johnson, J. R., and Kirwin, E. O.: The long-term results of fusion in situ for severe spondylolisthesis. J. Bone Joint Surg. 65B:43–46, 1983.
40. Johnson, R. M., and McQuire, E. J.: Urogenital complications of anterior approaches to the lumbar spine. Clin. Orthop. 154:114–118, 1981.
41. Kaneda, K., Satoh, S., Nohara, Y., and Tadanori, O.: Distraction rods instrumentation with posterolateral fusion in isthmic spondylolisthesis: 52 cases followed for 18–89 months. Spine 10:383–389, 1985.
42. Kettlekamp, D. B., and Wright, G. D.: Spondylolysis in the Alaskan Eskimo. J. Bone Joint Surg. 53A:563–566, 1971.
43. Lafond, G.: Surgical treatment of spondylolisthesis. Clin. Orthop. 22:175–179, 1962.
44. Lance, E. M.: Treatment of severe spondylolisthesis with neural involvement. J. Bone Joint Surg. 48A:883–891, 1966.
45. Laurent, L. E.: Spondylolisthesis. Acta Orthop. Scand. 35(suppl.):9–45, 1958.
46. Laurent, L., and Einola, S.: Spondylolisthesis in children and adolescents. Acta Orthop. Scand. 31:45–64, 1961.
47. Laurent, L. E., and Osterman, K.: Operative treatment of spondylolisthesis in young patients. Clin. Orthop. 117:85–91, 1976.
48. Lenke, L. G., Bridwell, K. H., Bullis, D., et al.: Results of in-situ fusion for isthmic spondylolisthesis. J. Spinal Disord. 5:433–442, 1992.
49. Louis, R., and Maresca, C.: Stabilization chirugicale avec reduction des spondylolyses et des spondylolisthesis. Int. Orthop. 1:215–225, 1977.
50. Louis, R.: Reconstitution isthmique des spondylolyses par plaque vissee greffes sans arthrodese. A propos de 78 cas. Rev. Chir. Orthop. 74:549–557, 1988.
51. McKee, B. W., Alexander, W. J., and Dunbar, J. S.: Spondylolysis and spondylolisthesis in children: A review. J. Can. Assoc. Radiol. 22:100–109, 1971.
52. McPhee, I. B., and O'Brien, J. D.: Reduction of severe spondylolisthesis: A preliminary report. Spine 4:430–434, 1979.
53. McQueen, M. M., Court-Brown, C. M., and Scott, J. H.: Stabilization of spondylolisthesis using Dwyer instrumentation. J. Bone Joint Surg. 68B:185–188, 1986.
54. Matthiass, H. H., and Heine, J.: The surgical reduction of spondylolisthesis. Clin. Orthop. 203:34–44, 1986.
55. Meyerding, H. W.: Spondylolisthesis: Surgical treatment and results. Surg. Gynecol. Obstet. 54:371–377, 1932.
56. Monticelli, G., and Ascani, E.: Spondylolysis and spondylolisthesis. Acta Orthop. Scand. 46:498–506, 1975.
57. Morscher, E., Gerber, B., and Fasel, J.: Surgical treatment of spondylolisthesis by bone grafting and direct stabilization of spondylolysis by means of a hook screw. Arch. Orthop. Trauma 103:175–178, 1984.
58. Nachemson, A.: Repair of the spondylolisthetic defect and intertranverse fusion for young patients. Clin. Orthop. 117:101–105, 1976.
59. Newman, P. H., and Stone, K. H.: The etiology of spondylolisthesis. J. Bone Joint Surg. 45B:39–59, 1963.
60. Nicol, R. D., and Scott, J. H.: Lytic spondylolysis repair by wiring. Spine 11:1027–1030, 1986.

61. Pavlovcic, V.: Surgical treatment of spondylolysis and spondylolisthesis with a hook screw. Int. Orthop. 18:6–9, 1994.
62. Pederson, A. K., and Hagen, R.: Spondylolysis and spondylolisthesis. Treatment by internal fixation and bone grafting of the defect. J. Bone Joint Surg. 70A:15–24, 1988.
63. Pizzutillo, P. D., Mirenda, W., and MacEwen, G. D.: Posterolateral fusion for spondylolisthesis in adolescence. J. Pediatr. Orthop. 6:311–316, 1986.
64. Poussa, M., Schlenzka, D., Seitsalo, S., et al.: Surgical treatment of severe isthmic spondylolisthesis in adolescents. Reduction or fusion in-situ. Spine 18:894–900, 1993.
65. Roca, J., Moretta, D., Fuster, S., and Roca, A.: Direct repair of spondylolysis. Clin. Orthop. 246:86–91, 1989.
66. Rombold, C.: Treatment of spondylolisthesis by postero-lateral fusion. J. Bone Joint Surg. 48A:1282–1300, 1966.
67. Salib, R. M., and Pettine, K. A.: Modified repair of a defect in spondylolysis or minimal spondylolisthesis by pedicle screw, segmental wire fixation, and bone grafting. Spine 18:440–443, 1993.
68. Scaglietti, O., Frontino, G., and Bartolozzi, P.: Technique of anatomical reduction of lumbar spondylolisthesis and its surgical stabilization. Clin. Orthop. 117:164–175, 1976.
69. Schoenecker, P. L., Cole, H. O., Herring, J. A., et al.: Cauda equina syndrome after in-situ arthrodesis for severe spondylolisthesis at the lumbosacral junction. J. Bone Joint Surg. 72A:369–377, 1990.
70. Schwend, R. M., Waters, P. M., Hey, L. A., et al.: Treatment of severe spondylolisthesis in children by reduction and L4–S4 posterior segmental hyperextension fixation. J. Pediatr. Orthop. 12:703–711, 1992.
71. Seitsalo, S.: Operative and conservative treatment of moderate spondylolisthesis in young patients. J. Bone Joint Surg. 72B:908–913, 1990.
72. Sevastikoglou, J. A., Spangfort, E., and Aaro, S.: Operative treatment of spondylolisthesis in children and adolescents with tight hamstrings syndrome. Clin. Orthop. 147:192–199, 1980.
73. Sherman, F. C., Rosenthal, R. K., and Hall, J. E.: Spine fusion for spondylolysis and spondylolisthesis in children. Spine 4:59–67, 1979.
74. Sijbrandij, S.: A new technique for the reduction and stabilization of severe spondylolisthesis. A report of nine cases. Int. Orthop. 9:247–253, 1985.
75. Simper, L. B.: Spondylolysis in Eskimo skeletons. Acta Orthop. Scand. 57:78–80, 1986
76. Snijder, J. G. N., Seroo, J. M., Snijder, C. J., and Schijvens, A. W. M.: Therapy of spondylolisthesis by repositioning and fixation of the olisthetic vertebra. Clin. Orthop. 117:149–155, 1976.
77. Steiner, M. E., and Micheli, L. J.: Treatment of symptomatic spondylolysis and spondylolisthesis with the modified Boston brace. Spine 10:937–943, 1985.
78. Stewart, T. D.: The age incidence of neural arch defects in Alaskan natives considered from the standpoint of etiology. J. Bone Joint Surg. 35A:937–950, 1953.
79. Turner, R. H., and Bianco, A. J., Jr.: Spondylolysis and spondylolisthesis in children and teenagers. J. Bone Joint Surg. 53A:1298–1306, 1971.
80. van Rens, J. G., and van Horn, J. R.: Long-term results in lumbosacral interbody fusion for spondylolisthesis. Acta Orthop. Scand. 53:383–392, 1982.
81. Ver der Werf, G. J. I. M., Tonino, A. J., and Zeggers, W. S.: Direct repair of lumbar spondylolisthesis. Acta Orthop. Scand. 56:378–379, 1985.
82. Verbiest, H.: The treatment of lumbar spondyloptosis or impending lumbar spondyloptosis accompanied by neurologic deficit and/or neurogenic intermittent claudication. Spine 4:68–77, 1979.
83. Wertzberger, K. L., and Peterson, H. A.: Acquired spondylolysis and spondylolisthesis in the young child. Spine 5:437–440, 1980.
84. Wiltse, L. L.: Spondylolisthesis in children. Clin. Orthop. 21:156–163, 1961.
85. Wiltse, L. L., and Hutchison, R.: Surgical treatment of spondylolisthesis. Clin. Orthop. 35:116–135, 1964.
86. Wiltse, L. L., Widell, E. H., Jr., and Jackson, D. W.: Fatigue fractures: The basic lesion in isthmic spondylolisthesis. J. Bone Joint Surg. 57A:17–22, 1975
87. Wiltse, L. L., and Jackson, D. W.: Treatment of spondylolisthesis and spondylolysis in children. Clin. Orthop. 117:92–100, 1976.
88. Wiltse, L. L., Newman, P. H., and Macnab, I.: Classification of spondylolysis and spondylolisthesis. Clin. Orthop. 117:23–29, 1976.
89. Winter, M., and Jani, C.: Results of screw osteosynthesis in spondylolysis and low-grade spondylolisthesis. Arch. Orthop. Trauma 108:96–99, 1989.

Surgical Treatment of Isthmic and Dysplastic Spondylolisthesis in the Adult

■

DAVID S. BRADFORD

Isthmic and dysplastic spondylolisthesis are frequently thought of as problems of the juvenile or adolescent patient. However, as a better understanding of the natural history of spondylolisthesis has evolved, it has become increasingly apparent that previously untreated patients may present in the adult period with symptomatic spondylolisthesis unresponsive to conservative management. Furthermore, patients for whom previous surgery, with or without instrumentation, failed may require salvage reconstruction in adulthood.

Saraste[49] followed untreated patients with spondylolisthesis into adulthood and noticed a striking frequency of symptoms. Of 255 patients followed for a mean of 53 years, 18% presented with neurologic deficits, one with paralysis, 91% with low back pain, 55% with sciatica, and 5% with slip progression. Harris and Weinstein[23] also found that, in a series of untreated patients with high-grade slips, 45% avoided heavy lifting, 36% believed their spinal deformity had influenced their job choice, and half of the patients had recurrent back symptoms; one was totally disabled. Other investigators have documented neurologic claudication and autoamputation of the S1 nerve root in severe spondylolisthesis.[21] Magnetic resonance imaging (MRI) studies have suggested that disc degeneration at the space above the defect is more likely among adults who have had spondylolisthesis than among the general population.[25]

In Saraste's[49] study, adults with spondylolisthesis were more likely to have symptoms if the slippage exceeded 25% and if the patients had a low lumbar index at L5 or if there was early disc degeneration. Defects at L4 had a much more guarded prognosis than defects at L5. Progression of the slippage is unusual in adulthood. Fredrickson and associates[16] conducted a prospective study and concluded that progression of spondylolisthesis is unlikely after adolescence. Several researchers have suggested that late progression may result from degeneration of the caudad disc.[46, 49] Progression does occur in adults who have undergone extensive laminectomy without fusion, especially if they have had a discectomy with a laminectomy.[15]

PATHOGENESIS AND ETIOLOGY

The incidence of spondylolisthesis in adult Caucasians is reported as 5% to 6% in men and 2% to 3% in women.[4, 48] The incidence appears to vary by race from as low as 3% in blacks to as high as 50% in Inuit.[34, 48, 55, 58] Numerous theories have been advanced regarding the etiology. A congenital predisposition seems to be the most likely explanation for type I, or dysplastic, spondylolisthesis. Type II, or isthmic, spondylolisthesis is thought to be the result of repetitive trauma (e.g., a fatigue fracture of the pars interarticularis). It is known that persons with lumbar hyperlordosis (e.g., gymnasts, new military recruits, weight lifters, football linemen, dancers, and competitive young athletes) have an increased incidence of isthmic spondylolisthesis. Thus, isthmic spondylolisthesis probably represents a stress or fatigue fracture of the pars interarticularis caused by repetitive microtrauma.[36, 44, 48, 62, 63]

Biomechanical evidence for the stress fracture theory is provided by polarized light stress analysis of the lumbar spine.[50] These studies show that the greatest stress concentration is at the level of the pars. Patients with increased lumbar lordosis and thoracic hyperkyphosis would be expected to have a greater stress placed on the pars interarticularis at L5, and they also have a higher incidence of spondylolisthesis.[45]

After a pars fracture or repetitive microtrauma with abortive attempts at repair of the pars, fibrocartilaginous callus develops to bridge the defect in the pars. This callus may become markedly hypertrophic and may extend anteriorly to impinge on the inferior aspect of the pedicle and the exiting nerve root.[1] Depending on the duration of the lysis, there may be marked osteophytic changes on the superior facet of the next caudal vertebra. In adults, secondary bony changes take place with further narrowing of the intervertebral disc from degeneration with a large uncinate spur formation of the posterior body of L5, further narrowing the intervertebral foramen. Furthermore, at the level of L5–S1, the dural sac may be tented across the posterior-superior margin of the S1 vertebral body, particularly with high-grade slips, and this, coupled with some posterior extrusion of the L5-S1 disc, may result in an impending or frank cauda equina syndrome.[34, 40, 57] Evidence from MRI scanning suggests an increased rate of disc degeneration at the level of the slippage.[25] As mentioned, the cumulative effects of these changes produce mild to moderate lateral, foraminal, and even central canal stenosis. This degenerative process can be ongoing and thus account for the symptoms of spondylolisthesis, even if low-grade slippage occurs after the patient is skeletally mature.

Complicating the local anatomic changes that produce symptoms of back and radicular pain are mechanical changes that take place proximally and distal to the spondylolisthesis. Higher grades of spondylolisthesis can alter the sagittal spinal alignment and shift the body's center of gravity anteriorly.[4, 7, 58] Flexion and shear forces occurring at the level of the deformity may lead to progression. In adults, compensatory hyperlordosis develops above the level of the lumbosacral kyphos in an attempt to balance the spine in the sagittal plane. Occasionally, hyperlordosis may extend from the lumbar spine into the upper thoracic spine, creating a kyphos at the cervical thoracic junction. Furthermore, with increased slippage, the segmental kyphosis at the lumbosacral joint is exacerbated. Consequently, the pelvis becomes retroverted and the sacrum attains a vertical orientation. With this pelvic malrotation, the hip and the femur undergo obligate rotation until the knee joint cannot be placed beneath the trunk unless the patient bends markedly forward. The patient then must flex the knees and hyperextend the spine further to stand. This position is fatiguing and disabling, leads to chronic back pain, and is associated with symptomatic spinal stenosis. This severe lumbosacral kyphosis is the most disabling aspect of spondylolisthesis. If a patient is unable to obtain normal sagittal balance, the kyphos must be addressed.

PATIENT EVALUATION

Evaluation of the patient with spondylolisthesis is similar to the evaluation of any patient with an orthopedic or neurosurgical spinal disorder. Not only is thorough assessment of the musculoskeletal system and evaluation of posture, gait, and truncal balance important, but a complete and thorough motor-sensory and reflex examination must also be carried out. Patients should be queried about any symptoms of a neurologic compromise, as well as any evidence of bowel or bladder dysfunction. The incidence of neurologic abnormality in adults is high. Saraste[49] found an incidence of 18%, and Harris and Weinstein[23] reported an incidence of 45%. Rarely, the patient may present with subtle cauda equina dysfunction or even a cauda equina syndrome. Under these circumstances, a rectal examination and urodynamic studies should be carried out. Patients presenting with spondylolisthesis may also have associated scoliosis secondary to olisthesis at the slippage site or an idiopathic curvature above the spondylolisthesis.[7, 24, 37, 40]

Imaging with plain radiographs is helpful not only in the standing anteroposterior and lateral planes but also in the oblique plane. Whereas spondylolisthesis is obvious on x-ray studies, diagnosis of spondylolysis can be more elusive. On the anteroposterior x-ray film, asymmetry of the neural arch, unilateral wedging of the vertebral body, and sclerosis of the contralateral pars all suggest the diagnosis. Oblique x-ray films usually demonstrate a pars defect; however,

20% of patients have only a unilateral defect.[36, 44, 47, 58]

Computed tomographic (CT) scanning is most helpful in ruling out spondylolysis. A bone scan or a single-photon emission computed tomographic (SPECT) bone scan is helpful in identifying a local area that may be evaluated further with a CT scan. In the presence of any neurologic deficit or suggestion of cauda equina compression, an MRI scan is the most helpful study (Fig. 1). Often, a better delineation of the neural canal, the dural sac, and the surrounding bony elements is possible with a CT-myelographic scan. Myelography alone is not a useful study. Lateral tomography may be useful in the presence of high-grade slips to determine whether spontaneous interbody fusion has formed. Sagittal reconstructed CT scans may give similar information.

An accurate description and reproducible evaluation of the spinal deformity demands a standard measurement technique. Although no technique is entirely satisfactory, standing lateral x-ray films of the spine should always be used for these measurements. The author routinely calculates the percentage of slippage as well as the lumbosacral kyphosis (slip angle).[7, 56] Additional measurements, such as sagittal rotation and sacral inclination, are also helpful when one attempts to follow the natural history of a high-grade slip.[7]

TREATMENT OF SPONDYLOLISTHESIS

Conservative Management

Nonoperative treatment of spondylolisthesis is reviewed elsewhere in this volume. The cornerstone of treatment at the author's institution consists of activity and lifestyle modification, administration of nonsteroidal antiinflammatory medication, a well-supervised physical therapy program, and occasionally, the use of temporary bracing (a flexion-molded thoracolumbosacral orthosis [TLSO]). Occasionally, epidural blocks, facet joint blocks, and injections into the fractured pars interarticularis provide temporary relief. Supervised physical therapy is a mainstay of nonoperative treatment and may help the patient to avoid surgery. This is particularly true when patients have pain in the absence of a neurologic deficit.

Operative Treatment

Adult patients with spondylolisthesis are candidates for surgery if they have continued severe, disabling, low back pain despite conservative management, if they present with symptoms of stenosis or radiculopathy, if they have neurologic deficits or cauda equina symptoms, or if they are unable to stand or walk because of severe sagittal plane imbalance.[7, 24, 37, 63] Furthermore, patients with L1 to L4 spondylolysis or spondylolisthesis generally have a poor prognosis. Continued back pain, in spite of nonoperative modalities, is common in these patients, and at the author's institution surgery is aggressively pursued after failure of an initial course of conservative treatment.[7]

The surgical management of adults with spondylolysis and spondylolisthesis consists of spinal fusion and decompression.

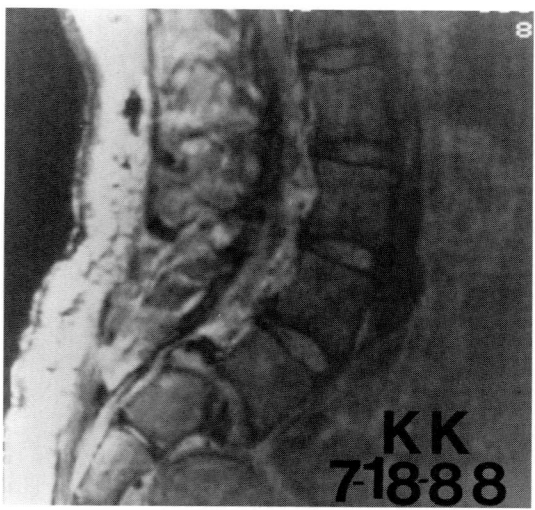

Figure 1. This sagittal MRI scan shows the sizeable posterior disc bulge that can develop at the caudad disc space in spondylolisthesis. In this young woman with a grade II spondylolisthesis of L5 on S1, the combination of sagittal deformity and disc bulge contributed to compression of the cauda equina. She was asymptomatic preoperatively, and underwent a bilateral lateral fusion. Cauda equina syndrome developed postoperatively. Partial reduction had occurred spontaneously under anesthesia. Emergency decompression with fixation was then carried out. She subsequently had total return of neurologic function. Orthopedists should remain aware that soft tissue changes may be far more dramatic than the bony changes in spondylolisthesis.

Decompression is usually required as part of the procedure in the adult population. Decompression alone is less likely to produce as satisfactory an outcome as decompression with fusion.[15, 20]

Decompression

Total laminectomy, removal of the loose posterior arch, does not adequately decompress the neuroforamen. Indeed, if the patient presents with radicular pain, with or without a neurologic deficit, and there is evidence of nerve root compression in the foramen, adequate decompression necessitates removal of the attenuated pars interarticularis and residual callus down to the base of the pedicle. Merely taking off the posterior arch may leave portions of fibrous cartilaginous material as well as an osteophytic ridge on the pedicle that compresses the nerve root. At times, to furnish adequate decompression, it may even be necessary to remove the medial inferior portion of the pedicle as well as the transverse process. In patients with high-grade slippage and cauda equina compression, removal of the dome of the sacrum anterior to the dural sac may be necessary to relieve compression of the cauda equina. Furthermore, the fifth root may be compressed laterally by the bulge of the sacral dome, and removing the disc and edge of the dome laterally facilitates decompression. Although decompression alone has been advocated by some investigators as providing adequate treatment,[26] it has been the author's experience that optimum results are achieved with the addition of spinal fusion. In fact, further slippage may occur even in adults after laminectomy.[15, 52]

It is particularly significant that in patients who have a mild degenerative lumbar scoliosis in association with spondylolisthesis, decompression may lead to progressive scoliosis deformity. This is best avoided by fusion in association with decompression (Fig. 2).

Spinal Fusion

The gold standard for surgical treatment of spondylolisthesis is lumbosacral fusion.[32, 45] For optimum results, the fusion is usually carried out posterolaterally; if it is associated with a decompression, the posterolateral procedure should be done through a midline incision. If decompression is thought to be unnecessary, the procedure may be performed through bilateral muscle-splitting incisions. The optimum bone graft is autologous material from the patient's iliac crest. Postoperative immobilization is controversial. There is little evidence to suggest that, in the absence of a reduction procedure, immobilization in a brace is preferable to the use of a lumbosacral corset or no immobilization at all. In general, if reduction has been carried out, the author prefers a rigid TLSO incorporating one thigh in extension for 3 to 4 months, depending on the radiographic quality of the fusion. There is some evidence that cigarette smoking and the use of antiinflammatory medications impede bone healing, and patients are encouraged to avoid these in the postoperative period.

Repair of the Spondylolysis Defect

Repair of spondylolysis and spondylolisthesis has been proposed by Kimura,[35] Buck,[11] Bradford and colleagues,[8–10] Morscher and associates,[43] and Jeanneret.[30] In general, the technique is best applied for defects from L1 to L4 as well as in younger, skeletally immature patients. However, Jeanneret[30] noted that adults are likely to achieve relief of their symptoms, provided the intervertebral disc is normal on the MRI scan and the slippage is not too great (<25%). In older patients (older than 20 years of age) in whom surgical repair of the defect is contemplated, it is essential to decompress the neuroforamen adequately at the time of defect repair. Repair of the defect narrows the neuroforamen, thus leading to greater nerve root compression, if decompression is not carried out.[9]

Posterior Fusion In Situ

Fusion in situ is the most commonly performed surgery for treating spondylolisthesis. This is true for the child as well as for the adult. Traditionally, fusion levels have been chosen according to the amount of translational displacement of the spondylolisthesis.[42] That is, for Meyerding classifications of grade I and grade II (25% to 50%), fusion over one motion segment is believed to be sufficient. For slippage greater than 50% (Meyerding grades III and IV), it has

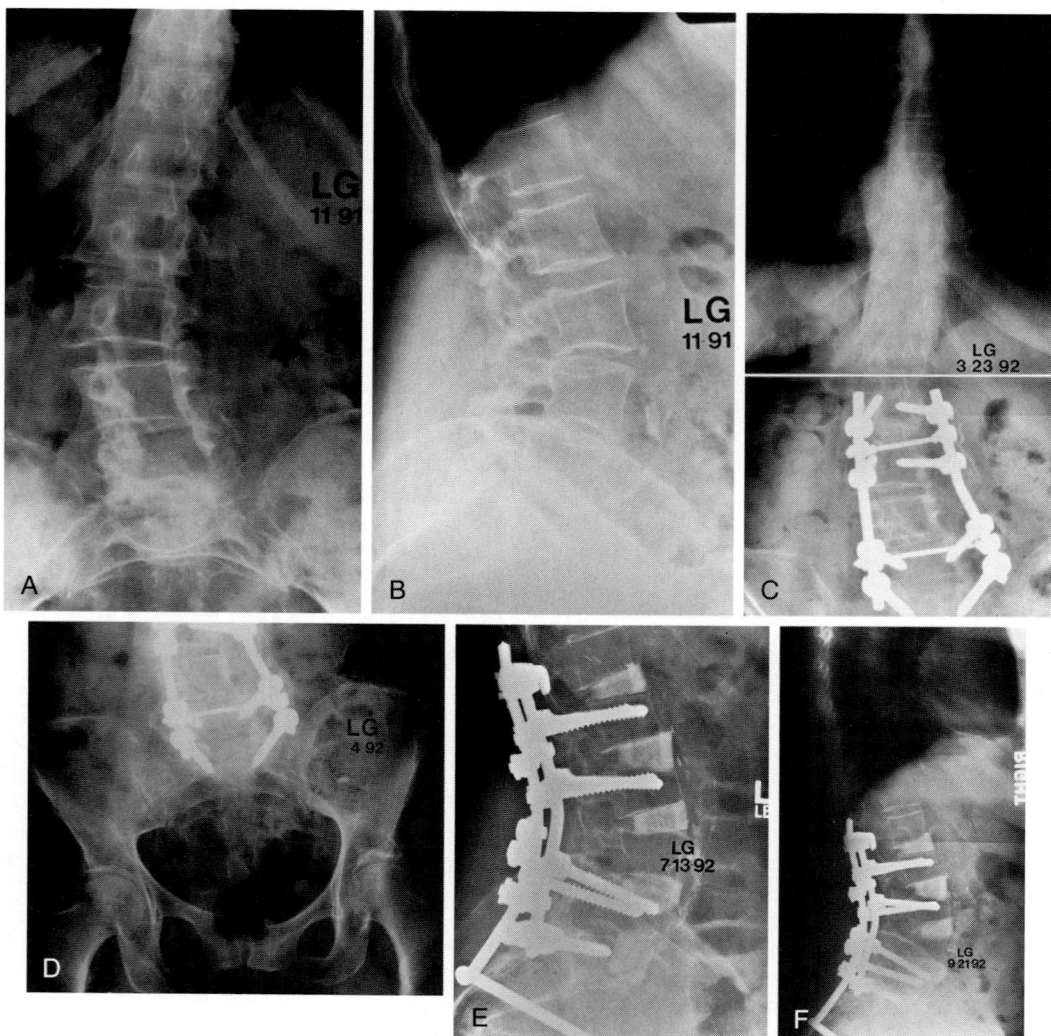

Figure 2. A 74-year-old woman with known degenerative spondylolisthesis (*A, B*) underwent wide decompressive laminectomy. Over the ensuing 6 months, increasing back and groin pain developed, accompanied by an obvious lumbar spine deformity. This case illustrates a phenomenon that should be more widely recognized. Subsequent to wide decompression for degenerative spondylolisthesis, patients may develop a pars fracture causing iatrogenic scoliosis. This patient initially underwent fusion posteriorly from L2 to S1 and had screw loosening and pain (*C, D*). She required revision anterior-posterior instrumentation from L2 to the ilium, using both a transpedicular and Galveston rod technique (*E*). After this final surgery, fusion was successful, and the patient resumed normal activities (*F*).

generally been proposed that the fusion should extend up to the L4 vertebra and down to the sacrum for a spondylolisthesis at L5. This may not always be necessary, and the extent of fusion depends not only on the presence or absence of lumbosacral kyphosis but also on the use of an implant posteriorly.

Surgery for posterior fusions in situ may be performed through either a midline skin incision or bilateral skin incisions for a bilateral lateral approach. The author generally prefers a single midline incision even for bilateral lateral approaches because the cosmetic result is superior. A transverse incision is not desirable. Great care should be taken to denude carefully and to decorticate the transverse processes, the ala, and the facet joints.[27] In the presence of moderate degrees of slippage (i.e., <50%), it is desirable to bridge cancellous bone grafts just ventral to the transverse process of L5 to small slots cut into the sacrum. This prevents postoperative graft dislodgment and furnishes a satisfactory base for additional bone grafts. With higher degrees of slip (>50%), this technique is less desirable because nerve root compression of L5 may occur if grafts are placed anterior or ventral to the transverse process of L5 (Fig. 3). The rate of successful fusion is reported to range from 70% to 90% and may depend on the magnitude of the slippage and the associated decompression procedure, the use of spinal implants, the use of primary versus salvage procedures, the presence of infection, or history of smoking.* Patients who are obese are at risk for incomplete fusions and unsuccessful outcomes.[3] Immediate postoperative cauda equina syndrome has been described in patients who have undergone posterior fusion in situ.[55]

Instrumentation

Instrumentation for managing spondylolisthesis has proved extremely useful, and in the author's experience, is an appropriate form of treatment, particularly in adult patients. Transpedicular fixation devices are biomechanically superior to traditional instrumentation. They provide not only rigid fixation[6, 14, 54] but also enhanced fusion rates and outcomes.[41, 64] In a study by Zdeblick,[64] 124 patients (56 with spondylolisthesis) undergoing lumbar fusion were treated by fusion, fusion with semirigid instrumentation, or fusion with rigid internal fixation. Radiographs of the patients with isthmic spondylolisthesis showed a successful fusion rate of 80% for those without instrumentation, 89% for those with semirigid instrumentation, and 100% for those with rigid instrumentation.

At the author's center, transpedicular instrumentation is preferred when performing posterior spinal fusion in adult patients with spondylolisthesis. In patients with lumbosacral kyphosis, for whom reduction is not indicated, placement of an S1 pedicle screw across the vertebral end plate and into the body of L5 has provided optimum distal fixation. Routine indications for combined anterior and posterior fusion in this group of patients cannot yet be identified. The current literature does not support routine use of combined anterior and posterior surgery in the management of patients with spondylolisthesis. Consequently, the author favors posterior spinal fusion with transpedicular fixation (with or without decompression, depending on the patient's symptoms, physical examination findings, and radiographic images) followed by anterior fusion at a later date if delayed union or nonunion occurs. A combined approach is considered in patients who have had multiple operations and who have large laminectomy defects or pseudarthroses or in patients who have high-grade slips (>75%) in whom reduction is not planned. The anterior strut graft can be accomplished through either a posterior interbody approach or a transperitoneal or retroperitoneal approach using a fibula strut graft (see below).

Anterior Fusions In Situ

Anterior fusion was first suggested for spondylolisthesis by Capener[13] in 1932. In 1933, Burns[12] performed the first anterior operation through a transperitoneal approach. Freebody and associates[17] in 1971 reported that 252 patients underwent arthrodesis by a transperitoneal approach; 84% achieved solid fusion and 92% were believed to have good or excellent clinical outcomes. van Rens and van Horn[60] (1982) also reported good outcomes from anterior interbody fusion: 21 of 24 patients had pain relief and one had a pseudarthrosis.

The anterior interbody fusion may be obtained from either a posterior approach or an anterior approach. The anterior approach was popularized by Verbiest,[61] who used a fibular graft placed from L4 to the sacrum through the body of L5. This technique has been most useful for spondylolisthesis. The posterior interbody approach as reported by Bohlman and Cook[5] relies on a fibular strut graft placed from the sacrum posteriorly at the S1–S2 level into the body of L5 after L5–S1 laminectomy. The techniques used by Verbiest[61] and Bohlman and Cook[5] are best applied to high-grade slips with significant lumbosacral kyphosis.

For high-grade slippage in which reduction is not indicated but stabilization is essential, the Bohlman technique can be coupled with internal fixation and a bilateral lateral fusion. The author recommends the use of either fibular autograft or fresh frozen

---

*References 7, 9, 18, 24, 32, 37, 47, and 50.

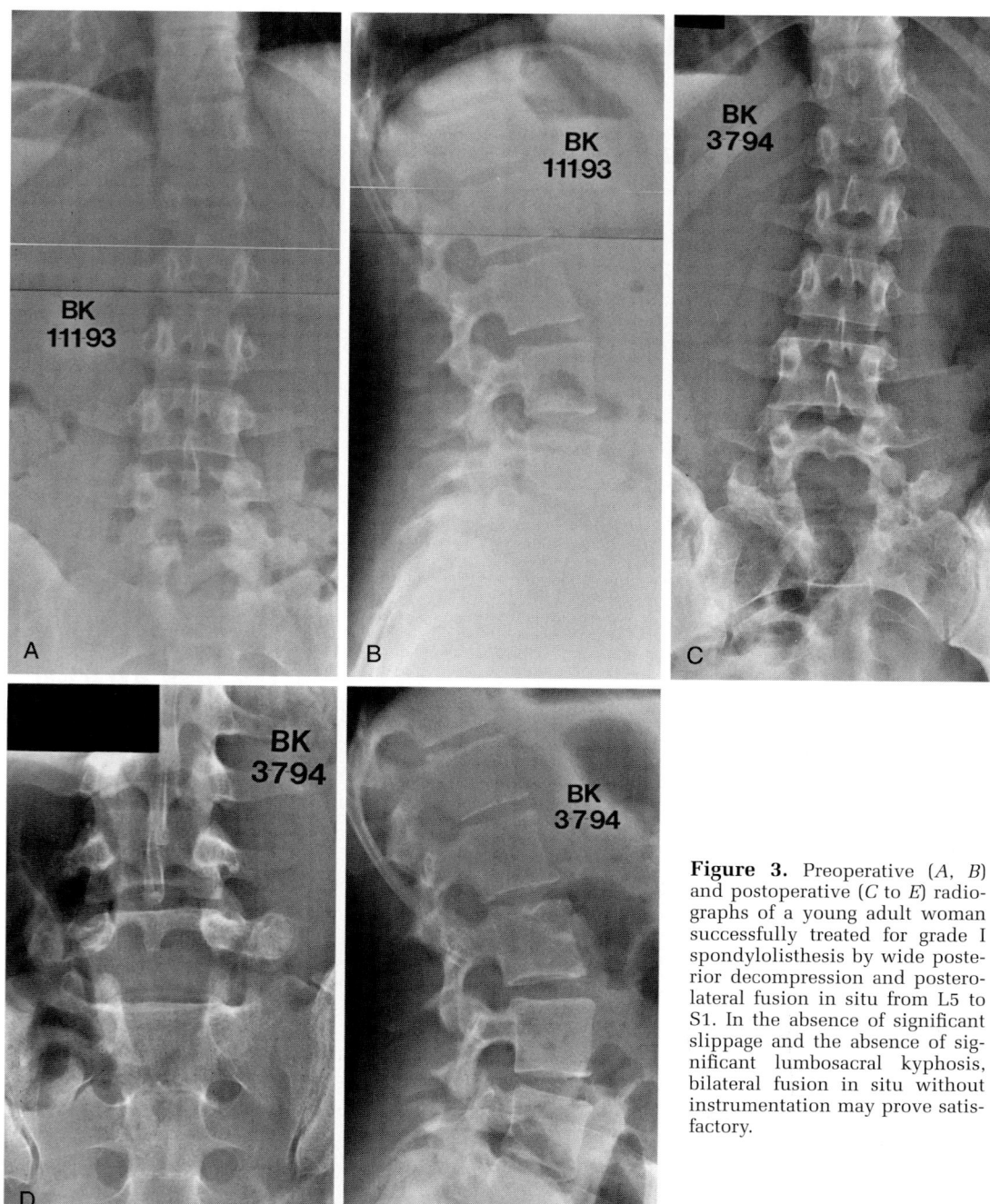

Figure 3. Preoperative (*A*, *B*) and postoperative (*C* to *E*) radiographs of a young adult woman successfully treated for grade I spondylolisthesis by wide posterior decompression and posterolateral fusion in situ from L5 to S1. In the absence of significant slippage and the absence of significant lumbosacral kyphosis, bilateral fusion in situ without instrumentation may prove satisfactory.

fibula because the fatigue characteristics are superior to those of freeze-dried bone. During anterior surgery, care must be taken to avoid damage to the presacral sympathetic nerves, which may result in retrograde ejaculation in men[33] (Fig. 4).

Reduction of Spondylolisthesis

Reduction of spondylolisthesis was first described by Jenkins[31] in 1936. Because of technical difficulties, poor results, and neurologic complications, interest in these techniques and procedures lagged until recent years. Fusions in situ have reported rates of nonunions ranging up to 44% in some series, along with progression of the slip, even in adult patients. Furthermore, fusion in situ does not alter sagittal plane imbalance and deformity. These findings have provided a stimulus for surgeons searching for improved alternative techniques.

The question of whether to reduce spondylolisthesis is difficult. The goals of any treatment should be (1) to prevent progression, (2) to relieve pain, (3) to reverse neurologic deficit, and (4) to improve function. Correction of spondylolisthesis is indicated only if it promotes these goals. The primary indication for reduction is a high-grade slip (>grade III or IV) that is associated with extreme degrees of kyphosis and that leads to loss of sagittal plane balance. These patients are unable to stand fully upright with their knees and hips extended. Furthermore, they often present with spinal stenosis and neurologic compromise that requires decompression. Reduction restores sagittal plane balance and mechanically improves the possibility of achieving a solid fusion. The chance of fusion is improved because the fusion mass is under compression forces rather than tensile forces, which arise from residual lumbosacral kyphosis. If reduction is contemplated, it appears to be more logical to perform it in adults younger than 35 years of age, although there are no supporting data. Advanced age with consequent osteopenia and disc degeneration appears to place older patients at greater jeopardy than younger patients for implant failure and neurologic dysfunction after reduction.

Current methods of obtaining reduction in adult spondylolisthesis fall into three broad

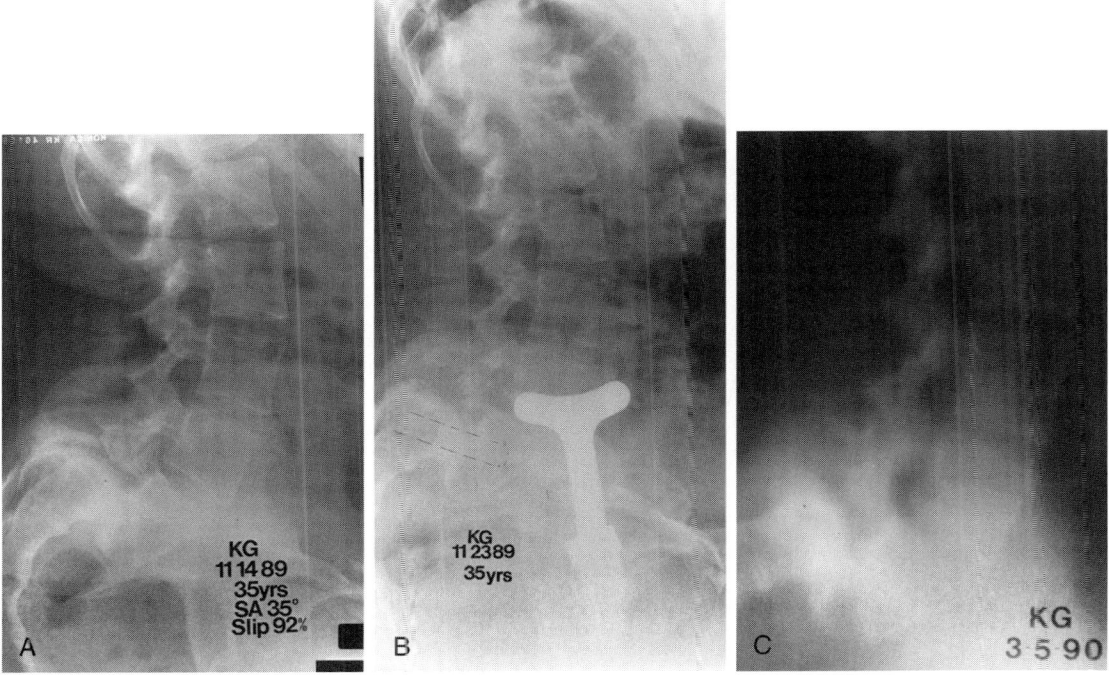

Figure 4. A 35-year-old woman had a grade IV spondylolisthesis and reported intractable back pain (A). Her sagittal balance was remarkably good. She reported excellent symptom relief after posterior decompression and posterolateral fusion in situ combined with anterior interbody fusion achieved by a fibular graft placed through the posterior approach (B, C).

categories: posterior instrumented approaches, combined anterior and posterior approaches, and vertebral body resections. For all three techniques, the utmost vigilance is required to prevent neurologic injury. The author conducts numerous wake-up tests during a reduction. Somatosensory evoked potentials may also be desirable to obtain. These measures notwithstanding, only surgeons with extensive training and experience in complex spine surgery should attempt these procedures and should do so only after obtaining hands-on experience.

POSTERIOR REDUCTION TECHNIQUES

Spondylolisthesis reduction performed by a posterior approach is the most frequently used technique. One advantage of this procedure is that it can be completed in a single stage. The author considers this procedure to be indicated in patients with slips greater than 50% or lumbosacral kyphosis greater than 45 degrees who have intractable back pain or sciatica.[28, 39] Thorough decompression before reduction is critical. The author recommends performing a laminectomy of L5 with extensive bilateral foraminotomy of L5 and a resection of the sacral dome for all patients. As with any spinal kyphosis, distraction instrumentation is contraindicated. It may be used temporarily to facilitate decompression and reduction, but it must be converted to an alternative construct before completion of surgery, with certainty that lumbar lordosis is maintained. Transpedicular instrumentation is the implant of choice. Obtaining adequate fixation at the lumbosacral junction may be problematic, and fixation to the ilium may be necessary to prevent implant failure. Neurologic monitoring is essential during the procedure and is best carried out with multiple wake-up tests, and/or somatosensory evoked potentials. Anatomic reduction, however, is not essential, and must be avoided if neurologic changes are noted either by somatosensory evoked potentials or wake-up test findings. Correction of kyphosis is more important than correction of translation. Residual translation (>50% to 75%) may require a second-stage anterior procedure with strut grafting to stabilize partial reduction.

Several researchers have reported their results with posterior reduction techniques.[2, 6, 39, 53, 54] Admundson and colleagues[2] cited a report by Edwards and associates on a series of 180 cases from the Spinal Fixation Study Group. Their population included patients of varying ages and varying degrees of slippage. Posterior instrumented reduction achieved a 90% correction and a successful fusion rate of 88% in this study. The reduction was complicated by radiculopathy in 3% of patients.

Steffee and associates[53, 54] reported their experience with reduction and fusion for spondylolisthesis in 1988 and again in 1993. In the initial report in 1988, Steffee and Sitkowski[53] followed 14 patients with grade III and grade IV spondylolisthesis who underwent posterior instrumented reduction. Complete reduction was achieved in all cases. The initial three patients underwent bilateral lateral fusion after reduction. All three of these patients eventually had recurrent deformity and required anterior fusion. After this initial experience, the remaining patients underwent fusion both posteriorly and anteriorly. In this series, three patients had hardware failure and one patient had a severe sciatica postoperatively, which eventually resolved.[53]

In 1993, Steffee and Brantigan[54] published a large follow-up study of patients undergoing posterior spinal fusion with the variable screw placement spinal fixation system. In this report of 250 patients, 51 patients from an original cohort of 57 patients with spondylolisthesis were available for evaluation. A clinical outcome scale with scoring systems for pain and functional capacity was used to evaluate results. Clinical success was obtained in 86% of patients with spondylolisthesis, and fusion success was obtained in 92%. More specifically, the preoperative clinical score was good or excellent for 7 of 51 patients with spondylolisthesis, and the postoperative score was good or excellent for 42 of 51 patients. Unfortunately, the complications reported in this surgical study were not divided according to the cause of the spinal disorder.[54]

Basic biomechanical research studies of instrumentation systems have shown improved fatigue life in rod-based systems as compared with plate-based systems. Consequently, the author has abandoned the use of screw-plate instrumentation systems in favor of screw-rod systems.[14]

Boos and colleagues[6] reported a series of

10 patients with grade III and grade IV spondylolisthesis who underwent instrumented posterior surgical reduction. The average follow-up was 56 months. Mean preoperative slip was 79%, which was reduced to 40% postoperatively. The slippage angle was a mean of 43 degrees preoperatively, which was reduced to 17 degrees postoperatively. Eighty-three percent of patients who underwent bilateral lateral posterior fusion alone had implant failure and a subsequent diagnosis of pseudarthrosis. Boos and colleagues[6] recommended anterior and posterior spinal arthrodesis when spondylolisthesis reduction is undertaken. Additionally, 2 of 10 patients had postoperative footdrop that resolved in both cases.

Hu and associates[28] reported on 16 patients with grade III or greater spondylolisthesis who underwent instrumented posterior reduction utilizing the Edwards rods (Scientific Spinal Limited). The average patient age in this study was 20 years. Four of the 16 patients had concomitant anterior spinal fusion. Reduction maneuvers were successful. Mean preoperative slippage of 89% was reduced to 38%, and mean preoperative slip angle of 56 degrees was reduced to 28 degrees. Three patients demonstrated neurologic complications. Two patients demonstrated postoperative footdrops. One case completely resolved, and one partially resolved. A third patient demonstrated lumbar plexus palsy, which reduced after revision surgery, which allowed some loss of correction. The postoperative clinical result was considered excellent in 10 cases, good in five cases, and fair in one case (Figs. 5 and 6).

What is apparent in these reports is that reduction is possible. It is best carried out slowly. Rod-screw combinations are preferable to plate-screw constructs. Although neurologic complications occur, they usually resolve.

COMBINED ANTERIOR AND POSTERIOR REDUCTION

Differences of opinion exist among recognized experts in spine surgery regarding the appropriate role for combined anterior-posterior surgery in the reduction of spondylolisthesis. Although the author believes that bilateral lateral fusion alone is sufficient if an appropriate reduction of the sagittal alignment is achieved, other researchers disagree The studies reported by Steffee and Sitkowski[53] and Boos and coworkers[6] suggest that fusion rates and maintenance of long-term correction of deformity are improved after posterior reduction and fusion supplemented by anterior fusion These results may, in part, be indicative of the type of implant used (plate-screw).

In patients undergoing their first surgical procedure for the correction of spondylolisthesis, the author recommends combining anterior spinal fusion with posterior spinal fusion only if reduction of the spondylolisthesis is incomplete. This means failure to reduce the slipped vertebra to less than 75% slippage or the presence of residual lumbosacral kyphosis. In this situation, the placement of an anterior fibular graft from L5 to the sacrum is advocated to augment the previous posterior instrumented fusion.

The value of combined anterior and posterior reconstruction in spondylolisthesis has been clearly demonstrated for patients undergoing revision surgery. In a series of 16 patients undergoing revision surgery by the authors,[10] the preoperative slippage of 98% and slippage angle of 74 degrees were corrected to 56% and 11 degrees, respectively. In eight patients in this revision series, postoperative neuropathy developed; it resolved completely in five and partially in one. All patients had relief of pain and correction of deformity (Fig. 7).

Another technique for the reduction of spondylolisthesis is that reported by Harms and associates.[22] Their technique involves an initial posterior decompression with placement of transpedicular instrumentation. Distraction force is then applied from the third lumbar vertebral body to the sacrum using Harrington instrumentation. Simultaneously, a surgeon applies a posterior correction force to the cephalad vertebra. The transpedicular screws are joined to rods and the Harrington rod is removed. After closure, the patient undergoes an anterior approach to the spine and L5–S1 interbody fusion using autogenous bone graft. No posterior fusion is employed. In detailing their technique, Harms and coworkers[22] reported on a series of 230 patients with spondylolisthesis who were treated with this reduction maneuver. One hundred sixty-three of these patients had isthmic and dysplastic spondylolisthesis. Follow-up at 1 year was

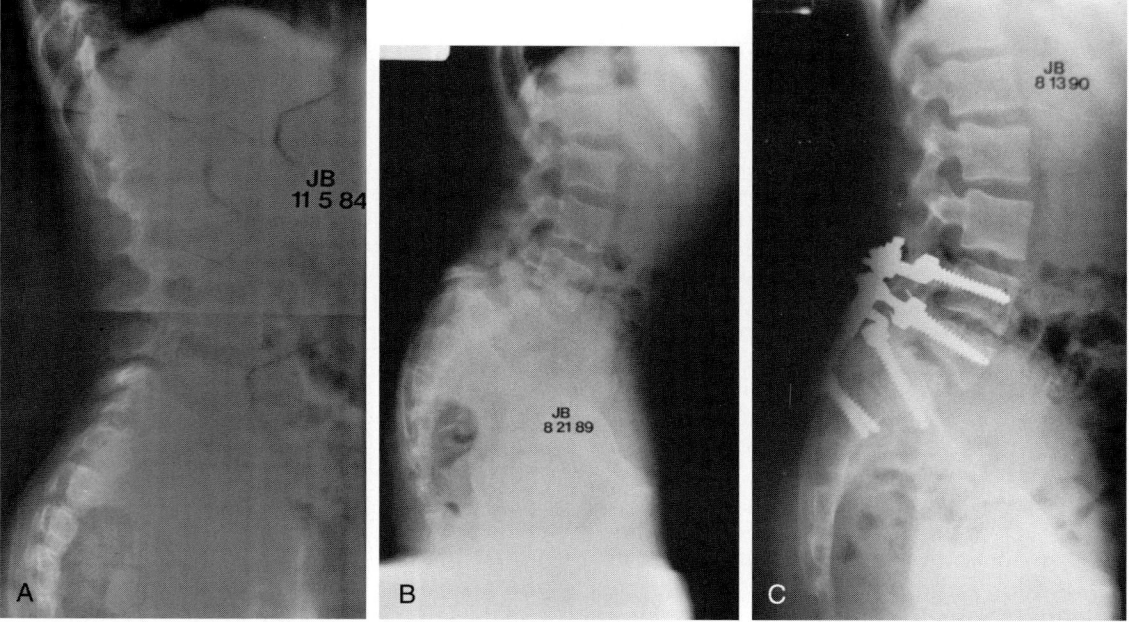

Figure 5. A 30-year-old man presented with symptomatic grade IV spondylolisthesis and significant sagittal plane decompensation (*A*, *B*). Excellent symptom relief and restoration of sagittal balance were accomplished via a posterior instrumented reduction and fusion of the spondylolisthesis utilizing Edwards rods (Scientific Spinal Limited) (*C*).

available for 180 patients from the entire series. Of these 180 patients, there were two with pseudarthroses, one with deep wound infection, five with deep venous thromboses, and none with neurologic complications.

VERTEBRAL BODY RESECTION

Several investigators have suggested that reduction of spondyloptosis might be facilitated by resection of the L5 vertebral body.[19, 38] They postulated that this results in shortening of the spinal column. Theoretically, this enhances the surgeon's ability to reconstruct the normal sagittal alignment and decreases the chance of neurologic complication from stretching of the neural elements. The author believes that resection is better described as a translational procedure for spinal reconstruction. Although the spine is shortened by resection in patients with a portion of L5 remaining superior to the S1 end plate, the spine maintains the same length or is actually lengthened during resection-reduction in cases in which the L5 body rests anterior to and inferior to S1. Additionally, the interposition of bone or a device anteriorly after resection may lengthen the spinal column, thus putting neurologic function at risk.

The technique of L5 vertebrectomy and reduction of L4 onto the sacrum has been reported by Gaines and Nichols[19] and by Huizenga.[29] Gaines and Nichols[19] reported on two patients who underwent L5 vertebral resection for spondyloptosis and instrumented reduction of L4 onto the sacrum. One patient had a delayed union; however, there were no neurologic complications. Lehmer and colleagues[38] reported the results of this technique in 16 patients. All underwent staged L5 vertebral body resection followed by posterior instrumented reduction and fusion of L4 to the sacrum. In this series, all 16 patients achieved a solid arthrodesis, although three patients required regrafting for delayed union and another patient had hardware failure with loss of reduction that required revision surgery. Average preoperative sagittal rotation of 48 degrees and sacral inclination of 26 degrees improved to −5 degrees and 39 degrees, respectively. Mean postoperative slippage of L4 on S1 was 11%. A subjective patient outcome questionnaire showed that postop-

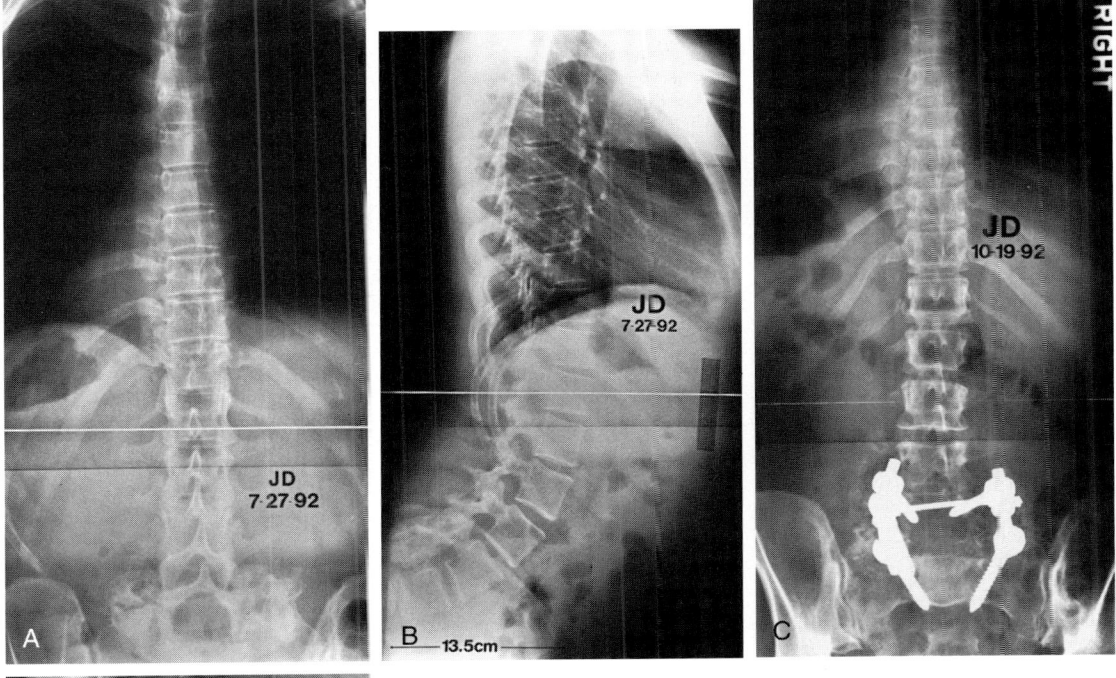

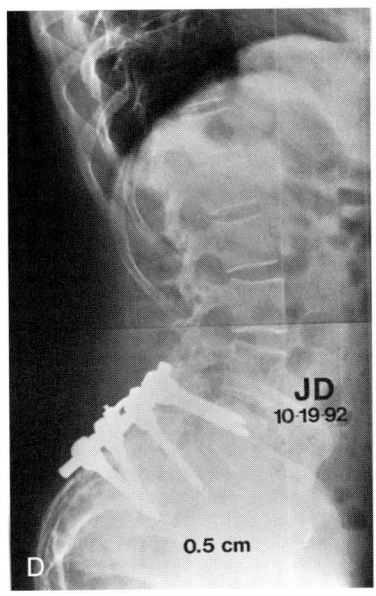

Figure 6. A 30-year-old woman had previously undergone posterior fusion in situ from L4 to S1 for grade II spondylolisthesis. Postoperatively, the patient had increasing low back pain with radiation to the buttocks. Additionally, she had difficulty with ambulation because of sagittal decompensation. X-ray films at her initial office visit showed questionable evidence of fusion from L4 to S1 (*A*). In addition, the patient demonstrated marked sagittal decompensation (*B*). Although the slippage angle was within normal limits, there was marked loss of sagittal balance. Tomograms suggested pseudarthrosis at L4–L5 and L5–S1. Surgical revision by decompression, instrumentation and fusion from a posterior approach was undertaken. At the time of surgery, pseudarthroses were identified and repaired. Osteotomy was performed through the existing fusion mass to allow an increase in lordosis with subsequent improvement in sagittal balance. Postoperatively, the patient had successful healing of the fusion and resolution of her symptoms (*C, D*).

eratively the patients were pleased with the procedure and had improved scores for pain, function, and appearance. The complication rate was high. Twelve of 16 patients had early postoperative neurologic deficits. Although seven of these patients had had a preoperative deficit, the study does not compare the preoperative and postoperative deficits. Five of the 12 patients (32%) had persistent motor deficits at follow-up.[38]

This study suggests that, although there may be a role for resection in carefully selected patients, the high complication rate precludes wide application of this technique. Resection should be employed only by surgeons with extensive experience. The author has performed 10 L5 vertebrectomies for symptomatic spondylolisthesis (Fig. 8). All cases have been followed for at least 1 year postoperatively. Four of these patients

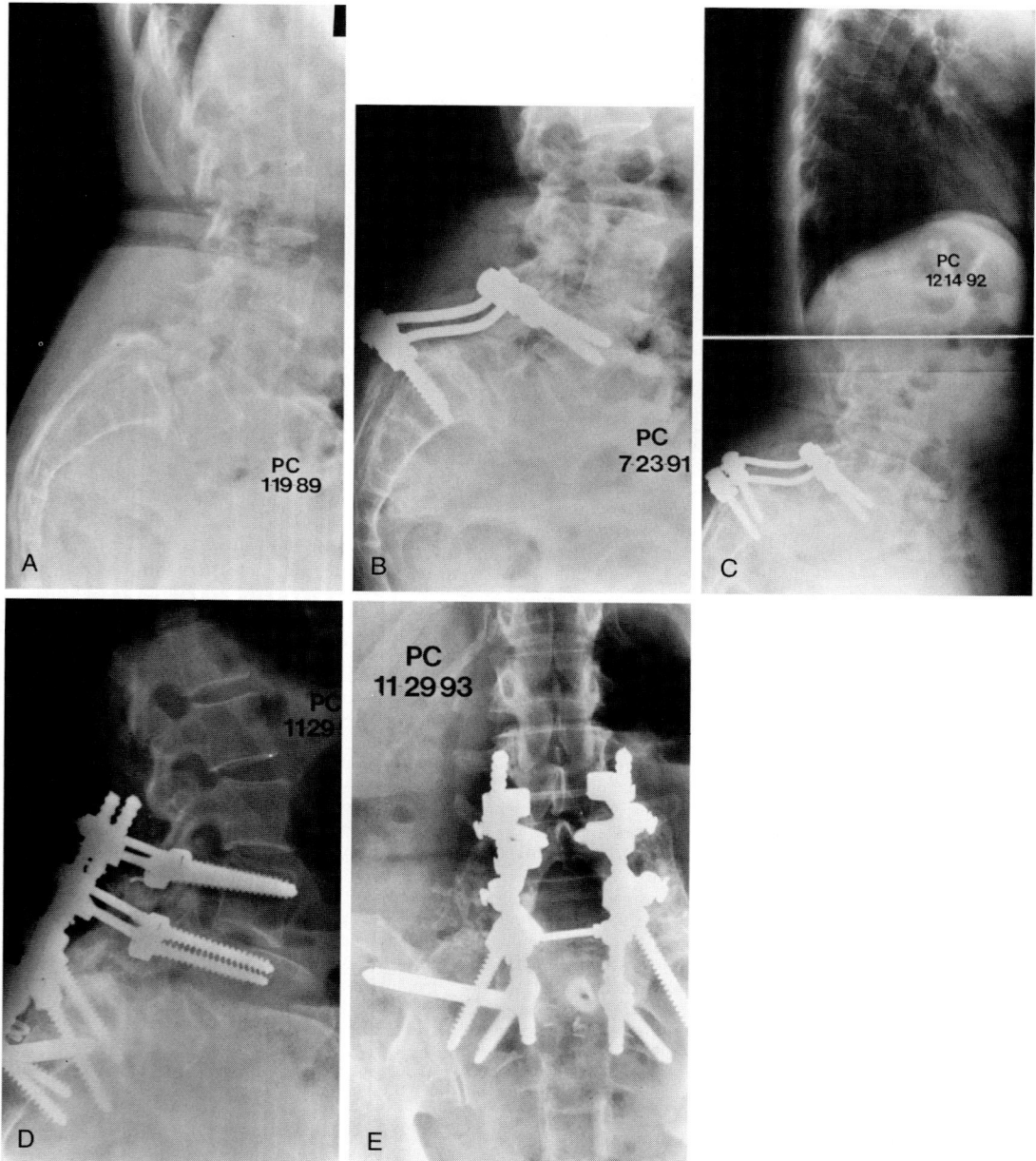

Figure 7. The case of a 48-year-old woman demonstrates the pitfalls associated with attempting posterior spine fusion with inadequate fixation in the presence of lumbosacral kyphosis. At the age of 44 years, she had the insidious onset of back pain with radiation to both legs (A). She underwent a posterior decompression and fusion from L4 to S1, with interpedicular fixation (B). Her initial postoperative course showed excellent relief; however, approximately 3 months after surgery, she began to experience a recurrence of symptoms. At that time a nonunion was diagnosed and an attempt was made to heal the fusion with an external bone stimulator. Despite the recommendations of her treating physician to undergo revision surgery, the patient refused and was lost to follow-up for approximately 2 years. When she was seen by the author, radiographic evidence of nonunion of the fusion was noted, along with marked lumbosacral kyphosis, progression of spondylolisthesis to grade IV, and marked compensatory lumbar hyperlordosis (C). Revision surgery consisted of hardware removal, decompression, and instrumentation. One week later, an anterior interbody fibular grafting procedure was carried out because of residual translation. One year postoperatively, the fusion appears to be solid both clinically and radiographically, and the patient has returned to her normal activities (D, E).

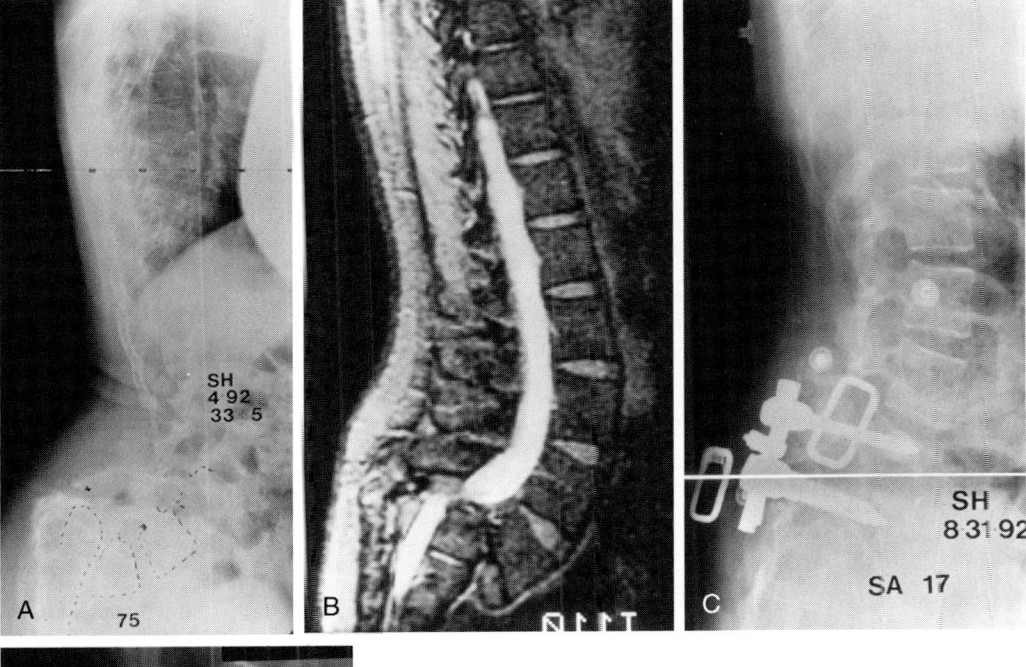

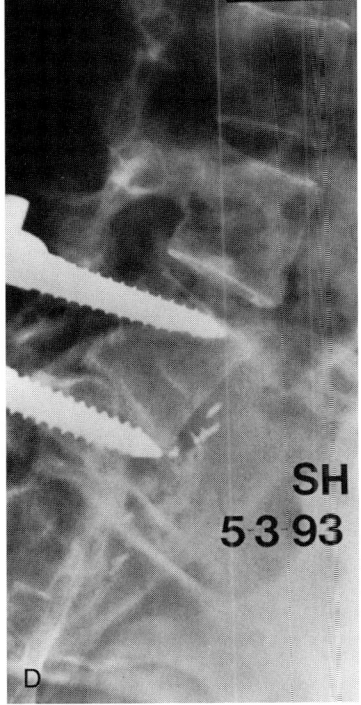

Figure 8. A 31-year-old woman presented with severe pain, sagittal imbalance, and lower extremity neurologic deficits with early cauda equina syndrome. Her preoperative x-ray film and MRI scan demonstrate spondyloptosis of L5, a slip angle of 75 degrees, and marked compression of the dural sac over the dome of S1 (*A, B*). The patient underwent anterior and posterior resection of the L5 vertebral body and translational reduction of L4 onto S1 with posterior instrumentation and fusion (*C*). Postoperatively, profound L5 and S1 radiculopathy developed bilaterally. However, over the ensuing year, her neurologic deficit has improved to better than preoperative status. The cauda equina syndrome has been relieved, and the fusion is solid (*D*). The patient has returned to her profession.

developed postoperative neurapraxia; one recovered completely, and two partially recovered.

Resection is occasionally indicated for patients who are skeletally mature, have disabling stenosis, are unresponsive to conservative management, and have severe sagittal imbalance. Even though it may theoretically be a spine-shortening procedure, the primary corrective force is that of spinal translation. This may prove risky because the lumbar plexus may be under excessive stretch after L4 is repositioned on the sacrum.[59]

Acknowledgment

I am indebted to Paul T. Rubery, M.D., for his significant role in the research and writing of this chapter.

REFERENCES

1. Adkins, E. W. O.: Spondylolisthesis. J. Bone Joint Surg. 37B:48–62, 1955.
2. Amundson, G., Edwards, C. C., and Garfin, S. R.: Spondylolisthesis. In Rothman, R. H., and Simeone, F. A. (eds.): The Spine. Philadelphia, W. B. Saunders, 1992, pp. 913–969.
3. Andreshak, T. G.: Lumbar spine surgery in the obese patient. Transactions of the 61st Annual Meeting of the American Academy of Orthopaedic Surgeons, New Orleans, LA, February 24–March 1, 1994.
4. Baker, D. R., and McHollick, W.: Spondylolysis and spondylolisthesis in children. J. Bone Joint Surg. 38A:933–934, 1956.
5. Bohlman, H. H., and Cook, S. S.: One-stage decompression and posterolateral and interbody fusion for lumbosacral spondyloptosis through a posterior approach. A report of two cases. J. Bone Joint Surg. 64A:415–418, 1982.
6. Boos, N., Marchesi, D., Zuber, K., and Aebi, M.: Treatment of severe spondylolisthesis by reduction and pedicular fixation: A 4–6 year follow-up study. Spine 18:1655–1661, 1993.
7. Boxall, D., Bradford, D. S., Winter, R. B., and Moe, J. H.: Management of severe spondylolisthesis. J. Bone Joint Surg. 61A:479–495, 1979.
8. Bradford, D. S.: Repair of spondylolysis or minimal degree of spondylolisthesis by segmental wire fixation and bone grafting. Orthop. Trans. 6:1–2, 1982.
9. Bradford, D., and Iza, J.: Repair of the defect in spondylolysis or minimal degrees of spondylolisthesis by segmental wire fixation and bone grafting. Spine 10:673–679, 1985.
10. Bradford, D. S., and Gotfried, Y.: Staged salvage reconstruction of grade-IV and V spondylolisthesis. J. Bone Joint Surg. 69A:191–202, 1987.
11. Buck, J. E.: Further thoughts on direct repair of the defect in spondylolysis. Proceedings and reports of universities, colleges, councils and associations. J. Bone Joint Surg. 61B:123, 1979.
12. Burns, B. H.: An operation for spondylolisthesis. Lancet 1:1233, 1933.
13. Capener, N.: Spondylolisthesis. Br. J. Surg. 19:374–386, 1932.
14. Cunningham, B. W., Sefter, J. C., Shono, Y., and McAfee, P. C.: Static and cyclical biomechanical analysis of pedicle screw spinal constructs. Spine 18:1677–1688, 1993.
15. Davis, I. S., and Bailey, R. W.: Spondylolisthesis: Long-term follow-up study of treatment with total laminectomy. Clin. Orthop. 88:46–49, 1972.
16. Fredrickson, B. E., Baker, D., McHolick, W. J., et al.: The natural history of spondylolysis and spondylolisthesis. J. Bone Joint Surg. 66A:699–707, 1984.
17. Freebody, D., Bendall, R., and Taylor, R. D.: Anterior transperitoneal lumbar fusion. J. Bone Joint Surg. 53B:617–627, 1971.
18. Freeman, B. L., III, and Donati, N. L.: Spinal arthrodesis for severe spondylolisthesis in children and adolescents: A long-term follow-up study. J. Bone Joint Surg. 71A:594–598, 1989.
19. Gaines, R. W., and Nichols, W. K.: Treatment of spondyloptosis by two-stage L5 vertebrectomy and reduction of L4 onto S1. Spine 10:680–686, 1985.
20. Gill, G. G., Manning, J. G., and White, H. L.: Surgical treatment of spondylolisthesis without spine fusion. J. Bone Joint Surg. 37A:493–520, 1955.
21. Gill, G. G., and Binder, W. F.: Autoamputation of the first sacral nerve roots in spondyloptosis. Spine 5:295–297, 1980.
22. Harms, J., Boehm, H., and Zielke, K.: Surgical treatment of spondyloptosis: The Harms technique. In Bridwell, K. H., and Dewald, R. L. (eds.): The Textbook of Spinal Surgery. Philadelphia, J. B. Lippincott, 1991, pp. 585–592.
23. Harris, I. E., and Weinstein, S. L.: Long-term follow-up of patients with grade III and IV spondylolisthesis. J. Bone Joint Surg. 69A:960–969, 1987.
24. Hensinger, R. N., Lang, J. R., and MacEwen, G. D.: Surgical management of spondylolisthesis in children and adolescents. Spine 1:207–216, 1976.
25. Henson, J., McCall, I. W., and O'Brien, J. P.: Disc damage above a spondylolisthesis. Br. J. Radiol. 60:69–72, 1987.
26. Herron, L. D., and Trippi, A. C.: L4–5 degenerative spondylolisthesis: The results of treatment by decompressive laminectomy without fusion. Spine 14:534–538, 1989.
27. Hibbs, R. H.: An operation for progressive spinal deformities. N. Y. J. Med. 93:1013–1016, 1911.
28. Hu, S. S., Bradford, D. S., Transfeldt, E. E., and Cohen, M.: Reduction of high-grade spondylolisthesis using Edwards instrumentation. Transactions of the 61st Annual Meeting of the American Academy of Orthopaedic Surgeons, New Orleans, LA, February 24–March 1, 1994.
29. Huizenga, B. A.: Reduction of spondyloptosis with 2-stage vertebrectomy. Orthop. Trans. 7:21, 1983.
30. Jeanneret, B.: Direct repair of spondylolysis. Acta Orthop. Scand. Suppl. 251:111–115, 1993.
31. Jenkins, J. A.: Spondylolisthesis. Br. J. Surg. 24:80–85, 1936.
32. Johnson, J. R., and Kirwan, E. O.: The long-term results of fusion in situ for severe spondylolisthesis. J. Bone Joint Surg. 65B:43–46, 1983.
33. Johnson, R. M., and McQuire, E. J.: Urogenital complications of anterior approaches to the lumbar spine. Clin. Orthop. 154:114–118, 1981.
34. Kettlekamp, D. B., and Wright, G. D.: Spondylolysis in the Alaskan Eskimo. J. Bone Joint Surg. 53A:563–566, 1971.
35. Kimura, M.: My method of filling the lesion with spongy bone in spondylolysis and spondylolisthesis. Orthop. Surg. 19:285–295, 1968.
36. Krenz, J., and Troup, J. D. G.: The structure of the pars interarticularis of the lower lumbar vertebrae and its relation to the etiology of spondylolysis, with a report of the healing fracture in the neural arch of a fourth lumbar vertebra. J. Bone Joint Surg. 55B:735–741, 1973.
37. Laurent, L. E., and Osterman, K.: Operative treatment of spondylolisthesis in young patients. Clin. Orthop. 117:85–91, 1976.

38. Lehmer, S., Steffee, A. D., Gaines, R. W., Jr.: Treatment of L5–S1 spondyloptosis by staged L5 resection with reduction and fusion of L4 onto S1 (Gaines procedure). Spine 19:1916–1925, 1994.
39. Matthiass, H. H., and Heine, J. The surgical reduction of spondylolisthesis. Clin Orthop. 203:34–44, 1986.
40. Mau, H.: Scoliosis and spondylolysis-spondylolisthesis. Arch. Orthop. Traumatol. Surg. 99:29–34, 1981.
41. McGuire, R. A., and Amundson, G. M.: The use of primary internal fixation in spondylolisthesis. Presented at the Scoliosis Research Society Meeting, Kansas City, 1992.
42. Meyerding, H. W.: Spondylolisthesis. Surg. Gynecol. Obstet. 54:371–377, 1932.
43. Morscher, E., Gerber, B., and Fasel, J.: Surgical treatment of spondylolisthesis by bone grafting and direct stabilization of spondylolysis by means of a hook screw. Acta Orthop. Traumatol. Surg. 103:175–178, 1984.
44. Murray, R. D., and Colwill, M. R.: Stress fractures of the pars interarticularis. Proc. R. Soc. Med. 61:555–557, 1968.
45. Ogilvie, J. W., and Sherman, J.: Spondylolysis in Scheuermann's disease. Spine 12:251–253, 1987.
46. Osterman, K., Lindholm, T. S., and Laurent, L. E.: Late results of removal of the loose posterior element (Gill's operation) in the treatment of lytic lumbar spondylolisthesis. Clin. Orthop. 117:121–128, 1976.
47. Porter, R. W., and Park, W.: Unilateral spondylolysis. J. Bone Joint Surg. 64B:344–348, 1982.
48. Rowe, G. G., and Roche, M. B. The etiology of separate neural arch. J. Bone Joint Surg. 35A:102–110, 1953.
49. Saraste, H.: Long-term clinical and radiological follow-up of spondylolysis and spondylolisthesis. J. Pediatr. Orthop. 7:631–638, 1987.
50. Schlüter, K.: Form und Struktur des normalen und des pathologisch veränderten Wirbels. Stuttgart, Hippokrates-Verlag, 1965.
51. Schoenecker, P. L., Cole, H. O., Herring, J. A., et al.: Cauda equina syndrome after in situ arthrodesis for severe spondylolisthesis at the lumbosacral junction. J. Bone Joint Surg. 72A:369–377, 1990.
52. Seitsalo, S., Osterman, K., Hyvarinen, H., et al.: Severe spondylolisthesis in children and adolescents: A long-term review of fusion in situ. J. Bone Joint Surg. 72B:259–265, 1990.
53. Steffee, A. D., and Sitkowski D. J.: Reduction and stabilization of grade IV spondylolisthesis. Clin. Orthop. 227:32–39, 1988.
54. Steffee, A. D., and Brantigan, J. W.: The variable screw placement spinal fixation system: Report of a prospective study of 250 patients enrolled in Food and Drug Administration clinical trials. Spine 18:1160–1172, 1993.
55. Stewart, T. D.: The age incidence of neural arch defects in Alaskan natives, considered from the standpoint of etiology. J. Bone Joint Surg. 35A:937–950, 1953.
56. Taillard, W.: Les spondylolisthesis chez l'enfant et l'adolescent. Acta Orthop. Scand. 24:115–144, 1955.
57. Taillard, W.: Les spondylolisthesis. Paris, Masson & Cie, 1957.
58. Tower, S. S., and Pratt, W. B.: Spondylolysis and associated spondylolisthesis in Eskimo and Athabascan populations. Clin. Orthop. 250:171–175, 1990.
59. Transfeldt, E. E., Dendrinos, G. K., and Bradford, D. S.: Paresis of proximal lumbar roots after reduction of L5–S1 spondylolisthesis. Spine 14:884–887, 1989.
60. van Rens, J. G., and van Horn, J. R.: Long-term results in lumbosacral interbody fusion for spondylolisthesis. Acta Orthop. Scand. 53:383–392, 1982.
61. Verbiest, H.: The treatment of lumbar spondyloptosis or impending lumbar spondyloptosis accompanied by neurologic deficit and/or neurogenic intermittent claudication. Spine 4:68–77, 1979.
62. Wiltse, L. L., Widell, E. H., and Jackson, D. W.: Fatigue fracture: The basic lesion in isthmic spondylolisthesis. J. Bone Joint Surg. 57A 17–22, 1975.
63. Wiltse, L. L., Newman, P. H., and Macnab, I.: Classification of spondylolysis and spondylolisthesis. Clin. Orthop. 117:23–29, 1976.
64. Zdeblick, T. A.: A prospective randomized study of lumbar fusion. Spine 18:983–991, 1993.

Surgical Treatment of Adult Degenerative Spondylolisthesis

RICHARD A. BALDERSTON
ALEXANDER R. VACCARO

With the increasing longevity of the populations of most countries, degenerative diseases will be seen more commonly by physicians.[2, 24] Degenerative spondylolisthesis, as a cause of symptoms of back and radicular pain, is a disorder that will be increasingly prevalent in the next several years and beyond.

DEFINITION AND PATHOANATOMY

Degenerative spondylolisthesis was first described in the German literature by Junghanns[10] in 1930 as a pseudospondylolisthesis, meaning no identifiable defect was noted in the posterior neural arch. Macnab[15] in 1950 was the first to report this entity in the English literature. Newman[17] further clarified the actual pathologic process of this disorder by describing the associated posterior facet arthrosis at the level of the listhesis, formally introducing the term degenerative spondylolisthesis.

Anatomically, degenerative spondylolisthesis describes an anterior translation of one vertebra compared with the subjacent vertebra. The specific amount of translation required to define degenerative spondylolisthesis varies with different studies, but the lower limit is between 2 and 5 mm, with the maximum percentage of slippage rarely exceeding 30%.[7] In the lumbar spine, the most common level of translation is at the L4–L5 disc space. Slippage at this level occurs approximately six times more frequently than at the L3–L4 disc space. Degenerative spondylolisthesis has also been described at the L2–L3 and L5–S1 disc space levels.[14] Plain x-ray films, including oblique films, demonstrate an intact neural arch and pars intraarticularis. Plain x-ray studies are used to differentiate spondylolisthesis with an intact neural arch from isthmic spondylolisthesis, in which there is an abnormality of the vertebrae at the level of the pars.

With anterior translation of one vertebra on another, the posterior elements of the superior vertebra are closer to the posterior vertebral body of the inferior vertebra, producing the possibility of spinal stenosis or narrowing of the neural tube at this level. In the early stages of disc and facet joint degeneration with horizontal vertebral translation at the level of the L4–L5 disc space, an anterior shift of the L4 inferior articular process as it passes across the superior posterior rim of the L5 vertebral body may cause constriction of the L5 nerve roots.[21]

Common anatomic changes include facet joint expansion due to degeneration, resulting in an overall increase in facet joint surface areas. As this process continues, osteophyte formation or gradual expansion of the L5 superior articular process, with slight posterior bulging of the L4–L5 disc, may cause further thecal sac encroachment.[20] Facet joint hypertrophy at the level of degenerative spondylolisthesis thus may affect the spinal nerves centrally, at the area of the lateral recess of the pedicle of the inferior vertebra. It also may affect the spinal nerve exiting through the foramen beneath the pedicle of the superior vertebra. With anterior translation of one vertebra on another, the loading characteristics of the facet joints change and become more dysfunctional. Dysfunctional loading of the facet joints, in an effort to counteract the pathologic forces, again leads to hypertrophy. Some facets may increase to 4 to 6 cm in diameter. Some degree of annular failure must also be present as the vertebral end plate on one side of the disc translates forward. This effect contributes to a vicious circle with respect to pressure at the disc level, as constant axial force produces more shear during cyclic loading.

Abnormalities of the ligamentum flavum are also seen, including thickening in the area of the central canal. This change may be due to degeneration or to volumetric changes induced by shortening of the spinal segment.

In addition to the anterior translation of the superior vertebra, there may be additional deformities. The superior vertebra may also be translated to the right or the left. There may be rotatory changes such that the vertebrae are aligned differently in the transverse plane. This is a result of greater asymmetric degeneration and therefore creates potential for instability of one facet joint over the other at the same level.[14] Also, there may be scoliosis with a Cobb angle of greater than 10 degrees in the coronal plane.

ETIOLOGY AND PATHOPHYSIOLOGY

Most researchers believe that degenerative spondylolisthesis occurs because of differential mobility between the spinal segments.[19] Usually, the inferior vertebra is L5, and either L5–S1 motion is limited or the L5 vertebra, as it relates to the sacrum, is supported in a more comprehensive way within the pelvis. The most obvious cause of this increased stability is a hemisacralization of L5, which is reported four times more frequently in patients with degenerative spondylolisthesis than in normal patients.[14]

If the intercrestal line drawn between the superior aspect of the iliac crest passes through the body of L5, there may be increased stress at the L4–L5 disc with flexion-extension. In the aging population, a more common cause of altered stress distribution in the lumbar spine may be advanced disc degeneration at L5–S1 that causes the L5–S1 disc to become less mobile, so that increased force is transmitted to the L4–L5 disc. Other anatomic findings in patients with degenerative spondylolisthesis include a mild to moderate decrease in lumbar lordosis and an increase in the sagittal orientation of the posterior facet angle noted on transaxial computed tomographic imaging (approximately 59 degrees versus 40 degrees).[4]

EPIDEMIOLOGY

Valkenburg and Haanen[24] noted a 10% prevalence of degenerative spondylolisthesis in women older than 60 years. Rarely is this entity reported in patients younger than 40 years of age.[14] Many of these patients are asymptomatic. Several studies have demonstrated that women are affected approximately five times more frequently than men, and that women who have undergone oophorectomy are at greater risk.[14] Also, patients with diabetes mellitus constitute a higher than normal percentage of patients in most series.

CLINICAL SYMPTOMS AND PHYSICAL EXAMINATION

Back pain is the most common chief symptom in patients with degenerative spondylolisthesis. The course of the back pain in the patient's history may be highly variable and is usually unrelated to trauma. The back pain is usually mechanical and may be relieved with rest. Back pain is usually noted early as the superior vertebral body translates anteriorly with forward displacement of its inferior articular processes.[21] Also, during the course of the day, pain usually worsens with increasing level of activity.

The second most common presenting symptom is neurogenic claudication. This results from further thecal sac compression by the posterior articular facets, as well as posterior displacement of the intervertebral disc at the level of listhesis.[7] The pain is usually diffuse in the lower extremities, involving dermatomes and muscles innervated by the L4, L5, and S1 nerves. Another type of presentation is a monoradicular nerve pain pattern usually involving an L5 spinal nerve. The pain in the legs is almost always accentuated by walking and is relieved with rest.

Patients may also describe lumbar flexion strategies that allow them to have increased endurance. For example, many patients notice that they lean forward while walking.

While shopping in a supermarket, many patients lean on the shopping cart, producing flexion of the lumbar spine, which allows flexion of the diseased segment. At the same time, symptoms are usually exacerbated by any maneuver that produces extension of the lumbar spine. Patients may feel they lose control of their legs while walking down stairs. Patients may also relate that they sense a paradoxical loss of function when they attempt to walk down a slight incline; function is improved when they attempt to walk up a slight incline. Function is related less to oxygen expenditure than to the anatomic relationship of relative flexion or extension of the lumbar spine while performing a specific activity.

The patients may also note sudden episodes of weakness, altered gait, or numbness. The pain may be progressive and incapacitating and may occur much more frequently with positional changes of the lumbar spine unrelated to significant exertion. For example, during sleep, a patient may inadvertently extend the lumbar spine and produce such severe pain that significant sleep disturbance results.[14, 25] Progressive motor weakness and symptoms and signs of cauda equina syndrome are indications for emergent decompressive surgery.

Cauda equina syndrome is extremely unlikely in this patient population. However, careful questioning with respect to subtle changes in bladder function are warranted. In many patients, urologic evaluation and cystometrographic analysis are warranted.

The physical examination findings in patients with degenerative spondylolisthesis, as in patients with spinal stenosis, may be nonspecific. In the standing position, the patient may decompensate anteriorly to allow a more flexed position of the lumbar spine. Inspection and palpation of the lumbar spine may reveal a palpable stepoff at the level of the listhesis. The iliolumbar ligaments, sacral iliac joints, sciatic notches, other spinous processes, and trochanteric bursae should all be palpated and the presence of symptoms should be noted.

Range of motion of the lumbar spine is usually normal, and many patients can flex forward without difficulty. The examiner should attempt to extend the lumbar spine fully and, if possible, to produce hyperextension. At this point, the patient should be asked whether the symptoms are being reproduced.

The neurologic examination may reveal a focal nerve deficit. The quadriceps tendon reflex may be reduced with an L4 radiculopathy. Less commonly, there is quadriceps weakness and possibly atrophy. With an L5 spinal nerve abnormality, extensor hallucis longus weakness may also be encountered. However, most commonly, the results of the neurologic examination are nonspecific, with symmetric motor findings and symmetrically depressed reflexes noted in the elderly population.

RADIOLOGIC EVALUATION

The diagnosis of degenerative spondylolisthesis is confirmed with a lateral lumbar roentgenogram, which demonstrates forward displacement of L4 on L5, the most common level at which this disorder occurs. Isthmic spondylolisthesis may also occur at this level, and plain films should help to rule out this entity. Concomitant degenerative changes include disc space narrowing, end-plate irregularities, sclerosis, osteophytes, and traction spurs about the disc. Facet sclerosis and hypertrophy should all be noted on the plain x-ray film. Flexion-extension views may be obtained but rarely demonstrate significant additional translational instability. Several researchers have suggested recumbent supine or prone lateral flexion-extension radiographs for patients who are too uncomfortable to endure standing dynamic x-ray studies.[25]

For patients with predominantly mechanical back pain that responds to the usual conservative modalities, further roentgenographic evaluation is not warranted. However, if significant back pain persists that is unresponsive to conservative means or if significant radicular pain intervenes, magnetic resonance imaging (MRI) is the next study of choice. Typically there is a diminished cross-sectional area at the level of the spondylolisthesis. There may also be hypertrophy of the superior facet with subarticular entrapment of the L5 nerve. Soft tissue abnormalities include thickening of the ligamentum flavum and, possibly, posterior translation of a disc fragment. Another useful study is postmyelography computed tomography.

Technetium bone scanning was more commonly ordered before the advent of MRI scanning to rule out possible metastatic disease. Currently, however, bone scanning is less commonly used in the initial evaluation of patients with degenerative spondylolisthesis.

DIFFERENTIAL DIAGNOSIS

Epidemiologic studies have demonstrated that degenerative spondylolisthesis is most often an asymptomatic roentgenographic finding. Numerous spinal entities can give rise to similar symptoms, including spinal stenosis, central disc herniation, and degenerative scoliosis. One study demonstrated that a high percentage of patients with degenerative scoliosis also had degenerative spondylolisthesis.[17] In patients with coronal plane abnormalities, who are frequently elderly, neurologic symptoms may suggest multilevel involvement.

Not uncommonly in the elderly population, degenerative disease of the cervical spine produces symptoms that radiate to the lower extremities. In all patients who are being evaluated, especially for surgery, cervical abnormalities should be ruled out with flexion-extension plain radiographs and possibly an MRI scan of the cervical spine if the physical examination raises any question of cervical abnormality.

Osteoarthritis of the hip is present in one sixth of patients with degenerative spondylolisthesis. Pain from a degenerated hip commonly radiates to the anterior thigh and may mimic an L4 radiculopathy. Also, medial knee pain from degenerative disease or a torn meniscus may simulate an L4 radiculopathy and produce considerable confusion for the clinician.

Peripheral vascular disease is common in elderly persons, who are also predisposed to degenerative spondylolisthesis. Pain with ambulation is a typical finding, but it is much more closely related to decreased oxygen-carrying capacity of circulation to the lower extremities than to activity. Patients with vascular disease typically have more problems walking uphill than do patients with degenerative spondylolisthesis or spinal stenosis. In addition, patients with peripheral vascular disease typically have increased pain when riding a stationary bicycle, whereas patients with spinal stenosis typically are able to ride a stationary bicycle for a prolonged period because they can flex the lumbar spine. Patients with peripheral vascular disease need only to stop walking to alleviate their symptoms; patients with degenerative spondylolisthesis often must sit down and flex the lumbar spine to produce symptom relief

Unfortunately, many patients in the elderly age group have both diseases. Doppler studies should be performed if there is any question of diminished blood flow to the lower extremities. With equal degrees of vascular and neural involvement from spinal stenosis, the vascular problem is usually addressed first with surgical management.

Diabetic neuropathy rarely produces a painful radiculopathy. Electromyelographic and neural conduction studies should be performed in patients with diabetes mellitus. The surgical outcome for radiculopathy may not be as good in diabetic patients as in nondiabetic patients.

Other disorders that may mimic the symptoms of spondylolisthesis include metastatic disease of the spine or the presence of retroperitoneal tumor.

TREATMENT

Conservative Management

Nonoperative treatment of degenerative spondylolisthesis is similar to the nonoperative management of other mechanical disorders of the lumbar spine. In patients who have predominantly back pain, the usual conservative modalities of appropriate rest, the use of antiinflammatory nonsteroidal medication, paraspinal and abdominal strengthening exercises, appropriate aerobic conditioning, and weight reduction may have a significant beneficial impact. Management of concomitant osteopenia usually related to osteoporosis is also appropriate at this time.

Many studies suggest that radicular pain is much less amenable to the same nonoperative management strategies that are applicable when radiculopathy is related to a herniated disc. In general, patients with predominantly leg pain require a longer trial of nonoperative care to evaluate the efficacy of treatment. For patients with significant leg pain, administration of epidural steroids may be an appropriate temporizing measure.[9]

Operative Treatment

The major indication for surgery in patients with degenerative spondylolisthesis is radicular pain radiating to the leg that is unresponsive to nonoperative management. Studies have shown that patients who manifest signs of neurologic dysfunction prior to surgery tend to report a better outcome than do patients with solely radicular pain.[4] Fortunately, only about 10% to 15% of patients treated nonoperatively for degenerative spondylolisthesis eventually undergo surgery as a result of failed conservative treatment.[4]

Great care must be taken in patients in whom back pain is the predominant symptom. Some investigators have advocated a primary in situ posterior lateral intertransverse process fusion for patients in their fifth and sixth decades of life with degenerative spondylolisthesis and mechanical low back pain with demonstrable single-level instability but without neurologic involvement.[4] In most of these patients, concomitant disc degeneration at other levels may be a significant contributing factor. In the authors' opinion, a spinal fusion for relief of mechanical low back pain in this setting is less than satisfying to both the patient and the surgeon as the longevity of follow-up increases. Also, iliolumbar ligament pain is also a contraindication to posterior lumbar fusion.

The primary goal of surgery for leg symptoms related to degenerative spondylolisthesis is decompression of the neural elements at the level of the deformity.[12, 16] The majority of surgical candidates tend to be frail and elderly with concomitant medical problems; therefore, a thorough preoperative medical evaluation is required prior to surgery.[25] The use of epidural anesthesia lessens the potential for blood loss. Special attention to patient positioning to avoid undue pressure on bony prominences and neurovascular pressure points should also be observed.[4]

The surgical approach is a midline muscle-splitting approach that divides the paraspinal muscles at the level of the spinous processes and the lamina of the two involved vertebral bodies. In addition, the facet joint between the vertebra and the transverse processes of the two involved vertebrae must be completely visualized. The spinous processes are removed, usually at L4 and L5, and a decompressive laminectomy is performed beginning at the L5 level. Until the pedicles of L5 are reached, there is usually minimum compressive pathologic change of the cauda equina. However, at the level of the superior aspect of the lamina at L5, the surgeon usually notes a narrowing of the dural sac. Care must be taken to free adhesions at the level of the ligamentum flavum and bone before proceeding. The midline laminectomy is carried to the level of the pedicle of L4.

At this point, the subarticular recesses are decompressed just medial to the pedicle of L4 and, more importantly, the pedicle of L5. The anterior medial portion of the inferior articular process of L4 is removed to decompress the exiting nerve roots at this level.[14] This exposes the superior articular process of L5, which is undercut flush with the medial border of the L5 pedicle to relieve pressure on the traversing L5 nerve roots.[4] A probe must demonstrate adequate space for the L4 and L5 nerves bilaterally. The L4–L5 disc on both sides is next checked for disc herniation. If the disc annulus is intact, discectomy is not routinely performed.

During the last 20 years, there has been considerable controversy about the necessity of performing concomitant spinal arthrodesis after posterior decompression for degenerative spondylolisthesis. Most studies attesting to the benefits of posterior decompression without fusion have been retrospective and have not had sufficient control groups for comparison. Rosomoff[20] supported the concept of performing adequate posterior decompression with concomitant total facetectomy and laminectomy, on the grounds that further postoperative slippage was part of the natural history of degenerative spondylolisthesis without any adverse effect on the final outcome. Dall and Rowe[1] reported that 83% of patients obtained pain relief with total facetectomy, compared with only 36% of patients undergoing wide foraminotomy with preservation of the articular facets. These investigators and others[14] believed that any postoperative slippage would stabilize after 1 year and should not pose a problem in terms of patient discomfort at follow-up.

Herron and Tripp[7] reviewed a series of 24 patients who underwent decompressive laminectomy and partial facetectomy without fusion in the setting of L4–L5 degenerative spondylolisthesis. They stressed the importance of maintaining the structural integrity of the L4 pars interarticularis and preserving as much of the L4–L5 facet joints as possible. Eighty-three percent of patients in their series had a good result, with 84% of patients reporting an improvement in back pain and 92% reporting an improvement in leg pain. No patient in this series had greater than 2 mm of translation on preoperative lateral plain flexion-extension radiographs, and only four patients had an increase in slippage greater than 2 mm in the postoperative period that was unrelated to outcome.

Although these investigators and others have attested to a satisfactory outcome after adequate surgical decompression without surgical fusion in 60% to 96% of patients, many studies have reported consistently unsatisfactory results when the structural integrity of the involved pars interarticularis and intervening facet joints is compromised.[14] Residual back pain was reported in as many as 73% of patients who have undergone decompression without fusion.[6] The presence of a postoperative slippage with resultant mechanical instability and recurrent spinal stenosis is thought to be responsible for such symptoms.

Lombardi and coworkers[14] retrospectively evaluated three different surgical approaches in 47 patients treated with symptomatic degenerative spondylolisthesis. Patients treated with wide decompression and complete sacrifice of the articular processes were found to have good to excellent results in 33% of cases at follow-up. Patients who underwent adequate posterior decompression with preservation of the articular processes with bilateral foraminotomies were found to have good to excellent result in 80% of cases. Ninety percent of patients who had adequate posterior decompression with preservation of the articular facets followed by intertransverse process fusion were found to have 90% good to excellent results overall.[14]

Many researchers have cited certain ill-defined indications for fusion in patients with degenerative spondylolisthesis, including radiographic evidence of instability on dynamic flexion-extension films; decompression in young, active patients; the presence of a large disc space; a previous wide posterior decompressive laminectomy and facetectomy resulting in instability; severe osteoporosis in patients with coexisting compression fractures; and disc excision performed during posterior decompression.[7, 25]

The role of fusion in a patient who has undergone decompression for degenerative spondylolisthesis was clarified by a superb, controlled, prospective randomized study by Herkowitz and Kurz[6] comparing two well-matched patient groups, both of which underwent similar decompressive procedures. Ninety-six percent of patients who underwent a bilateral intertransverse fusion experienced good to excellent results compared with only 46% who had good to excellent results when posterior fusion was not performed. In addition, 96% of patients in the group without fusion demonstrated progressive slippage in the postoperative period, compared with slippage among 28% of patients in the fusion group.[6]

At the very minimum, the authors perform bilateral floating fusion with grafted bone from the iliac crest placed over the decorticated transverse processes of L4 and L5 (Fig. 1). The remaining facet joint at L4–L5 is not routinely packed with bone graft. In some elderly patients with significant comorbidity, fusion surgery may not be elected if increased rate of complications is anticipated.

Various researchers have described different types of fusion for degenerative spondylolisthesis. Transverse process fusion is the most common procedure, although posterior interbody and anterior interbody fusions have also been advocated.[5] Proponents of posterior interbody fusion attest to the frequent findings of small or atrophic transverse processes in the setting of compromised facet joints after surgical removal, both of which compromise the available surface area for an intertransverse process fusion. An interbody fusion takes advantage of the large surface area for graft contact of both contiguous vertebral end plates, assists in maintaining or improving disc space height, and allows placement of the graft under compression, which biomechanically

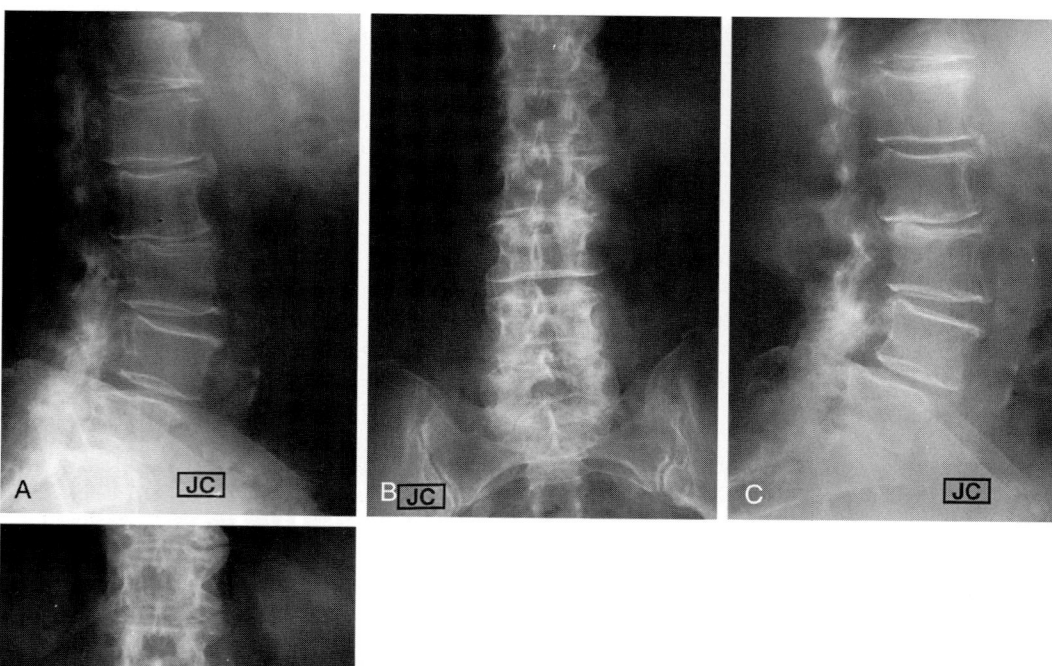

Figure 1. *A, B,* A 70-year-old woman had a 10-year history of right leg pain radiating to the posterior thigh and to her calf and heel. Because of progressive use of antiinflammatory medication, peptic ulcer disease had developed. MRI demonstrated severe spinal stenosis at the L4–L5 level with degenerative spondylolisthesis. *C, D,* Operative treatment included L4 and L5 laminectomy with medial facetectomy at L4–L5 bilaterally. Bilateral lateral fusion was accomplished from L4 to L5. At follow-up, significant relief of back and leg pain had been realized.

is a more suitable environment for graft maturation. The disadvantage of this technique is the potential for dural sheath or nervous tissue injury from medial dural sheath retraction during graft placement as well as graft extrusion into the cauda equina.[25]

To overcome some of these disadvantages, several investigators have reported satisfactory results with anterior interbody fusion. Although this involves an anterior retroperitoneal approach along with its attendant complications (e.g., the risk of autonomic system dysfunction in a male patient as well as the possibility of vascular injury), better decompression of the disc space can be performed and a structural graft of larger size can be safely placed than through the posterior approach.[25]

Inoue and associates[8] performed cadaveric and animal studies using microradiographic techniques. They concluded that the pathoanatomy of degenerative spondylolisthesis was related to anterior disc degeneration with resultant intersegmental instability and rotational strain in the posterior facet complex, leading to disc and facet failure and advanced osteoarthritic changes. Osteoarthritic changes in the articular processes, with concomitant localized slippage of vertebrae, lead to central as well as lateral recess stenosis. Inoue and coworkers[8] performed anterior interbody fusion for 36 patients to remove the diseased intervertebral disc and reported a correction in sagittal malalignment with restoration of disc space height in the majority of patients. Fusion was successful in all single-level fusions and in 85% of double-level fusions.

Takahashi and associates[23] confirmed rotational malalignment in this disorder in 9 of 22 patients who underwent thin-section computed tomographic evaluation and subsequent interbody fusion. Using a Kaplan-Meier survivorship analysis at an average follow-up of 12 years 7 months, Takahashi and colleagues[23] reported a 76% rate of satisfactory fusion at 10 years, a 60% rate of satisfactory fusion at 20 years, and a 52% rate of satisfactory fusion at 30 years.

Satomi and associates[21] compared the results of anterior interbody fusion with or without AO screws and wire supplementation to patients who underwent posterior decompression, with or without a posterior fusion. Seventy-seven percent of patients were found to be clinically improved in the group undergoing anterior interbody fusion compared with only 56% of patients in the group undergoing posterior decompression. The average percentage of vertebral slippage improved from 18.5% preoperatively to 7.4% postoperatively in the anterior interbody fusion group compared with a worsening of vertebral slippage of 1.7% in the posterior decompression group.

A drawback of an isolated anterior interbody fusion for degenerative spondylolisthesis is the frequently reported complication of nonunion in single- and multiple-level fusion attempts.[3] This has led some authors to prescribe combined anterior and posterior fusion, with or without instrumentation, in patients considered at risk for nonunion. Kim and associates[13] reported on 20 patients treated surgically for degenerative spondylolisthesis, eight of whom underwent combined anterior and posterior lateral fusion with posterior instrumentation. They reported good to excellent results in 95% of cases at an average follow-up of 4 years, with an overall fusion success rate of 95% in their patient population.

There is significant evidence that internal fixation with pedicle screw techniques increases the fusion rate in degenerative spondylolisthesis (Fig. 2). Sedgewick and colleagues,[22] in a retrospective review, reported a 96% fusion success rate with the absence of postoperative slippage in patients surgically treated for degenerative spondylolisthesis and spinal stenosis using pedicle screw fixation. This compared with only an 18% fusion success rate with frequent progression of vertebral translation in patients without instrumentation.

Kabins and associates[11] reported on 15 patients with degenerative spondylolisthesis who underwent posterior decompression and fusion with variable screw placement (VSP) instrumentation. At follow-up, no patients had progression in the degree of slippage. This is in contrast to the reported 96% incidence of slip progression in patients who did not undergo fusion and a 28% incidence of slippage in patients who underwent fusion without instrumentation in the landmark study by Herkowitz and Kurz.[6]

In October 1994, the largest retrospective historical cohort study of pedicle screw fixation in spinal fusions was reported.[26] A total of 2684 patients with surgically treated degenerative spondylolisthesis were reviewed. The study found a statistically higher rate of fusion in patients who underwent pedicle screw fixation to supplement their fusion than in noninstrumented patients (82.5% versus 74.5%). In addition, patients who underwent pedicle screw fixation had a better clinical outcome with less overall pain, better function, and greater neurologic recovery at follow-up. At present, there are few well-designed, controlled prospective studies evaluating the efficacy of pedicle screw fixation.

Zdeblick[27] reported a prospective study evaluating the efficacy of rigid and semirigid pedicle screw fixation in 124 patients with degenerative conditions of the lumbar spine, 26 of whom were considered to have degenerative spondylolisthesis. Patients who underwent posterior lateral fusion with autogenous bone grafting but without instrumentation were found to have a 65% fusion success rate, with 71% of patients reporting a good to excellent result at follow-up. Eighty-nine percent of the patients treated with a semirigid pedicle screw device had a good to excellent result, and the fusion success rate was 77%. Patients treated with a rigid pedicle screw fixation device had 95% fusion success rate, with 95% of results being good to excellent.

Overall, the results of surgical management of radiculopathy are 70% to 85% successful. Relief of low back symptoms is much less predictable over the long term. Increased age and associated comorbidities are significant risk factors for an unsatisfac-

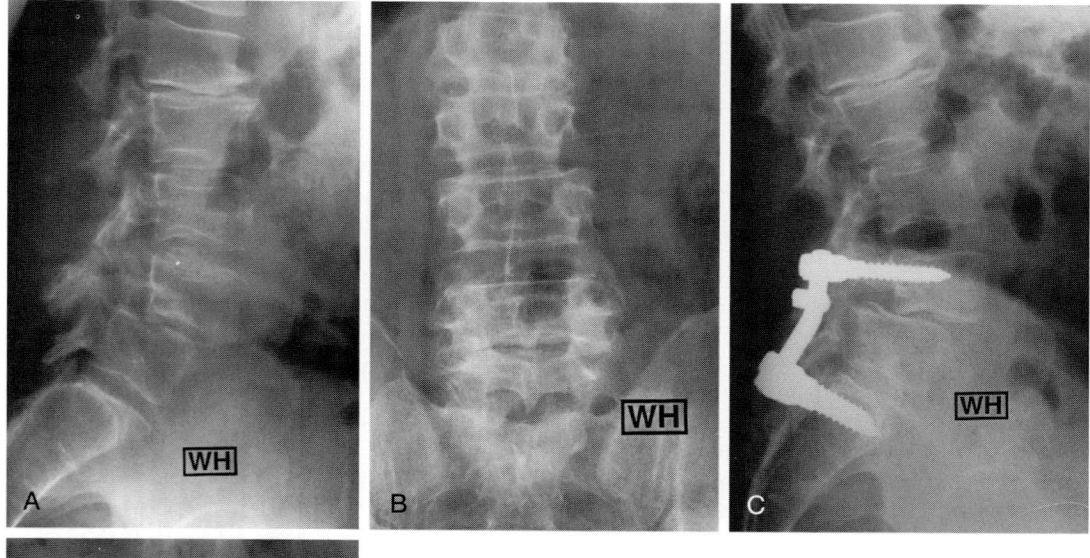

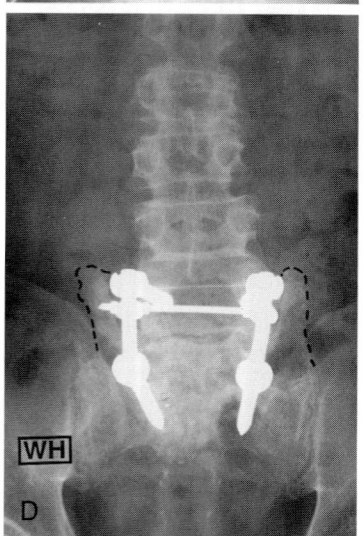

Figure 2. *A, B,* A 67-year-old man had a 3-year history of progressive leg pain on the left side greater than on the right. The pain radiated down his buttock to his posterior thigh and calf. His walking tolerance was less than one block. The myelogram demonstrated a complete block with spinal stenosis at the L4–L5 level. *C, D,* Operative treatment entailed an L5 and L4 laminectomy with medial facetectomy at L4–L5 bilaterally. Bilateral lateral fusion from L4 to the sacrum was augmented with Cotrel-Dubousset instrumentation. At 2-year follow-up, the patient continued to have significant improvement of back and leg pain.

tory outcome. Also, studies have demonstrated that a longer duration of surveillance may increase the risk of a long-term unsatisfactory result. However, many patients in these studies were treated by laminectomy without fusion, which has been shown to have an increased risk of unfavorable outcome. Deyo and coworkers[2] demonstrated that as many as 25% of elderly patients may have significant orthopedic and systemic complications that compromise long-term results. The importance of patient selection cannot be stressed enough in order to anticipate a successful long-term outcome after surgery in patients with degenerative spondylolisthesis.

REFERENCES

1. Dall, B. E., and Rowe, D. E.: Degenerative spondylolisthesis: Its surgical management. Spine 10:668–672, 1985.
2. Deyo, R. A., Cherkin, D. C., Loeser, J. D., et al.: Morbidity and mortality in association with operations on the lumbar spine: The influence of age, diagnosis and procedure. J. Bone Joint Surg. 74A:536–543, 1992.
3. Flynn, J. C., and Hogue, M. A.: Anterior fusion of the lumbar spine. J. Bone Joint Surg. 61A:1143–1150, 1979.
4. Grobler, L. J., and Wiltse, L. L.: Classification, nonoperative, and operative treatment of spondylolisthesis. *In* Frymoyer, J. W. (ed.): The Adult Spine: Principles and Practice. New York, Raven Press, 1991, pp. 1655–1704.
5. Grobler, L. J., Robertson, P. A., Novotny, J. E., and

Ahern, J. W.: Decompression for degenerative spondylolisthesis and spinal stenosis at L4–5: The effects on facet joint morphology. Spine 18:1475–1482, 1993.

6. Herkowitz, A. N., and Kurz, L. T.: Degenerative lumbar spondylolisthesis with spinal stenosis: A prospective study comparing decompression and decompression and intertransverse process arthrodesis. J. Bone Joint Surg. 73A:802–808, 1991.

7. Herron, L. D., and Tripp, A. C.: L4–5 degenerative spondylolisthesis: The results of treatment by decompressive laminectomy without fusion. Spine 14:534–538, 1989.

8. Inoue, S., Watanabe, T., Goto, S., et al.: Degenerative spondylolisthesis pathophysiology and results of anterior interbody fusion. Clin. Orthop. 227:90–98, 1988.

9. Johnsson, K. E., Rosen, I., and Uden, A.: The natural course of lumbar spinal stenosis. Clin. Orthop. 279:82–86, 1992.

10. Junghanns, H.: Spondylolisthesis. Ohne spalte im zwischenbelenkstu ("Pseudo-spondylolisthesen"). Arch. Orthop. Unfall-Chir. 29:118–127, 1930.

11. Kabins, M. B., Weinstein, J. N., Spratt, K. F., et al.: Isolated L4–L5 floating fusions using the variable screw placement system: Unilateral vs. bilateral. J. Spinal Disord. 5:39–49, 1992.

12. Katz, J. N., Lipson, S. J., Larson, M. G., et al.: The outcome of decompressive laminectomy for degenerative lumbar stenosis. J. Bone Joint Surg. 73A:809–816, 1991.

13. Kim, S. S., Denis, F., Lonstein, J. E., and Winter, R. B.: Factors affecting fusion rate in adult spondylolisthesis. Spine 15:979–984, 1990.

14. Lombardi, J. S., Wiltse, L. L., Reynolds, J., et al.: Treatment of degenerative spondylolisthesis. Spine 10:821–827, 1985.

15. Macnab, I.: Spondylolisthesis with an intact neural arch: The so-called pseudo-spondylolisthesis. J. Bone Joint Surg. 32:325–333, 1950.

16. Nakai, O., Ookawa, A., and Yamaura, I.: Long-term roentgenographic and functional changes in patients who were treated with wide fenestration for central lumbar stenosis. J. Bone Joint Surg. 73A:1184–1191, 1991.

17. Newman, P. H.: The etiology of spondylolisthesis. J. Bone Joint Surg. 45B:39–59, 1963.

18. Pritchett, J. W., and Bortel, D. T. Degenerative symptomatic lumbar scoliosis. Spine 18 700–703, 1993.

19. Rosenberg, N. J.: Degenerative spondylolisthesis: Predisposing factors. J. Bone Joint Surg. 57A:467–474, 1975.

20. Rosomoff, H. L.: Lumbar spondylolisthesis: Etiology of radiculopathy and role of the neurosurgeon. Clin. Neurosurg. 27:577–590, 1980.

21. Satomi, K., Hirabayashi, K., Toyamo, Y., and Fujimura, Y.: A clinical study of degenerative spondylolisthesis radiographic analysis and choice of treatment. Spine 17:1329–1336, 1992.

22. Sedgewick, T. A., Bridwell, K. H., Lenke, L. G., and Baldus, C.: Surgical treatment of degenerative spondylolisthesis with associated spinal stenosis. Presented at the Annual Meeting of the Scoliosis Research Society, Minneapolis, MN, September 27, 1991.

23. Takahashi, K., Kitahara, H., Yamagata, M., et al.: Long-term results of anterior interbody fusion for the treatment of degenerative spondylolisthesis. Spine 15:1211–1215, 1990.

24. Valkenburg, H. A., and Haanen, H. C. M.: The epidemiology of low back pain. In White, A. A., III, and Gordon, S. L. (eds.): American Academy of Orthopaedic Surgeons Symposium on Idiopathic Low Back Pain. St. Louis, C. V. Mosby. 1982, pp. 9–22.

25. Whiffen, J. R., and Neuwirth, M. G.: Degenerative spondylolisthesis. In Bridwell, K. H., and Dewald, R. L. (eds.): The Textbook of Spinal Surgery, Vol. 2. Philadelphia, J. B. Lippincott, 1991, pp. 657–674.

26. Yuan, H. A., Garfin, S. R., Dickman, C. A., and Mardjetko, S. M.: A historical cohort study of pedicle screw fixation in thoracic, lumbar, and sacral spinal fusions. Spine 19:2279S–2296S, 1994.

27. Zdeblick, T. A.: A prospective, randomized study of lumbar fusion. Spine 18:983–991, 1993.

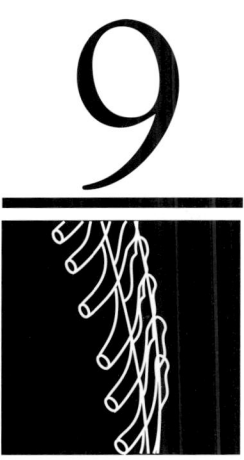

9

Lumbar Spinal Stenosis

Development of the Vertebral Canal

■

RICHARD W. PORTER

CLINICAL RELEVANCE OF THE VERTEBRAL CANAL

There is no doubt about the clinical relevance of a shallow vertebral canal. Subsequent to the early papers of Sarpyener,[21] Verbiest,[26] Van Gelderen,[25] and other investigators confirmed that a variety of back pain syndromes are related to spinal pathologic conditions in the presence of an already small canal.[5, 9, 12, 13, 20, 27] Edward and La Rocca[4] showed that 71% of patients with back pain and degenerative change have sagittal diameters that are less than the mean. Kornberg and Rechtine[10] demonstrated an inverse relationship between the size of the vertebral canal and the symptoms of disc protrusion. Forsberg and Wallœ[7] reported that patients who made a poor recovery from disc surgery had canals that were narrower than those of patients who recovered uneventfully.

The size and shape of the vertebral canal have long been neglected factors in back pain, but it is now known that a disc prolapse into a restricted space can produce more troublesome symptoms than does a protrusion into a wider canal. A canal with the trefoil shape is particularly troublesome in the presence of a posterolateral disc protrusion. A far-lateral disc protruding into the root canal, of course, quickly involves the root, irrespective of the size and shape of the central canal (Fig. 1).

In the presence of segmental instability, an adequate canal may ensure that the neural contents are not compromised, but stenotic symptoms can arise with segmental deformation if the canal is small.[6] The size and shape of the vertebral canal is undoubtedly a risk factor in many back pain syndromes.

RELATIVE IMPORTANCE OF THE BONY AND SOFT TISSUE COMPONENTS OF THE VERTEBRAL CANAL

The intersegmental region of the vertebral canal is the most important area in which pathologic changes affect the cauda equina and nerve roots. The anterior boundary of the canal indents the dura at disc level in older patients. The chronically affected disc tends to bulge into the canal and to be sand-

711

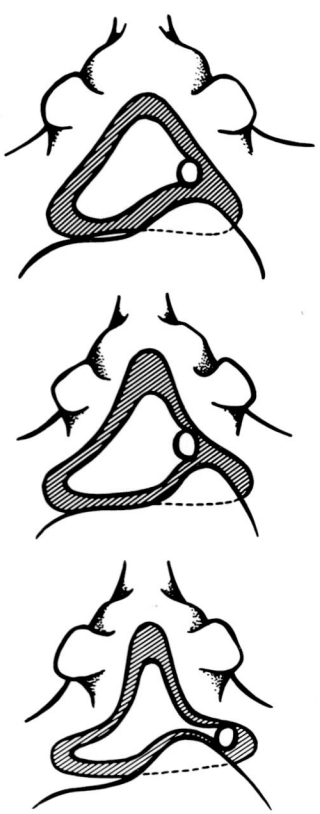

Figure 1. A disc protrusion into a large triangle-shaped canal merely displaces the root, whereas an equal-sized protrusion into a trefoil-shaped canal can quickly compromise the root.

wiched between two prominent vertebral bars of the vertebrae above and below. Posteriorly, the attachment of the ligamentum flavum to the cranial end of the lamina also indents the canal. In addition, the thickened capsule around the apophyseal joint can compromise the contents of the canal at the same level. Thus, the soft tissue constitutes the immediate boundaries of the canal at the intersegmental level. However, that does not diminish the importance of the bony boundaries of the canal. A person who has a stenotic bony canal also has limited space at the intersegmental level, even though much of this is composed of soft tissue, whereas large bony diameters ensure more adequate space for the soft tissue contents. In addition, the cranial end of the lamina forms an important bony constriction in central canal stenosis, as do the superior apophyseal joints in both central and root canal stenoses. The importance of soft tissues does not negate the relevance of a constitutionally small bony canal.

WHEN DOES THE BONY CANAL REACH MATURITY?

The author previously examined 155 juvenile and 836 adult archaeologic vertebrae, observing changes in shape and size with advancing age. It is difficult to obtain archaeologic spines of children younger than 4 years of age, but in the specimens examined, the mean midsagittal diameters were 10% larger than the mean adult midsagittal diameter at each of the lumbar levels. The reduction in size of the midsagittal diameter later in childhood is a result of the changing shape of the posterior aspect of the vertebral body, from concave to convex. The area of the vertebral canal was mature at 4 years of age (Fig. 2). In infants, the interpedicle diameter was 85% of the adult interpedicle diameter and increased steadily up to puberty.

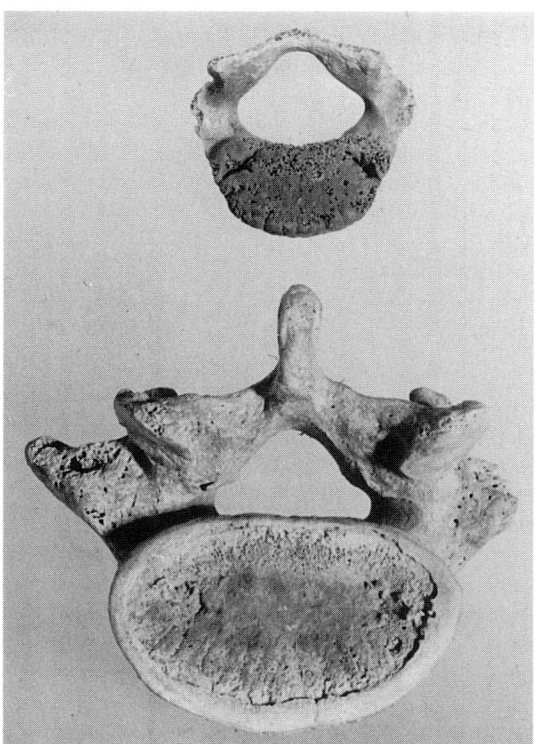

Figure 2. Two fifth lumbar vertebrae. The upper vertebra is from a 4-year-old child, and the lower from an adult. The cross-sectional area of the child's vertebral canal is similar to that of the adult.

Further studies were performed by Papp and Porter[11a] on more than 700 skeletons from the Spitalfield Collection of the Natural History Museum in London, for which the accurate date of death is known. By 1 year of age, the area of the vertebral canal of the upper four lumbar vertebrae was noted to be of adult size. In the four proximal lumbar vertebrae, there was no significant difference between the midsagittal diameter of the canal at 1 year of age and that in an adult spine. At L5, the sagittal diameter is mature by 6 years of age. Thus the vertebral canal growth takes place early indeed.

The upper lumbar vertebrae mature first. The shape of the canal changes throughout childhood, the trefoil shape not being apparent before 16 years of age and being present in about 15% of adult fifth lumbar vertebrae.[14] Trefoilness seems to increase throughout life.

FACTORS AFFECTING DEVELOPMENT OF THE VERTEBRAL CANAL

Anthropometric measurements provide a clue to the development of the vertebral canal. The vertebral canal was examined in archaeologic specimens and compared with the length of other bones in the skeleton. There was a useful correlation between the length of the femur and the interpedicle diameter: in tall subjects, the transverse diameter of the vertebral body is large and the pedicles are widely spaced. There were not many useful correlations between the midsagittal diameter of the canal and other bony measurements. There was a weak correlation between the anteroposterior and lateral diameters of the skull and the midsagittal diameter of the canal, but this clinically important canal diameter is largely independent of other skeletal growth.

Clark and coworkers[2] suggested that the size of the lumbar vertebral canal may be affected by factors that impair childhood development. They examined two archaeologic populations and found that a malnourished population tended to have shallow vertebral canals. The author examined the adult spines of two other archaeologic populations, comparing the canal size with four physiologic stress indicators (cribra orbitalia, porotic hyperostosis, dental hypoplasia, and Harris lines).[16] Dental hypoplasia correlated with a small interpedicle diameter at L1–L2 and L3; Harris lines correlated with a small midsagittal diameter at L1–L3 and L5, a small area at L5, and a more trefoil-shaped canal at L4 and L5. There was supportive evidence that an adverse environment in early life is associated with a shallow canal. No doubt, genetic factors influence the canal size but an adverse environment is probably important to impairing its growth.

Trefoil-Shaped Canal

The differential growth of the canal in the midsagittal and interpedicle planes makes possible a hypothesis about trefoil development. The Spitalfield study suggested that trefoil-shaped canals have a smaller midsagittal diameter ($p = .029$) and a larger interpedicular diameter ($p = .049$) than do non–trefoil-shaped canals at L5.[11a] Impaired neuroosseous development in infancy can result in a permanently small midsagittal diameter. In the absence of catch-up growth, the canal remains shallow. An improved environment can permit an adequate stature, with the vertebral bodies enlarging, and the pedicles widening. The interpedicle diameter increases, and the canal develops a trefoil configuration.

Relative Size of the Vertebral Canal and Its Contents

It might be expected that a person with a small canal is at no greater disadvantage than an individual with larger canal dimensions because of the relative size of the canal contents, that is, a small canal housing a small cauda equina. In utero, however, when the conus is in the sacral canal, the epigenetic influence of the spinal cord on the surrounding bony structures causes the size of the cord and the canal to be related. Impaired neuroosseous development results in a small spinal canal and small-sized contents. In infancy, as the conus rises to L2, improved nutrition may be too late to benefit the sagittal diameter of the canal, but with improving stature, longer limbs, good muscles, and large peripheral nerves, the cauda equina is relatively large within a

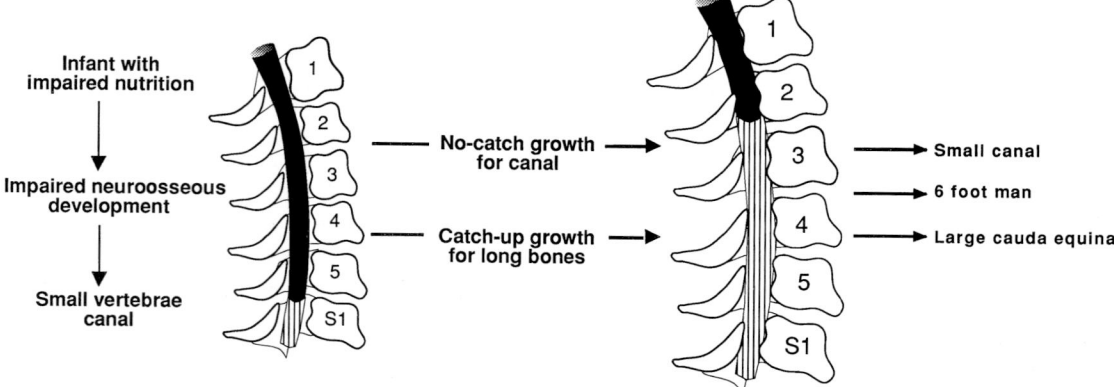

Figure 3. The vertebral canal's capacity in utero is probably influenced by the size of the cord. In childhood when the conus rises to L2, the cauda equina may become large after some catch-up growth. However, the small cross-sectional area of the vertebral canal remains, producing a cauda equina at risk.

shallow canal (Fig. 3). This can be a clinically dangerous situation if that canal is pathologically compromised. Unless there is a disparity between canal size and contents, it is difficult to explain the body of literature on the clinical relevance of the small canal.

SPINA BIFIDA AND SPONDYLOLYSIS

The neural tube develops in a craniocaudal manner and is usually complete at the 26th day of gestation. Failure of the neural tube to close results in spina bifida overta, and failure of the neural arch to close results in spina bifida occulta. Some evidence suggests that spina bifida occulta is not a single segmental lesion but that its presence is related to changes in the more proximal vertebrae. In an examination of the size of the vertebral canal proximal to the spina bifida occulta in affected skeletons, a significant increase in the midsagittal diameter at the two more proximal levels ($p < .01$) was found.[18] In the Spitalfield collection studies,

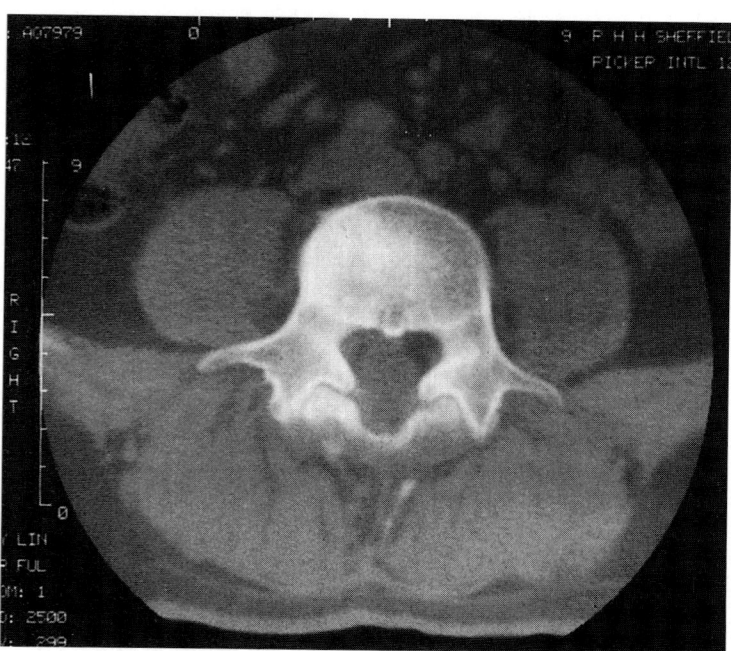

Figure 4. A CT scan of a patient with isthmic spondylolisthesis at L5, showing a large midsagittal diameter.

the cross-sectional area of the lumbar canal proximal to the spina bifida was significantly larger than that in unaffected spines ($p = .041$). A delay in closure of the neural arch influences at least the two more proximal vertebrae, leaving them wider than those of other skeletons without dysraphism.

Neural tube defects are probably related to periconception vitamin deficiencies,[22] particularly folic acid deficiency.[8] If spina bifida occulta and overta were related, it might be assumed that a vitamin deficiency was responsible also for spina bifida occulta, with a delay in closure of the neural arch with a wide canal proximally. However, evidence suggests that the occult and overt lesions are independent conditions.[22]

Vertebral displacement in isthmic spondylolisthesis widens the sagittal diameter of the central vertebral canal as the floating lamina is left behind, articulating with the next caudal segment (Fig. 4). Usually the pars interarticularis is elongated and the canal is dome shaped. The trefoil configuration is unusual in the presence of spondylolisthesis. For this reason, it is unusual to find an isthmic spondylolisthesis in patients with a symptomatic disc lesion or neurogenic claudication.[15] The large vertebral canal protects the cauda equina. Vertebrae with unilateral spondylolysis are asymmetric in shape, and the asymmetry of the canal provides some understanding of the changes observed in bilateral spondylolysis. Elongation of the pars, horizontal orientation of the lamina, and asymmetry of the inferior apophyseal joints and the posterior elements are found. The combination of these effects produces a rotation of the spinous process away from the side where the lesion occurs, and the inferior apophyseal joint on the side of the defect is placed more dorsally than the superior joint. This produces a unilaterally capacious vertebral canal (Fig. 5).

NEUROOSSEOUS DEVELOPMENT AND THE IMMUNE SYSTEM

Clark[1] suggested that infantile malnutrition not only might impair the development of the vertebral canal but also may similarly affect the developing immune and central nervous systems. It is believed that interfer-

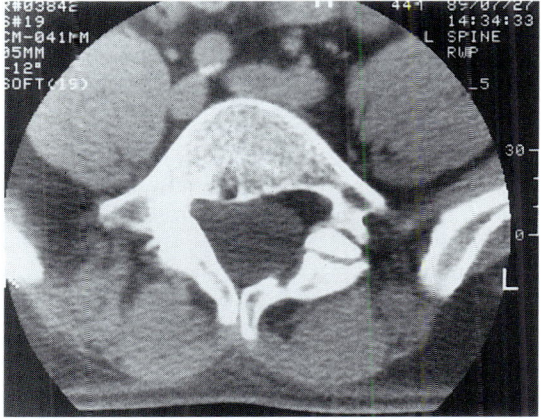

Figure 5. A CT scan of a unilateral spondylolysis at L5, with asymmetric increase in the canal.

ence with a baby's development during sensitive periods has permanent effects on programming of later development. If the hypothesis is correct, it might be expected that a small vertebral canal in an adult, being a marker of deficient early development, would also be associated with poor function of the immune and central nervous systems in that adult. The growth curves of the thymus and of the central nervous system are similar to that for the spinal neuroosseous development; they have the same sensitive periods and they are likely to be simultaneously affected by an adverse environment.

A relationship exists between the size of the vertebral canal and the thymus hormone thymosin α_1.[3] This is supported by the observation that adults with spinal stenosis more frequently have infections in childhood and in later adulthood than do subjects with wider canals.[17]

A comprehensive medical examination was conducted on two groups of patients with back pain. The first group had vertebral canals wider than the mean at L5, and the second group had canals smaller than the mean. Those with smaller canals had significantly more cardiovascular symptoms ($p = .04$) and significantly more gastrointestinal diseases ($p = .048$) than did those with wider canals, but there was no difference in the frequency of respiratory symptoms.[19]

There is also evidence that the academic performance of children with wider vertebral canals at 16 years of age is better than that of their peers with smaller canals; this may, of course, be a reflection of their socioeconomic status rather than of their early neurologic development. In a study of patients with back pain who had wider and narrower canals, those with narrower canals had fewer college and university qualifications than did those with wider canals ($p = .04$) and their poorer performance in vocabulary tests approached significance.

Evidence is accumulating, suggesting that subjects with spinal stenosis are disadvantaged, not only in relation to back pain, but also in their general health and academic status. A search for factors that affect spinal growth is likely to have significance beyond the investigation of back pain. The search should probably concentrate on the most rapid phase of growth, from the 8th to 16th weeks in utero, when the crown-rump length of the fetus increases from about 5 cm to 15 cm.[24] Specific insults to the sensitive enzyme systems at this stage are likely to be more significant than maternal malnutrition, to which the fetus is remarkably resistant.[11] A study of the relationship of such factors to the subsequent canal size could be rewarding, and their recognition may have considerable medical, social, and economic impact.

REFERENCES

1. Clark, G. A.: Heterochrony, Allometry and Canalization in the Human Vertebral Column: Examples from Prehistoric Amerindian Populations. Thesis. Boston, Graduate School of the University of Massachusetts, 1985, pp. 375–381.
2. Clark, G. A., Panjabi, M. M., and Wetzel, F. T.: Can infant malnutrition cause adult vertebral stenosis? Spine 10:165–170, 1985.
3. Clark, G. A., Hall, N. R., Aldwin, C. M., et al.: Measures of poor early growth are correlated with lower adult levels of thymosin α_1 J. Human Biol. 60:436–451, 1988.
4. Edward, W. C., and La Rocca, S. H.: The developmental segmental sagittal diameter in combined cervical and lumbar spondylosis. Spine 10:42–49, 1985.
5. Epstein, J. A., Epstein, B. S., and Levine, I.: Nerve root compression associated with narrowing of the lumbar spinal canal. J. Neurol. Neurosurg. Psychiatry 25:165–176, 1982.
6. Farfan, H. F., and Gracovetsky, S.: The nature of instability. Spine 9:714–719, 1984.
7. Forsberg, L., and Walloe, A.: Ultrasound in sciatica. Acta Orthop. Scand. 53:393–395, 1982.
8. Harris, R.: Vitamins and neural tube defects. Br. Med. J. 296:80–81, 1988.
9. Heliovaara, M., Vanharanta, H., Korpi, J., and Troup, J. D. G.: Herniated lumbar disc syndrome and vertebral canals. Spine 11:433–435, 1986.
10. Kornberg, M., and Rechtine, G. R.: Quantitative assessment of the fifth lumbar spinal canal by computed tomography in symptomatic L4/L5 disc disease. Spine 10:328–330, 1985.
11. Ounstead, M. C.: On fetal growth rate. Clin. Dev. Med. 46:9–16, 1973.
11a. Papp, T., and Porter, R. W.: The growth of the lumbar vertebral canal. Spine 19:2270–2273, 1994.
12. Porter, R. W., Wicks, M., and Hibbert, C.: The size of the lumbar spinal canal in the symptomatology of disc lesion. J. Bone Joint Surg. 60B:485–487, 1978.
13. Porter, R. W., Hibbert, C., and Wellman, F.: Backache and the lumbar spinal canal. Spine 8:99–105, 1980.
14. Porter, R. W., and Hibbert, C.: Relationship between the spinal canal and other skeletal measurements in a Romano-British population. Ann. R. Coll. Surg. Engl. 63:437, 1981.
15. Porter, R. W., and Hibbert, C. S.: Symptoms associated with lysis of the pars interarticularis. Spine 9:755–758, 1984.
16. Porter, R. W., and Pavitt, D.: The vertebral canal: I. Nutrition and development, an archaeological study. Spine 12:901–906, 1987.
17. Porter, R. W., Drinkall, J. N., Porter, D. E., and Thorp, L.: The vertebral canal: II. Health and academic status, a clinical study. Spine 12:907–911, 1987.
18. Porter, R. W., Mills, C., and Powers, R.: Is Spina bifida a bonus? Presented to the International Society for the Study of the Lumbar Spine Meeting, Miami, 1988.
19. Porter, R. W., and Oakshott, G.: Spinal stenosis and health status. Spine 19:901–913, 1994.
20. Salibi, B. S.: Neurogenic claudication and stenosis of the lumbar spinal canal. Surg. Neurol. 5:269–272, 1976.
21. Sarpyener, M. A.: Congenital stricture of the spinal canal. J. Bone Joint Surg. 27:70–79, 1948.
22. Schweitzer, M. E., Balsam, D., and Weiss, R.: Spina bifida occulta. Incidence in parents of offspring with spina bifida cystica. Spine 18:785–786, 1993.
23. Smithells, R. W., Sheppard, S., and Schorah, C. J.: Apparent prevention of neural tube defects by periconceptional vitamin supplementation. Arch. Dis. Child. 56:911–918, 1981.
24. Thompson, D. W.: Maximum velocity of growth at 4th month intrauterine life. In Growth and Form, 2nd Ed. London, Cambridge University Press, 1942.
25. Van Gelderen, V.: Ein orthotisches (lordotisches) Kaudasyndrom. Acta Psychiatr. Neurol. 23:57–68, 1958.
26. Verbiest, H.: A radicular syndrome from developmental narrowing of the lumbar vertebral canal. J. Bone Joint Surg. 36B:230–237, 1954.
27. Winston, K., Rumbaugh, C., and Colucci, V.: The vertebral canals in lumbar disc disease. Spine 9:414–417, 1984.

Pathophysiology of Neurogenic Claudication

RICHARD W. PORTER

The term claudication of the spinal cord was first used by DeJerine[10] when describing three patients with claudication symptoms but normal peripheral pulses. Van Gelderen[31] reported the case of a patient with symptoms of lumbar root compression that appeared on walking and were relieved by rest. Van Gelderen believed that the compression was the result of thickening of the ligamentum flavum. Bergmark[2] described intermittent spinal claudication, attributing a neurospinal origin to the walking pains of two patients. Verbiest in 1954[32] recognized that structural narrowing of the vertebral canal could compress the cauda equina and produce claudication symptoms. Since that time, it has become apparent that the etiology is multifactorial.

CAUSATIVE FACTORS

Developmental Stenosis

Neurogenic claudication is invariably associated with a shallow vertebral canal. The term spinal stenosis has unfortunately become synonymous with neurogenic claudication, whereas a shallow canal is only one factor in the pathologic process, and spinal stenosis can be an important factor in other back pain syndromes. Other factors must be involved because symptoms of claudication develop after middle life, and yet there is no evidence that the vertebral canal becomes much narrower with age. There may be a little encroachment into the canal from hypertrophy of the apophyseal joints and from the formation of marginal osteophyte, into both the root canal and the central canal. Also, posterior vertebral bar formation on the lower and upper posterior margins of the vertebral bodies can reduce the sagittal diameter to some degree. In general, however, the central canal retains the same cross-sectional diameter throughout life. A person with spinal stenosis and neurogenic claudication therefore has had a narrow canal for many years before the development of leg symptoms,[1, 9, 27] and many patients with stenotic canals never have claudication pain. Magnetic resonance imaging studies of asymptomatic subjects older than 60 years of age show spinal stenosis in 21%.[5] The size of the canal is therefore but one factor in the pathologic process.

Degenerative Stenosis

A second factor in neurogenic claudication is degenerative disease of the lumbar spine, which is often associated with manual work. Many patients with neurogenic claudication have been involved in heavy physical work. Few have been sedentary workers. It seems that the cumulative effects of the mechanical stress of laboring play a part in a multiple-segment pathologic state and is a more likely cause than the degenerative process from one disc insult in the earlier life of a sedentary worker. The high incidence of neurogenic claudication in men may be a result of the heavier manual work performed by men or it may indicate that hormonal factors are significant. Thickening of the ligamentum flavum[28] or ossification[14, 15] may be responsible for stenosis. Diffuse idiopathic spinal hyperostosis (DISH) can precipitate stenosis when it is associated with a developmentally small canal. Neurogenic claudication is unusual in children, but Birkensfeld and Kasdon[3] described it in two adolescent boys with congenital lumbar ridges that produced ventral defects on myelograms.

Vertebral Displacement

Vertebral displacement with an intact neural arch critically narrows an already small canal (Fig. 1). Degenerative spondylolisthesis effectively reduces the canal size at the level of displacement.[25, 33] Although degenerative spondylolisthesis is more common in women, half of the men with neurogenic claudication in one series had a degenerative spondylolisthesis.[22] Women with degenerative spondylolisthesis rarely have claudication symptoms, but many patients with unilateral claudication and lumbar scoliosis are women. Displacement of a stenotic spine is therefore only one factor among many.

Abnormal Nerve Function

The neuropathologic process is probably the result of inadequate oxygenation or accumulation of metabolites in the cauda equina in patients with claudication. Nerve function is just adequate at rest but inadequate during exercise. The effect of nerve compression has been extensively studied in animal experiments,[11, 19, 26] but how this is related to chronic stenosis and symptoms during walking has so far been purely speculative.

Central Canal Stenosis at One Level

Central stenosis at one level does not account for the symptoms. Although it is not possible to make the diagnosis of neurogenic claudication without central canal stenosis, there are a number of clinical reasons why central stenosis alone does not explain the mechanism. First, a steadily progressing spinal tumor can completely block the central vertebral canal without producing claudication. Second, a large central disc protrusion can block the canal without claudication. Third, a single-level central stenosis from degenerative changes at L3–L4 or L4–L5 may almost occlude the dural sac and yet produce only back pain. Furthermore, imaging studies of asymptomatic subjects confirm that stenosis is common, and patients who have claudication must have had asymptomatic stenotic canals for many years. Again, it is surprising that in canine studies a single-level experimental stenosis constricted the cauda equina by 25% without causing neurologic deficit.[11] In addition, why claudicating patients frequently have multiple-level central stenosis (Fig. 2) and associated root canal stenosis must be explained.

Root Canal Stenosis

If central canal stenosis does not explain the symptoms of neurogenic claudication, can root canal stenosis be responsible? A number of investigators have thought that root canal stenosis or foraminal stenosis had etiologic significance.[6, 8, 13, 18] However, isolated stenosis of the root canal might be asymptomatic or might sometimes be responsible for symptoms of root entrapment. If root canal pathologic processes are important, why do patients with neurogenic claudication invariably have a central canal stenosis? It is now apparent that the pathophysiology of neurogenic claudication can be explained only in terms of pathologic conditions at multiple levels.

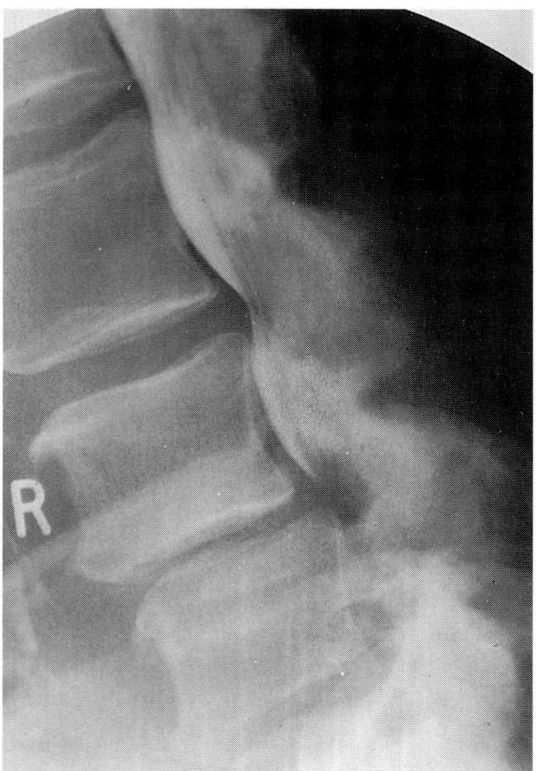

Figure 1. Lateral myelogram of a patient with bilateral neurogenic claudication. There is a degenerative spondylolisthesis at L3–L4, causing a total block to the flow of metrizamide, and a subtotal block at L2–L3.

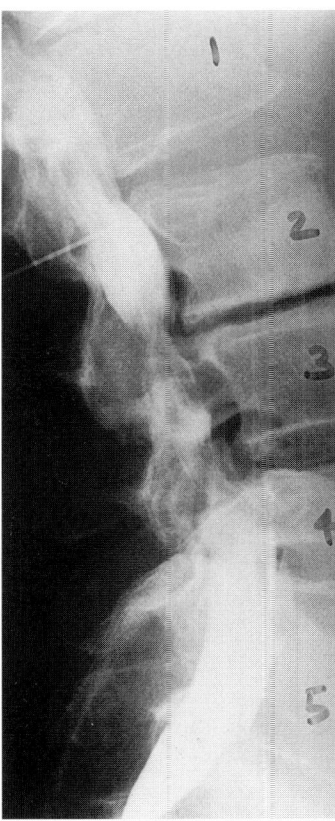

Figure 2. Lateral myelogram of a patient with bilateral neurogenic claudication showing a double-level total block at the L2–L3 and L3–L4 levels.

Two-Level Low-Pressure Stenosis—Venous Pooling

One of the radiologic features of neurogenic claudication is the high frequency of multiple-level stenosis. In myelographic and computed tomographic studies of 50 patients with neurogenic claudication, 47 patients had spinal stenosis at two or more levels.[23] There was either a two-level central stenosis or central stenosis associated with root canal stenosis. Two of the three patients with a single-level central stenosis had a lumbar scoliosis and unilateral claudication. The third patient had marked associated peripheral vascular disease. Clinically, a two-level stenosis is an important component of neurogenic claudication.

A two-level stenosis hypothesis agrees with the previously reported clinical observations of pathologic processes at multiple levels in claudicating patients. It agrees also with the observations of McGuire and colleagues,[16] who observed two claudicating patients with intradural spinal tumors who also had preexisting spinal stenosis at a second level.

The anatomic characteristics of the root veins make the roots vulnerable to venous congestion at the uncompressed segment between the two blocks. The veins of the roots (which do not anastomose between roots) drain distally to the foramen or, if this is blocked, proximally to the conus. A single block affects only a small section of root, but there is congestion and pooling in a larger segment between two blocks. The arterioles continue to feed the segment at the higher arterial pressure, but impaired drainage reduces the blood flow, oxygen supply, and nutrition, with a buildup of metabolites in the uncompressed segment between the two blocks.

This hypothesis is compatible with the findings of experimental studies. A single-level compression of 10 mmHg in a porcine cauda equina model had little effect on function, whereas a two-level compression of 10 mmHg caused a reduction of blood flow by 64%[30] and significantly reduced protein transport and nerve conduction.[20] A hypothesis of two-level compression below arterial pressure is also supported by the findings of myeloscopy studies, which showed a congested cauda equina in claudicating patients.[21]

A two-level stenosis hypothesis must include at least one level of central canal stenosis, but the stenosis at the second level can be in either the central canal or the root canal. Two levels of central stenosis cause venous congestion in all the roots of the cauda equina (Fig. 3). Central canal stenosis at one level and bilateral root canal stenosis at the lower level congests two roots. However, proximal central canal stenosis and distal unilateral root canal stenosis produce only a single root congestion (Figs. 4 and 5). This explains why the symmetric displacement at a degenerative spondylolisthesis usually produces bilateral and not unilateral claudication. The degenerative process is symmetric, with central canal stenosis at one level and symmetric bilateral root canal stenosis at a second level. Asymmetric degeneration produces root claudication (Fig. 6). Women are probably not as vulnerable as men to neurogenic claudication because of

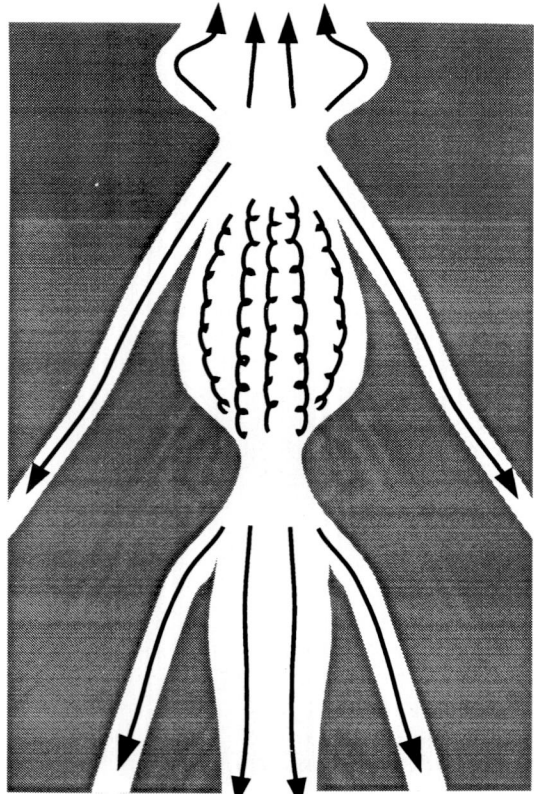

Figure 3. Diagram showing how a double-level central canal stenosis at low pressure (10 mmHg) will cause venous pooling of the cauda equina in the intervening segment (a situation often present in bilateral claudication).

volved. First, there is localized vasodilation of the radicular arteries in response to exercise. Exercising the single limb of a mouse produces vasodilation of the ipsilateral region of the spinal cord.[4] In addition, the selective paralysis in poliomyelitis is probably related to the vasodilation of the anterior horn in response to muscular activity in the preparalytic stage of the disease.[7] Blood flow to the nerve roots is also increased with peripheral nerve stimulation.[29] It therefore might be expected that the arteries of the cauda equina dilate with exercise and, if space is already at a premium, increases the stenosis block to above venous pressure. With exercise, localized vascular swelling then precipitates a venous block. This arterial vasodilation, however, probably fails in patients with claudication.

The author's group[1a] has used the porcine model of Olmarker and colleagues[20] to measure blood flow in the cauda equina. Stimu-

its multisegmental pathologic processes. Women, who have degenerative spondylolisthesis more frequently than men, rarely have bilateral claudication because their pathologic condition is unisegmental. Men with degenerative spondylolisthesis, however, frequently have a multiple-level pathologic condition and bilateral claudication symptoms.

Dynamics of Walking

Many factors are responsible for neurogenic claudication, with stenosis at various levels and the variable degree of segmental motion producing different patterns of symptoms.

Failed Arterial Response

Claudication is related to the dynamic activity of walking. Several factors are in-

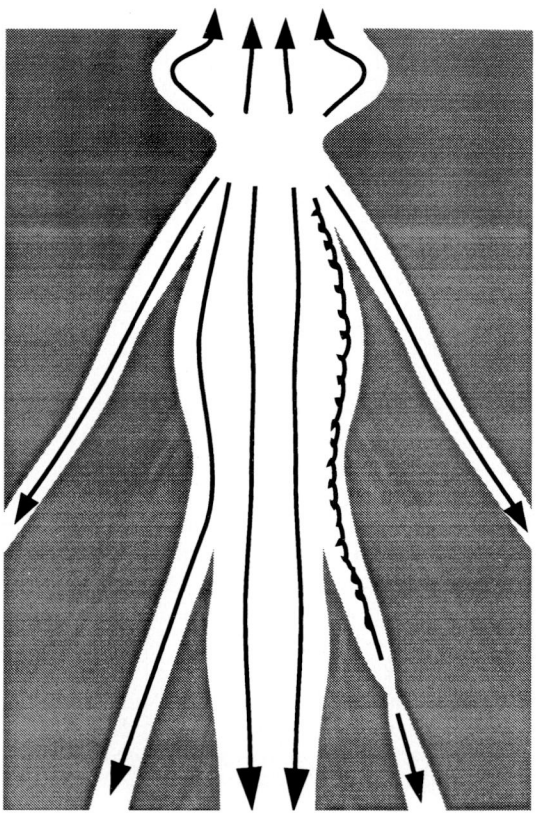

Figure 4. Diagram showing how a central canal stenosis and a more distal root canal stenosis will cause venous congestion of a single root (a situation often present in unilateral claudication).

lation of the proximal cauda equina electrically, causing tail muscle activity, rapidly increases the blood flow to approximately 300% of resting levels. This was maintained during 30 minutes of stimulation. After applying a double-level low-pressure (10 mmHg) compression, without stimulation, the blood flow in the intervening segment of cauda equina fell to approximately 36% of the precompression level. When the cauda equina was then stimulated electrically, the flow increased to 100% above the original resting level, but this rise was slow and was not maintained. Within 5 minutes, blood flow fell to 40% of the original resting flow. If this phenomenon occurs in patients with a double-level low-pressure stenosis, claudi-

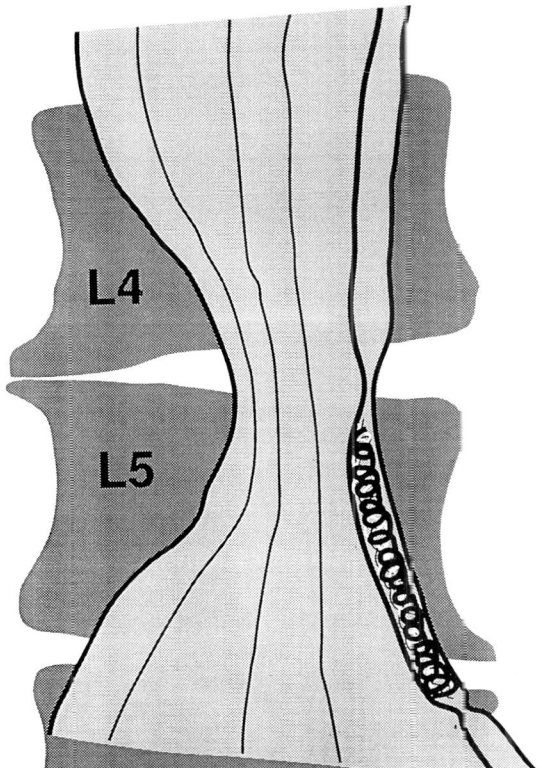

Figure 6. Diagram showing how a degenerative lumbar scoliosis produces a central canal stenosis at one level and a root canal stenosis distally, causing venous congestion of one root.

cation may result from failure of the arteriolar vasodilation response to exercise. In the presence of venous pooling, the arterial vasodilation may be short lived, followed by a failure of motor activity in the legs.

An arterial component to the pathophysiology of neurogenic claudication would explain the common association between neurogenic claudication and peripheral arterial disease.[12, 15] It would also account for the observation that neurogenic claudication generally occurs in only the age group in which arteriosclerosis is common. Arteriosclerosis of the cauda equina vessels may contribute to failed vasodilatation during exercise in the presence of venous pooling.

Segmental Rotation

Segmental rotation, which accompanies walking, reduces the available space in an already narrow canal, especially in the presence of segmental instability. This may be

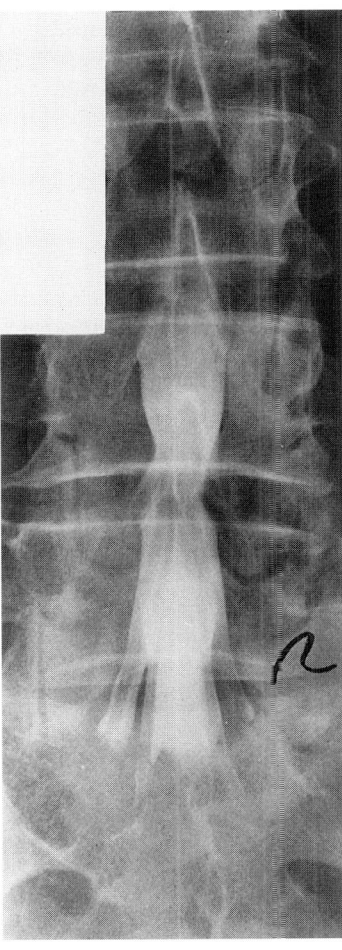

Figure 5. Myelogram of a patient with unilateral claudication. There is a central canal stenosis at L4–L5 and lack of filling of the L5 root in the root canal at L5–S1. A CT scan is preferable for demonstrating root canal stenosis.

more significant in the root canal, where the degenerated capsule of the facet joint limits available space for the nerve root complex.

Baston Venous Plexus

Increased venous return from the exercising lower limbs is accompanied by engorgement of the pelvic veins and of the Baston venous plexus, thereby reducing the available space for the cauda equina. Extradural venous engorgement then contributes to the block pressure.

Lumbar Artery Shunt

A lumbar artery shunt may exist, which when the patient is walking shunts blood from the lumbar vertebrae to the cauda equina. Vasoconstriction of the intraosseous arterial branches of the lumbar arteries may shunt blood to the radicular branch. In addition, a reduced arterial supply to the vertebral body is then associated with a reduced venous return and low pressure in the extradural venous plexus. If this shunt fails as a result of a bony degenerative process, symptoms of neurogenic claudication might develop in times of physiologic stress if there is restricted space in the vertebral canal. The arterial supply to the roots is impaired, and the Batson extradural plexus is congested.

Cerebrospinal Fluid

As yet, we do not know the importance of the cerebrospinal fluid (CSF) in the normal function of the cauda equina. It is possible that CSF contributes to the mechanics of neurogenic claudication. The cauda equina probably needs to be bathed in a free circulation of CSF for its nutrition, for the removal of metabolites, and for insulation. When the amount of fluid is deficient because of reduced space in the canal, and especially when there is a closed sac of fluid, the CSF circulation is inadequate and the roots are vulnerable to the effects of venous congestion. Magnaes[15] recorded a high CSF pressure in claudicating patients caudal to a stenosed segment and related to posture, with block pressure being relieved by flexion. This could explain a situation in which a claudicating patient stops after a few hundred yards and leans forward on a wall for a minute, and as the fluid above the stenosis is permitted to exchange with the closed sac below, the discomfort rapidly clears from the legs.

Lower Limbs

Although the primary pathologic process of neurogenic claudication is multiple-level spinal stenosis with venous pooling of the cauda equina and a failed arterial vasodilatory response in the cauda equina, the nociceptive source is possibly in the lower limbs. The symptoms of neurogenic claudication are so like those of intermittent claudication that they may share a common pain source—muscle ischemic pain. Muscle arterioles may not dilate in intermittent claudication because of pathologically affected arteries. In neurogenic claudication, they may not dilate because of neurogenic failure. The finding of initial studies of lower limb blood flow with positron emission tomography neither support nor refute this hypothesis.

SUMMARY

The evidence to date suggests that neurogenic claudication occurs when there is a double-level low-pressure stenosis. A two-level central canal stenosis tends to be associated with bilateral claudication. A central canal stenosis and a more distal root canal stenosis are associated with unilateral claudication. Venous pooling occurs with double-level low-pressure stenosis, but this alone does not cause claudication. There are no symptoms at rest; however, during the activity of walking, the normal arterial vasodilatory response fails. With that failure, there is impaired nerve conduction, producing the symptoms of claudication. This is compounded by the activity of walking, which increases the pressure at the site of the stenosis (1) from arterial dilatation within the dura, (2) from a rise in extradural venous pressure, and (3) from the mechanical rotatory effect of walking. Arteriosclerosis probably contributes to the arterial component of the syndrome.

REFERENCES

1. Ami Hood, S., and Weigl, K.: Lumbar spinal stenosis: Surgical intervention for the older person. Isr. J. Med. Sci. 19:169–171, 1983.

1a. Baker, A., Porter, R. W., Kidd, C., and Collins, T.: Failure of the vasodilatation of the cauda equina in a double level compression in a pig model. Spine (in press).
2. Bergmark, G.: Intermittent spinal claudication. Acta Med. Scand. Suppl. 246:30–36, 1950.
3. Birkensfield, R., and Kasdon, D. L.: Congenital lumbar ridge causing spinal claudication in adolescents. J. Neurosurg. 49:441–444, 1978.
4. Blau, J. N., and Rushworth, G.: Observations of blood vessels of the spinal cord and their responses to motor activity. Brain 81:354–363, 1958.
5. Boden, S. D., Davis, D. O., Dina, T. S., et al.: Abnormal magnetic resonance scans of the lumbar spine in asymptomatic subjects. A positive investigation. J. Bone Joint Surg. 72A:403–408, 1990.
6. Bose, K., and Balasybramaniam, P.: Nerve root canals of the lumbar spine. Spine 9:16–18, 1984.
7. Buchtal, F.: Problems of the pathologic physiology of poliomyelitis. Am. J. Med. 6:587–591, 1949.
8. Ciric, L., Michael, A., Mikhael, M. D., et al.: The lateral recess syndrome. A variant of spinal stenosis. J. Neurosurg. 53:433–443, 1980.
9. Critchley, E. M. R.: Lumbar spinal stenosis. Br. Med. J. 284:1588–1589, 1982.
10. DeJerine, J.: La claudication intermittente de la molle epiniere. Presse Med. 19:981, 1911.
11. Delmarter, R. B., Bohlman, H. H., Dodge, L. D., and Biro, C.: Experimental lumbar spinal stenosis. J. Bone Joint Surg. 72A:110–120, 1990.
12. Johansson, J. E., Barrington, T. W., and Amelie, M.: Combined vascular and neurogenic claudication. Spine 7:150–158, 1992.
13. Kirkaldy-Willis, W. H., Wedge, T. H., Yang-Hing, K., et al.: Lumbar spine nerve lateral entrapment. Clin. Orthop. 169:171–178, 1982.
14. Kurihara, A., Tanaka, Y., Tsumura, N., and Iwasaki, Y.: Hyperostotic lumbar spine stenosis. Spine 13:1308–1316, 1988.
15. Magnaes, B.: Clinical recording of pressure on the spinal cord and cauda equina. J. Neurosurg. 57:57–63, 1982.
16. McGuire, R. A., Brown, M. D., and Green, B. A.: Intradural spinal tumors and spinal stenosis. Spine 12:1062–1066, 1987.
17. Miyamoto, S., Takaoka, K., Yonenobu, K., and Ono, K.: Ossification of the ligamentum flavum induced by bone morphogenic protein. J. Bone Joint Surg. 74B:279–283, 1992.
18. Naylor, A.: Factors in the development of the spinal stenosis syndrome. J. Bone Joint Surg. 61B:306–309, 1979.
19. Olmarker, K.: Spinal nerve root compression. Nutrition and function of the porcine cauda equina compressed in vivo. Acta Orthop. Scand. Suppl. 242:1–27, 1991.
20. Olmarker, K., Holm, S., and Rydevik, B.: Single versus double level nerve root compression. An experimental study on the porcine cauda equina with analyses of nerve impulse conduction properties. Clin. Orthop. 279:35–39, 1992.
21. Ooi, Y., Mita, F., and Satoh, Y.: Myeloscopic study on lumbar spinal canal stenosis with special reference to intermittent claudication. Spine 15:544–549, 1990.
22. Porter, R. W., and Hibbert, C.: Calcitonin in treatment of neurogenic claudication. Spine 8:585–592, 1983.
23. Porter, R. W., and Ward, D.: Cauda equina dysfunction: The significance of multiple level pathology. Spine 17:9–15, 1992.
24. Postacchini, F.: Lumbar Spine Stenosis New York, Springer-Verlag, 1988, p. 141.
25. Rosenberg, N. J.: Degenerative spondylolisthesis. Clin. Orthop. 117:112–120, 1976.
26. Rydevik, B. L., Pedowitz, R. A., Hargens, A. R., et al.: Effects of acute, graded compression on spinal nerve root function and structure. Spine 16:487–493, 1991.
27. Salibi, B. S.: Neurogenic claudication and stenosis of the lumbar spinal canal. Surg. Neurol. 5:269–272, 1976.
28. Schonstron, N. R., and Hansson, J. H.: Thickness of the human ligamentum flavum as a function of load: An in vitro experimental study. Clin. Biomech. 6:19–24, 1991.
29. Takahashi, K., Nomura, S., Tomita, K., and Matsumoto, T.: Effects of peripheral nerve stimulations on the blood flow of the spinal cord and the nerve root. Spine 13:1278–1283, 1988.
30. Takahashi, K., Olmarker, K., Holm, S., et al.: Double level cauda equina compression: An experimental study with continuous monitoring of intraneural blood flow in the porcine cauda equina. J. Orthop. Res. 11:104–109, 1993.
31. Van Gelderen, C.: Ein orthotisches (lordotisches) Kaudasyndrom. Acta Psychiatr. Neurol. 23:57–68, 1948.
32. Verbiest, H.: A radicular syndrome from developmental narrowing of the lumbar vertebral canal. J. Bone Joint Surg. 36B:230, 1954.
33. Wilson, C. B., and Brill, F. R.: Spinal stenosis. The narrow lumbar spinal canal syndrome. Clin. Orthop. 122:244–248, 1977.

Classification and Treatment of Spinal Stenosis

History and Classification of Spinal Stenosis
PIETER VAN AKKERVEEKEN

HISTORY

The first description of a narrow vertebral canal was given in 1803 by Portal,[20] a French anatomist, who reported cord compression and paralysis in children severely deformed by rickets. Interestingly, he also mentioned the possibility of a narrow vertebral canal without a neural deficit, in particular when the narrowness developed slowly.

Sarpyener[24] is often quoted as the first one reporting on narrow vertebral canals; he noted narrow vertebral canals in children with congenital deformities of the spine. However, it was Sumita[27] who, 45 years earlier in 1910, described narrow vertebral canals in achondroplastic dwarfs. In 1949, Verbiest[32] published a remarkable observation: a narrow vertebral canal in patients without any disease or pathologic condition in the classic sense. The narrowness was caused by an isolated growth disturbance of the vertebral arch. He therefore coined the term "developmental stenosis." His way of thinking was new: normal structures, not pathologic processes, were causing symptoms. Only a difference in the dimension of the spinal canal and of its contents leads to symptoms.

In 1891, Gowers[10] (a neurologist in London) considered the possibility of lateral stenosis, obviously without using this term. He concluded from observations of the vertebrae of old people that "narrowing of the foramina may damage the nerve roots" and that "radiating pains may be produced, sometimes even a descending neuritis." He too mentioned the concept of asymptomatic pathologic states in lateral stenosis, writing "it has occasionally been found out at the postmortem examination without being suspected during life."

Putti, professor of Orthopedics in Bologna, wrote extensively in the 1920s about nerve root entrapment caused by degenerative changes of the facet joints. After his presentation of the Lady Jones lecture in London,[22] these concepts became well known in Europe. History, however, follows an unpredictable course. After the work of Mixter and Barr[16] was published, World War II intervened, and the knowledge of Putti was forgotten. It took nearly 30 years before these concepts were rediscovered. In 1955, Schlesinger[25] published reports of entrapment of the first sacral nerve root in a "lateral bony recess." Epstein[7] expanded on this concept and described in 1960 the clinical, radiologic, and pathoanatomic features of "lateral recess stenosis." Subsequently, Hadley,[11] a radiologist, correlated pathologic changes and radiologic observations of a narrow lumbar intervertebral foramen. Without using these terms, he described what was later called by Ray[23] and by Burton[3] up-down and front-back stenosis. Also, owing to the work of Crock,[5] Getty and colleagues,[9] Kirkaldy-Willis and Yong Hing,[13] Macnab,[14,15] and others,[4,18,21,28,29,31] knowledge about lateral stenosis evolved systematically. For an extensive overview of the historical developments the monographs of Verbiest[33] and Nixon[18] are recommended.

DEFINITIONS

The term stenosis is derived from an old Attic Greek word στενοσ or στεγνοσ and related to the Ionic Greek word στινοσ. These words are best translated as "being narrow." In medical terminology, a prefix, in this case steno-, may indicate pathologic conditions or anthropologic, biologic, or morphologic properties, whereas the suffix -osis always means a pathologic condition.

Verbiest[34,35] concluded that in the 19th century the term stenosis was used mainly to indicate impeded transport of fluid through channels in the circulatory, urogenital, and gastrointestinal tracts. In his opinion, the term narrowness is, in relation to the spine, linguistically preferable to the term stenosis.

Stenosis is defined by Verbiest[35] as an abnormal narrowness of cavities, tubular organs, orifices, or valves and is capable of producing disease through its influence on the contents. Stenosis is subdivided into transport stenosis and compressive stenosis. Transport stenosis is related to fluids and gases, whereas compressive stenosis causes symptoms by compression of living tissue. Lumbar stenosis is obviously a subclass of compressive stenosis. Compression of nervous tissue in the spine may occur at two opposite sides of that tissue or may be circumferential.

When dura and cauda equina are compressed in a narrow vertebral canal, canal stenosis is present. This entity is also often called central stenosis. The latter term should not be used, because as Verbiest[35] stated, "stenosis always reduces the periphery of an enclosed space and therefore the term central is a misnomer."

Lateral stenosis is an entity in which a nerve root, a dorsal root ganglion, or a spinal nerve is entrapped in its pathway.[28] This entity includes lateral recess stenosis and the far-lateral syndrome (see under Taxonomy). The term stenosis describes a morphologic condition and does not per se include symptoms. Symptoms and signs make up the clinical presentation and include neurogenic intermittent claudication, nerve root compression, radiculopathy, and atypical leg pain (see below).

Verbiest[33, 35] defined neurogenic intermittent claudication as "the onset of pain, tension and weakness upon walking in one or both legs, progressively increasing until walking becomes impossible and subsequent disappearance of symptoms after a period of rest." Scrutinizing this definition, one notes that symptoms should not be present before walking but should occur during walking and should disappear after a short rest. Furthermore, pain, tension, and weakness must be present in combination. In a great number of patients, however, only pain restricts the walking distance. For these patients and for patients in whom the leg pain decreases during sitting but does not completely disappear, the term atypical leg pain was introduced.[28]

Patients with a so-called radicular syndrome have nerve root compression. The clinical presentation is characterized by pain in one or both legs, often in a segmental pattern. Positive signs of nerve root compression such as positive findings on the Lasègue test are observed during examination.

Patients with a neural deficit of one nerve root have radiculopathy. Radiculopathy may occur in an isolated fashion, thus without signs of nerve root compression. This may be the case in lateral stenosis but also in a number of other diseases causing polyneuropathy, often without pain.

The term sciatica is derived from the neolatin word ischialgia. Ischialgia is composed from the Attic Greek words αλγοσ, pain, and ισχιον, buttock or hip. Sciatica literally means pain in the lower buttock and the upper part of the thigh.

The term sciatica is often applied to patients with referred pain in a leg. This pain pattern is not a sign of nerve root entrapment and therefore should not be called sciatica. This term is a misnomer and instead the term radicular pain or syndrome has to be used for patients with signs of nerve root compression.[30] To avoid confusion in terminology, sciatic neuralgia, radicular pain, and somatic referred pain should be distinguished.[30] Because the latter radiates into a leg, it is often called pseudoradicular pain, again a misnomer that should not be used. Referred pain is caused by stimulation of certain tissue in the back such as muscles, ligaments, facet joint capsules, and dura.

NATURAL HISTORY

Only one study has been found on the natural history of lumbar spinal stenosis: Johnsson and coworkers[12] observed 32 patients with a mean follow-up of 4 years: 24 patients had neurogenic claudication, four had radicular compression, and four had mixed symptoms. All had stenosis at least at one level. Multilevel stenosis was observed in 11 patients, with a complete block occurring in four patients. At late follow-up, patients were examined, an interview was conducted by using a standard questionnaire with visual analog scales. Three patients were dead at the time of follow-up and two refused to participate. At examination, the walking distance had decreased in eight patients, was unchanged in 9 and increased in 10. The walking distance of the group as a whole, however, did not significantly change. Although symptoms and signs at follow-up were nearly unchanged, symptoms were less severe in many cases.

Johnson and coworkers[12] concluded that the condition of the majority of patients with lumbar stenosis who were treated conservatively remained unchanged over a period of 4 years. However, the patients did not improve either, so surgical decompression may be an option as decompression of the symptomatic level yields a high rate of improvement.

TAXONOMY

Canal Stenosis

Verbiest[33-35] differentiated absolute and relative stenosis. Absolute stenosis is defined by a midsagittal diameter of 10 mm or less. This entity generally results in symptoms and signs as soon as the bony skeleton is mature. Only rare subjects with radiologically absolute stenosis but without symptoms have been described.

The emphasis on bony dimensions is historically understandable, but, in view of modern imaging techniques, is no longer justified. Schönström[26] found a poor correlation in patients with symptoms and signs between the size of the dural sac and the bony dimensions of the lumbar canal. However, a significant difference was observed in the cross-sectional area of the lumbar canal in these patients compared with asymptomatic subjects. This relationship was also experimentally investigated by placing a clamp around the dura of a porcine model and applying gradual constriction while pressure and cross-sectional area were measured in the thecal sac proximally from the clamp and under the clamp.[19] At the moment of pressure rise, the so-called critical size was found (75 ± 13 mm^2). In patients, the cross-sectional area as measured on computed tomographic (CT) scans was 90 ± 35 mm^2. This seems to correlate well with the animal experiments. Additional changes resulting from a change of posture and load to the spine were also measured in axial load, the critical size was 50 ± 30 mm^2; in maximum flexion and extension, it was 40 ± 20 mm^2. This phenomenon may explain the occurrence of symptoms during standing and walking, while symptoms disappear when the patient bends forward or sits. Microcirculatory changes have also been observed in these experiments. Finally, in patients with a cross-sectional area of less than 50 mm^2, a complete block at caudography was seen at that level.

In 1976, a classification of lumbar spinal stenosis[2] was agreed on by a group of pioneers and became widely used. However, this classification is not logical from different points of view and, to prevent confusion and errors in treatment, should not be used:

1. As Verbiest[35] stated in the previous edition of this book, acquired stenosis is "a property of a different pathologic condition and may even be an accidental rather than an essential property of that other condition. Therefore it makes more sense to consider acquired stenosis as a property of that primary abnormality or disease. In the taxonomy of such disease stenosis can be used as an objective indicating a category under the generic name of the underlying disease. For instance, although spondylolisthesis may produce clinically stenotic symptoms and signs, a rational treatment aims at reduction of the slip and stabilization and so corrects the stenosis. This entity should therefore be classified as spondylolisthesis with stenosis (see outline below for secondary stenosis).

2. Verbiest[35] gave a second example of why this classification may lead to errors: in nine patients with degenerative spondylolisthesis, absolute stenosis was present at other levels. By classifying these patients as having acquired stenosis, the possibility of developmental stenosis at a different level may be overlooked. Therefore, a taxonomy including a morphologic and an etiologic classification is desirable.

3. The combination of lateral stenosis and canal stenosis in one classification may also lead to errors in diagnosis and treatment. It is preferable to use classifications for each subclass in the knowledge that clinically these may occur simultaneously at the same or at different lumbar segments. For example, in older patients, degenerative changes may be seen in addition to relative canal stenosis and cause entrapment of a nerve root in its pathway, maybe even on a different segment. Entrapment of a nerve root in the intervertebral canal has been known since the early years of the 20th century

by the terms telescoping articular processes, widening of the joint space with relative forward movement of the superior articular process, vertebral osteophytes impinging on nerve roots, osteophytes of joints, small shifts of vertebral bodies, and nerve root kinked by pedicles.

4. The combined category is also a misnomer as a subcategory of acquired stenosis because congenital or developmental stenosis is already there; the other agents such as degenerative changes, deformity, and tumor are nothing more than additional compressive factors and have to be classified as such.

Postacchini[21] differentiated primary and secondary stenosis. The latter is present in patients with symptoms and signs of stenosis but with normal dimensions of the original vertebral canal. As stated above, the name of the disease causing the stenosis in a given patient with a normal-sized canal has to be used for purposes of classification with the term stenosis as an adjective.

On the basis of these reflections, the following taxonomy of canal stenosis is proposed:

I. Primary Stenosis
    A. Classification of etiology
        1. Congenital
            a. Spinal dysraphism
            b. Failure of vertebral segmentation
            c. Intermittent stenosis, or d'Anquin syndrome
        2. Developmental
            a. Inborn errors of bone growth
                (i) Achondroplasia
                (ii) Morquio disease
                (iii) Hereditary multiple exostosis
            b. Idiopathic
                (i) With bony hypertrophy of the vertebral arch
                (ii) In the absence of this hypertrophy (rare)

Additional factors such as degenerative changes and thickening of the ligamentum flavum may increase the stenosis.

    B. Classification of morphology
        1. Absolute stenosis
        2. Relative stenosis

Until recently, the midsagittal diameter was the diagnostic measure. Because of the work of Olmarker and colleagues,[19] Schönström,[26] and others, this dichotomy seems to be outdated and a continuous scale based on the cross-sectional area and on pressure recordings seems preferable. This needs further research before it can be used clinically.

II. Secondary Stenosis
    1. Spondylolisthesis
        a. Isthmic
        b. Degenerative
    2. Postfusion
        a. On the level of the fusion
        b. Level adjacent to the fusion
    3. Postdiscectomy
        a. Surgically by interlaminar approach
        b. Postchemonucleolysis
    4. Postlaminectomy
    5. Postfracture
    6. Systemic bone diseases
    7. Tumor
        a. Primary
        b. Secondary

Whether stenosis can occur without pre-existing relative stenosis is still controversial. Detailed morphologic studies are needed.

Congenital Stenosis

Stenosis is present at birth as part of a malformation. On the basis of the work of Sarpyener[24] and Nelson,[17] congenital lumbar stenosis was classified by Verbiest[35] as follows:

1. Spinal dysraphism. Symptoms and signs are often caused not only by the narrowness but also by myelodysplasia and other pathologic conditions such as a lipoma.

2. Failure of vertebral segmentation. This entity occurs often in combination with hypoplasia of the facet joints and synostosis of the lamina or spinous processes. Verbiest did not observe different symptoms and signs in these patients as compared with patients with idiopathic developmental stenosis.

3. Intermittent stenosis, or d'Anquin syndrome. In this entity, the spinous process of S1 is absent and the lamina of S1 has a large defect in the middle portion. A piece of bone, probably the hypoplastic spinous process, may be present in this defect. The

downward hooklike elongation of the spinous process of L5 may press on this rudimentary piece of bone, decreasing the midsagittal diameter of the vertebral canal and causing pain in the legs during standing and walking but disappearing when sitting owing to the relief of pressure.

Developmental Stenosis

Developmental stenosis may be due to inborn errors of bone growth.

1. Achondroplasia. The centers of ossification of the vertebral body fuse prematurely with those of the vertebral arches, resulting in short pedicles leading to a narrow canal. The narrowing is increased by thick vertebral arches from excessive periosteal bone apposition after birth. Additional factors such as a bulging disc and osteophytic reactions at the posterior aspect of the vertebral body may cause further narrowing. Disc protrusions increase the narrowing rather frequently. The kyphos resulting from wedge deformities of vertebral bodies may contribute to a gradually increasing neural deficit. Because the pathologic process shows a wide variation, a subclassification can only be broad: (1) upper cervical stenosis—in combination with a narrow foramen magnum and invagination of the odontoid process early death may occur, sometimes even shortly after birth; (2) stenosis at different levels of the cervical, thoracic, or lumbar spine; and (3) stenosis in only one area of the thoracolumbar or lumbar spine. Because of this wide variation, clinical symptoms may occur at about 10 years of age or, at the other end of the scale, older than 40 years. However, in the majority of patients, symptoms develop in the third decade. Verbiest[35] stated that a large percentage of patients face a danger of becoming paraplegic. Neural deficits have been found at careful neurologic examination of asymptomatic achondroplastic dwarfs. Therefore, patients should not be subjected to decompressive surgery before neurologic and radiologic examination of other regions than the suspected segment of the spine. Prophylactic decompression and, in particular, correction of spinal deformity, such as a kyphos should be performed at the same time or soon after decompression of the symptomatic stenotic area.

2. Morquio disease. This entity occurs in the majority of cases with progressive severe spinal deformities such as atlantooccipital instability and odontoid hypoplasia. These deformities frequently cause early death or at least severe neural deficits such as tetraparesis. When the stenosis develops in the lumbar area, this is a better situation because it is not an immediate life-threatening problem.

3. Hereditary multiple exostosis. In this entity, a particular exostose may cause lumbar stenosis. Verbiest[35] differentiated this from the presence of an isolated exostosis in patients with idiopathic developmental stenosis.

Lateral Stenosis

Terminology

According the definition of lateral stenosis, only one nerve root is involved and not the entire cauda equina as in canal stenosis. To describe the location of the entrapment, the term pathway has been introduced[28] because the nerve root, the dorsal root ganglion, and the spinal nerve are located partly inside the vertebral canal, partly in the intervertebral canal, and partly outside. This pathway begins at the point where the nerve root sheath comes off the dural sac and ends lateral to the intervertebral foramen where the spinal nerve merges into the lumbosacral plexus. The nerve root pathway can be divided into four parts: the entrance zone, the middle zone, the exit zone, and the far-lateral zone (Table 1).

1. The entrance zone is located medial to the superior articular process. It has no me-

Table 1

Nerve Root Pathway Terminology	
Term	Synonyms
Entrance zone	Lateral recess, ostium internum, or subarticular zone
Middle zone	Pedicle zone
Exit zone	Ostium externum
Far-lateral zone*	

*Strictly speaking, not part of the pathway of the nerve root but of the spinal nerve.

dial or lateral walls. The often-used term lateral recess is synonymous with this zone.

2. The middle zone is located in the area of the pars interarticularis medial and caudal to the pedicle. The anterior wall is formed by the posterior aspect of the vertebral body; the lateral wall, by the pedicle; and the posterior wall, by the pars interarticularis. A medial wall is lacking.

3. The exit zone is located at the lateral aspect of the pedicle. The anterior wall is formed by the posterior part of the two adjacent vertebral bodies and the intervertebral disc; the posterior wall, by the lateral margin of the inferior articular process of the vertebra above and the superior articular process of the vertebra below; the upper wall, by the caudal margin of the pedicle above; and the lower wall by the cephalad margin of the pedicle below.

4. The far-lateral zone as defined by Wiltse and coworkers[37] is located outside the exit zone.

The term intervertebral foramen is a two-dimensional concept and therefore should not be used.

Clinical Presentation

When patients demonstrate a neurologic deficit related to one nerve root, the diagnosis is made easily. However, the majority of patients with lateral stenosis caused by degenerative changes have no neurologic signs, only pain.[5, 9, 28]

Because lateral stenosis has been observed radiologically in many older subjects who have no symptoms whatsoever,[8, 23, 36] the diagnosis can be difficult in patients with only pain and no localizing signs. The differentiation in these patients between symptomatic and asymptomatic nerve root entrapment is possible by diagnostic nerve root sheath infiltration (see Chapter 3) or by neurophysiologic examination.[6] In the majority of these patients, however, the results of the latter are, in the experience of the author, normal and therefore not helpful in locating the symptomatic nerve root. The diagnostic value of nerve root sheath infiltration, however, has been proven, in particular in multi-level involvement.[4, 14, 28, 29, 31]

In patients with suspected symptomatic lateral stenosis, 4 questions must be answered: (1) What is the cause of the stenosis? (2) In which zone of the nerve root pathway does the stenosis occur? (3) Do the symptoms and signs presented by the patient correlate with the morphologic findings? and (4) Which tissue at that location causes the stenosis? To address these different variables, a taxonomy for each of these criteria has been advocated.[1, 28]

1. Classification based on etiology
    a. Congenital: spinal dysraphism, failure of segmentation
    b. Developmental: uncommon variation in shape, size, or orientation of the articular processes
    c. Degeneration: degenerative spondylolisthesis, osteophyte formation, and loss of disc height with telescoping facets; intraforaminal disc protrusion.
    d. Trauma: burst fracture of the vertebral body leading to a narrow lateral recess; fracture of the superior articular process with dislocation
    e. Tumor: metastases in pedicle and posterior aspect of the vertebral body
2. Classification based on the localization of abnormal narrowing
    a. Ostium internum, or entrance zone (lateral recess)
    b. Pedicle zone, or middle zone
    c. Ostium externum, or exit zone
    d. Far-lateral zone (strictly speaking, no narrowing)
3. Classification based on the clinical presentation
    a. Pain present at rest: atypical leg pain or nerve root compression
    b. Pain only on walking: neurogenic intermittent cladication
    c. Negative findings on Lasègue tests, and so on: atypical leg pain
    d. Positive findings on Lasègue tests and so on: nerve root compression
    e. Impaired nerve root function present at rest: radiculopathy
    f. Impaired nerve root function only on walking: neurogenic intermittent claudication
    g. A combination
4. Classification based on the pathologic anatomy of the narrowness (one factor or a combination of factors)
    a. Ligaments
        (i) Ligamentum flavum: hypertrophy, calcification, ossification
        (ii) Ligamentum longitudinale posterius: calcification

b. Disc
      (i) Bulging annulus in the case of severe degeneration
      (ii) Severe loss of disc height
      (iii) Protrusion
   c. Facet joint
      (i) Synovitis with synovial hypertrophy and effusion
   d. Bone
      (i) Articular process: osteophyte formation, uncommon shape and orientation
      (ii) Vertebral body: osteophyte formation posteriorly or laterally
      (iii) Lamina: hypertrophy spondylolysis with granulation tissue
5. Classification based on pathobiomechanics of the lumbar motion segment as a whole
   a. Fixed rotational deformity
   b. Segmental hypermobility, "dynamic stenosis"

REFERENCES

1. Andersson, G. B. J., and McNeill, T. W.: Lumbar Spinal Stenosis. St. Louis, Mosby–Year Book, 1992.
2. Arnoldi, C. C., Brodsky, A. E., Cauchoix, J., et al.: Lumbar spinal stenosis and nerve root entrapment syndromes, definition and classification. Clin. Orthop. 115:4–6, 1976.
3. Burton, C. V.: On the diagnosis and surgical treatment of lumbar subarticular and "far out" lateral spinal stenosis. In Watkins, R. G., and Collins, J. S. (eds.): Lumbar Discectomy and Laminectomy. Rockville, MD, Aspen, 1987.
4. Castro, W. H. M., and van Akkerveeken, P. F.: Der diagnostischen Wert der selektiven lumbalen Nervenwurzelblockade. Z. Orthop. 129:374–379, 1991.
5. Crock, H. V.: Normal and pathological anatomy of the lumbar spinal nerve root canals. J. Bone Joint Surg. 63B:487–490, 1981.
6. Dvorak, J., Herdmann, J., Theiler, R., and Grob, D.: Magnetic stimulation of motor cortex and motor roots for painless evaluation of central and proximal peripheral motor pathways. Normal values and clinical application in disorders of the lumbar spine. Spine 16:955–960, 1991.
7. Epstein, J. A.: Diagnosis and treatment of neurological disorders caused by spondylosis of the lumbar spine. J. Neurosurg. 17:991–1001, 1960.
8. Falconer, M. A., McGeorge, M., and Begg, A. C.: Observations on the cause and mechanism of symptom production in sciatica and low back pain. J. Neurol. Neurosurg. Psychiatry 11:13–26, 1948.
9. Getty, C. J. M., Johnson, J. R., Kirvan, E. O., and Sullivan, M. F.: Partial undercutting facetectomy for bony entrapment of the lumbar nerve root. J. Bone Joint Surg. 638B:320–335, 1981.
10. Gowers, W. R.: A Manual of Diseases of the Nervous System, 2nd Ed., Vol. 1. London, Churchill, 1891, pp. 263–264.
11. Hadley, M. D.: Anatomico-roentgenographic Studies of the Spine. Springfield, IL, Charles C Thomas, 1964.
12. Johnsson, K. E., Udén, A., and Rosén, I.: The effect of decompression on the natural course of spinal stenosis. A comparison of surgically treated and untreated patients. Spine 16:615–619, 1991.
13. Kirkaldy-Willis, W. H., and Yong Hing, K.: Lateral recess, lateral canal and foraminal stenosis. In: Watkins, R. G., and Collins, J. S. (Eds.): Lumbar Discectomy and Laminectomy. Rockville MD, Aspen, 1987.
14. Macnab, I.: Negative disc exploration. J. Bone Joint Surg. 53A:891–903, 1971.
15. Macnab, I.: The pathogenesis of spinal stenosis. In Hopp, E. (Ed.): Spinal Stenosis. Philadelphia, Hanley & Belfus, 1987.
16. Mixter, W. J., and Barr, J. S.: Rupture of the intervertebral disc with involvement of the spinal canal. N. Engl. J. Med. 211:210–215, 1934.
17. Nelson, M. A.: Spinal stenosis in achondroplasia. Proc. R. Soc. Med. 65:1028–1029, 1972.
18. Nixon, J. E.: Spinal Stenosis. London, Edward Arnold, 1991.
19. Olmarker, K., Rydevik, B., Hansson, T., and Holm, S.: Compression induced changes of the nutritional supply of the porcine cauda equina. J. Spinal Disord. 3:25–29, 1990.
20. Portal, A.: Cours d'anatomie médicale ou éléments de l'anatomie de l'homme. Tome premier. Paris, Baudoin, 1803, p. 299.
21. Postacchini, F.: Lumbar Spinal Stenosis. Vienna, Springer-Verlag, 1988.
22. Putti, V.: The Lady Jones lecture: On new conceptions in the pathogenesis of sciatic pain. Lancet 2:53–60, 1927.
23. Ray, C. D.: Far lateral decompression for stenosis, the paralateral approach to the lumbar spine. In White, A. H., Rothman, R. H., and Ray, C. D. (eds.): Lumbar Spine Surgery. St. Louis, C. V. Mosby, 1987.
24. Sarpyener, M. A.: Congenital stricture of spinal canal. J. Bone Joint Surg. 27:1–15, 1945.
25. Schlesinger, P. T.: Incarceration of the first sacral nerve in a lateral bony recess of the spinal canal. J. Bone Joint Surg. 37A:115–124, 1955.
26. Schönström, N.: The Narrow Lumbar Spinal Canal and the Size of the Cauda Equina in Man. A Clinical and Experimental Study. Thesis. Göteborg, Sweden, University of Göteborg, 1988.
27. Sumita, M.: Beitrage zur Lehre von der Chondrodystrophia foetalis und osteogenesis imperfecta met besonderer Berucksichtigung der anatomischen und klinischen differential Diagnose. Dtsch. Z. Chir. 107:1–110, 1910.
28. van Akkerveeken, P. F.: Lateral Stenosis of the Lumbar Spine. Ph.D. thesis. Utrecht, the Netherlands, University of Utrecht, 1989.
29. van Akkerveeken, P. F.: The symptomatic level in multilevel lateral lumbar stenosis. Presented at the 2nd Annual Meeting of the European Spine Society, Rome, 1991.
30. van Akkerveeken, P. F.: On pain patterns of patients with lumbar nerve root entrapment. Neuro-Orthopedics 14:81–102, 1993.
31. van Akkerveeken, P. F.: The diagnostic value of nerve root sheath infiltration. Acta Orthop. Scand. (Suppl. 251):61–63, 1993.
32. Verbiest, H.: Sur certaines formes rares de compres-

sion de la queue de cheval. I. Les sténoses osseuses du canal vertébral. *In* Hommage à Clovis Vincent. Paris, Maloine, 1949.
33. Verbiest, H.: Neurogenic Intermittent Claudication. New York, North Holland/American Elsevier, 1976.
34. Verbiest, H.: Fallacies of the present definition, nomenclature and classification of the stenosis of the lumbar vertebral canal. Spine 1:217–225, 1976.
35. Verbiest, H.: Lumbar spinal stenosis: Morphology, classification, and long term results. *In* Weinstein, J. N., and Wiesel, S. W. (Eds.): The Lumbar Spine. Philadelphia, W. B. Saunders, 1990, pp. 546–589.
36. Wiesel, S. W., et al.: The incidence of positive CT scans in an asymptomatic group of patients. Spine 9:549–552, 1984.
37. Wiltse, L. L., Guyer, R. D., Spencer, C. W., et al.: Alar transverse process impingement of the L5 nerve: The far out syndrome. Spine 9:31–41, 1984.

Clinical, Radiologic, and Electrodiagnostic Diagnosis of Degenerative Lumbar Stenosis

LAWRENCE T. KURZ
JIRI DVORAK

The clinical diagnosis of degenerative lumbar stenosis (DLS) is based on a history and the findings on physical examination. The majority of patients relate a history of radicular pain in one or both legs, whereas other patients may additionally report paresthesias, numbness, or weakness. Urinary and bowel elimination problems may also be mentioned. The examining physician must inquire about all these symptoms and investigate the conditions under which they occur.

HISTORY OF PRESENT ILLNESS

An evaluation of pain must include its anatomic location, timing, precipitating factors, and quality. Pain is the most common symptom of patients with DLS. Although the majority of patients do have low back pain, this pain is not usually amenable to surgical treatment. Low back pain arises from degenerative disc and joint disease and spondylolisthesis of the lumbar spine, a combination of which nearly always accompanies DLS. Because these conditions tend to occur more often and with more severity in the lower part of the lumbar spine, that region is where this pain is usually experienced. It tends to be an aching type of pain,[3] which is not usually felt as sharp or burning. It tends to be exacerbated or aggravated by walking, standing, bending, or any activity that increases the load on the lumbar spine. As would be expected from any mechanical problem, the pain tends to be diminished by rest, especially in the supine or the lateral decubitus position.

The other type of pain is a radicular type of pain, usually caused by direct compression or tension on the neural structures. Usually occurring down one or both legs, this pain may include or even be limited to the buttock region.[18] Although sharp pains are usually absent, occasionally a jolting pain is felt down the legs after acute hyperextension of the lumbar spine; this jolting pain is caused by a quick and deliberate compression of the neural structures. Most frequently, however, this pain is described as aching or dysesthetic. Classically, it worsens with walking, standing for prolonged periods, hyperextending the lower back,[28, 35] or walking down an incline and is diminished by walking up an incline,[22] sitting, or flexing the lower back. These changes may occur because, as the spine moves from flexion to extension, the spinal canal shortens, nerve tissue and ligamentum flavum shorten and broaden, the disc bulges posteriorly, and there is interference with the microcirculation of the nerve roots and cauda equina.[6]

The anatomic location of the radicular pain usually depends on the location and type of the offending agent producing the DLS. Patients with central stenosis caused by compression from the ligamentum flavum, bilateral posterolateral facet joint osteophytes, central disc protrusions, or spondylolisthesis usually report bilateral and symmetric leg symptoms,[11, 21] classically termed neurogenic claudication. Although typically the pain radiates down the posterolateral aspect of both legs, it usually is not in a specific dermatomal distribution. Although the pain is frequently associated with paresthesias or numbness, gait disturbances and weakness occur less often.

Patients with lateral recess stenosis (LRS) more frequently have a dermatomal component to their pain, even if it occurs bilaterally. This is commonly seen with the LRS that may accompany lumbar spondylolisthesis. Because this occurs most frequently at L4–L5, most patients have symptoms in the L5 distribution. This is because the lateral recess that is encroached on is the lateral recess that contains the L5 nerve root, and it is this compression that is worsened by the tension caused by the spondylolisthesis.

The symptoms of the previous two groups of patients, those with central stenosis and those with LRS, frequently are gradual in onset and may wax and wane over months or years. If the physician elicits a history of these symptoms' occurring while the patient is at rest, the possibility of DLS being the causative agent should not be discounted. The symptoms of these two groups of patients may progress in severity, and neural ischemia may reach such a degree that changes in position no longer relieve symptoms. This is a particularly bad prognostic sign.

The third group of patients have displacement of a lumbar disc as the inciting cause of their stenosis. They have an underlying LRS from osteophyte or facet overgrowth, spondylolisthesis, or simply bilateral central stenosis. Most often, they are asymptomatic until disc displacement occurs. The displacement is usually in the form of a protrusion, although extrusions and sequestrations are seen. Although these patients might have experienced symptoms from their disc displacement anyway, the occurrence of symptoms is usually earlier, more severe and intense, or simply prolonged because of their underlying stenosis. Although central disc displacements do occur in this group, asymmetry is much more common, as evidenced by mostly unilateral radicular pain.

PAST HISTORY

Obtaining a history of medical or surgical problems in the past is also important. Information regarding the present use of prescription medication should be elicited. The amount of pain medication being taken may inform the physician of the severity of symptoms that the patient is experiencing and their impingement on his or her lifestyle. Some antihypertensive medications adversely affect the course of symptoms of DLS. On the other hand, some drugs that counteract congestive heart failure have simultaneously improved neurocirculatory perfusion, thereby diminishing symptoms.

Diabetes mellitus, alcoholism, and other metabolic abnormalities may induce a peripheral neuropathy. Symptoms of peripheral burning[32] or painful dysesthesias are frequently seen and may be confused with symptoms of DLS. Peripheral neuropathy can be differentiated from DLS because it usually begins distally, progresses proximally, is not radicular, and is specifically unaffected by position or activity.

As alluded to above, cardiac disease may contribute to the symptoms of DLS by decreasing neurocirculatory perfusion. Peripheral vascular disease[7] may cause similar symptoms through the same mechanism and occurs in the same age group as patients with DLS. However, symptoms of peripheral vascular disease are usually unaffected by changes in body position. The classic bicycle test[9] may produce positive findings in peripheral vascular disease but negative ones in DLS. Pedaling a bicycle in a sitting position increases the need for arterial blood flow to the lower extremities and therefore leg symptoms are exacerbated in patients with peripheral vascular disease. On the other hand, patients with DLS do not report leg symptoms on the bicycle because the sitting position keeps the lumbar spine flexed, thereby reducing neural compression and ischemia, as previously described.[6, 9]

Knowledge of previous lumbar spine surgery is essential. Postsurgical causes of symptoms similar to those of DLS include spondylolisthesis, arachnoiditis, recurrent stenosis, postfusion stenosis, spinal instability, spinal deformity, infection, and epidural fibrosis.

These elderly patients frequently have other unrelated causes of urinary and bowel elimination dysfunction. Older women frequently have stress incontinence, whereas men frequently have prostatic obstruction. Both groups are prone to constipation because of inactivity, poor eating habits, and medication use. In general, however, excretory dysfunction is not a frequent accompaniment of DLS.[27]

PHYSICAL EXAMINATION

Although a neurologic examination is essential in the evaluation, its findings frequently are unremarkable. Motor weakness, objective sensory deficits, and the presence of reflexes indicative of a pathologic state are all distinctly unusual findings in patients with DLS.[22, 25] However, a number of patients may reveal deficits after exercise or muscular stress.[30]

Although reflexes frequently are diminished or absent, these findings are not useful for clinical diagnosis because the elderly population commonly exhibits these findings, even in the absence of DLS. Straight leg raising test results are usually negative, although an acute disc displacement, superimposed on an underlying stenosis, may lead to a positive finding.

The presence of atrophy of the lower extremity musculature is also not helpful because many elderly patients exhibit muscle wasting in the absence of DLS. On the other hand, diminished distal pulses and hair loss on the legs are frequent accompaniments of peripheral vascular disease, and their presence may indicate arterial disease either concomitant with, or exclusive of, DLS.

Palpable tenderness may be helpful only in differentiating DLS from neurologic symptoms referable to fractures, peripheral tumor masses, or venous thromboses. Gait testing is important in differentiating DLS from myelopathic states (spastic gait), hip and knee arthritides (antalgic gait), and intracerebral or metabolic abnormalities (shuffling or tremorous gait).

Although range of motion testing of the lumbar spine is helpful only when extension exacerbates symptoms, range of motion testing of the hips and knees is always important. Patients in the same age group as those with DLS frequently have concomitant osteoarthritis of the hips and knees. Demonstrating limited or painful range of motion of one or more of these joints may indicate an alternative cause of the patient's symptoms.

The patient's back should be viewed in the standing position as well as in the forward bending position. In this way, scoliosis and kyphosis, the deformity and subluxation of which can cause DLS, can be detected. Knowledge of the direction and magnitude of curves may be helpful in determining the need for appropriate imaging studies, as well as in the planning of surgery.

RADIOLOGIC DIAGNOSIS

Confirmation of a clinical diagnosis of DLS is best accomplished radiologically. Imaging techniques available include plain radiography, myelography, computed tomography (CT), and magnetic resonance imaging (MRI). Each has its own advantages and disadvantages when compared with the others, based on the ability of each to display appropriate pathologic details. The pathologic process in patients with DLS is located in the central canal, the lateral recess, or the neural foramen. Offending agents include ligamentum flavum, enlarged facets, vertebral body or facet osteophytes, displaced discs, narrowed disc spaces, intraspinal synovial cysts, and vertebral subluxations and deformities. All four imaging modalities are compared and contrasted in relation to their ability to demonstrate the appropriate pathologic details and to produce images of certain regions of the spine where the pathologic process occurs.

Plain Radiography

Every patient being evaluated for DLS should have at least three radiographs: anteroposterior pelvis and standing anteroposterior and lateral lumbar spine films. Although classically deemed unhelpful in enhancing the clinical examination, plain radiographs can show some important pathologic entities and may be helpful in ruling out other causes in the differential diagnosis of DLS. An anteroposterior pelvis radiograph can be used to rule out any obvious disease of the hip and sacroiliac joints. As previously stated, hip arthritis is prevalent in this age group. Anteroposterior and lateral lumbar spine radiographs are obtained with the patient standing to accentuate any deformity (scoliosis or kyphosis) or subluxation (usually anterior or lateral listhesis). Rotational abnormalities and disc space narrowing may also be seen. The midsagittal canal diameter can also be measured. Knowledge of its magnitude may indicate an underlying developmental or congenital bony stenosis. Bending or flexion-extension radiographs also allow the stiffness or correctability of deformities and subluxations to be measured. The disadvantages of plain radiographs lie in their inability to demonstrate neural structures, disc material, ligamentum flavum, osteophyte impingement, and the lateral recess. In addition, some radiation exposure is inevitable.

Myelography

The technique of lumbar myelography consists of the injection of a water-soluble contrast agent into the subarachnoid space, usually through a lumbar puncture, distal to the conus medullaris. The dye mixes with the cerebrospinal fluid (CSF) and outlines the neural elements within the thecal sac and nerve root sheaths. It is a sensitive test in detecting DLS. One study[2] found myelography to be more accurate than CT: 93% versus 89%, respectively. The radiographic image displayed with central stenosis is classically described as an hourglass constriction.[24, 31, 33] The image displayed with LRS or posterolateral facet or osteophyte impingement is nerve root cutoff (amputation of the column of dye in the nerve root sheath).

Myelography has a number of advantages over other imaging modalities. The entire lumbar spine is routinely visualized, and therefore lesions of the conus may be detected. Unsuspected (and less frequently occurring) levels of stenosis proximal to L3 may also be detected. The ability to run the dye proximally allows other possible levels of stenosis in the thoracic and cervical spine to be visualized. Extensive clinical experience is available with myelography because for many years it was the gold standard. Hyperextension may be performed during myelography to exacerbate or accentuate underlying but not readily detectable stenosis, thus providing the only dynamic imaging tool for evaluating DLS. Last, samples of CSF can be obtained to rule out other causes in the differential diagnosis, such as demyelinating diseases or intradural tumors.

On the other hand, the disadvantages of myelography are numerous. Although the incidence of arachnoiditis has markedly diminished because water-based contrast has virtually replaced oil-based dye, other complications have not been eradicated completely. Headaches, nausea, seizures, and rarely, infections may occur. Allergic reactions, although minimized by pharmacologic pretreatment, may still occur because the contrast is iodinated. Although central stenosis is visualized well with myelography, the pathologic entity is seen only indirectly, and the offending agent must be inferred from the abnormal appearance of the contrast column. Furthermore, stenosis in the lateral recess and foramen is visualized poorly, if at all. A previous disadvantage of myelopathy, the need for hospital admission, is almost completely eliminated, because it is now routinely performed on an outpatient basis.

Computed Tomography

CT provides direct visualization of all three major regions where pathologic processes are found in DLS: the central canal, the lateral recess, and the neural foramen. In addition, using both bone and soft tissue windows, it allows direct visualization of the offending agents, such as disc herniations, osteophytes, enlarged facets, ligamentum flavum, and intraspinal synovial cysts. Neural structures such as the thecal sac and the nerve roots are fairly well visualized. Some enhancement of visualizing soft tissue and neural structures may be achieved by changing machine settings for contrast and slice thickness. Further advantages are gained with CT scanning because a three-dimensional "feel" for the anatomy present can be achieved when axial images are used. It is noninvasive and is usually performed on an outpatient basis. Loss of epidural fat, a classic criterion for the diagnosis of DLS, is usually fairly well delineated. A CT scan may also provide identifying information regarding pathologic states distal to a complete myelographic block.[15]

CT does, however, have some disadvantages. Without contrast, it poorly visualizes the spinal cord itself. In fact, conus lesions are frequently missed. Routine scanning is from L3 to S1, and it therefore may miss pathologic entities proximal to L3. Older machines may give misinformation because of the inability to change the gantry to obtain images parallel to each disc space. Distortion may also be caused by a partial volume effect from large slice thicknesses. This can sometimes be resolved with reformatting in a sagittal plane.[5, 12] Finally, images of severely obese patients may be grainy because of the thickness of their soft tissues.

Intrathecal contrast medium–enhanced CT scanning does not increase the diagnostic accuracy of DLS. In a review of surgical patients with DLS, the accuracy of CT scanning alone was 83%, of myelography alone was 76%, and of the two combined was 91%.[34] However, the results were not statistically significant. Therefore, there appears to be no well-documented advantage in combining the studies.

Magnetic Resonance Imaging

MRI produces an anatomic image through the use of radiowaves absorbed and reemitted from protons rotating about their axis in a magnetic field. Its accuracy in diagnosing DLS is at least equal to that of CT scanning, contrast-enhanced CT scanning, or myelography.[4, 26, 29] For DLS, the T1-weighted image is useful in evaluating the size and contour of the foramen and conus. The T2-weighted image gives an accurate assessment of the extradural-CSF interface and central canal dimensions.

MRI has many distinct advantages. The patient receives no ionizing radiation, and the test is noninvasive and performed on an outpatient basis. As with myelography, the entire lumbar spine is imaged (at least in the sagittal plane), and soft tissue evaluation of the conus, cauda equina, and nerve roots is better than with CT scanning. Axial and even coronal images may be obtained to enhance diagnosis. Visualization of offending agents such as ligamentum flavum, disc herniations, and intraspinal synovial cysts is superior to that of all other imaging modalities. Specifically, delineating the loss of epidural fat is superior to that with CT scanning and myelography and is extremely useful. Diagnosis of LRS is nearly as good as with CT scanning. Foraminal stenosis is well visualized on sagittal images and renders this technique more useful than CT scanning of pathologic processes occurring in the foramen. MRI usually produces a better image than CT scanning in obese patients.

The disadvantages of MRI are few. Cortical bone (osteophytes) is poorly delineated, which may be important in diagnosing LRS. Patients with nontitanium metal in their lumbar spine; metal shavings around the eyes, brain, or spinal cord; those with pacemakers; and those with severe claustrophobia should be excluded from undergoing MRI. Last, machines with magnets less than 1.5 T or older models may yield low-quality images and render MRI less useful.

For a patient suspected of having DLS, a CT scan from L2 to S1 is probably the appropriate screening test. If it is interpreted as abnormal and surgical treatment is proposed, MRI should be performed. If the results of the CT scan are normal, then MRI is also the appropriate next imaging study if further work-up is indicated. Although an MRI scan might be used as the initial screening test, it is slightly more expensive than a CT scan. Even if MRI were to be used as the screening test, it probably would be followed by a CT scan prior to surgery. This is because universal guidelines for stenosis on sagittal MRI scans are not yet widely accepted. Lumbar myelography may be used in cases in which CT and MRI results are equivocal or when imaging of the entire spine is desired. Lumbar myelography is especially useful in the work-up of patients with DLS secondary to scoliosis or listhesis. In these cases, axial images parallel to disc spaces are difficult to obtain. Furthermore, stenosis from neural tension and distortion (rather than compression) is difficult to demonstrate on CT or MRI studies.

ELECTRODIAGNOSTIC DIAGNOSIS

Electromyography

Electromyography (EMG) evaluates the physiology of nerve roots, which is useful in the evaluation of diseases of the lower motor neuron units, such as DLS. It is performed by inserting an electrode into the desired muscle and recording the muscle's electrical activity at rest and with stimulation. EMG studies in patients with DLS frequently show bilateral multiradicular findings, even when symptoms are only unilateral.[10] Johnsson and coworkers[19] showed a positive correlation between the degree of myelographic block and EMG findings. On the other hand, they also demonstrated that EMG was not a useful predictor of surgical outcome.

Although it is extremely useful in differentiating between peripheral neuropathy and DLS, EMG has some disadvantages. A minimum of 10 days to 6 weeks from the onset of symptoms may be required for abnormalities to be detected. In addition, false-negative results may occur because of overlap in the lumbar and sacral plexus. Involved lower extremity muscle groups may be multiply innervated. Furthermore, EMG measures motor nerve potentials, and thus sensory disturbances are not evaluated.[14] Finally, a significant number of patients with DLS have normal or nonspecific findings on EMG, rendering this test less than helpful.

Nerve Conduction Studies

A nerve conduction velocity test measures the speed at which the nerve impulse travels. It is most helpful in differentiating peripheral neuropathy from radiculopathy.[17]

Somatosensory Evoked Potentials

Somatosensory evoked potentials represent electrical responses of the nervous system to sensory stimulation. The spinal evoked potential is transmitted through the dorsal columns and is mediated by large myelinated fibers sensitive to both mechanical compression and ischemia.[13] The technique involves stimulation of a peripheral nerve, with the signal being picked up by scalp electrodes in preset locations and recorded by a microprocessor.[16]

A number of studies[1, 8, 20, 23] have shown varied results in their ability to diagnose DLS. At present, somatosensory evoked potentials have limited ability to localize stenotic lesions accurately and reproducibly with regard to the type and location of the pathologic process involved.

SUMMARY

Making the diagnosis of DLS is rendered easier by conducting a thorough investigation and paying strict attention to details. The investigation should begin with obtaining a history of the present illness and past medical or surgical conditions, continue with a physical examination, on occasion use electrodiagnostic aids, and conclude with imaging studies. A wise physician makes use of all the information derived to formulate a diagnosis, thereby allowing him or her to offer an appropriate plan for treatment.

REFERENCES

1. Aminoff, M. J., Goodin, D. S., Barbaro, N. M., et al.: Dermatomal somatosensory evoked potentials in unilateral lumbosacral radiculopathy. Ann. Neurol. 17:171–176, 1985.
2. Bell, G. R., Rothman, R. H., Booth, R. E., et al.: A study of computer assisted tomography: Comparison of metrizamide myelography and computed tomography in the diagnosis of herniated lumbar disc and spinal stenosis. Spine 9:552–556, 1984.
3. Blau, J. N., and Logue, V.: Intermittent claudication of the cauda equina. Lancet 1:1081–1086, 1961.
4. Bowden, S., Davis, D., Dina, T., et al.: Abnormal MRI scans of the lumbar spine in asymptomatic subjects. J. Bone Joint Surg. 72A:403–409, 1990.
5. Braun, I., Lin, J. P., George, A. E., et al.: Pitfalls in the computed tomographic evaluation of the lumbar spine in disc disease. Neuroradiology 26:15–20, 1984.
6. Brieg, A.: Biomechanics of the Central Nervous System. Stockholm, Almquist & Wiksell, 1960.
7. Dodge, L., Bohlman, H., and Rhodes, R.: Concurrent lumbar spinal stenosis and peripheral vascular disease. Clin. Orthop. 230:141–148, 1988.
8. Dvonch, V., Scoff, T., Bunch, W. H., et al.: Dermatomal somatosensory evoked potentials: Their use in lumbar radiculopathy. Spine 9:291–293, 1984.
9. Dyke, P., and Doyle, J.: "Bicycle test" of Van Gelderen in diagnosis of intermittent cauda equina compression. J. Neurosurg. 46:667–670, 1977.
10. Epstein, J. A., Epstein, B. S., Rosenthal, A. D., et al.: Sciatica caused by nerve root entrapment in the lateral recess. J. Neurosurg. 36:584–589, 1972.
11. Evans, J.: Neurogenic intermittent claudication. Br. Med. J. 2:985–987, 1964.
12. Glenn, W. V., Jr., Rhodes, M. L., Altschuler, E. M., et al.: Multiplanar display computerized body tomography applications in the lumbar spine. Spine 4:282–352, 1979.
13. Gonzales, E., Hajdu, M., Bruno, R., et al.: Lumbar spine stenosis. Analysis of pre- and post-operative somatosensory evoked potentials. Arch. Phys. Med. Rehabil. 66:11–15, 1985.
14. Haldeman, S.: The electrodiagnostic evaluation of nerve root function. Spine 9:42–48, 1984.
15. Herkowitz, H. N., Garfin, S. R., Bell, G., et al.: The use of computerized tomography in evaluating

novisualized vertebral levels caudad to a complete block on a lumbar myelogram. J. Bone Joint Surg. 69A:218–224, 1987.
16. Herron, L., Trippi, A., and Gonyeau, M.: Intraoperative use of dermatomal somatosensory evoked potentials in lumbar stenosis surgery. Spine 12:379–383, 1987.
17. Hirsch, L. F.: Diabetic polyradiculopathy simulating lumbar disc disease. J. Neurosurg. 60:183–186, 1984.
18. Joffe, R., Appleby, A., and Arjona, V.: Intermittent ischemia of the cauda equina due to stenosis of the lumbar canal. J. Neurol. Neurosurg. Psychiatry 29:315–318, 1966.
19. Johnsson, K. E., Rosen, I., and Udén, A.: Neurophysiologic investigation of patients with spinal stenosis. Spine 12:483–487, 1987.
20. Keim, H. A., Hajdu, M., Gonzalez, E. G., et al.: Somatosensory evoked potentials as an aid in the diagnosis and intraoperative management of spinal stenosis. Spine 10:338–344, 1985.
21. Kirkaldy-Willis, W. H., Paine, K. W. E., Cauchoix, J., et al.: Lumbar spinal stenosis. Clin. Orthop. 99:30–50, 1974.
22. Lipson, S.: Clinical diagnosis of spinal stenosis. Semin. Spine Surg. 1:143–144, 1989.
23. Machida, M., Asai, T., Sato, K., et al.: New approach for diagnosis in herniated lumbosacral disc. Spine 11:380–384, 1986.
24. McIvor, G. W. D., and Kirkaldy-Willis, W. H.: Pathologic and myelographic changes in major types of spinal stenosis. Clin. Orthop. 115:72–76, 1976.
25. Macnab, I.: Spondylolisthesis with an intact neural arch—the so-called pseudospondylolisthesis. J. Bone Joint Surg. 32B:325, 1950.
26. Modic, M. T., Masaryk, T., Boumphrey, F., et al.: Lumbar herniated disc disease and canal stenosis: Prospective evaluation by surface coil MR, CT and myelography. AJR 147:757–765, 1986.
27. Nelson, M. A.: Lumbar spinal stenosis. J. Bone Joint Surg. 55B:506–512, 1973.
28. Rosenberg, N. J.: Degenerative spondylolisthesis. J. Bone Joint Surg. 57A:467–474, 1975.
29. Schnebel, B., Kingston, S., Watkins, R., et al.: Comparison of MRI to contrast CT in the diagnosis of spinal stenosis. Spine 14:332–337, 1989.
30. Spengler, D. M.: Degenerative stenosis of the lumbar spine. J. Bone Joint Surg. 69A:305–308, 1987.
31. Teng, P., and Papatheodorou, C.: Myelographic findings in spondylosis of the lumbar spine. Br. J. Radiol. 36:122–128, 1963.
32. Thomas, P. K.: Clinical features and differential diagnosis. In Dyck, P. J., Thomas, P. K., Lambert, E. H., et al. (Eds.): Peripheral Neuropathy, 2nd Ed. Philadelphia. W. B. Saunders, 1984, pp. 1169–1190.
33. Udén, A., Johnsson, K. E., Jonsson, K., and Petterson, H.: Myelography in the elderly and the diagnosis of spinal stenosis. Spine 10:171–174, 1985.
34. Voelker, J. L., Mealey, J., Eskridge, J., et al.: Metrizamide enhanced computed tomography as an adjunct to metrizamide myelography in the evaluation of lumbar disc herniation and spondylosis. Neurosurgery 20:379–384, 1987.
35. Wiltse, L. L., Kirkaldy-Willis, W. H., McIvor, G. W. D.: The treatment of spinal stenosis. Clin. Orthop. 115:83–91, 1976.

Surgery for Spinal Stenosis

NANCY E. EPSTEIN
JOSEPH E. EPSTEIN

SURGERY FOR THE DIFFERENT TYPES OF LUMBAR STENOSIS

Laminectomy

Before lumbar surgery, older patients are placed in a hard cervical collar to facilitate both intubation and operative positioning. Because of the greater frequency of chronic but often unrecognized prostatism or partially neurogenic bladders, Foley catheters are inserted before procedures for lumbar stenosis in older individuals so that bladder overdistention and urosepsis can be avoided. Patients are subsequently routinely monitored with end-tidal carbon dioxide analyzers, pulse oximeters, and an electrocardiogram, whereas the use of central venous and arterial catheters and Swan-Ganz catheters are reserved for patients with cardiopulmonary and other medical problems.

Laminectomy, rather than the more restricted fenestration procedure, is more typically chosen for older patients in whom the sagittal diameter of the canal is severely compromised over many levels.[2] The laminectomy may especially be warranted in cases in which hypertrophied inferior articular processes markedly impinge on the midline. The presence of severe paraparesis before surgery may also warrant a complete laminectomy to ensure that adequate decompression is achieved. Laminectomy, however, ensures decompression of the central canal alone and must therefore be supplemented with sufficient unroofing of the lateral recesses if concomitant radicular symptoms are also to be relieved.

Except where hip, knee, or other skeletal pathologic states (including replacements) prohibit it, single- or multiple-level laminotomies, hemilaminectomies, or complete laminectomies are performed with the patient in the knee-chest position. The most common alternative is the use of the Cloward saddle, which is available for both normal and overweight individuals. Advantages of the knee-chest position include reversal of the lumbar lordosis, which opens the spinal canal and facilitates intracanalicular dissection, and a reduction of intraabdominal pressure, which mitigates intraoperative blood loss through the Batson plexus and nearly eliminates the need for transfusion.

The wound is initially infiltrated with 30 ml of 0.5% bupivicaine containing a 1:200,000 dilution of epinephrine. This injection at the outset of the procedure not only diminishes intraoperative blood loss but also reduces the intraoperative anesthetic requirements, allowing anesthesia to be more readily reversed after the surgery. A free fat graft may be harvested immediately after the incision is made and placed in kanamycin (Kantrex) solution, or a pedicle fat graft may be fashioned just before closing the incision. With the electrocautery, a periosteal elevator, and vaginal packing, subperiosteal dissection of the lumbodorsal fascia from the spinous processes is then accomplished. Retraction is subsequently achieved with combinations of Taylor or Collis retractors, with Addson suboccipital retractors being routinely placed at either end. In selected instances, the Grossman apparatus may be substituted, particularly in cases of extreme stenosis in which lateral purchase for the Taylor and Collis systems is limited.

Laminectomy, accomplished in an en face fashion, is then initiated with a Leksell rongeur. First, the spinous processes and protruding caudal edges of the lamina are removed. The operating surgeon should then start on the most symptomatic side for two reasons. One, bone tends to be more extensively removed on the side of opening, and two, should an emergency arise and urgent closure become warranted, the most symptomatic side has been decompressed. The introduction of the Midas Rex drill has shortened operative time, because it may be readily employed to shave down hypertrophied laminae, particularly where the bone is hard and thick or where the stenosis is so extreme that the introduction of a rongeur is prohibited. Drill bits employed vary from the acorn to smaller cutting burs for superficial dissection, diamond bits being reserved for dissection closer to the neural and soft tissue contents of the spinal canal. However, after the laminae have been shaved down, direct removal of the remaining bony lip is effected by hand with small rongeurs and is not accomplished with the foot-plate B1 drill as advocated in some of the Midas Rex courses. The risk of neural injury and dural laceration is considered too high for the use of such instrumentation under the circumstances described. Rather, the remaining ligamentum flavum may be dissected away from the underlying nerve root and cauda equina with a small curet. Because stenosis is typically most severe and most common at the L4–L5 level, entry into the canal at a higher or lower level, if not precluded by the presence of additional cephalad and caudal pathologic processes, may be both simpler and safer.[22] An added safety maneuver includes leaving the ligamentum flavum until after the bone has been excised, because this affords greater protection for the underlying dura and neural tissues.

Routinely, a lateral intraoperative x-ray film is obtained to document accurately the location of surgical decompression. This is done even when the sacrum can be directly visualized or palpated because lumbosacral anomalies abound, including transitional lumbar vertebrae, abnormalities of segmentation, and anomalous sacral foramina. Unfortunately, operating at the wrong level, without x-ray confirmation, still accounts for perhaps the greatest number of failures encountered in lumbar stenosis surgery.

An angulated Kerrison rongeur, thin and filed down, may be used to complete an initial laminotomy, following which the ligamentum flavum and lamina may be resected. Excision of bone is accomplished in both lateral gutters and extended to the neural foramina. Leksell rongeurs may be employed to thin the leading edge of the inferior lamina continuously as the laminectomy progresses. Using this technique, the laminectomy may be readily accomplished in a classic caudad-to-cephalad fashion. Hemostasis is achieved by placing hemostatic agents successively in the lateral gutters as decompression proceeds to limit intraoperative epidural bleeding and to facilitate visualization. Microfibrillar collagen (Avitene) hemostat has proved to be far more effective than absorbable gelatin sponge (Gelfoam) or other agents.

After the laminectomy has been completed, medial facetectomies and foraminotomies must be done to expose each nerve root carefully. The neural foramina are best identified by following the contour of the resected lamina. With a Penfield elevator or a Woodson dissector, the assistant from the opposite side of the table, may readily define neural foramina obliterated by hypertrophied bone or soft tissue elements in the lateral recesses. Small Kerrison rongeurs are then used in an undercutting technique to complete medial facetectomies and foraminotomies, which preserve the lateral two thirds of the facet joints. Turning the table obliquely to himself or herself, the surgeon then inclines the Kerrison punch another 30 degrees to best enter the foramen. These maneuvers facilitate foraminal decompression while also ensuring that more facet is preserved along with the pars interarticularis. Occasionally, dissection in a tight foramen requires the use of the smallest of up-biting curets, with sequentially larger curets being employed before an attempt is made to introduce the Kerrison rongeurs. Resection of accompanying osteophytes may or may not be needed after adequate lateral recess decompression has been achieved. Additionally, large spurs may have to be either tamped down or resected with down-biting Epstein curets.

After the multiple foraminotomies have been inspected, more rigorous evaluation is carried out beneath the individual nerve roots, looking for attendant disc herniations, limbus vertebral fractures, or other pathologic processes. A No. 4 Penfield elevator is most often employed to gently retract the individual nerve roots. This is replaced by a bayoneted nerve root retractor if more protracted retraction is required, such as during discectomy.

After lumbar stenosis with or without disc (or other) excision has been completed, the operative bed is checked with intraoperative ultrasonography. Montalvo and colleagues,[27] evaluating 104 patients with lumbar stenosis or disc disease, showed that intraoperative ultrasonography helped guarantee adequate disc removal and sufficient stenosis decompression.[27] Residual disc herniations, which are found in 41% of cases, and additional canal stenosis, which is observed in 23% of patients, can then be addressed before operative closure, thereby averting the need for a second operation after a failed procedure.

Routinely, except where the dura has been lacerated, a medium suction drain (Hemovac) is used and brought out through a cephalad stab incision. If there is a CSF leak, however, as occurs in 5% of first and 10% of second lumbar decompressions, direct suturing of the leak site is required and no drain is used because active suction tends both to maintain and to enlarge the fistula.

Dural repair is then done with 6–0 Prolene suture on a fine, round needle. A running suture or interrupted repair may prove appropriate in different circumstances. A free muscle graft, free fat graft, or pedicled muscle or fat graft is then used over the repair site to ensure CSF fistula closure. If a leak has been created beneath the dura, either centrally or peripherally, and cannot be directly repaired, generous application of microfibrillar collagen (Avitene) hemostat, muscle, and or fat is employed until a Valsalva maneuver no longer readily demonstrates CSF. If this is not the case, more stringent attempts should be made to place at least interrupted sutures along the edges of the dural tear, interspersing either a muscle, fascial, or fat graft. After the major CSF leak has been closed, the muscle and fascia are closed with two interrupted layers of 0 synthetic absorbable polyglactin 910 suture coated with polyglactin 370 and calcium stearate; this closure is supplemented with a running back-and-forth unlocked 0 absorbable suture. A routine subcutaneous closure with 2–0 absorbable suture then follows. If a good closure of the fistula has been attained, subcuticular closure is accomplished with a resorbable polydioxanone (PDS) No. 3 suture, and Steri-Strips are placed on the skin. Alternatively, if there is some doubt regarding the repair, staples or interrupted or running nylon suture may be used for skin closure. As soon as closure is completed, the anesthesiologist may immediately reverse the anesthesia so that the patient can be examined while still on the table or an adjacent stretcher before leaving the operating room.

Fenestration Procedures in Sagittal Stenosis

Central canal stenosis is occasionally managed with wide fenestration techniques consisting of bilateral laminotomies over single or multiple segments, with resection of the medial portion of the articular facet joint and the ligamentum flavum. Such fenestration techniques are more useful in younger patients with diffuse, congenital spinal stenosis, in whom extensive laminectomy carries a greater risk for instability. Nakai and coworkers,[29] treating 34 patients with stenosis over a mean interval of 5½ years, noted not only that fenestration procedures produce lasting symptomatic relief, but also that new bony deposition at previously operated segments contributed to stability and not to recurrent stenosis.

Expansive Laminoplasty Versus Laminectomy

Frequently used to treat patients with cervical stenosis and myelopathy, the expansive laminoplasty may also be adapted for the management of lumbar stenosis. In treating younger patients with low back pain and sciatica associated with primary stenosis or in treating those with secondary stenosis associated with lumbar ossification of the posterior longitudinal ligament, Tsuji and colleagues[43] found that the lumbar laminoplasty provided adequate decompression of the spine while ensuring continued stability. Matsui and coworkers[26] similarly studied the results of expansive lumbar laminoplasty during a mean interval of 3 years in 18 manual laborers with lumbar stenosis and two other patients with spinal tumors. They determined with postoperative non–contrast-enhanced CT examinations in 10 patients that a 119% enlargement of the canal had been maintained, along with an overall rectangular configuration, and that the laminoplasty had reinforced stability. These findings additionally correlated with a 73% degree of improvement of the mean postoperative Japanese Orthopedic Association (JOA) scores.

Fenestration Procedures for Lateral Recess Stenosis

Single- or multiple-level bilateral fenestration procedures constitute the major surgical alternative to decompressive laminectomy in the management of multilevel lateral recess stenosis of the lumbar spine.[22, 47] Focal laminotomies, accompanied by medial facetectomies and foraminotomies, provide operative decompression of the nerve root in the lateral recesses while also facilitating excision of overhanging tissues, including hypertrophied lamina, ligamentum flavum, and degenerated facet joints. Employing a microsurgical fenestration technique spares the spinous processes, the interspinous and supraspinous ligaments, medial portions of the yellow ligaments, and the major weight-bearing aspects of the lateral facets. Maintaining the integrity of the pars interarticularis further preserves the facet joints and limits the degree of postoperative instability.

Both single laminotomies and bilateral fenestration procedures may be technically facilitated with Midas Rex instrumentation. However, such dissection must be performed in a carefully graded, piecemeal fashion, preferably with the AM No. 8 diamond bit, because often the nerve roots are deviated laterally in tight lateral recesses. Unfortunately, overzealous and vigorous dissection in this area may produce inadvertent root damage. If sequestrated disc fragments have migrated cephalad or caudad to the interspace, these laminotomies may be extended through an undercutting technique, with great care being taken to preserve as much of the laminar margin, facet, and pars interarticularis as possible. When Aryanpur and Ducker[2] performed fenestration procedures during a mean period of 5 years in 32 patients with lateral recess stenosis, they determined that the fenestration technique was less destructive, required less operative time, and resulted in a 90% incidence of excellent postoperative results.

Secondary Surgery for Recurrent Lumbar Stenosis

Success rates of 80% for initial lumbar decompressions for stenosis, with or without fusion, may deteriorate to below 50% when second operations are conducted.[8, 9] In the authors' series of 857 patients operated on for differing types of spinal stenosis, 53 (6%) required additional surgery. Second lumbar procedures may address combinations of residual, recurrent, or new stenosis at previously decompressed or more cephalad, untouched levels. Repeated surgery may also require the excision of new or recurrent disc fragments and occasionally decompression and fusion for facet fractures.[32]

For patients who have previously had lumbar surgery, accurate preoperative assessment with MRI scans, myelograms, and CT-myelographic examinations is critical to the success of second procedures. However, MRI scans with or without gadolinium–diethylenetriamine pentaacetic acid (DPTA) enhancement tend to underestimate stenotic and other changes while providing good soft tissue detail, and are helpful in distinguishing between recurrent disc and scar. Alternatively, non–contrast-enhanced CT scans provide good bony detail but poor soft tissue detail, with the intravenously enhanced examination less clearly distinguishing disc from scar. Ultimately, CT-myelographic studies best define newly recurrent or residual cauda equina or nerve root impingement and thereby provide the best template for repeated surgical intervention.

When a second laminectomy is conducted, either at levels previously operated on or at new levels, an intraoperative film to document location is critical because prior multilevel laminectomies with their resultant prolific scar formation may make determination of the location of a new or recurrent disc protrusion more difficult. Further alterations in alignment, including progression of a scoliotic deformity, make the confirmation of level even more essential.

When second procedures are conducted in patients who have previously undergone surgery, a CSF fistula resulting from damage to the cauda equina, nerve roots, and dura may best be avoided by maintaining close contact with the lateral bony margins while dissecting from normal to abnormal tissues. Identifying and following these lateral bony contours with a curet, a Penfield elevator, or a dental tool allows careful dissection of these elements away from the underlying residual lamina and facet joints. After the lateral margin of the laminectomy is identified and its inferior edge freed from underlying soft tissues, small curets succeeded by larger and larger Kerrison punches may afford a new lateral margin of canal decompression. If a fat graft has survived from the original surgery, adhesions may be minimal, but even in the presence of some viable fat grafts, adhesions abound and require meticulous dissection of dura from scar with blunt instruments, e.g., a No. 4 Penfield elevator. If a new CSF leak is incurred, direct repair is mandated in the fashion previously described. Closure may consist of not only closure of the muscle and fascia in two layers with 0 absorbable polyglactin 910 suture coated with polyglactin 370 and calcium stearate, but also repair with a running back-and-forth 0 absorbable suture.

Disc Disease with Lumbar Stenosis

The incidence of disc herniations accompanying lumbar stenosis is markedly varied in the literature. Disc herniations with spinal stenosis appeared in 15% of patients in the series of Hall and colleagues,[16] in 33% of the 49 patients involved in Heath's[17] study, and in 392 (45%) of the authors' series of 857 patients with spinal stenosis. The frequency of disc herniations with degenerative spondylolisthesis was 20% in the series of 50 patients reported by Alexander and coworkers,[1] with Tsou and Hopp[42] finding a significantly lesser occurrence of only 4.3%.

Far-Lateral Discs and Far-Lateral Stenosis with Lumbar Stenosis

Located beyond the neural foramen, the far-lateral compartment's cephalad border consists of the pedicle, its anterior border, the disc, its caudal border, a portion of the vertebral body and the leading edge of the superior articular facet, and laterally, fat. Far-lateral disc herniations or spondylotic stenosis produces extremely severe radicular symptoms that involve the nerve root that exits superiorly rather than the one that exits inferiorly. Because most of the far-lateral compartment is located beyond the dural sleeve, myelography and CT-myelographic studies fail to provide details as good as those provided by an MRI scan or a non–contrast-enhanced CT evaluation alone. Nevertheless, in 72% of cases, these studies may identify attendant stenosis at the same or adjacent levels that warrants more extensive surgical decompression.[13] Janes intertransverse procedure, designed for the resection of far-lateral lesions, includes removal of the superolateral aspect of the facet joint, while carefully preserving the pars interarticularis. Even though this maintains the integrity of the facet joint, the risk of postoperative facet fracture, which is a common source of acute or delayed postoperative discomfort, is increased.

Limbus Vertebral Fractures with Lumbar Stenosis

Four types of limbus vertebral fractures, often mimicking disc herniations, may contribute to or accompany lumbar stenosis[14] (Figs. 1 and 2). To avoid overretraction and neural injury in the removal of these lesions, resection must be accomplished with a down-biting curet, tamp, and mallet technique directed ventral to the thecal sac and beneath either superiorly or inferiorly exiting nerve roots. Medial displacement of the thecal sac with a bayoneted nerve root retractor and lateral dissection of the nerve root with a Penfield dissector facilitate the introduction of small and then successively larger bayoneted curets via the axilla of the nerve roots. Right-angle tamps may next be introduced to initiate removal of the inferior margin of most limbus fractures. After the inferior portions of these fractures are débrided, the disc space is entered. This provides the room needed for subsequent ventral dissection and superior limbus fracture excision. Direct manipulation of limbus

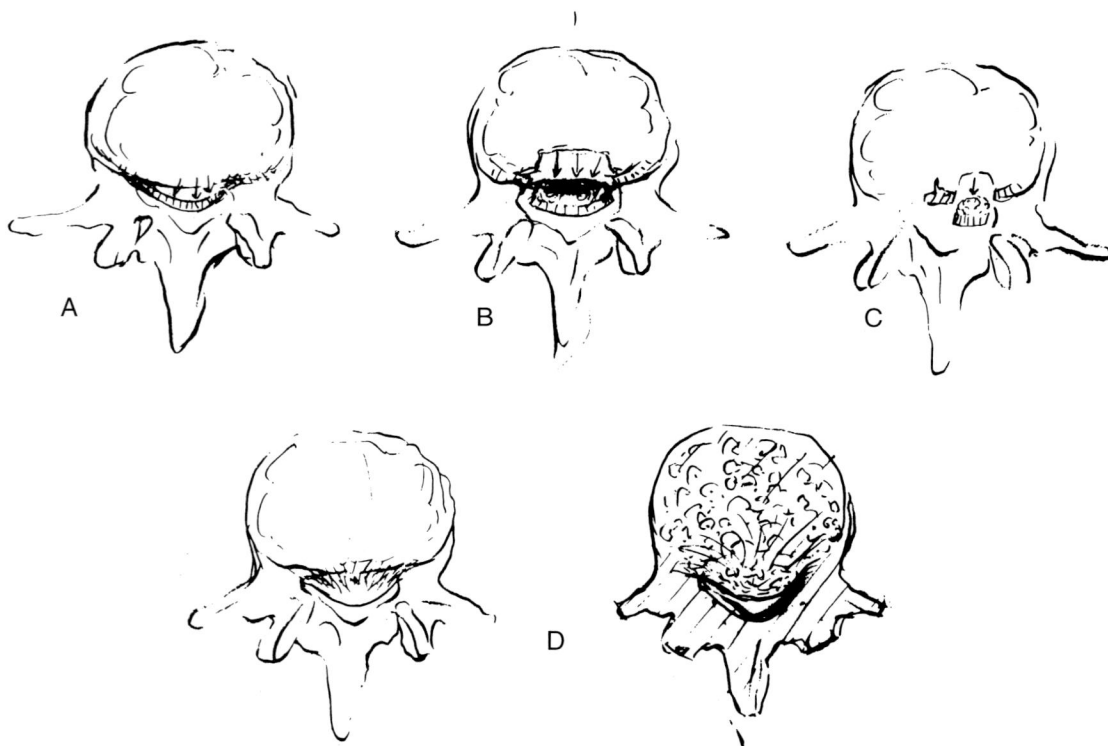

Figure 1. The transaxial appearance of the four types of limbus vertebral fractures. *A*, A type I limbus fracture consisting of a cortical shell of the posterior vertebral end plate contributing to both medial and lateral canal compromise. *B*, A type II fracture in which central cortical and cancellous bony fragments are more responsible for compromise of the central thecal sac than for compromise of the lateral recess. *C*, A type III fracture in which lateral cortical and cancellous chip fractures predominantly produce lateral recess compromise. *D*, Type IV limbus fractures, consisting of both cortical and cancellous bone, span the entire length and breadth of the vertebral bodies, from one disc space to another. The fracture in *A* is at the disc space itself, and the fracture in *B* is at the midvertebral level. Note the extreme medial and lateral canal compromise produced by the type IV lesions in *D*.

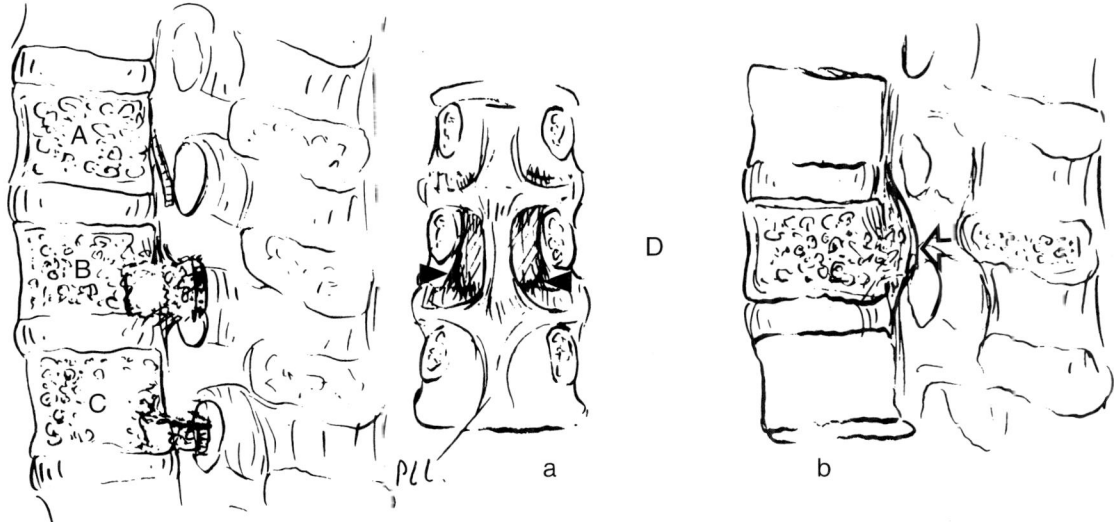

Figure 2. Sagittal and posteroanterior views of the four types of limbus fractures. *A*, A midline sagittal view of a type I limbus fracture consisting of only a posteriorly extending, convex shell of cortical bone. Arising from either the superior or inferior vertebral margins, adjacent to the disc spaces, these fractures contribute to marked central thecal sac compression and lesser degrees of lateral nerve root intrusion. *B*, A type II limbus fracture consisting of both cortical and cancellous bone produces more isolated midline ventral cauda equina compromise. *C*, A type III lateral chip fracture, including both cortical and cancellous bone originates from the superior or inferior vertebral end plates. If they originate superiorly, they can be found in the axilla of the nerve root that exits superiorly at the superior midpedicle level. Alternatively, if they occur inferiorly, they are critically located in the axilla of the inferiorly exiting nerve root at the inferior midpedicle level. *D*, Coronal posteroanterior *(a)* and lateral *(b)* views of a type IV limbus fracture demonstrate the massive extension across the entire posterior vertebral margin, from one interspace to another. On both the coronal posteroanterior *(a)* and sagittal *(b)* studies, the type IV lesion balloons beyond the confines of the posterior longitudinal ligament *(arrowheads)*, producing its maximum canal compromise at the midvertebral level *(arrow)*.

fractures and the soft discs frequently associated with them may then be completed with down-biting curets, tamps, and mallets, which succeed in breaking off smaller and smaller portions of the limbus fracture. Once delivered into the inferior interspace, these cartilage, soft tissue, and bone fragments may be safely removed with pituitary rongeurs in a piecemeal fashion, all dissection taking place away from the overlying neural elements.

All four types of limbus vertebral fractures may be removed using modifications of the techniques just described.[14] Type I fractures, composed of a thin shelf of posterior cortical bone, extend the full breadth of the disc space and simulate large central disc herniations in both size and location. Type II lesions, consisting of both cortical and cancellous bone and being found more centrally at the interspaces, contribute to more midline thecal sac compression. For both the type I and type II fractures, dissection must first be carried out medial to the nerve root that exits inferiorly or in its axilla, followed by lateral manipulation, if injury to that root is to be avoided.

Type III limbus fractures, which are best described as lateral cortical and cancellous chip fractures found either above or below the disc spaces approaching their respective cephalad or caudad pedicle, may appear calcified or noncalcified on MRI and CT studies. Neither the noncalcified fractures, which are most easily mistaken for soft disc herniations, nor the more calcified variants are found through the restricted laminotomies used for most discectomies. For instance, if the fracture originates cephalad to an interspace, it is actually located in the axilla of the nerve root that exits superiorly. To remove it, an extended superior laminotomy must be conducted. In a comparable manner, an inferiorly located type III lesion, located in the axilla of the nerve root that exits inferiorly at the midpedicle level, mandates a more inferior laminar exposure. Type III lesions, unlike disc protrusions or other types of limbus fractures, are not found at the interspaces and are therefore not resectable using typical discectomy techniques. Those arising from the superior vertebra must be removed from within the axilla of the nerve root that exits superiorly, whereas those originating from the inferior vertebral body, located at the distal pedicle, must be resected from within the inferior nerve root's axillary sleeve. Penfield elevators and small bayoneted microcurets successively replaced with increasingly larger curets and tamps allow resection to proceed in the piecemeal fashion described.

Unlike the other three types of fracture, type IV limbus lesions span the entire length and breadth of the vertebral body, from interspace to interspace.[14] Composed of cancellous and cortical bone and a thickened posterior longitudinal ligament, these fractures may produce superior and inferior bilateral nerve root compression or frank cauda equina syndromes. The onset of symptoms may be acute, subacute, or chronic. They are removed with a bilateral fenestration procedure or a single-level laminectomy, which must expose the cephalad and caudal nerve roots and the thecal sac. Resection is then similarly accomplished with the down-biting curet, tamp, and mallet technique in a piecemeal fashion.

Degenerative Spondylolisthesis with an Intact Neural Arch and Acquired Lumbar Stenosis

Degenerative spondylolisthesis with an intact neural arch, which is a secondary form of lumbar stenosis, is most frequently found at the L4–L5 level, followed in descending order by occurrence at the L3–L4, the L2–L3, and the L5–S1 interspaces.[5, 10, 23, 45, 46] More prevalent in women than men by a 2:1-to-10:1 ratio, degenerative spondylolisthesis most often appears in patients in their late 50s or early 60s through their 80s and 90s.[3, 34] Evaluation of 60 of the authors' patients with degenerative spondylolisthesis revealed that 56 had L4–L5, two had L3–L4, and another two had L5–S1 involvement.[12] The L4–L5 level was thought most vulnerable because progressive degenerative changes of the lumbar facet joints, consisting of the loss of their normal coronal configuration in favor of a more oblique orientation, left them uniquely susceptible to olisthesis. This resulted in the typical grade I slip, comprising one fourth of the vertebral body length, with further olisthesis usually being limited by a spontaneous locking of hugely hypertrophied posterior facet joints.[11] On the contrary, the absence of slippage at L5–S1 and its continued stability were attributed to its usual location below the intercrestal line, where added support was afforded by the longer transverse processes and iliotransverse ligaments.

Neurologic compromise associated with degenerative spondylolisthesis is attributed to the progressive scissoring effect of the grade I olisthesis created ventrally by the slip and posteriorly by markedly intruding hypertrophied facet joints. Together, both contribute to cauda equina compression and inferior nerve root compression more than to superior nerve root compression. Disc degeneration and rarely herniation may contribute to up to a 33% incidence of grade I olistheses.[35]

Symptoms more typically evolve over decades rather than months, with only 50% of patients exhibiting minor, late neurologic signs often initially consisting of neurogenic claudication and being only slowly succeeded by asymmetric radiculopathy. Later in the disease course, motor and sensory findings become evident without significant attendant mechanical findings.

Single-level degenerative spondylolisthesis, which produces focal lateral recess stenosis rather than central stenosis, is surgically addressed with a bilateral fenestration approach. Many younger patients can have adequate decompression with these bilateral procedures consisting of interlaminar laminotomies, medial facetectomies, and foraminotomies with undercutting of the subarticular zones and lateral recesses, in the absence of fusion. Getty and colleagues[15] successfully conducted partial undercutting facetectomies while preserving the pars interarticularis in 78 patients, with root entrapment managed with decompression alone without fusion.

However, most instances of degenerative spondylolisthesis produce both central and lateral recess stenosis and deserve either a generous coronal hemilaminectomy, involving resection of half of the adjacent superior and inferior laminae, or a full two-level laminectomy. Forty of the authors' patients underwent multilevel laminectomies, 14 had coronal hemilaminectomies, and only six had fenestration procedures for degenerative spondylolisthesis.[12] Safe removal of the diving lamina at the level of olisthesis with the Midas Rex AM No. 8 cutting bit followed by a diamond bur avoided placing any instrument, even a small, filed-down Kerrison punch, under the lamina at the maximally stenotic level.

The remainder of the dissection, including extensive foraminal decompression, was accomplished with the undercutting technique at the level of maximum olisthesis. Using a typical laminectomy, great attention was paid to preservation of the facet joints. Unique to patients with degenerative spondylolisthesis is their greater foraminal compromise, which is magnified by the slip. Occasionally, retrospondylolisthesis of the inferior vertebral body, which is responsible for the protrusion on the inferiorly exiting nerve root, has to be either tamped down or directly resected away from the ventral aspect of the nerve root or thecal sac. This often requires the removal of portions of the hypertrophied pedicles also contributing to nerve root torsion. If only unilateral symptoms are present, contralateral decompression can be more restricted to help preserve stability. Spontaneous vertebral body fusion at the levels of olisthesis also limits fusion considerations. Additionally the authors' experience was that an extremely low 3.7% of 191 patients with degenerative spondylolisthesis required fusion, consisting of only four primary and three secondary fusion procedures.[12]

Assessment of preoperative stability in these patients is more critical than in those with stenosis alone because olisthesis more frequently progresses. Fusion is rarely warranted when plain x-ray films document a fixed fusion at the level of olisthesis, but it should be strongly considered for those whose erect flexion and extension x-ray films document abnormal motion in the presence of severe mechanical back pain. From a different vantage point, Wiltse and Rothman[46] advocated more generous fusions for patients with spondylolisthesis. Bolesta and Bohlman[3] further advocated decompression and posterolateral fusion for patients with degenerative spondylolisthesis with or without demonstrated motion, believing that the slip would progress without such stabilization. Sano and colleagues[33] similarly advocated universal, instrumented stabilization for presumed micromotion independent of any radiographic abnormalities at the level of olisthesis in patients who previously had undergone surgery for degenerative spondylolisthesis.

Good to excellent outcomes have been observed for over 80% of patients with degenerative spondylolisthesis in most series. Fifty-three of 60 of the authors' patients exhibited good to excellent outcomes, with only seven showing poor results.[12] Four with recurrent symptoms between 5 months and 3 years postoperatively needed second procedures, which consisted of only one discectomy; the others required more extended laminectomies for decompression; no fusion was needed.

Spondylolisthesis with Lysis Contributing to Acquired Lumbar Stenosis

Typically occurring at the L5–S1 level in young adults, spondylolisthesis with lysis is treated with the Gill procedure and a posterolateral fusion, with or without instrumentation. Exceptions to the fusion requirements include instances in which no active motion is demonstrated radiographically or in which, for older individuals, the degree of olisthesis, even with the lysis, is fixed. In the Gill procedure, the free-floating lamina is removed along with epidural scar encompassing the inferiorly exiting nerve root, which becomes stretched over the slip at the pseudarthrotic level. Here, because of the larger baseline size of the central canal, sagittal stenosis is rare, the stenosis being largely confined to the lateral subarticular recesses and foramen. The nerve root that exits superiorly may also become confined as it slips below the cephalad pedicle and makes its way through the neural foramen into the far-lateral compartment.

After the lamina at the level of lysis has been excised, bilateral lateral in situ fusions are conducted, most frequently involving fusion of the L5 transverse processes to the sacrum, with or without instrumentation. Such in situ posterolateral fusions were performed in the adults in the series of Vanden Berghe and coworkers,[44] in which the spondylolisthetic defect was deemed responsible for increased anterior displacement or progressive symptoms.[44] Over a 7-year period, good to excellent outcomes were achieved in 13 (72%) of 18 patients managed with posterolateral in situ fusions without laminectomy, except where severe neural compression existed. No olisthetic defects were actively reduced. Failures were attributed to pseudarthrosis, most frequently involving the L4–L5 level.

On the other hand, isthmic spondylolisthesis can be successfully treated with posterior or anterior decompression combined with instrumentation. With microsurgical techniques, the Louis plate fixation system is used for grade I olisthesis and the Cotrel-Dubousset device for grade II lesions, Markwalder and coworkers[24] treated 72 patients with isthmic spondylolisthesis. Excellent results were achieved in 82% of patients; good outcomes, in 14%; and poor outcomes, in 4% of patients. Similarly, treating 50 consecutive patients with spondylolisthesis and spondylolysis with the Cotrel-Dubousset system over a 25-month period, Boos and colleagues[4] achieved a 76% incidence of good clinical responses and a 96% frequency of solid fusions in 32 of 44 patients managed with in situ procedures, with 12 being treated with combined slip reduction and neural decompression. Kim and Kim[21] observed a comparable 77% frequency of success with anterior interbody fusions in 75 patients, 87% of whom continued to be asymptomatic with good to excellent outcomes 1 year later.

Degenerative Scoliosis with Lumbar Stenosis

The rotational and conformational narrowing of the spinal canal in degenerative scoliosis, which is attributed to degenerative changes of the discs, vertebral bodies, and posterior facet joints, contributes to asymetric nerve root and cauda equina compression.[36, 40] Marked vertebral body rotation, resulting in a progressive loss of alignment, may inadvertently lead the surgeon to perform a complete rather than a more limited medial facetectomy, particularly when dissection is proceeding on the concave side of the curve in the presence of the most profuse spondyloarthrotic changes of the facets and exit foramina.

Whereas many surgeons advocate laminectomy and foraminotomy for the decompression of degenerative scoliotic stenosis, other surgeons proceed with fusions. For example, when Simmons and Simmons[37] simultaneously used instrumentation and fusion in 40 patients with lumbar stenosis and scoliosis, they converted an 83% incidence of preoperative back pain to a 93% frequency of postoperative pain relief over a mean postoperative interval of 44 months.[37] Laminectomy and pedicle screw fixation techniques included the Zielke device (24 patients), the Cotrel-Dubousset apparatus (eight patients), and the Texas Scottish Rite Hospital (TSRH) system (eight patients). They incurred no deaths, no instrument failures, no pseudarthroses, and an average deformity correction of 19 degrees.

Posttraumatic Lumbar Stenosis

Trauma-induced stenosis of the thoracolumbar or lumbar spinal canal may be responsible for radicular deficits, cauda equina syndromes, paraparesis, or frank paraplegia.[20, 25] In the series of 80 consecutive patients with acute thoracic, lumbar, or thoracolumbar fractures reported by Keene and colleagues[20], the degree of neurologic dysfunction did not directly correlate with CT-documented severity of canal compromise. Burst fractures and lumbar spinal injuries, although often resulting in the greatest degree of canal compromise, were nevertheless most frequently associated with the least severe neurologic deficits because at lumbar levels the cauda equina rather than the cord was threatened.

Crutcher and coworkers,[6] studying thoracolumbar burst fractures in 44 patients, attempted to determine whether posterior distraction-instrumentation could provide sufficient, indirect reduction of retropulsed bone fragments. Using the Denis classification system, which divided all except two patients into type A (13 patients) and type B (29 patients) fracture types, they noted that posterior distraction with instrumentation alone could reduce the severity of canal stenosis by 50%. Neither the severity of the original kyphotic deformity nor the extent of initial vertebral collapse influenced these results. Additionally, the degree of neurologic compromise most closely correlated with the original preoperative severity of canal stenosis but did not reflect the extent of canal narrowing remaining after distraction and instrumentation. Patients with even the most severe distal L5 canal compromise attributed to isolated L5 burst fractures or other injuries typically incurred minimum neurologic deficits, surgery rarely being indicated because these injuries were often considered stable.

COMPLICATIONS OF SURGERY FOR LUMBAR STENOSIS

Complications Related to Age

Morbidity and mortality after lumbar surgery for stenosis and disc disease are more frequent in the geriatric population, which is defined as those persons older than 70 to 75 years of age. Of 78 patients undergoing lumbar laminectomy for either stenosis or discectomy without attendant fusion, Smith and Hanigan[39] found that 23 (85.2%) of 27 patients having discectomy did well, as did 35 (81.4%) of 43 with stenosis. However, postoperative complications were significantly more likely if patients exhibited three or more major preoperative medical risk factors such as cardiovascular compromise, pulmonary disease, diabetes, and hypertension. Deyo and coworkers[7] confirmed that when 84% of 18,122 patients with herniated discs or spinal stenoses were evaluated, those older than 75 years of age exhibited an 18% frequency of complications and a 7% occurrence of discharges to nursing homes.[7] Risks for hospitalized patients and hospital charges increased with advancing years. Fusions accompanying stenosis operations in these older patients most significantly added to morbidity and demanded the greatest hospital resources, in contrast to the case with decompressions alone, in which morbidity and the need for additional resources were reduced. Last, those with disc herniations had the fewest complications and required fewer hospital-based services.

On the other hand, Quigley and colleagues[31] came to very different conclusions following their study of 143 geriatric (>70 years old) patients who underwent 155 operations. The average age was 74.9 years. Thirty-two patients had surgery for disc herniations only, 29 had surgery for disc disease with stenosis, and 94 had operations for stenosis alone. Neither the average hospital stay of 7.5 days nor the average 6.9% frequency of major morbidity without mortality was increased by advanced age. Even long-term follow-up 34.3 months later revealed that 66.6% had no or minimum symptoms and 77.3% still had good postoperative outcomes.

Factors Related to Psychosocial Phenomena

One of the most common reasons for surgical failure in lumbar stenosis is poor patient selection. Psychosocial and financial factors may prove to be the most relevant, outstripping real neurologic and neurodiagnostic findings in importance. Certainly, some of the poorest surgical candidates are those with vague reports of back pain with poorly defined neurologic symptoms and signs.[28] Compensation or litigation, as emphasized by Herron and Mangelsdorf,[18] may be the most significant factors responsible for a failure to achieve postoperative symptom relief in certain patients.

Cerebrospinal Fluid Fistulas and Pseudomeningoceles

The most frequent complications encountered after lumbar decompressions for stenosis, with or without fusion, include cauda equina or nerve root deficits caused by direct or indirect injury (e.g., postoperative clot), infection, and CSF fistulas. Such CSF leaks are an inevitable consequence of operating on patients with severe lumbar stenosis, because the dura, which is often severely tethered to overlying structures, becomes increasingly atretic or paper thin. Although the incidence of CSF fistulas is lower at first operations, the frequency at successive procedures increases because of adhesions. From the authors' series of 357 patients undergoing surgery for stenosis during the past 20 years, the surgeons incurred a 4.6% incidence of CSF fistulas at first procedures and a 9.8% frequency when second operations were performed.

A significant additional source of CSF leakage both intraoperatively and postoperatively is a lumbar puncture site from a recent myelogram. Because these fistulas may persist for up to several weeks after myelography, the authors perform myelography well before surgery. If the lumbar puncture site is directly visualized, direct, watertight repair with a 6-0 Prolene suture on a round needle is appropriate. A fat or muscle graft over the site of direct water-tight dural repair further enhances leak obliteration but does not substitute for adequate direct closure. Testing of the repair with several Valsalva maneuvers helps to confirm the adequacy of the repair while decreasing the likelihood that a second operation for a failed repair will become necessary. After the closure is completed, microfibrillar collagen (Avitene) hemostat and/or absorbable gelatin sponge may be applied along with the routine free or pedicled fat graft. Most important at this juncture is to close the wound without a drain, because the drain potentiates fistula formation. Blood left in the wound also forms a "blood patch" at both the surgical level and adjacent levels, the latter being more critical when the original lumbar puncture site could not be identified in the operative bed. Nevertheless, all attempts should be made to achieve adequate hemostasis because the intraoperative loss of CSF from the thecal sac diminishes the hemostatic role of a tight dural tampon and thereby enhances the chance of a postoperative hematoma. Routine closure should additionally be supplemented with a tight, back-and-forth running, unlocked, absorbable (e.g., 0 Vicryl) suture placed in the lumbodorsal fascia above the two underlying muscle and fascial layers completed with interrupted 0 Vicryl. The patient is then kept supine for a 24- to 48-hour period, after which ambulation is initiated.

Persistent postoperative CSF fistulas are rare because most leaks occurring intraoperatively can be immediately identified and repaired. Exceptions may include lacerations incurred along the central midline dura or critically located below or along nerve roots that exit laterally. If the degree of seepage is marked, a lumbar drain placed in the wound but brought out through a tunneled, cephalad incision may sufficiently divert CSF away from the wound to allow adequate wound healing. This maneuver may also be used in instances in which the entire distal thecal sac is so lacerated and atretic that no attempt at direct repair is feasible. In such cases, superficial application of a lyophilized fascial graft or even absorbable gelatin sponge may facilitate closure.

Nevertheless, despite the measures enumerated above, postoperative CSF pseudomeningoceles or frank fistulas may form. They may prove to be either symptomatic or asymptomatic, depending on their size, pressure gradients, and extent through epidural, muscle, fascial, subcutaneous, or subcuticular compartments. Only a few actually extend to the surface and pose a significant risk of infection. These collections are best initially studied with an MRI scan with gadolinium-DTPA enhancement to help rule out infection. In the absence of external leakage, multiple transcutaneous taps with a 20-gauge needle, pressure dressings, and bed rest often suffice. During this period, antiinflammatory agents with antiplatelet aggregate effects are prohibited to facilitate healing. More than 95% of postoperative CSF collections should respond to these measures. If they fail, a blood patch may be applied to a known leakage site. Alternatively, if the collection increases rather than decreases in size and becomes responsible for progressive neurologic symptoms and signs, or if CSF continues to leak through the skin, repeated surgical intervention becomes necessary. If the ball-valve source of the pseudomeningocele is unknown, a preparatory preoperative CT-myelographic study facilitates direct operative closure.

Recurrent Stenosis Related to Postoperative Bone Regrowth

Postoperative stenosis attributed to the regrowth of bone is another common contributor to recurrent symptoms in patients who have previously undergone surgery for lumbar stenosis or degenerative spondylolisthesis. To quantitate the frequency and the severity of recurrent postoperative bony stenosis, Postacchini and Cinotti[30] evaluated 50 patients over 8.6 years. Of these 50 patients, 34 had laminectomies or fenestration procedures for stenosis, whereas 10 of 16 with degenerative spondylolisthesis had laminectomies with fusions. Patients were then divided into four groups depending on the severity of bony regrowth responsible for recurrent stenosis. The 12% in group I showing minimum regrowth and the 48% in group II exhibiting mild bony regrowth were asymptomatic, whereas the 28% in group III demonstrating moderate regrowth and the 12% in group IV exhibiting marked regrowth were symptomatic. Furthermore, patients with degenerative spondylolisthesis who did not undergo fusion experienced a much greater increase in their recurrent stenosis compared with those who had undergone primary fusion. In short, the best long-term results after surgery for lumbar stenosis were achieved when bony regrowth was limited, such as by performing a primary fusion in patients with degenerative spondylolisthesis.

Postoperative Lumbar Facet Fractures

Pain in patients after lumbar surgery may also be attributed to postoperative and often undiagnosed lumbar facet fractures. Rosen and colleagues[32] evaluated CT studies in 50 patients with persistent postoperative pain resulting from lumbar facet fractures and compared them with appropriate control subjects over an average of 3.2 years. They documented that the greater extent of bony removal in the former group most likely contributed to these fractures.[32] More than half of the pars immediately above the inferior articular facet had been resected at surgery for patients with fractures, whereas the control population showed only one quarter of this extent of bony resection. Meticulous attention must therefore be paid to limiting the extent of facetectomy and to maintaining the integrity of the pars interarticularis if such facet fractures are to be avoided.

Additional Cephalad Involvement

Because fusion increases the stresses transmitted to adjacent levels, any patient who has had a distal lumbar fusion is at increased risk for developing more cephalad stenosis, spondyloarthrosis, and disc herniation.

Infection

Infections of the lumbar spine, which are divided into the osteomyelitis, discitis, and granulomatous infection categories, may contribute to spinal stenosis through progressive loss of disc space height and vertebral body collapse. Certainly, the majority of postoperative superficial and deep infections result from direct intraoperative inoculation. Deep infections include discitis, epidural or transdural empyema leading to meningitis and adhesive arachnoiditis, osteomyelitis, and paraspinal abscess formation. Superficial processes may range from minor intercuticular suture irritation to subcuticular, subcutaneous, subfascial, or intramuscular involvement. Symptoms, often delayed for 6 weeks or longer, may vary from nondescript and difficult to categorize to exquisitely focal, producing searing and disabling pain.

Neurodiagnostic confirmation of infection is best effected with an MRI scan with gadolinium-DTPA enhancement or a tagged white blood cell nuclear medicine study because the bony alterations perceived on plain x-ray films or CT studies often require up to 6 weeks to appear.

In the presence of deep wound infections, culturing blood or examining Craig needle biopsy specimens may identify the inciting organism, whereas with more superficial processes, culture of subcutaneous, subcuticular, or actively draining fluid may allow organism identification.

The single most reliable laboratory study indicating the presence of a deep wound infection is not the white blood cell (WBC) count, as anticipated, but rather an erythrocyte sedimentation rate (ESR) acutely *and* persistently elevated to a level 2 standard deviations above the mean value normally seen in the first 2 weeks postoperatively in uninfected individuals.[19] To establish this, Jonsson and coworkers[19] studied the WBC counts and ESRs of 110 uninfected patients after lumbar operations, observing their ESRs and WBC counts before surgery and 2 days, 4 days, and 1, 2, 6, and 16 weeks postoperatively.[19] The ESR in the absence of infection maximally increased by the fourth postoperative day but returned to normal levels in 2 weeks, whereas the WBC count was never markedly elevated. Of interest, a greater ESR increase was noted 4 days after fusions (ESR of 102 mm/h) compared with discectomies (ESR of 75 mm/h). Comparison with five other patients with deep wound infections showed that the latter patients developed acute postoperative increases of their ESR, which persisted at markedly elevated levels (plus 2 standard deviations) for months, compared with the lesser elevations, which normalized over 2 weeks. No comparable significant elevations were noted in the WBC counts of patients from either group, the five infected patients showing only mild increases.

Surgical management of an infected postoperative wound has to be dictated by the extent of involvement (i.e., superficial or deep) and the type of surgery originally performed (e.g., laminectomy with or without fusion). Thalgott and coworkers[41] conducted a multicenter study designed to enhance classification of deep postoperative lumbar wound infections for patients with spinal implants. The extent of osteomyelitis involvement (Cierny scheme) was categorized into groups I to III, reflecting the severity of the infection, and the class A to C, indicating the host's capacity to respond. Group I patients had single-organism superficial or deep infections; group 2 patients had multiple-organism deep infections; and group 3 patients had both multiple-organism invovlement and myonecrosis. Class A persons had normal host defenses; class B patients exhibited localized, multisystem compromise and cigarette smoking; and class C individuals were frankly immunocompromised. Thalgott and colleagues[41] found that group I patients could be successfully managed with a single wound débridement and primary reclosure supplemented with suction drainage systems; group 2 patients required an average of three reoperations for irrigation and wound débridement, the best results being achieved with inflow and outflow suction and irrigation systems; and group 3 patients, with the poorest outcomes, warranted multiple reoperations. Comparably, those with the best host defenses (class A) exhibited the best prognoses for overcoming infections compared with the more susceptible and less resistant class B and C categories.

Vascular Injury

The possibility of an intraoperative vascular injury must always be entertained in patients undergoing lumbar surgery for stenosis and disc disease.[38] In some instances, acute symptoms arising with direct aortic or iliac puncture warrant immediate laparotomy in the presence of exsanguination. Alternatively, subacute postoperative hypotension and unexplained, postoperative high-output cardiac failure or more chronic swelling of one leg may forecast an underlying traumatic arteriovenous fistula, which in stable patients, should be evaluated with a distal aortogram. Better outcomes for these vascular injuries correlate with early diagnosis and treatment, preferably instituted on the first or second postoperative day.[38]

These injuries are best avoided by ensuring, particularly during discectomy, that pituitary rongeurs are immediately opened once introduced below the level of the annulus in the disc space. Constant awareness of the depth of these and any other instruments, such as down-biting curets, is critical. Additional attention should be paid to possibly encountering vascular structures when dissecting far laterally, particularly on the left side.

CASE REPORTS

CASE ■ 1

A 64-year-old man exhibited a persistent right L4 root syndrome and increased neurogenic claudication 1 year after an L4–S1 laminectomy for lumbar spinal stenosis. This surgery was done at an outside institution. Quadriceps weakness (3 to 4/5), a loss of the patellar response, and decreased pin appreciation in the L4 distribution correlated with MRI and CT-myelographic findings of a right-sided far-lateral (extraforaminal) L4–L5 disc herniation, mild recurrent L4–L5 stenosis, and more marked new cephalad L3–L4 and L2–L3 stenosis (Figs. 3 to 5). Because the flexion and extension x-ray films revealed no evidence of instability at the L4–L5 level, an L2–S1 decompression without fusion was conducted, along with removal of a right far-lateral disc herniation with preservation of the pars interarticularis and facet. After wearing a thoracolumbosacral orthosis (TLSO) for 3 months postoperatively, the patient became symptom free and remained so 1 year later.

CASE ■ 2

During the previous year, a 78-year-old man developed the more rapid exacerbation of neurogenic claudication accompanied by a right-sided footdrop. MRI and CT-myelographic examina-

Figure 3. Case 1. A lateral myelogram obtained one year after an L4–S1 laminectomy revealed residual or new L2–L4 stenosis *(arrowheads)*, mild recurrent L4–S1 stenosis *(double white arrows)*, and a new right-sided, L4–L5 far lateral disc herniation *(black arrow)*.

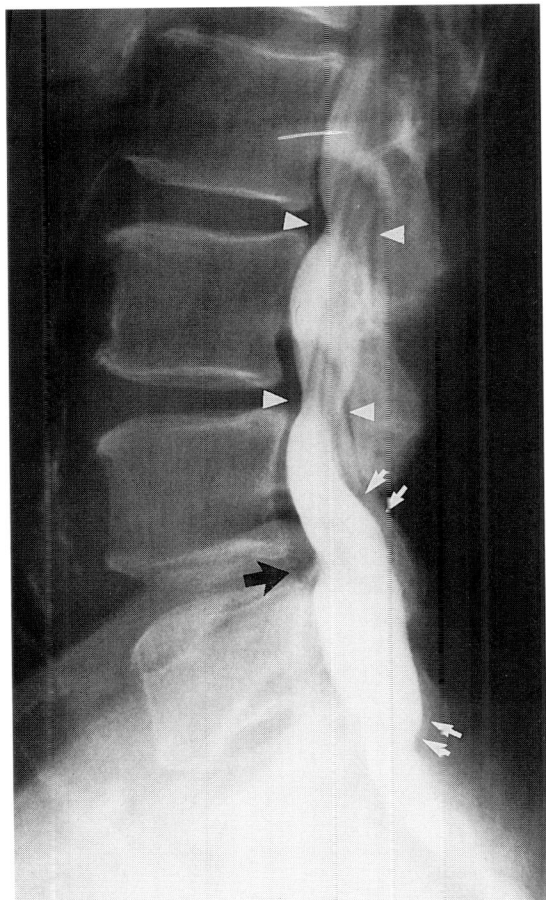

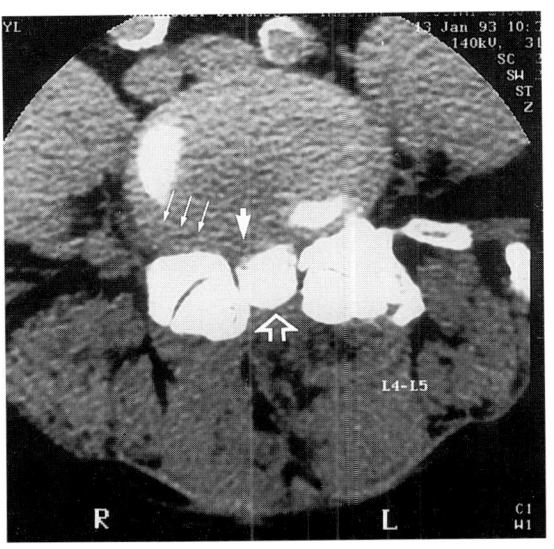

Figure 4. Case 1. One year after an L4–S1 laminectomy, a transaxial CT-myelographic examination at the L4–L5 level demonstrated adequate decompression of the thecal sac *(open arrow)*, minimum postoperative stenosis, and excellent preservation of the facet joints bilaterally. Note the lateral *(solid filled arrow)* and far lateral *(small multiple arrows)* disc herniation on the right side.

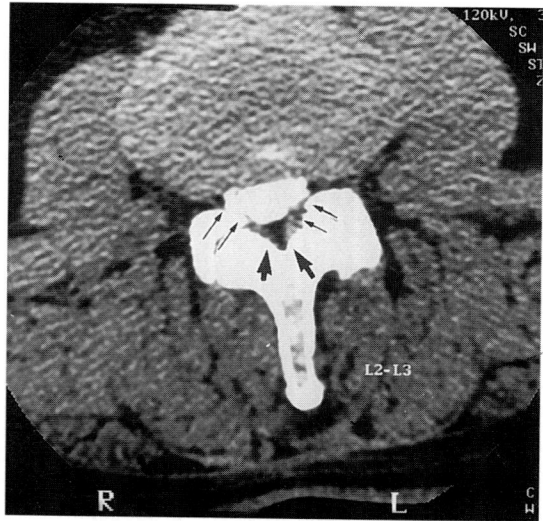

Figure 5. Case 1. A transaxial CT-myelographic scan of the L2–L3 level revealed moderate spinal stenosis composed of sagittal compression of the thecal sac *(large arrows)* and bilateral lateral recess stenosis *(small arrows)*.

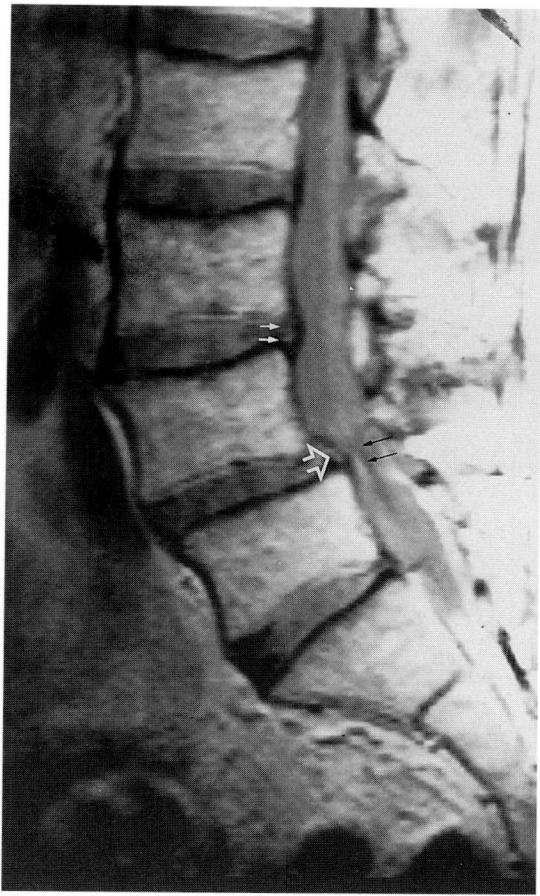

Figure 6. Case 2. A sagittal T1-weighted MRI scan revealed severe lumbar stenosis attributed to the grade I degenerative spondylolisthesis at the L4–L5 level. Dorsolateral compression was produced by a combination of the leading edge of the L4 lamina, hypertrophied L4–L5 facet joints, and ligamentum flavum *(small black arrows)*, whereas ventral intrusion primarily consisted of the vertebral olisthetic slip *(open white arrow)* rather than frank disc herniation. Early degenerative changes were also present at the L3–L4 disc level *(small white arrows)*.

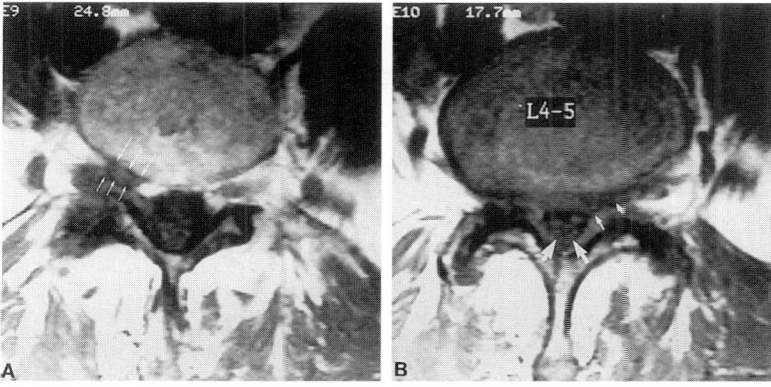

Figure 7. Case 2. *A,* A transaxial T1-weighted MRI scan of the L4–L5 disc space revealed a right-sided far-lateral (extraforaminal) disc herniation *(arrows)*. *B,* A subsequent transaxial study, obtained just below the interspace, demonstrated marked L4–L5 spinal stenosis and severe sagittal compromise of the thecal sac *(large arrows)* and lateral recess *(small arrows),* which were magnified by the degenerative grade I slip.

tions demonstrated L4–L5 degenerative spondylolisthesis with a complete block, plus more cephalad L3–L4 stenosis (Figs. 6 to 8). A right-sided far-lateral disc herniation was also noted. An L3–S1 laminectomy with medial facetectomy and foraminotomy was done to decompress the stenosis, and the extraforaminal disc was removed using the intertransverse approach. After surgery, although the patient was neurologically intact, persistent urinary retention developed, which warranted a transurethral prostatectomy. An incidental subcutaneous collection of CSF was tapped once and resolved with the application of pressure dressings for 3 weeks. Two years later the patient remained symptom free.

CASE ■ 3

With an 8-year history of increasing pain radiating down both lower extremities to the calves and ankles, a 67-year-old woman stated that she could no longer tolerate to traverse a room. On examination, she exhibited more right-sided (4/5) than left-sided (4 to 5/5) weakness of the ex-

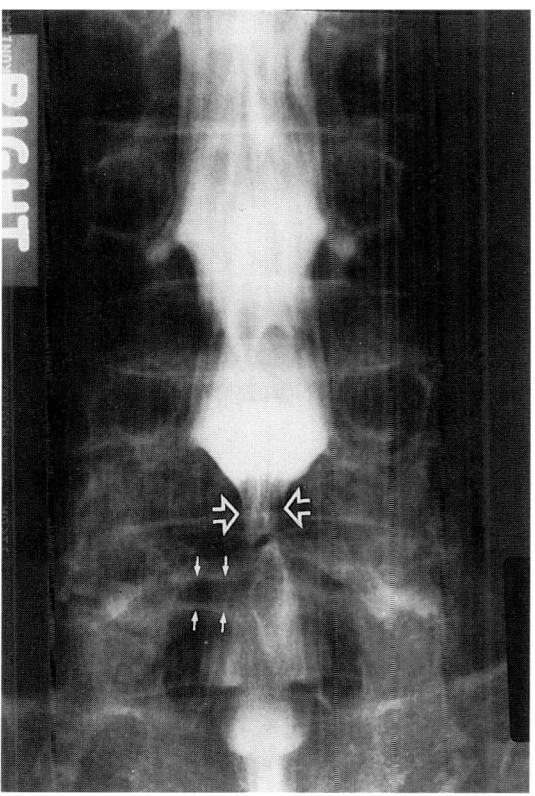

Figure 8. Case 2. The bilateral "napkin ring" intrusions and a near-complete obstruction of intrathecal contrast material at the L4–L5 level seen on this posteroanterior myelogram were attributed to grade I degenerative spondylolisthesis *(open arrows).* Marked angulation of the diving L5 lamina at the level of olisthesis accounted for its foreshortened appearance *(small arrows).*

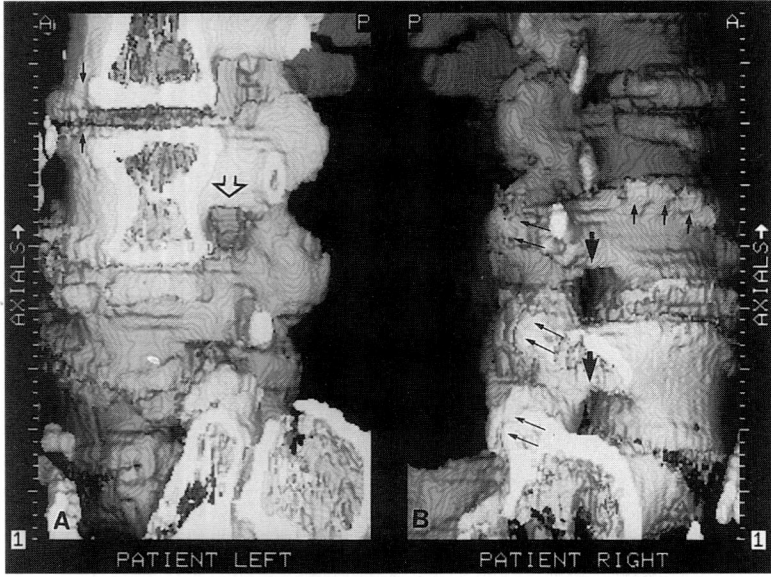

Figure 9. Case 3. *A*, A left oblique three-dimensional lumbar CT study demonstrated the L2–S1 laminectomy defect. Marked degenerative changes were evident in the neural foramina *(open arrow)* and were accompanied by osteophytic lipping of the apposing vertebral edges *(small arrows)*. *B*, A right oblique three-dimensional lumbar CT scan revealed osteophytic intrusion into compromised neural foramina *(large arrows)* and diffuse arthrotic changes of the facet joints *(thin double arrows)* and vertebral end plates *(small arrows)*.

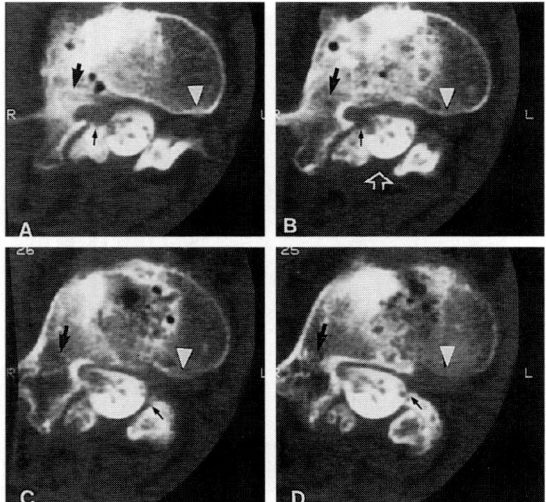

Figure 10. Case 3. *A*, The severe scoliotic deformity accounted for simultaneous visualization of the L4 pedicle on the right *(large arrow)* and the L3–L4 disc space on the left *(arrowhead)* on this transaxial CT-myelographic scan at the L3–L4 level. The L4 root was trapped in the right lateral recess beneath the hypertrophied L3–L4 facet joint *(small arrow)*. *B*, At the L3–L4 level, but with 2 mm added inferiorly, marked scoliosis still contributes to the rotational deformity that allowed the L4 pedicle on the right *(large black arrow)* to be seen at the same time as the disc space *(arrowhead)* on the left. The margins of the laminar decompression *(open arrows)* and the persistent right lateral recess compromise *(small black arrow)* were also evident. *C*, On this third, lower image, more of the L4 pedicle *(small arrow)* can be seen on the right *(large arrow)*, along with the L3–L4 disc on the left *(arrowhead)*. Note how the lateral recess compromise was now greater on left *(small arrow)*. *D*, This view, obtained at the midpedicle level of L4 on the right *(large arrow)*, and the disc space on the left *(arrowhead)*, illustrated the severity of rotatory scoliosis. Left-sided intrusion by the superior facet of L4 now compromised the lateral recess and the L4 nerve root exiting inferiorly *(small arrow)*.

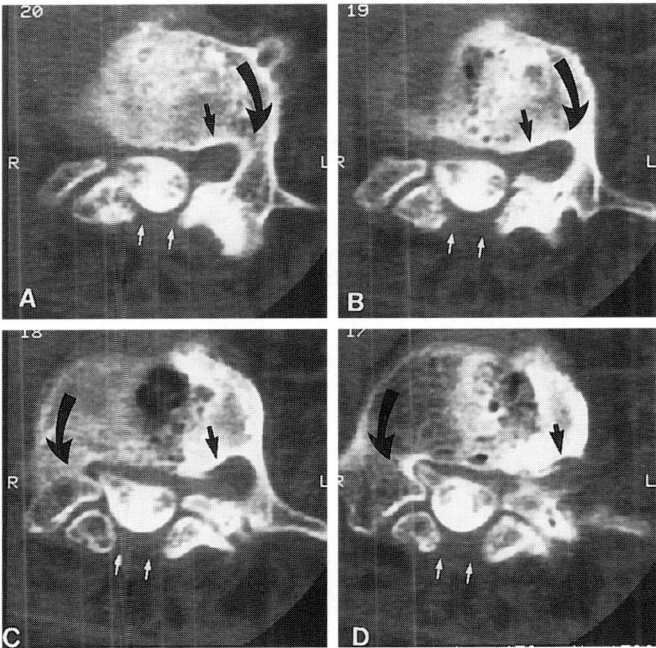

Figure 11. Case 3. *A,* The extreme degree of scoliotic rotation at the L5–S1 level allowed the disc space to be visualized on this transaxial L5–S1 image on the right. At the same time, the L5 pedicle could be seen on the left *(curved arrow).* The soft tissue density in the left lateral recess *(black arrow)* extending intraforaminally and far laterally impinged on the exiting L5 nerve root. The decompression of the central stenosis was adequate *(white arrows). B,* The left-sided soft tissue mass continued to extend into the superior aspect of the left L5–S1 neural foramen *(small black arrow).* The rotational deformity allowed the right L5–S1 disc space to appear on the same image as the left L5 pedicle *(curved arrow).* Note that the sagittal stenosis was adequately decompressed at the first surgery *(white arrows). C,* The right S1 pedicle was now visible *(curved arrow)* on the same image as the right L5–S1 neural foramen with its persistent disc material *(black arrow).* Note how the decompression for the central stenosis with its carefully preserved facet joints was still adequate *(white arrows). D,* The right S1 pedicle was now extensively visualized on the right *(curved arrow),* whereas on the left, the far-lateral disc herniation *(black arrow)* could be seen. The central stenosis was still sufficiently decompressed *(white arrows),* despite the appearance of some mild, recurrent stenotic changes in the left lateral recess.

tensor hallucis longus and dorsiflexors, bilaterally absent Achilles responses, and a loss of pin appreciation bilaterally in the L5 distributions. The original plain films, MRI, myelogram, CT-myelogram, and three-dimensional CT scans revealed diffuse, rotatory lumbosacral degenerative stenosis with scoliosis with a near-complete block at the L4–L5 level, with more moderate changes being noted at L2–L3, L3–L4, and L5–S1. Before the first operation, a fusion was considered because of the extensive deformity. However, the patient's advanced age, the presence of osteoporosis, the presence of marked spondylotic changes with bridging osteophytes, and evidence of spontaneous multilevel fusion led to a limited coronal hemilaminectomy of L2 with laminectomies through L5–S1.

For the first 2 postoperative months, while still wearing a TLSO with bar brace, she reported continued discomfort and new left radicular pain but showed no new motor or sensory deficits. Postoperative flexion and extension films failed to demonstrate active subluxation, and an MRI scan with gadolinium showed anticipated postoperative scarring without significant focal abnormalities.

Nevertheless, 8 months later, she acutely developed a flail left foot (2 to 3/5), loss of the Achilles response, and decreased pin appreciation in both the L5 and S1 distributions. The anteroposterior, lateral, flexion, and extension x-ray films showed no changes at the prior laminectomy site, no new progression of scoliosis, or instability. However, a myelogram, CT-myelogram, and three-dimensional CT scans with intrathecal contrast enhancement showed the wide L2–S1 laminectomies, a new right-sided L2–L3 synovial cyst with facet arthritis, and a far-lateral, left-sided L5–S1 disc (Figs. 9 to 11). The second operation included resection of the more cephalad L1 lamina and L2 hemilamina, with dissection being carried down to S1. Bilateral multilevel foraminotomies were conducted for resection of scar tissue, along with neurolysis and dura lysis from L1–L2 through L5–S1. The far-lateral left L5–S1 disc was also excised through an intertransverse approach and the facet joint was preserved. Postoperatively, again after wearing a TLSO brace for 3 months, she slowly began to regain function. Three years later she had no residual deficit.

REFERENCES

1. Alexander, E., Jr., Kelly, D. L., Davis, C. H., et al.: Intact arch spondylolisthesis: A review of 50 cases and description of surgical treatment. J. Neurosurg. 63:840–844, 1985.
2. Aryanpur, J., and Ducker, T.: Multilevel lumbar laminotomies: An alternative to laminectomy in the treatment of lumbar stenosis. Neurosurgery 26:429–432, 1990.
3. Bolesta, M. J., and Bohlman, H. H.: Degenerative spondylolisthesis. Instr. Course Lect. 38:157–165, 1989.
4. Boos, N., Marchesi, D., and Aebi, M.: Treatment of spondylosis and spondylolisthesis with Cotrel-Dubousset instrumentation: A preliminary report. J. Spinal Disord. 4:472–479, 1991.
5. Cauchoix, J., Benoist, M., and Chassaing, V.: Degenerative spondylolisthesis. Clin. Orthop. 115:122–129, 1976.
6. Crutcher, J. P., Jr., Anderson, P. A., King, H. A., and Montesano, P. X.: Indirect spinal canal decompression in patients with thoracolumbar burst fractures treated by posterior distraction rods. J. Spinal Disord. 4:39–48, 1991.
7. Deyo, R. A., Cherkin, D. C., Loeser, J. D., et al.: Morbidity and mortality in association with operations on the lumbar spine. The influence of age, diagnosis and procedure. J. Bone Joint Surg 74A:536–543, 1992.
8. Ehni, G.: Significance of the small lumbar spinal canal: Cauda equina compression syndromes due to spondylosis: Part I: Introduction. J. Neurosurg. 31:490–494, 1969.
9. Ehni, G.: Effects of certain degenerative disease of the spine, especially spondylosis and disk protrusion on the neural contents, particularly in the lumbar region: Historical account. Mayo Clin. Proc. 50:327–338, 1975.
10. Epstein, B. S., Epstein, J. A., and Jones, M. D.: Degenerative spondylolisthesis with an intact neural arch. Radiol. Clin. North Am. 15:227–239, 1977.
11. Epstein, J. A., Epstein, B. S., Rosenthal, A. D., et al.: Degenerative lumbar spondylolisthesis with an intact neural arch (pseudospondylolisthesis). J. Neurosurg. 44:139–147, 1976.
12. Epstein, N. E., Epstein, J. A., Carras, R., and Lavine, L. S.: Degenerative spondylolisthesis with an intact neural arch: A review of 60 cases with an analysis of clinical findings and the development of surgical management. Neurosurgery 13:555–561, 1983.
13. Epstein, N. E., Epstein, J. A., Carras, R., and Hyman, R.: Far lateral lumbar disc herniations and associated structural abnormalities: Evaluation in 60 patients of the comparative value of CT, MRI, and Myelo-CT in diagnosis and management. Spine 15:534–539, 1990.
14. Epstein, N. E.: Lumbar surgery for 56 limbus fractures emphasizing non calcified type III lesions. Spine 17:1489–1496, 1992.
15. Getty, C. J. M., Johnson, J. R., Kirwan, E. O'G., and Sullivan, M. F.: Partial undercutting facetectomy for bony entrapment of the lumbar nerve root. J. Bone Joint Surg. 63B:330–335, 1981.
16. Hall, S., Bartelson, J. D., Onofrio, B. M., et al.: Spinal stenosis: Clinical features, diagnostic procedures, and results of surgical treatment in 68 patients. Ann. Intern. Med. 103:271–275, 1985.
17. Heath, J. M.: The clinical presentation of lumbar spinal stenosis. Ohio Med. 85:484–487, 1989.
18. Herron, L. D., and Mangelsdorf, C.: Lumbar spinal stenosis: Results of surgical treatment. J. Spinal Disord. 4:26–33, 1991.
19. Jonsson, B., Soderholm, R., and Stromqvist, B.: Erythrocyte sedimentation rate after lumbar spine surgery. Spine 16:1049–1950, 1991.
20. Keene, J. S., Fisher, S. P., Vanderby, R., Jr., et al.: Significance of acute posttraumatic bony encroachment of the neural canal. Spine 14:799–802, 1989.
21. Kim, N. H., and Kim, D. J.: Anterior interbody fusion for spondylolisthesis. Orthopedics 14:1069–1076, 1991.
22. Lin, P. M.: Internal decompression for multiple levels of lumbar spinal stenosis: A technical note. Neurosurgery 11:546–549, 1982.
23. Lombardi, J. S., Wilste, L. L., Reynolds, J., et al.: Treatment of degenerative spondylolisthesis. Spine 10:821–827, 1985.
24. Markwalder, T. M., Saager, C., and Reulen, H. J.: "Isthmic" spondylolisthesis—an analysis of the clinical and radiological presentation in relation to intraoperative findings and surgical results in 72 consecutive cases. Acta Neurochir. (Wien) 110:154–159, 1991.
25. Masaryhk, T. J., and Modic, M. T.: The lumbar spine. In Stark, D. D., Bradley, W. G. (Eds.): Magnetic Resonance Imaging. St. Louis, C. V. Mosby, 1988, pp. 666–682.
26. Matsui, H., Tsuji, H., Sekido, H., et al.: Results of expansive laminoplasty for lumbar spinal stenosis in active manual workers. Spine 17(Suppl. 3): S37–S40, 1992.
27. Montalvo, B. M., Quencer, R. M., Brown, M. D., et al.: Lumbar disk herniation and canal stenosis: Value of intraoperative sonography in diagnosis and surgical management. AJR 154:821–830, 1990.
28. Nachemson, A. L.: Newest knowledge of low back pain. A critical look. Clin. Orthop. 279:8–20, 1992.
29. Nakai, O., Ookawa, A., and Yamaura, I.: Long-term roentgenographic and functional changes in patients who were treated with wide fenestration for central lumbar stenosis. J. Bone Joint Surg. 73A:1184–1191, 1991.
30. Postacchini, F., and Cinotti, G.: Bone regrowth after surgical decompression for lumbar spinal stenosis. J. Bone Joint Surg. 74B:862–869, 1992.
31. Quigley, M. R., Kortyna, R., Goodwin, C., and Maroon, J. C.: Lumbar surgery in the elderly. Neurosurgery 30:672–674, 1992.
32. Rosen, C., Rothman, S., Zigler, J., and Capen, D.: Lumbar facet fracture as a possible source of pain after lumbar laminectomy. Spine 16(Suppl.):S234–S238, 1991.
33. Sano, S., Yukukura, S., Nagata, Y., and Young, S. Z.: Unstable lumbar spine without hypermobility in postlaminectomy cases. Mechanism of symp-

toms and effect of spinal fusion with and without spinal instrumentation. Spine 15:1190–1197, 1990.
34. Satomi, K., Hirabayashi, K., Tomaya, Y., and Fujimura, Y.: A clinical study of degenerative spondylolisthesis. Radiographic analysis and choice of treatment. Spine 17:1329–1336, 1992.
35. Scoville, W. B., and Corkill, G.: Lumbar spondylolisthesis with ruptured disc. J. Neurosurg. 40:529–534, 1974.
36. Simmons, E. H., and Jachson, R. P.: The management of nerve root entrapment syndromes associated with the collapsing scoliosis of idiopathic lumbar and thoracolumbar curves. Spine 4:533–541, 1979.
37. Simmons, E. D., Jr., and Simmons, E. H.: Spinal stenosis with scoliosis. Spine 17(Suppl. 6):S117–S120, 1992.
38. Smith, D. W., and Lawrence, B. D.: Vascular complications of lumbar decompression laminectomy and foraminotomy. A unique case and review of the literature. Spine 16:387–390 1991.
39. Smith, E. B., and Hanigan, W. C.: Surgical results and complications in elderly patients with benign lesion of the spinal canal. J. Am. Geriatr. Soc. 40:867–870, 1991.
40. Spengler, D. M.: Current concepts review: Degenerative stenosis of the lumbar spine. J. Bone Joint Surg. 69A:305–308, 1987.
41. Thalgott, J. S., Cotler, H. B., Sasso, R. C., et al.: Postoperative infections in spinal implants. Classification and analysis—a multicenter study. Spine 16:981–984, 1991.
42. Tsou, P. M., and Hopp, E.: Postsurgical instability in spinal stenosis. *In* Hopp, E (ed.): Spine: State of the Art Reviews. Philadelphia, Hanley & Belfus, 1987, pp. 533–550.
43. Tsuji, H., Itoh, T., Sekido, H., et al.: Expansive laminoplasty for lumbar spinal stenosis. Int. Orthop. 14:309–314, 1990.
44. Vanden Berghe, L., Maes, G., Fabry G., and Hoogmartens, M.: In situ posterolateral fusion for spondylolisthesis. Acta Orthop. Belg. 57(suppl. I):214–218, 1991.
45. Wiltse, L. L.: Salvage of failed lumbar spinal stenosis surgery. *In* Hopp, E. (ed.) Spine: State of the Art Reviews. Philadelphia, Hanley & Belfus, 1987, pp. 421–450.
46. Wiltse, L. L., and Rothman, S.: Lumbar and lumbosacral spondylolisthesis: Classification, diagnosis, and natural history. *In* Weinstein, J. W., and Wiesel, S. W. (Eds.): The Lumbar Spine. Philadelphia, W. B. Saunders, 1990, pp. 471–499.
47. Young, S., Veerapen, R., and O'Laoire, S.: Relief of lumbar canal stenosis using multilevel subarticular fenestrations as alternative to wide laminectomy: Preliminary report. Neurosurgery 23:628–633, 1988.

Role of Arthrodesis

HARRY N. HERKOWITZ

The previous sections outline the indications for, techniques of, and results of decompressive laminectomy. The success rate for patients with clinical symptoms of spinal stenosis and a confirming imaging study who undergo decompression of the involved segment or segments is 75% to greater than 90%.[12, 14, 17, 22, 31, 32]

The difficulty arises in deciding which patients would benefit from a concomitant arthrodesis. The decision to add an arthrodesis at the time of the decompressive laminectomy, is based on two factors. The first is the preoperative structural integrity of the lumbar spine. The second is the structural changes that may occur during the surgical procedure. The significant preoperative structural alterations are (1) the presence of degenerative spondylolisthesis along with spinal stenosis; (2) scoliosis and/or kyphosis, along with spinal stenosis; and (3) recurrent spinal stenosis at a previously decompressed spinal level with or without iatrogenic spondylolisthesis. The significant intraoperative changes are (1) excessive removal of lumbar facets and (2) radical excision of the intervertebral disc at the level of decompression.

PREOPERATIVE STRUCTURAL ALTERATIONS

Degenerative Spondylolisthesis

Until the early 1990s, there was no consensus for adding an arthrodesis in patients undergoing decompressive laminectomy when an associated degenerative spondylolisthesis was present (Fig. 12). Numerous articles appeared in the literature advocating no arthrodesis, whereas others supported arthrodesis at the time of the decompressive laminectomy.* Herkowitz and

---

*References 2, 4, 7, 8, 10, 11, 15, 16, 25, and 32.

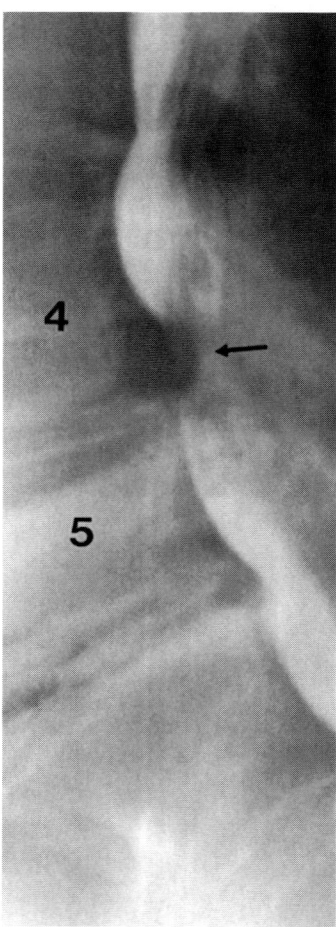

Figure 12. Lateral lumbar myelogram demonstrating spinal stenosis and degenerative lumbar spondylolisthesis at L4–L5.

Kurz[15] published a prospective study comparing decompressive laminectomy with decompressive laminectomy combined with intertransverse arthrodesis in 50 patients with single-level spinal stenosis associated with degenerative spondylolisthesis. The results of that study demonstrated statistically significantly better results in those patients undergoing a concomitant arthrodesis. On the basis those data, the authors recommended arthrodesis for patients undergoing decompressive laminectomy with an associated degenerative spondylolisthesis (Fig. 13). Since then, other articles have supported the addition of an arthrodesis when the stenotic segment was associated with a degenerative spondylolisthesis.[5, 28, 29]

Postacchini and Cinotti[28] reported on the occurrence of laminar regrowth after decompressive laminectomy for spinal stenosis. They reviewed the cases of 40 patients with an average follow-up of 8.6 years. Degenerative spondylolisthesis was present preoperatively in 16 of the 40 patients. Six of these 16 had a decompression alone; 10 had an added arthrodesis. Patients without an arthrodesis had more bone regrowth, contributing to recurrent stenosis, and a significantly poorer clinical outcome than did the group with the arthrodesis.

Further support for the addition of an arthrodesis when spinal stenosis is associated with a degenerative spondylolisthesis was reported by Satomi and colleagues.[29] In their series, 27 patients underwent anterior lumbar interbody fusion, and an additional 14 patients had a posterior decompression only. Excellent and good results were achieved in 93% and 72%, respectively. Although in the arthrodesis group, the spine was fused anteriorly rather than through the traditional posterolateral approach, superior results with an arthrodesis were demonstrated.

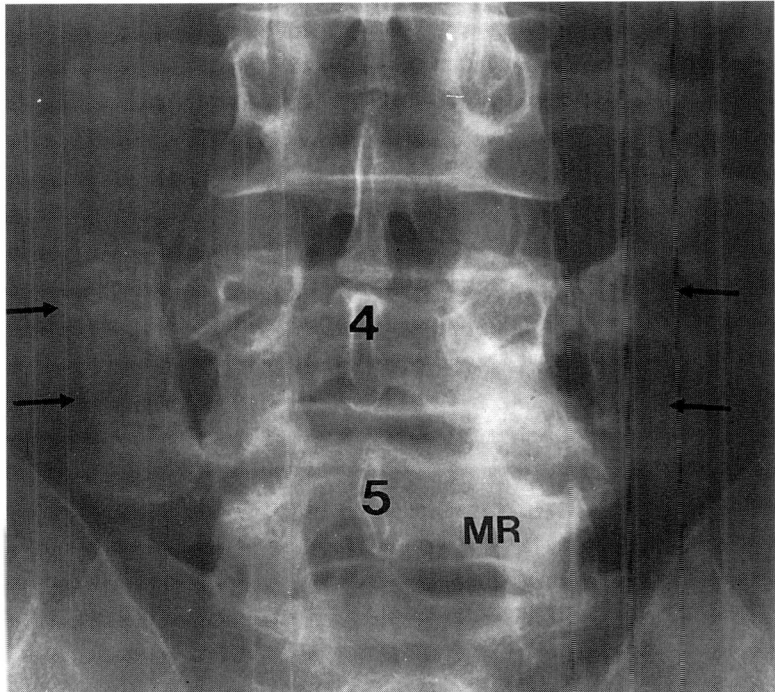

Figure 13. Postoperative anteroposterior radiograph demonstrating solid posterolateral arthrodesis at L4–L5 *(arrows)*.

Caputy and Lessenhop[5] reported on 96 patients undergoing decompression alone for spinal stenosis. At 5 years postoperatively, the procedure was considered a failure for 26 patients. Sixteen of the 26 patients had recurrent leg pain, five of whom had a preexisting degenerative spondylolisthesis. Ten of the 26 patients were considered to have failed procedures because of recurrent low back pain. Five of these 10 patients had a preexisting degenerative spondylolisthesis at the stenotic level. On the basis of their study, Caputy and Lessenhop[5] recommended the addition of an arthrodesis for all patients undergoing surgery for degenerative spondylolisthesis associated with spinal stenosis.

In summary, the data regarding spondylolisthesis in association with spinal stenosis strongly support the addition of a posterolateral arthrodesis at the time of the decompressive laminectomy. The decompression addresses the stenosis, whereas the arthrodesis addresses the instability of the spondylolisthesis.

Scoliosis or Kyphosis

The surgical management of spinal stenosis in association with preexisting idiopathic or degenerative lumbar scoliosis is not as clear-cut as that of degenerative spondylolisthesis (Fig. 14). Prior studies have focused on retrospective analysis of surgical technique without comparative reviews of various surgical options.[23, 26, 27, 30]

Not all patients with surgically significant spinal stenosis within a lumbar scoliosis or kyphosis require a concomitant arthrodesis. The author uses the following criteria for adding an arthrodesis:

1. Curve flexibility. On side bending films, the curve demonstrates at least 50% correction. A decompressive laminectomy alone would most likely increase the risk of curve progression unless arthrodesis is added when a flexible curve exists.

2. A documented preoperative history of curve progression. This alone is an indication for arthrodesis.

3. Scoliosis with a predominant radiculopathy within the concavity of the curve (Fig. 15). In this case, a partial facetectomy may not be sufficient to alleviate nerve root compression in the concavity that may be due to root compression between the pedicles of the concavity. Thus, partial correction of the deformity to reduce pedicular kinking is indicated.

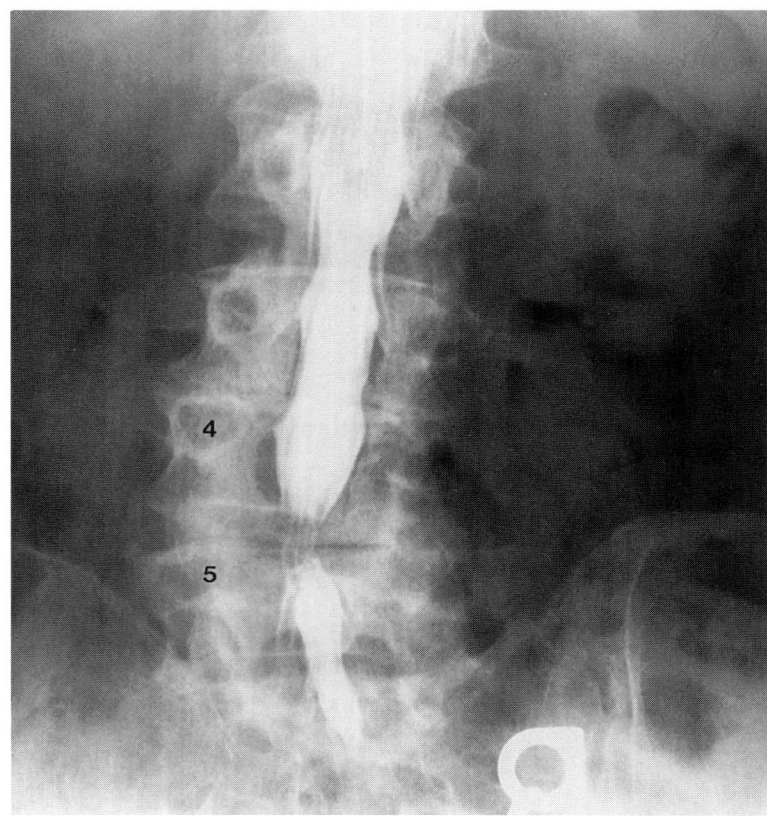

Figure 14. An anteroposterior radiograph of spinal stenosis in association with degenerative lumbar scoliosis.

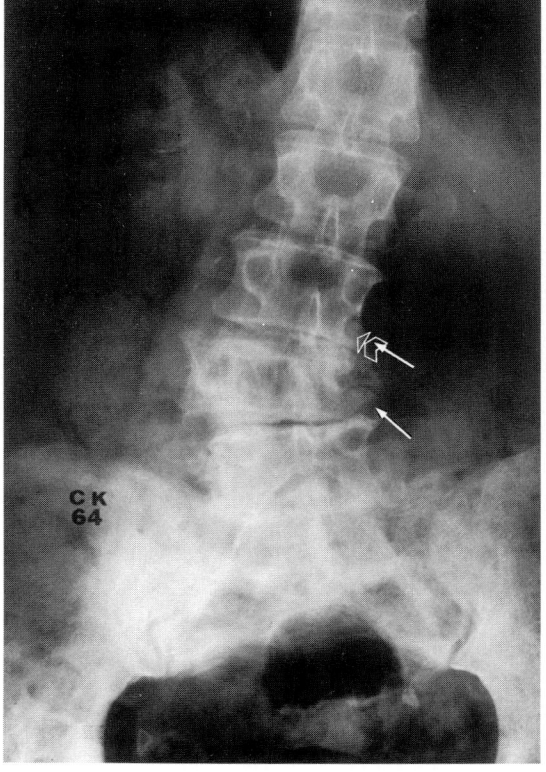

Figure 15. An anteroposterior radiograph depicting scoliosis and spinal stenosis in a 66-year-old woman with right lumbar radiculopathy *(arrows)*.

4. Loss of lumbar lordosis such that the patient is in sagittal imbalance, which is defined from a standing lateral x-ray film including the base of the skull to the sacrum. On this film, a plumb line is drawn inferiorly from the odontoid process. This line normally passes through the posterior half of the vertebral body of L5. In a patient with sagittal imbalance, this line passes anterior to this point (Fig. 16). Persistence of a flat back may lead to increasing back pain postoperatively.

5. Lateral spondylolisthesis. Lateral listhesis that demonstrates correction on side bending films is an indication of a hypermobile segment, which may become more unstable after a decompression alone.

The magnitude of the scoliotic curve itself is not a sufficient reason to recommend arthrodesis without the presence of the other preexisting factors outlined. As an example, a 60-degree rigid lumbar curve with satisfactory sagittal balance and three-level spinal stenosis requires only a decompressive laminectomy.

Recurrent Spinal Stenosis at the Same Segment

Patients who require a second decompressive laminectomy at the same segment are candidates for an arthrodesis. Further compromise of the facet joints is usually necessary to accomplish decompression of the central canal and lateral recesses in these cases. Sacrificing more than 50% of each facet joint renders that motion segment unstable, especially when the facet joints lie in a sagittal orientation.[1, 13]

Segmental instability may be detected on

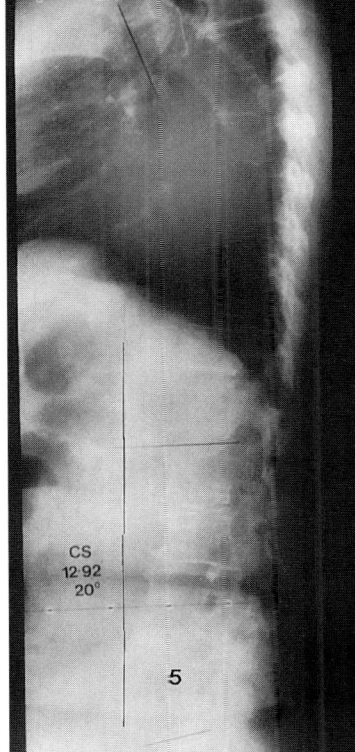

Figure 16. Standing lateral lumbar radiograph demonstrating loss of lumbar lordosis with the plumb line in front of the L5 vertebral body (lordosis of 20 degrees).

lateral flexion-extension radiographs. Excessive translational or angular movement of the motion segment is defined as greater than 4 mm of translational movement (Fig. 17A, B) or greater than 10 degrees of angular change measured at the end plate when compared with that of the adjacent vertebrae (Fig. 18).

Patients in whom a recurrent stenosis develops in conjunction with an iatrogenic spondylolisthesis also require concomitant arthrodesis because further instability is produced after the second surgery.[18, 20, 21, 24, 34] Patients who develop stenosis above a previous posterior fusion require decompression only unless criteria for instability are present.

INTRAOPERATIVE STRUCTURAL ALTERATIONS

Loss of Structural Support: Excessive Removal of the Facet Joints

Abumi and coworkers[1] demonstrated in cadaveric specimens the importance of the lumbar facet joints for the structural stability of the motion segment. After performing progressive facetectomies of the lumbar motion segment and subjecting the specimens to cyclic loading in an Instron machine, they concluded that removal of greater than 50% of each facet joint led to unacceptable movement of that motion segment (defined as greater than 50% of each facet joint). Therefore, when excessive facet excision occurs during surgery, posterolateral arthrodesis should be added to prevent postoperative instability.

Disc Excision

The prevalence of disc herniation in conjunction with spinal stenosis has been reported to be from 5% to 25%.[12, 14] Most disc herniations that occur in this group represent extrusions or free fragments of disc at the level of the foramen. In those cases, simple removal of the disc fragment at the time of decompressive laminectomy is all that is required. Radical disc excision means removal of as much disc material as possible. This may lead to an iatrogenic spondylolisthesis because it destabilizes the anterior column after the posterior column has been compromised by the decompressive laminectomy.[8] If a radical discectomy was thought to be necessary, a posterolateral arthrodesis should be added.

SPINAL INSTRUMENTATION

The goals of internal fixation are (1) deformity correction, (2) spinal stabilization, (3)

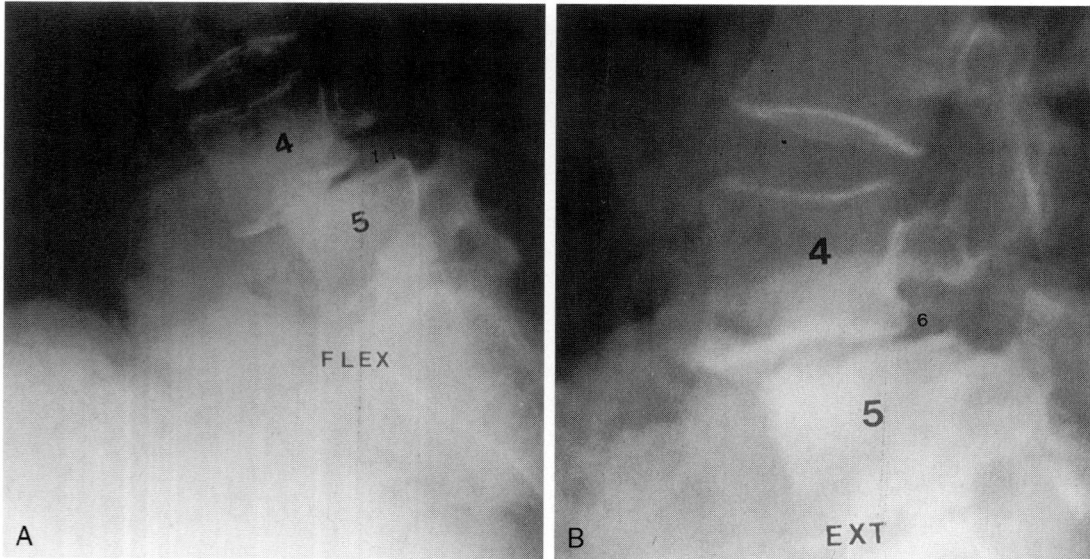

Figure 17. A, Lateral flexion radiograph showing 11 mm of forward translation. B, Lateral extension radiograph showing 6 mm of residual translation. A total of 5 mm of translational motion is present.

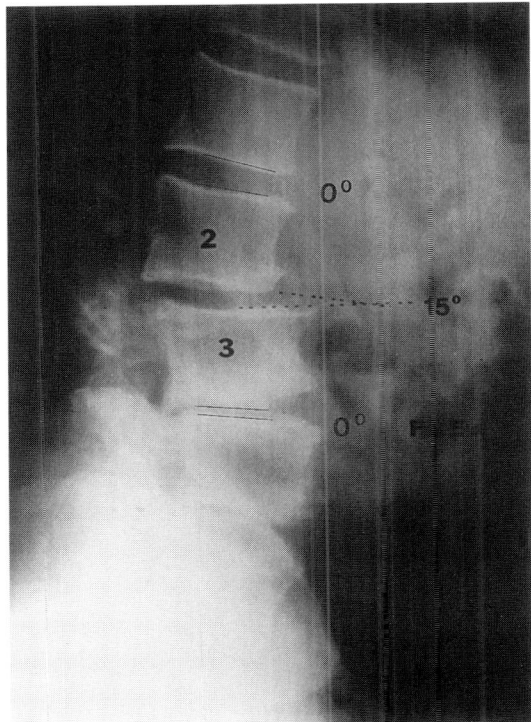

Figure 18. Lateral flexion radiograph demonstrating excessive angular motion at L2–L3 after a prior decompressive L2–L3 laminectomy.

protection of the neural elements, (4) improvement in the rate of fusion, (5) a reduction in the number of segments requiring arthrodesis by preserving as many distal lumbar segments as possible, and (6) a reduction in rehabilitation time.

Fixation of the lumbar and lumbosacral spine presents unique considerations, especially when dealing with an aged population. Lumbar spinal instrumentation in the older age population must address osteoporosis and the lack of lamina available for fixation that occurs following the decompressive laminectomy. The use of traditional posterior distraction systems such as Harrington rods and Knodt rods often leads to a loss of lumbar lordosis. The maintenance of lumbar lordosis is a critical factor in long-term surgical success, because failure to maintain lumbar lordosis is a significant cause of recurrent back or leg pain.

Fixation into the pedicle appears to solve the technical problems of the traditional implant systems. It places the fixation points through the lumbar pedicle, which is the strongest part of the osteopenic vertebra,[36] and allows segmental fixation, which improves torsional stability and aids in maintaining lumbar lordosis (Fig. 19A,B). In addition, segmental fixation may reduce the number of motion segments requiring arthrodesis, thus preserving distal lumbar segments, which is an important factor in reducing the incidence of low back pain. Pedicle screw systems also improve the ability to achieve adequate sacral fixation over conventional hook and rod systems.[3]

Balancing the advantages of pedicle fixation are its disadvantages. First, a significant learning curve exists, even for experienced spine surgeons.[33, 35] Failure to place the pedicle screw in the correct location may lead to neurologic deficit or loss of fixation.[9] In addition, the longevity of pedicle fixation systems is being evaluated.[3] Boos and colleagues[3] evaluated the AO internal fixator and the Cotrel-Dubousset system after their implantation for degenerative disorders of the lumbar spine. At more than 2 years after surgery, only 70% of the implants remained intact.

The negative factors of pedicle fixation must be weighed against their advantages so that the surgeon can make an informed decision about whether an implant system is necessary at the time of arthrodesis. With

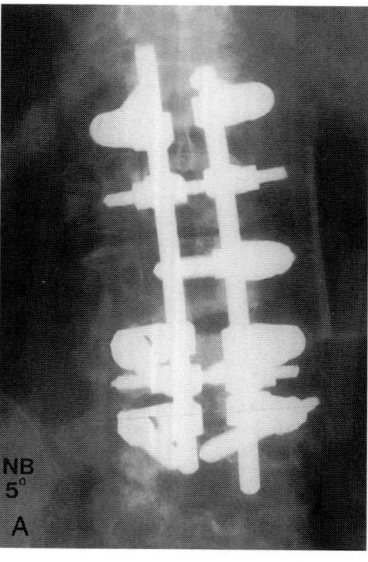 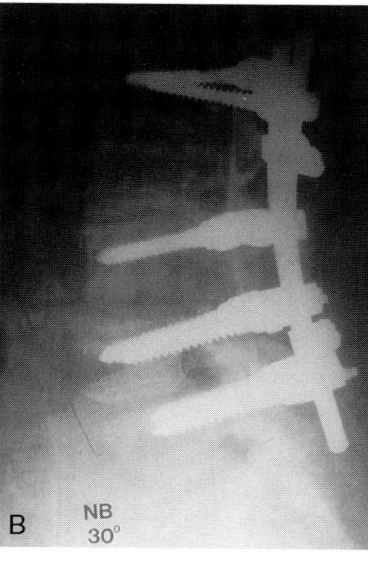

Figure 19. Anteroposterior *(A)* and lateral *(B)* radiographs of pedicle fixation.

the increasing efforts surgeons must make to control costs, this becomes even more important.

A surgeon contemplating the addition of a spinal implant to the arthrodesis in patients with spinal stenosis is faced with the lack of hard scientific data are to assist in making an informed decision. In many cases, the purpose of adding instrumentation after decompression and arthrodesis is most often to improve the chance for a solid arthrodesis and to correct a preexisting deformity.

The occurrence of pseudarthrosis after posterolateral fusion is inversely proportional to the number of levels that are being fused. The rates of pseudarthrosis for one-level, two-level, and three-level fusions are 3.5% to 10%, 15% to 20%, and 25% to 33%, respectively.[19] In addition, the pseudarthrosis rate increases if segmental instability at that motion segment is present (e.g., a prior decompressive laminectomy produced translational or angular instability). Therefore, placing the arthrodesis when these conditions are present aids in obtaining a successful fusion.

The indications for the addition of instrumentation following spinal stenosis decompression and arthrodesis are (1) correction of scoliosis or kyphosis, (2) arthrodesis of two or more motion segments with an associated decompressive laminectomy, (3) recurrent spinal stenosis with iatrogenic spondylolisthesis, (4) translational motion greater than 4 mm in flexion and extension, and (5) angular motion greater than 10 degrees when compared with the adjacent levels in flexion and extension. Is the addition of instrumentation indicated for a one-level arthrodesis in degenerative spondylolisthesis following decompressive laminectomy or if excessive facet excision has occurred at the time of the one-level laminectomy? The answer to these questions is not as yet present in the literature.

SUMMARY

In summary, this discussion outlines the indications for arthrodesis and spinal instrumentation in degenerative lumbar spinal stenosis. It has not attempted to detail surgical technique. Analysis of the various implant systems, along with their advantages and disadvantages, has been omitted because it is beyond the scope of this discussion.

Much needs to be clarified regarding arthrodesis and instrumentation for lumbar degenerative disorders. Only prospective controlled studies will answer these questions so that patients can receive the most effective and long-lasting surgical treatment.

REFERENCES

1. Abumi, K., Panjabi, M., Kramer, K., et al.: Biomechanical evaluation of lumbar spinal stability after graded facetectomies. Spine 15:1142–1147, 1990.
2. Bolesta, M., and Bohlman, H.: Degenerative spon-

dylolisthesis: The role of arthrodesis. Presented at the American Academy of Orthopaedic Surgery Annual Meeting, Las Vegas, February, 1989.
3. Boos, N., Marchesi, D., and Aebi, M.: Survivorship analysis of pedicular fixation systems in the treatment of degenerative disorders of the lumbar spine. J. Spinal Disord. 5:403–409, 1992.
4. Brown, M., and Lockwood, W.: Degenerative spondylolisthesis. Instr. Course Lect. 28:162–169, 1983.
5. Caputy, A., and Lessenhop, A.: Long term evaluation of decompressive surgery for degenerative lumbar stenosis. J. Neurosurg. 77:669–676, 1992.
6. Carlson, G. D., Abitbol, J. J., Anderson, D. R., et al.: Screw fixation in the sacrum. Spine 17:S196–S203, 1992.
7. Chang, K. W., and McAfee, P. Degenerative spondylolisthesis and degenerative scoliosis. J. Spinal Disord. 1:247–256, 1989.
8. Dall, B., and Rowe, D.: Degenerative spondylolisthesis: Its surgical management. Spine 10:668–672, 1985.
9. Davne, S., and Myers, D.: Complications of lumbar spinal fusion with transpedicular instrumentation. Spine 17:S184–S189, 1992.
10. Feffer, H., Wiesel, S., Cuckler, J., and Rothman, R. H.: Degenerative spondylolisthesis. To fuse or not to fuse. Spine 10:287–289, 1985.
11. Fitzgerald, J. A. W.: Degenerative spondylolisthesis. J. Bone Joint Surg. 58B:184–192, 1976.
12. Garfin, S., Glover, M., Booth, R., et al.: Laminectomy: A review of the Pennsylvania Hospital experience. J. Spinal Disord. 1:116–133, 1988.
13. Grobler, L., Robertson, P., Novotny, J., and Pope, M.: Etiology of spondylolisthesis: Assessment of the role played by lumbar facet joint morphology. Spine 18:80–91, 1993.
14. Herkowitz, H. N., and Garfin, S. R.: Decompressive surgery for spinal stenosis. Semin. Spine Surg. 1:163–167, 1989.
15. Herkowitz, H. N., and Kurz, L. T.: Degenerative lumbar spondylolisthesis with spinal stenosis. A prospective study comparing decompression with decompression and intertransverse process arthrodesis. J. Bone Joint Surg. 73A:802–808, 1991.
16. Herron, L., and Trippi, P.: Degenerative spondylolisthesis. Spine 14:534–538, 1989.
17. Herron, L., and Mangelsdorf, C.: Lumbar spinal stenosis: Results of surgical treatment. J. Spinal Disord. 4:26–33, 1991.
18. Hopp, E., and Tsou, P.: Postdecompression lumbar instability. Clin. Orthop. 227:143–151, 1988.
19. Jackson, R. K., Boston, D. A., and Edge, A. J.: Lateral mass fusion: A prospective study of a consecutive series with long term follow-up. Spine 10:828–832, 1985.
20. Johnsson, K. E., Wilner, S., and Johnsson, K.: Postoperative instability after decompression for lumbar spinal stenosis. Spine 11:107–110, 1986.
21. Johnsson, K., Wilner, S., and Petterson, H.: Analysis of instability after decompression for lumbar spine stenosis. Spine 11:63–67, 1986.
22. Katz, J. N., Lipson, S. J., Larson, M. G., et al.: The outcome of decompressive laminectomy for degenerative lumbar stenosis. J. Bone Joint Surg. 73A:809–816, 1991.
23. Kostuik, J., Errico, T., and Gleason, T.: Lucque instrumentation in degenerative conditions of the lumbar spine. Spine 15:318–321, 1990.
24. Lee, C. K.: Lumbar spine instability (listhesis) after extensive posterior spinal decompression. Spine 8:429–433, 1983.
25. Lombardi, J. S., Wiltse, L., Reynolds, J., et al.: Treatment of degenerative spondylolisthesis. Spine 10:821–827, 1985.
26. Marchesi, D., and Aebi, M.: Pedicle fixation devices in the treatment of adult lumbar scoliosis. Spine 17:S304–S309, 1992.
27. Nasca, R.: Rationale for spinal fusion in lumbar spinal stenosis. Spine 14:451–454, 1989
28. Postacchini, F., and Cinotti, G.: Bone regrowth after surgical decompression for lumbar spinal stenosis. J. Bone Joint Surg. 74B:862–869, 1992.
29. Satomi, K., Hirabayahi, K., Toyama Y., and Fujimura, U.: A clinical study of degenerative spondylolisthesis. Spine 17:1329–1336, 1992.
30. Simmons, E. D., Jr., and Simmons, E. H.: Spinal stenosis in scoliosis. Spine 17:S117–S120, 1992.
31. Spengler, D.: Degenerative stenosis of the lumbar spine: Current concepts review. J. Bone Joint Surg. 69A:305–308, 1987.
32. Tile, M., McNeil, S. R., Zarins, R. K., et al.: Spinal stenosis: Results of treatment. Clin Orthop. 115:104–108, 1976.
33. Weinstein, J., Spratt, K., Spengler, D., et al.: Spinal pedicle fixation: Reliability and validity of roentgenogram-based assessment and surgical factors on successful screw placement. Spine 13:1012–1018, 1988.
34. White, A., and Wiltse, L.: Postoperative Spondylolisthesis in Lumbar Spondylosis. Diagnosis, Management, and Surgical Treatment. Chicago, Year Book, 1977, pp. 184–194.
35. Whitecloud, T., Skalley, T., Crooks, S., and Morgan, E.: Roentgenographic measurement of pedicle screw penetration. Clin. Orthop. 245:57–68, 1989.
36. Zindrick, M., Wiltse, L., Widell, E., et al.: A biomechanical study of intrapedicular screw fixation in the lumbosacral spine. Clin. Orthop. 203:99–112, 1986.

Long-Term Results

FRANCO POSTACCHINI

Many authors have analyzed the results of the surgical treatment of lumbar stenosis. It is, however, difficult to compare the results in the different series. Some investigators, in fact, do not provide a precise definition of the term stenosis and thus of the nature of the pathologic conditions included in the clinical series. Furthermore, there are contrasting concepts of stenosis as well as various classifications of the stenotic conditions. These difficulties are further increased by the lack of uniformity in the postoperative clinical evaluation of patients and in the qualitative definition of the results. On the other hand, in some series no distinction is made between patients who have not previously undergone spine surgery and patients previously operated on, the results for whom may be influenced by the earlier surgical treatment.

The author previously reported a definition and classification of lumbar stenosis.[50] The latter includes developmental, degenerative, and combined (developmental and degenerative) stenosis. In each of these conditions, there may be spinal canal stenosis, isolated nerve root canal stenosis, and stenosis of the intervertebral foramen. The former two types of stenosis correspond, respectively, to the so-called central stenosis and lateral stenosis. Stenosis of the intervertebral foramen, which is a fairly rare condition, is mostly associated with one of the two other types of stenosis.

NATURAL HISTORY

Little is known about the clinical evolution of an untreated lumbar stenosis. Jones and Thomson[33] reported on three untreated patients. One of them improved, the condition of one was unchanged, and one was not followed. Blau and Logue[3] followed two untreated patients. One had a slow progression of symptoms during a 10-year period, while the other remained unchanged over 7 years. Johnsson and colleagues[32] compared 19 untreated patients with 30 patients who underwent surgery. They were followed for a mean period of 31 and 53 months, respectively; all patients in both groups had lumbar stenosis of moderate severity. About one third of the untreated patients were improved and two thirds were unchanged or had worsened. Porter and coworkers[49] reviewed 169 patients with radicular canal stenosis, most of whom had not undergone treatment. At the last follow-up (2 years on average), 78% of patients still reported radicular symptoms, but in almost all cases (90%), symptoms had improved or were so mild as to require no treatment. In the vast majority of the patients, however, there was no evidence of neurologic deficits, and in no instances was clinical diagnosis confirmed by imaging or neurophysiologic studies.

In degenerative spondylolisthesis, progression of slipping was observed in 30% of 40 patients followed for longer than 5 years, but the progression was not necessarily associated with deterioration of the patient's condition.[43]

Twelve untreated patients with central lumbar stenosis were followed for 3 to 12 years (mean of 5.2 years). There were five men and seven women, aged 52 to 74 years. All patients underwent myelography, CT scanning and MRI, and six, at the time of diagnosis, had weakness of muscles innervated by one or more nerve roots. Stenosis was at a single intervertebral level in seven cases and at two or more levels in five cases. Compression of the neural structures was severe in seven cases and moderate in five cases. Radicular symptoms worsened over time in two cases, remained unchanged in six, and improved or disappeared in four. Of the latter four patients, three had a moderate compression of the neural structures. Muscle weakness increased in one patient, did not change in three, and improved partially or completely in two. These findings indicate that, in most patients with central lumbar stenosis, symptoms tend to remain unchanged or to worsen, particularly when stenosis is severe. However, improvement may occur and persist, even in the long term, in the presence of moderate stenosis.

CONSERVATIVE TREATMENT

Few studies have analyzed the results of conservative treatment in lumbar spinal stenosis.

Tile and colleagues[67] obtained unsatisfactory results in 11 of 14 patients treated with conventional conservative therapy. Excellent results were observed only in patients with developmental stenosis, whereas the results were poor for almost all patients with degenerative spondylolisthesis. However, the severity of stenosis and the length of follow-up were not reported. Similar considerations are valid for some 150 patients with degenerative spondylolisthesis treated with conservative measures by Rosenberg.[58] Most of his patients had mild symptoms that, although not improved by conservative therapy, were not severe enough to require surgical treatment.

Of the 23 patients treated conservatively by Hasue and coworkers,[23] more than half had an improvement of symptoms, but almost none showed recovery from neurologic deficits, when present. Hawkes and Roberts[24] found that six of nine patients had a remission of symptoms with the use of a lumbar corset.

Of the 41 patients with intermittent claudication treated with calcitonin by Porter and Hibbert,[48] 11 showed lasting improvement both of radicular symptoms at rest and of walking capacity. Before treatment most of the improved patients had a walking capacity of less than 1 mile and reported leg pain and paresthesias. Most of these patients, however, had no neurologic deficits, and myelography, when performed, usually showed a relatively mild compression of the neural structures, as the case reports appear to indicate.

In the author's experience, most patients with severe central spinal stenosis do not improve or show temporary relief after conventional conservative treatment. Conversely, patients with central stenosis causing posterior or posterolateral compression of the thecal sac, but no significant nerve root compression in the radicular canal, often show a significant improvement, which is probably due to the natural course of the disease rather than the conservative therapy. This holds true also for lateral stenosis; if narrowing of the radicular canal is marked and responsible for significant neurologic changes, conservative treatment does not usually yield any appreciable improvement, particularly in the long term.

SURGICAL TREATMENT

Overall Results

Spinal Canal Stenosis

Of the 29 patients reported by Teng and Papateodorou,[66] 25 showed a significant clinical improvement, but only 18 were asymptomatic at long-term follow-up. In the series of Tile and coworkers,[67] satisfactory results were observed in 83% of the 18 patients with developmental stenosis and in 82% of the 29 cases of degenerative stenosis (with or without spondylolisthesis) after a mean follow-up of 5 years.

Paine[47] evaluated 150 patients with spinal stenosis alone and 119 in whom stenosis was associated with herniation of the nucleus pulposus 1 to 15 years after surgery. Results were rated as satisfactory in 75% of patients in the former group and in 82% in the latter group. When three levels or more were involved, only 60% had a good to excellent outcome, compared with 85% who had a good to excellent result with one or two levels of involvement.

Of the 92 patients followed by Verbiest[73] for periods ranging from 1 to 20 years, 62 (68%) were completely relieved of preoperative symptoms and neurologic deficits. In the remaining 29 cases, low back pain was the most frequent persisting symptom (18 cases); none of 29 patients reported radicular pain, but in 10 cases, sensory or motor deficits persisted. The highest rate of complete recovery from preoperative symptoms and signs was obtained in cases with pure absolute stenosis (i.e., with the most marked narrowing of the bony vertebral canal), whereas the patients showing the least favorable results were those with milder stenosis.

In one series,[14] more than 80% of the patients showed clinical improvement. Of the two achondroplastic dwarfs included in the series (both previously unsuccessfully operated on), one had no improvement of preoperative paraplegia and disturbances in micturition despite extensive decompression from T10 to the sacrum, whereas in the other, disturbances in micturition and radicular pain were relieved after laminectomy of the last two thoracic vertebrae. Similarly, in the other two cases of achondroplastic stenosis[1] that were submitted to extensive decompressive laminectomy as far as the last thoracic vertebrae, only a partial improvement of symptoms and signs was obtained.

Hasue and coworkers,[23] in a follow-up study of 58 patients, observed complete relief of the preoperative symptoms and signs in 52% of cases and partial improvement in 36%. Results were excellent in 55% of the 20 patients with a radicular syndrome, in 61% of the 31 patients with intermittent claudication, and in none of the seven patients with multiple radicular paralysis, five of whom, however, showed partial improvement.

Getty[21] followed 31 patients for a mean period of 3½ years after surgery. The results were good in 55% of the cases, fair in 20%, and poor in 16%. Four patients, who had previously undergone total laminectomy at multiple levels, were operated on again because of a poor clinical result, probably because of persistent stenosis of the lateral portions of the spinal canal. The clinical result improved in two cases and remained unchanged in the other two cases.

In a review of 50 patients with degenerative stenosis, most of whom had a redundancy of the caudal nerve roots, a marked improvement of symptoms was observed in 36% of cases and a moderate improvement in 57%.[68] No significant relationship was found between the degree of nerve root redundancy and the quality of the result. However, patients with a considerable improvement more frequently showed a mild or no redundancy than a marked redundancy.

Lassale and coworkers[39] evaluated 128 patients 2 to 14 years after surgery using a grading scale of 0 to 20. Satisfactory results were found in 83% of patients. Severe neurologic deficits resolved completely in 60% of the cases. On the grading scale, four recovery profiles were identified: a stable result (60%), regular improvement (14%), improvement with episodic aggravation of symptoms (19%), and subsequent worsening (8%).

In a prospective study of 140 patients, an average leg pain improvement of 82% and back pain improvement of 71% was found a mean of 3 years after surgery. Considerable improvement (75% or more) of leg pain was obtained by 80% of patients and of back pain by 67%.[28]

In a metaanalysis of the literature,[69] the mean proportion of good to excellent results at long-term follow-up was 64%. No statistically significant relationship emerged between outcomes and patient characteristics such as age, sex, presence of claudication, and prior back surgery.

Isolated Nerve Root Canal Stenosis

Proportions of satisfactory results ranging from 79% to 93% were obtained by several investigators using laminotomy[2, 11, 15, 67] or total laminectomy.[37] In one series,[37] the patients in whom a disc herniation was associated with stenosis had a higher proportion of excellent outcomes (69%) than did those with stenosis alone (25%). Venner and Crock[72] reviewed 45 patients with stenosis of the S1 nerve root canal in the presence of isolated resorption of the fifth lumbar disc an average of 45 months after surgery. An excellent result was obtained by 62% and a good result by 25% of patients.

In a review of 62 patients with atypical leg pain caused by lateral stenosis and defined by positive results on nerve root sheath infiltration testing, a success rate of 90% as objectively assessed and 80% as subjectively evaluated by the patients was found.[72] Decompression of only the symptomatic nerve root in the presence of entrapment of more than one root yielded satisfactory results in 93% of the cases.

Results were satisfactory in 83% of 43 cases followed for 3 years on average.[51] Good to excellent outcomes were observed in 90% of patients with preoperative motor deficits or reflex changes and in 71% of those without neurologic deficits. The proportion of satisfactory results was lower in patients with normal myelographic findings (66%) than in those in whom myelography showed evidence of compression of the clinically involved nerve root (88%).

Stenosis of the Intervertebral Foramen

Epstein and colleagues[16] reported on 12 patients treated surgically, three of whom had degenerative spondylolisthesis. In five of the 12 patients, there was also spinal canal stenosis, whereas in seven cases, stenosis of the intervertebral foramen was apparently isolated. Six patients had an excellent result, five had a fair to good outcome, and one remained disabled. Instability due to facet removal alone was not observed. Two patients with degenerative spondylolisthesis, however, underwent spinal fusion at the time of decompression.

Degenerative Spondylolisthesis

Numerous studies have selectively analyzed the results of surgical treatment in degenerative spondylolisthesis. Rosenberg[58] followed 26 patients, of whom 11 had been submitted to monolateral or total laminectomy. Satisfactory results were obtained in only 54% of the patients in the first group, whereas considerable improvement of symptoms was achieved by all patients in the second group. High proportions of satisfactory results after decompression alone are also reported by other researchers. Cauchoix and coworkers[9] found satisfactory outcomes in 85% of 26 patients who underwent total laminectomy associated or not associated with arthrectomy. In another study, 53 (87%) of 60 patients followed for 1 month to 7 years obtained good to excellent results and seven (13%) had a poor outcome.[17] Herron and Trippi[29] observed 85% satisfactory results in 26 patients followed for an average of 3 years after surgery.

In the past 2 decades, vertebral fusion, without or with (nontranspedicule) instrumentation, has been performed more and more often in addition to decompression.* The proportions of satisfactory results have ranged from 85% to 100%. Few studies, however, have compared patients with fusion and patients without fusion. Feffer and colleagues,[19] in a retrospective analysis of a small series of cases, observed a significantly higher proportion of satisfactory results in patients who had undergone fusion. In one study, good to excellent outcomes were found in 80% of patients who had undergone total laminectomy with partial arthrectomy and in 90% of those who also had intertransverse fusion.[42] Herkowitz and Kurz,[27] in a prospective study comparing 25 patients without fusion and 25 patients with fusion (without instrumentation) followed for a mean of 3 years, found satisfactory results in 44% of the first group and in 96% of the second group. In the fusion group, however, the rate of solid fusion was 64%. In other studies analyzing patients who had undergone noninstrumented arthrodesis, the percentage of solid fusion ranged from 91% to 100%.[19, 20, 42, 52]

Screw fixation has become the system of internal fixation most widely used in degenerative spondylolisthesis. Nevertheless, few data are available on the results of this type of instrumented fusion. The fusion rate has ranged from 87% to 100% when autograft was used.[5, 10, 34] The clinical results were found to be satisfactory in 33% of the cases reported by Bridwell and colleagues[5] and in 88% of those reported by Chang and McAfee.[10] Not only was an increase in olisthesis rarely observed, but also a decrease of slipping was often obtained with pedicle screw fixation.[10]

The results of anterior interbody fusion not associated with posterior decompression were analyzed an average of 12 years after surgery in 34 patients examined postoperatively at intervals of about 5 years.[65] The results were satisfactory in 67% of the cases for 10 years, in 60% for 20 years, and in 52% for 30 years. The good results lasted longer in patients undergoing surgery before 50 years of age, but no convincing explanation was found for the deterioration of the results with increasing patient age and time since surgery. Furthermore, no information is reported on the degree of preoperative stenosis.

Postoperative Instability

Removal of a large portion of the posterior vertebral arch may be responsible for postoperative instability. However, the data on the incidence of instability after total laminectomy are not uniform. In patients with no preoperative olisthesis, postsurgical ver-

---

*References 9, 19, 20, 22, 27, 35, 38, 42, and 75.

tebral slipping at the operated levels was observed in 4% to 32% of the cases.[30, 32, 61] Iida and coworkers[31] found evidence of instability (vertebral slipping and/or hypermobility on functional radiographs) at the operated levels in 27% of the cases; however, the proportion reached 90% when the adjacent levels were also examined. It is interesting to note that these researchers found evidence of instability at the operated level and/or adjacent levels in 40% of patients who had undergone laminotomy.

A postoperative increase of slipping in patients with preoperative degenerative spondylolisthesis has been found in proportions ranging from 46% to 100%.[27, 29, 32, 40, 64] An increase in slipping was found in both patients without fusion and patients with fusion. However, in the patients without fusion, the incidence and the amount of increase in olisthesis were generally greater than those in patients who had undergone fusion.[27, 42] In most reports, new olisthesis or increases in existing olisthesis were more often observed in women at the L4–L5 level after a radical decompression and in patients with preoperative hypermobility on flexion-extension radiographs.

Contrasting results have been obtained when vertebral hypermobility, new olisthesis, or an increase in existing olisthesis was related to postoperative clinical symptoms. In some studies, no significant relationship was found.[29, 42, 64] In other studies, patients with postoperative instability (vertebral hypermobility or slipping) reported pain or more severe pain more frequently than did patients with a stable spine.[27, 31, 32]

The matter is further complicated by the still poor understanding of instability. Some researchers have identified two types of instability: radiologic (hypermobility on functional radiographs or CT scans) and clinical (no radiologic hypermobility, but the presence of symptoms of instability). The existence of the latter type of instability is proved by the disappearance of back pain and even leg pain after vertebral fusion in patients who were previously operated on and who showed no radiologic evidence of instability. Sano and colleagues[59] reported on 20 such patients, most of whom had good clinical results after spinal fusion.

Method and Extent of Decompression

Until few years ago, total laminectomy was the standard method of decompression for central lumbar stenosis. In 1988, Senegas and coworkers[60] described an alternative to total laminectomy, the so-called "recalibrage" of the spinal canal. This procedure, consisting of bilateral laminectomy and partial

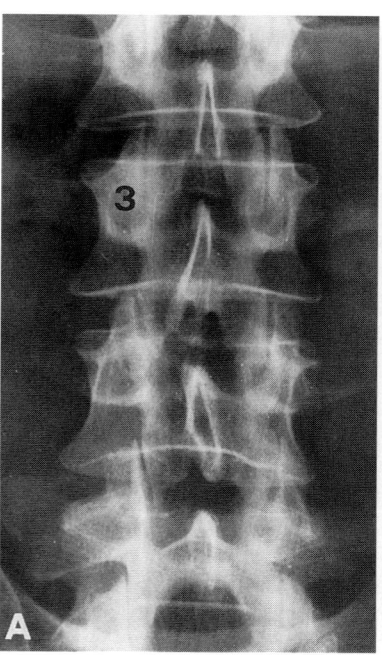
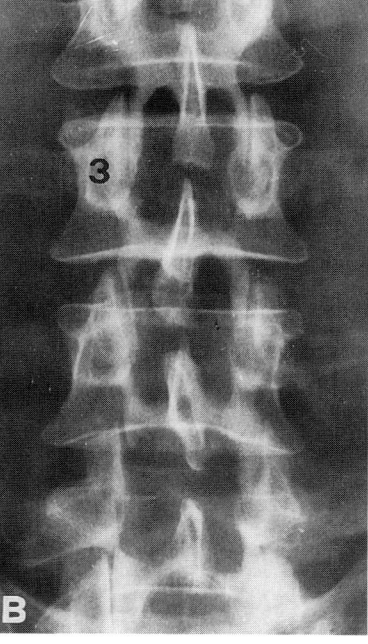

Figure 1. Example of multiple laminotomy in a patient with developmental stenosis. *A*, Preoperative radiograph. *B*, Postoperative radiograph showing bilateral laminotomies at L2–L3 to L4–L5.

arthrectomy performed only at the level of the intervertebral space, gave satisfactory results in 88% of the cases. In only one case did postoperative instability occur.

Surgical techniques preserving a larger part of the posterior vertebral arch than does laminectomy have been developed with the aim of reducing the risks of postoperative instability. Lin,[41] Young and coworkers,[76] and Postacchini and colleagues[55] have described the use of multiple laminotomy in central lumbar stenosis (Fig. 1). Nakai and colleagues[45] described a procedure called wide fenestration, consisting of the removal of only the medial part of the inferior facets and the adjoining ligamentum flavum. Satisfactory results were observed in 91% of 32 patients undergoing laminotomies[76] and 75% of 32 patients undergoing wide fenestration.[45] In the latter series, three patients had recurrent stenosis and five had segmental instability an average of 5 years after surgery.

Postacchini and colleagues[55] studied prospectively and followed for an average of 3 years 67 patients with central stenosis assigned to undergo either multiple laminotomy or total laminectomy. The protocol, however, allowed multiple laminotomy to be changed to total laminectomy if, during surgery, it was realized that the former procedure might not provide adequate neural decompression. This occurred in seven patients with severe stenosis. Bilateral laminotomy at two or three levels required a longer mean operative time than did total laminectomy at an equal number of levels. The mean blood loss at surgery and the clinical results did not differ significantly in the two groups (81% and 78% of patients having satisfactory outcomes, respectively). The mean subjective improvement score for low back pain was significantly higher in patients with laminotomies, but there was also a higher incidence of postoperative radicular deficits in this group. No patient undergoing laminotomies had postoperative vertebral instability, whereas this occurred after laminectomy in three patients who had lumbar scoliosis or degenerative spondylolisthesis preoperatively (Fig. 2).

Arthrectomy may be total (or subtotal) or partial and vertical or oblique. Dall and Rowe[13] reported that, in 26 cases of degenerative spondylolisthesis reviewed an average of 20 months after surgery, the proportion of

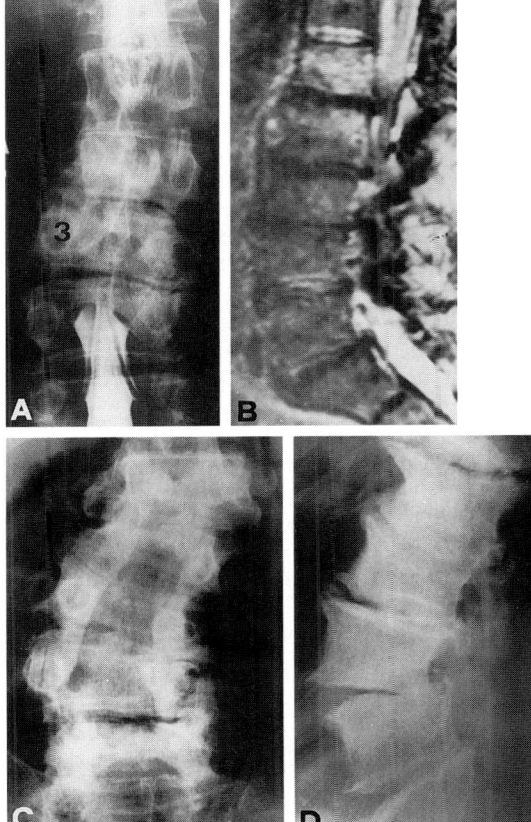

Figure 2. Postoperative instability after multilevel total laminectomy for severe stenosis at L1 to L5, as shown by an anteroposterior myelogram (A) and MRI scan (B). Four years after surgery (C and D), there is an increase in lumbar scoliosis, anterior and lateral slipping of the L4 vertebra, and a kyphotic deformity at the upper lumbar levels.

satisfactory results was significantly higher (83%) in patients for whom laminectomy and total arthrectomy were performed than in those who had undergone laminectomy and partial facetectomy. Opposite results were observed by Reynolds and Wiltse.[57] They obtained satisfactory results in 78% of patients with degenerative spondylolisthesis who had undergone partial arthrectomy and only in 33% of those who had had total arthrectomy. Consistent with these findings are numerous reports[8, 25, 30, 61, 62] indicating that a subtotal or total arthrectomy may cause postoperative instability in patients with no preoperative vertebral slipping and particularly in those with preoperative olisthesis. It should be emphasized, on the other hand, that a too-limited removal of the articular processes may lead to persistence or recurrence of radicular symptoms because of insufficient nerve root decompression.[21, 51, 53]

Oblique (or so-called undercutting) facetectomy[21] has become widely used because of its potential ability to allow adequate decompression of the emerging nerve roots while preserving vertebral stability to a larger extent than does straight facetectomy. However, no studies have compared the two procedures. No sound conclusion can thus be reached, considering that similar proportions of satisfactory results have been obtained with the two methods.

The clinical results seem to be influenced by the number of levels decompressed, but contrasting findings have been reported. Katz and colleagues[36] found a single-level decompression to be frequently associated with poor results. However, in other studies,[8, 47, 64] patients operated on at three levels or more were found to have a higher risk of surgical failure.

Type and Severity of Stenosis

It is difficult to determine from the data in the literature whether the etiologic type of stenosis (developmental, degenerative, and combined) influence the results of surgery. Most studies analyzing selectively the outcomes of surgery in different types of stenosis refer to patients treated in the era before computed tomography, when the distinction between the types of stenosis was difficult or impossible, based on measurements of the spinal canal made on myelograms or during surgery. Paine[47] found a lower rate of satisfactory results in developmental (62%) than in combined (68%) or degenerative (79%) stenosis. Similar rates of satisfactory outcomes were reported by other investigators, who analyzed developmental (68%)[73] or developmental (69%) and degenerative (76%)[56] stenosis. In some studies, however, no differences in outcome were found between different types of stenosis,[46, 67] or patients with developmental stenosis were found to have better results.[21]

Conflicting data have been reported on the influence of the severity of stenosis on the quality of the long-term results of surgery. In a few studies, better results were obtained in patients with milder stenosis.[47, 64] In other investigations, no differences were found between patients with mild and those with marked stenosis,[28, 71, 74] or the latter condition was found to be more often associated with a satisfactory outcome.[51, 73]

Age at Operation

Advanced age does not seem to have a negative influence on the quality of the clinical result. Of the 19 elderly patients reviewed postoperatively by Fast and Robin,[18] 18 had sufficient improvement to return to normal daily activities. Similar findings obtained in other studies indicate that surgical decompression also may offer significant relief to patients older than 70 years.[28, 32, 36, 47]

Length of Follow-up

Katz and colleagues[36] analyzed the results of surgery in 72 patients with degenerative lumbar stenosis 1 year (by review of the patient chart) and an average of 4 years (by questionnaire completed by the patient) after surgery. At 1 year, 13% of patients had severe pain or had undergone a second operation. At the latest follow-up, 43% were considered to have an unsatisfactory outcome. They reported persistent severe pain or had had a repeated operation for instability or stenosis.

In one study,[46] 72 patients were assessed at 1 month and at long-term follow-up (4 years on average). Forty-two percent stated that there had been no change in or absence of radicular pain between the two assessments, and 53% stated that their back pain or lack of it was unchanged. A gradual improvement in radicular pain or back pain was reported by 39% and 21% of patients, respectively. The remaining 19% and 26% reported a gradual deterioration of leg or back pain, respectively. In another study, 108 patients were followed for an average of 6 years and reevaluated 12 years (on average) after surgery.[26] At 6-year follow-up, 69% of patients had satisfactory results. This reached 75% at the latest follow-up. Repeated surgery had been performed in 9% of patients an average of 7 years after the initial operation, mostly because of recurrent stenosis.

Postacchini and coworkers[54] followed 64

patients for 6 months and reassessed them at a mean of 8 years after surgery. Of the 54 who had a satisfactory result at short-term follow-up, 76% still had a satisfactory result at long-term follow-up. Of the 15 patients with degenerative spondylolisthesis, those who had had an arthrodesis showed a higher proportion of satisfactory outcomes (80%) than did those who had not (40%).

Previous Surgery

Surgery for spinal stenosis tends to give less favorable results in patients who previously underwent decompressive procedures in the lumbar spine.[4, 21, 28, 44] This holds true particularly when stenosis is at the same level or levels at which the previous surgery for disc herniation or spinal stenosis had been performed.[51] The rates of solid fusion or satisfactory clinical results after arthrodesis for postoperative instability are slightly lower than those generally found after primary fusion.[9, 30, 59]

Effects of Comorbidity

In only one study was the influence of comorbidity on the quality of the clinical results throughly analyzed.[33] A high rate of comorbid illnesses (orteoarthrosis, cardiac disease, rheumatoid arthritis, and chronic pulmonary disease) was found to be inversely related to the rate of satisfactory results.

One study compared the long-term results of surgery in 24 diabetic and 22 nondiabetic patients.[63] In the group of diabetic patients, there was a 41% rate of satisfactory results, compared with 90% in the nondiabetic patients. The poor results in diabetics were thought to be related to coexisting diabetic neuropathy, microvascular disease affecting the spinal nerve roots, or failure of the nerve roots to recover after decompression. Different results, however, were observed by Cinotti and colleagues,[12] who followed 25 diabetic and 25 nondiabetic patients for a mean of 3 years. The preoperative symptoms were similar in the two groups, except that an abrupt onset of symptoms, the presence of night pain, and the absence of any posture-related pain relief were recorded only by diabetic patients. Nerve conduction velocity was slowed in 80% of the diabetic and in 25% of the nondiabetic patients. The outcome of surgery was satisfactory in 72% of the diabetic and 80% of the nondiabetic patients. Neither the duration of diabetes before surgery nor its type correlated with the final outcome. A mistaken preoperative diagnosis was found to be the main cause of failure in diabetic patients, in whom diabetic neuropathy or angiopathy may mimic the symptoms of lumbar stenosis.

Recurrence of Stenosis

Few studies have reported on stenotic patients operated on a second time for symptoms related to a stenotic condition, and often, it is not clear whether the reason for the repeated operation was an insufficient decompression at the initial surgery or a recurrence of stenosis.[6, 21, 36, 45, 59, 67] Recurrence is generally due to regrowth of posterior vertebral arch in the years after surgery. This was briefly mentioned by Brodsky[6] and then incidentally observed by other investigators.[59, 73]

Postacchini and Cinotti,[53] in reviewing 40 patients an average of 8 years after surgery for lumbar stenosis, found evidence of bone regrowth in 35 cases. Of these, 54% showed mild, 31% showed moderate, and 14% evidenced marked regrowth of the posterior vertebral arch (Fig. 3). The regrowth had usually occurred in the first few years after surgery. A few patients, however, showed a progressive increase of new bone formation with increasing time after the operation. All patients with degenerative spondylolisthesis showed bone regrowth, which was milder in those who had undergone fusion. The clinical results of surgery were significantly better in patients with mild or no bone regrowth than in those with moderate or marked regrowth. Two of the latter underwent repeated surgery for recurrent stenosis with good results.

GUIDELINES TO SURGICAL TREATMENT ON THE BASIS OF LONG-TERM RESULTS

Indications

Central Spinal Stenosis

Surgical treatment is usually indicated in patients with moderate or marked compres-

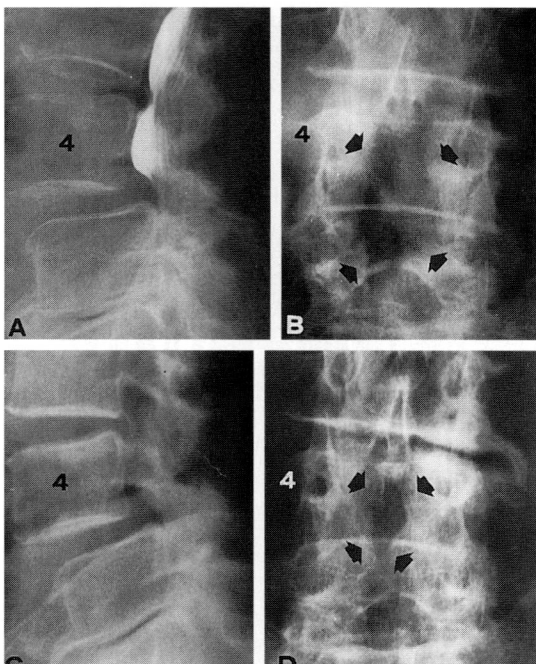

Figure 3. *A*, Marked regrowth of the posterior vertebral arch in a patient with degenerative spondylolisthesis *(A)* after total laminectomy *(B)*. Eight years after surgery, a lateral radiograph *(C)* showed no increase in olisthesis; an anteroposterior radiograph *(D)* revealed an almost complete regrowth of the posterior arch. The arrows in *B* and *D* point to the border of the laminectomy.

sion of the caudal nerve roots. In the author's experience, the greater the degree of compression of the neural structures is, the higher the chances of obtaining a satisfactory result, provided that the motor deficits, when present, are not extremely severe and long-standing.[51] In these cases the symptoms may improve considerably or disappear, but the motor deficits often resolve only partially or remain unchanged.

In patients with a narrow but not stenotic (responsible for compression of the neural structures) spinal canal, there are no indications for surgery. The latter, on the other hand, is rarely indicated in patients with mild to moderate posterior or posterolateral indentations in the thecal sac (even if they become slightly more marked in extension of the spine) in the absence of any compression of the nerve roots in the radicular canals. This holds particularly true when back pain prevails over leg symptoms in the absence of any evidence of spinal instability; the leg symptoms are vague and inconstant; or the main symptom is claudication, but the walking distance is several hundred meters or longer. In these patients, it is difficult or impossible to exclude extraspinal conditions or spinal conditions other than stenosis as being responsible for the symptoms. Consistent with these observations are the findings indicating that patients with atypical leg pain, in whom preoperative nerve root block is needed to confirm or make the diagnosis, have high probabilities of obtaining an unsatisfactory result.

A concomitant disc herniation in the stenotic area does not influence the indications for surgery. However, the presence of multiple, markedly bulging discs associated with only mild posterolateral compression of the neural structures exposes the patient to the risk of persistent anterior compression of the nerve roots after a posterior decompression.

The best candidate for surgery is the patient with marked osteoligamentous compression of the neural structures, severe leg symptoms, moderate or no neurologic deficits, and, excluding patients with degenerative spondylolisthesis, mild or no back pain. In degenerative spondylolisthesis, back pain may be the most prominent symptom. Nevertheless, excellent results can be obtained with decompression and fusion, particularly when olisthesis is at a single level and the slipped vertebra is hypermobile on flexion-extension radiographs.

Isolated Nerve Root Canal Stenosis

Surgery is indicated when clinical findings or imaging studies clearly indicate compression of the nerve root in the stenotic radicular canal. This often occurs only in the presence of a disc protrusion, which causes a clinically silent osteoligamentous compression of the nerve root to be symptomatic. Isolated disc resorption is associated with compression of the emerging nerve root only exceptionally; thus, it does not normally represent an indication for surgery.

Stenosis of the Intervertebral Foramen

Stenosis of the neuroforamen is often seen on CT or MRI scans. However, in the vast majority of cases, narrowing of the foramen causes no compression of the nerve root.

Osteoligamentous decompression for foraminal narrowing is rarely indicated, unless protrusion or marked bulging of the intervertebral disc coexists.

Comorbidity

Increased comorbidity is associated with higher risks of a poor outcome and functional limitations. However, this problem is not peculiar to lumbar stenosis. In this condition, the illness exposing the patient to the highest risks of poor results after surgery is diabetes, because its clinical manifestations may mimic those of spinal stenosis. The presence of diabetes does not appear to affect the outcome in patients treated by lumbar decompression.[12] The main cause of failure of surgical treatment is a mistaken preoperative diagnosis in patients whose leg symptoms are caused by diabetic neuropathy rather than by lumbar stenosis.

Planning of Surgery

Method of Decompression

Surgery for lumbar stenosis is aimed at adequately decompressing the neural structures, particularly the nerve roots in the extrathecal course, with no significant compromise of vertebral stability. Preservation of spinal stability is paramount because the disappearance of leg symptoms may not make the patient satisfied if back pain appears or worsens after surgery. This is especially true for patients in middle age or early senile age.

In the past few years, the technique of multiple laminotomy or its variants, has become widely used in the treatment of central spinal stenosis because it preserves vertebral stability better than total laminectomy does. However, a major role is still maintained by total laminectomy, which often allows a more effective decompression of the nervous structures. Analysis of long-term results of surgery[55] indicates that multiple laminotomy is the treatment of choice for developmental stenosis because the patients are usually middle aged, the stenosis is rarely severe, and disc excision is often necessary in addition to decompression. Multiple laminotomy is also preferred for degenerative or combined stenosis when narrowing of the spinal canal is mild or moderate, particularly if disc excision has been planned. Total laminectomy is usually more effective for severe stenosis, provided that the involved segments are stable preoperatively (Fig. 4). When this is not the case, the choice is between multiple laminotomy and total laminectomy with fusion of the decompressed segments.

Degenerative Spondylolisthesis

There are conflicting opinions on whether decompression alone yields a similar rate of satisfactory results to decompression and fusion. In the author's experience, both procedures have a role in the treatment of the condition. Bilateral laminotomy, or even total laminectomy, may be carried out with no concomitant fusion in patients with mild olisthesis, no vertebral hypermobility on functional radiographs, mild central stenosis or any degree of isolated radicular canal stenosis, and mild or no back pain. Similarly, in elderly patients with moderate olisthesis and marked resorption of the discs below, no vertebral hypermobility, and severe stenosis requiring total laminectomy, there may be no indication for fusion. On the other hand, patients with moderate or severe olisthesis, vertebral hypermobility even of mild degree, and/or severe central stenosis should undergo decompression and fusion. In these instances, the association of an arthrodesis allows the surgeon to decompress the neural structures as widely as necessary without the risk of symptomatic post-

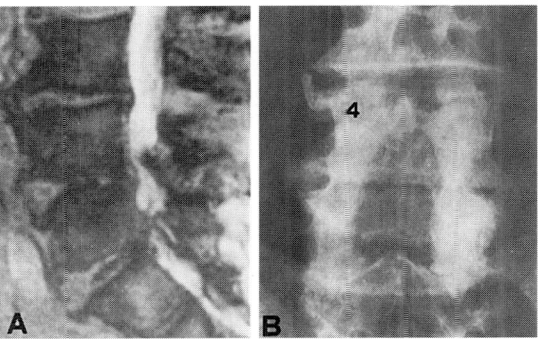

Figure 4. Total laminectomy in a patient with severe L4–L5 lumbar stenosis. *A*, Preoperative MRI scan. *B*, Postoperative radiograph. In this patient with resorbed discs and osteophytes joining the vertebral bodies, there is no risk of instability after total laminectomy.

operative instability, which may necessitate further surgery. A further reason for performing an arthrodesis is that most patients with fusion have less severe postoperative back pain, even in the absence of a clear evidence of instability, than patients undergoing total laminectomy alone.

In isolated degenerative spondylolisthesis of L4 or higher levels, arthrodesis may be performed only at the involved level or the lumbosacral joint may be included in the fusion. Extension of the fusion to the sacrum puts greater mechanical stresses on the vertebra above the fusion, which subsequently may easily become unstable (Fig. 5). On the other hand, a floating fusion has the same chances to become solid as an extended fusion, particularly when internal fixation with pedicle screws is used,[6, 34] and should thus be preferred.

Transpedicle fixation is aimed at increasing the chances of fusion and avoiding rigid and prolonged postoperative immobilization, which is badly tolerated by patients older than 50 years of age. Internal fixation may be bilateral or unilateral. The former provides a greater vertebral stability, but it is also likely to cause higher functional stresses on the adjacent unfused motion segments. Unilateral instrumentation, which

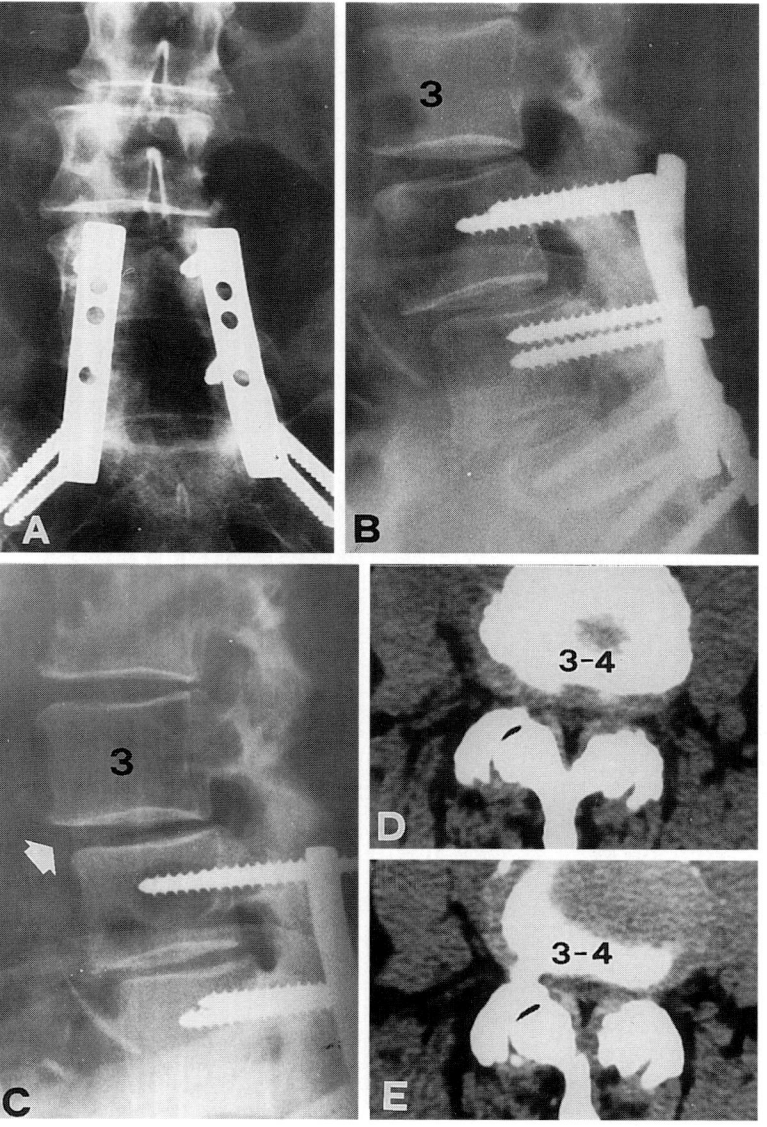

Figure 5. This 54-year-old woman underwent total laminectomy and instrumented fusion at L4–S1 (*A* and *B*) for degenerative spondylolisthesis of L4 and lumbar stenosis at the L4–L5 level. Four year later, a lateral radiograph *(C)* showed spondylolisthesis of L3 *(arrow)* and CT scans *(D, E)* revealed spinal stenosis at L3–L4. The L3 vertebra showed mild hypermobility on flexion-extension radiographs.

possibly decreases the potential morbidity of the more rigid bilateral system, was found to give nearly identical results in terms of fusion rate as the bilateral fixation.[34] The author carried out bilateral bone grafting and unilateral fixation in 16 patients, all of whom obtained a solid fusion. Although a larger experience is needed to reach sound conclusions, it appears that, in many cases of degenerative spondylolisthesis, unilateral instrumentation can be as effective as bilateral, with the advantage of decreased operative time and decreased risks of neurologic complications. The patients in whom unilateral instrumentation may be indicated are those with no or mild preoperative hypermobility (Fig. 6). Instead, bilateral fixation should always be performed in patients with marked vertebral hypermobility (Fig. 7). Reduction of vertebral slipping does not seem to influence in any respect the clinical results of surgery in patients with degenerative spondylolisthesis.

Scoliosis

Lumbar scoliosis, particularly of the degenerative type, is not rarely associated with spinal stenosis. In patients with both conditions, total laminectomy may be not sufficient to relieve compression of the caudal nerve roots when their compromise is related to pedicle and facet migration and rotation. Furthermore, in scoliotic patients, decompressive surgery may lead to an aggravation of the curve and/or lateral vertebral slipping. Laminectomy alone may thus yield poor outcomes because of increased deformity or instability. These risks should lead one to limit the indications for decom-

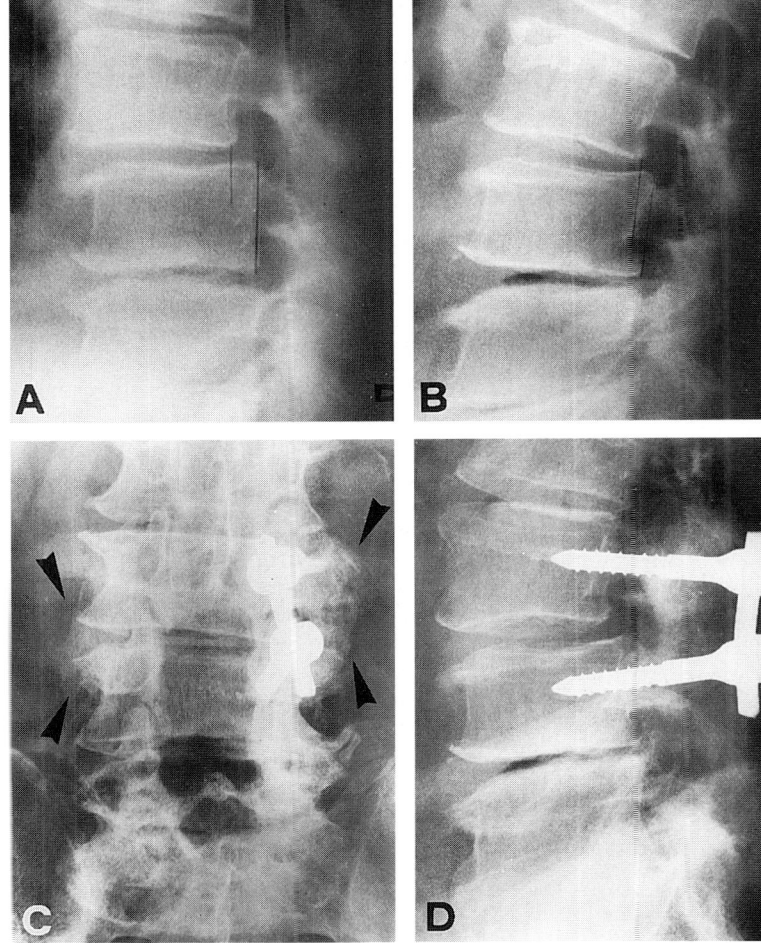

Figure 6. This 62-year-old patient with severe L3–L5 central lumbar stenosis had degenerative spondylolisthesis of L3 with mild hypermobility of the olisthetic vertebra *(A and B)*. He underwent total laminectomy at the L3–L5 level and intertransverse process arthrodesis with a unilateral compact Cotrel-Dubousset system at L3–L4. Five months after surgery *(C and D)*, the fusion was solid *(arrowheads)*.

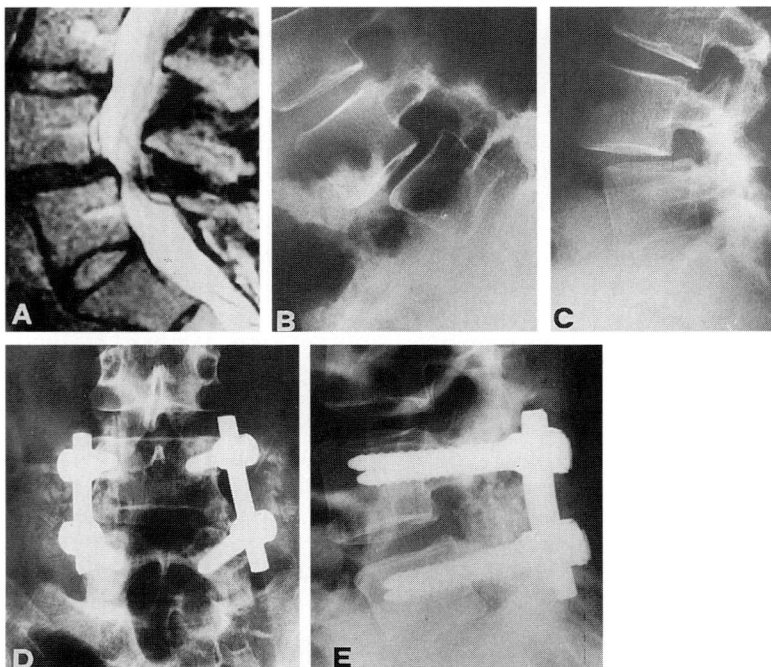

Figure 7. Degenerative spondylolisthesis of L4 with spinal stenosis and marked hypermobility of the olisthetic vertebra on flexion-extension radiographs *(A–C)*. Total laminectomy and intertransverse process fusion with a bilateral compact Cotrel-Dubousset system was performed *(D and E)*.

pressive surgery or, if surgery is undertaken, to carry out concomitantly a spinal fusion after correction of the scoliotic curve using a segmental rod (or plate) with transpedicle fixation systems.

Prophylactic Decompression

In patients with multilevel stenosis, it may be difficult to determine with certainty whether only one or all stenotic levels are responsible for the patient's symptoms and signs. When this is the case, all stenotic levels should be decompressed. In some patients, however, one or two levels contiguous to an area of marked stenosis are clearly asymptomatic because of the mildness of neural compression or the site of stenosis (posterior indentations of the thecal sac with no or mild narrowing of the radicular canal). In these cases, a prophylactic decompression in the areas of asymptomatic stenosis may be considered.

The indication for decompression is based on the evaluation of several factors, such as the patient's age, the site and severity of stenosis, the presence of disc abnormalities, and the extent of vertebral stability. In elderly patients, it is usually unnecessary to extend the decompression to areas of asymptomatic stenosis. On the other hand, in middle-aged or early-old-age patients, it is generally preferable also to decompress the areas of milder stenosis (Fig. 8); in these patients, in fact, there are higher chances that stenosis will become symptomatic as a result of degenerative changes related to the aging process. This holds particularly true if there is no specific risk of vertebral instability after decompression (e.g., scoliosis, spondylolisthesis, and late sequelae of vertebral fractures). The author reoperated on three middle-aged patients for lumbar stenosis at levels untreated at the initial surgery. Stenosis had progressively increased in severity and had become symptomatic 4 to 11 years after the original operation. Three other patients with a similar clinical history declined further surgical intervention.

Surgical Technique

Multiple Laminotomy

It is necessary to be extremely cautious in performing laminotomies when the spinal

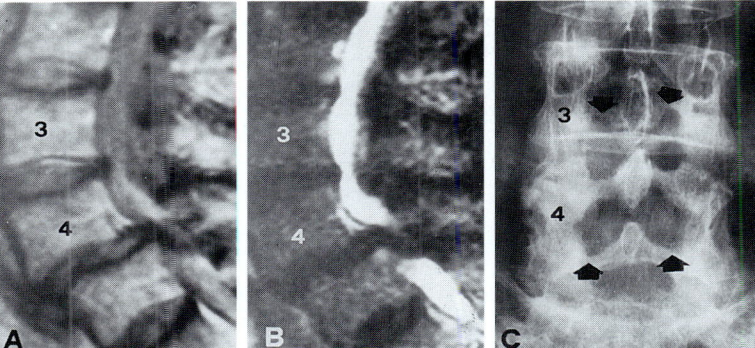

Figure 8. MRI scans *(A and B)* of this 54-year-old woman showed degenerative spondylolisthesis of L4, severe central spinal stenosis at L4–L5, and mild stenosis at L3–L4. Flexion-extension radiographs showed no vertebral hypermobility. Bilateral laminotomy *(C)* was performed at both L3–L4 and L4–L5 levels *(arrows)* because of the relatively young age of the patient.

canal is markedly stenotic or disc excision is required, because the nerve roots emerging from the thecal sac are more easily injured when the spinal canal is approached from the lateral side.[55] The use of an operating microscope may decrease the risks of nerve root injuries. Young and colleagues[76] reported a 9% incidence of dural tears with the microsurgical technique. In the author's experience, the incidence of dural tears also is less with use of the microscope than with conventional technique.

Laminotomy should be extended to total laminectomy when the surgeon realizes that the procedure provides inadequate decompression of the neural structures. This may easily occur in degenerative spondylolisthesis, in which case the thecal sac may be compressed between the central portion of the posterior arch and the upper border of the vertebra below.

Care should be taken not to fracture the pars interarticularis. This complication, which occurs more easily when one is performing contiguous laminotomies than a total laminectomy, may cause greater instability than that produced by excision of the central portion of the posterior arch. If both partes interarticulares of a single vertebra are fractured, the residual portion of the posterior arch should be excised and spinal fusion considered.

Extent of Decompression

The long-term results of surgical treatment may deteriorate with time because of gradual regrowth of the resected portion of the posterior arch.[53] This is more likely to occur when a narrow decompression is performed. The author strongly believes that decompression should be as wide as possible in the lateral portion of the spinal canal, while at the same time preserving vertebral stability. In the longitudinal direction, decompression should extend as far as half of the height of the vertebrae above and below the stenotic area.

Partial arthrectomy can be performed with rongeurs or osteotomes. The latter are preferable when performing total laminectomy because they allow an undercutting facetectomy to be performed more easily. This technique of facetectomy is always preferred. However, in severe stenosis, it may be difficult to perform an undercutting facetectomy without risk to the emerging nerve root. In these circumstances, the inferior facet may be excised with an osteotome and the superior facet with rongeurs in such a way as to remove the facet obliquely.

Discectomy

A traditional concept in spinal surgery is that discectomy should not generally be performed in spinal stenosis because removal of the posterior longitudinal ligament and annulus fibrosus increases the potential for instability. In the author's experience, a standard discectomy performed unilaterally does not usually increase the risks of instability in a preoperatively stable spine. Discectomy should be avoided when the disc is hard and does not bulge significantly in the spinal canal. However, disc excision should be carried out in the presence of marked bulging of an abnormally soft disc to avoid the risk of persistence or recurrence of radicular symptoms. This holds particularly for developmental central stenosis and isolated nerve root canal stenosis when a bulging or herniated disc contributes significantly to the compression of the neural structures.

REFERENCES

1. Alexander, E.: Significance of the small lumbar canal: Achondroplasia. Part 5. J. Neurosurg. 31:513–519, 1969.
2. Aryanpur, J., and Ducker, T.: Multilevel lumbar laminotomies: An alternative to laminectomy in the treatment of lumbar stenosis. Neurosurgery 26:429–433, 1990.
3. Blau, J. N., and Logue, V.: The natural history of intermittent claudication of the cauda equina: A long term follow-up study. Brain 101:211–222, 1978.
4. Boccanera, L., Pelliccioni, S., and Laus, M.: Stenosis of the lumbar vertebral canal (a study of 25 cases operated on). Ital. J. Orthop. Traumat. 10:227–236, 1984.
5. Bridwell, K. H., Sedgewick, T. A., O'Brien, M. F., et al.: The role of fusion and instrumentation in the treatment of degenerative spondylolisthesis with spinal stenosis. J. Spinal Disord. 6:461–472, 1993.
6. Brodsky, A. E.: Post-laminectomy and post-fusion stenosis of the lumbar spine. Clin. Orthop. 115:130–139, 1976.
7. Brodsky, A. E., Hendricks, R. L., Khalil, M. A., et al.: Segmental ("floating") lumbar spine fusions. Spine 14:447–450, 1989.
8. Caffinière, J. Y., de la: Evaluation du risque de glissement vertébral après traitement chirurgical d'une stenose lombaire. Rev. Chir. Orthop. 72:73–80, 1986.
9. Cauchoix, J., Benoist, M., and Chassaing, V.: Degenerative spondylolisthesis. Clin. Orthop. 115:122–129, 1976.
10. Chang, K. W., and McAfee, P. C.: Degenerative spondylolisthesis and degenerative scoliosis treated with a combination segmental rod-plate and transpedicular screw instrumentation system: A preliminary report. J. Spinal Disord. 1:247–256, 1989.
11. Choudury, A. R., and Taylor, J. C.: Occult lumbar spinal stenosis. J. Neurol. Neurosurg. Psychiatry 40:506–510, 1977.
12. Cinotti, G., Postacchini, F., and Weinstein, J. N.: Lumbar spinal stenosis and diabetes. Outcome of surgical decompression. J. Bone Joint Surg. 76B:215–219, 1994.
13. Dall, B. E., and Rowe, D. E.: Degenerative spondylolisthesis. Its surgical management. Spine 10:668–672, 1985.
14. Dick, P.: Intermittent cauda equina compression syndrome. Its surgical management. Spine 2:75–81, 1977.
15. Epstein, J. A., Epstein, B. S., and Rosenthal, A. D.: Sciatica caused by nerve root entrapment in the lateral recess: The superior facet syndrome. J. Neurosurg. 36:584–589, 1972.
16. Epstein, J. A., Epstein, B. S., Lavine, L. S., et al.: Lumbar nerve root compression at the intervertebral foramen caused by arthritis of the posterior joints. J. Neurosurg. 39:362–369, 1973.
17. Epstein, N. E., Epstein, J. A., Carras, R., et al.: Degenerative spondylolisthesis with an intact neural arch: A review of 60 cases with an analysis of clinical findings and the development of surgical management. Neurosurgery 13:555–561, 1983.
18. Fast, R., and Robin, G. C.: Surgical treatment of lumbar spinal stenosis in the elderly. Arch. Phys. Med. Rehabil. 66:149–151, 1985.
19. Feffer, H. L., Wiesel, S. W., Cuckler, J. M., et al.: Degenerative spondylolisthesis. To fuse or not to fuse. Spine 10:287–289, 1985.
20. Fitzgerald, J. A. W., and Newman, P. H.: Degenerative spondylolisthesis. J. Bone Joint Surg. 58B:184–192, 1976.
21. Getty, C. J. M.: Lumbar spinal stenosis. The clinical spectrum and the results of operation. J. Bone Joint Surg. 62B:481–485, 1980.
22. Hanley, E. N.: Decompression and distraction-derotation arthrodesis for degenerative spondylolisthesis. Spine 11:269–276, 1986.
23. Hasue, M., Kida, H., Inoue, K., et al.: Lumbar spinal stenosis. A clinical study of symptoms and therapeutic results. Int. Orthop. 1:133–137, 1977.
24. Hawkes, C. H., and Roberts, G. M.: Lumbar canal stenosis. Br. J. Hosp. Med. 23:498–505, 1980.
25. Hazlett, J. W., and Kinnard, P.: Lumbar apophyseal process excision and spinal instability. Spine 7:171–176, 1982.
26. Herno, A., Airaksinen, O., and Saari, T.: Long-term results of surgical treatment of lumbar spinal stenosis. Spine 18:1471–1474, 1993.
27. Herkowitz, H. N., and Kurz, L. T.: Degenerative spondylolisthesis with spinal stenosis. A prospective study comparing decompression with decompression and intertransverse process arthrodesis. J. Bone Joint Surg. 73A:802–808, 1991.
28. Herron, L. D., and Mangelsdorf, C.: Lumbar spinal stenosis: Results of surgical treatment. J. Spinal Disord. 4:26–33, 1991.
29. Herron, L. D., and Trippi, A. C.: Degenerative spondylolisthesis. The results of treatment by decompressive laminectomy without fusion. Spine 14:534–538, 1989.
30. Hopp, E., and Tsou, P. M.: Postdecompression lumbar instability. Clin. Orthop. 227:143–151, 1988.
31. Iida, Y., Kataoka, O., Sho, T., et al.: Postoperative lumbar spinal instability occurring or progressing secondary to laminectomy. Spine 15:1186–1189, 1990.
32. Johnsson, K. E., Udén, A., and Rosén, I.: The effect of decompression on the natural course of spinal stenosis. A comparison of surgically treated and untreated patients. Spine 16:615–619, 1991.
33. Jones, R. A. C., and Thomson, J. L. G.: The narrow lumbar canal. J. Bone Joint Surg. 50B:595–605, 1968.
34. Kabins, M. B., Weinstein, J. N., Spratt, K. F., et al.: Isolated L4–L5 fusions using the variable screw placement system: Unilateral versus bilateral. J. Spinal Disord. 5:39–49, 1992.
35. Kaneda, K., Kazama, H., Satoh, S., et al.: Follow-up study of medial facetectomies and posterolateral fusion with instrumentation in unstable degenerative spondylolisthesis. Clin. Orthop. 203:159–167, 1986.

36. Katz, I. N., Lipson, S. J., Larson, M. G., et al.: The outcome of decompressive laminectomy for degenerative lumbar stenosis. J. Bone Joint Surg. 73A:809–811, 1991.
37. Kirkaldy-Willis, W. H., Wedge, J. H., Yong-Hing, K., et al.: Lumbar spinal nerve lateral entrapment. Clin. Orthop. 169:171–178, 1982.
38. Knox, B. D., Harvell, J. C., Nelson, P. B., et al.: Decompression and Luque rectangle fusion for degenerative spondylolisthesis. J. Spinal Disord. 2:223–228, 1989.
39. Lassale, B., Deburge, A., and Benoist, M.: Resultats à long terme du traitement chirurgical des stenoses lombaires operées. Rev. Rheum. Ed. Fr. 52:27–33, 1985.
40. Lee, C. K.: Lumbar spinal instability (olisthesis) after extensive posterior spinal decompression. Spine 8:429–433, 1983.
41. Lin, P. M.: Internal decompression for multiple levels of lumbar spinal stenosis: A technical note. Neurosurgery 11:546–549, 1982.
42. Lombardi, J. S., Wiltse, L. L., Reynolds, J., et al.: Treatment of degenerative spondylolisthesis. Spine 10:821–827, 1985.
43. Matsunaga, S., Sakov, T., Morizono, Y., et al.: Natural history of degenerative spondylolisthesis. Pathogenesis and natural course of the slippage. Spine 15:1204–1210, 1990.
44. Nasca, R. J.: Rationale for spinal fusion in lumbar spinal stenosis. Spine 14:451–454, 1989.
45. Nakai, O., Ookawa, A., and Yamaura, I.: Long-term roentgenographic and functional changes in patients who were treated with wide fenestration for central lumbar stenosis. J. Bone Joint Surg. 73A:1184–1191, 1991.
46. Nixon, J. E.: Results of surgical treatment. In Nixon, J. E. (ed.): Spinal Stenosis, London, Edward Arnold, 1991.
47. Paine, K. W. E.: Results of decompression for lumbar spinal stenosis. Clin. Orthop. 115:96–100, 1976.
48. Porter, R. W., and Hibbert, C.: Calcitonin treatment for neurogenic claudication. Spine 8:585–592, 1983.
49. Porter, R. W., Hibbert, C., and Evans, C.: The natural history of root entrapment syndrome. Spine 9:418–421, 1984.
50. Postacchini, F.: Lumbar spinal stenosis and pseudostenosis. Definition and classification of pathology. Ital. J. Orthop. Traumatol. 3:339–351, 1983.
51. Postacchini, F.: Lumbar Spinal Stenosis. Vienna, Springer-Verlag, 1989.
52. Postacchini, F., Cinotti, G., and Perugia, D.: Le spondilolistesi degenerative lombari. 2. Trattamento chirurgico. Giorn. Ital. Ortop. Traumatol. 17:479–489, 1991.
53. Postacchini, F., and Cinotti, G.: Bone regrowth after surgical decompression for lumbar spinal stenosis. J. Bone Joint Surg. 74B:862–869, 1992.
54. Postacchini, F., Cinotti, G., Gumina, S., et al.: Long-term results of surgery in lumbar stenosis. 8-year review of 64 patients. Acta Orthop. Scand. Suppl. 251:78–80, 1993.
55. Postacchini, F., Cinotti, G., Perugia, D., et al.: The surgical treatment of central lumbar stenosis. Multiple laminotomy compared with total laminectomy. J. Bone Joint Surg. 75B:386–392, 1993.
56. Reale, F., Delfini, R., Gambacorta, D., and Cantore, G. P.: Congenital stenosis of lumbar spinal canal: Comparison of results of surgical treatment for this and other causes of lumbar syndrome. Acta Neurochir. 42:199–207, 1978.
57. Reynolds, J. B., and Wiltse, L. L.: Surgical treatment of degenerative spondylolisthesis. (Abstract.) Spine 4:148–149, 1979.
58. Rosenberg, N. J.: Degenerative spondylolisthesis. Surgical treatment. Clin. Orthop. 117:112–120, 1976.
59. Sano, S., Yokokura, S., Nagata, Y., et al.: Unstable lumbar spine without hypermobility in postlaminectomy cases. Mechanism of symptoms and effect of spinal fusion with and without spinal instrumentation. Spine 15:1190–1197, 1990.
60. Senegas, J., Etchevers, J. P., Vital, J. M., et al.: Le recalibrage du canal lombaire alternative à la laminectomie dans le traitement des stenoses du canal lombaire. Rev. Chir. Orthop. 74:15–22, 1988.
61. Shenkin, H. A., and Hash, C. J.: Spondylolisthesis after multiple bilateral laminectomies and facetectomies for lumbar spondylosis. Follow-up review. J. Neurosurg. 50:45–47, 1979.
62. Sienkiewicz, P. J., and Flatley, T.: Postoperative spondylolisthesis. Clin. Orthop. 221:172–180, 1987.
63. Simpson, J. M., Silveri, C. P., Balderston, R. A., et al.: The results of operations on the lumbar spine in patients who have diabetes mellitus. J. Bone Joint Surg. 75:1823–1929, 1993.
64. Surin, V., Hedelin, R., and Smith, L.: Degenerative lumbar spinal stenosis. Acta Orthop. Scand. 53:79–85, 1982.
65. Takahashi, K., Kitahara, H., Yamagata, M., et al.: Long-term results of anterior interbody fusion for treatment of degenerative spondylolisthesis. Spine 15:1211–1215, 1990.
66. Teng, P., and Papateodorou, C.: Lumbar spondylosis with compression of cauda equina. Arch. Neurol. 8:221–229, 1963.
67. Tile, M., McNeil, S. R., Zarins, R. K., et al.: Spinal stenosis. Results of treatment. Clin. Orthop. 115:104–108, 1976.
68. Tsuji, H., Tamaki, T., Itoh, T., et al.: Redundant nerve roots in patients with degenerative lumbar spinal stenosis. Spine 10:72–82, 1985.
69. Turner, J. A., Ersek, M., Herron, L., et al.: Surgery for lumbar spinal stenosis: Attempted meta-analysis of the literature. Spine 17:1–8, 1992.
70. van Akkerveeken, P. F.: Lateral Stenosis of the Lumbar Spine. Ph.D. Thesis. Utrecht, the Netherlands, University of Utrecht, 1989.
71. Udén, A., Johnsson, K. E., Jonsson, K., et al.: Myelography in the elderly and the diagnosis of spinal stenosis. Spine 10:171–174, 1985.
72. Venner, R. M., and Crock, H. V.: Clinical studies of isolated disc resorption in the lumbar spine. J. Bone Joint Surg. 63B:491–194, 1981.
73. Verbiest, H.: Results of surgical treatment of idiopathic developmental stenosis of the lumbar vertebral canal. A review of twenty-seven years experience. J. Bone Joint Surg. 59B:181–188, 1977.
74. Weir, B., and De Leo, R.: Lumbar stenosis Analysis of factors affecting outcome in 81 surgical cases. Can. J. Neurol. Sci. 8:295–298, 1981.
75. Wiltse, L. L., Kirkaldy-Willis, W. H., and McIvor, G. W. D.: The treatment of spinal stenosis. Clin. Orthop. 115:83–91, 1976.
76. Young, S., Veerapen, R., O'Laoire, S. A.: Relief of lumbar canal stenosis using multilevel subarticular fenestration as an alternative to wide laminectomy: Preliminary report. Neurosurgery 23:628–633, 1988.

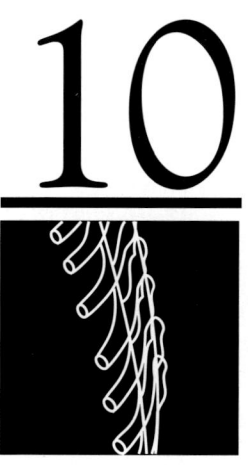

10

Segmental Instability

JOHN W. FRYMOYER
MALCOLM H. POPE
DAVID G. WILDER

Thirteen years ago Professor William Kirkaldy-Willis,[29] then President of the International Society for the Study of the Lumbar Spine, convened a symposium on degenerative segmental instability. He posed three challenging questions: (1) What is the precise definition of the term instability? (2) How can one diagnose this phase of the degenerative process? (3) How can one formulate treatment on a rational basis? Clinicians are not yet able to answer his three challenges with any precision. At the same time, segmental instability constitutes one of the most common indications for lumbar spine fusion.

DEFINITION

The American Academy of Orthopaedic Surgeons[3] defined segmental instability as an abnormal response to applied loads, characterized by movement in the motion segment beyond normal constraints. The engineering model is loss of stiffness of a functional spinal unit resulting in increased and/or abnormal motions in response to applied loads.[51] However, there has been difficulty in translating this definition into criteria that can reliably be applied to clinical diagnosis and treatment decisions (Figs. 1 and 2). Frymoyer and Krag[18] defined segmental instability as a loss of spinal motion segment stiffness, such that force application to that motion segment produces greater displacement than would be seen in a normal structure. This results in a painful condition with the potential for progressive deformity and places neurologic structures at risk. This is consistent with White and Panjabi's[66] definition based on studies of the sectioned sequential ligaments and facet joints of cadaver specimens.

PATHOLOGY

The conceptual model advanced by Kirkaldy-Willis[29] is still the most popular explanation of degenerative instabilities. In his model, degeneration starts with a phase of dysfunction followed by instability and then restabilization. During the unstable phase, the disc becomes degenerative and less mechanically competent, the ligaments and facet capsules are lax, and the facet joints are degenerative. Later, osteophyte formation as well as alterations in the chemical composition and water content of the disc may restabilize the affected functional spinal unit.[44]

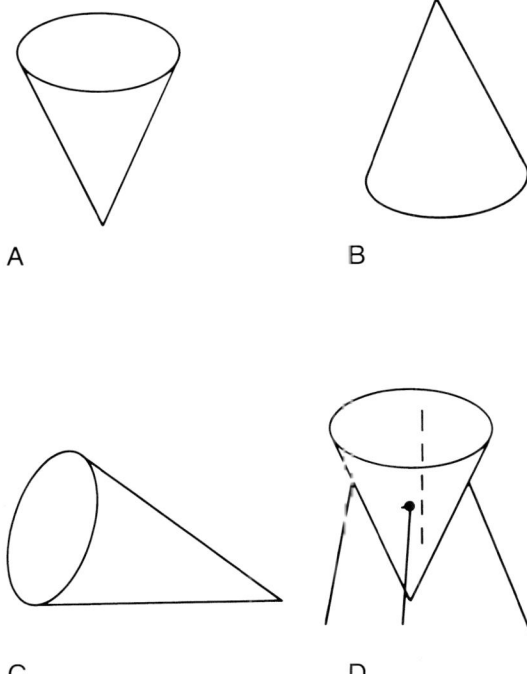

Figure 1. Stable and unstable equilibrium conditions. A, If slightly displaced, cone A moves into a new position of equilibrium (unstable equilibrium). B, Cone B returns to the same position (stable = equilibrium). C, Cone C stays in the displaced position (neutral equilibrium). D, The unstable cone has been made stable by the addition of guy wires to hold it in position. (From Pope, M. H., and Panjabi, M.: Biomechanical definitions of spinal instability. Spine 10:255–256, 1985.)

BIOMECHANICS

Many of the models of instability are based on in vitro testing of the mechanical characteristics of functional spinal units and other structures, such as facets, after sequential sectioning of the spinal ligaments.[52] Similarly, in models studied in vivo, the ligaments, joints, or experimentally created fractures are removed, and then spinal stiffness is measured over time.[60, 61] The results of these latter experiments have been varied. Sullivan and associates[61] reported that mobility increased following removal of the facet joints and that increased spinal degeneration occurred over time. In contrast, Stokes and coworkers[60] showed that acute instability was followed by restabilization over time (Fig. 3), with no evidence of acceleration of disc degeneration.

These models have less relevance[26, 27] to degenerative instability[1, 36] than do cyclic loading experiments. Dependent on the magnitude, direction, and number of applied cycles, a variety of anatomic changes can be produced including annular tears, distortions of the lamellae of the annulus fibrosus, lumbar disc herniations, and facet or vertebral body fractures.[69, 70]

Additional experiments have yielded the concept of the balance point. Tencer and Ahmed[63] are credited with originally describing the balance point as the point or line at which compressive load application minimizes coupled flexion-extension rotations. Later, Wilder and associates[66, 70] were able to define the balance point within fairly narrow limits. After exposing specimens to vibrational loads of from 330 to 410 N at 5 Hz for as many as 18,000 load cycles, they found that some specimens exhibited nonlinear buckling, loss of stiffness, and sometimes dramatic rapid rotations and displacements (Figs. 4 to 8). Other researchers have used the term neutral zone and have assessed laxity within that zone to measure spinal instability.

Attempts have also been made to measure spinal stiffness in living humans.* To quantify relatively small displacements, a variety of anatomic landmarks or implanted tantalum balls have been used as fiduciary mark-

---

*References 2, 4, 6, 19, 30, 35, 47, 48, and 62.

Figure 2. A typical load deflection curve of a stable material (S) and an unstable material (U), manifested by loss of stiffness. The stiffness of material U is L/d_2. (From Pope, M. H., and Panjabi, M.: Biomechanical definitions of spinal instability. Spine 10:255–256, 1985.)

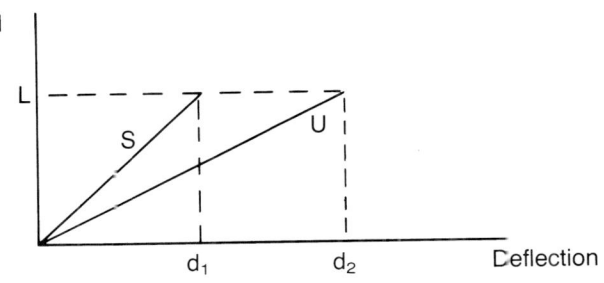

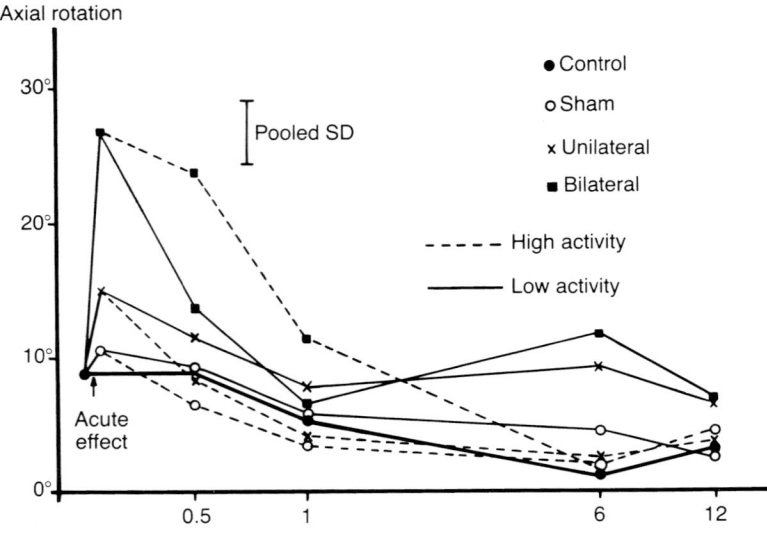

Figure 3. The degrees of axial rotation in the four experimental conditions (i.e., control, sham, unilateral facetectomy, and bilateral facetectomy) are illustrated as a function of time. Note that the initial instability in the facetectomized animals tends to become restored and to approach sham and control at 1, 6, and 12 months. (From Stokes, I. A. F., Counts, D. C., and Frymoyer, J. W.: Experimental instability in the rabbit lumbar spine. Spine 14:68–72, 1989.)

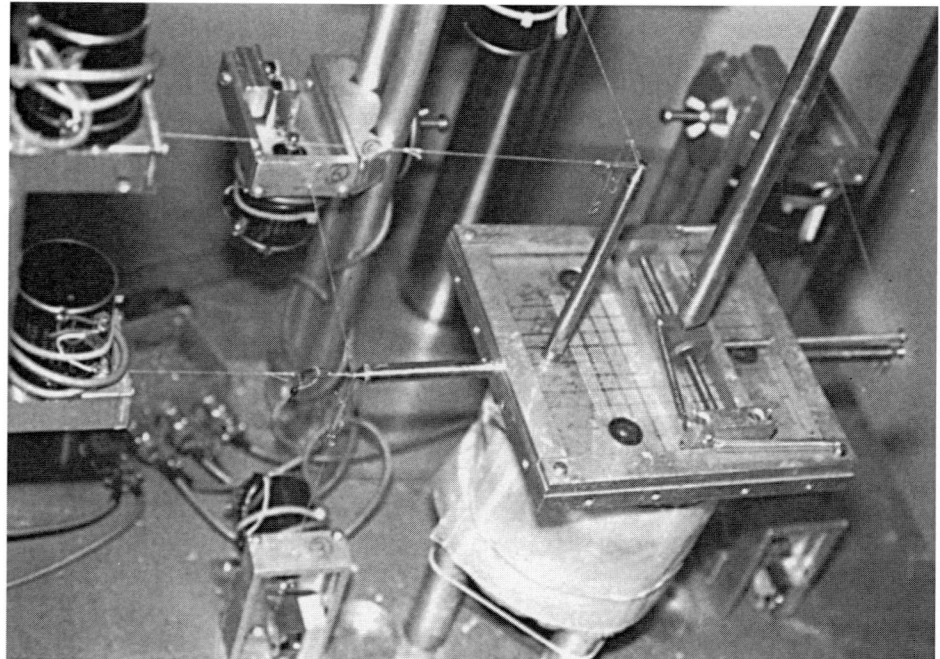

Figure 4. Motion sensor in place on materials testing apparatus. Note notches in ends of posts. Kevlar loops fit in notches and are connected to displacement potentiometers. Also, note two-dimensional adjustability of load application point (at end of load application link) for determining balance point location. (From Wilder, D. G., Pope, M. H., and Frymoyer, J. W.: The biomechanics of lumbar disc herniation and the effect of overload and instability. Winner of 1987 American Back Society's Annual Competition. Presented at the Spring Symposium on Back Pain, American Back Society, Anaheim, CA, May 1987. Am. Back Soc. Newsletter 3:10–11, 1987; J. Spinal Disord. 1:16–32, 1988.)

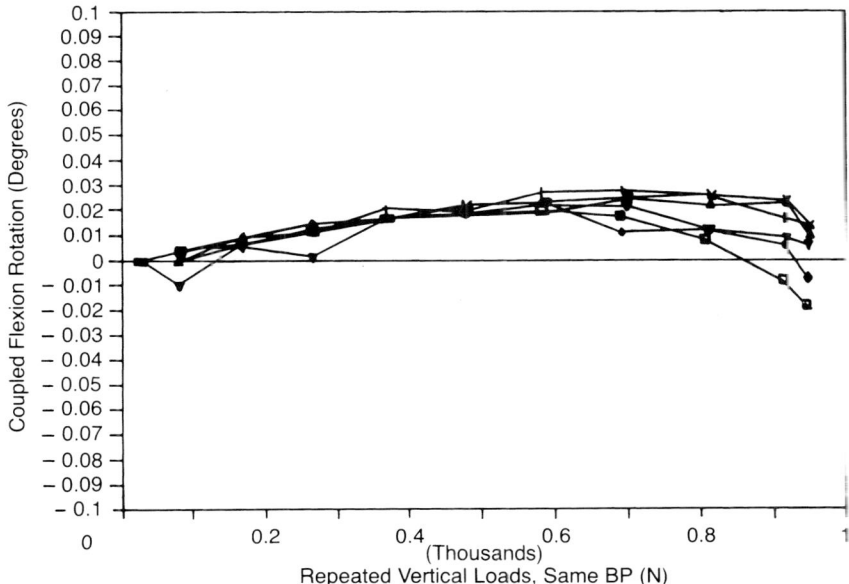

Figure 5. Coupled flexion-rotation response resulting from a vertical load applied at the balance point. The load was applied six times. Note the consistency and small magnitude of the response. (From Wilder, D. G., Pope, M. H., and Frymoyer, J. W.: The biomechanics of lumbar disc herniation and the effect of overload and instability. Winner of 1987 American Back Society's Annual Competition. Presented at the Spring Symposium on Back Pain, American Back Society, Anaheim, CA, May 1987. Am. Back Soc. Newsletter 3:10–11, 1987; J. Spinal Disord. 1:16–32, 1988.)

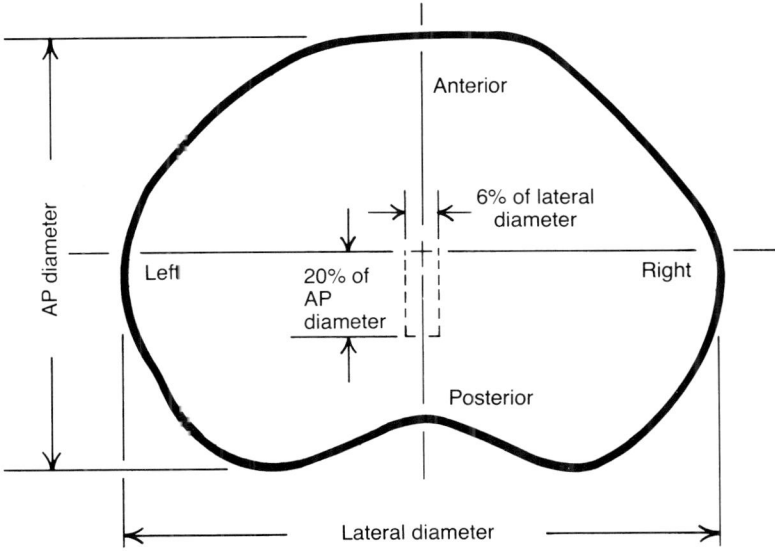

Figure 6. This diagram shows the region in which the projections of the balance points were located in the midtransverse plane. Most of the balance points found were located in a rectangular region of the disc. The region is very thin (6% of the lateral diameter of the endplate) but relatively long (20% of the anteroposterior (AP) diameter of the end plate). It is bilaterally symmetric but is located posterior to the geometric center shown. (From Wilder, D. G., Pope, M. H., and Frymoyer, J. W.: The biomechanics of lumbar disc herniation and the effect of overload and instability. Winner of 1987 American Back Society's Annual Competition. Presented at the Spring Symposium on Back Pain, American Back Society, Anaheim, CA, May 1987. Am. Back Soc. Newsletter 3:10–11, 1987; J. Spinal Disord. 1:16–32, 1988.)

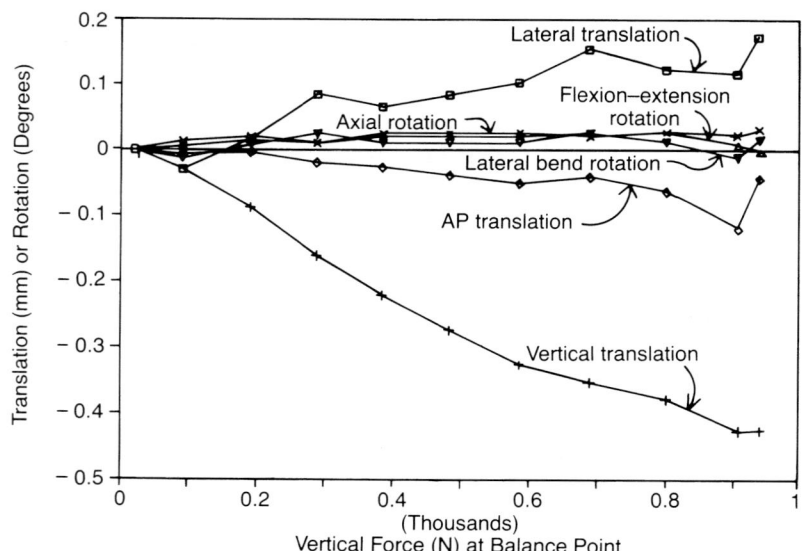

Figure 7. Segment response to load—main and coupled effects. Graph shows typical translation and rotation responses of a motion segment (L2–L3) to a compressive load applied at the original balance point. Note the virtually negligible rotations resulting from vertical load applied at the balance point. (From Wilder, D. G., Pope, M. H., and Frymoyer, J. W.: The biomechanics of lumbar disc herniation and the effect of overload and instability. Winner of 1987 American Back Society's Annual Competition. Presented at the Spring Symposium on Back Pain, American Back Society, Anaheim, CA, May 1987. Am. Back Soc. Newsletter 3:10–11, 1987; J. Spinal Disord. 1:16–32, 1988.)

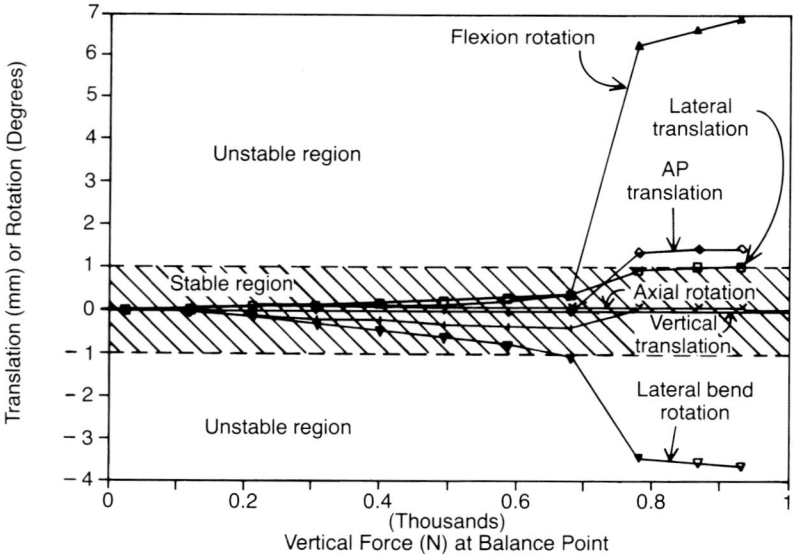

Figure 8. This graph shows the stable and unstable translation-load and rotation-load responses of an L2–L3 motion segment tested by using a 100-second load ramp. Note the sudden unstable or buckling response. This response occurred after a 1-hour intervention of vibration loading, loaded at the original balance point. (From Wilder, D. G., Pope, M. H., and Frymoyer, J. W.: The biomechanics of lumbar disc herniation and the effect of overload and instability. Winner of 1987 American Back Society's Annual Competition. Presented at the Spring Symposium on Back Pain, American Back Society, Anaheim, CA, May 1987. Am. Back Soc. Newsletter 3:10–11, 1987; J. Spinal Disord. 1:16–32, 1988.)

ers. Most studies have employed highly sophisticated biplanar motion radiographs.[49, 58, 68] Although these systems have proved useful in measuring the progression of spinal fusions, they have not been helpful in clinical diagnosis.

Other anatomic and mechanical studies have focused on specific segments of the lumbar spine and on the role of muscles in spinal stability and instability. In general, the L4–L5 segment is thought to be at greater risk for instability, because it has fewer anatomic constraints. MacGibbon and Farfan,[38] Fitzgerald,[13] and Allbrook[2] evaluated the position of L4–L5 relative to the intercristal line and concluded that an elongated L5 transverse process and a deeper-seated L5 vertebral body conferred relative stability on the motion segment.[42]

The analysis by Leong and colleagues[34] of the iliolumbar ligament has reenforced the general concept that these structures protect the L5 intervertebral level.

CLINICAL SYMPTOMS AND SIGNS

Despite substantial efforts, there are no agreed-upon clinical criteria. Kirkaldy-Willis and Farfan[28] concluded that segmental instability should be suspected when minor perturbations produce acute low back pain. "Catching" sensations and the "instability catch" are often mentioned as clinical attributes, but a well-defined, consistent syndrome has yet to be identified.[43]

In the clinical examination, intermittent scoliosis and intermittent neurologic symptoms and signs are cited as important attributes of instabilities, yet the sensitivity and specificity of these observations have not been quantified. Some clinicians surmise that they can palpate abnormal motions, but interobserver and intraobserver studies continue to show poor reliability of this method[51] (Nelson, T., personal communication).

RADIOGRAPHIC SIGNS

There are no certain signs demonstrable on static anteroposterior and lateral spinal radiographs (Fig. 9). Disc space narrowing, traction spurs, and spinal malalignments[21]

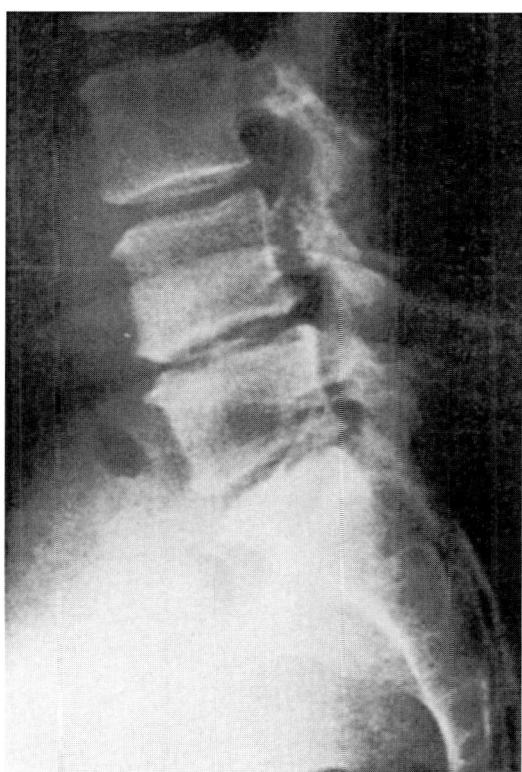

Figure 9. Lateral radiograph demonstrating traction spurs at L3–L4 and L4–L5 levels. Note that the spurs are separated from the vertebral end plate by greater than 3 mm, thus fulfilling Macnab's criterion. (From Frymoyer, J. W., Newberg, A., Pope, M. H., et al.: Spine radiographs in patients with low-back pain. J. Bone Joint Surg. 66A:1048–1055, 1984.)

(Fig. 10) are commonly cited correlates of instability[16, 40, 64] (Farfan, H. F., personal communication). Frymoyer and Krag[18] argued that radiographic evidence of instability can be assured only when a deformity progresses over time and is accompanied by pain and/or neurologic symptoms. Ito and coworkers[23] proposed that the degree of instability can be predicted statistically from the disc deformation. The segmental instability is given by the ratio of the radiographic residual of the abnormal discs to the standard deviation. These investigators also calculated the strain resultant in the abnormal discs.[23]

ROLE OF MOTION RADIOGRAPHY

The earliest descriptions of segmental instability, advanced by Knutsson,[30] were

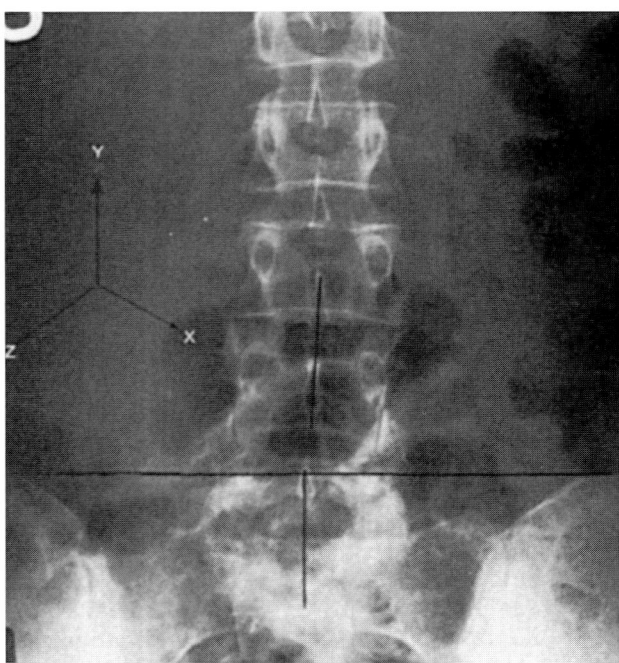

Figure 10. Anteroposterior radiograph demonstrates discontinuity of the L4–L5 spinous process line, one possible sign of a rotational instability. (From Frymoyer, J. W., and Selby, D. K.: Segmental instability. Rationale for treatment. Spine 10:280–286, 1985.)

based on motion radiography. When translations of greater than 3 mm were observed, he concluded that disc degeneration was likely. Since that time, there have been numerous attempts to measure accurately abnormal motions and displacements under conditions of spinal flexion and extension, lateral bend, and rotation[2, 9, 35, 62] (Fig. 11). As an alternative to motion radiography, Freiberg[14] used plain films taken after the application of compressive loads and traction. This is a more sophisticated method but one similar to that proposed by Lowe and associates.[37]

A variety of sophisticated radiographic measurement techniques have been proposed, including biplanar radiographs using bony landmarks or implanted fiduciary markers.[22] MRI analyses have attempted to correlate bone marrow changes with suspected degenerative instability.[23]

All of these studies can be summarized as follows:

1. Abnormal stresses can be identified (Fig. 12), principally as shear in the spinal levels thought to be unstable.
2. Abnormal coupling of spinal motion can also be observed in these same segments.
3. Abnormal and/or increased motions occur independent of current or previous history of back pain.
4. The rates of interobserver and intraobserver errors are high, particularly when standard radiographic techniques are used.[67]

OTHER TESTS OF INSTABILITY

On the premise that the symptoms of instability relate to abnormal movements or displacements, relief of pain by immobilization has been cited as a useful clinical test. Immobilization by spinal orthoses, or casts and spica casts, is used by many clinicians as a prefusion test.[7, 12] A more dramatic test is the use of temporary external fixators.[46] With these devices, the linkage systems can be perturbated by the investigator and the pain responses measured. The results of these analyses are mixed in determining which patients will benefit from a lumbar spine fusion. Although complications are reported to be low in the hands of experts, widespread use of these tests seems premature in routine clinical analyses.

KNOWLEDGE ABOUT LUMBAR DEGENERATIVE INSTABILITY

In the past years since Kirkaldy-Willis'[29] challenge, knowledge has advanced primar-

Segmental Instability 789

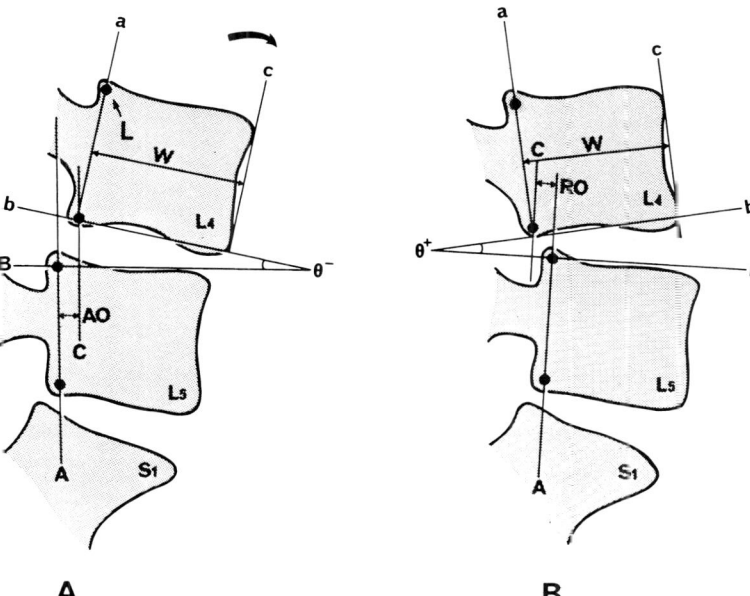

Figure 11. *A, B,* Radiographic method of Dupuis and coworkers for the calculation of horizontal and angular displacement in flexion-extension views. (From Dupuis, P. R., Yong-Hing, K., Cassidy, J. D., and Kirkaldy-Willis, W. H.: Radiologic diagnosis of degenerative lumbar spinal instability. Spine 10:262–276, 1985.)

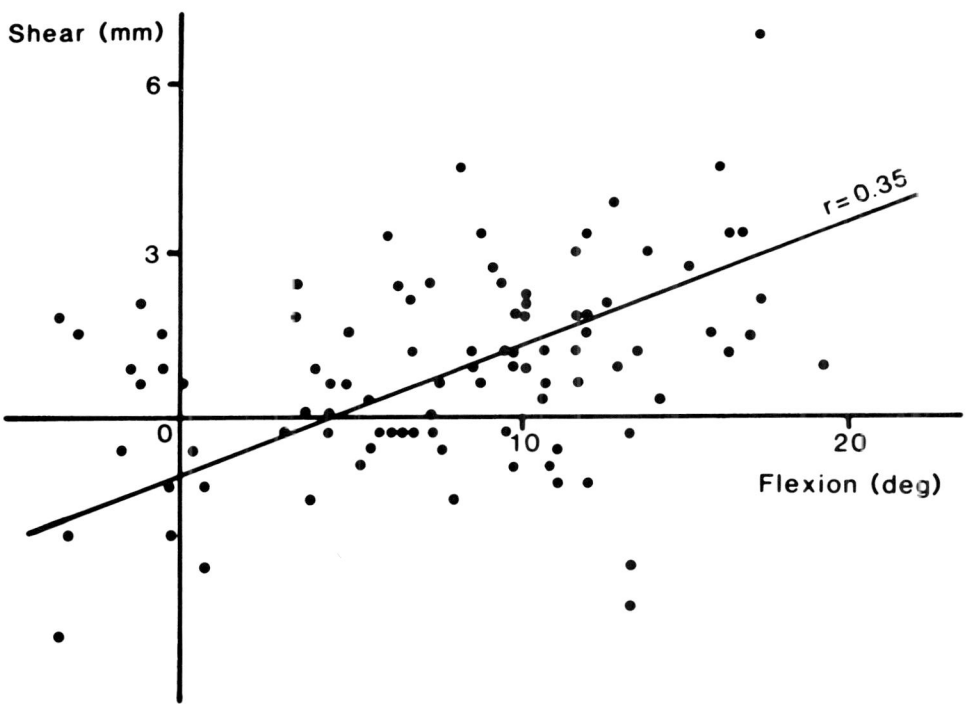

Figure 12. The relationship between shear at vertebral levels and range of motion at these levels. Note that increased motion is associated with increased shear. (From Stokes, I. A. F., and Frymoyer, J. W.: Segmental motion and instability. Spine 12:688–691, 1987.)

ily from biomechanical studies. Unfortunately, it is difficult to define clinical syndromes in clear and reproducible ways.

Frymoyer and associates[17,18] attempted to create a classification system, but the authors acknowledge that it is a conceptual model with unproven utility. The principles that govern this conceptual model are based on the assumption that instability can be suspected when the following evidence is present:

1. A deformity can be observed on plain radiographs and can be seen to progress over time, accompanied by pain.
2. Progression of deformity is accompanied by other signs and symptoms that correlate with the suspected level or levels of instability. Among these clinical signs and symptoms, neurologic symptoms and confirmatory clinical signs are most reliable.
3. A less reliable symptom is referred pain in the expected distribution to a sclerotome. A suggestive symptom is the history of repeated episodes of back pain brought on by decreasing mechanical overloads.
4. The more focal the lesion, the greater is the probability of successful treatment.

Table 1

Lumbar Segmental Instabilities

I. Fractures and fracture-dislocation
II. Infections involving anterior columns with
   A. Progressive loss of vertebral body height and deformity despite antibiotic treatment
   B. Progressing neurologic symptoms, despite appropriate antibiotic treatment, if accompanied by criterion IIA
III. Primary and metastatic neoplasms with
   A. Progressive loss of vertebral body height and deformity
   B. Progressing neurologic symptoms, if symptoms are not the result of direct tumor involvement of the spinal cord, cauda equina, or nerve roots, but result from the conditions of IIIA
   C. Postsurgical symptoms after resection of neoplasms
IV. Spondylolisthesis
   A. Isthmic spondylolisthesis
     1. L5–S1 progressive deformity in a child, particularly when accompanied by the radiographic risk signs of Wiltse; rarely an unstable lesion in the adult.
     2. L4–L5 lesion, probably an unstable lesion in the adult
V. Degenerative
VI. Scoliosis—any progressive deformity in a child

Table 2

Degenerative Segmental Instabilities

Primary Instabilities
I. Axial rotational instability
II. Translational instability
III. Retrospondylolisthetic instability
IV. Progressing degenerative scoliosis
V. (?) Internal disc disruption

Secondary Instabilities
I. Post disc excision—subclassified according to the pattern of instability as described under primary instabilities.
II. Post decompressive laminectomy
   A. Accentuation of preexistent deformity
   B. New deformity (i.e., no deformity existed at the time of original decompression); further subclassified as for primary instabilities
III. Post spinal fusion
   A. Above or below a spinal fusion, subclassified as for primary instabilities
   B. Pseudarthrosis
   C. Acquired spondylolisthesis

This approach has a number of drawbacks. A patient must be observed over a period of time sufficient to demonstrate focal radiographic changes and to correlate these changes with clinical symptoms and signs. It also implies an inability to address Kirkaldy-Willis' original conceptual model,[29] in which the symptomatic instability phase is expected to antedate any significant deformity.

CLASSIFICATION

Within the constellation of spinal instability (Table 1), degenerative instability can be divided into primary and secondary types (Table 2). In primary instabilities, the patient has no history of prior surgical intervention, whereas in secondary instabilities, symptoms follow some recent or remote lumbar spine operation. The underlying mechanical principle is that the spine functions in six degrees of freedom with three rotations and three translations along the three mutually perpendicular axes. The classification given in Table 1 is an expansion of a classification first proposed by Frymoyer and Selby in 1985.[17]

Primary Instabilities

Type I. Axial Rotational Instability

It remains uncertain whether type I and type II (translational) instabilities are the

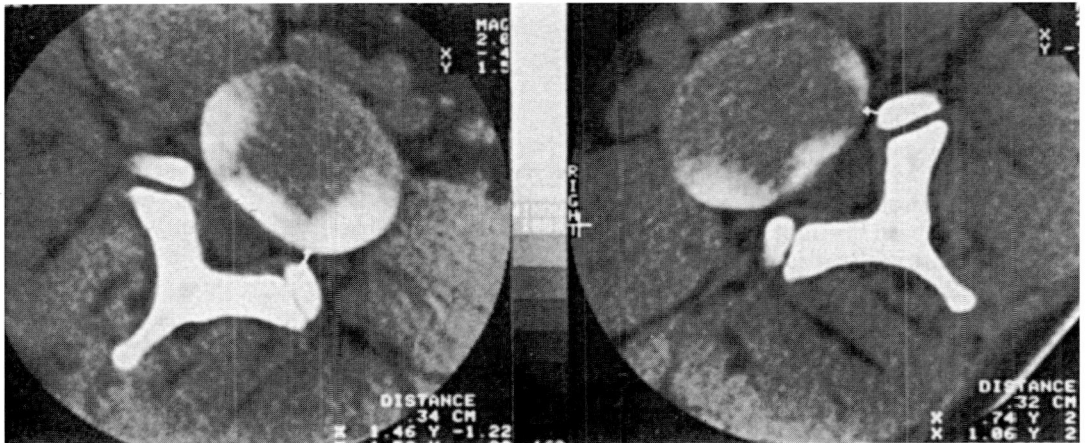

Figure 13. Computed tomographic scans of spine taken with rotational stresses. According to the authors, increased movement and gapping of the facet joints should be observed. (From Kirkaldy-Willis, W. H., and Farfan, H. F.: Instability of the lumbar spine. Clin. Orthop. 165:110, 1982.)

same (Fig. 13). Both are included because the studies by Farfan[10] demonstrated rotational deformities in pathologic specimens of degenerative spondylolisthesis and because, in some animal studies of torsional instability, accelerated degeneration can be identified. The role of torsional instability is also an attractive conceptual model because of the ability of static and cyclic torsional overloads to produce radial annular tears. This instability is most common at L4–L5 because this level is often less well protected anatomically. Farfan[10] also identified a pedicle-to-pedicle myelographic defect (Fig. 14), which he believes arises from the rotational deformity. A derotation facet fusion was proposed by him.

Type II. Translational Instability

The prototype of degenerative instability is degenerative spondylolisthesis. This can be shown to progress over time at the rate of 2 mm/year, often (but not always) accompanied by clinical symptoms and signs that indicate instability at the L4–L5 level.* Analysis of computed tomographic scans suggests that progression is more likely when the facets are oriented more sagittally. This prototype is of particular interest because it is the one example in which prospective, controlled studies have shown efficacy of lumbar spine fusion in treatment. A nondegenerative condition, L4–L5 ischemic spondylolisthesis, also has the same propensity to progress in adults, unlike the L5–S1 ischemic lesion. This again demonstrates the greater risk of instability at the L4–L5 level.

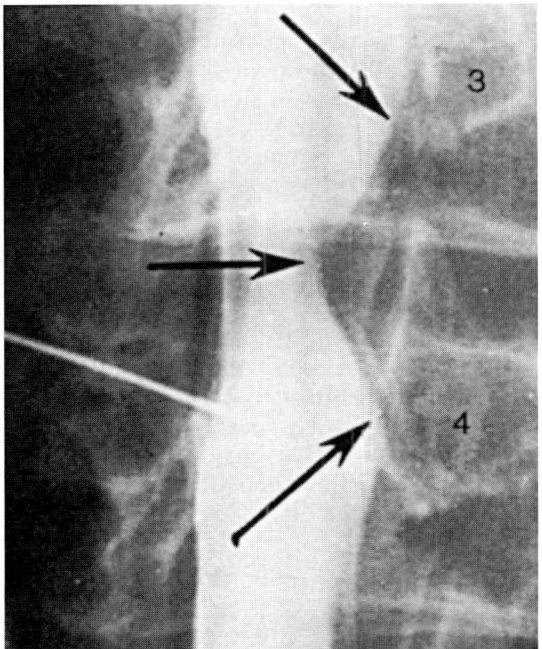

Figure 14. A pedicle-to-pedicle defect seen in myelography in a patient with rotational deformity. (From Frymoyer, J. W., and Selby, D. K.: Segmental instability. Rationale for treatment. Spine 10:280–286, 1985.)

---

*References 11, 20, 25, 37, 39, 45, 54, 56, 65, and 71.

Type III. Retrospondylolisthetic Instability

In the historical literature, retrospondylolisthetic deformity was thought to be most common at L5–S1 and a frequent cause of lateral spinal stenosis affecting S1.[32] This lesion can be seen at any level, and typically, it is associated with radiographic evidence of advanced disc degeneration. The authors have proposed fusion in flexion as the most logical approach to this lesion or, alternatively, the use of interbody techniques that can reduce the retrospondylolisthetic deformity.

Type IV. Progressing Degenerative Scoliosis

Scoliotic deformities typically involve multiple levels. The most common pattern is accompanied by a laterally directed translational deformity and rotation, usually centered at L4–L5. Degenerative spondylolisthesis is often present.

Because multilevel nerve root involvement and symptoms of spinal stenosis often occur, determining how many levels should be decompressed is frequently difficult. Accurate diagnosis often requires multiple studies including electromyograms, somatosensory evoked potentials, selective nerve root blocks, and sometimes, the use of graded spinal anesthetics. Although debate continues, the authors advocate fusion, particularly in patients who require wide decompression. One or another internal fixation device seems appropriate, but their efficacy has been debated.

Type V. Internal Disc Disruption

The conceptual model of the etiology of disc disruption is of (1) a compressive overload sufficient to cause disruption of the end plates and (2) the ingrowth of neovascular tissue and its accompanying nociceptors. Whether this condition belongs in a classification of segmental instability can be debated. The experts believe that this condition, whether or not it is unstable, is best treated by anterior interbody fusion. Their premise is that the symptoms arise from the disc and that continued micromovement of solid posterior fusions may lead to continued symptoms. There is increasing demand for combined anterior and posterior procedures. The rationale for that approach is the premise that a painful disc can be eliminated only by absolutely rigid immobilization and fusion.

Secondary Instabilities

Type I. Post Disc Excision

Back pain after lumbar disc excision is common. Not surprisingly, fusions are often recommended. Analyses of the failures of disc excision indicate that the original diagnosis of lumbar disc herniation was based on symptoms other than sciatica and that the imaging studies were often equivocal. It is doubtful whether the majority of these patients fulfill the criteria for instability. However, some patients with apparent instability are asymptomatic. For example, 20% of patients who had undergone disc excision at least 10 years previously had a positive Knuttson sign.[15] As originally defined by Knuttson, this radiographic finding was more than 3 mm of translation as measured by flexion-extension radiographs. The cases progressed to frank degenerative spondylolisthesis. Typically, patients were women. L4–L5 was the level operated on most frequently. Many patients with radiographic signs had no symptoms.

Three percent of patients with these findings required a later fusion. It has been argued that L4–L5 instability is common after discectomy, and some investigators have recommended primary fusion. Attempts to select patients for fusion by attempting to measure intraoperative instability have not been consistently reliable.

A second condition, less well studied, is collapse of the disc space with a retrospondylolisthetic deformity. Disc space narrowing almost always follows lumbar disc excision; particularly at the L5–S1 level, this may be accompanied by later lateral recess stenosis similar to that observed in primary type III deformities.[57]

Type II. Post Decompressive Laminectomy

The risk of instability after laminectomy is directly related to the amount of facet joint removed.[5, 24, 31] Laboratory studies show that removal of one entire facet or more than 50% of both facets alters the stiffness of the motion segment. Additionally, violation of the pars, or overzealous removal of facets, can also lead to later facet fracture and presumed secondary instability. This latter condition is more common than was previously believed.

ACCENTUATION OF PREEXISTENT DEFORMITY

This problem is seen most commonly in patients who have undergone decompression for degenerative spondylolisthesis. Other important factors reported are the preoperative extent of the deformity, the presence of osteophytes, incision or excision of the disc, and the height of the disc. Reynolds and Wiltse,[54] Johnsson and associates,[24] and Feffer and associates[11] noted that all patients had progression of their deformities after decompression although the degree of progression did not reliably correlate with the symptoms. Other researchers have noted that failures are most common when progression occurs. As noted, the evidence derived from careful prospective studies favors fusion as the operation of choice.

NEW DEFORMITY

This problem is most commonly seen in younger patients after extensive multilevel decompression for spinal stenosis. A variety of instability patterns may be observed. In Lee's[31] small series, only 3.7% of patients had this event but Johnsson and coworkers[24] observed it as a common cause of failure (Fig. 15).

At the current time, the optimum method of stabilization is still under debate. Some experts use only pedicle fixation, whereas others argue for pedicle fixation in combination with posterior interbody fusion.

Type III. Post Spinal Fusion

ABOVE OR BELOW A FUSION

That spine fusion increases shear stresses at the next adjacent mobile spinal levels seems clear, based on biomechanical and clinical observations.[53, 55] In long-term follow-up studies, evidence of translational instability was observed in 20% of patients

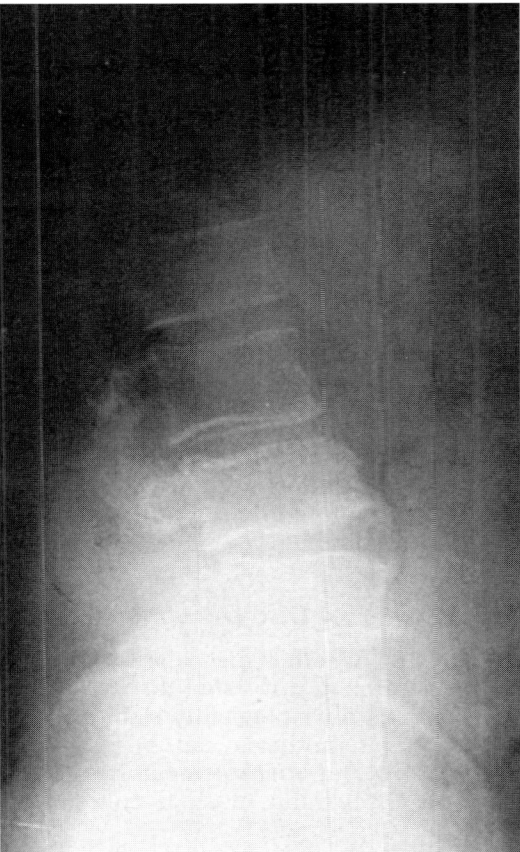

Figure 15. This 55-year-old man had multilevel decompressions for severe congenital spinal stenosis with superimposed degeneration. More than one third of the facets were sacrificed. Note the vertebral displacements that have occurred. The patient has disabling low back pain.

followed for 10 years or longer by Frymoyer and coworkers[15] and in 45% of the cohort followed for more than 20 years by Lehmann and associates.[33] All of these patients had undergone fusion from L4 to the sacrum, but many had no symptoms. Ultimately, 4% of Frymoyer and coworkers'[15] patients required an extension of the fusion because of progressing pain. In the smaller group of patients who underwent fusion from L5 to the sacrum in the past, 20% required a later operation for symptoms at the L4–L5 level. This seems consistent with the observations that L4–L5 is inherently less stable. In comparison, Brodsky[5] reported that later instability is not a problem after floating L4–L5 fusion. In patients with degenerative spondylolisthesis, fusions usually can be limited to the single level of the lesion. Because of the increased shear loads above a fusion, the authors favor the use of pedicle fixation.

PSEUDARTHROSIS

It has been well established that pseudarthrosis[8] per se correlates poorly with signs and symptoms of spinal pain. However, most studies in which pseudarthrosis was reported were in patients who had undergone fusion as an adjunct to lumbar disc excision, rather than as the treatment of an instability. It is a challenge to determine which patients have a symptomatic pseudarthrosis or indeed whether a pseudarthrosis is present in patients with metal implants. Methods for diagnosis include local anesthesia injections, discography,[41] tomography, and reexploration. The diagnosis of continued pain is difficult, as reflected in the generally poorer results that follow repair of even established pseudarthroses.

ACQUIRED SPONDYLOLISTHESIS

This is a rare condition that follows prior midline fusions. It is reported to occur in 1% of patients.[15] Whether this represents a fatigue fracture or a fracture produced by overzealous decortication of the pars remains uncertain.

CONCLUSIONS

Ten years after Kirkaldy-Willis issued a challenge to be precise in defining the symptoms and signs and formulating treatment of degenerative lumbar instability, clinicians are still groping for reliable criteria to guide clinical decisions. During these 10 years, advances in biomechanical knowledge have continued. However, accompanying clinical studies have yet to define symptoms that can be used reliably by the clinician. This is particularly so when a deformity has yet to develop and one relies on the uncertain signs of motion radiography. The diagnostic classification given here has significant limitations, but it offers an approach that may be of use in the management of patients with intransigent debilitating low back pain.

REFERENCES

1. Adams, M. A., and Hutton, W. C.: Prolapsed intervertebral disk: A hyperflexion injury. Spine 7:184–191, 1982.
2. Allbrook, D.: Movements of the lumbar spine column. J. Bone Joint Surg. 39B:339–345, 1956.
3. American Academy of Orthopaedic Surgeons: A glossary on spinal terminology. Chicago, American Academy of Orthopaedic Surgeons, 1985, p. 34.
4. Arkin, A. M.: The mechanism of rotation in combination with lateral deviation in the normal spine. J. Bone Joint Surg. 32A:180–188, 1950.
5. Brodsky, A. E.: Post-laminectomy and post-fusion stenosis of the lumbar spine. Clin. Orthop. 115:130–139, 1976.
6. Brown, R. H., Burstein, A. H., Nash, C. L., and Schock, C. C.: Spinal analysis using a three-dimensional radiographic technique. J. Biomechan. 9:355–366, 1976.
7. Brown, T., Hansen, R. J., and Yorra, A. J.: Some mechanical tests on the lumbosacral spine with particular reference to the intervertebral discs: A preliminary report. J. Bone Joint Surg. 39A:1135–1164, 1957.
8. DePalma, A. F., and Rothman, R. H.: The nature of pseudarthrosis. Clin. Orthop. 59:113–118, 1968.
9. Dupuis, P. R., Young-Hing, K., Cassidy, J. D., and Kirkaldy-Willis, W. H.: Radiologic diagnosis of degenerative lumbar spinal instability. Spine 10:262–276, 1985.
10. Farfan, H. F.: The pathological anatomy of degenerative spondylolisthesis: A cadaver study. Spine 5:412, 1980.
11. Feffer, H. L., Wiesel, S. W., Cuckler, J. M., and Rothman, R. H.: Degenerative spondylolisthesis. To fuse or not to fuse. Spine 10:287–289, 1985.
12. Fidler, M. W., and Plasmans, C. M. T.: The effect of four types of support on the segmental mobility of the lumbosacral spine. J. Bone Joint Surg. 65A:943, 1983.
13. Fitzgerald, J. A. W.: Degenerative spondylolisthesis. J. Bone Joint Surg. 58B:184–192, 1976.
14. Friberg, O.: Lumbar instability: A dynamic approach by traction-compression radiography. Spine 12:119–129, 1987.
15. Frymoyer, J. W., Hanley, E. N., Howe, J., et al.: A comparison of radiographic findings in fusion and non-fusion patients ten or more years following lumbar disc surgery. Spine 4:435, 1979.
16. Frymoyer, J. W., Newberg, A., Pope, M. H., et al.: Spine radiographs in patients with low-back pain. J. Bone Joint Surg. 66A:1048–1055, 1984.
17. Frymoyer, J. W., and Selby, D. K.: Segmental instability. Rationale for treatment. Spine 10:280–286, 1985.
18. Frymoyer, J. W., and Krag, M. H.: Spinal stability and instability: Definitions, classification, and general principles of management. In Dunsker, S. B., Schmidek, H. H., Frymoyer, J. W., and Kahn, A. (eds.): The Unstable Spine. New York, Grune & Stratton, 1986.
19. Gertzbein, S. D., Seligman, J., Holtby, R., et al.: Centrode patterns and segmental instability in degenerative disc disease. Spine 10:257–261, 1985.
20. Goldner, J. L.: The role of spine fusion: Question 6. Spine 6:293, 1981.
21. Gonnella, C., Paris, S., and Kutner, M.: Reliability

in evaluating passive intervertebral motion. Phys. Ther. 62:437, 1982.
22. Hallgren, R. C., Reynolds, H. M., Soutas-Little, R. W., et al.: 3-D analysis and display of sequential position data in the lumbar spine. J. Clin. Engineer. (in press).
23. Ito, M., Tadano, S., and Kaneda, K.: A biomechanical definition of spinal segmental instability taking personal and disc level differences into account. Spine 18:2295–2304, 1993.
24. Johnsson, K.-E., Willner, S., and Johnsson, K.: Postoperative instability after decompression for lumbar spinal stenosis. Spine 11:107–110, 1986.
25. Junghanns, H.: Spondylolisthesen ohne Spalt in Zwischengelenkstuck. Arch. Orthop. Unfall-chir. 29:118–267, 1930.
26. Kaleps, I., Kazarian, L. E., and Burns, M. L.: Analysis of compressive creep behavior of the vertebral unit subjected to a uniform axial loading using exact parametric solution equations of Kelvin-solid models—part II. Rhesus monkey intervertebral joints. J. Biomech. 17:131–136, 1984.
27. Kazarian, L. E.: Creep characteristics of the human spinal column. Orthop. Clin. North Am. 6:3–18, 1975.
28. Kirkaldy-Willis, W. H., and Farfan, H. F.: Instability of the lumbar spine. Clin. Orthop. 165:110, 1982.
29. Kirkaldy-Willis, W. H.: Presidential Symposium on Instability of the Lumbar Spine, introduction. Spine 10:254, 1985.
30. Knutsson, F.: The instability associated with disc degeneration in the lumbar spine. Acta Radiol 25:593–609, 1944.
31. Lee, C.: Lumbar spinal instability (olisthesis) after extensive posterior spinal decompression. Spine 8:426–433, 1983.
32. Lehmann, T., and Brand, R.: Instability of the lower lumbar spine. Orthop. Trans. 7 97, 1983.
33. Lehmann, T. R., Spratt, K. F., Tozzi, J. E., et al.: Long-term follow-up of lower lumbar fusion patients. Spine 12:97–104, 1987.
34. Leong, J. C. Y., Luk, K. D. K., Chow, D. H. K., and Woo, C. W.: The biomechanical functions of the iliolumbar ligament in maintaining stability of the lumbosacral junction. Spine 12:669–674, 1987.
35. Lindahl, O.: Determination of the sagittal mobility of the lumbar spine. Acta Orthop. Scand. 37:241–254, 1966.
36. Liu, Y. K., Goel, V. K., DeJong, A., et al.: Torsional fatigue of the lumbar intervertebral joints. In Proceedings of the International Society for the Study of the Lumbar Spine, Cambridge, England, April 8, 1983.
37. Lowe, R. W., Hayes, T. D., Kaye, J., et al.: Standing roentgenograms in spondylolisthesis. Clin. Orthop. 117:80–84, 1976.
38. MacGibbon, B., and Farfan, H. F.: A radiologic survey of various configurations of the lumbar spine. Spine 4:258, 1979.
39. Macnab, I.: Spondylolisthesis with an intact neural arch—the so-called pseudo-spondylolisthesis. J. Bone Joint Surg. 32B:325–333, 1950.
40. Macnab, I.: The traction spur: An indication of segmental instability. J. Bone Joint Surg. 53A:663, 1971.
41. Macnab, I., and Johnson, R. G.: Localization of symptomatic lumbar pseudarthroses by use of discography. Clin. Orthop. 197:164–170, 1985.
42. McGlashen, K. M., Miller, J. A. A., Schultz, A. B., and Andersson, G. B. J.: Load displacement behavior of the human lumbo-sacral joint. J. Orthop. Res. 5:488–496, 1987.
43. Nachemson, A.: Lumbar spine instability. A critical update and symposium summary. Spine 10:290–291, 1985.
44. Nathan, H.: Osteophytes of the vertebral column. An anatomical study of their development according to age, race, and sex with considerations as to their etiology and significance. J. Bone Joint Surg. 44A:243–268, 1962.
45. Newman, P. H., and Stone, K. H.: The etiology of spondylolisthesis. J. Bone Joint Surg. 45B:39–59, 1963.
46. Olerud, S., Sjostrum, L., Karlstrom, G., and Hamberg, M.: Spontaneous effect of increased stability of the lower spine in cases of severe chronic back pain—the answer of an external transpeduncular fixation test. Clin. Orthop. 203:67–74, 1986.
47. Olsson, T. H., Selvik, G., and Willner, S.: Kinematic analysis of posterolateral fusion in the lumbosacral spine. Acta Radiol. (Diagn.) 17:519, 1976.
48. Olsson, T. H., Selvik, G., and Willner, S.: Kinematic analysis of spinal fusions. Invest. Radiol. 11:202–209, 1976.
49. Olsson, T. H., Selvik, G., and Willner, S : Mobility in the lumbosacral spine after fusion studied with the aid of roentgen stereophotogrammetry. Clin. Orthop. 129:181–190, 1977.
50. Paris, S. V.: Physical signs of instability. Spine 10:277–279, 1985.
51. Pope, M. H., and Panjabi, M.: Biomechanical definitions of spinal instability. Spine 10:255–256, 1985.
52. Posner, I., White, A. A., Edwards, W. T., et al.: A biomechanical analysis of the clinical stability of the lumbar and lumbosacral spine. Spine 7:374–389, 1982.
53. Quinnell, R. C., and Stockdale, H. R.: Some experimental observations of the influence of a single lumbar floating fusion on the remaining spine. Spine 6:263–267, 1981.
54. Reynolds, J. B., and Wiltse, L. L.: Surgical treatment of degenerative spondylolisthesis. Spine 4:148–149, 1979.
55. Rolander, S. D.: Motion of the lumbar spine with special reference to the stabilizing effect of posterior fusion. An experimental study on autopsy specimens. Acta Orthop. Scand. Suppl. 90:1–144, 1966.
56. Rosenberg, N. J.: Degenerative spondylolisthesis; predisposing factors. J. Bone Joint Surg. 57A:467, 1975.
57. Selby, D.: Internal fixation with Knodt's rods. Clin. Orthop. 203:179–184, 1986.
58. Stokes, I. A. F., Wilder, D. G., Frymoyer, J. W., and Pope, M. H.: Assessment of patients with low back pain by biplanar radiographic measurement of intervertebral motion. Spine 6:233, 1981.
59. Stokes, I. A. F., and Frymoyer, J. W.: Segmental motion and instability. Spine 12:688–691, 1987.
60. Stokes, I. A. F., Counts, D. C., and Frymoyer, J. W.: Experimental instability in the rabbit lumbar spine. Spine 14:68–72, 1989.
61. Sullivan, J. D., Farfan, H. F., and Kahn, D. S.: Pathologic changes with intervertebral joint rotational instability in the rabbit. Can. J. Surg. 14:71–79, 1971.

62. Taylor, J., and Twomey, L.: Sagittal and horizontal plane movement of the human lumbar vertebral column in cadavers and in the living. Rheumatol. Rehabil. 19:223–232, 1980.
63. Tencer, A. F., and Ahmed, A. M.: The role of secondary variables in the measurement of the mechanical properties of the lumbar intervertebral joint. ASME J. Biomech. Engineer. 103:129–137, 1981.
64. Torgerson, W. R., and Dotter, W. E.: Comparative roentgenographic study of the asymptomatic and symptomatic lumbar spine. J. Bone Joint Surg. 58A:850–853, 1976.
65. Valkenburg, H. A., and Haanen, H. C. M.: The epidemiology of low back pain. In White, A. A., III, and Gordon, S. L. (eds.): American Academy of Orthopaedic Surgeons Symposium on Idiopathic Low Back Pain. St. Louis, C. V. Mosby, 1982.
66. White, A. A., III, and Panjabi, M. M.: Kinematics of the spine. In White, A. A., III, and Panjabi, M. M. (eds.): Clinical Biomechanics of the Spine. Philadelphia, J. B. Lippincott, 1978.
67. Wiesel, S. W., Tsourmas, N., Feffer, H. I., et al.: A study of computer-assisted tomography. I. The incidence of positive CAT scans in an asymptomatic group of patients. Spine 9:549–551, 1984.
68. Wilder, D. G., Seligson, D., Frymoyer, J. W., and Pope, M. H.: Objective measurement of L4–5 instability: A case report. Spine 5:56, 1980.
69. Wilder, D. G.: On Loading of the Human Lumbar Intervertebral Motion Segment. Dissertation. University of Vermont, 1985. Abstract: Dissertation Abstracts International 46:4328-5, 1986; Manuscript no. DA8529728, Ann Arbor, University Microfilms International, 1986.
70. Wilder, D. G., Pope, M. H., and Frymoyer, J. W.: The biomechanics of lumbar disc herniation and the effect of overload and instability. Winner of 1987 American Back Society's Annual Competition. Presented at the Spring Symposium on Back Pain, American Back Society, Anaheim, CA, May 1987. Am. Back Soc. Newsletter 3:10–11, 1987; J. Spinal Disord. 1:16–32, 1988.
71. Wiltse, L. L., and Winter, R. B.: Terminology and measurement of spondylolisthesis. J. Bone Joint Surg. 65A:768–772, 1983.

11

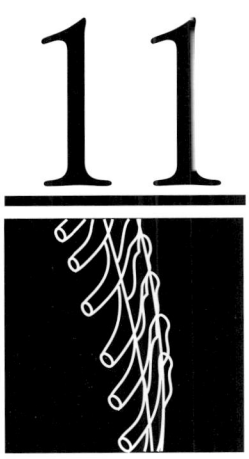

Inflammatory Disorders

Inflammatory Spondyloarthropathies

MICHEL BENOIST

DEFINITION AND HISTORICAL REVIEW

The term inflammatory spondyloarthropathies refers to a group of diseases originally considered to be variants of rheumatoid arthritis (RA). It is now well established that this group is a separate entity, clearly distinct from RA. These disorders include ankylosing spondylitis (AS) and its variants, which are enteropathic arthritis (ulcerative colitis and Crohn disease), psoriatic arthritis, and reactive arthritis (postenteric and postvenereal arthritis). The inflammatory spondyloarthropathy group is characterized by varying inflammatory involvement of the axial skeleton (sacroiliac and spinal joints), peripheral synovial and cartilaginous joints, and the entheses, bursae, and tendon sheaths. These disorders share the absence of immunoglobulin M–agglutinating rheumatoid factor and a familial aggregation, suggesting a genetic susceptibility. The crucial discovery that HLA-B27 was strongly associated with IS and the frequent overlapping of these various inflammatory disorders has justified their identification in a unified group. Moreover, extraarticular (ocular, mucocutaneous, and genital) symptoms are often encountered in the course of the spondyloarthropathies. The triggering role of infectious agents in some cases of HLA-B27–related arthritis has strongly stimulated the research for both immunogenetic and environmental factors.

Historically, AS was described first. Three eminent neurologists, Von Strümpel, Bechterew, and Pierre Marie, accomplished pioneering work at the beginning of the 20th century. Later, major contributions were made by Forestier and coworkers[29] and by Scandinavian authors, especially Romanus and Yden.[68]

Primary AS remains the major and central part of the inflammatory spondyloarthropathy group. AS secondary to enteropathic, psoriatic, and reactive arthritis was subsequently linked to primary AS because of interrelated clinical and radiologic features and because of a common immunogenetic background.

ANKYLOSING SPONDYLITIS

Primary AS is a chronic inflammatory disease of the axial skeleton, often associated with a varying involvement of the peripheral joints and entheses.

Pathology

The main pathologic feature of AS is its tendency to affect the insertion of joint capsules and ligaments into bone (i.e., entheses). In these sites, the inflammation is usually mild and leads to fibrotic and osseous proliferation. Involvement of peripheral joints, bursae, and tendon sheaths is characterized by inflammation of the synovium, usually milder than that observed in RA. These pathologic changes explain the major features of AS: syndesmophytes, bony ankylosis, and reactive proliferative changes.[17]

Anatomically, the sacroiliac joints are initially involved. Sacroiliitis is the hallmark of the disease, which subsequently spreads to the spinal joints.

Diagnostic Criteria

The diagnosis of AS is based on the association of characteristic clinical and radiologic features. Episodes of low back pain radiating to the buttocks and the sciatic territory are predominant late at night. Morning stiffness that subsides with exercise is also highly suggestive of the diagnosis. The pain usually starts insidiously in young people, and it spreads progressively to the thoracic and cervical spine. The physical examination may show a decrease of spinal mobility in both anterior and lateral planes, which can be measured by the Schober test. However, the restriction of spinal mobility as well as the loss of lumbar lordosis can be absent in early or mild cases. In this classic form, the diagnosis is usually confirmed by the radiologic demonstration of sacroiliitis and syndesmophytes. Nevertheless, the diagnosis can be difficult early in the course of the disease, when the sacroiliac changes are minimum and doubtful.

Criteria for the diagnosis of AS were formulated at a conference in Rome in 1961 (Table 1) and revised in New York in 1966 (Table 2). However, these criteria have been regarded as too restrictive. To encompass the wider spectrum of undifferentiated spondyloarthropathy, a more inclusive set of criteria has been proposed.[20] These criteria for spondyloarthropathy are based on statistical analysis and clinical reasoning (Table 3).

Positive results of HLA-B27 testing are helpful in difficult diagnoses. However, this should not be considered a diagnostic test. The HLA-B27 antigen, although found in the great majority of Caucasian patients with AS, can be absent, especially in non-Caucasian patients. On the other hand, a certain number of HLA-positive patients never have the disease.

Other laboratory findings are nonspecific. The erythrocyte sedimentation rate is usually, but not consistently, elevated. High elevations are found, especially in the active forms of the disease, with involvement of

Table 1

Rome Clinical Criteria for Ankylosing Spondylitis

Low back pain and stiffness for more than 3 months
Pain and stiffness in the thoracic region
Limited motion in the lumbar spine
Limited chest expansion
History or evidence of iritis or its sequelae
Ankylosing spondylitis present if bilateral sacroiliitis is associated with any one of the above clinical criteria

Data from Calin, A.: Ankylosing spondylitis. Clin. Rheum. Dis. 11:41–60, 1985.

Table 2

New York Clinical Criteria for Ankylosing Spondylitis

1. Limitation of motion of the lumbar spine in all three planes (anterior flexion, lateral flexion, and extension)
2. A history of pain or the presence of pain at the dorsolumbar junction or in the lumbar spine
3. Limitation of chest expansion to 1 inch (2.5 cm) or less, measured at the level of the fourth intercostal space

Definite ankylosing spondylitis present if:
  Grade 3–4 bilateral sacroiliitis associated with at least one clinical criterion
  Grade 3–4 unilateral or grade 2 bilateral sacroiliitis associated with clinical criterion 1 or with both clinical criteria 2 and 3

Probable ankylosing spondylitis present if:
  Grade 3–4 bilateral sacroiliitis without any clinical criteria

Data from Calin, A.: Ankylosing spondylitis. Clin. Rheum. Dis. 11:41–60, 1985.

Table 3

European Spondyloarthropathy Study Group Criteria for Classification of Spondyloarthropathy

Inflammatory spinal pain *or* **Synovitis**
- Asymmetric or
- Predominantly in the lower limbs

and

One or more of the following:
- Positive family history
- Psoriasis
- Inflammatory bowel disease
- Urethritis, cervicitis, or acute diarrhea within 1 month before arthritis
- Buttock pain alternating between right and left gluteal areas
- Enthesopathy
- Sacroiliitis

Data from Dougados, M., van der Linden, S., Juhlin, R., et al.: The European Spondyloarthropathy Study Group preliminary criteria for the classification of spondyloarthropathy. Arthritis Rheum. 34:10, 1991.

the peripheral joints. Anorexia with loss of weight and fever can be observed in these patients, particularly during untreated initial acute episodes. Synovial fluid in the involved peripheral joints is inflammatory, with a predominance of lymphocytes. Histologic examination of the synovium reveals the following nonspecific inflammatory changes similar to those observed in RA: hyperplasia of the cells lining the synovium, plasma cells, and lymphocyte infiltrates, with occasional lymphoid follicle formation. However, in most cases synovial inflammation remains mild.[14]

Radiology

Radiology of AS has recently been reviewed.[44] The diagnosis of AS relies on suggestive history and clinical symptoms but is mainly based on radiographic findings involving the sacroiliac joints and the spine.

The most important diagnostic criterion of AS is bilateral sacroiliitis affecting the superior and posterior part of the sacroiliac joint. In advanced cases, the radiologic diagnosis is obvious when symmetric bilateral changes are observed, including erosion and widening of the joint space with a reactive, poorly limited band of subchondral bony sclerosis, sometimes progressing to a partial or total bony ankylosis. However, the early changes can be minimum and doubtful. Sacroiliitis may be unilateral early in the course and may be restricted to mild periarticular osteoporosis with minimum erosions.

In difficult cases, computed tomographic examination may reveal erosions and subchondral sclerosis that are not apparent on standard radiographs of the sacroiliac joint. Computed tomographic examination appears to be the best diagnostic imaging tool in detecting early subtle sacroiliac abnormalities.[48] It should be performed in cases in which the history and clinical findings are suggestive of AS. On the other hand, quantitative bone scintigraphy has proved to be less reliable in patients with normal or doubtful radiographic findings. Numerous causes of errors have been detected, depending on the effects of age, sex, and laterality.[30]

Radiologic demonstration of sacroiliitis is the major diagnostic criterion of AS. Table 4 summarizes the five grades of sacroiliac changes introduced in the New York diagnostic criteria. AS with a persisting absence of sacroiliitis is extremely rare. In exceptional cases, the diagnosis relies on characteristic clinical symptoms, association with uveitis and peripheral arthritis, typical syndesmophytes, and apophyseal joint involvement.

Radiologic abnormalities of the spine are well explained by basic pathology. As mentioned, AS predominantly affects the insertion of ligaments and capsules into bone. Chronic inflammation with bone resorption takes place at the discovertebral junction, where the outer part of the annulus fibrosus inserts into the vertebral body. At this site,

Table 4

Sacroiliac Changes According to New York Criteria

Grade 0	Normal
Grade 1	Doubtful
Grade 2	Minimal sacroiliitis (discrete blurring—minimal erosions)
Grade 3	Moderate sacroiliitis (definite blurring—erosions and sclerosis)
Grade 4	Ankylosis

Data from Calin, A.: Ankylosing spondylitis. Clin. Rheum. Dis. 11:41–60, 1985.

bone resorption progresses to erosion and sclerosis. Osseous proliferation, the hallmark of the reparative process, leads to ossification of the outer fibers of the annulus fibrosus (syndesmophytes). According to this pathologic process, the initial radiographic finding is erosion with subsequent bony formation at the discovertebral junction, usually occurring at the central part or at the corners of the vertebral body. Syndesmophytes are vertically oriented and follow the outer part of the annulus fibrosus. They are easy to distinguish from osteophytes and from the hyperostotic formations seen in Forestier disease (diffuse idiopathic skeletal hyperostosis). Syndesmophytes are usually bilateral and are originally detected at the thoracolumbar region. In advanced stages, the ossification can bridge the intervertebral space, creating the classic bamboo spine, related to extensive syndesmophytosis. Central and/or lateral discovertebral erosion and destruction with bony sclerosis similar to an infectious spondylodiscitis can occasionally be seen. Inflammation and localized fracture with pseudarthrosis are the speculative explanations of this rare radiologic feature.

Involvement of the apophyseal joints with erosions and subchondral sclerosis may progress to bony ankylosis of the facets. This is a frequent finding in the cervical spine. Additional radiologic features include discal calcification and ballooning, and calcification of supraspinous and interspinous ligaments. Involvement of the atlantoaxial joint is not a common feature in AS but is occasionally observed. Relatively little is known about the frequency of atlantoaxial and subaxial dislocations. Axial cartilaginous joints, including the symphysis pubis and the manubriosternal joints, are commonly involved. Bony erosions, adjacent sclerosis, and proliferation often lead to complete disappearance of the joints and to ankylosis.

Peripheral Joint Involvement

Peripheral joint disease occurs in approximately 25% of patients. The proximal joints (shoulders and hips) are most frequently involved. Erosions, joint space narrowing, osteophytosis, and sometimes bony ankylosis are the main radiologic features. In the shoulder, disruption of the rotator cuff is often associated with articular abnormalities. Other joints (knee, temporomandibular joint) may also be involved, sometimes late in the evolution of the disease when the axial inflammation has disappeared.[44]

Enthesopathies

The main pathologic feature of AS is inflammation of the enthesis. This is manifested radiologically by osseous erosion, bony sclerosis, and proliferation at the site of insertion of the involved tendons or ligaments. Enthesopathies may be seen in axial sites such as the ischial tuberosity and the iliac crest. The most common peripheral insertional lesions include plantar fasciitis, Achilles tendinitis, and dactylitis. Involvement of the calcaneus is a frequent finding.

Fractures

Fractures through the vertebral body or the ossified disc space often occur after minor trauma. They are a major source of mortality and morbidity, including respiratory complications. The cervical spine is frequently involved, with a high rate of neurologic deficits. Conservative management is often successful in achieving union and complete or partial neurologic recovery. Surgery is indicated to stabilize unstable fractures. Decompression may be mandatory in cases with major evolving neurologic lesions.[31]

Systemic Aspects

Extraspinal and extraarticular manifestations may occur during the course of the disease, clearly indicating that AS is a systemic disorder. For references, see a review by Bourgeois.[14]

Uveitis. Nongranulomatous anterior uveitis is observed in approximately 25% of patients with AS. It can be an early manifestation of the disease and sometimes precedes the spinal and articular symptoms. Iritis may also develop years after the onset of AS when the spinal disease is inactive. Uveitis is usually mild but can be severe and relapsing. It requires prompt and adequate treatment, including general and/or local steroid therapy. Uveitis is predominantly seen in HLA-B27–positive patients with peripheral joint involvement.

Cardiovascular Involvement. Cardiovascular symptoms occur in 1% to 10% of patients with AS. The symptoms occur most often in the severe evolutionary and relapsing forms of the disease, especially those associated with uveitis and peripheral joint disease.

Aortic incompetence is the most frequent and most severe cardiovascular manifestation. Pericarditis is usually latent. Defects in cardiac conduction are observed in 5% to 8% of patients. They often consist of incomplete first-degree block, discovered by electrocardiography. However, complete atrioventricular blocks with Adams-Stokes syndrome and cardiac insufficiency may develop. Inflammation and subsequent fibrosis and scar tissue formation primarily affect the aortic valve cusps and the root of the aorta. The lesions progress toward the septum and the main mitral valve, with direct inflammatory involvement of the conduction tissue.

Pulmonary Disease. Involvement of the lung is observed in approximately 1.3% of patients with longstanding AS. Lymphocytic inflammatory infiltrates and progressive interalveolar fibrosis are responsible for the radiographic changes seen mainly in the upper lobe of the lungs but sometimes progressing to the other lobes. The radiographs reveal extensive fibrosis with cyst formation and tissue destruction resembling tuberculosis. The lung involvement is often latent but is occasionally revealed by cough, dyspnea, and hemoptysis. Subsequent *Aspergillus* invasion is a major complication.

Neurologic Manifestations. Cauda equina syndrome is a rare complication of AS, but it may occur in a longstanding form of the disease after the spinal inflammation has become inactive. After an insidious onset, the syndrome is revealed by low back and leg pain with reflex, sensory, and sphincter impairment. The motor symptoms usually remain discrete. The myelographic examination reveals enlargement of the dural sac and lumbar diverticula without signs of nerve root compression. Anatomic lesions consist of thickening and fibrotic proliferation of the epidural space and the meningeal envelopes. Surgical treatment may be necessary, but it is difficult and not always rewarding.

A few patients with vertebral cord compression at the thoracic level, accompanied by similar histologic lesions probably secondary to arachnoiditis, have been reported.

Amyloidosis. Amyloidosis is a rare but serious complication of AS. It occurs in the severe form of the disease after a long period of evolution. There are numerous relapsing acute episodes, including involvement of the peripheral joints. Often, the disease starts in childhood or adolescence. Amyloid is found in the liver, spleen, and kidneys. Renal involvement may be a cause of death.

The prevalence of amyloidosis in AS is still under discussion. It varies from 4% to 8%. In one study, three of 35 patients had amyloid on rectal biopsy.[14]

The Kidney Disorders. Glomerular renal function is not impaired in AS. However, vascular abnormalities were found in 11 of 14 renal biopsy specimens from patients with AS. In another study, three cases of renal papillary necrosis were associated with AS. Cases of immunoglobulin A γ nephropathy have also been reported.

Ankylosing Spondylitis in Women

Ankylosing spondylitis has long been regarded as a male disease. Studies have shown that the frequency of AS in women is higher than traditionally thought. AS in female patients is also usually regarded as milder than that in men. However, a review of the literature clearly demonstrated that the natural history and clinical course of primary AS in women appears similar to that in men.[32] Clinical expression, including age at onset, initial symptoms, frequency of peripheral arthritis, and restriction of spinal mobility, is comparable. Similarly the radiologic manifestations, including sacroiliitis, frequency of spinal involvement, presence of bamboo spine, and cervical spine involvement, do not demonstrate any significant differences between men and women. Systemic manifestations and frequency of HLA-B27 are also similar. Pregnancy usually has no effect on the clinical course of AS. However, remissions may occur in some pregnant women whereas other pregnant patients experience exacerbation.[32]

Epidemiology

The epidemiology of AS has been reviewed.[33] The increased frequency of AS in families of patients with AS compared with that in the general population is now well established. In 1961, de Blecourt and coworkers,[13] studying a series of 7405 patients, found that the disease was detected 22.6 times more frequently in families of patients with AS than in those of control subjects. In another study, 16% of the first-degree relatives of 76 patients with AS had sacroiliitis.[24]

In 1973, Brewerton and coworkers[15] and Schlosstein and associates[70] independently described the high frequency of HLA-B27 in patients with AS and their families. The fact that half of the first-degree relatives of patients with AS were HLA-B27 positive explained this familial aggregation. *HLA-B27* is genetically transmitted as an autosomal codominant characteristic. The link between *HLA-B27* and spondyloarthropathies is discussed below.

Primary AS commonly begins in young persons at about 25 years of age, sometimes earlier. Classically, there is a striking predominance in males with a male/female ratio of 10:1. However, as mentioned above, studies have shown that AS is much more frequent in women than was thought before, with a prevalence in women approaching the frequency in men.[18]

An interesting study has investigated the interrelated effect of phenotypic expression (primary AS, or disease secondary to psoriasis or inflammatory bowel disease) and age at onset, sex, and inheritance of responsible genes in cases of AS (sporadic or familial). Sex ratio and age at onset were shown to be influenced both by each other and by such factors as disease type and familial versus sporadic occurrence. For example, the sex ratio for the entire group of 1949 subjects with AS was 2.6:1 in favor of men. However, although AS due to inflammatory bowel disease had an equal sex distribution, AS due to psoriasis resulted in a male dominance of 4.1:1.[43]

The prevalence of AS in the general population is still under discussion. It is generally estimated to be between 0.5 and 4 per 1000 population.[53]

AS develops much more frequently in Caucasians than in other populations. The disease is rare in black Africans and the Japanese. The rarity of HLA-B27 in these two populations provides a reasonable explanation.[19]

Etiology

The cause of primary AS is unknown. The association with HLA-B27 is well established, but its link with clinical manifestations remains speculative. Involvement of infective agents is still under study. A high fecal carriage of *Klebsiella pneumoniae* in patients with active disease led to speculation that this agent was involved in the pathogenesis.[23] However, other conflicting data, including the absence of lymphocyte transformation to *K. pneumoniae*, have kept the debate open.[45]

Prognosis

Severity of evolution is difficult to predict on an individual level. However, in western countries, extensive spinal disease with peripheral joint and systemic involvement is rare. Proper management usually enables most patients to enjoy normal lives. However, severe forms of disease, with total ankylosis and major extraspinal involvement, are sometimes encountered. A higher frequency of severe AS with juvenile onset is noted in some geographic regions (e.g., North Africa).[8] Comparison of patients with AS in various populations with similar genetic backgrounds suggests a modulation of the severity of the disease according to the age of exposure to an infectious agent in predisposed individuals. The mortality of patients with AS is 1.6 to 1.9 times higher than in the general population. Causes of death from AS are secondary amyloidosis and cardiovascular complications.[55]

Treatment

Patient and family education concerning the course of the disease, the prognosis, and the aims and possibilities of therapy are most important. Each patient should be properly informed that there is no definitive cure for the disease but that relief of pain and maintenance of good posture and activity can be expected with proper management.

Nonsteroidal antiinflammatory drug (NSAID) therapy usually relieves inflammation and pain. Phenylbutazone is classically the most effective agent and is sometimes the only efficacious one. However, its potential long-term toxicity or patient intolerance limits its use. Indomethacin and the newer NSAIDs are often effective. Whatever drug is used, the dosage regimen should be adapted according to the severity of the disease. A high dosage should be used to decrease inflammation during severe flareups and then carefully tapered during nonevolutionary periods of disease. If the disease becomes dormant, continuous therapy does not seem to be necessary.

Aspirin and corticosteroids have a small place in the treatment of AS. Neither gold nor penicillamine has demonstrated efficacy. Treatment of AS has traditionally included exercise and nonsteroidal antiinflammatory drugs.

Sulfasalazine has been assessed as a disease-modifying drug. Sulfasalazine is an antibiotic with demonstrated efficacy in the treatment of inflammatory bowel diseases. Sulfasalazine also has a beneficial effect on intestinal permeability as well as an immunomodulating effect. As discussed below, the role of gastrointestinal infection and inflammation in the etiology of AS has been suggested.[60] A few double-blind, randomized, placebo-controlled studies have been conducted to evaluate the effect of sulfasalazine in patients with active AS.[27, 46, 65] A clinical benefit is observed in patients with recurrent extraspinal problems, including peripheral arthritis and iritis. No definite or significant benefit in increasing spine mobility or decreasing back pain and sleep disturbance was disclosed in the group of patients with principally spinal symptoms.

The other major aim of therapy is to avoid ankylosis and curvature. Maintaining good posture and function by extension exercises, swimming, physiotherapy, and adequate attention to day and night position is an important part of the therapeutic regimen.

Vertebral wedge osteotomy may be necessary in patients with severe deformities. Spinal fractures or neurologic manifestations require careful neurosurgical evaluation. Hip arthroplasty, when necessary, contributes to maintaining proper posture and activity.

REACTIVE ARTHRITIS

The term reactive arthritis has been proposed to designate aseptic arthritides, which develop after an infection elsewhere in the body, without entry of the microorganism into the joint.[3]

Historically, Reiter syndrome, which in its complete form associates arthritis with intestinal or genitourinary symptoms, was the first example of reactive arthritis to be described. *Shigella* was the first suspected agent associated with Reiter disease.[28] Subsequently, other postenteric or postvenereal infectious triggering agents have been identified. Table 5 illustrates the frequency of the bacteria identified in 352 cases of reactive arthritis, disclosed in a survey by the French Society of Rheumatology.[6]

Epidemiology of these agents may vary according to the endemic areas. Complete Reiter syndrome, including arthritis, conjunctivitis, and urethritis, may develop after either an enteric infection or a sexually transmitted infection. In both cases, there is a striking association with HLA-B27.[13, 41]

On the other hand, incomplete Reiter syndrome (i.e., reactive arthritis without extraarticular manifestations) after a triggering infection has also been closely associated with HLA-B27. Moreover, a group of HLA-B27–positive patients have a disease exactly resembling reactive arthritis, although they show no evidence of a recent infection.[59]

In the postvenereal form of HLA-B27–

Table 5

Bacteria Identified in 352 Cases of Reactive Arthritis

Bacteria	Identification	
	Serology	Culture
Chlamydia trachomatis	61	25
Yersinia enterocolitica	46	3
Yersinia pseudotuberculosis	24	0
Shigella flexneri		
Klebsiella pneumoniae	29	2
Neisseria gonorrhoeae		2
Ureaplasma urealyticum		6
No bacteria identified in 50% of cases		7

National Survey by the French Society of Rheumatology.
Data from Amor, B., Bouchet, H., and Delrieu, F.: Enquête nationale sur les arthrites réactionnelles de la Société Française de Rhumatologie. Rev. Rhum. Mal. Osteoartic. 50:733, 1983.

associated reactive arthritis, *C. trachomatis* is considered the main etiologic agent.[7,47] Serologic studies and cultures of urethral smears have demonstrated a recent chlamydial infection in 40% to 70% of patients with postvenereal reactive arthritis. Results from electron microscopic studies of the synovium and the synovial fluid and from molecular biologic techniques led to the assumption that postvenereal Reiter syndrome may not be a reactive arthritis, but rather a septic arthritis due to *C. trachomatis* infection.[12]

In the postenteric form, *Shigella, Salmonella, Yersinia,* and *Campylobacter jejuni* infections have been the main triggering agents. However, in some cases, these pathogens cannot be identified, and it is likely that other still unknown etiologic Enterobacteriaceae may also be implicated.[2-4]

Postenteric reactive arthritis affects only a fraction of the HLA-B27–positive population, although the pathogens found in arthritic and nonarthritic patients do not differ. This clearly indicates the importance of the host response. However, the capacity of the Enterobacteriaceae to trigger arthritis appears to differ in some microbial strains. For example, *Shigella flexneri* is arthritogenic and *S. sonnei* is not. *Y. enterocolitica* type 03 and type 09, found in Scandinavia, is associated with reactive arthritis. In contrast, *Y. enterocolitica* type 08 is not arthritogenic.[3,8]

Rheumatic fever after pharyngeal streptococcal infection is another example of reactive arthritis with no link to the HLA-B27 antigen. Its incidence has dramatically decreased in western countries. Reactive arthritis can also follow meningococcal, gonococcal, or brucellar infections.

Clinical Picture

The present description addresses only postenteric and postvenereal forms of HLA-B27–associated reactive arthritis, which represent by far the vast majority of the group with reactive arthritis.

Articular Symptoms

The onset of the articular symptoms usually begins 1 week to 3 weeks after the infection. The lower extremities are first and almost always affected. Involvement of the upper limbs is not consistently present. Synovial inflammation appears in the involved joints in rapid succession. There is a predilection for large joints, although feet and hand joints may also be involved. Acute asymmetric oligoarthritis is the typical clinical picture. In approximately one third of patients, an inflammatory type of back pain and peripheral enthesopathy are observed. These manifestations link reactive arthritis to the other forms of inflammatory spondyloarthropathies.

Postvenereal arthritis is predominantly observed in young men. It has been suggested that some cases of the self-limited seronegative oligoarthritis of unknown cause observed in women may be misdiagnosed episodes of reactive arthritis. Nongonococcal venereal infection is frequently asymptomatic in women. Postenteric arthritis can be observed at all ages, with no difference in the sex distribution.

Extraarticular Symptoms

Urethritis is the triggering infection in the postvenereal form, and it is probably reactive and less frequent in the postdysenteric form.

Ocular lesions, including conjunctivitis and less frequently uveitis, are part of the complete Reiter syndrome and a common extraarticular feature.[3]

Keratoderma blennorrhagicum is usually seen in patients with a definite diagnosis of Reiter syndrome and appears on the soles and palms, sometimes with a circinate balanitis. Clinically and histologically, keratoderma is indistinguishable from pustular psoriasis. These skin lesions provide a strong link between HLA-B27–reactive arthritis and psoriatic arthritis. Moreover, epidemiologic studies have shown a high prevalence of psoriasis in the relatives of male patients with reactive arthritis.[54] On the other hand, clinical observations have demonstrated that Reiter syndrome could be followed by typical psoriatic arthritis.[73]

Cardiovascular manifestations, including valvulitis, are rare and, with the exception of myocarditis, are usually asymptomatic.[40]

Fatigue and fever are common at the onset of joint inflammation, especially in the postenteric form.

Evolution

Reactive arthritis usually subsides within a few weeks or months. The self-limited course of the acute attack can be followed by recurrences. This is especially true in the postvenereal form because of new genital infections or because of the spontaneous recurrence of nongonococcal urethritis.[41] In some cases, chronic deformities with erosive arthritis and cutaneous lesions follow the acute recurrences. In chronic Reiter disease, sacroiliitis is a common finding. The sacroiliac changes are often unilateral or asymmetric. Spondylitis can occur in chronic Reiter syndrome but is less frequent than in psoriasis. The paravertebral ossifications are nonmarginal, identical to those described in psoriatic spondylitis, and clearly different from the classic syndesmophytes of primary AS. They randomly affect the lower thoracic and upper lumbar vertebrae.[44]

Long-term follow-up studies also indicate that AS with bilateral sacroiliitis may develop in patients with reactive arthritis, especially in those with postvenereal Reiter syndrome or *Shigella* infection.[69]

Diagnosis

The diagnosis of reactive arthritis is based on the clinical history and physical examination findings and on identification of the triggering agent. As shown in Table 5, demonstration of the enteric bacteria from the stools is rare. The usual absence of direct bacteriologic evidence is attributable to the fact that cultures are often started too late after the beginning of symptoms, when identification of the bacteria from the stools is no longer possible.

Levels of antibodies for the suspected infectious agent are the second laboratory criterion. The antibody titer has usually reached its peak at the time of the first blood examination and can be expected to show a progressive reduction in subsequent weeks or months.

The search for *Chlamydia* in posturethritis reactive arthritis is not always successful. On the other hand, *Chlamydia* can be identified in asymptomatic patients, especially in females. Immunoglobulin G γ *Chlamydia* antibodies are also found in control subjects for long periods after infection. It is thus sometimes difficult to appreciate the significance of the laboratory findings at an individual level.[8]

Furthermore, as shown in Table 5, in half of patients with arthritis that closely resembles reactive arthritis, no evidence of recent infection can be demonstrated.[6]

Treatment

Treatment of the infection when the germ has been identified is still a matter of debate.[12] The use of antibiotics in the postvenereal disease was previously not recommended, as their use did not seem to have any influence on the duration of joint symptoms or the prevention of recurrences. This opinion was based on studies using antibiotic treatment of short duration. However, a double-blind, controlled study of 3 months of treatment with tetracyclines has shown significant shortening of the articular manifestations.[51] Another study has also demonstrated that the incidence of relapses was significantly reduced by the administration of antichlamydial antibiotics.[51] It seems therefore advisable to treat the postvenereal disease with long-term antibiotic therapy. It is also appropriate to treat the patient's sexual partner. Patients with postenteric arthritis should be treated only at the beginning of the infection, in instances of persistent diarrhea, fever, and positive stool cultures.

NSAIDs and local injections of corticosteroids are usually efficacious and can control the disease during its self-limited evolution. Certain patients with severe chronic or relapsing Reiter syndrome do not respond to this conventional therapy. Gold and penicillamine have been administered without any demonstrated effect. In those cases, the use of methotrexate seems advisable.[50]

PSORIATIC SPONDYLOARTHROPATHY

An association between psoriasis and seronegative spondyloarthropathies has been demonstrated by family and epidemiologic studies.[72] The studies have also shown that psoriasis and psoriatic spondyloarthropathy are more frequent in the families of patients with psoriatic arthritis. Although a strong genetic factor has been established, its expression is not yet clearly understood. No etiologic or environmental factor has been recognized.

Clinical Picture

The skin and nail symptoms usually precede or accompany the arthritis. However, in about 10% of patients, the skin disease appears later than the joint manifestations.[10]

Numerous classifications of psoriatic arthritis have been proposed. They illustrate the heterogeneity of the disease and the various clinical patterns of peripheral and axial joint involvement. The classification by Moll and Wright[61] provides a satisfactory clinical framework (Table 6).

Sacroiliac and Spinal Involvement

The association of psoriasis and AS, with or without peripheral seronegative arthritis, is well established. The clinical and radiologic symptoms may be identical to those of primary AS. However, some features often differentiate psoriatic spondylitis from definite AS.

Sacroiliitis develops in approximately 30% to 40% of patients with psoriatic arthritis.[35] Moreover, about 20% of patients with severe psoriasis have abnormal sacroiliac joints. The radiologic features include erosion, widening of the joint space, and sclerosis. Ankylosis is rare. Asymmetric or unilateral involvement may be encountered. Psoriatic sacroiliitis is often asymptomatic and found isolated without spondylitis.[44]

Two types of spondylitis associated with psoriasis have been distinguished. One is clinically and radiologically similar to primary AS. It is considered a chance association of the two diseases.

The second group appears to be different, on both clinical and radiologic grounds.[52] The vertebral symptoms appear at an older age and are usually milder than in primary AS. Typical syndesmophytes may be observed but are often replaced by nonmarginal syndesmophytes developing in paravertebral tissues. These ossifications are distant from the vertebral margins and the disc, are more voluminous, and may be unilateral with an asymmetric distribution. Lower thoracic and upper lumbar segments are usually affected, but involvement of the cervical spine may be predominant and is sometimes exclusive. Cervical spinal abnormalities, including paravertebral ossifications and arthritis of the facets, are usually seen in the lower cervical region, but involvement of the atlantoaxial joint may also be observed. These paravertebral ossifications due to calcification of the spinal ligaments are similar to those observed in Reiter spondylitis. However, nonmarginal spondylitis is usually less extensive in Reiter syndrome than in psoriasis.[44] In general, the clinical spinal symptoms, including pain and stiffness, are less marked in psoriatic spondylitis than in primary AS.[52]

Peripheral Involvement

The peripheral clinical patterns are characterized by an inflammatory arthritis, including pain, morning stiffness, articular swelling, and deformities. Radiologically, bone resorption and proliferation are the two important hallmarks of psoriatic arthritis.[52]

Bone resorption often begins at the joint margins and progresses centrally. Destruction of the subchondral bone sometimes leads to the classic pencil-in-cup deformity. The interphalangeal joints, and the metacarpophalangeal and metatarsophalangeal joints of the hands and feet are the usual targets. Severe acroosteolysis of the phalanges, metatarsi, or metacarpi is characteristic of arthritis mutilans. Bony proliferation often accompanies osseous subchondral destruction, producing a spiculated appearance. Periostitis of the epiphysis and metaphysis of the hand and foot bones are frequent, sometimes preceding joint destruc-

Table 6

Classification of Psoriatic Arthritis

Category	% of Cases
Pauci, asymmetric arthritis	70%
Symmetric polyarthritis	15%
Arthritis mutilans	5%
Asymmetric and exclusive involvement of distal interphalangeal joints	5%
Ankylosing spondylitis	5%

Based on data from Moll, J. M. H., and Wright, V.: Psoriatic arthritis. Semin. Arthritis Rheum. 3:55, 1973.

tion. Bony proliferation can also produce the so-called ivory appearance of the phalanx and may lead to fusion of the distal interphalangeal and the proximal interphalangeal joint. Finally, enthesopathies with calcification at the site of insertion of tendons and ligaments may be seen in the same areas as in primary AS, including the ischial tuberosity, the calcaneus, and the trochanters on the iliac side.[44]

Extraarticular Involvement

The most severe cases of peripheral arthritis and spondylitis are usually seen in patients with widespread skin disease. However, the psoriatic lesions may be discrete and unnoticed by the patient. They should be carefully looked for, especially in the scalp and the perineum. In patients with a typical picture of seronegative spondyloarthropathy and an absence of skin lesions, the discovery of nail changes is an important diagnostic aid.

Anterior uveitis occurs in approximately 15% of patients with spinal and sacroiliac involvement, but with a much lower frequency in patients with pure peripheral arthritis.[53]

Laboratory Findings

No specific laboratory abnormalities occur in psoriatic seronegative spondyloarthropathy. Psoriasis is associated with HLA-B13 and HLA-B17, but not with HLA-B27. Psoriatic peripheral arthritis is usually seen in the absence of HLA-B27, but 45.5% of the patients are HLA-B38 positive.[25] In contrast, HLA-B27 is found in approximately 70% of patients with sacroiliitis, with or without peripheral involvement. The prevalence of HLA-B27 is higher, approximately 80% in patients with both sacroiliitis and spondylitis.[22]

Prognosis and Therapy

As already mentioned, axial disease is less severe in psoriatic spondylitis than in primary AS. The loss of motion and pain is less marked and can usually be controlled by proper management. However, severe psoriatic spondylitis is occasionally seen with pulmonary complications and a fatal outcome.[67]

Severe evolution of peripheral arthropathy with joint destruction and functional incapacity is observed in about 15% of patients, especially those with arthritis mutilans.[52]

The treatment of psoriatic spondyloarthropathy must be adapted to the clinical pattern of the disease and to its severity. The management of psoriatic spondylitis is the same as for primary AS, including the administration of NSAIDs, exercises, and physiotherapy. The use of NSAIDs with local injections of corticosteroids usually relieves inflammation and pain in asymmetric oligoarticular arthritis of mild severity. In the serious polyarticular forms, with or without arthritis mutilans, the management can be difficult. NSAID administration and local forms of treatment are not sufficient to control the disease activity and prevent deformations and erosions. In these patients, gold preparations and D-penicillamine have been used with conflicting results.[21] Cytotoxic drugs such as azathioprine have proved beneficial. Methotrexate is the most effective in controlling both the cutaneous and articular manifestations.[26, 49] As already mentioned, the vertebral symptoms of psoriatic spondyloarthropathy are usually milder than those in primary AS. Methotrexate should be used only in patients with associated active peripheral arthritis

INFLAMMATORY BOWEL DISEASE

Inflammatory bowel diseases including ulcerative colitis, Crohn disease, and Whipple disease, may be associated with peripheral arthritis and axial symptoms. Many studies have confirmed the prevalence of seronegative inflammatory spondyloarthropathies in this group of disorders. The same studies have demonstrated that these arthropathies are clearly different from and not coincidental with RA.[1, 9, 16, 34, 62]

Ulcerative Colitis

Peripheral arthritis occurs in approximately 10% of patients with ulcerative colitis.[62] The acute synovial inflammation usually starts in one joint, primarily affecting the large joints of the lower limbs. However, the hands and feet are sometimes involved. The synovitis often remains monoarticular or oligoarticular and disappears spontaneously within a few weeks or months. Radiologic changes are usually not seen. The arthropathy is primarily observed in patients with widespread and chronic bowel involvement. The synovitis is often associated with exacerbations of intestinal disease. Moreover, the peripheral arthropathy is particularly frequent in patients with colitis with local or general complications. Surgical removal of the colon has a dramatic beneficial effect on the articular symptoms.[74]

AS may also be associated with ulcerative colitis. It sometimes precedes the appearance of the bowel symptoms. Later, there is no relationship between the course of the intestinal disease and the evolution of the spondylitis, which is not affected by colectomy. The sacroiliitis and the spinal changes are exactly the same as those seen in primary AS.[58, 75]

Family studies have shown a strong genetic influence in the development of ulcerative colitis. These studies have also demonstrated an increased prevalance of AS in first-degree relatives of patients with colitis, especially those with spondylitis.[56] Histocompatibility studies have shown the presence of the HLA-B27 antigen in approximately 65% of patients with ulcerative colitis and AS.[57]

Crohn Disease

The peripheral arthritis associated with Crohn disease closely resembles the arthropathy already described in ulcerative colitis. Seronegative oligoarthritis, affecting primarily the lower limbs, may antedate the bowel symptoms by many years. The temporal relationship between the articular and the intestinal exacerbations is not as striking as in ulcerative colitis.[36]

The spinal disease comprises sacroiliitis with or without spondylitis. The clinical and radiologic features of the axial involvement are similar to those encountered in primary AS.[37, 62] There is no correlation between flare-ups of Crohn disease and the evolution of spondylitis, which is unaffected by intestinal surgery.

Family studies have demonstrated a strong genetic factor in Crohn disease.[36] They have also shown a genetic association between ulcerative colitis and Crohn disease. HLA-B27 is found in about 53% of patients with Crohn disease–associated spondylitis.[38]

Whipple Disease

Whipple disease is a rare form of inflammatory bowel disease produced by an interplay of an infectious agent with host factors. The exact nature of the enterogenic organism is not well established. However, the infectious origin of the disease has been demonstrated by the efficacy of antibiotic therapy.

Peripheral arthritis and spondylitis identical to those found in ulcerative colitis and Crohn disease are seen in a substantial proportion of cases of this rare disease.[42, 66]

SAPHO SYNDROME

A syndrome of synovitis, acne, pustulosis, hyperostosis, and osteitis (SAPHO syndrome) has been identified. References are presented in a review by Kahn and Chamot.[39] SAPHO syndrome designates a group of frequently combined manifestations, of which the most common is osteitis of the anterior chest wall. These aseptic hyperostotic lesions can also be observed in the spine. The radiologic abnormalities are numerous; they can be isolated but are most often associated. The main features are as follows:

1. Sclerosis of the vertebral body, unifocal or multifocal, without involvement of the discs or of the end plates.
2. Discovertebral erosion and destruction similar to the aseptic spondylodiscitis sometimes complicating AS. One or several levels may be involved.
3. Paravertebral ossifications different from the typical syndesmophytes. They are voluminous, are nonmarginal, and are similar to the ossifications seen in psoriatic arthritis.
4. In children, vertebral plana have been observed.

The physiopathology of the vertebral lesions is not known. The few vertebral biopsies performed have shown nonspecific inflammation. No definite organism was found.

Inclusion of SAPHO syndrome in the group of spondyloarthropathies is justified by the frequent sacroiliac involvement. Sacroiliitis may resemble that seen in AS. However, it is more often unilateral, and an unusual osteosclerosis is frequently observed on the two edges of the sacroiliac joint. The link between this condition and seronegative spondyloarthropathies is further underlined by the possible combination with chronic inflammatory bowel diseases and the increased prevalence of HLA-B27 as compared with that in the general population. Moreover, although SAPHO syndrome is usually seen with palmoplantar pustulosis and acne, a weak association exists between psoriasis and the bone lesions.

ETIOLOGY AND PATHOGENESIS

A close interrelationship between the seronegative spondyloarthropathies is suggested by the numerous overlapping syndromes. Association of AS occurs with psoriatic arthritis and inflammatory bowel disease. As already mentioned, definite AS may follow chronic Reiter syndrome.[69] Other clinical overlaps strongly support the concept of a separate entity. They include an association between psoriatic arthritis and Reiter syndrome, between inflammatory bowel disease and psoriasis, and between ulcerative colitis and Reiter syndrome.[63, 74]

Moreover, a significantly increased frequency of one or more types of inflammatory spondyloarthropathy is found in the families of patients. Such clustering has been found in psoriatic arthritis, in Reiter syndrome, and in the inflammatory bowel disease group. For instance, there is an increased prevalence of spondylitis and inflammatory bowel disease in the families of patients with psoriatic arthritis.[71]

Finally, similar extraarticular involvement, including eye and skin lesions, can be found in any inflammatory spondyloarthropathy. The mucocutaneous lesions of Reiter syndrome can easily be confused with pustular psoriasis.[76] Anterior uveitis is a frequent manifestation of the entire inflammatory spondyloarthropathy group. The overlap of symptoms in the same patient and the evidence of familial associations strongly suggest a common genetic background. Genetic factors have indeed been recognized in each of the spondyloarthritides by family studies and HLA antigen investigations.[64] A close relationship between HLA-B27 and axial involvement has been demonstrated.[71] However, the frequency of HLA-B27 is not identical in each disease. HLA-B27 is present in 90% of patients with AS, 70% to 80% of patients with psoriasis and spondylitis, 50% to 60% of patients with inflammatory bowel disease and spondylitis, and 30% to 80% of patients with urogenital or Yersinia-reactive arthritis.*

The absence of HLA-B27 in about 10% of Caucasian patients with primary AS and in a greater proportion of patients with the other seronegative spondyloarthropathies strongly suggests the effect of other genes with polygenic inheritance. However, the strong association of primary AS with HLA-B27 makes it likely that this antigen is the major gene for AS.[71] It remains a hypothetic issue whether the HLA-B27 gene itself has a direct effect on pathogenesis or whether another gene in strong linkage disequilibrium with HLA-B27 is the actual disease-susceptibility gene.[5] On the other hand, subtypes of HLA-B27 have been recognized, clearly establishing the heterogeneity of the HLA-B27 gene.[40] However, the relationship of this heterogeneity to disease remains under intense study.

In addition to genetic predisposition, the importance of environmental factors is now well recognized. The triggering effect of gram-negative enteric bacteria and of genitourinary tract infections has been demonstrated in reactive arthritis.[8] The mechanism of the microbial triggering effect is still under discussion. However, the concept of molecular mimicry between HLA-B27 and the microbial antigens is currently the most attractive model. Other hypotheses have been formulated, such as an association of HLA-B27 with immune response genes or a modification of the HLA-B27 gene by a viral antigen.[8, 63]

No infective agent has been demonstrated in primary AS. The triggering role of K. pneumoniae is still a matter of debate. Inter-

---

*References 15, 18, 22, 38, 41, 57, and 70.

estingly, gut inflammatory lesions have been found by ileocoloscopies in 75% of a series of patients with primary AS, suggesting the role of an enterogenic infection.[60] As in inflammatory bowel disease, gut microorganisms could, in genetically predisposed patients, produce immune reactions leading to bowel lesions and extraintestinal symptoms, including peripheral and axial arthropathy.[62]

CONCLUSIONS

Clinical and epidemiologic studies and the investigations of HLA associations have shown that the seronegative types of inflammatory spondyloarthropathy can be classified as a distinct group of diseases. Genetic predisposition, especially regarding the role of *HLA-B27,* has been demonstrated.

However, many questions remain unresolved concerning the exact nature of the genetic constitution, the host's response, and the interaction between genetic factors and the suspected infectious agents.

One hopes that genetic studies, as well as the precise identification of the responsible infective agents, will improve the possibilities of therapy by methods other than symptomatic treatment.

REFERENCES

1. Acheson, E. D.: An association between ulcerative colitis, regional enteritis and ankylosing spondylitis. Q. J. Med. 29:489, 1960.
2. Aho, K., Ahvonen, P., and Lassus, A.: *Yersinia* arthritis and related diseases. *In* Dumond, D. C. P. (ed.): Infection and Immunology in the Rheumatic Diseases. Oxford, Blackwell, 1976.
3. Aho, K., Leirisalo-Repo, M., and Repo, H.: Reactive arthritis. Clin. Rheum. Dis. 11:25, 1985.
4. Ahvonen, P., Sievers, K., and Aho, K.: Arthritis associated with *Yersinia enterolitica* infection. Acta Rheum. Scand. 15:232, 1969.
5. Albert, E., and Scholz, S.: Immunogenetics and rheumatic disease. Clin. Exp. Rheumatol. 5(suppl. 1):29, 1987.
6. Amor, B., Bouchet, H., and Delrieu, F.: Enquête nationale sur les arthrites réactionnelles de la Société Francaise de Rhumatologie. Rev. Rhum. Mal. Osteoartic. 50:733, 1983.
7. Amor, B.: *Chlamydia* and Reiter's syndrome. *In* Ziff, M., and Cohen, S. B. (eds.): Advances in Inflammation Research. The Spondyloarthropathies. New York, Raven Press, 1985, p. 203.
8. Amor, B.: Suspected infectious agent and host environment interactions in spondyloarthropathies. Clin. Exp. Rheumatol. 5(suppl.):19, 1987.
9. Ansell, B. M., and Wigley, R. A. D.: Arthritic manifestations in regional enteritis. Ann. Rheum. Dis. 23:64, 1964.
10. Baker, H.: Epidemiological aspects of psoriasis and arthritis. Br. J. Dermatol. 78:249, 1966.
11. Bardin, T., Enel, C., and Lathrop, M.: Treatment by tetracycline or erythromycine of urethritides allows significant prevention of post-venereal arthritic flares in Reiter's syndrome patients (abstract). Arthritis Rheum. 33:S26, 1990.
12. Bardin, T., and Schumacher, H. R.: Should we treat postvenereal Reiter's syndrome by antibiotics? J. Rheumatol. 18:1780, 1991.
13. Blecourt, J. J. de, Polman, A., and de Blecourt-Meindersma, T.: Hereditary factors in rheumatoid arthritis and ankylosing spondylitis. Ann. Rheum. Dis. 20:215, 1961.
14. Bourgeois, P.: Aspects systémiques de la spondylarthrite ankylosante. *In* Kahn, M. F., and Peltier, A. P. (eds.): Maladies dites systémiques. Paris, Flammarion, 1982.
15. Brewerton, D. A., Caffrey, M., Hart, F. D., et al.: Ankylosing spondylitis and HLA B27. Lancet 1:904, 1973.
16. Bywaters, E. G. L., and Ansell, B. M.: Arthritis associated with ulcerative colitis. Ann. Rheum. Dis. 17:169, 1958.
17. Bywaters, E. G. L.: Pathology of the spondyloarthropathies. *In* Calin, A. (ed.): Spondyloarthropathies. Orlando, Grune & Stratton, 1984.
18. Calin, A., and Fries, J. F.: The striking prevalence of ankylosing spondylitis in healthy W27 positive males and females. A controlled study. N. Engl. J. Med. 293:835, 1975.
19. Calin, A.: Spondyloarthropathy in Caucasians and non-Caucasians. J. Rheumatol. 10 (suppl.):16, 1983.
20. Dougados, M., van der Linden, S., Juhlin, R., et al.: The European Spondyloarthropathy Study Group preliminary criteria for the classification of spondyloarthropathy. Arthritis Rheum. 34:10, 1991.
21. Dowart, B. B., Gall, E. P., Schumaker, H. R., et al.: Chrysotherapy in psoriatic arthritis. Arthritis Rheum. 21:513, 1978.
22. Eastmond, C. J., and Woodrow, J. C.: The HLA system and the arthropathies associated with psoriasis. Ann. Rheum. Dis. 36:112, 1977.
23. Ebringer, R. W., Cawdell, D. R., Cowling, P., et al.: Sequential studies in ankylosing spondylitis. Association of *Klebsiella pneumoniae* with active disease. Ann. Rheum. Dis. 37:146, 1978.
24. Emery, A. E., and Lawrence, J. S.: Genetics of ankylosing spondylitis. J. Med. Genet. 4:239, 1967.
25. Espinoza, L. R., Vasey, F. B., Wilkinson, O. R., et al.: Association between BW 38 and peripheral psoriatic arthritis. Arthritis Rheum. 21:72, 1978.
26. Espinoza, L. R., Zakraoui, L., Espinoza, C. G., et al.: Psoriatic arthritis: Clinical response and side effects to methotrexate therapy. J. Rheumatol. 19:872, 1992.
27. Ferraz, M. B., Tugwell, P., Goldsmith, C. H., et al.: Meta-analysis of Sulfasalazine in ankylosing spondylitis. J. Rheumatol. 17:1482, 1990.
28. Fiessinger, N., and Leroy, E.: Contribution a l'étude d'une épidémie de dysenterie dans la Somme. Bull. Soc. Med. Hop. Paris 40:20, 1916.
29. Forestier, J., Jacqueline, F., and Rotes-Querol, J.: La spondylarthrite ankylosante. Paris, Masson, 1951.
30. Goldberg, R. P., Genant, H. K., Shimshak, R., et al.: Applications and limitations of quantitative sacroiliac joint scintigraphy. Radiology 128:683, 1978.

31. Graham, B., and Van Peteghem, P. K.: Fractures of the spine in ankylosing spondylitis. Diagnosis, treatment and complications. Spine 14:803, 1989.
32. Gran, J. T., and Husby, G.: Ankylosing spondylitis in women. Semin. Arthritis Rheum. 19:303, 1990.
33. Gran, J. T., and Husby, G.: The epidemiology of ankylosing spondylitis. Semin. Arthritis Rheum. 22:319, 1993.
34. Hammer, B., Ashurst, P., and Naish, J.: Disease associated with ulcerative colitis and Crohn's disease. Gut 9:17, 1986.
35. Harvie, J. N., Lester, R. S., and Little, A. H.: Sacroiliitis in severe psoriasis. Am. J. Roentgenol. 127:579, 1976.
36. Haslock, I.: Arthritis and Crohn's disease. A family study. Ann. Rheum. Dis. 32:479, 1973.
37. Haslock, I., and Wright, V.: The musculo-skeletal complications of Crohn's disease. Medicine 52:217, 1973.
38. Huaux, J. P., Fiasse, R., Le Bruyere, M., et al.: HLA B27 in regional enteritis with and without ankylosing spondylitis or sacroiliitis. J. Rheum. 3(suppl. 4):60, 1977.
39. Kahn, M. F., and Chamot, A. M.: SAPHO syndrome. Rheum. Dis. Clin. North Am. 18:225, 1992.
40. Khan, M. A.: Immunogenetics of ankylosing spondylitis: Clinically oriented aspects. Clin. Exp. Rheumatol. 5(suppl. 1):49, 1987.
41. Keat, A.: Reiter's syndrome and reactive arthritis in perspective. N. Engl. J. Med. 309:1606, 1983.
42. Kelley, J. J., and Weisiger, B. E.: The arthritis of Whipple's disease. Arthritis Rheum. 6:615, 1963.
43. Kennedy, L. G., Will, R., and Calin, A.: Sex ratio in the spondyloarthropathies and its relationship to phenotypic expression, mode of inheritance and age at onset. J. Rheumatol. 20:1900, 1993.
44. Kerr, R., and Resnick, D.: Radiology of the seronegative spondyloarthropathies. Clin. Rheum. Dis. 11:113, 1985.
45. Kinsella, T. D., Lanteigne, C., Fritzler, M. J., et al.: Absence of impaired lymphocyte transformation to *Klebsiella* in ankylosing spondylitis. Ann. Rheum. Dis. 43:590, 1984.
46. Kirwan, J., Edwards, A., Huitfeldt, B., et al.: The course of established ankylosing spondylitis and the effects of sulphasalazine over 3 years. Br. J. Rheumatol. 32:729, 1993.
47. Kousa, M., Saikku, P., Richmond, S., et al.: Frequent association of chlamydial infection with Reiter's syndrome. Sex. Transm. Dis. 5:57, 1978.
48. Kozin, F., Carrera, G. F., Ryan, L. M., et al.: Computed tomography in the diagnosis of sacroiliitis. Arthritis Rheum. 24:1479, 1981.
49. Kragballe, K., Zachariae, E., and Zachariae, H.: Methotrexate in psoriatic arthritis. A retrospective study. Acta Dermatovener. 63:165, 1982.
50. Lally, E. V., and Ho, G.: A review of methotrexate therapy in Reiter syndrome. Semin. Arthritis Rheum. 15:139, 1985.
51. Lauhio, A., Leirisalo-Repo, M., Lähdevirta, J., et al.: Double-blind, placebo-controlled study of three-month treatment with lymecycline in reactive arthritis, with special reference to *Chlamydia* arthritis. Arthritis Rheum. 34:6, 1991.
52. Laurent, R.: Psoriatic arthritis. Clin. Rheum. Dis. 11:61, 1985.
53. Lawrence, J. S.: The prevalence of arthritis. Br. J. Clin. Pract. 17:699, 1963.
54. Lawrence, J. S.: Family survey of Reiter's disease. Br. J. Vener. Dis. 50:140, 1974.
55. Lehtinen, K.: Mortality and causes of death in 398 patients admitted to hospital with ankylosing spondylitis. Ann. Rheum. Dis. 52:174, 1993.
56. MacRae, I., and Wright, V.: A family study of ulcerative colitis with special reference to ankylosing spondylitis and sacroiliitis. Ann. Rheum. Dis. 32:16, 1973.
57. Mallas, E. G., MacKintosh, P., Asquith, P., et al.: Histocompatibility antigens in inflammatory bowel disease. Their clinical significance and their association with arthropathy with special reference to HLA-B27. Gut 17:906, 1976.
58. McEwen, C., di Tata, D., and Lingg, C.: A comparative study of ankylosing spondylitis and spondylitis accompanying ulcerative colitis, regional enteritis, psoriasis and Reiter's disease. Arthritis Rheum. 14:291, 1971.
59. Mayer, O., Vignalli, M., and Ryckewaert, A.: Rhumatismes inflammatoires inclassables avec HLA B27. Rev. Rhum. Mal. Osteoartic. 49:11, 1982.
60. Mielants, H., Veys, E. M., Cuvelier, C., et al.: Significance of gut inflammation in the seronegative spondyloarthropathies. Clin. Exp. Rheumatol. 5(suppl. 1):81, 1987.
61. Moll, J. M. H., and Wright, V.: Psoriatic arthritis. Semin. Arthritis Rheum. 3:55, 1973.
62. Moll, J. M.: Inflammatory bowel disease. Clin. Rheum. Dis. 11:87, 1985.
63. Moll, J. M. H.: Pathogenic mechanism of B27 related seronegative polyarthritis: Interplay between genetic and environmental factors. Clin. Exp. 5(suppl. 1):7, 1987.
64. Moller, P.: Genetics of ankylosing spondylitis, psoriatic arthritis and Reiter's syndrome. C in. Exp. Rheumatol. 5(suppl. 1):35, 1987.
65. Nissila, M., Lehtinen, K., Leirisalo-Repo, M., et al.: Sulfasalazine in the treatment of ankylosing spondylitis. Arthritis Rheum. 31:1111, 1988.
66. Paite, R. H., and Tesluk, H.: Whipple's disease. Am. J. Med. 19:383, 1955.
67. Roberts, M. E. T., Wright, V., Hill, A. G. S., et al.: Psoriatic arthritis. Follow-up study. Ann. Rheum. Dis. 35:216, 1976.
68. Romanus, R., and Yden, S.: Pelvo-spondylitis ossificans. Rheumatoid or ankylosing spondylitis. Copenhagen, Munskgaard, 1955.
69. Sairanen, E., Paronen, I., and Mahonen, H.: Reiter's syndrome. A follow-up study. Acta Med. Scand. 185:57, 1969.
70. Schlosstein, L., Teresaki, P. I., and Bluestone, R. T.: High associations of an HLA antigen W27, with ankylosing spondylitis. N. Engl. J. Med. 288:704, 1973.
71. Woodrow, J. C.: Genetic aspects of the spondyloarthropathies. Clin. Rheum. Dis. 11:1, 1985.
72. Wright, V.: Psoriatic arthritis. Ann. Rheum. Dis. 20 123, 1961.
73. Wright, V., and Reed, W. B.: The link between Reiter's syndrome and psoriatic arthritis. Ann. Rheum. Dis. 23:12, 1964.
74. Wright, V., and Watkinson, G.: The arthritis of ulcerative colitis. Br. Med. J. 5463:670, 1965
75. Wright, V., and Watkinson, G.: Sacro-iliitis and ulcerative colitis. Br. Med. J. 5463:675, 1965
76. Wright, V.: Skin and arthritis. Clin. Exp. Rheumatol. 5(suppl. 1):75, 1987.

Fibrosis, Chronic Inflammation, and Vascular Damage in Mechanical Back Pain Syndromes

MALCOLM I. V. JAYSON
ANTHONY J. FREEMONT

CLINICAL FEATURES

Back problems most commonly arise owing to mechanical disorders within the spine. Well identified are specific pathologic changes such as herniated intervertebral disc, spinal stenosis, and spondylolisthesis. However, in many patients, it is difficult to relate the identified pathologic alteration to the clinical pattern, and the objective evidence of mechanical damage provides only a limited explanation of the symptoms experienced. There is a poor correlation between the degrees of degenerative change and the development of back pain. Some patients with advanced damage may have limited back movements but be symptom free, and other patients with minimum change may experience severe and persistent symptoms. Studies using both plain radiography[16] and magnetic resonance imaging[2] have shown only a weak correlation of back symptoms with evidence of degenerative change in the spine. Garfin and colleagues[7] described four patients with nerve root pain in whom symptoms resolved despite persisting nerve root pressure. They suggested that some form of inflammatory reaction in the perineural tissues had been present and subsequently decreased.

In this context, it is important to note that the clinical pattern of mechanical back problems is one of fluctuating symptoms. Patients have acute episodes of pain, which remit, and then are symptom free or have only minor problems until the next episode. However, the degenerative change within the spine does not fluctuate. It therefore appears likely that there are other changes present and playing a role in the development of symptoms. This discussion reviews the contributions of vascular damage, fibrosis, and chronic inflammation associated with mechanical back problems and their relevance to the development of symptoms.

In a classical inflammatory rheumatic disorder involving the spine, such as ankylosing spondylitis, there is a characteristic history of pain and stiffness aggravated by rest and relieved by exercise. The mechanism by which this occurs is uncertain, but it may be due to the acculumation of edema in inflamed tissues. Many patients with mechanical back problems give a similar history. In particular, they describe a lot of aching and stiffness when they are in bed and stiffness when they first wake up or sit for a prolonged time in a chair. They obtain relief by getting up and moving around. In the patients who have this pattern of symptoms, antiinflammatory drug administration appears to be particularly effective. The work described below suggests that venous obstruction and engorgement occur in association with mechanical damage within the spine. Static posture is likely to aggravate this, and relief obtained by moving around could improve venous return and reduce venous hypertension. There is a striking analogy with symptoms in patients with varicose veins in whom standing still aggravates the problem and movement provides relief.

Examination of radiculograms of patients with herniated intervertebral discs can show evidence of edema with swelling of the affected nerve root. At surgery, an erythematous layer of vascular granulation tissue covering the nerve root is often observed[8] and is most marked when disc rupture is complete to the outer border of the annulus fibrosus.[11] Enhancement of computed tomographic scans or magnetic resonance im-

e this as an en-
f the prolapse,[5]
esent increased
eflecting the in-

nd the nerve
stologic exam-
ows hyperpla-
hronic inflam-
pinal stenosis,
nd around the
n[10] performed
animals and
matory action
later became
studies there-
only a tissue
e, and this in
t. The nature
e subject of

observations
ch there has
intervention,
scular dam-
natory cells.
ne previous
ery and oil-
natory cells
... and then the fibrotic reaction can be much more exuberant.

Defective Fibrinolysis in Association with Spine Problems

In the course of studies of fibrinolytic activity in patients with connective tissue disorders, the authors observed a defect in the fibrinolytic system in patients with severe chronic back pain syndromes. This led to detailed studied of the association of these defects with spine problems

Polymerization of fibrinogen to form fibrin is a normal physiologic response in damaged tissues. The clot formed stops the leakage of blood from damaged blood vessels. The fibrinolytic enzyme system is a complex cascade of reactions in which plasmin cleaves fibrin to form fibrin degradation products. Plasmin is formed from plasminogen, which in turn is activated by tissue plasminogen activator. There are several inhibitors of this system, including tissue plasminogen activator inhibitor. If the inhibitors are present in excess, there is defective fibrinolytic activity.

In response to trauma, there is normally a temporary decrease in the fibrinolytic enzyme activity, which gradually normalizes over the succeeding weeks. This means that the clearance of fibrin is relatively slow but eventually the tissue returns to a normal state. Innes and Sevitt[14] suggested that a defect of the fibrinolytic system with failure to clear fibrin can interfere with diffusion of oxygen and nutrients into the tissues and can be responsible for the development of chronic tissue damage.

In a series of patients with chronic back pain taken as a whole, the authors found a decrease in fibrinolytic activity compared with that in control subjects. In subgroups of patients with back pain, there were similar changes of varying degrees. The fibrinolytic defect was most severe and significant in patients with the worst back problems such as arachnoiditis, but there were similar trends in other groups of patients with back pain.[23] This change was not present in all patients but occurred much more frequently in those with the worst back problems. This defect was demonstrated by a significant increase in the euglobulin lysis time and a decrease in the fibrin plate lysis area and appears to be due to an excess of tissue plasminogen activator inhibitor.[3]

In part, this can explain the poor correlation of radiographic changes with back problems. When one compares patients with similar degrees of lumbar spondylosis with and without back pain, the fibrinolytic defect correlates with the presence of symptoms. In a prospective study of patients presenting with their first episodes of back pain and sciatica and then followed for 1 year, the changes in the fibrinolytic defect correlated with the clinical outcome, with a persistent defect being noted in those in whom the sciatica failed to resolve.[15] However, it has not been possible to correlate these fibrinolytic changes with individual clinical or imaging features.[3]

These findings suggest that the changes in fibrinolytic activity can be helpful as an objective marker of the severity of the back problem, although the authors did not find this abnormality in all subjects. The authors believe that it is a marker of vascular changes (described below), and it may then act as a secondary pathogenic mechanism in that failure to clear fibrin may contribute to the persistence of tissue damage. In this context, Haaland and associates[9] reported that defective fibrinolytic activity is an adverse prognostic marker in patients undergoing lumbar spine surgery. This is in keeping with the fibrinolytic defect's being a marker of the severity of the vascular lesion and possibly playing a pathogenic role.

Smoking is an identified risk factor for back pain.[1, 6] Smoking produces a defect in the fibrinolytic system,[18] which may well explain the association of smoking with coronary vascular disease. It is possible that smoking is associated with spine problems by a similar mechanism.

The authors have undertaken studies of stimulating the fibrinolytic enzyme system using stanozolol, which is an anabolic steroid of low virilizing potential. It has the specific effect of correcting the fibrinolytic defect. A pilot study suggested that it is helpful for milder chronic back problems,[19] but in more severe postsurgical cases, it was not of benefit despite normalizing fibrinolytic activity.[4] It is possible that this approach is incorrect. However, it more likely that the difficulty in the use of this agent is that the vascular damage has already taken place. In coronary thrombosis, fibrinolytic therapy with tissue plasminogen activator is effective only if it is administered within a few hours of vascular obstruction. If its administration is delayed, it is of no value. It seems likely that similar mechanisms have operated in the spine. The vascular damage is long-standing and irreversible by fibrinolytic enhancement. In this context, it is known that physical exercise is effective in stimulating the fibrinolytic system, and it is possible that some of the benefits obtained with exercise in preventing and treating back problems are by these means.

EXPERIMENTAL STUDIES

Effect of Compression on Nerve Roots

Rydevik and colleagues[20-22, 24] conducted a series of studies in animal models examining the effects of graded compression on nerve root structure and function. These studies were performed on the pig cauda equina, which resembes the human cauda equina in various respects.

At operation, an inflatable balloon was placed across the cauda equina and the effects of various pressures on nerve root blood flow, solute transport nerve conduction, and neural and vascular anatomy were determined.[21] Even slight compression of the nerve roots (about 5 to 10 mmHg) could induce changes of venous congestion in the intraneural microcirculation.[20] Pressures of 50 mmHg could induce edema formation.[22] This was more marked when the pressure was applied rapidly. With applied pressures of 50 to 75 mmHg, there were changes in both afferent and efferent nerve conduction.[25]

There is a difference in the vascular supply between the peripheral nerves and the nerve roots. The peripheral nerves have a much more developed network of arterioles and venules than do the nerve roots. The main vessels of the nerve roots are located superficially and are more easily exposed to mechanical deformation. They also have no regional arteriolar blood supply (see Etiology of Sciatic Pain and Mechanisms of Nerve Root Compression by Rydevik and colleagues in Chapter 3). This suggests that the nerve roots are at particular risk of vascular obstruction due to mechanical compression.

These experimental findings all suggest that compression of the nerve root, even at low pressures, is likely to cause venous obstruction and edema formation and to impair neurologic function. This pathogenic sequence is entirely consistent with observations in humans.

Pathogenesis of Vascular Damage

The authors have performed two major studies (cadaveric and biopsy) to investigate the role of vascular changes, inflammation, and perineural fibrosis in the genesis of low back pain.

Cadaveric Studies

A cadaveric study was performed on 125 persons. Twenty-five of these patients were symptomatic with long-standing low back pain of longer than 3 years' duration. This was well documented but in every case had been managed conservatively, the only invasive procedure being myelography, which had been performed in 14 cases. All 25 patients had died of conditions unrelated to the back pain. The other 100 individuals were a sequential group of patients coming to autopsy for the diagnosis of sudden death. Most had died from myocardial infarction, pulmonary embolism, or acute intracranial hemorrhage. Although these cases were sequential, criteria for inclusion in the control group of the study were that the patient should have had no history of venous hypertension, endocrine disease, spinal instrumentation, or any documented back pain sufficient to have necessitated seeing their general medical practitioner or a hospital specialist.

The lumbosacral spine was removed in every case and fixed in neutral buffered formalin. After fixation, it was cut longitudinally and tissue blocks incorporating the intervertebral root canal and the hemisected spinal canal were taken from alternate sides from L1–L2 to L5–S1. The blocks were decalcified and serially sectioned. Histologic

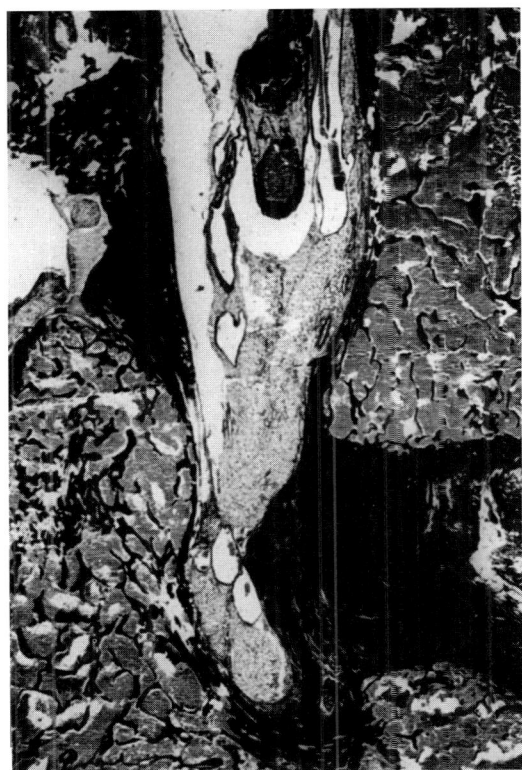

Figure 2. A disc protrusion associated with venous dilatation and periradicular fibrosis. (van Gieson, × 20).

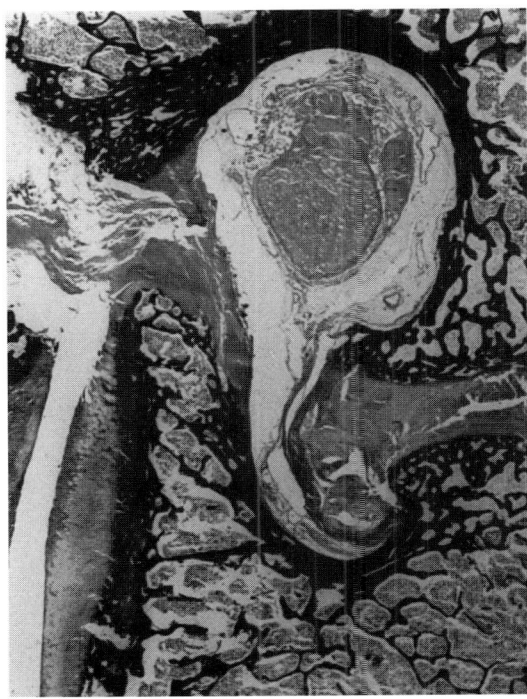

Figure 1. A large disc protrusion compressing structures in the lower pole of the intervertebral root canal at a distance from the nerve root. (Hematoxylin and eosin, × 15.)

analyses were performed, and the area of the intervertebral root canal occupied by the nerve complex and veins was calculated histomorphometrically. The proportion of the nerve root occupied by fibrous tissue and by neural tissue was also calculated.

Subjectively, there was little difference between the changes seen in either the symptomatic patients or members of the control group. Disc bulging, or frank sequestration, was seen in a high proportion of the specimens examined (41% of levels in the control group and 59% in the symptomatic group). The protruding disc impinged on vascular structures and fat within the intervertebral root canal (Fig. 1) and spinal canal, but only in the most severe sequestrations, usually associated with massive osteophyte formation, was direct nerve root compression seen. Vascular compression in the lower part of the intervertebral root canal was always associated with prominent dilatation of the vessels of the venous plexus in the intervertebral root canal (Fig. 2) and fibrosis around and within nerve roots and spinal nerves (Fig. 3). The area of the intervertebral root canal occupied by veins was directly related to the proportion of the adjacent nerve root complex occupied by perineural and intraneural fibrous tissue.

Further changes were seen in the soft tissues around the nerve. Frequently, the fat cells that occupy the majority of the intervertebral root canal showed the histologic changes associated with early fat necrosis. The microvessels around the nerve root were characterized by extensive thickening of their basement membranes, and where the meninges still covered the nerve roots, there was arachnoid cell proliferation and psammoma body formation.[13] In other tissues, these three changes are considered evidence of tissue ischemia.

In all cases of disc bulging and sequestration, there was degeneration within the disc. Typically, these degenerative changes included chondrocyte proliferation and myxoid change in the matrices. In addition, the

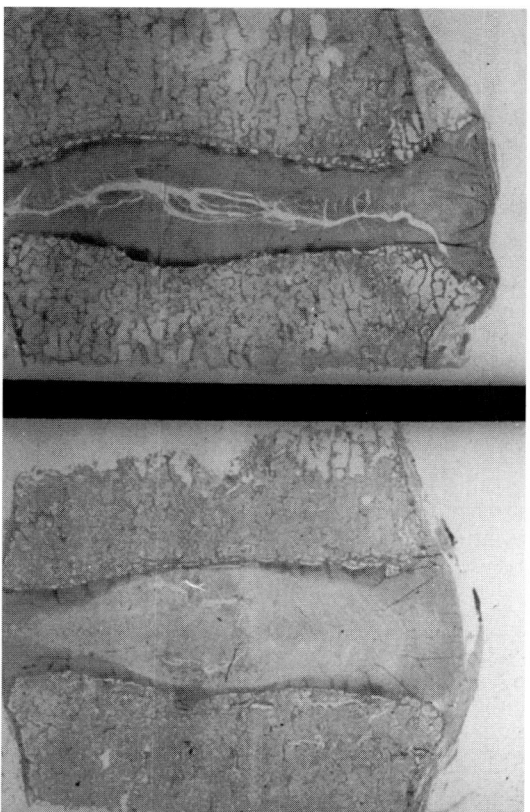

Figure 4. Top, A fissure within a degenerated disc. Bottom, A normal disc. (The posterior surface is to the right in both prints.) (Hematoxylin and eosin, × 20.)

disc frequently contained propagated intradiscal fissures. These were cracks or splits running through the disc, usually entering into and through the fibers of the posterior annulus, where they turned caudally to end at the vertebral end plate adjacent to the vertebral rim (Fig. 4). In these cases, there was usually damage to the vertebral end plate or rim manifest as defects in the bone and cartilage of the vertebral end plate or the bone of the rim. Through these defects, new vascular channels, accompanied by neural ingrowth, extended into the disc (Fig. 5) and propagated along the edges of the fissures (Fig. 6). Elsewhere within the biopsy specimens, high densities of nerves were seen in the longitudinal and intraspinous ligaments, the vertebral periosteum, and the walls of epidural and peridural veins.

A common finding was the presence of fibrin deposition within the dilated vascular channels of the intervertebral root canal

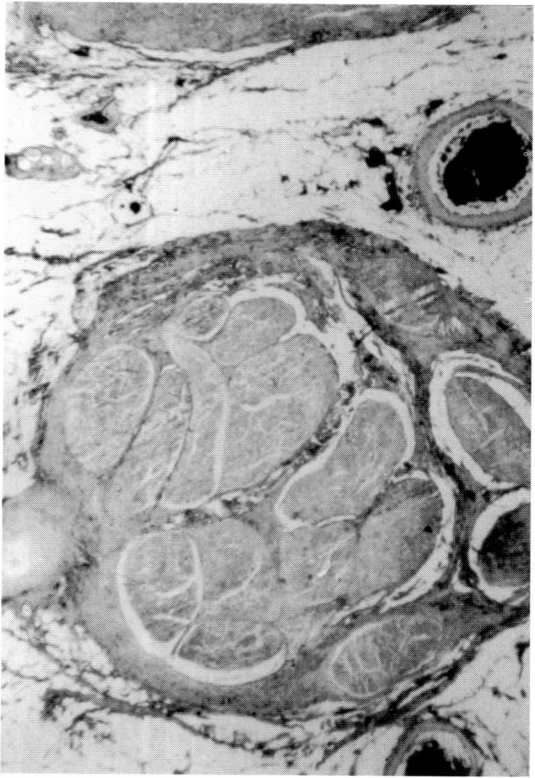

Figure 3. A spinal nerve showing extensive intraneural and perineural fibrosis. (Hematoxylin and eosin, × 40.)

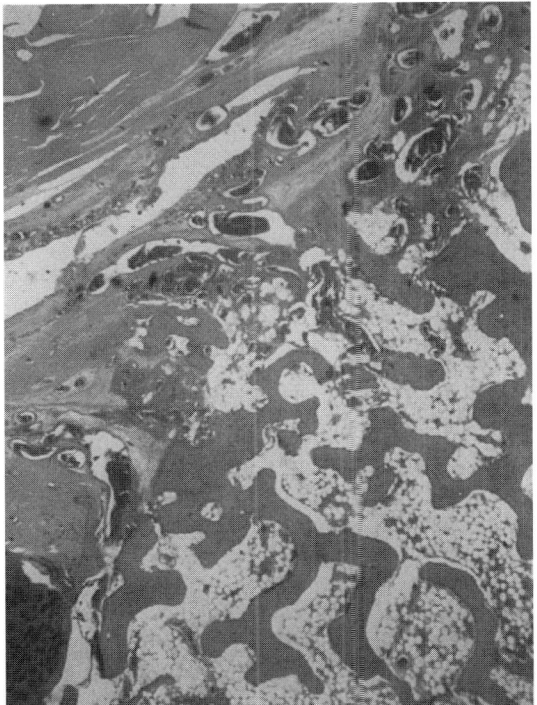

Figure 5. An end-plate lesion showing ingrowth of vessels from the marrow (right) into the disc (left). (Hematoxylin and eosin, × 100.)

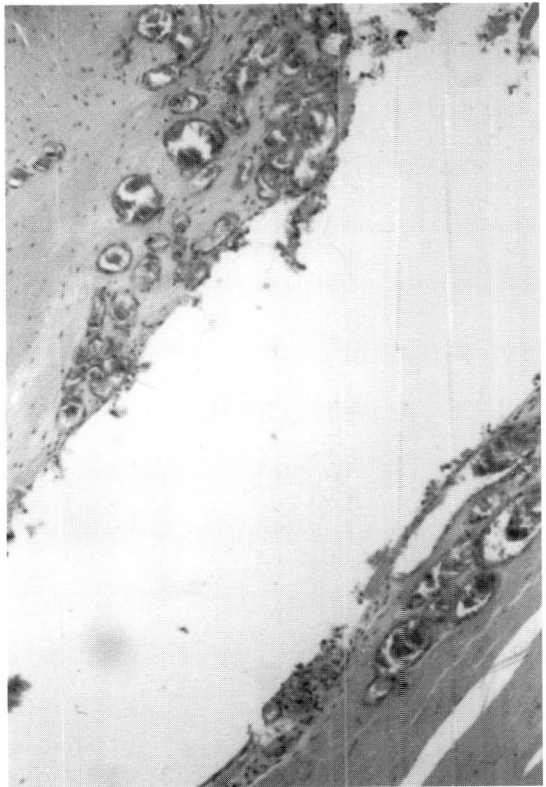

Figure 6. An intradiscal fissure lined by new blood vessels. (Hemotoxylin and eosin, × 150.)

(Fig. 7). In places, this amounted to occlusive thrombus formation showing organization (Fig. 8), which is absolute evidence that the thrombus had formed prior to death.[12]

In purely subjective terms there was no obvious difference in the type or extent of the pathologic changes in any one specimen from symptomatic and asymptomatic individuals. However, when the changes described above were analyzed over all five levels from each spine, differences appeared.

When spines from symptomatic and asymptomatic patients were compared, disc pathologic changes (disc protrusion or sequestration) were seen in the former in 96% of cases compared with 23% of the latter; venous dilatation, in 96% versus 47%; multiple-level venous dilatation, in 48% compared with 6%; periradicular fibrosis, in 84% versus 12%; and organizing thrombus, in 16% of systematic patients but only 5% of asymptomatic patients.

Histomorphometric analyses also disclosed two aspects of the pathologic alterations in which statistically defined differences could be identified between symptomatic and asymptomatic groups. Taken overall, the proportion of the area of the intervertebral root canal occupied by di-

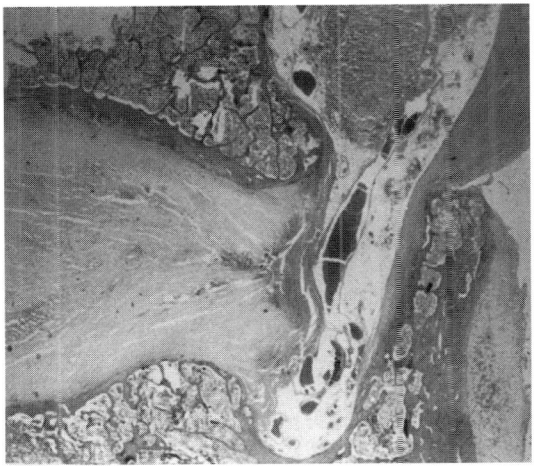

Figure 7. Thrombus within the dilated veins adjacent to a protruded disc. (Hematoxylin and eosin, × 20.)

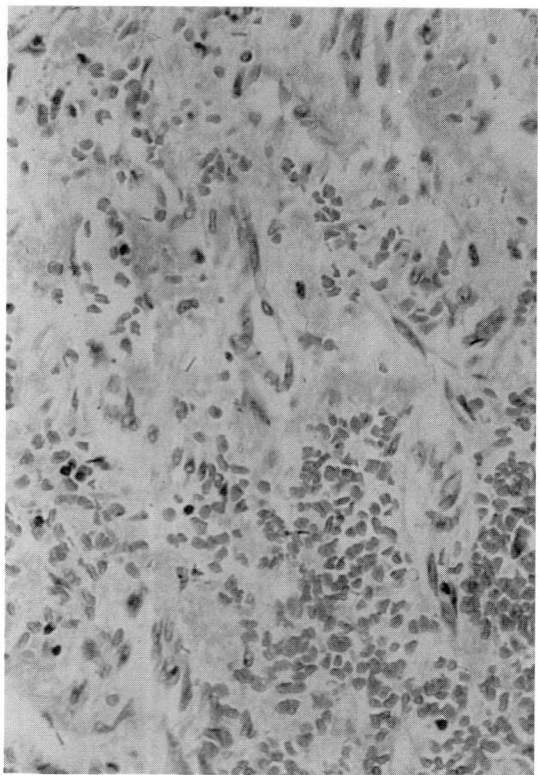

Figure 8. Organizing thrombus within the vessels seen in Figure 7. (Hematoxylin and eosin, × 200.)

lated veins was 28.8% ± 5.9% in symptomatic patients and 10.6% ± 3.8% in asymptomatic patients ($p = .001$). The proportion of the nerve root occupied by fibrous tissue was 35.1% ± 7.2% in symptomatic patients and 18.4% ± 6.6% in asymptomatic patients ($p = .005$).

A number of conclusions can be drawn from this study:

1. The presence of discal and associated pathologic changes is not necessarily associated with significant back pain.
2. The greater the number of spinal levels affected, the greater is the likelihood that back pain will develop.
3. Extensive vascular changes accompany pathologic alterations in the disc. These include venous dilatation and thrombosis, extensive ingrowth of vessels into dense connective tissues, and thickening of the basement membranes of exchange vessels (e.g., capillaries and venules).
4. Morphologic features usually suggestive of tissue ischemia accompany the discal and vascular changes in mechanical spinal disease.
5. Venous dilatation in the intervertebral root canal and periradicular and intraradicular fibrosis are linked.

Biopsy Studies

The second study involved histologic and in situ cell and molecular biologic observations on biopsy specimens taken from periradicular structures at the time of primary surgery for mechanical spinal disease. These biopsy specimens incorporated vascular fibrous and adipose tissue. When compared with normal periradicular tissue excised from fresh cadavers (within 4 hours of death) and similar specimens excised from organ donors at the time of donation, the spine surgical specimens showed extensive changes in the fibrous tissue and in the vessels.

At the morphologic level, the surgical specimens showed tissue fibrosis, fibrin deposition in thin-walled vascular channels, endothelial vacuolation, and neovascularization of a type not seen in control subjects.

The two tissue-probing techniques of immunohistochemistry and in situ hybridization have been used to explore the in situ cell and molecular biology of the vessels and connective tissue within the intervertebral root canal. Studies of von Willebrand factor (vWf), a product of endothelial cells whose release is associated with platelet aggregation and thrombus formation, showed loss of immunostainable vWf but increase in its messenger RNA (mRNA) in endothelial cells from the operative group. vWf is normally stored in endothelial cell cytoplasm within organelles called Weibel-Palade bodies. When the endothelial cell is stimulated, the vWf is discharged and is no longer immunodetectable. If stimulation continues, vWf mRNA is unregulated, increasing the detectable in situ hybridization signal, but because the gene product is continuously secreted under these circumstances, insufficient amount is available to be detected within the cell immunohistochemically (Fig. 9). Therefore, it follows that, in symptomatic patients with mechanical spinal disease, venous channels around nerve roots are subject to endothelial stimulation leading to release of vWf, which in turn causes platelet aggregation and throm-

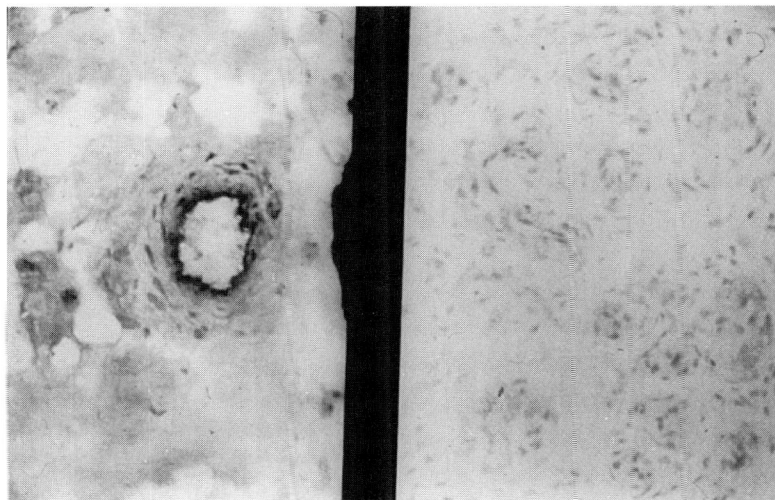

Figure 9. Immunohistochemical staining for vWf. Left, A vessel from a control biopsy specimen shows strong reaction. Right, The proliferating vessels from the periradicular tissues of a patient coming to spine surgery show a negative result. (× 200.)

bosis. In this study, upregulation of vWf mRNA was associated with an increase in intravascular accumulation of platelets detected by the presence of platelet glycoprotein IIa.

These studies also revealed other changes in endothelial function in the operated group of patients. These included endothelial cell expression of the fibrogenic cytokines transforming growth factor-β and interleukin-1 (Fig. 10). Fibroblasts within the fibrous tissue surrounding these vessels showed a marked increase in mRNA for type I collagen. Although it is not possible to quantify the absolute amount of protein or mRNA from the density of the immunohistochemical or in situ hybridization reaction products, the relative densities of staining suggested that the increase in type I collagen mRNA was directly proportional to the level of cytokine expression.

Both morphologic studies and histochemical probing of the tissue with antibodies directed toward cell surface antigens expressed only on B lymphocytes, T lymphocyte subsets, macrophages, and mast cells failed to reveal an inflammatory cell infiltrate in any specimen.

Unifying Hypothesis to Explain Some of the Tissue Changes

Although these studies showed an association among various types of pathologic change within the spines of patients with mechanical spinal disease, the only causal links that could even be inferred from these studies related vascular changes to radicular fibrosis. Piecing these data together indicates that disc disease leads to venous compression in the lower part of the intervertebral root canal and disturbed blood flow. In multilevel disease particularly, significant impairment of venous outflow from the spinal cord occurs as a consequence of disc disease and can lead to venous hypertension in the cord. This is manifested as venous dilatation. The poor blood flow causes tissue ischemia, endothelial dysfunction, and thrombus formation within the vessels of the intervertebral root canal. Simultaneous changes in endothelial function lead to the synthesis of fibrogenic cytokines. The contribution of new cytokine synthesis and tissue ischemia results in increased collagen synthesis by local fibroblasts.

At the same time, the trauma that caused disc disease results in morphologic evidence of tissue disruption of the disc and paracisal structures. This leads to an attempted repair process, with vascular ingrowth into the disc. The ingrowing vessels secrete matrix-degrading enzymes, which further weaken the disc connective tissues and are accompanied by nerves. This leads to a cycle of persistent or increasing tissue damage and potential pain induction.

Possible Associations Between Pathologic Appearances and Genesis of Low Back Pain

Although circumstantial evidence indicates a relationship between fibrosis and

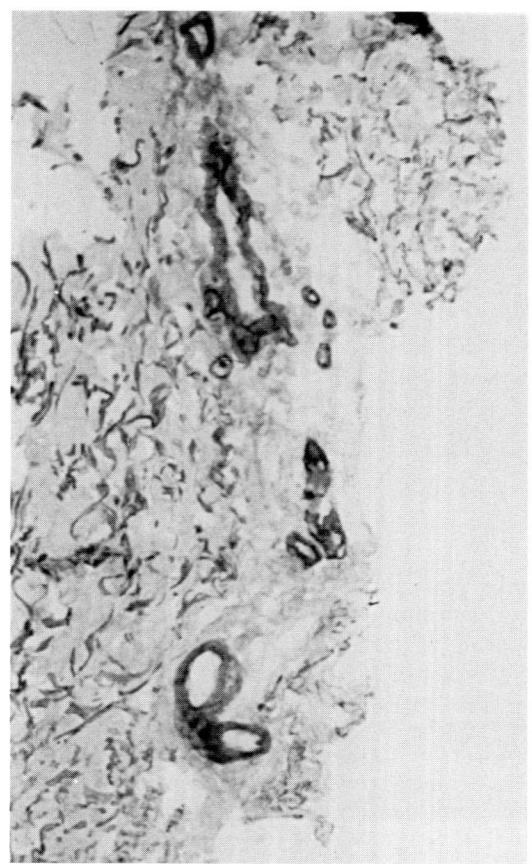

Figure 10. Immunohistochemical staining for interleukin-1 in vessels from a diseased spine. (× 150.)

pain, the authors' studies could only hint at potential mechanisms for pain induction associated with mechanical disease of the spine.

It has been proposed that direct nerve root compression causes pain. There is substantial evidence to support this in patients with acute disc prolapse, but the authors have been unable to show any significant association between chronic back pain and direct nerve root compression.

Inflammation has also been implicated in the genesis of pain, but in neither the cadaveric nor the biopsy study was it possible to identify any conventional inflammatory cell infiltrate morphologically or immunohistochemically within the soft tissues inside the spinal and nerve root canals. Furthermore, these studies suggest that the redness often noted at surgery in the peridural tissues and annulus, and reported as inflammation, is not a manifestation of inflammation as such but rather a consequence of vascular dilatation.

These investigations indicate another potential mechanism by which nerves might be stimulated in spinal disease, in addition to nerves penetrating the disc (which could be prone to physical stimulation under load). Dense aggregates of nerves are distributed around periradicular veins and are associated with vessels in traumatized and degenerated discs. These vessels show evidence of platelet aggregation and thrombus formation, and the adjacent tissues exhibit features usually associated with ischemia. Nociceptive nerve endings can be stimulated by a variety of chemical mediators, including the kinins, serotonin (5-hydroxytryptamine), prostanoids, lactic acid, and potassium ions. In the context of observations on blood vessels and the distribution of nerve endings, it is interesting to note that kinins are formed during coagulation, serotonin is released from activated aggregated platelets and prostanoids, and lactic acid and potassium ions are released from ischemic cells.

FUTURE STUDIES

The above observations represent only a crude beginning to understanding mechanisms of back pain, but they highlight how techniques might be employed to develop a better understanding of the significance of the tissue changes recorded in mechanical spinal disease. They also raise the possibility of novel methods of addressing the problem of low back pain. If some patients have pain consequent to disturbed vascular physiology, these patients at least might be helped by therapy aimed at normalizing endothelial function and/or intravascular flow. One would also predict that, because the apparent long-term consequences of this seem to be relatively permanent, a realistic strategy to redress the vascular lesion would have to be delivered early in the course of the disease.

REFERENCES

1. Battié, M. C., Bigos, S. J., Fisher, L. D., et al.: A prospective study of the role of cardiovascular risk factors and fitness in industrial back pain complaints. Spine 14:141–147, 1989.

2. Buirski, G., and Silbertstein, M.: The symptomatic lumbar disc in patients with low back pain. Magnetic resonance imaging appearances in both asymptomatic and control population. Spine 18:1808–1811, 1993.
3. Cooper, R. G., Mitchell, W. S., Illingworth, K. J., et al.: The role of epidural fibrosis and defective fibrinolysis in the persistence of postlaminectomy back pain. Spine 16:1044–1048, 1991.
4. Cooper, R. G., Mitchell, M. S., Illingworth, K. J., and Jayson, M. I. V.: Fibrinolytic enhancement by stanozolol fails to improve symptoms and signs in patients with post surgical back pain. Scand. J. Rheumatol. 20:414–418, 1991.
5. Firooznia, H., Kricheff, I. I., Rafii, M., and Golimbu, C.: Lumbar spine after surgery: Examination with contrast-enhanced CT. Neurophysiology 16:221–226, 1963.
6. Frymoyer, J. W., Pope, M. H., Clements, J. H., et al.: Risk factors in low back pain: An epidemiological study. J. Bone Joint Surg. 65A:213–218, 1983.
7. Garfin, S. R., Rydevik, B. L., and Brown, R. A.: Compressive neuropathy of spinal nerve roots. A mechanical or biological problem? Spine 16:162–166, 1991.
8. Goldie, I.: Granulation tissue in the ruptured intervertebral disc. Acta Pathol. Scand. 42:302–304, 1958.
9. Haaland, A. K., Graver, V., Ljunggren, A. E., et al.: Fibrinolytic activity as a predictor of the outcome of prolapsed intervertebral disc surgery with reference to background variables: Results of a prospective cohort study. Spine 17:1022–1027, 1992.
10. Hansen, H.-J.: A pathologic-anatomical study on disc degeneration in dogs. Acta Orthop. Scand. Suppl. 11:1–117, 1952.
11. Hirsch, C.: Studies on the pathology of low back pain. J. Bone Joint Surg. 41B:237–243, 1959.
12. Hoyland, J. A., Freemont, A. J., and Jayson, M. I. V.: Intervertebral foramen venous obstruction. A cause of periradicular fibrosis. Spine 14:558–568, 1989.
13. Hoyland, J. A., and Freemont, A. J.: The incidence and significance of psammoma bodies within nerve roots of lumbar spines. Neuro-Orthopaedics 11:83–89, 1991.
14. Innes, D., and Sevitt, S.: Coagulation and fibrinolysis in injured patients. J. Clin. Pathol. 17:1–13, 1964.
15. Klimiuk, P. S., Pountain, G. D., Keegan, A. L., and Jayson, M. I. V.: Serial measurements of fibrinolytic activity in acute low back pain and sciatica. Spine 12:925–928, 1987.
16. Lawrence, J. S.: "Disc Disorders" in Rheumatism in Populations. Oxford, Heinemann, 1977, pp. 68–97.
17. Lindhal, O., and Rexed, B.: Historical changes in spinal nerve roots of operated cases of sciatica. Acta Orthop. Scand. 20:215–225, 1951.
18. Meade, T. W., Chakrabarti, R., Haines, A. P., et al.: Characteristics affecting fibrinolytic activity and plasma fibrinogen concentrations. Br. Med. J. 1:153–156, 1979.
19. Mitchell, W. S., Illingworth, K. J., Jayson, M. I. V.: Fibrinolytic enhancement therapy in the treatment of severe chronic low back pain. Br. J. Rheumatol. A2:12, 1988.
20. Olmarker, K., Rydevik, B., and Holm, S.: Edema formation in spinal nerve roots induced by experimental, graded compression. An experimental study of pig cauda equina with special reference to differences in effects between rapid and slow onset of compression. Spine 14:569–573, 1989.
21. Olmarker, K., Holm, S., Rosenqvist, A.-L., and Rydevik, B.: Experimental nerve root compression. A model of acute, graded compression of the porcine cauda equina and an analysis of neural and vascular anatomy. Spine 16:61–69, 1991.
22. Pedowitz, R. A., Garfin, S. R., Massie, J. B., et al.: Effects of magnitude and duration of compression on spinal nerve root conduction. Spine 17:194–199, 1992.
23. Pountain, G. D., Keegan, A. L., and Jayson, M. I. V.: Impaired fibrinolytic activity in defined chronic back pain syndromes. Spine 12:83–86, 1987.
24. Rydevik, B. L., Pedowitz, R. A., Hargens, A. R., et al.: Effects of acute, graded compression on spinal nerve root function and structure. An experimental study of pig cauda equina. Spine 16:487–493, 1991.
25. Watanabe, A., and Parke, W. W.: Vascular and neural pathology of lumbosacral spinal stenosis. J. Neurosurg. 64:64–70, 1986.

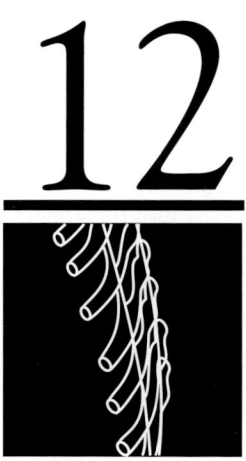

12

Fractures of the Lumbar Spine: Evaluation, Classification, and Treatment

STEVEN R. GARFIN
STANLEY GERTZBEIN
FRANK EISMONT

The goals in the treatment of patients with lumbar spinal injuries include preserving life and neurologic function, obtaining a healed and stable spine, and maintaining or restoring alignment. This includes minimizing the extent of fusion of spinal motion segments and preventing the development of late deformity and pain. These objectives are best accomplished when the treating physician understands the structural anatomy of the spinal column and the biomechanics involved in the injury (mechanism of injury), as well as the appropriate concepts of spinal stability and instability. The options for treating spinal column injuries have increased along with better understanding of the anatomy, physiology, and biomechanics of the spinal column and the introduction of instrumentation devices.

This chapter reviews the anatomy and biomechanics of the lumbar spine as related to spinal column injuries, the concepts of spinal instability, and the mechanisms of injury. Additionally, a discussion of classification schemes for lumbar injuries is included, as well as discussions on the clinical evaluation of patients with these injuries, the appropriate choice of diagnostic modalities, and the utility of various imaging studies.

RELEVANT ANATOMY AND BIOMECHANICS

The five lumbar vertebrae increase in size and strength progressively from L1 to L5. This increased strength is directly related to size rather than mineral content.[76] The vertebrae, as well as the discs, are somewhat larger anteriorly than posteriorly. This contributes to lumbar lordosis. The maintenance of lordosis is rather dependent on the bone's withstanding compression forces. The average lordosis in the lumbosacral spine is 50 degrees, with a range from 32 degrees to 84 degrees. In a study by Stagnara and associates,[74a] 92% of patients had a lordosis ranging from 42 to 74 degrees.

Flexion-extension motion measures 15 degrees across each lumbar motion segment, with a range from 12 to 20 degrees. Lateral bending is only 6 degrees at each level in the lumbar spine. Because of the sagittal alignment of the facets in the lumbar spine, axial rotation is markedly restricted (2 degrees of rotation at each level).[78, 79]

The center of gravity in the normal lordotic lumbar spine is located relatively posteriorly. The posterior elements provide approximately 30% of the weight-bearing support of the lumbar spine. This is in contradistinction to the case in the thoracic spine and the thoracolumbar junction, where the compressive forces are directed more anteriorly.[78, 79]

Similarly to the vertebral bodies, the pedicles increase in size as they progress caudally from the first lumbar to the fifth lumbar vertebra. Zindrick[84] and associates reported on pedicle isthmus widths and pedicle angles in the sagittal and transverse planes. At L1, the pedicle angle inclines medially (from posterior to anterior) approximately 11 degrees, increasing to approximately 30 degrees of medial inclination at L5. Over the same levels, the mean transverse width increases from approximately 7 mm to 17 mm.

The predominant neural element of the lumbar spine, usually below the L1–L2 disc space, is the cauda equina, which is composed of spinal nerve roots as opposed to the actual spinal cord. The conus medullaris usually begins at T11 and in the majority of persons ends at approximately the L1–L2 disc space. There is extensive collateral circulation from peripheral to proximal central along the nerve roots and from proximal to distal along the spinal cord. Because of this, the lumbar region is relatively protected from significant, catastrophic, irreversible, neurologic injuries. Trauma in this area occurs in a highly vascular area comprising primarily spinal nerve roots rather than the more unforgiving spinal cord, which is located more proximally and has segments with less vascularity.

Most lumbar spinal fractures fail in axial loading and/or axial flexion, rather than in rotation. The intervertebral discs transfer compressive loads from one vertebra to another through the nucleus pulposus and annulus fibrosus.[78] Increasing axial load may cause the nucleus pulposus to rupture through the endplates into the adjacent vertebra, resulting in a typical burst fracture.[10] Fredrickson and colleagues,[32] in experimental studies, showed a site of weakness in the vertebral bodies at the location where a leash of blood vessels enters through the posterior cortex. This usually occurs at the junction of the upper and middle third of a vertebra. Appropriate force transmitted across this stress riser leads to fragmentation of bone, often penetrating posteriorly into the spinal canal from this junctional position[32] (Fig. 1).

A number of investigators have shown that the ability of a vertebra to resist loads decreases with age.[7] This is related to alterations in mineral content and bone quality.[76] Cancellous bone transmits 55% of the axial load in persons younger than 40 years of age, but only 35% in persons older than 40 years.[71]

Vertebrae fail under compressive loading in three different modes.[51] In the first, there is a decrease in strength in the load deformation curve after loading to failure, which explains the progressive collapse observed when some lumbar fractures are axially loaded. In the second mode, vertebral strength is constant after failure, leading to the stability noted in the majority of compression fractures without significant cortical comminution. In the third mode, the vertebral strength actually increases with compression. This is most often seen in women younger than 40 years and is likely related to the concurrence of bone impaction and unyielding fluid compression (blood).

The integrity and stability of the spinal column are also related to the anterior longitudinal[4] and posterior longitudinal ligaments,[6] in addition to the bones and discs. These structures are uniaxial and resist tensile forces. The site of failure of these ligaments depends on the rate of loading, with

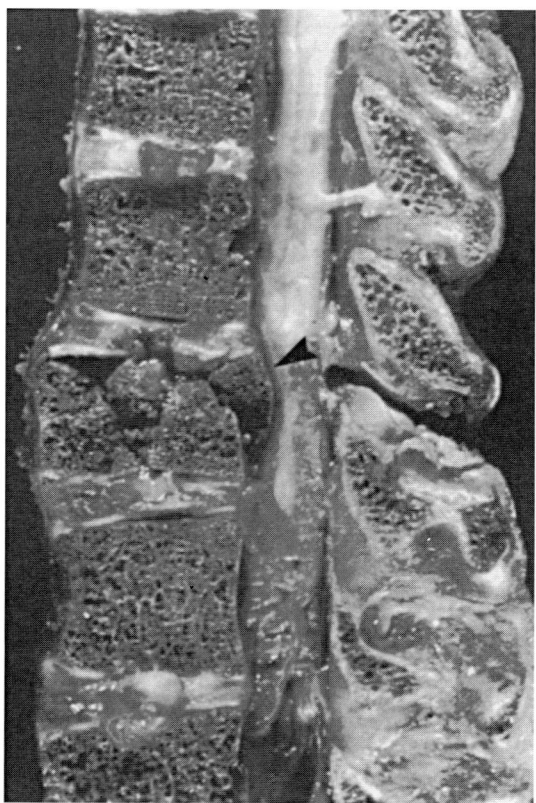

Figure 1. Cadaver specimen demonstrates a burst fracture with a fragment of bone penetrating the spinal canal at the junction of the upper and middle thirds of the posterior cortex *(arrow)*, a point of entry of a leash of blood vessels that acts as a stress riser. (Courtesy of Dr. B. Frederickson.)

bone failing at slow rates of loading and ligaments failing at rapid rates.[65]

SPINAL INSTABILITY

The concept of instability of the spinal column has been developed during the past 4 or 5 decades by a number of investigators. In 1949, Nicoll[63] suggested that the integrity of the interspinous ligaments was the major factor in maintaining stability. Later, Holdsworth[43] described instability as occurring when the entire posterior ligamentous complex was disrupted, along with the anterior portion of the spinal column. Bedbrook[4, 5] disagreed with this concept and pointed out that disruption of the posterior ligamentous complex was frequently carried out surgically (e.g., during laminectomies) without resulting in instability. He believed that the integrity of the disc and the integrity of the anterior longitudinal ligament were more important factors in maintaining stability than were the posterior ligamentous restraints.

The work of Holdsworth[43] was useful in providing an early understanding of the mechanisms of injury, but it did not recognize the significant instability associated with flexion-distraction injuries or burst fractures. Computed tomography (CT) has helped demonstrate that many spinal fractures are more extensive than formerly realized.[3] As radiographic studies improved, follow-up lengthened, and anatomy was better understood, more sophisticated concepts of spinal instability were developed. The two apparently disparate concepts of posterior (Bedbrook) and anterior (Holdsworth, Nicoll) restraint, or support, structures gradually merged into a two-column concept of spinal stability.

Whitesides and colleagues[47, 81] described the importance of the anterior weight-bearing column of vertebral bodies and discs, along with the substantial structural support supplied by the posterior column of neural arches and ligaments in resisting extension and supplying a tensile force to counteract flexion movements. These researchers believed that destruction of either of these columns (anterior or posterior) was enough to produce instability—late if not early. They employed this two-column model to describe and explain the often late-developing chronic instabilities and progressive kyphotic deformities seen after spinal injuries. However, the two-column model was unable to fully explain all instances of acute instability.

In 1983, Denis[20] further advanced the understanding of spinal stability by conceptualizing three columns of the spine in the support mechanism. The anterior column is the anterior two thirds of the vertebral body, the disc, and the anterior longitudinal ligament. The posterior column is composed of the spinous processes and associated ligaments, the facet joints, the lamina, and the pedicles. The middle column is the pericanal structures (i.e., the posterior portion of the vertebral bodies and disc, the posterior longitudinal ligament, the base of pedicles, and the transverse process [Fig. 2]). Unfortunately, in the original description, the neural

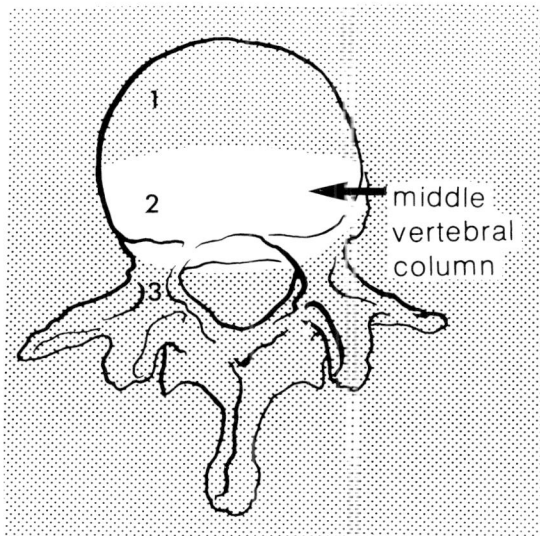

Figure 2. Axial cut of a typical lumbar vertebra demonstrates the anterior (1), middle (2), and posterior (3) columns. (Modified from Gertzbein, S. D., and Court-Brown, C. M.: Lumbar spinal fracture. In Floman, Y. (ed.): Disorders of the Lumbar Spine. Rockville, MD, Aspen, 1990, pp. 615–662.)

elements (i.e., spinal cord, conus medullaris, cauda equina, and spinal nerve roots) were not mentioned in the middle column, which was a significant omission. Denis classified spinal fractures according to the mechanism of the injury and the resulting fracture pattern. The three-column concept was a major advance, particularly because it included burst fractures. It categorized injuries related to the bone and ligamentous structures. However, as mentioned, it failed to emphasize the importance and significance of neurologic involvement.

The three-column concept helps to explain collapse as well as malalignment. Instability is present when two or three columns are disrupted. Therefore, in this configuration, when trauma to the posterior interspinous ligaments (posterior column) and posterior annulus fibrosus (middle column) occurs, instability in flexion results. Complete destruction of only the posterior ligamentous complex is not sufficient to create instability.[4, 66, 69] In the two-column concept, this is more difficult to explain and visualize.

Using the three-column categorization, Denis described fracture types that occur in four major spinal injuries and four minor injury patterns. None of the latter is unstable (Table 1).

MECHANISMS OF INJURY AND CONVENTIONAL CLASSIFICATION

The spine may fail in the following directions and modes: flexion-extension, rotation, side bending, anteroposterior (AP) or lateral shear, compression, distraction, or a combination of these. Well-recognized patterns of injury usually result. The forces and vectors applied to the spine have been related to the fracture patterns by Denis[20] (Table 1). This classification is the most practical and best accepted at this time, although a number of other classifications have been proposed.[28, 54, 56] For completeness, the conventional classification is discussed, followed by a consideration of a newer, more mechanistically derived treatment-oriented system.

Table 1
■

Modes of Failure of the Three Columns for the Four Major Spinal Injuries

Type	Column		
	Anterior	*Middle*	*Posterior*
Compression	Compression	None	None or distraction (severe)
Burst	Compression	Compression	None or splaying of pedicles
Flexion-distraction	None or distraction	Distraction	Distraction
Fracture-dislocation	Compression	Distraction	Distraction
	Rotation	Rotation	Rotation
	Shear	Shear	Shear

From Denis, F., Armstrong, E. W., Searls, K., et al: Acute thoracolumbar burst fractures in the absence of neurological deficit: A comparison between operative and non-operative treatment. Clin. Orthop. 189:142–149, 1984.

Compression Fractures

Compression fractures occur with eccentric axial loading. This load may be applied anterior to or lateral to the axis of rotation (Fig. 3), resulting in the common anterior wedge fracture (Fig. 3A,B) or a less common lateral compression fracture[20] (Fig. 3C).

On lateral radiographs, anterior compression fractures are characterized by a loss of height in the anterior column. There is usually no damage to the middle or posterior columns, although in younger patients who have had violent injuries, the posterior elements may be disrupted (Fig. 4).

Anterior compression fractures have four subtypes. In type A fractures both end plates are damaged; in the more common type B fracture, the superior end plate is fractured; the inferior end plate alone is fractured in

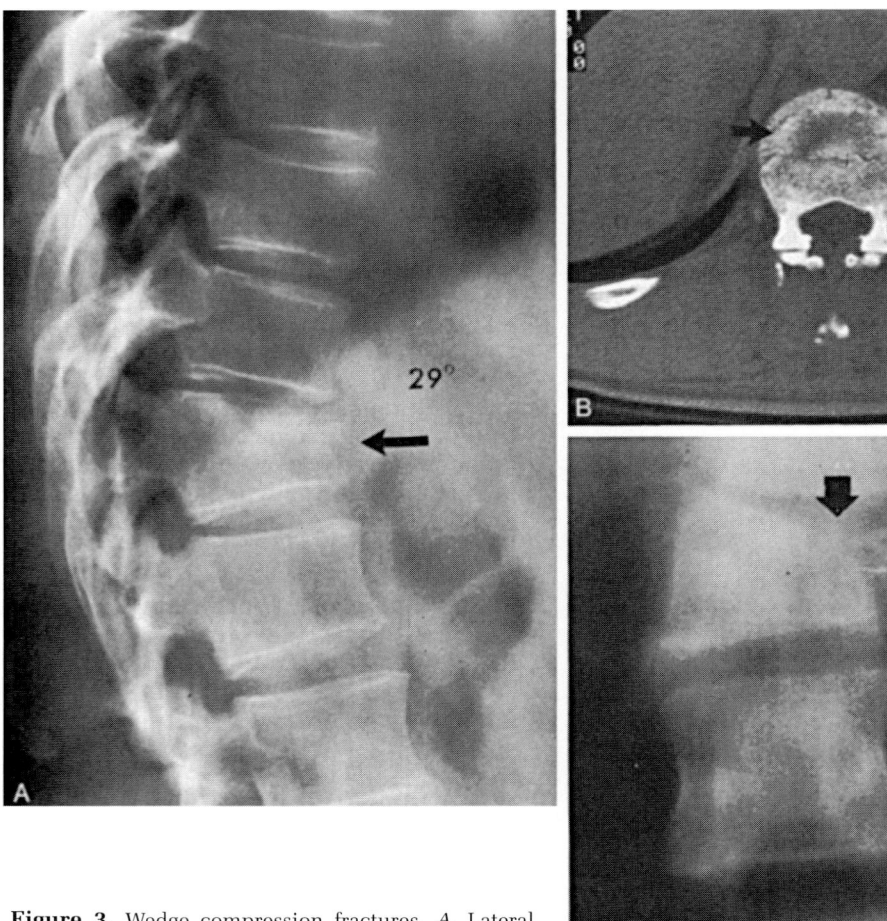

Figure 3. Wedge compression fractures. *A*, Lateral radiograph demonstrates anterior compression of the vertebral body *(arrow)* with posterior elements intact. *B*, CT scan shows the same patient with compression of the anterior column alone *(arrow)*. *C*, AP tomogram of the first lumbar vertebra in another patient demonstrates lateral wedge compression of 15 degrees *(arrow)*. (*A–C*, Modified from Gertzbein, S. D., and Court-Brown, C. M.: Lumbar spinal fracture. *In* Floman, Y. (ed.): Disorders of the Lumbar Spine. Rockville, MD, Aspen, 1990, pp. 615–662.)

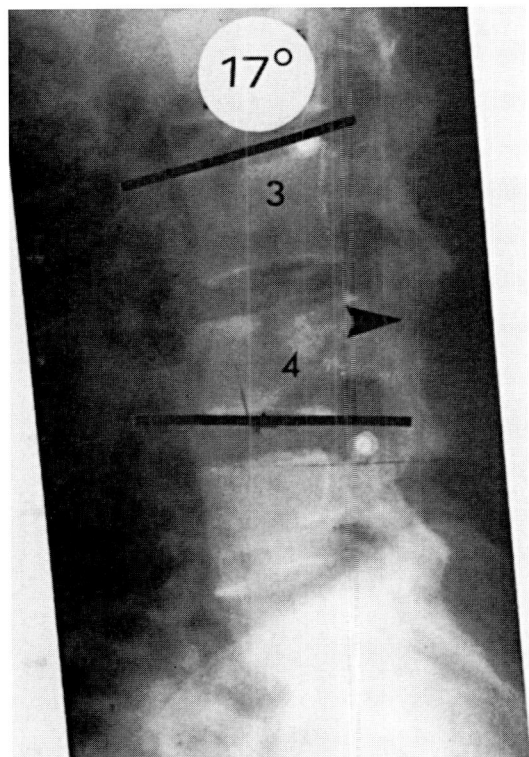

Figure 4. Anterior wedge compression fracture with widened spinous processes. Lateral radiograph shows anterior wedging of the body and widening of the interspinous space *(arrow)*. (Modified from Gertzbein, S. D., and Court-Brown, C. M.: Lumbar spinal fracture. *In* Floman, Y. (ed.): Disorders of the Lumbar Spine. Rockville, MD, Aspen, 1990, pp. 615–662.)

type C fractures; and in type D fractures, the end plates are intact, but the anterior vertebral cortex is compressed.

Burst Fractures

Burst fractures are caused by axial loading (Fig. 5). The end plates are damaged first, commonly during falls or traffic collisions, although other mechanisms such as rapid ejection from an aircraft, also result in this type of fracture.[78] The three types of end-plate fracture are (1) those involving the central portion of the end plate, (2) those occurring at the periphery of the end plate, and (3) those producing transverse cracks across the end plate.

The load-bearing capacity of a lumbar vertebra varies with changes in a number of factors, such as the magnitude of the applied axial load, the time over which the load is applied, the spatial orientation of the vertebral column, and the age of the bone.[7] Axially loaded vertebrae, in individuals older than 60 years of age, fail at approximately 4200 N, whereas in patients younger than 40 years, the average load to failure is 7600 N.[67] Increased loading causes propagation of a fracture in the end plate in different directions. This is followed by displacement of the disc into the vertebral body, at which stage the simple end-plate disruption changes to a burst fracture with loss of integrity of the vertebral body.

The importance of end-plate fractures is twofold. First, they are frequently missed and may be the source of back pain after trauma. Tomography or CT scanning may be required to facilitate the diagnosis. Second, they are the initial stage of both compression and burst fractures.

Willen and colleagues,[82] in a laboratory investigation of the cause of burst fractures, showed that they occur with an average load of 8000 N (range of 6000 to 10,000 N).[82] Comminution of the body with severe encroachment of the spinal canal occurs with an axial load of about 11,000 N. These workers distinguished between burst injuries with and without posterior element injury. The latter were referred to as burst fractures and the former as crush injuries. This definition is somewhat arbitrary, but it draws attention to the role of the facet joints in absorbing axial load. Damage to the facets depends to some extent on the spatial position of the spine during impact; 33% of the total load bearing of the spine is absorbed through the facet joints during full extension.[78] In addition, recognizing that the posterior elements can be damaged in burst fractures is important in determining the degree of instability. It is not uncommon for CT scans to show posterior element fractures, when plain radiographs do not indicate their presence (Fig. 5).

Relating these injuries to the three-column concept, Denis[20] stated (by definition) that in burst fractures, failure occurs through at least the anterior and middle columns. Failure of the middle column is demonstrated on a lateral radiograph by a fracture of the posterior wall of the vertebra, usually at the junction of the upper and middle thirds, a loss of posterior height, and retropulsion of a bony fragment into the spinal canal (Fig. 5).

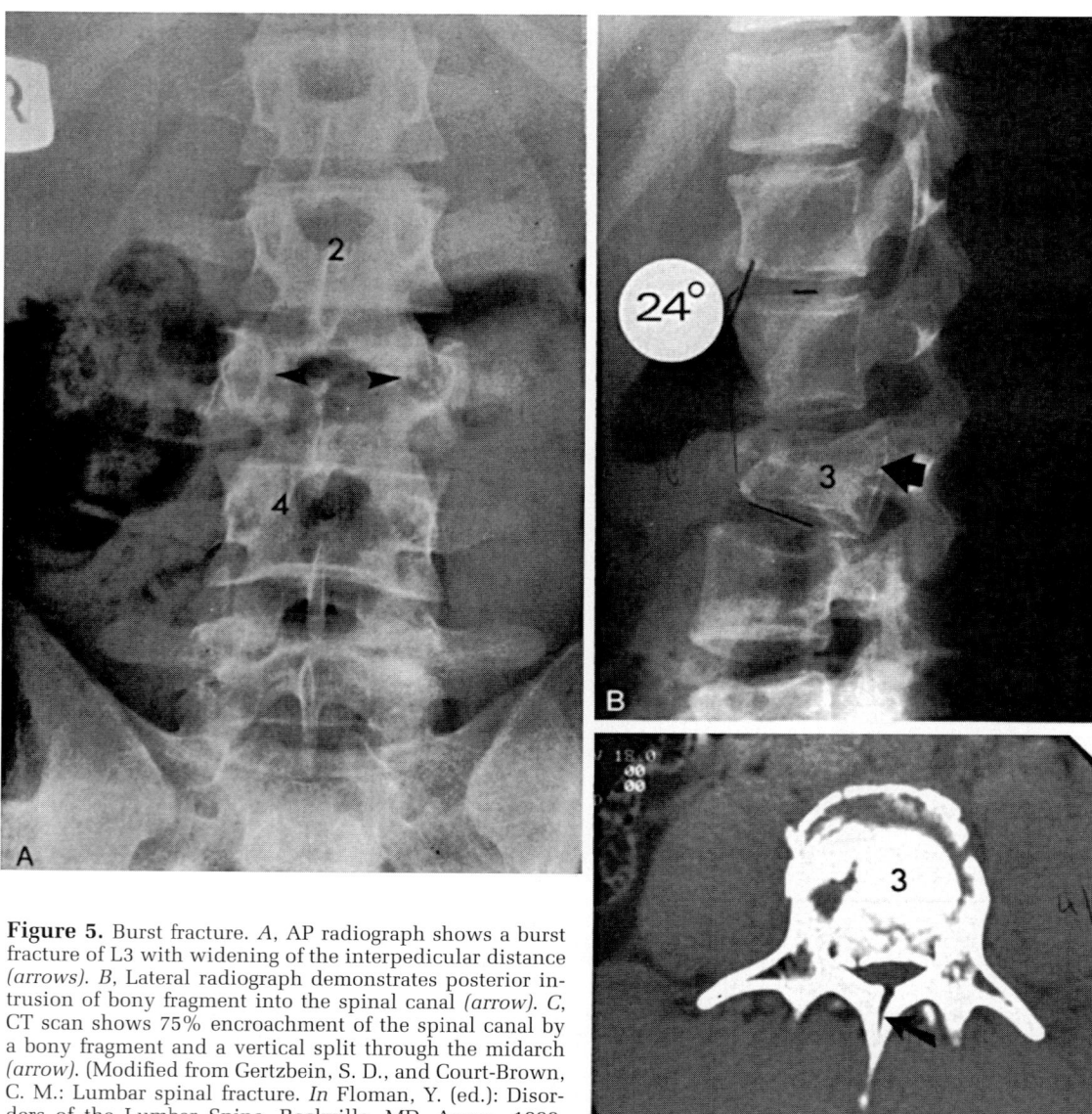

Figure 5. Burst fracture. *A*, AP radiograph shows a burst fracture of L3 with widening of the interpedicular distance *(arrows)*. *B*, Lateral radiograph demonstrates posterior intrusion of bony fragment into the spinal canal *(arrow)*. *C*, CT scan shows 75% encroachment of the spinal canal by a bony fragment and a vertical split through the midarch *(arrow)*. (Modified from Gertzbein, S. D., and Court-Brown, C. M.: Lumbar spinal fracture. *In* Floman, Y. (ed.): Disorders of the Lumbar Spine. Rockville, MD, Aspen, 1990, pp. 615–662.)

An AP radiograph usually, but not always, reveals an increase in the interpedicle distance. A CT scan confirms the diagnosis and also contributes additional information that may be lacking in conventional radiography and tomography. A CT scan highlights the extent of spinal canal intrusion and also demonstrates damage to the middle column, which may not have been severe enough to cause splaying of the pedicles (Fig. 5). Posterior column fractures may also be observed. The authors have noted a sagittal fracture of the lamina often to be a consistent injury. It resembles a broken wishbone[2, 12] (Fig. 5).

Flexion-Distraction Injuries

A flexion-distraction injury was first reported in 1948 by Chance.[14] He described a lesion entering the upper half of the spinous process, passing anteriorly through the pedicles, and emerging on the superior aspect of the vertebral body just anterior to the spinal canal. Smith and Kaufer[74] suggested that the fracture was caused by flexion around a fulcrum anterior to the anterior longitudinal ligament. The fulcrum is frequently an automobile seat belt forced against the abdominal wall, just anterior to the spinal column. The classification of Denis[20] includes four flexion-distraction types. Type A, type C, and type D are variations of the Chance fracture, and type B is essentially a dislocation through the ligamentous and soft tissue components of the motion segments.

Court-Brown and Gertzbein[16] subdivided flexion-distraction injuries into three categories related to the posterior element fracture, the anterior column fracture, and the state of the vertebral body (Fig. 6). They observed that the fracture could enter the posterior elements of the spine in three ways, in a fashion similar to that described by Gumley and colleagues.[40] Most commonly, the fracture is found to enter above the spinous process, although it may enter through the spinous process. A third type extends asymmetrically across the posterior elements, which is indicative of a rotational component.

The position of the disruption through the anterior column also varies. Three configurations are possible. First, the injury may pass through the disc space (type A) (Fig. 7). Second, the fracture may be similar to the one described by Howland and coworkers,[44] exiting at the anterior vertebral cortex (type B) (Figs. 7 and 8). Third, the fracture may be similar to that described by Chance, exiting through the superior end plate (type C1) or the inferior end plate (type C2)[14] (see Figs. 6 and 7).

It was shown in this[16] and other studies that flexion-distraction injuries may occur with a wedge compression fracture or a burst injury.[42] The explanation of the anterior body compression lies in the fact that most Chance fractures occur in high-speed motor vehicle collisions, in which victims are wearing seat belts. Begeman and coworkers,[6] in studying spinal loading that results

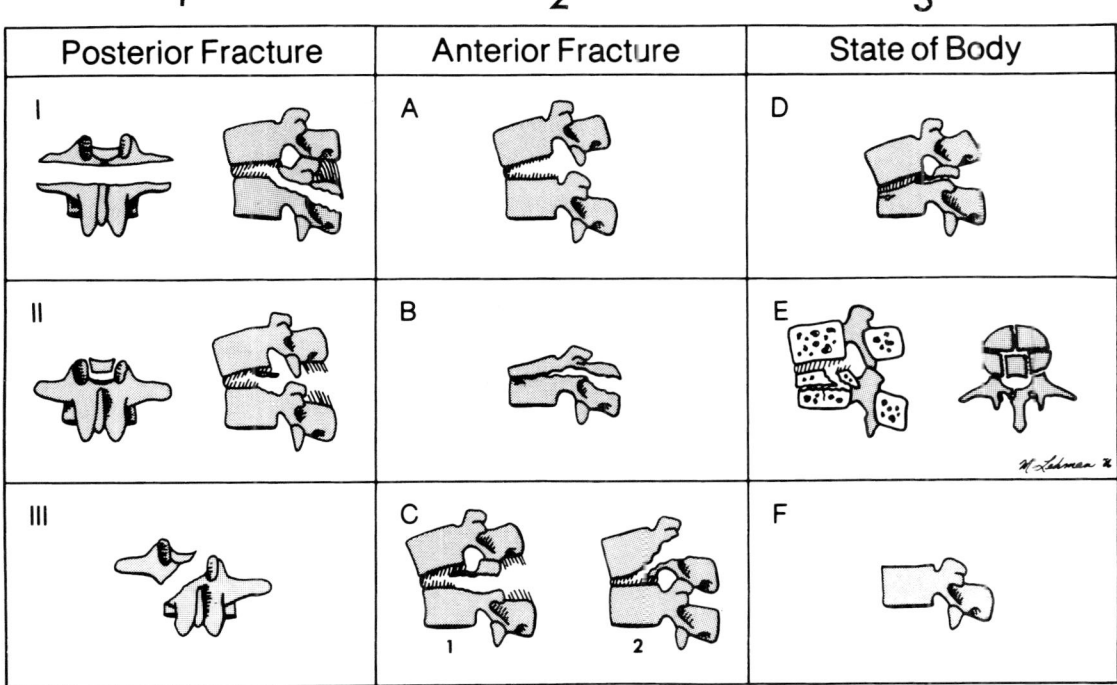

Figure 6. Diagrammatic schema of classification of flexion-distraction injuries represents the posterior (1) and anterior (2) components as well as the state of the vertebral body (3). (Modified from Gertzbein, S. D., and Court-Brown, C. M.: Lumbar spinal fracture. In Floman, Y. (ed.): Disorders of the Lumbar Spine. Rockville, MD, Aspen, 1990, pp. 615–662.)

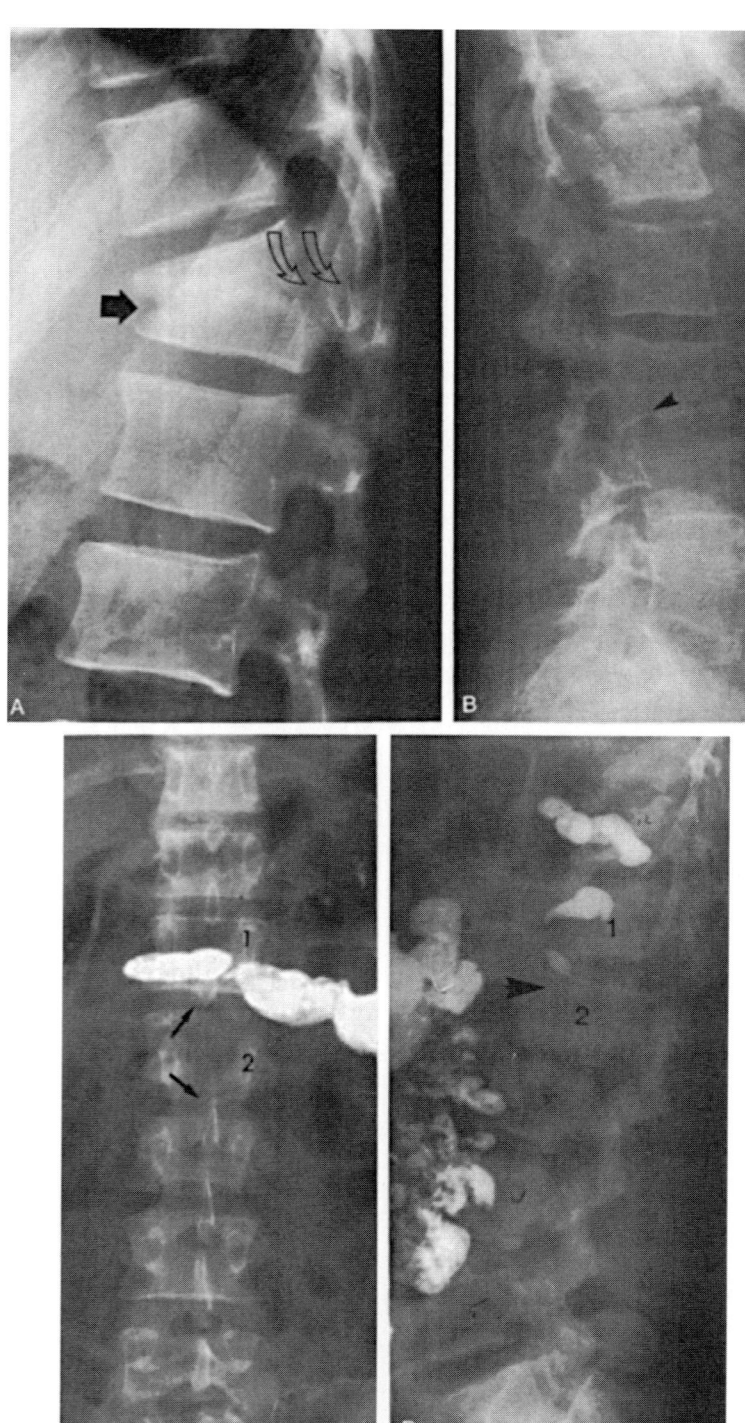

Figure 7. Flexion-distraction injuries. *A*, This injury extends through the posterior arch *(open arrows)* and through the vertebral body to the anterior cortex *(arrow)* and is classified as a type IB injury. *B*, A second example is this flexion-distraction type of injury, which passes between the spinous processes and extends from the midportion of the posterior cortex of the body, inferiorly to the disc space and anteriorly through the disc *(arrowhead)*. *C, D,* A third variant demonstrates a widening of the interspinous spaces *(arrows),* on the AP radiograph between L1 and L2, with a wedge compression component noted on the lateral radiograph *(arrowhead).* (Modified from Gertzbein, S. D., and Court-Brown, C. M.: Lumbar spinal fracture. *In* Floman, Y. (ed.): Disorders of the Lumbar Spine. Rockville, MD, Aspen, 1990, pp. 615–662.)

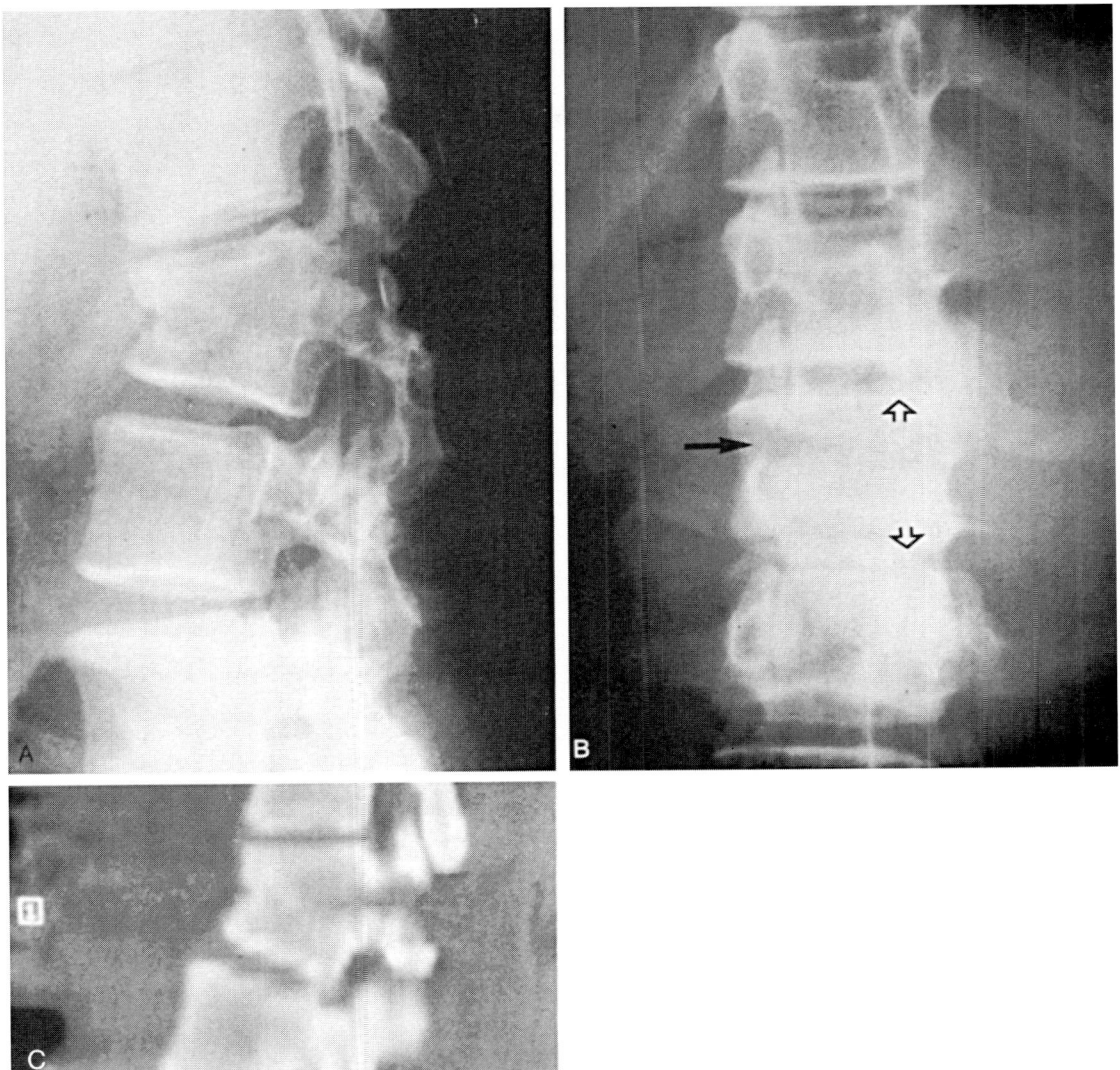

Figure 8. This patient sustained a seat belt flexion-distraction type of injury involving the second lumbar vertebra. She remained neurologically normal. *A*, Lateral roentgenogram shows the anterior compression of the L1 vertebral body and the distraction of the posterior vertebral body and spreading of the posterior elements. *B*, The AP roentgenogram shows a fracture of the pedicle of L2 *(filled arrow)* and spreading of the spinous processes *(open arrows)*. *C*, CT scan in the transverse plane reveals the fracture of the posterior elements. The sagittal reconstruction reveals the anterior vertebral body compression as well as the distraction of the posterior vertebral body and the split in the pedicle. The neural elements are poorly visualized on CT scans unless intrathecal contrast medium has been introduced.

Illustration continued on following page

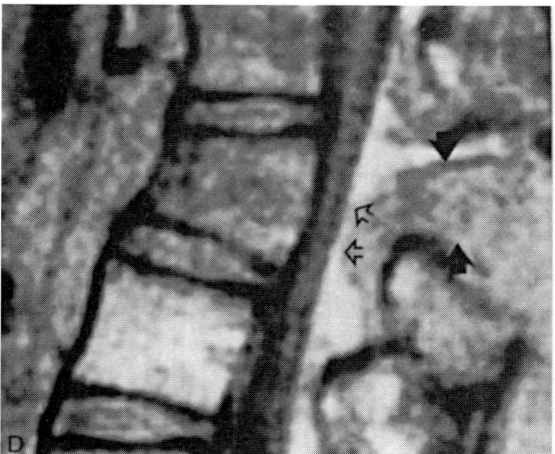 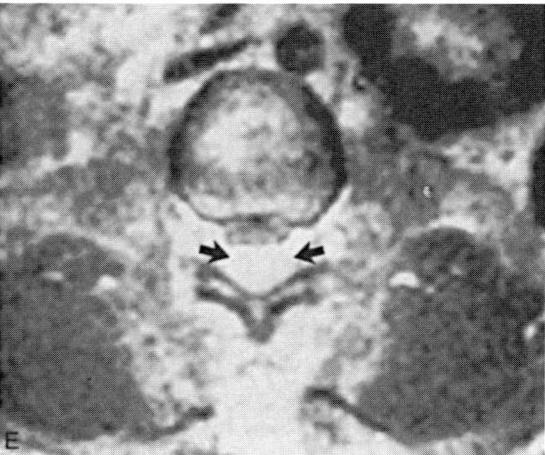

Figure 8. *Continued D,* A midsagittal MRI scan shows the bony pathologic condition poorly. The soft tissue visualization, however, is much better, and a hematoma extending from the posterior paraspinal region into the spinal canal *(filled arrows)* can be seen with the compression of the thecal sac *(open arrows). E,* The transverse MRI scan again clearly shows the neural compression secondary to hematoma extending to the spinal canal. (Hematoma is marked by arrows.)

from deceleration injuries, clearly showed that considerable axial loading of the spine occurs early during deceleration. The magnitude of the axial load depends on the g forces encountered during deceleration. In addition, an increase in the axial load occurs late in the deceleration phase as a result of the body's being lifted off the seat and then returning to the sitting position. This accounts for the vertebral body fracture. Distraction then occurs across the anteriorly located fulcrum (seat belt) with posterior and middle column failure.

In these injury patterns, AP radiographs show a gap between the posterior elements of the adjacent vertebrae that is caused by the distraction component of the fracture (see Figs. 6 and 7). There may be an associated anterior compression or burst fracture (see Figs. 6 and 7). CT scanning (with reconstruction) is often helpful in completely visualizing the injury pattern, particularly if an associated burst fracture is suspected.

Extension Fractures

Extension injuries are rare in the lumbar spine. They may occur with violent extension forces that cause tension loading anteriorly (Fig. 9). The injury pattern includes fractures of the posterior elements, retrolisthesis of the cephalad vertebra over the caudal one, and anterior lip (avulsion) fractures through a vertebral body.

Fracture-Dislocation Injuries

Fracture-dislocation of the lumbar spine occurs when there is failure of all three columns of the spine under compression, tension, rotation, shear, or a combination of these forces. It may be panligamentous, all bone, or a combination of hard and soft tissues. The essential feature of this injury is that the magnitude of the applied loads is sufficient to significantly, and possibly completely, disrupt the intrinsically stable anatomy. Disruption of the facet joints leads to subluxation or dislocation. Occasionally, a fracture-dislocation may spontaneously reduce, and the true nature of the lesion may be missed on conventional radiographs. CT scans often show the extent of bony injury. Fracture-dislocation injuries can be divided into three types on the basis of the direction of the loads applied.[20]

Flexion-Rotation Injuries

Flexion-rotation injury occurs when the posterior and middle columns fail under tension and rotation and the anterior column fails under compression and rotation. This leads to anterior wedging of the verte-

combination of flexion and distraction.[16] Failure occurs through the ligaments and/or bone in the posterior and middle columns and through the disc and/or bone in the anterior column. The anterior longitudinal ligament is stripped from the vertebra below (Fig 13).

Posterior Arch Fractures

Fractures of the posterior vertebral column are stable. They are commonly seen as fractures of the articular processes, the transverse processes, the spinous process, or the pars interarticularis (Fig. 14). Two mechanisms of injury are likely: flexion and axial rotation or extension. Sometimes, these injuries are difficult to identify on

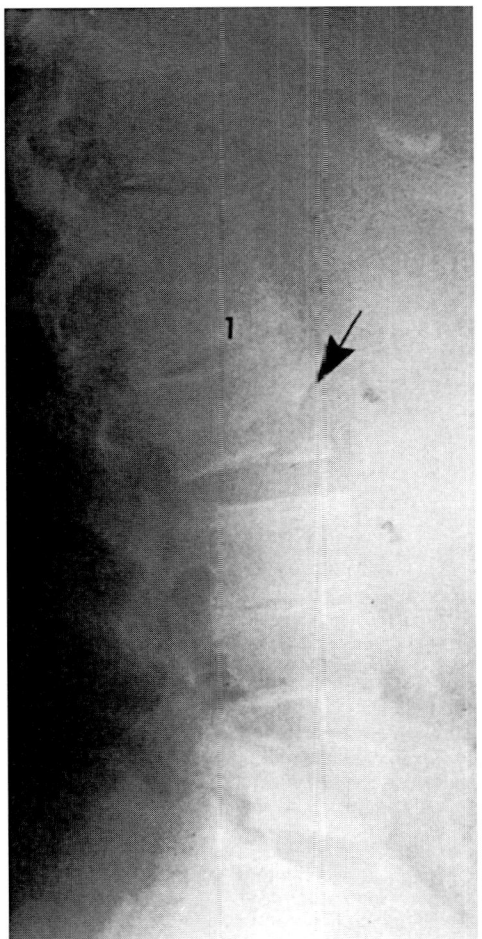

Figure 9. Extension fracture: This patient, with an old wedge compression fracture of L1, had an extension injury with a teardrop fracture noted at the anteroinferior corner *(arrow).*

bral body and stripping of the anterior longitudinal ligament from the vertebra below (Fig. 10).

Shear Injuries

All three columns are disrupted by shear injury, including the anterior longitudinal ligament. The shear force is usually applied in the lateral direction (Fig. 11), but may be applied in the AP direction (Fig. 12).[22]

Flexion-Distraction Burst Injuries

A flexion-distraction burst injury is a variant of the seat-belt injury produced by a

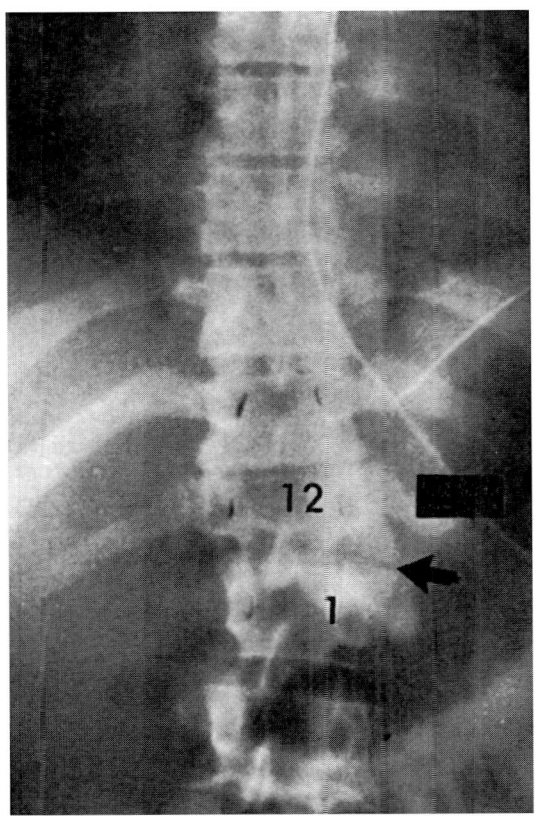

Figure 10. Fracture-dislocation of T12–L1 with significant lateral translation *(arrow)* as a result of rotational forces. (Modified from Gertzbein, S. D., and Court-Brown, C. M.: Lumbar spinal fracture. *In* Floman, Y. (ed.): Disorders of the Lumbar Spine. Rockville, MD, Aspen, 1990, pp. 615–662.)

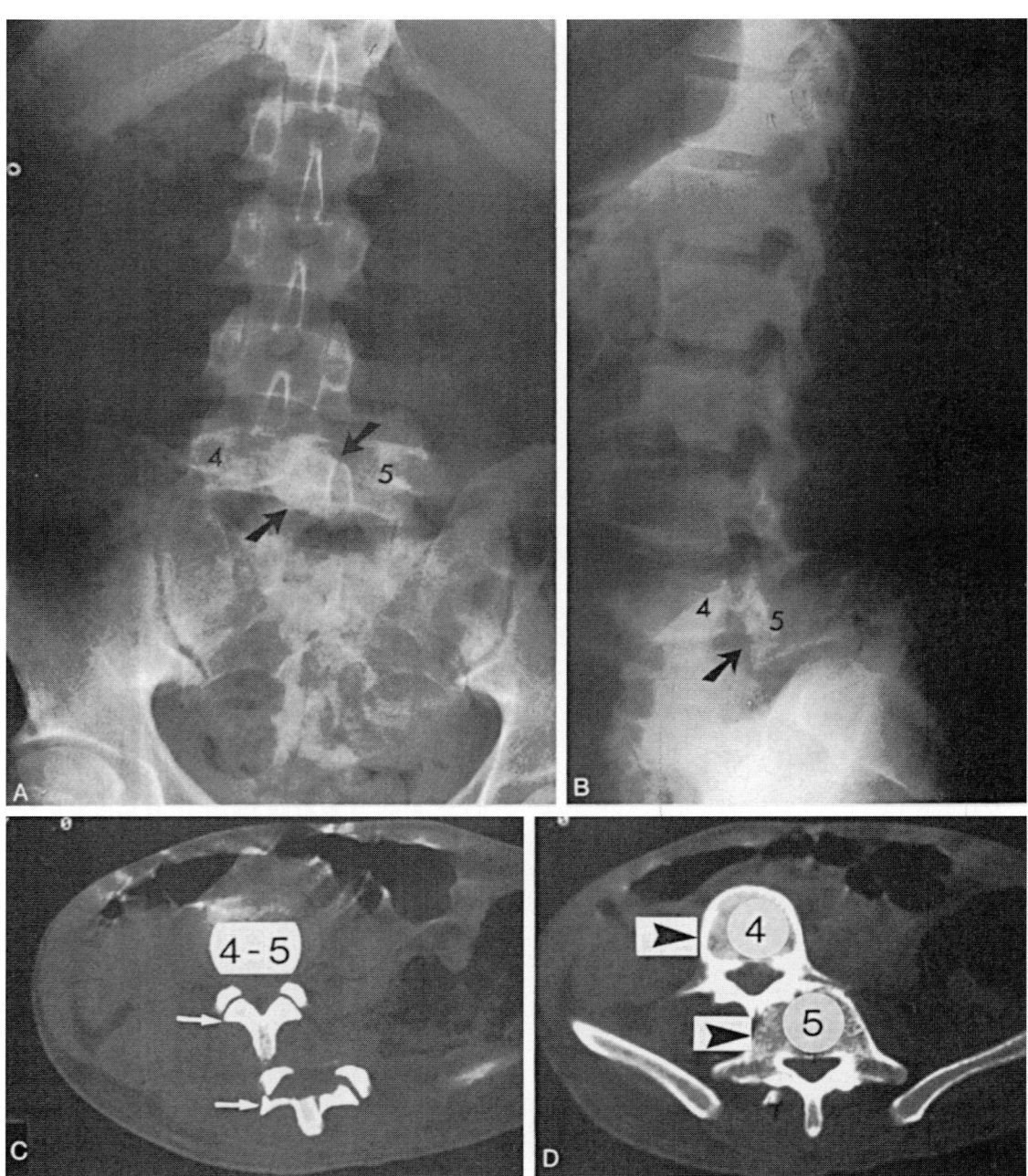

Figure 11. Shear injury. *A, B*, AP and lateral radiographs demonstrate displacement of the vertebral column to the right and anteriorly *(arrows)*. *C, D*, CT scans of the posterior elements *(white arrows)* and vertebral bodies *(arrowheads)*, respectively, seen in the same axial cuts. (Modified from Gertzbein, S. D., and Court-Brown, C. M.: Lumbar spinal fracture. *In* Floman, Y. (ed.): Disorders of the Lumbar Spine. Rockville, MD, Aspen, 1990, pp. 615–662.)

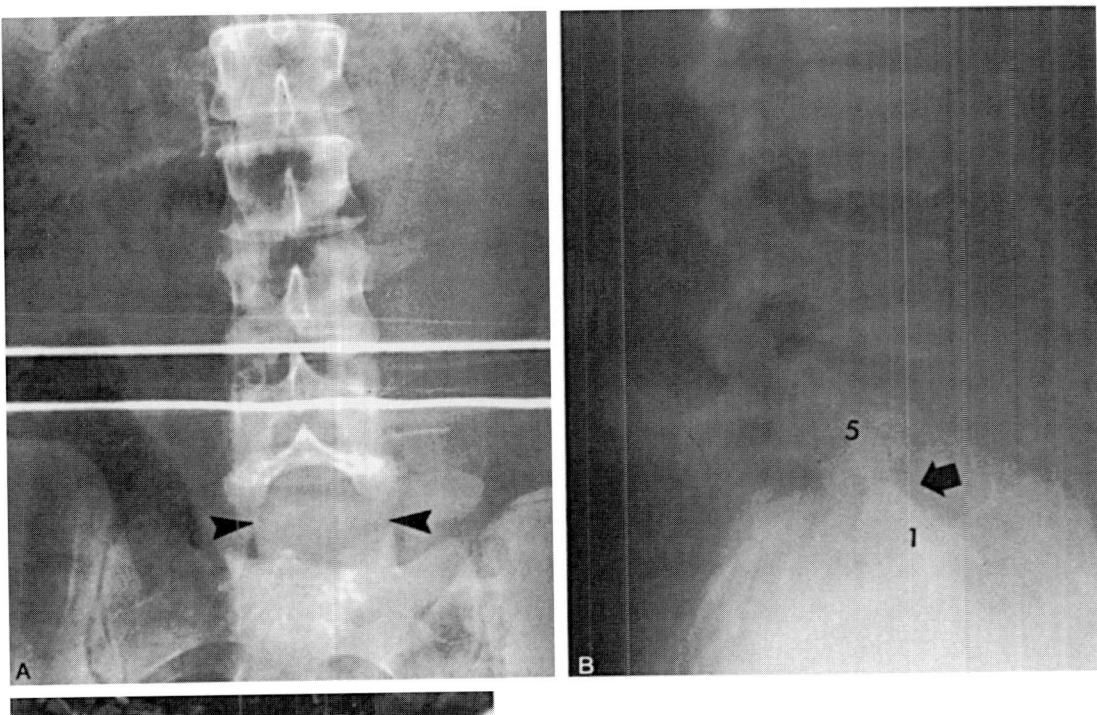
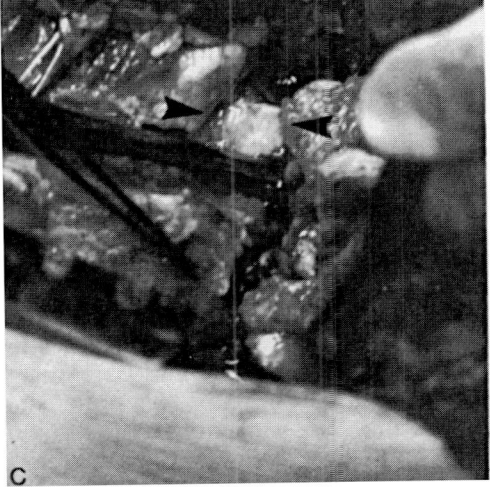

Figure 12. Posterior shear injury. *A, B,* AP and lateral radiographs of the lumbosacral junction show marked displacement of the L5 vertebra posteriorly on the sacrum and widening of the L5–S1 interspinous distance *(arrow)*. *C,* Severe posterior shear forces have disrupted the soft tissues as seen intraoperatively by a gap between L5 and S1 facets *(arrowheads)*.

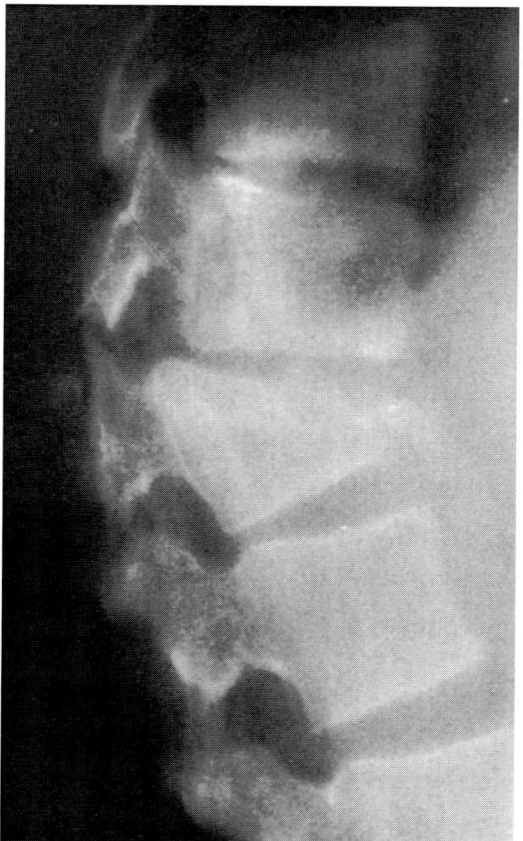

Figure 13. Flexion-distraction burst injury. This lateral tomogram demonstrates the combination of flexion-distraction and burst injury, representing a complex combination of forces.

COMPREHENSIVE CLASSIFICATION

The descriptions above are presented as one example of a commonly used mode of describing injury patterns. They are useful in planning treatment approaches, particularly surgery. However, not all observed injuries easily fall into the major or minor categories described by Denis.[20]

The extent of spinal instability occurs across a spectrum that increases with increasing involvement of each of the columns. Thus, a one-column injury is more stable than a two-column injury, and a three-column injury is the most unstable. The im-

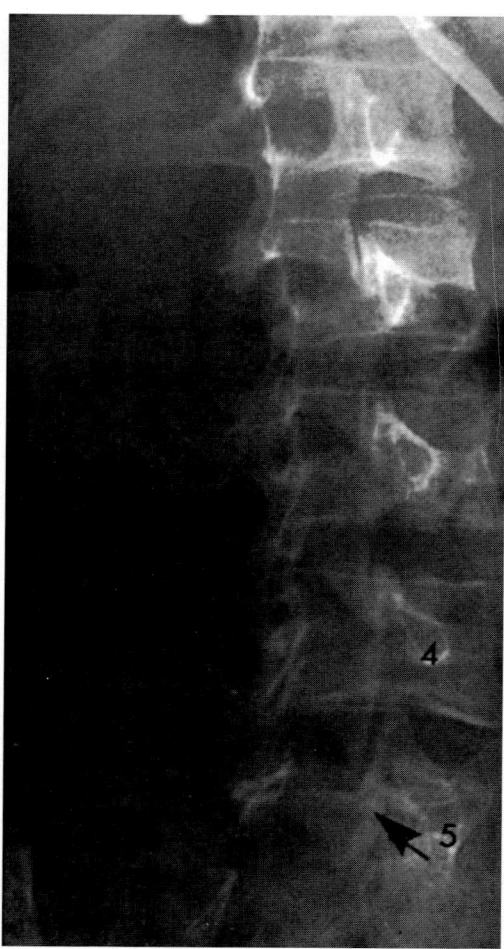

Figure 14. Posterior arch injuries. Fracture of the pars interarticularis *(arrow)* has resulted from hyperextension forces. (Modified from Gertzbein, S. D., and Court-Brown, C. M.: Lumbar spinal fracture. *In* Floman, Y. (ed.): Disorders of the Lumbar Spine. Rockville, MD, Aspen, 1990, pp. 615–662.)

plain radiographs, and CT scanning may be required for an accurate diagnosis.

Transverse process fractures often result from direct, blunt trauma to the spine or avulsion of the tip secondary to violent contraction of the attached (psoas) muscle. Fractures of the L5 transverse process may be associated with severe pelvic and sacral fractures and may provide a clue to the instability of the pelvis.[75] They may also be the direct result of violent lateral flexion. Transverse process fractures of the upper lumbar vertebrae may be associated with a large intramuscular hematoma, causing neurapraxia of the femoral nerve as the roots pass through the psoas muscle.[36]

Posterior element fractures commonly occur in association with more major spinal fractures; an associated occurrence rate as high as 39% has been noted with Chance fractures.[16]

plications relate to early as well as to late consequences. That is, in the early stages of instability, there is a risk of damage to the neural elements, whereas late instability leads to deformity, particularly kyphosis, and may be associated with chronic pain and possible neurologic deficit.[80]

When evaluating the number of columns involved, it is important to determine the soft tissue component of the injury as well as the bony one. For example, a burst fracture caused by a pure axial load (e.g., a fracture of the vertebral body) is a two-column injury. However, if a significant component of flexion is associated with the fracture, the soft tissues of the posterior column may rupture transversely. Even though the radiographs demonstrate a bony injury in only the anterior and middle columns (see Fig. 4), the posterior soft tissue lesion converts this bony, stable burst fracture to a three-column (very unstable) injury. Not only are the neural elements at risk with early mobilization, but as a late consequence, significant kyphosis may develop because of a loss of posterior support. Thus, the ability of a classification to identify logically the extent of instability, both early and late, provides a means of determining the prognosis and subsequently the management of patients with spinal injuries.

A newer classification proposed by Gertzbein and associates[33, 34, 53] attempts to be more comprehensive than other systems. It takes into account the morphologic appearance of the radiographs, the progressive severity of the injury, and the mechanisms of the injury, arranged within defined categories (Fig. 15). It can be applied to the thoracic spine as well as the lumbar spine.

This system defines common morphologic characteristics within each type, as well as the common primary force producing the injury pattern.

Within each categoric type are three groups of injuries, each with a specific fracture pattern. They are then ordered according to a configuration of progressively greater instability (Table 2). Soft tissue injury is accounted for within each group, which in turn provides a continuum for predicting the potential healing of the injuries (soft tissue injuries are known to heal less efficiently than pure bony injuries). Each group is further categorized into subgroups, with specific patterns also arranged according to the authors' assignment of severity, taking into consideration soft tissue trauma. The subgroup categories are included primarily for purposes of documentation and clinical research, but may offer treatment choices as well.

Primary Fracture Types

There are three broad fracture types: A, B, and C (Fig. 15). Type A injuries include fractures of the vertebral body with compression. These injuries are caused by *axial loading*, with or without an element of flexion. They are characteristically associated with a loss of vertebral height and are primarily fractures of the vertebral body alone. If a fracture of the posterior arch is present, it is a vertical split that does not substantially influence the stability of the injury. There is no disruption of the posterior soft tissues and no translation of one vertebral body on another.

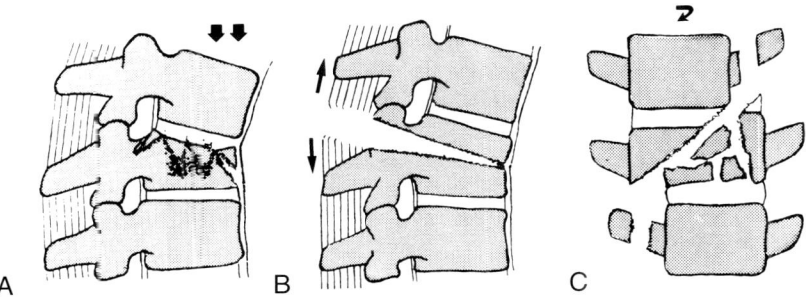

Figure 15. New classification of spinal fractures by type. *A*, Vertebral body compression. *B*, Anterior and posterior element injury with distraction. *C*, Anterior and posterior element injury with rotation. (From Gertzbein, S. D.: Classification of thoracic and lumbar fractures. *In* Gertzbein, S. D. (ed.): Fractures of the Thoracic and Lumbar Spine. Baltimore, Williams & Wilkins, 1992, pp. 25–57.)

Table 2

Classification of Thoracic and Lumbar Fractures

Type	Group	Subgroup
A. Vertebral body compression	1. Impaction fracture	1. End-plate infraction 2. Vertebral body collapse 3. Wedge impaction
	2. Split fracture	1. Sagittal split 2. Coronal split 3. Pincer fracture
	3. Burst fracture	1. Partial burst 2. Burst-split 3. Complete burst
B. Anterior and posterior element injury with distraction	1. Posterior disruption, predominantly ligamentous	1. With transverse disruption of the disc 2. With compression of the vertebral body
	2. Posterior disruption, including the arch	1. With transverse disruption through the vertebral body 2. With transverse disruption through the disc 3. With compression of the vertebral body
	3. Anterior disruption	1. With hyperextension subluxation of the facet joint 2. Hyperextension spondylolysis 3. With posterior facet dislocation
C. Anterior and posterior element injury with rotation	1. Vertebral body compression with rotation	1. Impaction 2. Split 3. Burst
	2. Distraction with rotation	1. Posterior disruption, predominantly ligamentous 2. Posterior disruption, including the arch 3. Anterior disruption of the disc
	3. Rotational shear	1. Slice fracture of the vertebral body 2. Oblique fracture of the vertebral body

From Magerl, F., Harms, J., Gertzbein, S. D., et al.: A new classification of spinal fractures. Presented at the Société Internationale Orthopédie et Traumatologie Meeting, Montreal, September 9, 1990.

Type B injuries involve the anterior and posterior elements through distraction forces. An *elongation* of the distance between portions of the vertebra or vertebrae caused by *distraction* is noted. This is due to disruption of the (soft) tissues in the *transverse* plane. Distraction may be initiated either posteriorly or anteriorly, depending on whether the forces are in flexion or extension, respectively. Most of these injuries involve disruption of the posterior elements caused by distraction and flexion forces. A small proportion of injuries in this category, however, result from distraction and extension. They initially cause anterior disruption, followed secondarily by a compression-type injury to the posterior elements.

When posterior disruption occurs through a flexion mechanism, it is seen as a transverse disruption of the posterior elements. Anteriorly, there may be a disruption of the disc as the vertebral bodies separate. If the transverse axis of rotation of the spine is within the vertebral body, axial loading occurs, resulting in vertebral body failure with loss of body height, comparable with any of the compression injuries noted in the type A category. Thus, the classification builds on itself with additional subgrouping of injuries identified from type A patterns. Many type B injuries include a significant posterior soft tissue component; radiographs should be evaluated for this component (see Fig. 4). Patterns of soft tissue disruption are determined by increased distance between the vertebrae, such as occurs with subluxations and dislocations. Separation of the posterior elements, as noted by increased interspinous distance, or perched or dislocated facets, may be seen. Translation may also occur in this type of injury pattern, but only in the sagittal plane, as is typically seen with dislocations. Because the posterior elements have been disrupted in the transverse plane, these injuries are unstable in two planes (i.e., sagittal as well as vertical).

In type C injuries, the anterior and posterior elements have been disrupted and there are associated signs of rotation (see Fig. 10). These are the most unstable of the three types, because there is loss of stability in three planes (i.e., vertical, sagittal, and axial). Generally, the injury patterns are similar to those described for type A and type B fractures, but with the additional component of rotation. Features of rotation, observed radiographically, include an offset of the vertebral bodies or spinous processes, fractures of the transverse processes or spinous processes, fractures of the transverse processes, unilaterally fractured or jumped facets (see Figs. 10 and 11), and in thoracic injuries, subluxation or dislocations of the rib heads and rib fractures.

Fracture Subgroups

Type A Groups

Within each type, there are three groups. In type A, in which loss of vertebral height is the common characteristic, a number of specific fracture patterns can be identified (Fig. 16).

Impaction fractures are injuries that result in compression of the cancellous bone because of axial loading. This may result in an end-plate infraction; symmetric collapse of the vertebral body, such as is seen in elderly patients with osteoporosis; or wedging of the vertebral body superiorly, inferiorly, or laterally (see Fig. 3).

A second group of fractures are referred to as *split fractures*. These also occur because of axial loading and result in a splitting of the vertebral body in the sagittal or coronal plane. These fractures may simply be hairline cracks, or there may be more displacement, as in the case of the pincer fracture in which the anterior corner of the vertebral body above the fracture rotates downward and backward, driving the nucleus pulposus into the subjacent injured vertebral body, imprinting its shape onto the vertebra immediately caudal to it. Concurrently, the nucleus pulposus from the disc below the fracture may herniate upward into the vertebral body, filling the vertebral body with disc material, which potentially may lead to a nonunion. Because characteristically the posterior wall of the vertebral body is undisturbed, this fracture is not usually associated with neurologic complications.

With larger axial loads, burst fractures may occur involving the upper or lower half of the vertebral body (see Fig. 5) or the entire body. Posteriorly, a bony fragment may pro-

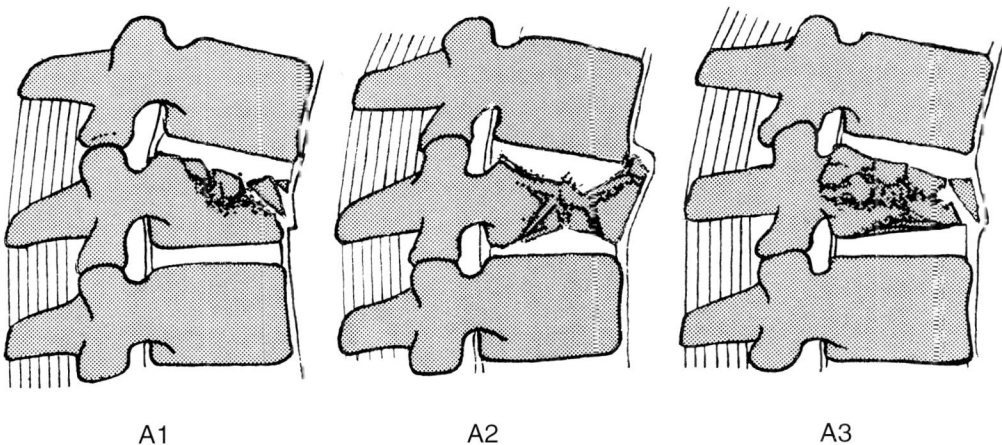

Figure 16. The three categories of type A fractures include impaction injuries *(A1)*, of which wedge fractures are commonly seen; split fractures *(A2)*, of which the pincer fracture is the typical injury, and burst fractures *(A3)*. (From Gertzbein, S. D.: Classification of thoracic and lumbar fractures. In Gertzbein, S. D. (ed.): Fractures of the Thoracic and Lumbar Spine. Baltimore, Williams & Wilkins, 1992, pp. 25–57.)

trude at the upper third of the vertebral body, often leading to a neurologic deficit. In some cases, a sagittal split may occur in the other half of the vertebral body, producing an injury referred to as a burst-split fracture (Fig. 17). If sufficient force is exerted on the vertebral body, both end plates may be involved, resulting in a complete burst fracture (Figs. 18 and 19). In the burst-split subgroup, as well as the complete burst fracture subgroup, there is usually a vertical split of the posterior arch with an increase in the interpedicle distance. These arch fractures, however, are not usually associated with a significant increase in instability.

Type B Groups

Type B injuries involve all three columns and are associated with distraction, either posteriorly or anteriorly (Fig. 20). In the first group of injuries, posterior disruptions occur predominantly through the soft tissues (i.e., through the interspinous ligaments, the capsular ligaments, and the ligamentum flavum [see Fig. 4]). Subluxations and dislocations of the facets are often seen. Anterior propagation of the injury results in either an anterior disc disruption (see Fig. 7) or a vertebral body fracture, as is also seen with type A injuries (see Figs. 4 and 7).

In the second group of type B injuries, there is posterior distraction due to a transverse disruption force extending through the bony posterior elements. Injuries in the bony arch include fractures that extend transversely through the pedicle, the pars interarticularis (producing a traumatic *flexion* spondylolysis), the lamina, and the transverse processes (see Fig. 7). As the injury propagates anteriorly, it may pass transversely through the vertebral body producing a characteristic fracture commonly (but incorrectly) referred to as a Chance fracture[13, 42] (see Fig. 7). Alternatively, the fracture through the arch may propagate anteriorly through the disc, or the injury may cause compression of the vertebral body, comparable with any of the injury patterns seen in type A fractures.

Distraction may also occur anteriorly and be associated with hyperextension forces. Although seen more commonly in the cervical spine, this mechanism may also occur in the thoracic and lumbar regions. Typically, the lesion passes through the disc anteriorly (Fig. 20, B3), although it may produce an avulsion fracture of an anterior vertebral body (see Fig. 9). As the injury extends posteriorly, it may pass through the bony arch, particularly the pars interarticularis, producing a hyperextension spondylolysis. If the pattern extends through the soft tissues, subluxation or posterior dislocation may occur (see Fig. 12).

Type C Groups

Type C injuries are identified by involvement of all three columns, with radiographic signs of rotation (Fig. 21). These signs include vertical fractures of the transverse processes, fractures or dislocations of the heads of the ribs, offset of the vertebral bodies or the spinous processes, and thoracic level injuries. A fracture of the corner of the vertebral body may also reflect a rotational component. If these signs are identified on the radiographs in association with what appears to be a type A or a type B injury, these lesions should be considered type C injuries because of the torsional component. The added plane of involvement results in the most unstable lesions with the highest frequency of neurologic deficit.[54]

The first two groups in the type C category include rotational compression fractures (see Fig. 17) and rotational distraction injuries (see Fig. 11). In addition, a third group of fractures is described that are caused by a rotational shearing force. They can be identified on radiographs as an oblique fracture line through the vertebral body. The first subgroup is the slice fracture, as described by Holdsworth,[43] in which a thin wedgelike slice of bone close to the superior end plate is sheared off because of torsional and flexion forces (Fig. 22). The second subgroup can be identified by an oblique fracture that extends from one corner of the vertebral body to the opposite corner, resulting in foreshortening and overlapping of the adjacent vertebral bodies (Fig. 23).

Sequence of the Classification

Because the classification progresses in severity with increasing involvement of the bony and soft tissue elements, and because it also builds on an increasing number of

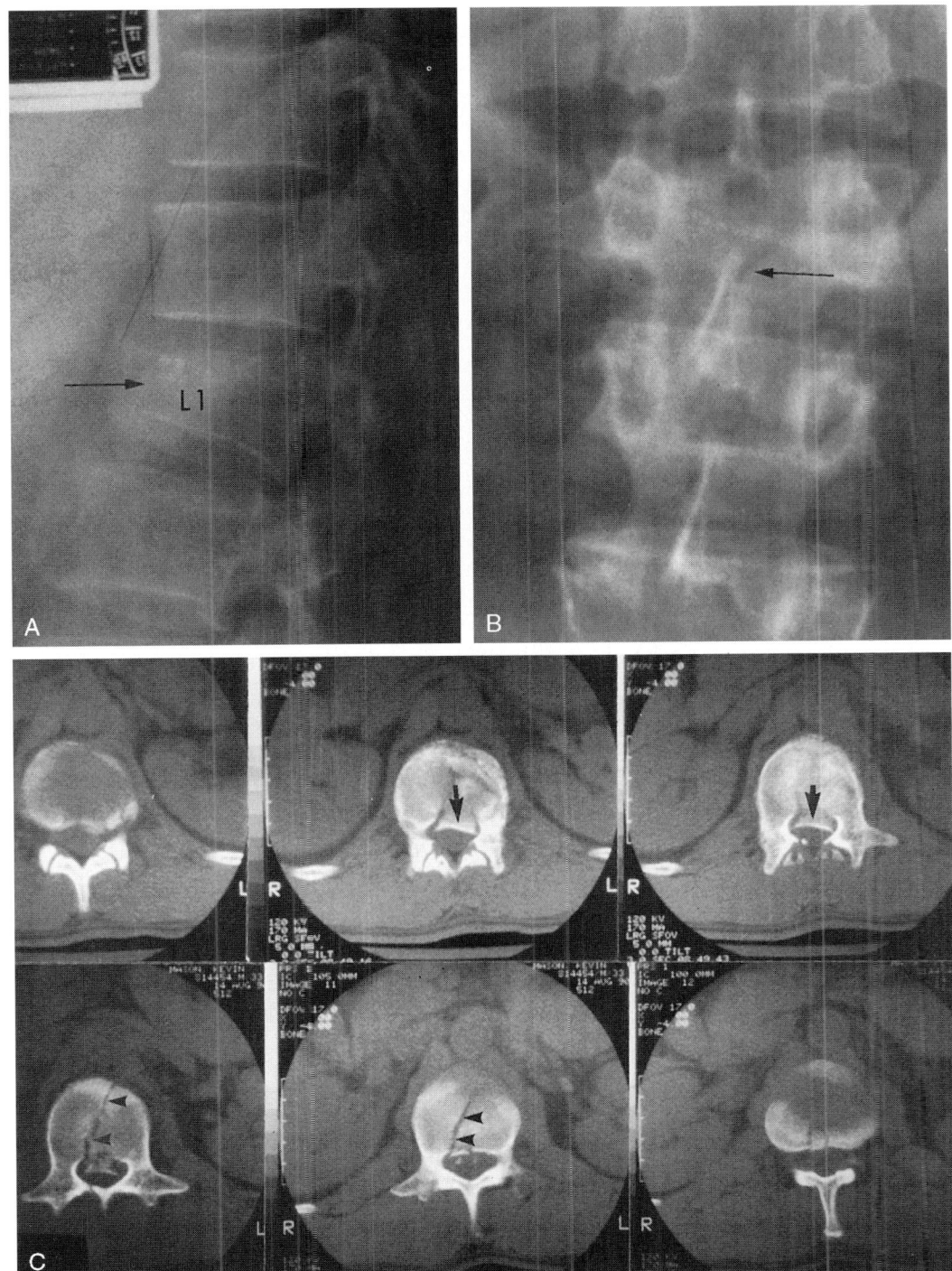

Figure 17. Burst-split fracture. *A, B,* AP and lateral radiographs, respectively, of a burst-split fracture of L1 demonstrating a split of the lamina posteriorly *(arrow)*. *C,* CT scans confirm the burst fracture with a posterior fragment in the spinal canal *(large arrow)* and a sagittal split *(small arrow)* extending into the inferior half of the vertebral body. (From Gertzbein, S. D.: Classification of thoracic and lumbar fractures. *In* Gertzbein, S. D. (ed.): Fractures of the Thoracic and Lumbar Spine. Baltimore, Williams & Wilkins, 1992, pp. 25–57.)

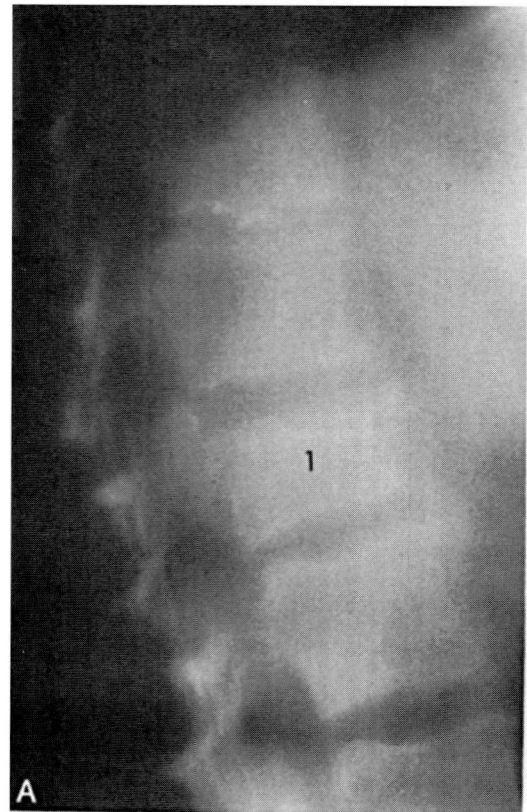
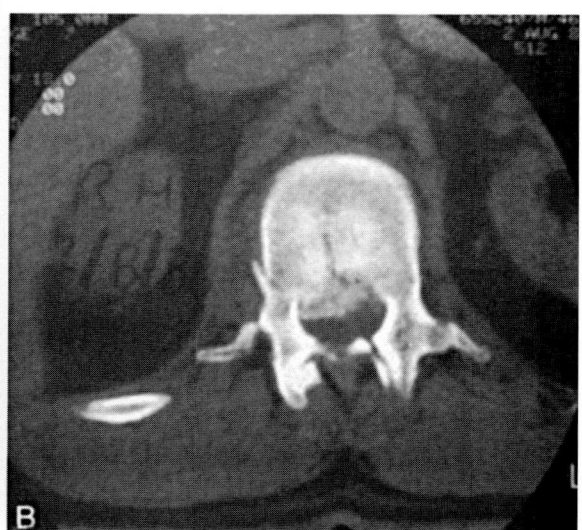

Figure 18. Burst fracture treated with AO internal fixator. *A*, Lateral tomogram of burst fracture at L1. *B*, CT scan with significant encroachment by a fragment in the spinal canal.

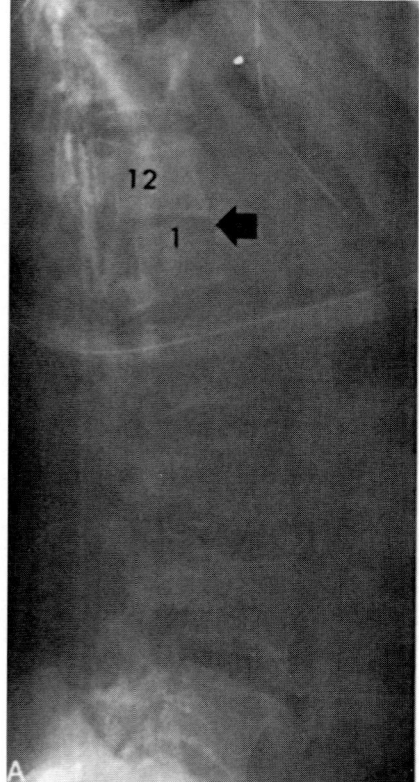
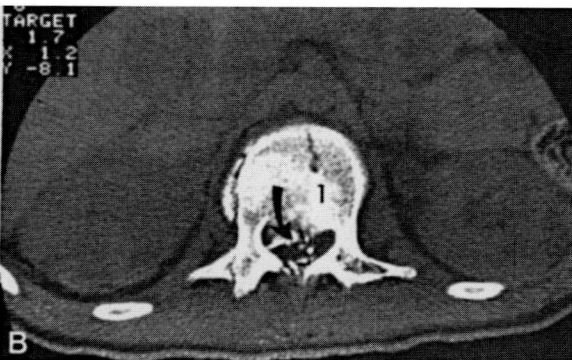

Figure 19. Burst fracture of both end plates. *A*, This 16-year-old girl developed a progressive neurologic deficit following a burst fracture of L1 seen on the lateral radiograph. *B*, Significant encroachment into the spinal canal by an intraspinal fragment *(arrow)*. (Modified from Gertzbein, S. D., and Court-Brown, C. M.: Lumbar spinal fractures. *In* Floman, Y. (ed.): Disorders of the Lumbar Spine. Rockville, MD, Aspen, 1990, pp. 615–662.)

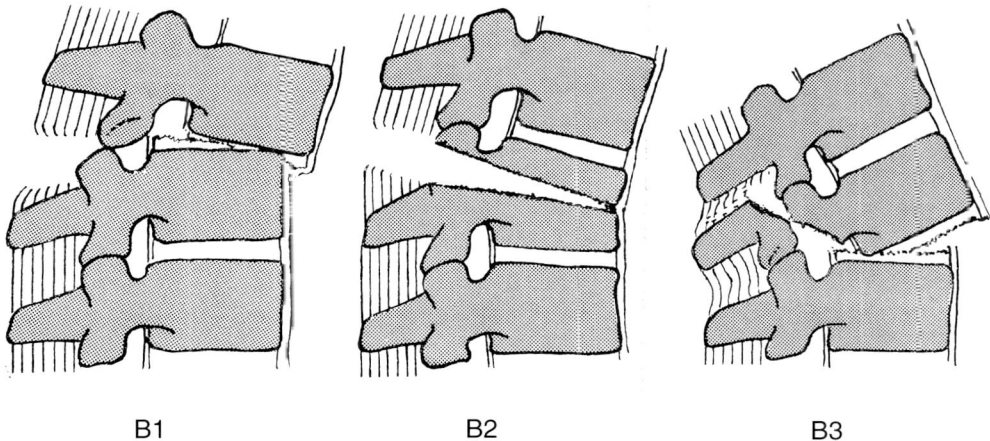

Figure 20. Type B injuries. Flexion and distraction injuries may result in disruption of the soft tissues posteriorly through the capsules of the facet joints *(B1)* or through the bony arch *(B2)*. If distraction and extension occur, anterior disruption through the disc often occurs *(B3)* with or without associated fractures or soft tissue injuries of the posterior elements. (From Gertzbein, S. D.: Classification of thoracic and lumbar fractures. *In* Gertzbein, S. D. (ed.): Fractures of the Thoracic and Lumbar Spine. Baltimore, Williams & Wilkins, 1992, pp. 25–57.)

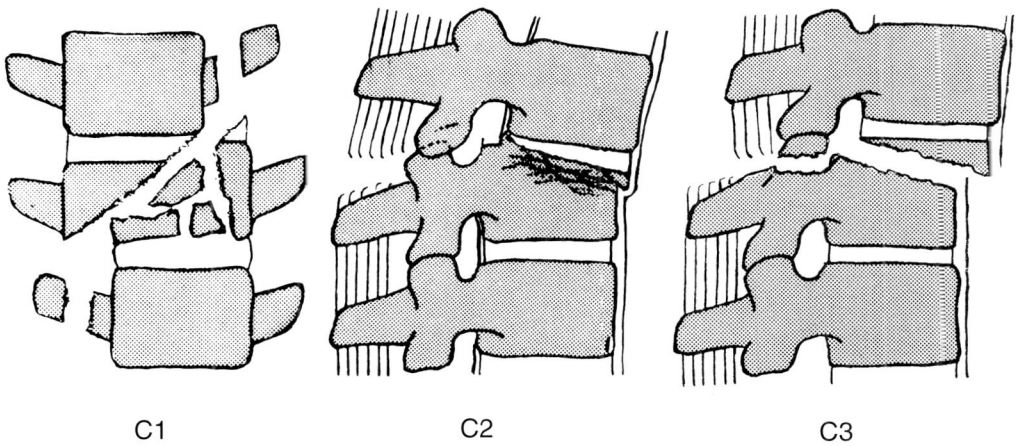

Figure 21. Type C injuries. The common features of these injuries are rotation associated with compression *(C1)*, distraction *(C2)*, and rotational shear *(C3)*. (From Gertzbein, S. D.: Classification of thoracic and lumbar fractures. *In* Gertzbein, S. D. (ed.): Fractures of the Thoracic and Lumbar Spine. Baltimore, Williams & Wilkins, 1992, pp. 25–57.)

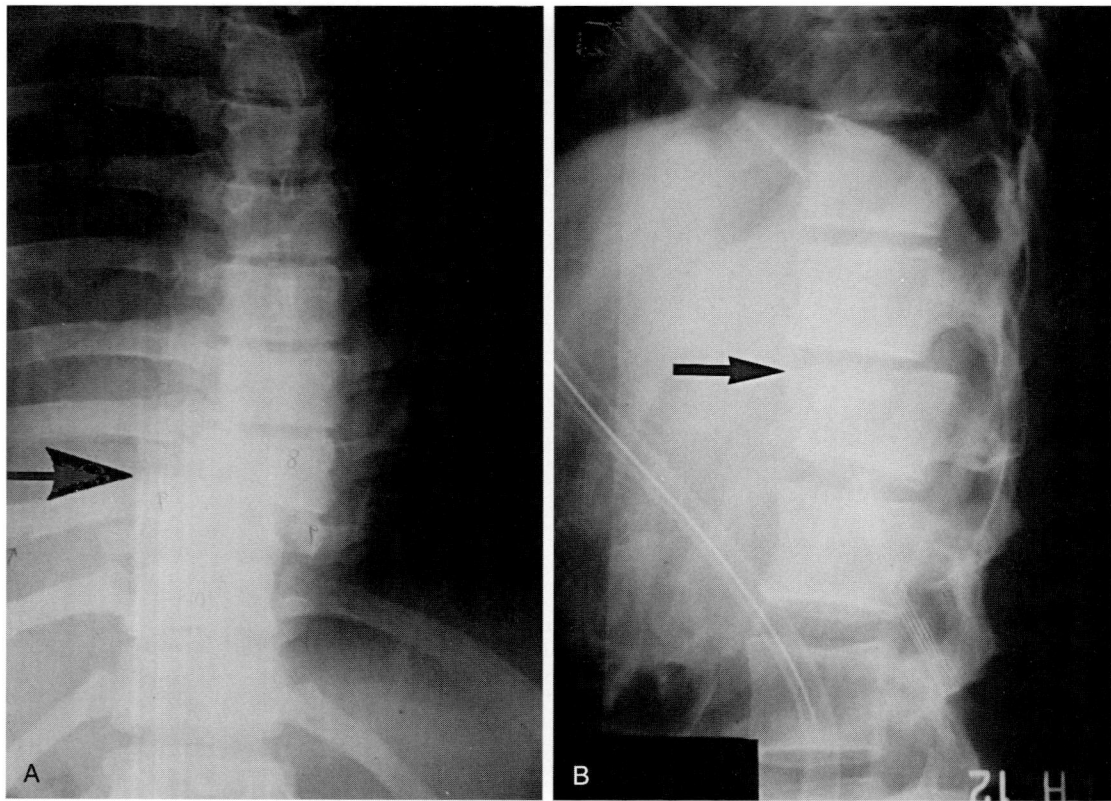

Figure 22. *A, B,* AP and lateral radiographs demonstrating a Holdsworth slice fracture with rotational shearing of the superior end plate *(arrows)*. (From Gertzbein, S. D.: Classification of thoracic and lumbar fractures. *In* Gertzbein, S. D. (ed.): Fractures of the Thoracic and Lumbar Spine. Baltimore, Williams & Wilkins, 1992, pp. 25–57.)

planes of deforming forces, the fractures are in general more unstable with progression along the classification. Furthermore, the resultant forces reflect the mechanisms of the injury and thereby determine the directions in which the failure of the spinal column occur. Because of the progressive instability, fractures further along the classification are more likely to be treated surgically. Of equal importance, the principles of management of the fracture can be established as better understanding and definition of the direction of the forces takes place.

In general, for type A injuries caused by axial loading with compression, the basic principle of surgical stabilization is to reverse the forces that caused the injury by applying distraction to the lesion to restore alignment through ligamentotaxis. On the other hand, in type B injuries, in which distraction is the primary component force producing the injury, corrective forces of compression are necessary. For type C injuries, the most unstable of all types, a rigid instrumentation system should be considered, not only to derotate the fracture, but also to provide greater stability. This may require fixation to vertebrae several levels above and below the injury instead of only adjacent to the injured levels. Alternatively, combined anterior and posterior approaches for stabilization may be considered for these injuries.

Algorithm for the Identification of Fracture Types

In evaluation of the radiographs of a patient with an injury to the spine (Fig. 24), the first step is to assess the vertebral body with particular reference to its height. If a fracture is identified, the posterior elements should then be examined for additional injuries. If no injury is observed, or only a vertical split is present, it is a type A frac-

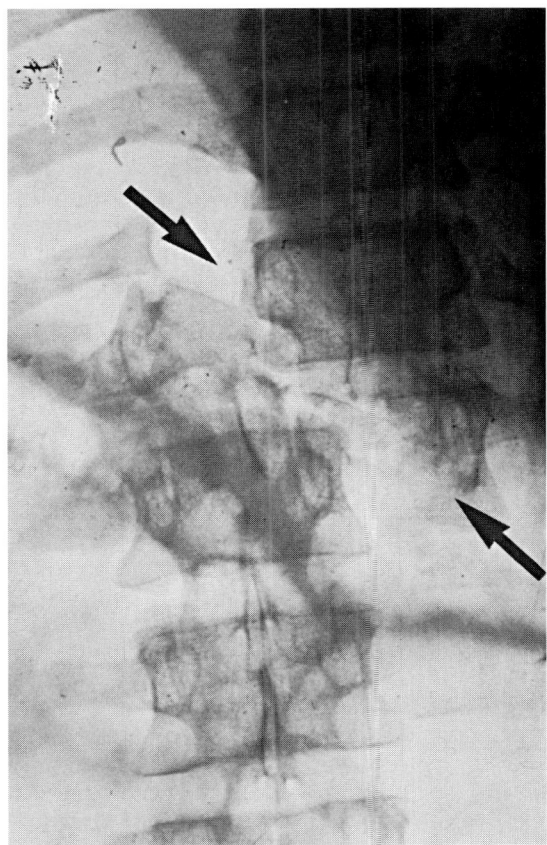

Figure 23. Oblique shearing fracture of L1 similar to a slice fracture but with greater obliquity to the fracture line through the vertebral body *(arrows)*. (From Gertzbein, S. D.: Classification of thoracic and lumbar fractures. *In* Gertzbein, S. D. (ed.): Fractures of the Thoracic and Lumbar Spine. Baltimore, Williams & Wilkins, 1992, pp. 25–57.)

plified to include only three major categories (types), each of which can be subdivided into three groups. For additional detail, each group can be further categorized into three subgroups. Progressive severity is seen for the types, groups, and subgroups, both in terms of the extent of bony and soft tissue involvement and in the increasing number of planes of disruption of the various components of the spinal columns. Thus, the severity and prognosis of the injury, as well as the mechanism of injury, can be determined by locating the fracture pattern within the classification, which in turn provides a basis for the management of these injuries.

CLINICAL EVALUATION OF PATIENTS WITH LUMBAR SPINAL FRACTURES

Evaluation includes obtaining a history of the injury. This often allows the examiner to determine the mechanism and energy involved in the injury. Questioning the patient about neurologic symptoms, even transient extremity weakness or paresthesias, often helps the physician to evaluate the extent of instability and neural compression. Associated injuries can often be detected from a carefully taken history.

The patient should be specifically asked about cramping pain in the legs, because it

ture. On the other hand, if there is *transverse* disruption of the posterior elements with no signs of rotation, the injury is a type B. If signs of *rotation* are present in the posterior elements, then the injury falls into the type C category.

On the other hand, if no vertebral body injury is identified, attention should be directed toward evaluating the intervertebral disc. If a disruption is noted the posterior elements must be scrutinized. If there is evidence of transverse disruption due to distraction, it is a type B injury. However, if features of rotation are seen in the posterior elements, the injury falls into the type C category.

In this scheme, the classification of spinal injury patterns has been intentionally sim-

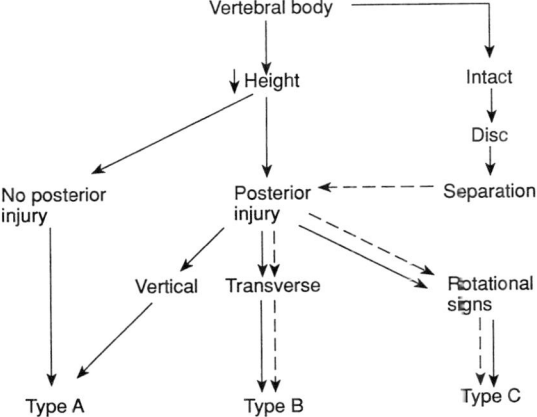

Figure 24. Algorithm for identifying spinal fracture types radiographically. (From Gertzbein, S. D.: Classification of thoracic and lumbar fractures. *In* Gertzbein, S. D. (ed.): Fractures of the Thoracic and Lumbar Spine. Baltimore, Williams & Wilkins, 1992, pp. 25–57.)

often indicates neural compression, just as it does with severe spinal stenosis or an impending cauda equina syndrome. Its presence should indicate to the clinician that the extent of neural compression may be significant, even if the patient is neurologically normal.

Examination should include an assessment of vital signs; gross examination of the head, trunk, and extremities; and palpation of the spine from the first cervical vertebra to the sacrum. Abdominal abrasions, if present, may indicate a seat belt injury and a flexion-distraction injury to the spine. The clinician should rule out associated intraabdominal injuries. The back should be inspected to be certain that there are no significant abrasions that may influence the decision to perform surgery or its timing.

The physical examination should include sensory and motor components with careful documentation of the findings. A perineal examination is most important and should include a rectal examination for baseline tone, voluntary sphincter contraction, and perineal sensation. The latter should include the ability to distinguish sharp from dull during testing with a pin. The examination is not complete until postvoid residual urine volume is assessed (if possible), with 50 to 100 ml being the upper limit of normal. The importance of perineal and bladder assessment cannot be overemphasized, because injuries to the conus medullaris or the S2–S4 nerve rootlets may be manifested only by isolated involvement of this area, with the remainder of the neurologic examination being entirely normal.

DIAGNOSTIC EVALUATION OF PATIENTS WITH LUMBAR SPINAL FRACTURES

When there is a suspected spinal injury, the patient should remain immobilized on a spine board until the clinical and radiologic assessment has been completed. Plain AP and lateral radiographs of the affected area of the spine should be obtained. If there is an associated paralysis or head injury or if the patient is noncooperative or noncommunicative, the entire spine below the level of injury (the head in the latter cases) should be studied, because there is a 5% or greater incidence of multiple levels of spinal injuries in this group of patients.[11]

CT scans are routinely obtained for further evaluation of lumbar spinal fractures, including scans at least one level above and one level below the injured vertebra. CT scans are most useful for assessing intrusion of bone fragments into the spinal canal and for studying the posterior elements, including facet and lamina fractures, often seen in conjunction with burst injuries.[12, 56, 57, 60]

The usefulness of CT scans is limited in the detection of transverse plane fractures. Significant Chance-type fractures may go undetected unless sagittal reconstruction is performed. Disc herniation may be visible on a plain CT scan; however, if there is an associated vertebral subluxation, a disc herniation may be misinterpreted as an averaging of the signal because of the subluxation (or vice versa). Another weakness of this modality is that the neural tissues are poorly visualized on a CT scan unless it is performed after a myelogram is obtained. When indicated, this can be safely done with the patient remaining immobilized and supine on the spine board; a lateral C1–C2 needle puncture is performed for introduction of the contrast material.[39] Myelograms and postmyelogram CT scans are usually reserved for those infrequent cases in which the clinical assessment of the patient does not correlate with the radiographic findings and further neural tissue visualization is needed. In this setting, however, a magnetic resonance imaging (MRI) scan may be more useful.

MRI is replacing myelography in the study of patients with spinal injuries (see Fig. 8). Its major advantages are that it provides much clearer soft tissue visualization than do other available tests and the spinal cord and cauda equina can be assessed for extrinsic compression as well as intrinsic changes. Some studies suggest that MRI may be helpful in predicting which spinal cord injuries are complete and which are incomplete and potentially reversible.[15] MRI is also helpful in assessing the continuity of the anterior and posterior longitudinal ligaments.[9] Further prospective studies are necessary to delineate better the role of MRI in acute lumbar spinal injuries. Unfortunately, this study is difficult to use in the acute trauma setting. It is not universally available. The MRI scanner is often in a separate location, and the study can be hampered by the presence of metal intravenous needles, metal splints, ventilatory support equipment, and so forth.

Ultrasonographic examination of the spine has been used to assess spinal canal size transcutaneously.[68] Unfortunately, the artifacts resulting from the intervening soft tissues and the blockage of the ultrasound signal by lamina limit its usefulness as a diagnostic test in preoperatively evaluating lumbar spinal injuries. It can, however, be used intraoperatively to assess the patency of the spinal canal[26, 27, 70] (Fig 25).

Any real-time ultrasonography machine that can be set at 7.5 MHz can be used. The tip of the ultrasound probe is covered with a surgical lubricant gel and then covered with a sterile shield, such as a plastic arthroscopy barrier, while care is taken to eliminate any air bubbles in the gel between the probe tip and the sterile barrier. The surgical wound is filled with isotonic irrigation solution, and the probe is submerged below the surface to eliminate totally any air interface between the spine and the probe (Fig. 25). A small laminotomy (1.5 × 1 cm) at the site of injury allows visualization of the thecal sac and its contents.[26] Any anterior neural compression by bone or disc fragments can be documented through the posterior approach to the spine. By rotating the probe 90 degrees, the surgeon can obtain either a sagittal or a transverse view of the spinal canal. This is a useful method in checking for persistent spinal canal compromise. It can be used during and after posterolateral decompression procedures. Because real-time ultrasonography provides direct visualization of the conus medullaris and cauda equina, the information is more

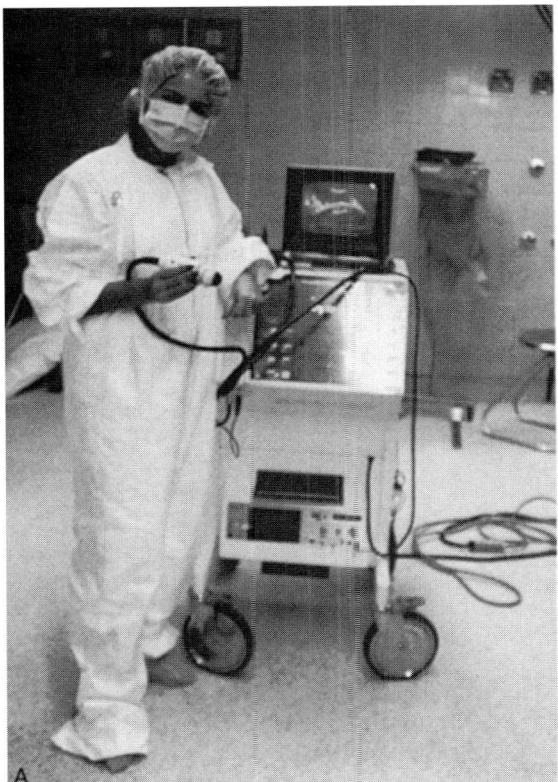 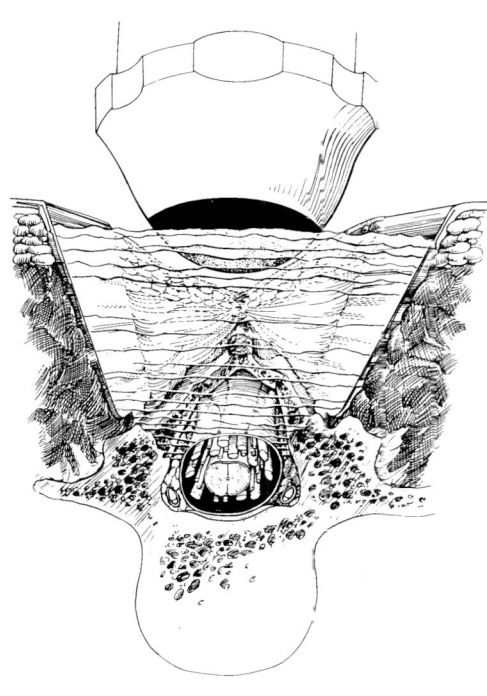

Figure 25. *A,* The ultrasonography equipment in the operating room to demonstrate that it is portable and to show the relative size of the probe, which is in the physician's hand. *B,* The posterior surgical incision with the patient in the prone position and the wound filled with saline. The probe tip, which has been covered with lubricating gel in a sterile barrier, is then submerged below the surface of the irrigation fluid. Turning the probe 90 degrees allows the surgeon to view the spinal canal in either the transverse plane or the sagittal plane.

Illustration continued on following page

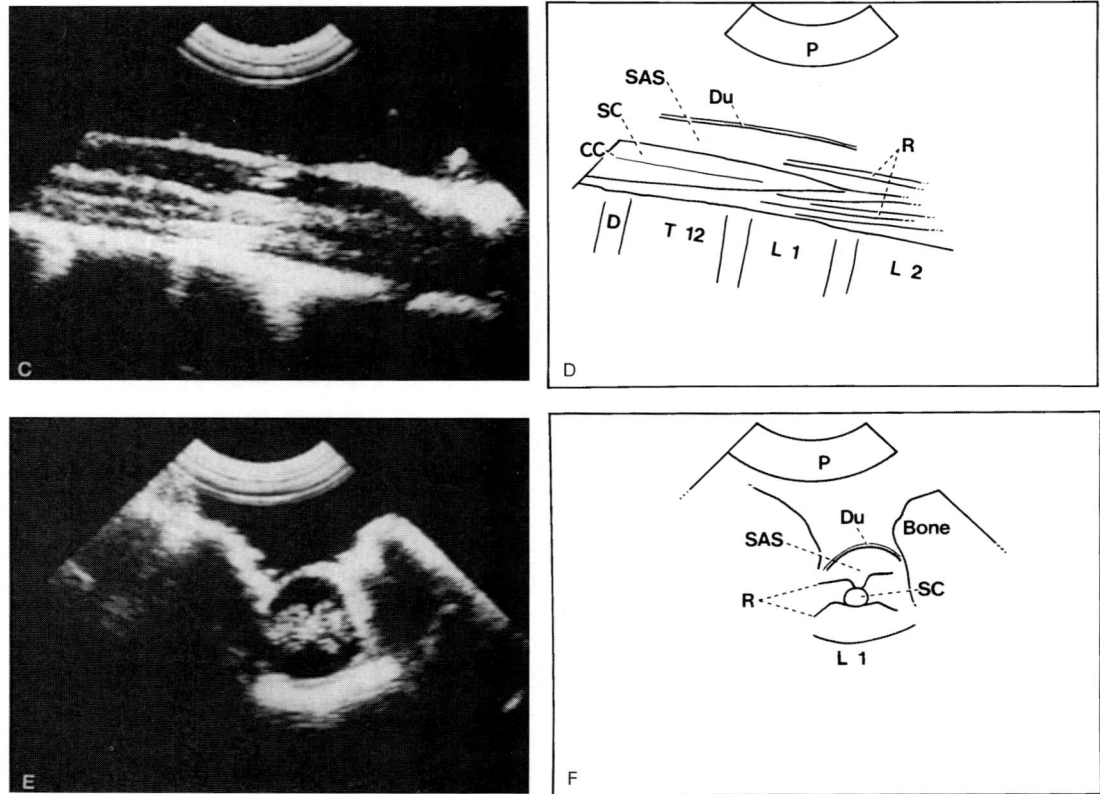

Figure 25 *Continued* C, In this sonogram, the patient has undergone a laminectomy over several levels at the thoracolumbar junction. Ultrasonography allows visualization of the spinal cord, the conus medullaris, and the posterior aspect of the vertebral body. D, The structures visualized in C. (CC, central canal within the spinal cord; D, intervertebral disc; Du, dura; L1, L1 vertebral body; L2, L2 vertebral body; P, ultrasound probe tip; R, nerve rootlets; SAS, subarachnoid space; SC, spinal cord; T12, T12 vertebral body.) E, This ultrasonogram at the L1 vertebral body level clearly shows the conus medullaris with lumbar and sacral nerve rootlets. The subarachnoid space is clearly visualized. F, The structures shown in the ultrasonogram in E. (A–F, From Eismont, F. J., Green, B. A., Berkowitz, B. M., et al.: The role of intraoperative ultrasonography in the treatment of thoracic and lumbar spine fractures. Spine 9:783–784, 1984.)

detailed than that obtained with an intraoperative myelogram.

MANAGEMENT OF LUMBAR SPINAL INJURIES

Aims of Treatment

The primary aims in treating lumbar spinal injuries are (1) restoring alignment and stabilizing the spinal column, (2) improving the patient's neurologic status, and (3) mobilizing and rehabilitating the patient as soon as possible. Although both nonsurgical and surgical means are capable of achieving these aims, there has been considerable debate regarding the merits of surgical and nonsurgical treatment for unstable fractures.[77] Interest in a surgical approach has increased, particularly regarding burst fractures of the lumbar spine. This is related to the improved management made possible by the advent of innovative, rigid internal fixation devices for both posterior and anterior fixation.[21]

The nonsurgical approach has been recommended by a number of investigators, who suggest that many fractures are best treated by postural reduction, a period of bed rest, and external immobilization.[19, 48, 49] Many years ago, Bedbrook[4, 5] stated that mobilization out of bed has little to recommend it, because in well-disciplined treatment units, mobilization and physical restoration can be applied equally well while the patient is in bed. This philosophy still holds true in many regional geographic areas today. It has also been demonstrated that fragments within the spinal canal may resorb with time if treated nonsurgically.[48, 49] Despite the relative success of the multidisciplinary team approach advocated by Bedbrook and others, the type of unit required is expensive in terms of both person-hours and financial resources, and the late outcome has not been as favorable as might be expected.[21, 45] In many countries, physicians and patients have found it to be an untenable concept. Late deformity and the sequelae of late pain are uncertain when nonsurgical techniques are used. However, in some reports, fewer than 5% of patients treated nonsurgically for unstable injuries eventually undergo surgical intervention because adequate reduction cannot be maintained.[5, 26, 31, 77]

The neurologic improvement in patients with incomplete neurologic deficits who are treated nonsurgically is not as great as that seen with surgical treatment. In patients treated nonsurgically, approximately 60% to 70% achieve a recovery of at least one Frankel grade, although Davies and colleagues[19, 31, 41, 83] reported an improvement rate of 95%. The literature related to patients undergoing surgery with a posterior approach reports a recovery rate somewhat higher, on the order of 80% to 85%.* In patients with incomplete neurologic deficit who undergo anterior decompression surgery with strut fusion, the rates of those who improve at least one Frankel grade are approximately the same.[24, 55, 59] Reduction of the intraspinal fragment by posterior distraction techniques has been shown to increase the diameter of the canal by 75%, if it is performed early.[1, 37, 82] It is not possible to determine whether the neurologic improvement differs statistically, because of inadequate measures for comparison, bias, and nonrandomization in patient selection. It appears, however, that there is a trend toward greater improvement with the surgical approach compared with the nonsurgical approach in patients with incomplete lesions, and certainly in those whose condition is neurologically deteriorating.

---

*References 22, 23, 25, 57, 59, 72, and 73.

Management of Specific Injuries

Surgical Versus Nonsurgical Treatment

In the treatment of nearly every spinal injury, there is almost always a nonsurgical option. This can range from the placement of an orthosis and early mobilization to prolonged bed rest. Lumbar orthoses provide varying degrees of stability and are usually not completely rigid.[29, 30, 50, 58, 61, 34] The decision to perform surgery, on the other hand, entails issues of instability and spinal cord injury. It is useful for rigidly stabilizing and realigning the spine, although it carries the risks inherent in all surgical procedures. The decision whether to operate depends on issues of instability, neurologic compromise, and the physician's confidence in his or her ability to treat the injury appropriately coupled with the patient's decisions and needs.

Minor Fractures

Minor fractures are relatively stable and include transverse process fractures, isolated fractures of the pars interarticularis (these are rare injuries), and spinous process fractures. In general, these injuries are related to a direct blow or avulsion (e.g., violent contraction of the psoas muscle leading to transverse process fractures) and can be treated symptomatically. Despite the benign appearance of these injuries on plain films, the authors recommend looking for concomitant injuries in the involved area on a CT scan. This is particularly true with transverse process fractures of L5, because they are frequently associated with sacral fractures and possibly bladder dysfunction from injury to the sacral nerve roots.

Compression Fractures (Type A Injuries)

A compression fracture usually is stable (acute or late). It primarily involves the anterior column (vertebral body) with minimal or no middle column component and an intact posterior column. When a flexion force is added to the compression (axial loading), posterior disruption may occur. This may lead to late instability because it produces a more unstable injury, with the potential for progressive collapse and deformity. This becomes a type B injury (see under Comprehensive Classification) and is more unstable than the common compression fracture. A kyphosis of more than 25 to 30 degrees or compression greater than 40% to 50% suggests that there has been posterior ligament disruption (or separation of the facet joints), particularly in young individuals (nonosteoporotic fractures). In these instances, because of the soft tissue component and the risk of potential collapse and deformity, surgery may be the best treatment choice.

If the injury is primarily to bone, with no suggestion of posterior element disruption, treatment with a rigid thoracolumbosacral orthosis (TLSO) or even a Jewett-type three-point extension brace often is adequate. The orthosis is worn for 6 to 12 weeks depending on the nature of the injury and the patient's symptoms.

If there is significant wedging anteriorly coupled with gaping of the spinous processes or if there is disruption of the facet joints posteriorly, surgery should be considered. To reestablish alignment and ensure stability, a posterior approach with insertion of instrumentation is generally indicated. In the lower lumbar spine, this includes the placement of pedicle screw fixation systems; in the upper lumbar spine, hooks (or pedicle screws) and rods with or without polyethylene sleeves may be used. Some of the goals of surgical treatment are to minimize the number of lower lumbar motion segments included in the construct to preserve neurologic function, to maintain (or reestablish) lumbar lordosis, and to mobilize the patient as early and as rapidly as possible. Because the posterior elements are disrupted and there is compression anteriorly, a distraction system with three-point fixation (e.g., Edwards or Harrington distraction rods or segmental systems, including Cotrel-Dubousset and newer variants) can be used. If the middle column is unquestionably intact, a compression system may be used from the posterior approach. However, compression systems may cause posterior protrusion of a bony fragment or disrupted disc if there has been undetected middle column disruption.

If the diagnosis is in doubt, a compression construct is best used along with intraoperative ultrasonographic examination. Additionally, posterolateral evaluation and decompression may be useful in avoiding neurologic compromise during compression. If surgery is chosen, one of the goals should be to realign the spine and to regain lordosis. Because of this, a neutralization system (noncontoured plates and screws, systems that lack three-point fixation, or those that do not supply an anteriorly directed vector force) should not be the first choice if other systems are available.

If surgery is being performed after the fracture (bone) has begun to consolidate and if most of the significant pathologic processes are in the anterior two columns, it is possible to use anterior instrumentation and fusion (Fig. 26). The available anterior instrumentation is strong enough to fix such injuries rigidly. An anterior fusion without instrumentation is not likely to be successful as an isolated procedure and often leads to an increased deformity. The treating physician should also appreciate that, as the posterior instability becomes more severe, even with the best available anterior instrumentation, it will still be necessary to add posterior instrumentation (Fig. 27).

Burst Fractures (Type A Injuries)

Burst fractures can be considered an extension of a compression injury, with definite involvement of the middle column. Additionally, posterior element fractures are frequently noted. The type of treatment depends on the severity of the injury.[46] Additionally, the percentage of spinal canal compromise, the degree of angulation present related to the injury, and the presence or absence of a neurologic deficit are important factors to be considered in managing the patient.

Not all patients with burst fractures benefit from surgery. Cantor and colleagues[13] as well as Mumford and coworkers[62] have shown in selected patients that it is not necessary to operate on a burst fracture when the injury pattern includes less than 40% canal compromise, there is no significant posterior column injury, and there is no neurologic deficit. Additionally, if there is relatively uniform compression and the angulatory (kyphotic) deformity is minimal, the use of a TLSO and early ambulation may be prescribed. However, surgery is useful and may be the preferred treatment in individuals with greater than 40% to 50% canal compromise, kyphosis related to the injury that

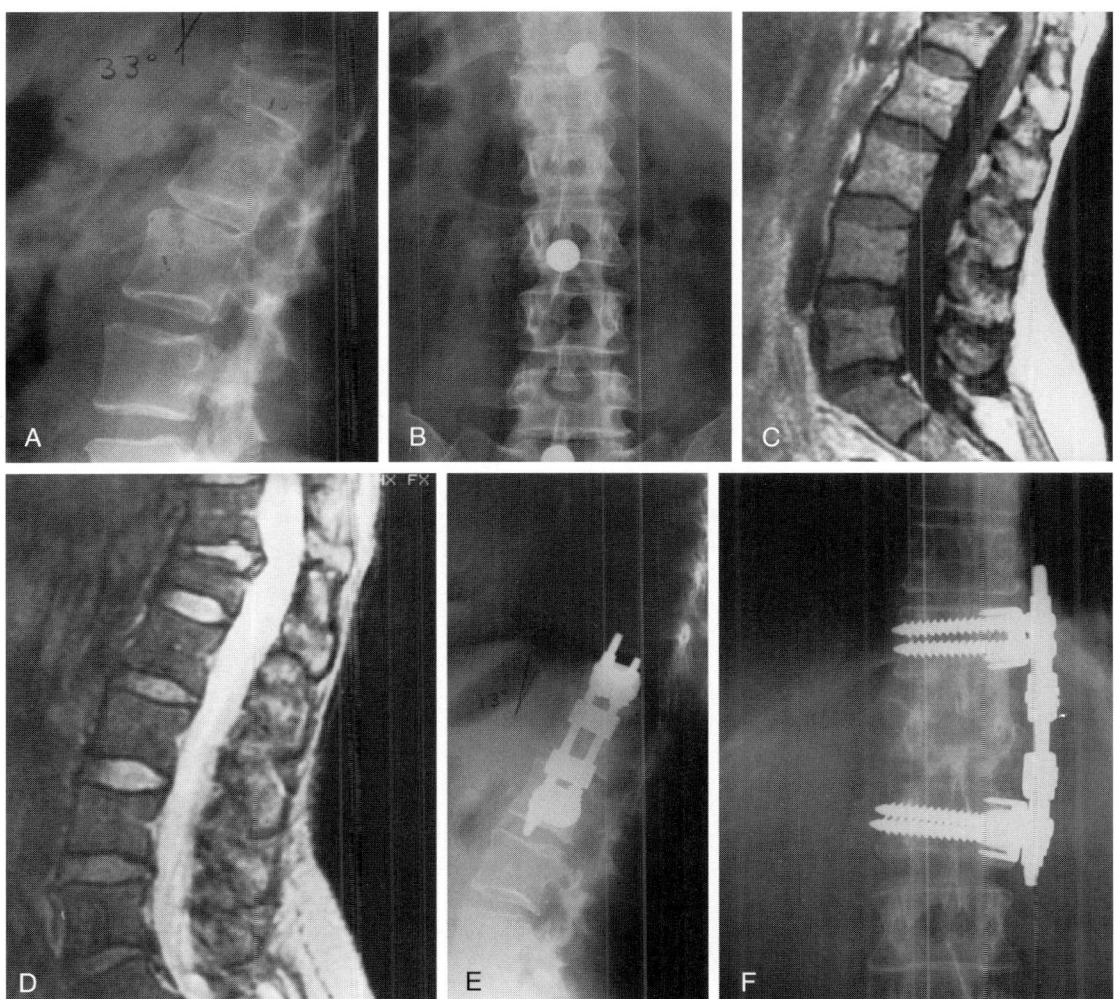

Figure 26. A 45-year-old woman was involved in an accident 10 years previously when she had a transient weakness of her legs that resolved with conservative treatment. The patient was seen 10 years later for pain at the thoracolumbar junction, which was gradually increasing in both frequency and intensity. She also had a feeling as though she was tipping forward. She was neurologically normal. A, A lateral x-ray film shows a 33-degree kyphosis centered at the L1 level. B, An AP x-ray film reveals only minimally increased posterior widening between the T12 and L1 spinous processes. C, A T1-weighted MRI scan reveals that the patient has adequate room at the level of her injury for the conus medullaris. D, A T2-weighted MRI scan again shows that the spinal canal is of adequate size and confirms that there is no retropulsion of bone or disc into the spinal canal. E, The patient was treated with an anterior discectomy with resection of the superior portion of the vertebral body at T12–L1 and a discectomy and fusion at L1–L2, followed by application of a Kaneda device to achieve correction and to maintain adequate reduction. The kyphosis was reduced to 13 degrees on this follow-up film obtained 6 months after the surgery. F, An AP x-ray film shows the Kaneda device in place 6 months postoperatively. She was treated in a TLSO brace for 5 months after the surgery, and at that time, the fusion was judged to be solid. At last follow-up (18 months postoperatively), she had no thoracolumbar spine pain and she felt her posture to be normal.

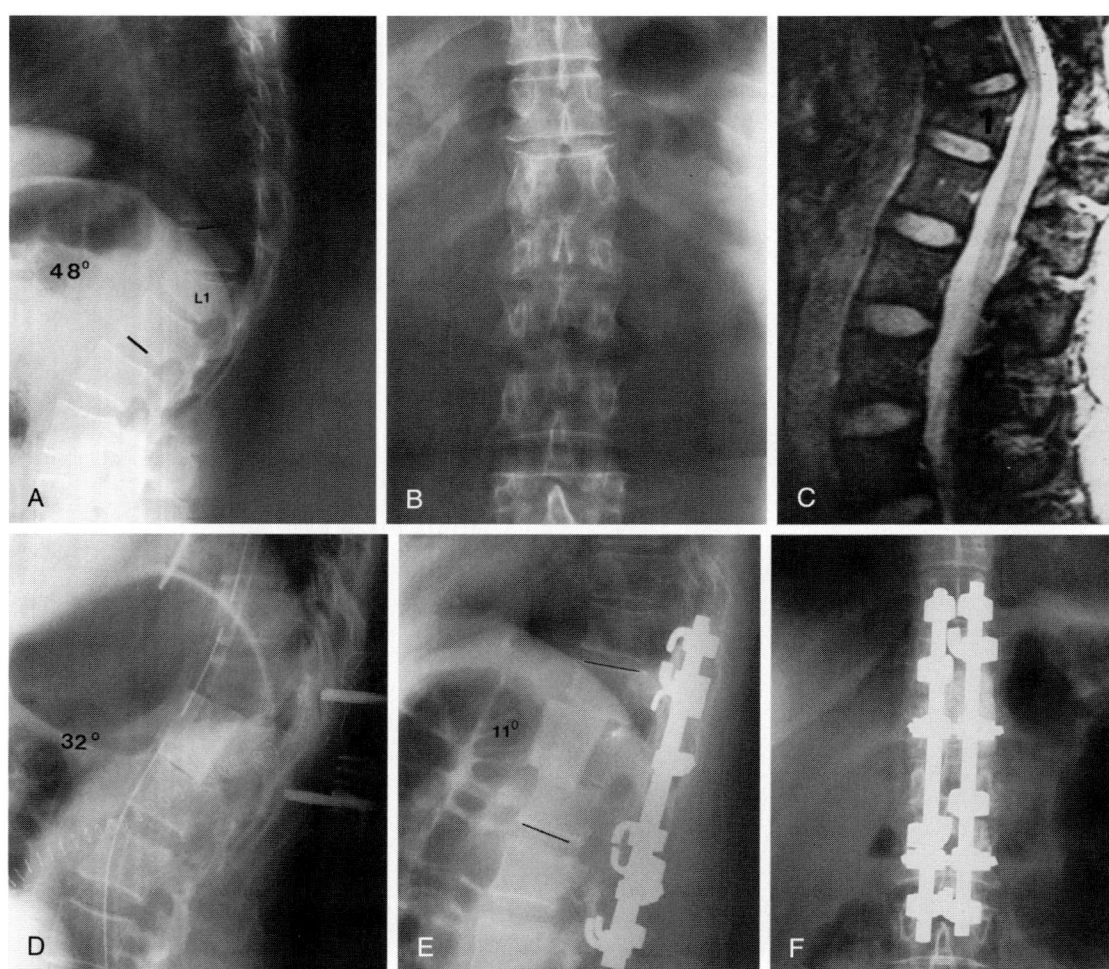

Figure 27. A 46-year-old woman had been injured 9 years previously and sustained a L1 compression fracture, which was treated nonsurgically. She was being seen 9 years later because of severe thoracolumbar spinal pain, which was progressive. She was neurologically normal. *A*, A lateral x-ray film reveals a 48-degree kyphosis centered at the L1 compression fracture. Because of the severe degree of kyphosis, it was assumed that there was posterior disruption present. *B*, An AP x-ray film shows a significant spread of the posterior elements, and it was assumed that the ligaments were torn at this level. *C*, A T1-weighted MRI scan reveals that, even though there is a severe kyphosis, there is adequate room for the neural elements. *D*, Because of the severe degree of the kyphosis preoperatively, and because this was a 9-year-old injury, it was decided to proceed with an anterior corpectomy of the L1 vertebra and to determine at that time how much correction could be achieved. The deformity could only be reduced to 32 degrees, and hence it was decided that same day to proceed with posterior instrumentation, reduction, and fusion. Adding anterior instrumentation at this same time would not have served any useful purpose. At the posterior surgery, it was found that the patient's facets were perched and were spontaneously fused in that position. It was necessary to perform an osteotomy to achieve reduction. *E*, A standing lateral x-ray film was taken 1 month postoperatively and shows that the deformity had been reduced to 10 degrees. The majority of the hooks for this segmental fixation were used in a compression mode, with some hooks used in distraction to prevent any type of hook pullout. *F*, An AP x-ray film again shows the hook pattern of segmental fixation. At the time, the patient felt as though her posture and her thoracolumbar pain were significantly improved.

is greater than 25 degrees, or a neurologic deficit. In the latter instance, the neurologic deficit often includes lower extremity dysfunction (motor and/or sensory). However, there may be normal lower extremity function but isolated alteration in bowel or bladder function. The physician should always attempt to evaluate the patient for postvoid residual urine and rectal sensation, function, and tone. Any deficits should be considered evidence of neurologic compromise.

The diagnosis of a burst fracture depends on a CT or MRI scan to visualize all the components of the injury. If possible, a sagittal reconstruction should be performed to visualize and elucidate the injury pattern better.

The nonsurgical treatment of burst fractures includes placing the patient in a TLSO for approximately 3 months for nearly 24 hours per day. The patient can ambulate and participate in controlled aerobic activities, as tolerated. However, for 6 to 12 weeks the patient should avoid (or minimize) riding in vehicles, activities that result in impact, and frequent bending or twisting activities related to the trunk. If, in the course of nonsurgical treatment, any changes occur in neurologic symptoms or signs to the lower extremities, including bowel or bladder function, the patient should be urgently re-evaluated and consideration given to decreasing activity or proceeding to surgery. Standing lateral radiographs should be obtained at frequent intervals to be certain that there has been no change in the angulation or degree of compression across the fractured vertebra.

Most lumbar burst fractures can be stabilized by means of posterior instrumentation.[43] This may include hooks and rods in the upper lumbar spine (Fig. 23) or pedicle screw–based systems in the upper lumbar and particularly in the lower lumbar spine (Fig. 29). The surgical approach may be dictated by the neurologic condition. In general, in a neurologically intact person with a lumbar burst fracture, adequate reduction, stabilization, and indirect decompression can be achieved with posterior instrumentation involving hooks and rods or pedicle screw devices. If there are large fragments of bone within the canal, posterolateral decompression can be performed at the time of instrumentation.

In general, fractures of L3, L4, or L5 are best treated with pedicle screw–based devices rather than hook-rod systems. There is a 5% to 20% hook dislodgment rate with distal hook fixation to L4, L5, and the sacrum.[17] Fractures treated surgically can be reduced and stabilized using any system that allows distraction and three-point or four-point fixation.

One of the authors (F.G.E.) has extensive experience with intraoperative ultrasonography in evaluating the indirect or direct reduction of retropulsed fragments. An alternative to this, if it is deemed critical in evaluating the spinal canal, is to obtain a postoperative CT scan. However, it is unlikely in the absence of a neurologic deficit that any further surgery is necessary. With reestablishment of lumbar lordosis and the passage of time, intracanal fragments tend to resorb, with improvement in intracanal capacity.[62]

A neutralization system may be adequate in the treatment of middle and lower lumbar burst fractures if the overall alignment has not been markedly altered. If there is a loss of lumbar lordosis, however, neutralization should not be employed. Additionally, compression constructs should not be used, because they increase the risk of further retropulsion of bone fragments, possibly leading to neurologic deterioration. Also, instrumentation that does not protect the spine from axial loading (e.g., Luque rods with sublaminar wires) should not be used, because there is an increased risk of further compression of the neural elements by bone owing to retropulsion of fragments into the spinal canal.

For a patient with lumbar fractures with neurologic deterioration, the recommended treatment is surgery, including active canal decompression (see Fig. 7A). The latter can occur indirectly (by realigning the spine) or directly through either a posterolateral or an anterior approach. When performing posterior stabilization procedures in patients with burst fractures, CT-documented laminar fractures, and a neurologic deficit, there is a greater than 50% chance that a dural laceration has occurred[12] (Figs. 29 and 30). This by itself need not direct the surgeon to a posterior approach. However, if a posterior approach is chosen, the surgeon should be aware that there is a high likelihood of encountering nerve roots entrapped within the laminar fracture, a dural tear (often com-

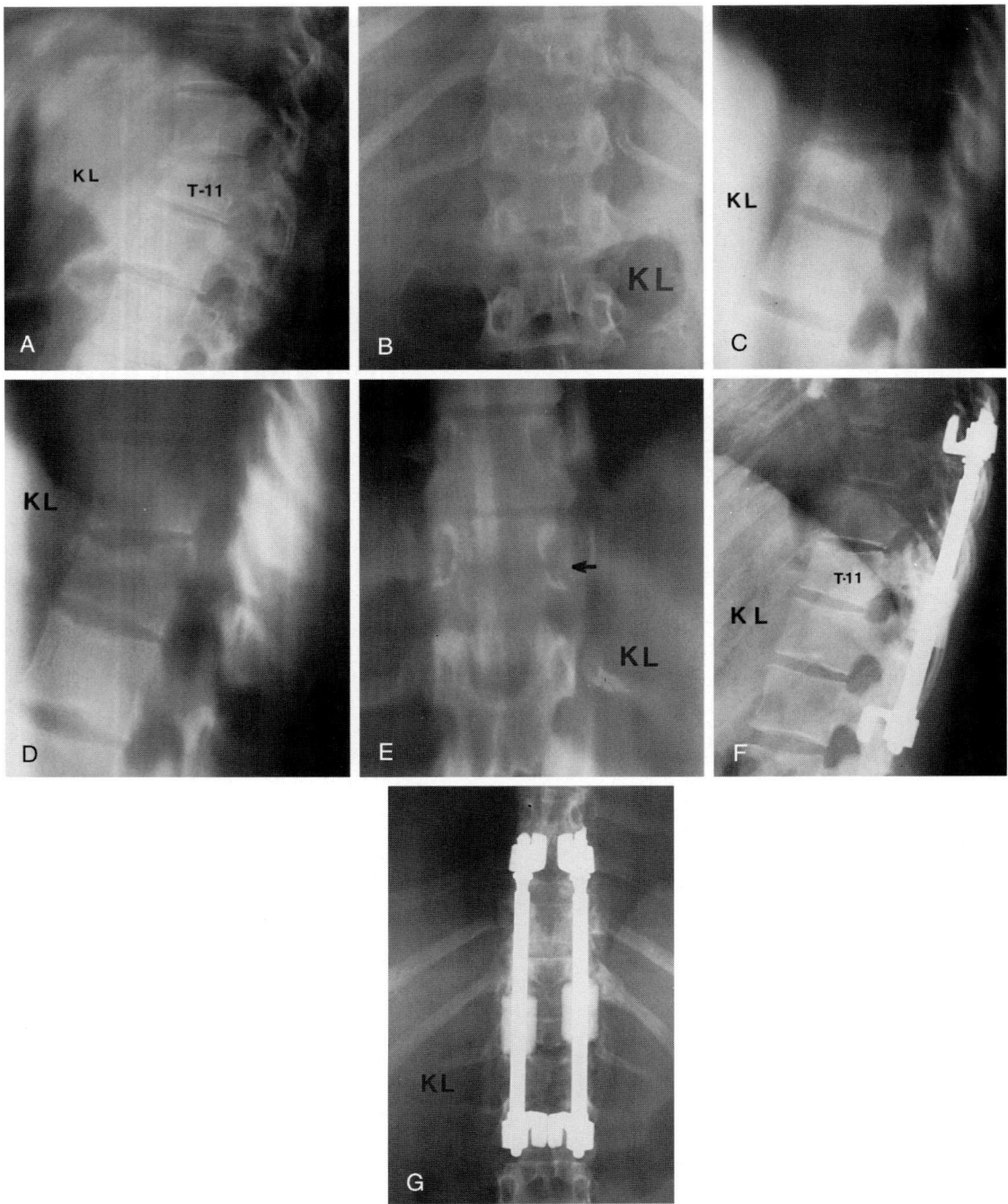

Figure 28. A 46-year-old woman was involved in a motor vehicle collision and was wearing a lap seat belt at that time. She was neurologically normal. *A*, A lateral x-ray film was interpreted initially as showing an anterior compression fracture. *B*, An AP x-ray film shows a suggestion of widening of the posterior elements. *C*, A lateral tomogram shows a fracture extending through the pedicle of T11. *D*, A lateral tomogram in the midline shows that this is associated with a burst component of the middle column. The posterior laminar fracture is also clearly seen. *E*, An AP tomogram shows the fracture line extending through the pedicles of T11. Because this injury was associated with a significant burst component and was at the level of the spinal cord, it was decided to proceed with surgery to stabilize the injury. Compression instrumentation could not be used with this injury because it would cause more retropulsion of the burst fragment into the spinal canal and may have resulted in paralysis. It was decided to treat this with an Edwards hook and rod-sleeve construct. The instrumentation was extended three levels above and two levels below the injury. At the thoracolumbar junction, the number of levels included in the instrumentation was not significant. *F*, A lateral x-ray film was taken approximately 18 months after the surgery. The patient had no problems with pain and was able to perform all of her normal activities. The reduction is excellent. *G*, An AP x-ray film at 1½ years postoperatively reveals a solid fusion.

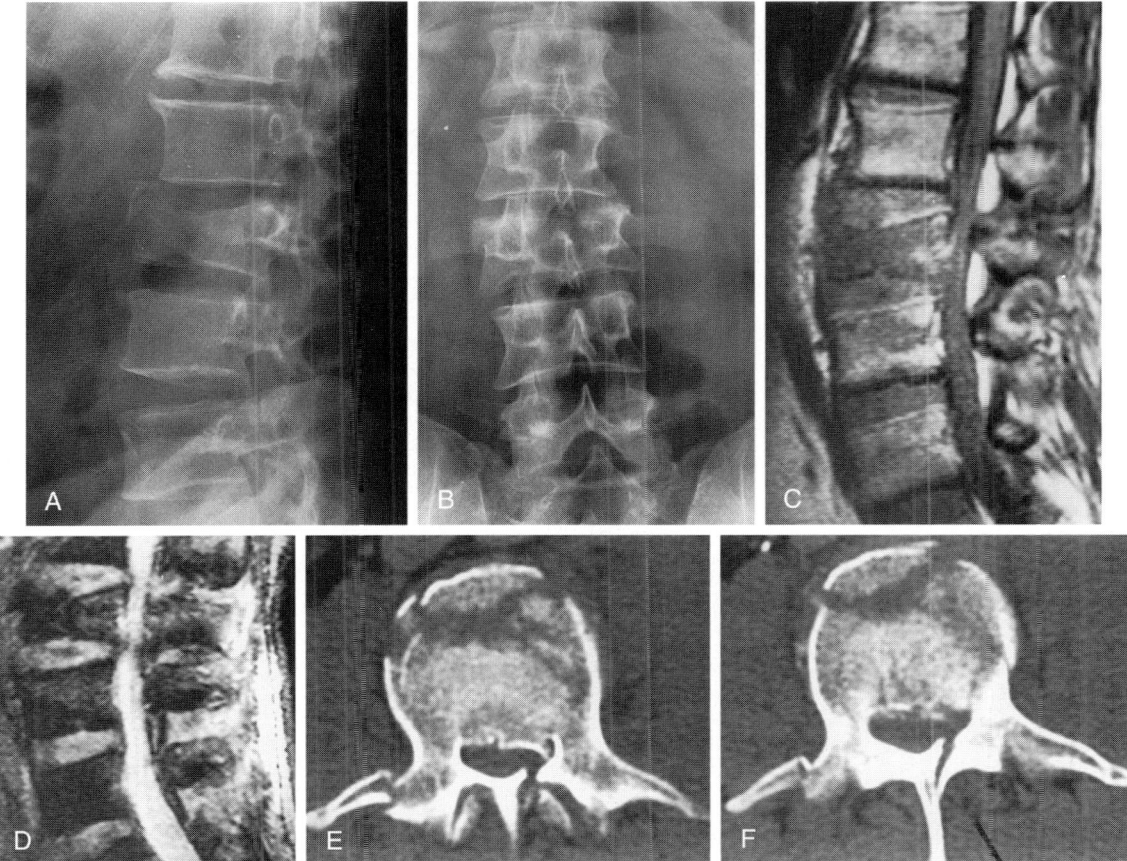

Figure 29. A 54-year-old man sustained an L3 fracture in a fall. He was neurologically normal but had severe pain in his left heel and left posterior calf. Over a period of several days, this progressed to a severe radicular pain and numbness in the L5 and S1 nerve root distribution. *A*, A lateral x-ray film shows the significant loss of height of the L3 vertebral body and suggests that there is a burst component to the injury. *B*, An AP x-ray film shows that there is a spread of the L3 pedicles consistent with a burst fracture. *C*, A T1-weighted MRI scan shows significant compromise of the spinal canal at the L3 level and reveals that he also has a moderate degree of stenosis at other levels of his spine. *D*, A T2-weighted MRI scan again reveals the extent of spinal canal compromise at L3 and also the stenosis at other levels of the spine. *E*, A CT scan at the upper level of the pedicles shows the burst component of the middle column, a left-sided posterior laminar fracture, and significant disruption of the facet joints posteriorly. *F*, A CT scan at a slightly lower level shows the continuation of the laminar fracture up into the spinous process. This type of greenstick fracture is commonly seen with this injury. This patient's clinical problem of severe pain in the left leg in the L5 and S1 nerve root distributions combined with the findings on the CT scan raises the possibility of a posterior dural tear and nerve roots entrapped in the laminar fracture.

Illustration continued on following page

plex), and the potential for persistent cerebrospinal fluid leakage, if the tear itself is not addressed.

In patients with incomplete neurologic deficit who are improving, posterior instrumentation using distraction techniques is usually sufficient. If this is performed within the first 3 or 4 days after injury, there is a high likelihood that fragments within the spinal canal can be indirectly reduced through ligamentotaxis. A laminotomy at the level of injury, with posterolateral decompression or intraoperative ultrasonographic examination, enables the surgeon to assess residual anterior neural compression. An alternative is to proceed with the posterior instrumentation and fusion and then to obtain a postoperative CT scan. If there is a residual neurologic deficit and residual bone within the canal, a delayed anterior decompression and fusion can be performed during the same hospitalization. This does

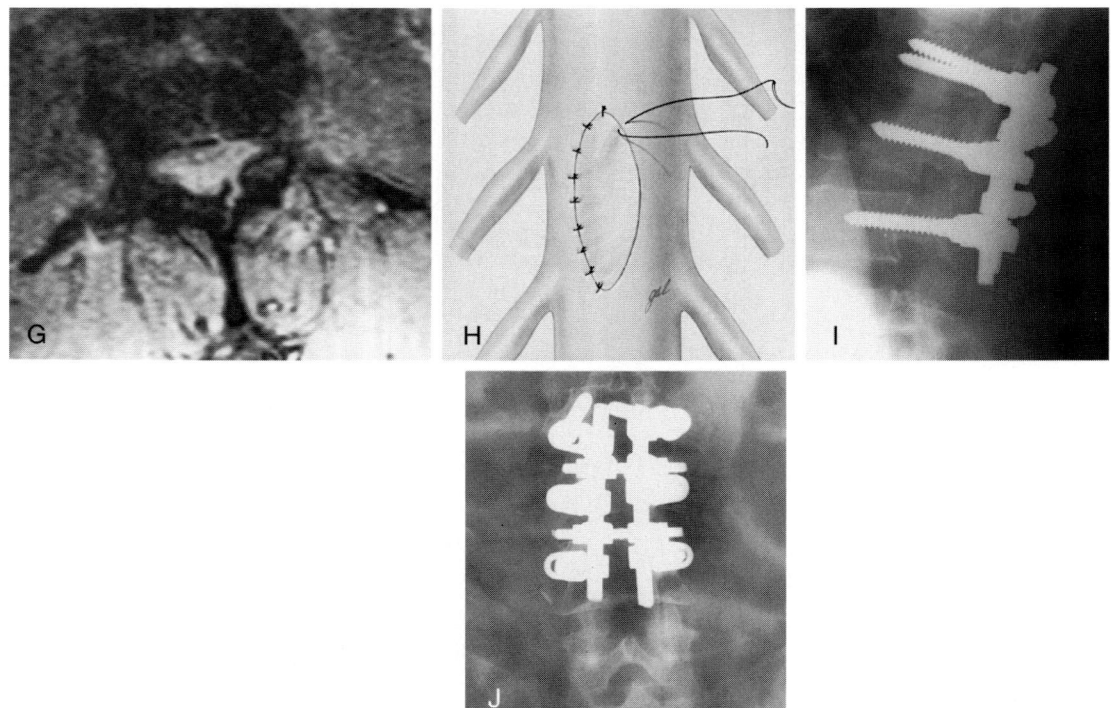

Figure 29 *Continued* *G*, A transverse MRI scan also reveals the posterior laminar fracture and suggests that there may be soft tissue entrapped within the fracture. The patient was taken to surgery for a laminectomy, and indeed, he had a large dural laceration and nerve rootlets were entrapped within the posterior laminar fracture. *H*, Because of the degree of swelling that was present within the nerve rootlets, it was not possible to put the nerve rootlets back into the dural sac and perform a primary repair. For this reason, it was necessary to use a freeze-dried dural patch graft to repair the dural laceration in a water-tight fashion. This allowed closure of the dura without any constriction of the nerve rootlets. (From Eismont, F. J., Weisel, S., and Rothman, R. H.: Treatment of dural tears associated with spinal surgery. J. Bone Joint Surg. 63A:1132–1136, 1981.) *I*, Pedicle screw fixation was used from L2 to L4 and adequate lordosis and fracture reduction were achieved with this instrumentation. Immediately following the surgery, the patient had complete relief of his leg pain and paresthesias. *J*, An AP x-ray film shows the instrumentation and crosslink that achieved solid fixation.

not compromise the long-term, eventual neurologic function. It does, however, necessitate two episodes of anesthesia and two procedures.

Anterior decompression and fusion may be the preferred primary treatment for patients who have a burst fracture and an incomplete neurologic deficit. This is probably the safest approach for individuals with significant neurologic compression (greater than 50% canal involvement and marked neurologic deficit). If surgery is delayed beyond 1 week, the anterior approach may be preferred, because indirect decompression is unlikely to occur with a delayed, isolated, posterior procedure. Anterior instrumentation, if available, is strong enough to supplement the strut fusion and to allow the patient to be mobilized. If the surgeon is not familiar with anterior instrumentation or if it is not available at the time of the anterior decompression and strut fusion, a posterior stabilizing procedure (compression or neutralization instrumentation) should be considered, either during the same session of anesthesia or 4 to 7 days later.[38]

Complete neurologic deficits are rarely encountered with lumbar burst fractures. Even if the injury occurs at the level of the conus and the patient initially appears to have a complete neural injury, there is still potential for recovery of the function of at least the adjacent nerve rootlets, which course past the conus and originate from undamaged spinal cord. The same consideration should be given to this patient as to a patient with an incomplete neurologic deficit.

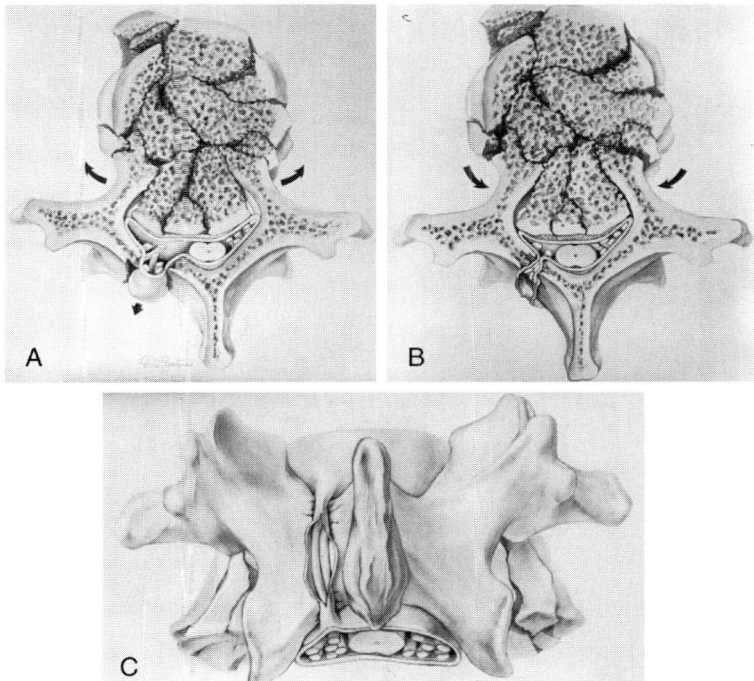

Figure 30. *A*, At the time of impact, when the pedicles are spread laterally, the dura and neural elements are forced out posteriorly through the laminar fracture. *B*, Immediately after injury, as the pedicles recoil medially, the dura and nerve rootlets are entrapped within the posterior laminar fracture. *C*, This posterior view of the spinous process and lamina demonstrates that, at the time of surgery, the dura and nerve rootlets may even be located posterior to the lamina. Great care must be taken in exposing this area. To free the neural elements safely, it is usually necessary to perform a laminectomy on the opposite side of the spinal canal, away from the fracture, and then to remove the midline posterior elements in one piece and tease the neural elements out of the fracture site. (From Cammisa, F., Eismont, F. J., and Green, B. A.: Dural laceration occurring with burst fractures and associated laminar fractures. J. Bone Joint Surg. 71A:1044–1052, 1989.)

Flexion-Distraction Injuries (Type B Injuries)

Flexion-distraction injuries mechanically result from a fulcrum for the applied force being situated anterior to the vertebral body (e.g., in an individual who is wearing a seat belt over the lower abdomen). With this anterior fulcrum, the flexion force leads to a disruption of the posterior and middle columns, which occurs in tension, with the anterior column acting as a hinge. Depending on the location of the fulcrum, there may be compression injuries anteriorly, avulsion through or fracture completely across bone, or separation through soft tissue only. Nonsurgical treatment may be appropriate if this is primarily a bony injury, as originally described by Chance.[14] However, surgery is more likely to be helpful and indicated in patients who have mainly ligamentous involvement. All of these injuries are acutely unstable, although those primarily through bone can heal without surgical intervention (but stabilization may be chosen because of the acute instability). In addition, many of these patients have multiple severe injuries, and spine surgery may be indicated to allow these patients with multiple trauma to be mobilized (Fig. 31).

Most flexion-distraction or seat belt injuries should be treated with posterior stabilization using compression instrumentation. As mentioned, the injury can occur primarily through bone, through bone and soft tissue, or entirely through soft tissue (Fig. 32). The likelihood of healing without surgery decreases as the amount of soft tissue involvement increases.[35] In general, hooks and rods over the injured motion segment, or one additional level depending on how much bone is involved (pars and/or facets), are usually sufficient. However, if

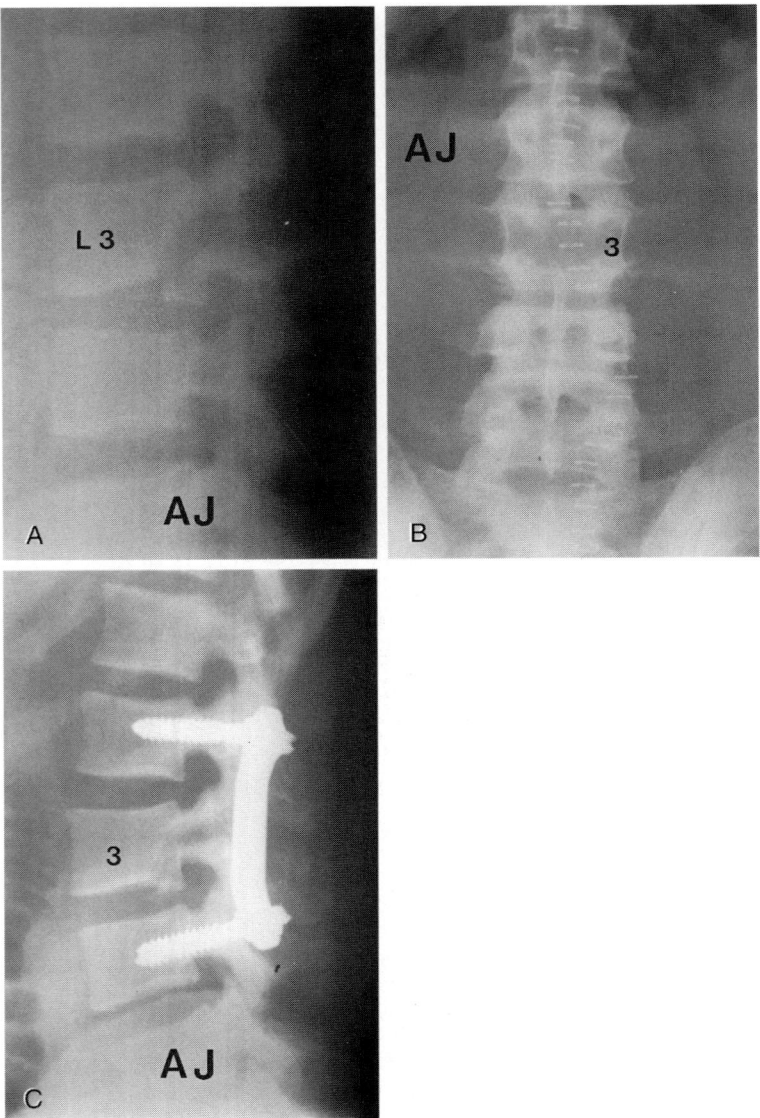

Figure 31. A young man was injured in a motor vehicle collision and sustained a seat belt injury of his spine. He also had a hollow viscus disruption that was acutely treated by general surgeons. Postoperatively, the patient reported significant lumbar spinal pain during attempts at mobilization. He was neurologically normal. *A*, A lateral x-ray film shows a typical seat belt fracture, which proceeds through the posterior elements, splits the pedicles, proceeds through the inferior portion of the L3 vertebral body, and into the L3–L4 disc space. *B*, An AP x-ray film shows that the flexion-distraction injury has disrupted the transverse processes bilaterally and has split the L3 posterior elements. The surgical clips that can be seen are from his anterior abdominal surgery to repair the bowel injury. At that time, the general surgeons believed that it was imperative to mobilize the patient. *C*, The patient was taken to surgery and, after he was placed prone on a four-poster frame, his fracture was completely reduced and pedicle screw instrumentation was used to stabilize the spine in this reduced position. As an alternative, it would have been possible to utilize a hook and rod compression system over these same levels. The patient was easily mobilized after this spine surgery and recovered uneventfully. At follow-up examination 2 years postoperatively, he had no pain and a normal range of motion of his lumbar spine.

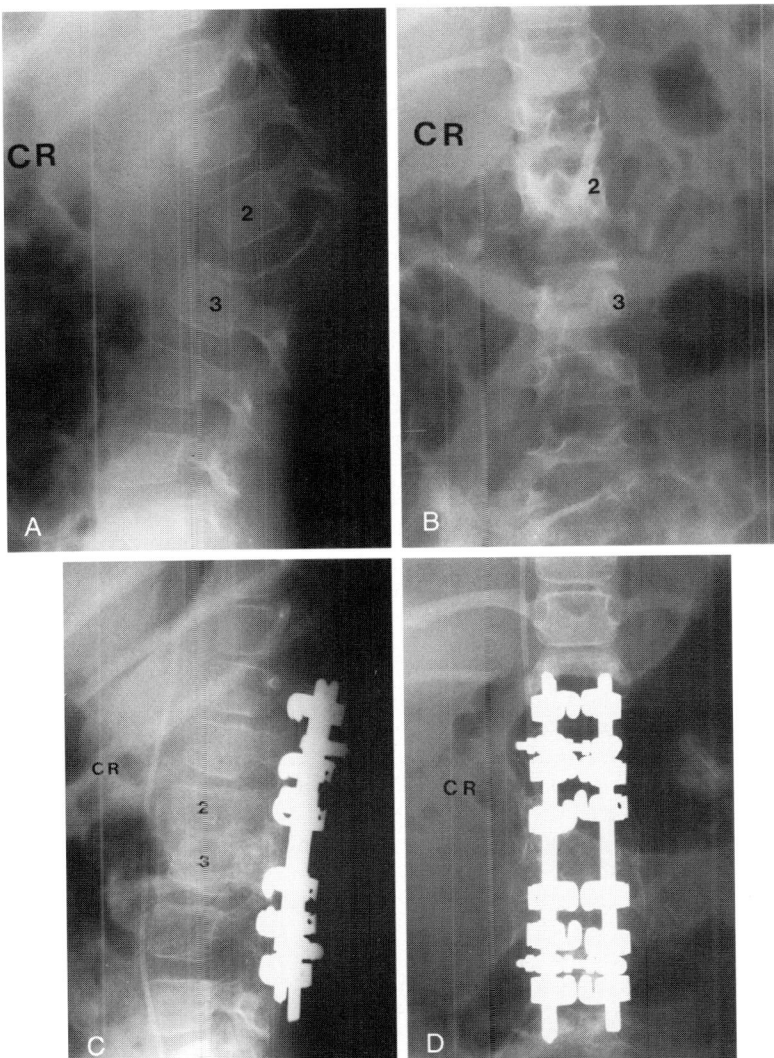

Figure 32. A 6-year-old girl was involved in a motor vehicle collision and sustained severe flexion-distraction injury of her lumbar spine. She was immediately rendered quadriplegic secondary to a neck injury. Because of extreme medical lability, it was not possible to surgically treat her lumbar spinal injury acutely. Her kyphosis created severe local problems, with skin breakdown over the prominence. A, A lateral x-ray film taken after several weeks reveals a line of callus at the level of injury. B, An AP x-ray film shows that there is no significant displacement in this plane. C, Surgical correction was performed through a posterior approach only and bilateral posterolateral approaches were used to remove the L2–L3 disc and end plates and the callus that had developed because of the injury. The L2 vertebral body was then placed directly on the L3 vertebral body and posterior segmental instrumentation was then used to hold the reduction. This follow up x-ray film was obtained at 1 year after injury. D, An AP x-ray film shows a solid fusion over the levels of instrumentation.

there is significant bony involvement, particularly through the pars interarticularis (Fig. 33), pedicle screw–based systems may be useful to decrease the number of motion segments that must be included in the instrumentation and fusion.

Nonsurgical treatment of patients with seat belt injuries includes extension bracing (molded body cast) until healing is observed radiographically. Again, if there is significant ligamentous involvement, it is unlikely that healing will occur, and this may not be the best treatment choice.

Fracture-Dislocation Injuries

Fracture-dislocations are the most unstable of all of the injury patterns because they almost always involve disruption of all three columns of the spine. The mechanism of injury involves flexion and rotation. The injury pattern can be through bone, leading to shear-type fractures, or through ligaments, leading to dislocations anteriorly or laterally, with significant translational changes of the cephalic vertebra and column relative to the caudic structures. In general, surgery is the only or best option available for these patients. It can be achieved most often through a posterior approach, particularly in a neurologically intact patient or a patient with minimum neurologic compromise. After realignment, rigid segmental fixation is necessary. Occasionally, because of complete anterior disruption, a subsequent anterior operation (usually interbody fusion) is necessary.

For surgery, intubation and positioning with the patient awake are helpful if the patient is neurologically intact or has an incomplete neurologic pattern. This allows the patient's own muscle tone to help to stabilize the spine during turning and allows the surgeon to monitor neurologic function after the positioning and before general anesthesia is induced. Most patients are able to tolerate this, particularly if the importance is explained to them preoperatively.

In most instances of flexion-rotation injuries as well as flexion-distraction injuries, the anterior longitudinal ligament is intact, although stripped from the vertebral body. This can therefore be used in reducing the deformity from the posterior approach. The reduction should be performed cautiously, however, because the anterior longitudinal ligament, if intact, may be stretched, and overdistraction can occur. Intraoperative radiographs should be obtained and evoked potential monitoring should be performed.

If necessary, reduction of the amount of distraction or the addition of a compression system (hook and rod over the segments of injury) or tension band wiring (interspinous process wiring) can help to minimize or to prevent overdistraction. After the injury is reduced, it should be stabilized posteriorly with rigid segmental fixation. If necessary, semirigid instrumentation used to reduce the deformity can be removed and converted to or replaced by a rigid neutralization device. Because of the forces involved, and the long lever arms above and below the injury, there is rarely a role for primary, acute, anterior decompression and reduction. In general, the anterior approach, if necessary, should be used concomitantly with the posterior reduction and stabilization procedure or performed as a second procedure to achieve additional decompression or bone grafting.

Lateral Wedge Injuries

Lateral compression fractures are rare. They are primarily bony, involving the anterolateral aspects of a vertebra, the vertebral body, and the facets. If there is sharp angulation, instrumented distraction across the concavity can be performed, with neutralization or compression on the convexity. However, the majority of patients with these injuries are adequately treated with the use of a TLSO and early mobilization.

Extension Injuries

Extension injuries are relatively rare in the lumbar spine. The mechanism of injury involves axial loading with the spine extended. This leads to posterior element fractures (spinous processes, laminae, and facets) with possible anterior disruption through the disc space or avulsion anteriorly through the superior or inferior lip of the vertebra. Generally, these can be treated nonsurgically with a flexion-type orthosis. If, however, there is significant disruption anteriorly or retrolisthesis of the cephalic vertebra on the subjacent one, surgery may

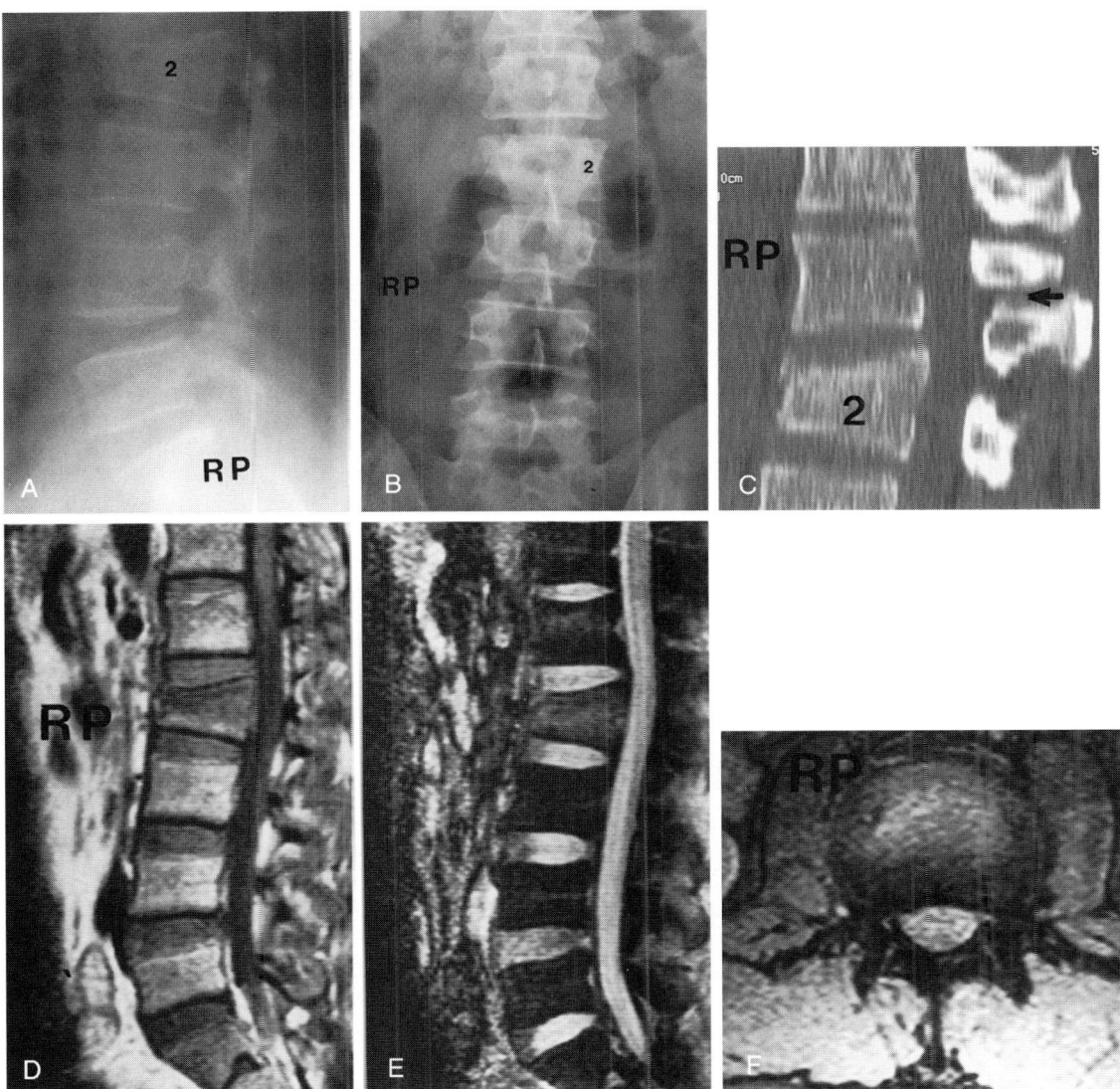

Figure 33. A 37-year-old man was injured in a fall. He was neurologically normal. *A*, A lateral x-ray film shows a 40% compression fracture of the L2 vertebral body and widening of the facet joint at L1–L2. *B*, An AP x-ray film shows that the spinous process of L1 is split and that a fracture line extends through the pars interarticularis. *C*, A midsagittal lateral tomogram shows the split in the spinous process and lamina of L1 *(arrow)*. *D*, A T1-weighted midsagittal MRI scan shows that there is no intrusion of bone or disc into the spinal canal at the level of injury. *E*, A midsagittal T2-weighted MRI scan confirms that there is no bone or disc protruding into the spinal canal but also reveals that the patient has a generally narrow spinal canal. *F*, A transverse MRI image confirms that there is generalized spinal stenosis. Considering this, pedicle screw instrumentation was used rather than hooks and rods, which would cause some intrusion into the spinal canal centrally.

Illustration continued on following page

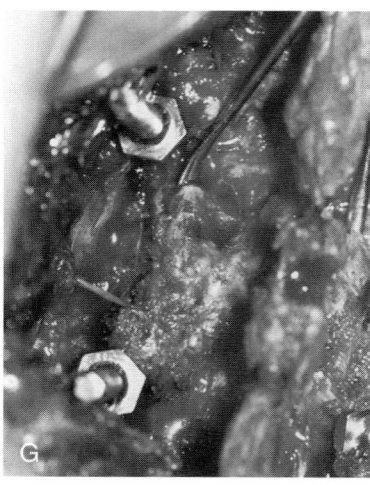
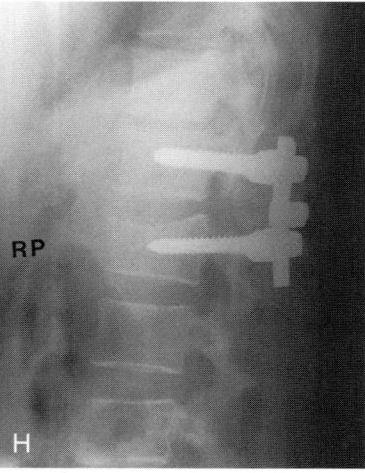

Figure 33 Continued G, At surgery, Penfield elevators were placed in the fractures of the pars interarticularis. Placing the patient prone on a four-poster frame achieved a significant reduction and closed the fracture site. H, A lateral postoperative x-ray film shows that the unstable L1–L2 segment has been adequately stabilized and that the anterior compression fracture of L2 has been partially corrected. At this time the patient was mobilized in a TLSO brace. A minimal number of levels were affected with this instrumentation.

be indicated. If this is done from a posterior approach, pedicle screw–based systems with slight distraction and flexion are best used to stabilize these injuries. Alternatively, if there is significant anterior disruption through soft tissue, an anterior approach with a bone graft and anterior compression instrumentation may be chosen.

Considerations in Surgical Stabilization

Technical Factors

The surgical approaches to the spine are as illustrated in other sections of this textbook. There are many instrumentation systems currently available to allow adequate anterior or posterior stabilization of the spine. In general, there is a trend toward instrumentation with greater rigidity, which allows shorter constructs. Other factors that need to be considered are the cost of the instrumentation, the risks associated with the procedure, and potential benefit to the patient.

In general, posterior compression techniques are indicated for significant compression fractures and flexion-distraction injuries, posterior distraction techniques or rigid anterior fixation techniques are best for burst fractures, and posterior segmental fixation with rods and multiple hooks or screws is indicated for fracture-dislocation injuries.

The length of the construct should be dictated by the degree of instability and the level of the injury. The more unstable an injury (e.g., a severe shear type of fracture-dislocation) is, the more often it is necessary to apply instrumentation to the spine at least two levels above and two levels below the injury. The more stable an injury (e.g., a simple flexion-distraction injury) is, the more likely it is that a one–motion segment fixation is adequate. In the thoracic and thoracolumbar spine, saving one motion segment is not important; in the middle and lower lumbar spine, however, it is essential to minimize the caudal extent of the instrumentation to preserve lower lumbar motion.

When considering the use of pedicle screws, the risk-benefit ratio must be considered. In the middle and lower lumbar spine and in the sacrum, the pedicles are relatively large and the adjacent neural structures are nerve rootlets and roots, which are relatively resistant to injury. Also, in the middle and lower lumbar spine it is more important to preserve motion segments. Hence, in the middle and lower lumbar spine, the use of pedicle screws as part of the stabilization construct is often justified. In the thoracic and thoracolumbar spine, however, the pedicles are smaller, the adjacent spinal cord is sensitive to injury, and the benefit of saving levels is minimal. Hence, unless there are other considerations, pedicle screws are not usually recommended for injuries at these levels and hook-rod constructs are usually the instrumentation of choice.

Finally, consideration must also be given

to cost. If two systems both give satisfactory results and one is substantially less expensive, the less expensive system can be used, even though it may not be the most modern system. Clinical function should be the primary consideration.

Some of the surgical techniques used to treat fractures and dislocations of the thoracolumbar and lumbar spine are illustrated: a simple hook-rod construct (Fig. 34), some of the hook patterns for segmental hook-rod constructs (Fig. 35), an example of pedicle screw–rod constructs (Fig. 36), and anterior decompression and stabilization techniques (Fig. 37). There are obviously many other types of instrumentation that can be used to treat these problems adequately and the author's recommendations are as generic as possible.

Techniques of Surgical Decompression

For anterior exposure of L1, either a transthoracic approach or a retroperitoneal approach can be used; the diaphragm and part of the crus must be detached from the spine with either approach. The transperitoneal surgical approach is best for anterior exposure of L5. A midline posterior approach

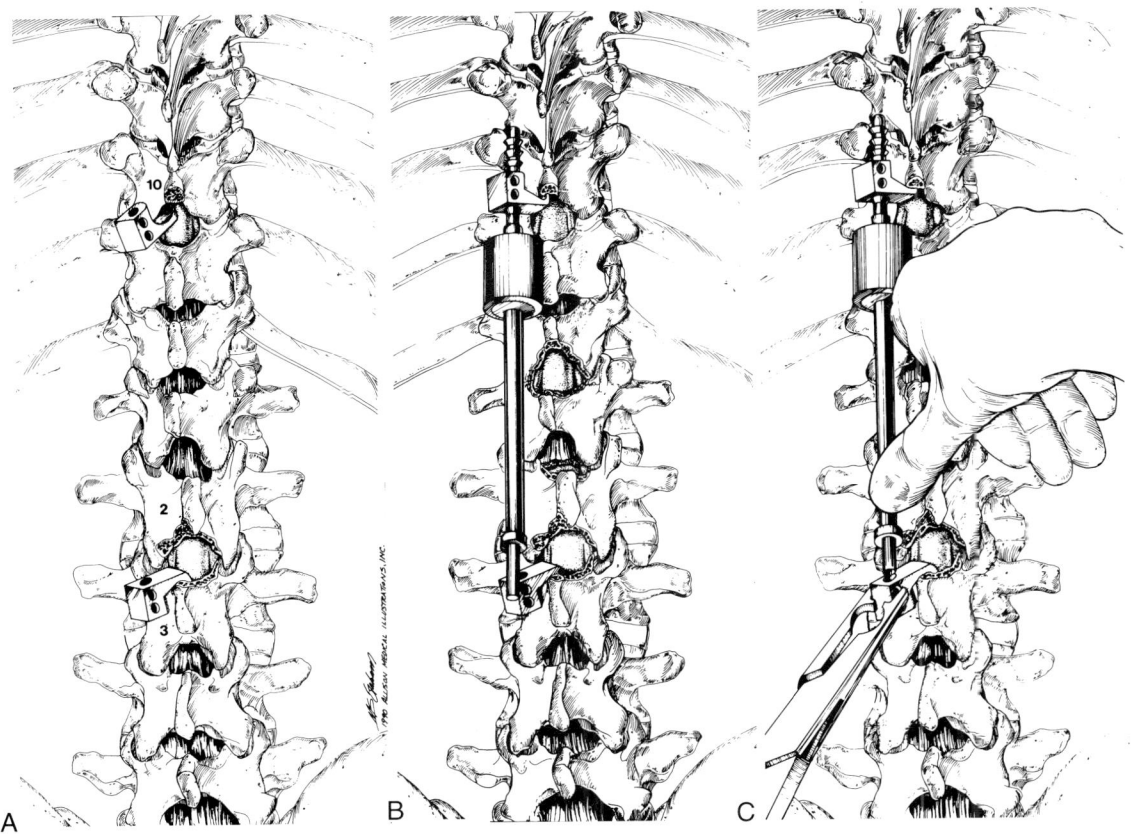

Figure 34. The technique for the Edwards distraction system using hooks, rod sleeves, and rods. In this example, the L1 vertebra has been fractured and is unstable. *A*, Laminotomies are performed at T10–T11 and at L2–L3. Care is taken to remove no bone from the lamina of T10, and the spinous process of T10 is trimmed only enough to allow insertion of the hook. No bone is removed from L3, and enough bone is removed from the inferior portion of L2 to allow placement of the hook under the lamina of L3. The laminotomy must be wide enough to allow placement of hooks bilaterally. Care must be taken to preserve the pars interarticularis of L2. *B*, A Harrington rod or Edwards rod of the appropriate length is selected and placed through the cephalic hook, and the rod sleeve is positioned either cephalad to the fracture or caudad to the fracture. *C*, The caudal hook is held with an Edwards hook holder and manual pressure is applied anteriorly to engage the distal end of the rod into the inferior hook. The posterior aspect of the L2 lamina may need to be trimmed with a bur to facilitate this.

Illustration continued on following page

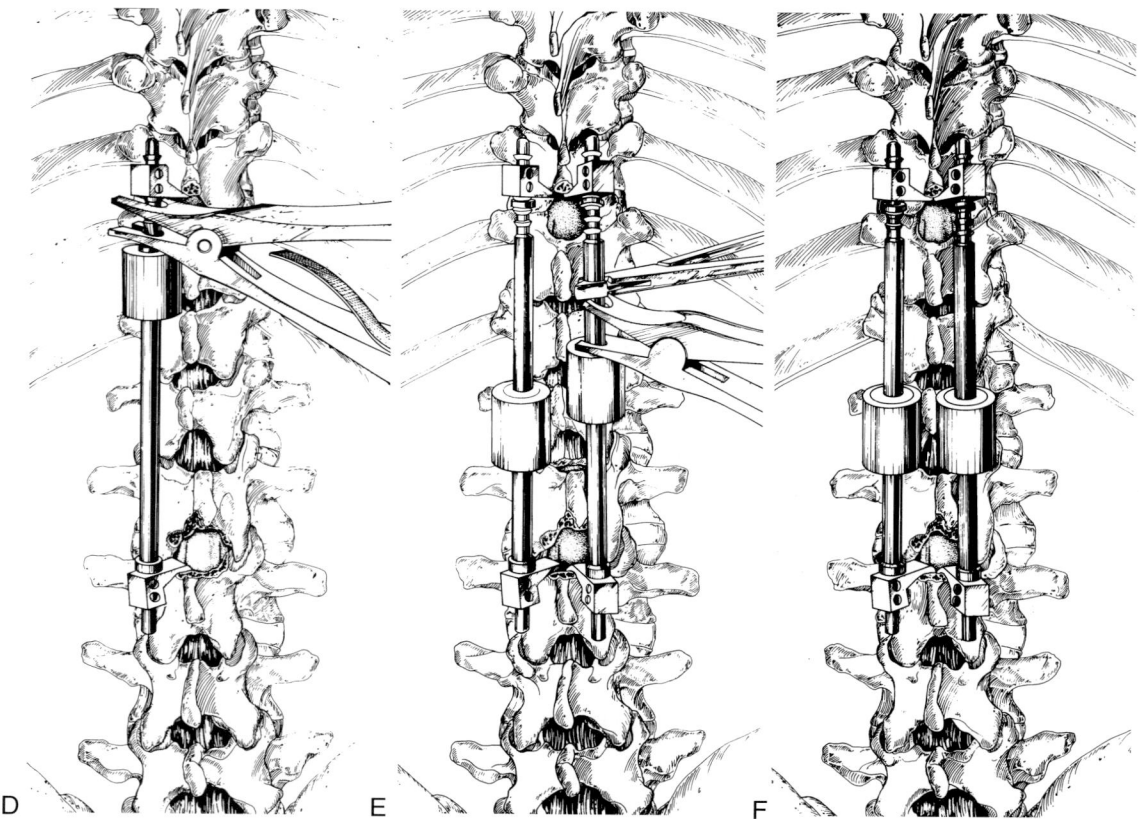

Figure 34 *Continued D*, The distractor is used at the cephalic end of the rod to apply appropriate distraction across the fracture site. The force is limited to three fingers on the distractor device. After several minutes, this tension can again be checked and often further distraction can be achieved while still using only the force of three fingers. *E*, The rod sleeves are advanced along the rod and should ideally be placed over the lamina and pedicle of the fractured vertebra. If there are associated laminar fractures, a bridging technique would be used with four rod sleeves, two placed on the lamina above the fracture and two placed on the lamina below the fracture. *F*, After the appropriate tension has been achieved in the rods and the sleeves are properly positioned, the locking washer is placed on the ratchets just below the cephalic hook to prevent inadvertent loss of distraction. A fusion is performed over the length of the instrumentation. This includes facet decortication and bone grafting over the posterior elements, including the transverse processes, the lamina, and the spinous processes. (From Eismont, F. J., Garfin, S. R., and Abitbol, J. J.: Thoracic and upper lumbar spine injuries. *In* Browner, B. D., Jupiter, J. B., Levine, A. M., and Trafton, P. G. (eds.): Skeletal Trauma. Philadelphia, W. B. Saunders, 1992, pp. 729–803.)

with a posterolateral decompression can be performed for any of the lumbar vertebrae.

When any decompression is performed, care must be taken to decompress the spinal canal across its entire width from pedicle to pedicle. For posterolateral approaches, the surgeon can use intraoperative ultrasonography to be certain that the decompression is adequate.[26, 27, 70] For anterior approaches, the surgeon must rely more on anatomic landmarks; the tendency is to decompress the spinal canal inadequately on the side opposite that on which the exposure is made.

The technique of posterolateral transpedicle decompression is illustrated in Figure 38. The patient is prone, and the spine is exposed through a midline incision. At the level of injury, a laminotomy is performed to expose the dura for a width of 1.5 cm and a length of 1 cm.[27] For most lumbar spinal injuries, this means removing the torn or attenuated ligaments and a thin rim of adjacent bone. Only the most medial portion of the facet joint is removed. Intraoperative ultrasonography is then used to visualize the anterior neural compression,[26] which most typically is bone retropulsed into the

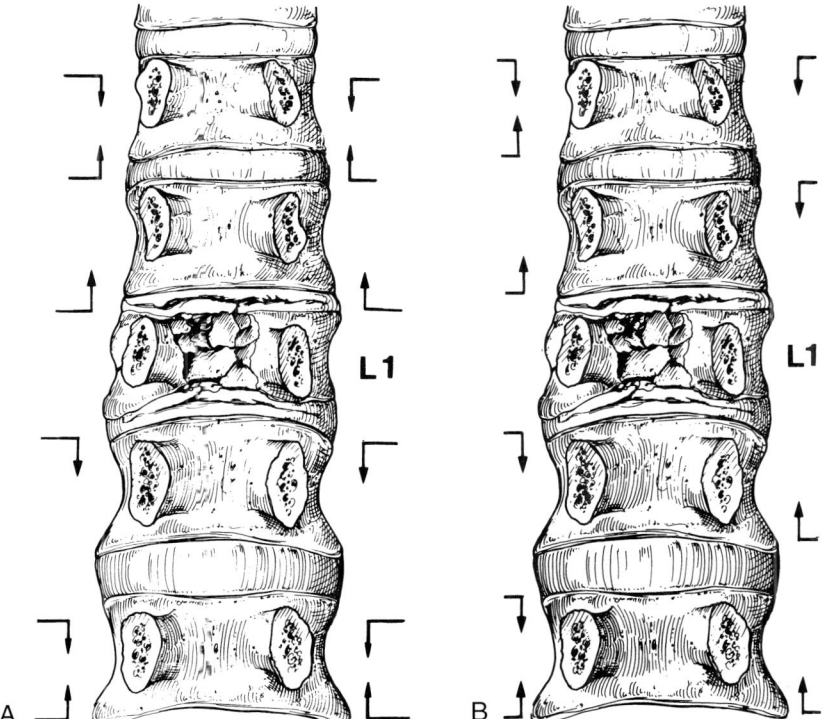

Figure 35. A, One of the possible arrangements for hook placement using segmental instrumentation with hooks and rods. This achieves adequate distraction and minimizes the chance of hook pullout. A, Special care should be taken in the placement of the hooks under the T12 lamina to be certain that no bone from the L1 fracture is protruding into the spinal canal at this same level. If this is a concern because of the fracture pattern, T12 can be eliminated from the construct and the hooks would then begin under T11 and would also include hook claws above and below T10. B, A typical hook pattern for compression instrumentation using segmental hooks and rods. The hooks do not necessarily have to be symmetric from one side to the other, but the construct does need to be balanced. (Redrawn from Eismont, F. J., Garfin, S. R., and Abitbol, J. J.: Thoracic and upper lumbar spine injuries. In Browner, B. D., Jupiter, J. B., Levine, A. M., and Trafton, P. G. (eds.): Skeletal Trauma. Philadelphia, W. B. Saunders, 1992, pp. 729–803.)

spinal canal at the level of the pedicle. In the case of an acute lumbar injury, instrumentation should be inserted initially to attempt neural decompression by fracture reduction; this can be visualized by ultrasonography. If the neural compression is not reduced with the instrumentation or if the fracture is not an acute injury, a posterolateral transpedicle decompression is performed. The superior portion of the lamina is resected to expose the cephalic two thirds of the pedicle. A power bur is then used to remove the central portion of the pedicle, and this tunnel is extended into the posterior portion of the vertebral body. A fine rongeur is used to remove the remaining medial cortex of the pedicle. Care is taken to protect the nerve root exiting the spinal canal below the level of the partially removed pedicle. Reverse-angle currets and a mallet are used to pack the bone fragments back into the vertebral body, away from the neural elements. Intraoperative ultrasonography is then used to assess the adequacy of decompression. Posterolateral transpedicular decompression is safest at the level of the cauda equina, but it can be performed at more cephalic levels with the help of ultrasonography and monitoring of somatosensory evoked potentials. Intraoperative myelography may be used to assess the canal patency if there is any concern regarding the decompression, if ultrasound is unavailable.

Spinal Orthoses

Basic research has been carried out on spinal orthoses, but these studies have

866 Fractures of the Lumbar Spine

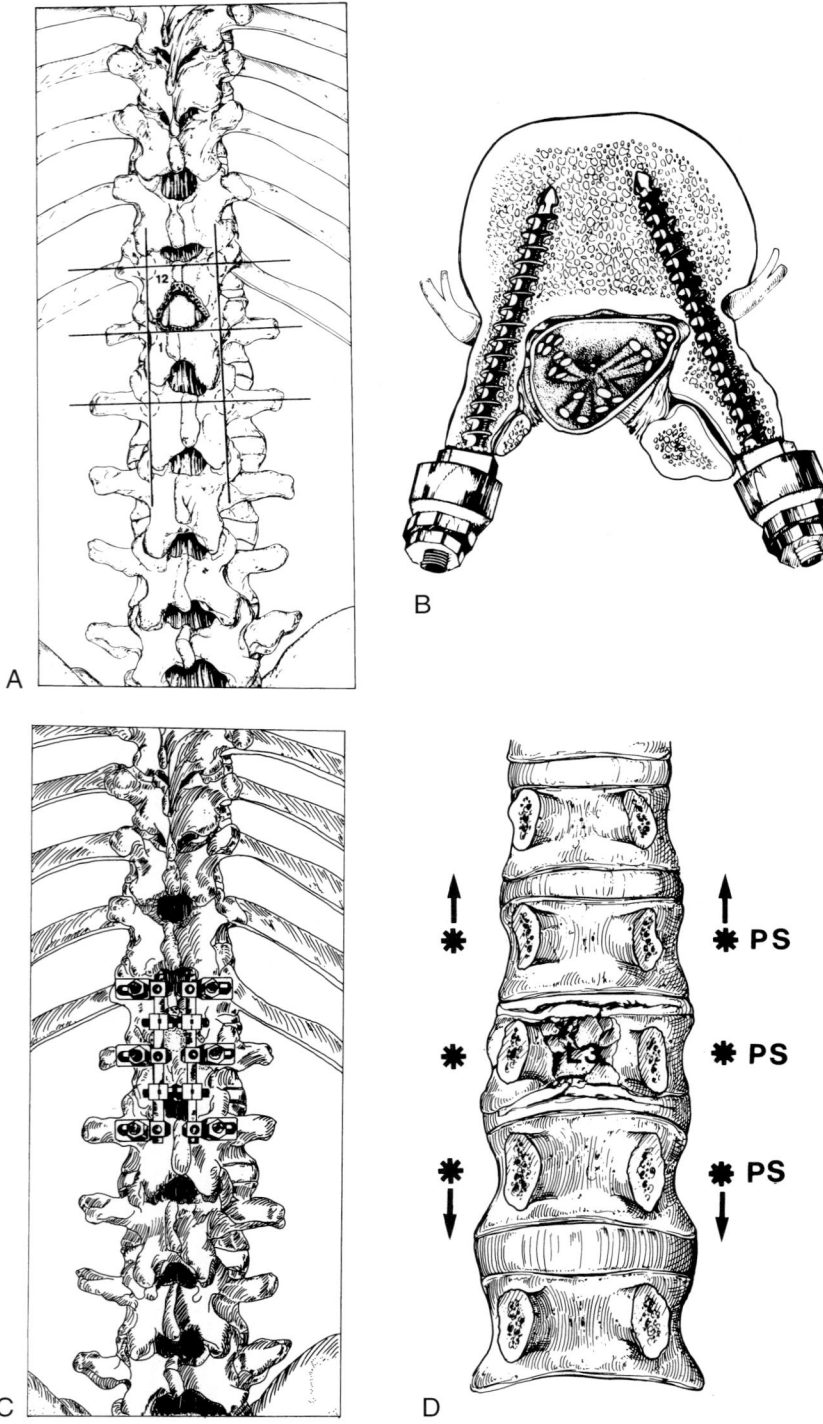

Figure 36 See legend on opposite page

tested devices in only small numbers of volunteers and most often with large variations in results among volunteers.[29, 52, 61, 64]

Some of the difficulties with research in this area have included exposure of volunteers to radiation[29, 61] and the requirement of invasive procedures such as placing Steinmann pins in the spinous processes of the volunteers.[52, 64] There has been no prospective clinical study of spinal orthoses in patients with spinal fractures that includes such information as the amount of motion allowed by the orthoses in different positions.

The available reviews show that braces can be effective in three different ways. First, they can physically restrain different spinal motions.[29, 30, 52, 64] Second, they can remind the patient to limit the spinal range of motion by causing discomfort over pressure points.[64] Third, braces can be effective by simply increasing the intraabdominal pressure, which tends to support the spine and divert weight-bearing forces away from the spine.[58, 61] Different braces apply different principles. A good general review has been published by the American Academy of Orthopaedic Surgeons.[30] Two disadvantages of all types of braces, over which the physician has little control, are patient obesity and patient compliance.

Three groups of patients with spinal fractures are commonly encountered. The first is the group with stable injuries for whom a brace is prescribed for comfort only. The second group, of greater clinical concern, consists of those who have minimum to moderate degrees of instability after a spinal injury and who can ambulate in a brace to minimize both the expense and the inconvenience of prolonged bed rest. The third group comprises those with moderate to severe degrees of spine instability who have undergone stabilization procedures and require a brace for protected mobilization. These three groups are now considered in relation to lumbar spinal injuries, including both the upper and lower lumbar spine.

Patients with Stable Spinal Fractures

In the group of patients with stable spinal fractures, braces may be prescribed to enhance comfort. For most, a wraparound type of lumbosacral orthosis is adequate to increase the patient's intraabdominal pressure and hence make the patient more comfortable.[61] This type of brace does not provide a significant degree of physical restraint. It may or may not provide pressure point discomfort to remind the patient to limit his or her range of motion.

Patients with Minimal to Moderate Degrees of Lumbar Spinal Instability

The group of patients with minimal to moderate degrees of spinal instability is of prime concern to clinicians. In addition to providing comfort for the patient, the goal is to prevent increasing spinal deformity and especially subsequent neurologic deterioration. Hence, this group of patients should be treated with braces that physically restrain the spine. For this purpose, a TLSO must be used. The clinician should determine the

---

Figure 36. The technique for pedicle screw instrumentation using the ISOLA system. *A*, The lines that proceed through the facet joints and adjacent to the pars interarticularis intersect with lines passed through the transverse processes to localize the center of the pedicles at each level. *B*, This transverse section shows the ideal location for the pedicle screws. It also shows the relationship of the screws to the neural elements both medial to and lateral to the pedicle screws. The inclination of each of these pedicles and screws changes depending on the level of the spine. There is normally 5 to 10 degrees of medial angulation at L1 and approximately 30 degrees of angulation at L5. (*A* and *B*, From Eismont, F. J., Garfin, S. R., and Abitbol, J. J.: Thoracic and upper lumbar spine injuries. *In* Browner, B. D., Jupiter, J. B., Levine, A. M., and Trafton, P. G. (eds.): Skeletal Trauma. Philadelphia, W. B. Saunders, 1992, pp. 729–803.) *C*, After the pedicle screws have been satisfactorily placed, the slotted connectors are placed over the screws and the rods are placed through the slotted connectors. Care must be taken that the slotted connector fits perfectly flush with each screw collar. Flat or angled washers may need to be used to achieve this. Appropriate lordosis should be applied to achieve a normal alignment of the spine. Nuts are tightened down over the slotted connectors loosely and the set screw connecting the rod to the slotted connector is then tightened securely, followed by a final tightening of the nut on the pedicle screw. The transverse connectors are then applied as shown. A final tightening of each screw and nut is then performed. *D*, This type of instrumentation is best for injuries of the middle and lower lumbar spine. Moderate distraction can then be achieved. Pedicle screws should be placed into the fractured vertebra whenever possible because this does add considerably to the strength of the construct.

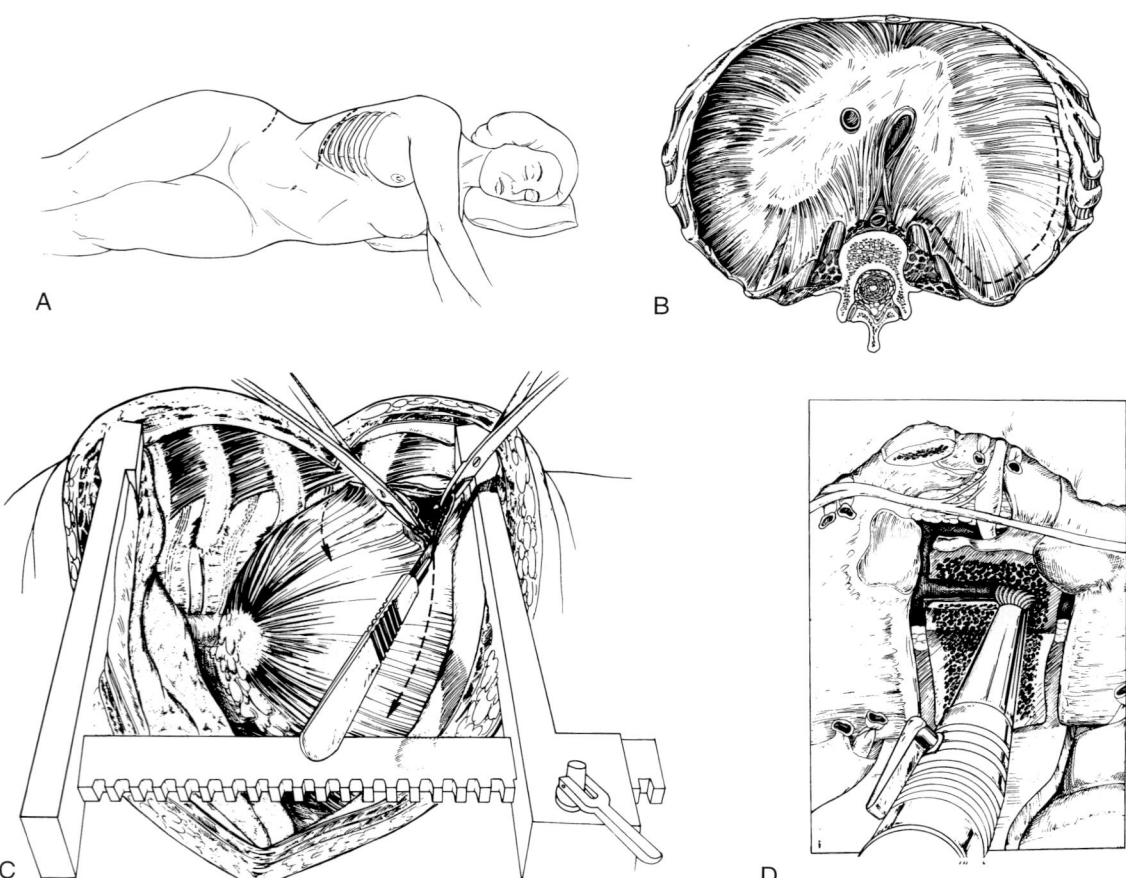

Figure 37. The anterior transthoracic approach to thoracolumbar and upper lumbar spinal injuries. *A*, The patient is positioned in the straight decubitus position. By having the patient straight up and not rolled to one side, the surgeon is always able to predict the position of the spinal canal in relation to the vertebral body and pedicles and hence to avoid inadvertent neural trauma because of disorientation. The incision is made over the 10th rib. The side of approach should be chosen on the basis of the preoperative CT scans. In most cases, a left-sided approach is easiest and safest. The pelvis is normally included in the operative field so an additional bone graft can be obtained if necessary. *B*, This transverse section looking down on the diaphragm shows how the diaphragm is cut approximately 1 cm from the chest wall to gain access to the retroperitoneal space. *C*, After the thoracotomy has been performed and a self-retaining retractor has been positioned, the incision in the diaphragm is made. This incision is normally made away from the spine and then advanced toward the spine. *D*, After the psoas muscle is retracted, the discs above and below the fractured vertebra are removed with a scalpel, curets, and rongeurs. The anteriormost portion of the vertebral body can be removed using gouges or osteotomes. The opposite side of the vertebral body can be left in place because this does not interfere with the decompression and facilitates bone healing afterward. After the posterior cortex has been approached and when the color of the bone within the vertebral body changes from red (cancellous) to white (cortical), the power bur is used to cut through the posterior vertebral body cortex into the spinal canal.

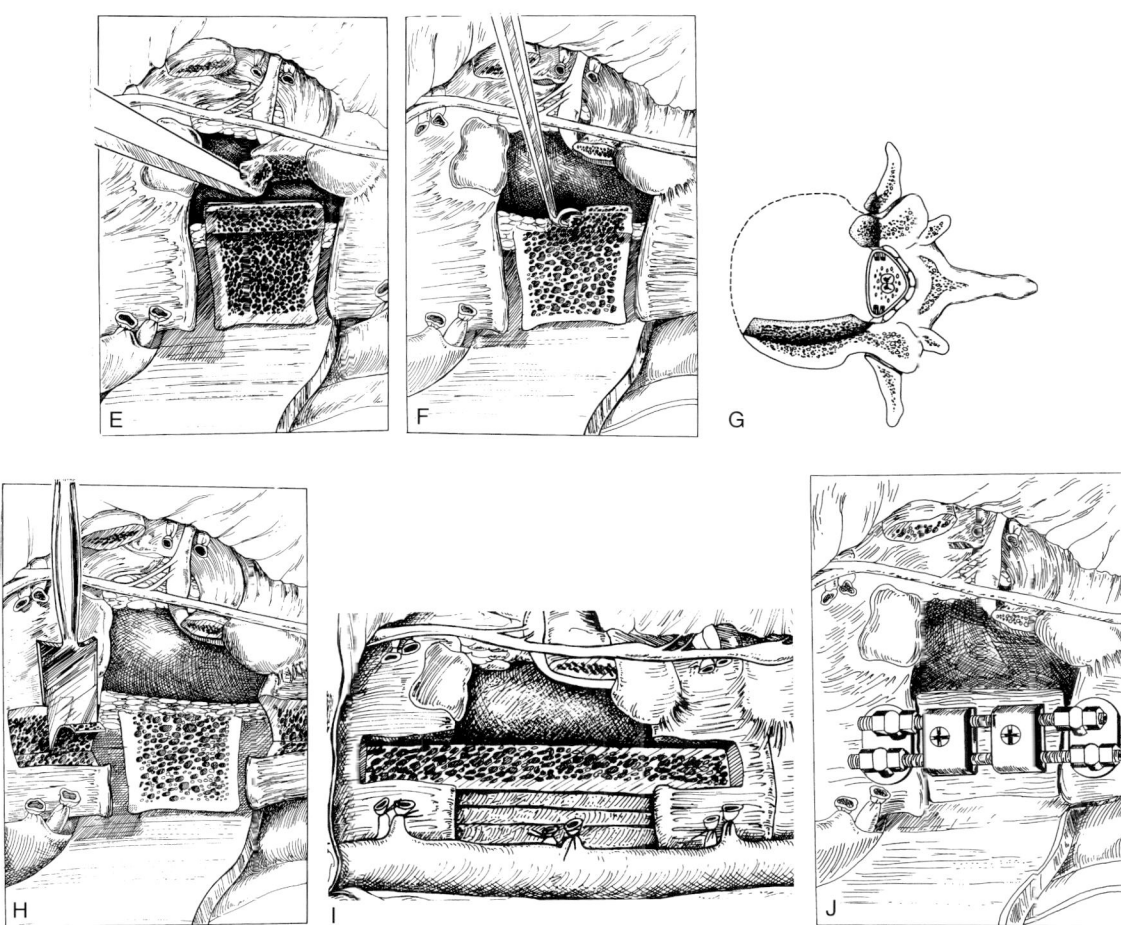

Figure 37 *Continued* E, Ninety-degree and 45-degree rongeurs are used to remove the bone from the spinal canal on the side from which the spine is approached. The pedicle can be located using an angled probe to orient the surgeon to the location of the nerve roots at that level. F, The opposite side of the spinal canal is decompressed using reverse-angle curets to scoop the bone away from the spinal canal. G, A transverse section at the level of decompression shows the extent of bone removal. Bone on the opposite side of the vertebral body can be left in place and facilitates eventual healing of the bone graft. The surgeon must be certain to decompress from pedicle to pedicle. The posterior longitudinal ligament is usually removed to be certain that the decompression is complete. H, If an in situ fusion is going to be performed, gouges or a power bur are used to cut a trough into the vertebral body above and the vertebral body below to lock the bone grafts in place. If instrumentation systems are going to be used anteriorly, these troughs into the vertebral bodies are not made because this significantly weakens the adjacent vertebral bodies. I, The bone graft after an in situ fusion is performed. A large iliac bone graft is placed in the posterior trough and impacted in place while pressure is applied posteriorly over the back of the spine to correct any kyphosis that might be present. The rib graft can be inserted anterior to the iliac graft as shown. (*A–I*, From Eismont, F. J., Garfin, S. R., and Abitbol, J. J.: Thoracic and upper lumbar spine injuries. *In* Browner, B. D., Jupiter, J. B., Levine, A. M., and Trafton, P. G. (eds.): Skeletal Trauma. Philadelphia, W. B. Saunders, 1992, pp. 729–803.) *J,* An anterior Kaneda device, which has been used to provide anterior rigid fixation after the decompression. A large full-thickness iliac graft is again used, but in this case it is not inserted into a trough in the cephalad and caudad vertebral bodies. Instead, after the vertebral body staples have been applied to the adjacent vertebrae and after the vertebral body screws have been inserted, a distractor is used to correct the kyphosis, and the adjacent cartilaginous end plates are removed, and a full-thickness iliac bone graft is inserted. Compression is then applied across the bone graft, and the uprights to the construct are then inserted. The posterior rod is first tightened, followed by the anterior rod. Two cross connectors are then applied from side to side to provide the needed rigidity. Plain films to assess the positioning of the staple and screws in the vertebral body, the reduction of the normal spinal alignment, and the positioning of the Kaneda device and bone graft are needed to ensure a satisfactory result.

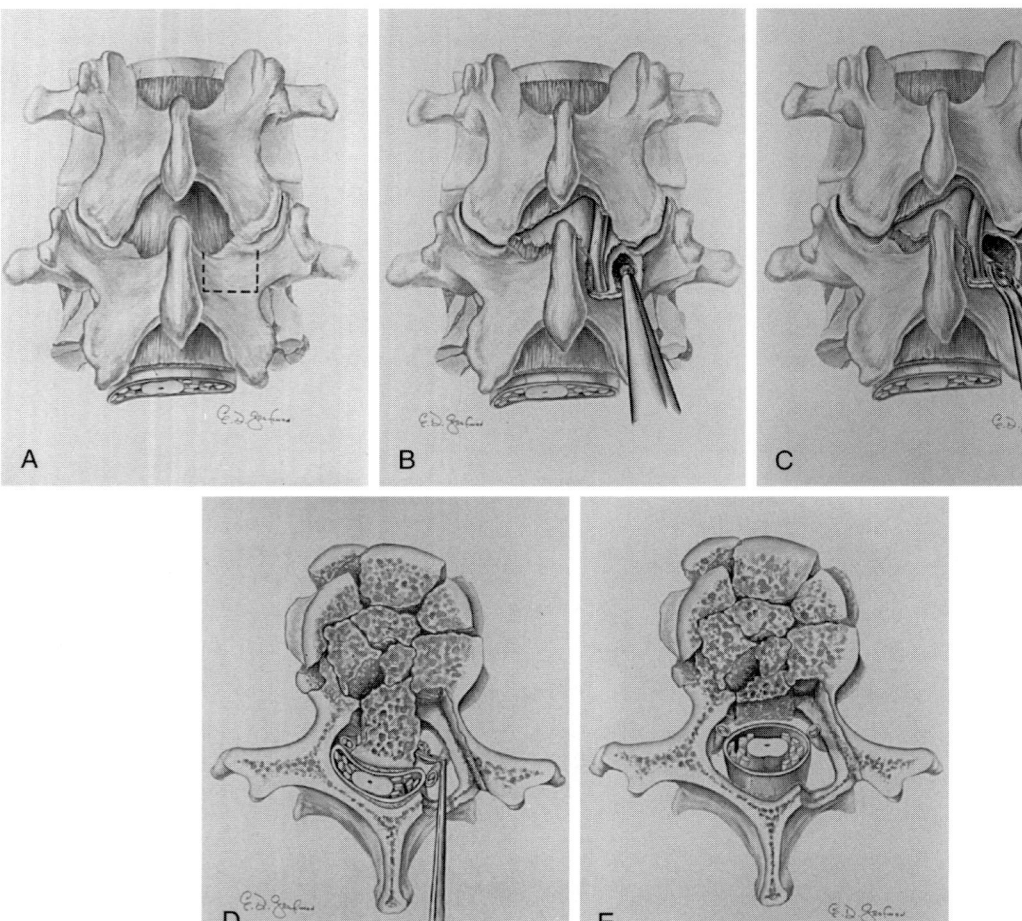

Figure 38. The technique for posterolateral decompression that would be used for treating an L1 burst fracture. *A*, Posterior elements of T12 and L1 are illustrated. The dotted lines indicate the bone that would be removed for a posterolateral decompression. *B*, Central laminotomy that has been performed to facilitate the use of intraoperative ultrasonography. The laminotomy has been extended into the L1 lamina on the side at which the decompression will be performed. After this laminotomy, a power bur is used to drill out the central portion of the pedicle, leaving a thin wall medially and a thicker wall laterally to maintain the continuity of the transverse process with the vertebral body. The drill hole is continued down into the vertebral body anteriorly. Care is taken to protect the nerve root exiting at the level of the pedicle. *C*, A fine rongeur is used to remove the remaining thin medial wall of the pedicle. Again, care is taken to identify and protect the nerve root exiting under that pedicle. *D*, A reverse-angled curet is introduced into the spinal canal lateral to the dural sac and the exiting nerve root. It is used to impact the bone fragments away from the neural elements. Intraoperative ultrasonography is useful to demonstrate whether there are residual bone fragments within the spinal canal and also to document whether the neural elements are being deformed by the bone fragments. *E*, The ideal final result, showing removal of all bone fragments from the spinal canal. The transverse process maintains continuity with the fractured vertebral body, which aids in achieving stability with a lateral fusion.

mechanism of injury from the patient's history, radiographic studies, and clinical examination, and the brace should be designed to prevent further deformity in the direction of injury. If a patient has a simple flexion injury, such as a compression fracture with no rotational instability, a TLSO flexion control brace such as a Jewett brace is adequate.

Many types of orthoses primarily utilize cloth with rigid stays; however these usually fail to provide adequate restraint.[30, 52, 64] The only brace that provides control of flexion, extension, lateral movement, and rotary movement is a TLSO made of a rigid synthetic, nonplastic material that has total contact over the rib cage, the lumbar spine posteriorly, and the pelvis inferiorly.[30] This can provide adequate support down to L4. Studies have indicated that to adequately immobilize the lumbosacral junction (and this should include significant L5 vertebral fractures), a thigh extension must be included to lock the hip in a neutral position.[29] Reviews have shown that if braces do not immobilize the hip joint, there may actually be compensatory increased movement at the lumbosacral junction with attempts at flexion and extension.[64] Disadvantages of the total-contact individually fitted TLSO are that it must be custom-made (and is therefore more expensive) and it usually requires several days for fabrication. Compared with the TLSO flexion control brace, it is also more difficult to remove and apply, and the patient may need assistance. In the past, emphasis has been placed on adequate relief at all bony prominences in patients with insensate skin. The authors have not found this to be a problem, even in patients with complete paralysis in the lumbar spine, because the skin sensation over the torso remains normal in these patients.

Moderate to Severe Instability in Patients Treated Surgically

The considerations that were discussed for patients with minimal to moderate degrees of instability to patients with moderate to severe instability also apply. If the surgeon is pleased with the degree of stability achieved intraoperatively, the brace may be prescribed for comfort only, in which case simply increasing the intraabdominal pressure may be adequate. Various degrees of physical restraint may also be required, in which case a TLSO flexion control brace, a total-contact TLSO, or even a total-contact TLSO with locked thigh extension may be required.

REFERENCES

1. Aebi, M., Etter, C., Kehl, T., and Thalgott, J.: Stabilization of the lower thoracic and lumbar spine with internal spinal skeletal fixation system. Indication, techniques and first results of treatment. Spine 12:544–551, 1987.
2. Armstrong, G.: Personal communication.
3. Ballock, R. T., MacKenzie, R. Abitbol, J. J., et al.: Can burst fractures be predicted from plain radiographs? J. Bone Joint Surg. 74B:147–153, 1992.
4. Bedbrook, G. M.: Stability of spinal fractures and fracture dislocations. Paraplegia 9:23–32, 1970.
5. Bedbrook, G. M.: Treatment of thoracolumbar dislocation and fractures with paraplegia. Clin. Orthop. 112:27–43, 1975.
6. Begeman, P. C., King, A. L., and Prasad, P.: Spinal injuries resulting from −Gx acceleration. In Proceedings of the 17th STAPP Car Crash Conference. New York, Society of Automotive Engineers, 1973, pp. 343–360.
7. Bell, G. H., Dunbar, O., Beck, J. S., and Gibb, A.: Variation in strength of vertebrae with change and their relation to osteoporosis. Calcif. Tissue Res. 1:75–86, 1987.
8. Bradford, D. S., and McBride, G. G.: Surgical management of thoraco-lumbar spine fractures with incomplete neurologic deficits. Clin. Orthop. 218:201–216, 1987.
9. Brightman, R. P., Miller, C. A., and Hunt, W. E.: MRI of spinal trauma: Imaging of the anterior and posterior longitudinal ligaments. Presented at the 14th Annual Scientific Meeting of the American Spinal Injury Association, San Diego, CA, May 2–4, 1988.
10. Brown, T., Hanson, R., and Yorra, A.: Some mechanical tests on the lumbosacral spine with particular reference to the intervertebral disc. J. Bone Joint Surg. 39A:1135–1164, 1957.
11. Calenoff, L., Chessare, J. W., Rogers, L. F., et al.: Multiple level spinal injuries: Importance of early recognition. AJR 130:665–669, 1978.
12. Cammisa, F. P., Eismont, F. J., and Green, B. A.: Dural laceration occurring with burst fractures and associated laminar fractures J. Bone Joint Surg. 71A:1044–1052, 1989.
13. Cantor, J. B., Lebwohl, N. H., Garvey, T., and Eismont, F. J.: Nonoperative management of stable thoracolumbar burst fractures with early ambulation and bracing. Spine 18:971–976, 1993.
14. Chance, G. Q.: Note on a type of flexion fracture of the spine. Br. J. Radiol. 21:452–453, 1948.
15. Cotler, H. B.: Magnetic resonance imaging in acute spinal cord injury. Presented at the 14th Annual Scientific Meeting of the American Spinal Injury Association, San Diego, CA, May 2–4, 1988.
16. Court-Brown, C. M., and Gertzbein, S. D.: Flexion/distraction injuries of the lumbar spine. Clin. Orthop. 227:52–60, 1988.
17. Court-Brown, C. M., and Gertzbein, S D.: Burst fractures of the fifth lumbar vertebra. Spine 12:305–312, 1987.
18. Davies, D. V. (Ed.): Gray's Descriptive and Applied Anatomy, 34th Ed. London, Longmans, Green and Co., 1967.
19. Davies, W. E., Morris, J. H., and Hill, V.: An analysis of conservative (non-surgical) management of thoracolumbar fractures and fracture/dislocations with neurological damage. J. Bone Joint Surg. 62A:1324–1328, 1980.
20. Denis, F.: Three column spine and its significance in the classification of acute thoracolumbar spinal injuries. Spine 8:817–831, 1983.
21. Denis, F., Armstrong, C. W., Searls, K., et al.: Acute thoracolumbar burst fractures in the absence of neurological deficit. A comparison between operative and non-operative treatment. Clin. Orthop. 189:142–149, 1984.
22. de Oliviera, J. C.: A new type of fracture/dislocation of the thoracolumbar spine. J. Bone Joint Surg. 68:481–488, 1978.

23. Dickson, J. H., Harrington, T. R., and Erwin, W. D.: Results of reduction and stabilization of the severely fractured thoracic and lumbar spine. J. Bone Joint Surg. 60A:799–805, 1978.
24. Dunn, H. K.: Anterior spine stabilization and decompression for thoracolumbar injuries. Orthop. Clin. North Am. 17:113–119, 1986.
25. Edwards, C. C., and Levine, A. M.: Early rod sleeve stabilization of the injured thoracic and lumbar spine. Orthop. Clin. North Am. 17:121–145, 1986.
26. Eismont, F. J., Green, B. A., Berkowitz, B. M., et al.: The role of intraoperative ultrasonography in the treatment of thoracic and lumbar spine fractures. Spine 9:782–787, 1984.
27. Eismont, F. J., Morse, B., Post, J. D., et al.: Intraoperative ultrasonography of the lumbar spine. Presented at the International Society for the Study of the Lumbar Spine Meeting, Montreal, June 3–7, 1984.
28. Ferguson, R. L., and Allen, D. L.: A mechanistic classification of thoracolumbar spine fractures. Clin. Orthop. 189:77–88, 1984.
29. Fidler, M. W., and Plasmans, C. M. T.: The effect of four types of support on the segmental mobility of the lumbosacral spine. J. Bone Joint Surg. 65A:943, 1983.
30. Fishman, S., Berger, N., Edelstein, J. E., and Springer, W. P.: Spinal Orthoses. In American Academy of Orthopaedic Surgeons. Atlas of Orthotics, 2nd Ed. St. Louis, C. V. Mosby, 1985, pp. 238–256.
31. Frankel, H. L., Hancock, D. O., Hyslop, G., et al.: The value of postural reduction in the initial management of closed injuries of the spine with paraplegia and tetraplegia. Paraplegia 7:179–192, 1969.
32. Fredrickson, B. E., Yuan, H. A., and Miller, H.: Burst fractures of the fifth lumbar vertebra. A report of four cases. J. Bone Joint Surg. 64A:1088–1094, 1982.
33. Gertzbein, S. D.: In Stauffer, E. S. (ed.): Thoracolumbar Fractures without Neurological Deficit. Chicago, American Academy of Orthopaedic Surgeons, 1993.
34. Gertzbein, S. D.: Classification of thoracic and lumbar fractures. In Gertzbein, S. D. (ed.): Fractures of the Thoracic and Lumbar Spine. Baltimore, Williams & Wilkins, 1993, Ch. 3.
35. Gertzbein, S. D., and Court-Brown, C. M.: Rationale for the management of flexion/distraction injuries of the thoracolumbar spine based on a new classification. Spine 13:892–895, 1988.
36. Gertzbein, S. D., and Evans, D. C.: Femoral nerve neuropathy complicating iliopsoas hemorrhage in patients without hemophilia. J. Bone Joint Surg. 54B:149–151, 1972.
37. Gertzbein, S. D., Court-Brown, C. M., Jacobs, R. R., et al.: Neurological outcome following surgery for fractures of the thoracic and lumbar spine. Spine 13:641–644, 1988.
38. Gertzbein, S. D., Jacob, R. R., Stoll, J., et al.: Decompression and circumferential stabilization of unstable spinal fractures. Spine 13:892–895, 1988.
39. Green, B. A., and Callahan, R. A.: A radiological approach to acute spinal cord injury. In Post, J. D. (ed.): Radiographic Evaluation of the Spine: Current Advances with Emphasis on Computed Tomography. New York, Masson, 1980, p. 3.
40. Gumley, G., Taylor, T. K. F., and Ryan, M. D.: Distraction fractures of the lumbar spine. J. Bone Joint Surg. 64B:520–525, 1982.
41. Guttman, L.: Spinal Injuries. Folia Traumatologica Geigy, 1972.
42. Hall, H. E., and Robertson, W. W.: Another Chance: A non–seat belt related fracture of the lumbar spine. J. Trauma 25:1163–1166, 1985.
43. Holdsworth, F. W.: Fractures, dislocations and fracture/dislocations of the spine. J. Bone Joint Surg. 45B:6–20, 1962.
44. Howland, W. J., Curry, J. L., and Buffington, C. B.: Fulcrum fractures of the lumbar spine. JAMA 193:140–141, 1965.
45. Jacobs, R. R., Asher, M. A., and Snider, R. K.: Thoracolumbar spinal injuries. A comparison study of recumbent and operative treatment in 100 patients. Spine 5:463–477, 1980.
46. Keene, J. S., Wackwitz, D. L., Drummond, D. S., and Breed, A. L.: Compression-distraction instrumentation of unstable thoraco-lumbar fractures: Anatomic results obtained with each type of injury and method of instrumentation. Spine 11:898–902, 1986.
47. Kelly, R. P., and Whitesides, T. E.: Treatment of lumbodorsal fracture-dislocations. Ann. Surg. 167:705–717, 1968.
48. Krompinger, W. J., Fredrickson, B. E., Mino, D. E., and Yuan, H. A.: Conservative treatment of fractures of the thoracic and lumbar spine. Orthop. Clin. North Am. 17:161–170, 1986.
49. Krompinger, W. J., Yuan, H. A., Fredrickson, B. E., et al.: Non-surgical management of thoracic and lumbar fractures in neurologically intact patients: CT evidence of reabsorption of bony canal compromise. In Transactions of the 12th Annual Meeting of the International Society for the Study of the Lumbar Spine, Sydney, Australia, April 14, 1985, p. 75.
50. Lavernia, C. J., Botte, M. J., and Garfin, S. R.: Spinal orthoses for traumatic and degenerative disease. In Rothman, R. H., and Simeone F. A. (eds.): The Spine, 3rd Ed. Philadelphia, W. B. Saunders, 1992.
51. Lindahl, O.: Mechanical properties of dried, defatted, spongy bone. Acta Orthop. Scand. 47:11–16, 1976.
52. Lumsden, R. M., and Morris, M. M.: An in vivo study of axial rotation and immobilization at the lumbosacral joint. J. Bone Joint Surg. 50A:1591–1597, 1968.
53. Magerl, F., and Harms, D.: Classification of thoracic and lumbar fractures. Presented at the Spine Trauma Section, Société Internationale de Chirurgie Orthopédie et Traumatologie, August, 1987, Munich, Germany.
54. Magerl, F., Harms, J., Gertzbein, S. D., et al.: A comprehensive classification of thoracic and lumbar injuries. Eur. Spine J. 3:184–201, 1994.
55. McAfee, P. C., Bohlman, H. H., and Yuan, H. A.: Anterior decompression of traumatic thoracolumbar fractures with incomplete neurological deficit using a retroperitoneal approach. J. Bone Joint Surg. 67A:89–104, 1985.
56. McAfee, P. C., Yuan, H. A., Fredrickson, B. E., et al.: The value of computed tomography in thoracolumbar fractures. An analysis of 100 consecutive cases and a new classification. J. Bone Joint Surg. 65A:461–473, 1983.
57. McAfee, P. C., Yuan, H. A., and Lasda, N. A.: The unstable burst fracture. Spine 4:365–373, 1982.

58. McCollough, N. C., III: Biomechanical analysis of the spine. In American Academy of Orthopaedic Surgeons, Committee on Prosthetics and Orthotics: Atlas of Orthotics, Biomechanical Principles and Application. St. Louis, C. V. Mosby, 1975.
59. McEvoy, R. D., and Bradford, D. S.: The management of burst fractures of the thoracic and lumbar spine: Experience in 53 patients. Spine 10:631–637, 1985.
60. Miller, C. A., Dewey, R. C., and Hunt, W. E.: Impaction fracture of the lumbar vertebrae with dural tear. J. Neurosurg. 53:765–771, 1980.
61. Morris, J. M., Lucas, D. B., and Bresler, B.: Role of the trunk in stability of the spine. J. Bone Joint Surg. 43A:327, 1961.
62. Mumford, J., Weinstein, J. N. Spratt, K. F., and Goel, V. K.: Thoracolumbar burst fractures: The clinical efficacy and outcome of nonoperative management. AcroMed Award Paper. Spine 18:955–970, 1993.
63. Nicoll, E. A.: Fractures of the dorsolumbar spine. J. Bone Joint Surg. 31B:376–394, 1949.
64. Norton, P. L., and Brown, T.: The immobilizing efficiency of back braces: Their effect on the posture and motion of the lumbosacral spine. J. Bone Joint Surg. 39A:111, 1957.
65. Noyes, F. R., Torvin, P. J., Hyde, W. B., and LeLucas, J. L.: Biomechanics of ligament failure: An analysis of immobilization, exercise and reconditioning effects in primates. J. Bone Joint Surg. 56A:1406–1418, 1974.
66. Panjabi, M. M., White, A. A., and Johnson, R. M.: Cervical spine mechanics as a function of transection of components. J. Biomech 8:327–336, 1975.
67. Perey, O.: Fractures of the vertebral end plate in the lumbar spine. Acta Orthop. Scand. 25(Suppl.): 237–238, 1957.
68. Porter, R. A., Hibbert, C. S., and Wicks, M.: The spinal canal in symptomatic lumbar disc lesions. J. Bone Joint Surg. 60B:485–487, 1978.
69. Purcell, G. A., Markolf, K. L., and Dawson, E. G.: Twelfth thoracic first lumbar vertebral mechanical instability of fractures after Harrington rod instrumentation. J. Bone Joint Surg. 53A:71–78, 1981.
70. Quencer, R. M., Montalvo, B. M., Eismont, F. J., and Green, B. A.: Intraoperative spinal sonography in thoracic and lumbar fractures: Evaluation of Harrington rod instrumentation. AJNR 6:353–359, 1985.
71. Rockoff, S. D., Sweet, E., and Bleustein, J.: The relative contribution of trabecular and cortical bone to the strength of human and lumbar vertebrae. Calcif. Tissue Res. 3:163–175, 1969.
72. Roy-Camille, R., Saillant, G., and Mazel, C.: Plating of thoracic, thoracolumbar and lumbar injuries with pedicle screw plates. Orthop. Clin. North Am. 17:147–159, 1986.
73. Ryan, M. D., and Taylor, T. K. F.: The early management of thoracolumbar fractures by ORIF. Aust. N. Z. J. Surg. 52:236–244, 1982.
74. Smith, W. S., and Kaufer, H.: Patterns and mechanisms of lumbar injuries associated with lap seat belts. J. Bone Joint Surg. 51A:239–259, 1969.
74a. Stagnara, P., Demauroy, J. V., Dran, G., et al.: Reciprocal angulation of vertebral bodies in a sagittal plane: Approach to references for the evaluation of kyphosis and lordosis. Spine 7:335–342, 1982.
75. Tile, M.: Fractures of the Pelvis and Acetabulum. Baltimore, Williams & Wilkins, 1984.
76. Weaver, J. K., and Chalmers, J.: Bone: Its strength and changes with aging and an evaluation of some methods for measuring its mineral content. J. Bone Joint Surg. 41A:935–941, 1961.
77. Weinstein, J., Collalto, P., and Lehmann, T.: Thoracolumbar burst fractures treated conservatively: A long-term followup. Spine 13:33–38, 1983.
78. White, A. A., and Panjabi, M. M.: Clinical Biomechanics of the Spine. Philadelphia, J. B. Lippincott, 1978.
79. White, A. A., and Panjabi, M. M.: The basic kinematics of the human spine—a review of past and current knowledge. Spine 3:12–20, 1978.
80. Whitesides, T. E., Jr.: Traumatic kyphosis of the thoracolumbar spine. Clin. Orthop. 128:78–92, 1972.
81. Whitesides, T. E., and Ali Shan, S. G. On the management of unstable fractures of the thoracolumbar spine: Rationale for use of anterior decompression and fusion and posterior stabilization. Spine 1:99, 1976.
82. Willen, J., Lindahl, S., Irstram, L., and Nordwall, A.: Unstable thoracolumbar fractures. A study by CT and conventional roentgenology of the reduction effect of Harrington instrumentation. Spine 9:214–219, 1984.
83. Young, J. S., and Dexter, W. R.: Neurological recovery distal to the zone of injury in 172 cases of closed, traumatic spinal cord injury. Paraplegia 16:39–49, 1978.
84. Zindrick, M. R., Wiltse, L. L., Doornik, A., et al.: Analysis of the morphometric characteristics of the thoracic and lumbar pedicles. Spine 12:160–166, 1987.

13

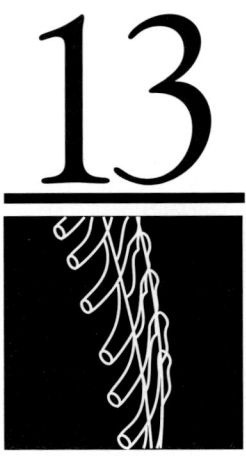

Spinal Infections

Pyogenic and Tuberculous Infections

JOHN C. Y. LEONG
KEITH D. K. LUK

The following discussion deals mainly with tuberculosis and pyogenic infections of the spine. Other rare or unusual infections occur, but only a short description of them is given here.

Infection of the spine is not an uncommon disease. The frequency of tuberculosis relative to pyogenic infection varies among countries. Poor social conditions, poor environmental hygiene, and a dense population tend to favor the development of tuberculosis. Pyogenic infection, on the other hand, is less influenced by such factors. Therefore, in so-called advanced countries tuberculosis is seen less often, but it does exist. Its relative rarity has unfortunately decreased the awareness of the condition and led to a marked delay in its diagnosis.[52] The disease has been emerging again because of immigration from third-world countries, chronically debilitating conditions such as alcoholism, and immunocompromised patients such as those with acquired immunodeficiency syndrome (AIDS). Pyogenic infections may present in otherwise healthy individuals, patients with a septic focus elsewhere in the body, and frequently in drug addicts.

The main controversies surrounding spinal infection are about conservative and surgical treatment; if surgical treatment is indicated, they are also about the extent of excision of the diseased focus and the use of bone grafts to achieve a solid fusion.

TUBERCULOSIS OF THE SPINE

Tuberculosis of the spine is a secondary infection. The primary lesion may be in the lung (Ghon focus), the alimentary tract, or the tonsil. The primary focus is small but evokes a marked regional lymph node response; together, these features are called the primary complex. This may occur in childhood with reactivation in adulthood, or it may occur in adulthood de novo.

Over 1000 cases of tuberculosis of the spine were studied from 1955 to 1960 at the University of Hong Kong. The distribution according to level of involvement is seen in Figure 1. Although the frequency per year has dropped to about 20 cases, the pattern

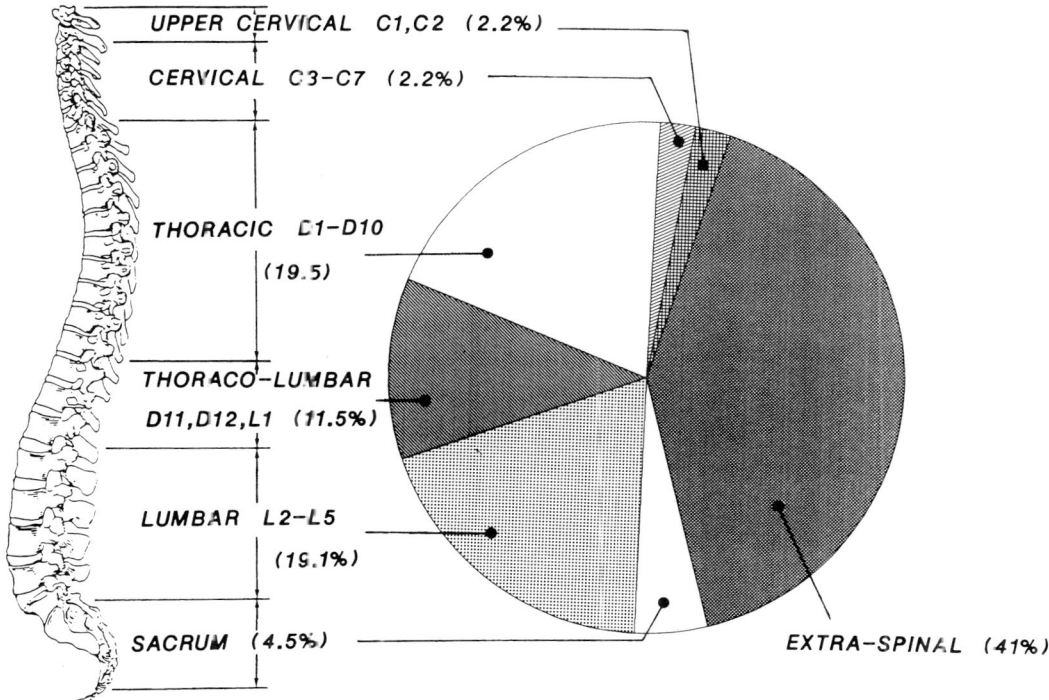

Figure 1. Distribution of spinal and extraspinal bone and joint tuberculosis by site in over 1000 cases studied from 1955 to 1960.

continues. The most common site is therefore the thoracolumbar region. The three main patterns of clinical presentation are as follows:

1. Typical presentation—The classic clinical features include back pain and a gibbus. Other features may be present, such as an abscess in the loin, groin, trochanteric area, or the buttock; paraplegia or paraparesis may occur, with or without bladder and bowel involvement. In young children with high thoracic involvement, a paraspinal abscess may lead to bronchial compression and irritation, and a symptom known as Millar asthma (simulating asthmatic bronchitis) occurs when the patient lies down at night.
2. Atypical presentation—Involvement of the neural arch alone, an epidural abscess, or extensive external pachymeningitis, without significant anterior vertebral involvement, is rare. The clinical features are significantly different. Paraparesis or paraplegia occurs much more commonly, and may be highly spastic, simulating a spinal cord tumor. External pachymeningitis with resulting arachnoiditis may produce a picture of fluctuating neurologic deficit.
3. Presentation with a difficult clinical problem.
   a. Kyphosis—Severe angular kyphosis occurs with marked pulmonary function restriction. It may be associated with paraplegia of spontaneous onset.
   b. Reactivation in old age[25]—Another difficult situation is one in which extensive spinal tuberculosis has occurred during early adulthood, a full course of antituberculous chemotherapy has been administered for conservative treatment, and the disease is deemed to be cured. Significant kyphosis has resulted because of the extent of the disease. Some 30 to 40 years later, the disease is reactivated, and there may or may not be cord compression. Patients in this age group have osteoporotic bone, and after surgical excision of the diseased tissue, the stable seating of bone grafts is extremely difficult to achieve.
   c. Disease affecting the lumbosacral

junction[42]—Surgical access is difficult to obtain in this area. On the other hand, conservative treatment is usually followed by a kyphotic deformity. Besides being unsightly, this leads to compensatory hyperlordosis above the junction, which is frequently associated with significant low back pain.

Pott Paraplegia

Sorrel and Sorrel-Dejerine[49] classified paraplegia or paraparesis due to tuberculosis of the spine into the following groups: (1) paraplegia of early onset and (2) paraplegia of late onset. Hodgson and Yau[19] proposed a classification based on the in vivo pathologic process. From direct observation of the pathologic process during anterior radical resection and spinal fusion, they classified patients as follows: (1) those with paraplegia of active disease and (2) those with paraplegia of healed disease.

In paraplegia of active disease, there is direct cord compression by the tuberculous abscess, caseous material, necrotic bone, and sometimes sequestered disc. Subluxation and concertina collapse of the vertebral body may also cause pressure. Spinal artery thrombosis may also cause paraplegia (*unrelated* to pressure). When there is external pachymeningitis, direct involvement of the dura and even of the spinal cord leads to a severe and spastic form of paraplegia.[16] This may sometimes be mistaken for a spinal cord tumor.

Paraplegia of healed disease has a different pathogenesis. In patients with significant destruction of the vertebral body, especially if more than one or two levels are affected, the spine tends to become markedly kyphotic. Even if healing occurs, either as a spontaneous process or as a result of conservative treatment with chemotherapy, the newly formed bone at the diseased site is soft, and the effect of gravity tends to exaggerate the kyphosis. There may also be

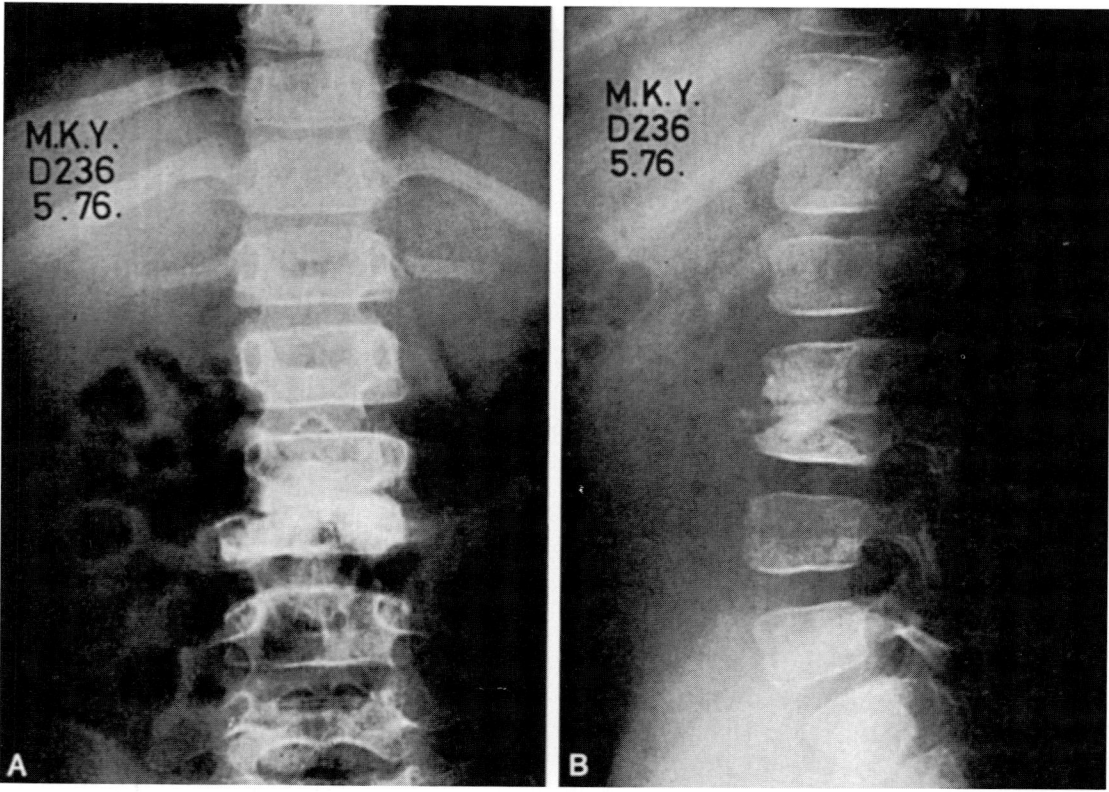

Figure 2. *A*, Anteroposterior x-ray film showing early disc narrowing in tuberculosis of the spine. *B*, Lateral x-ray film showing early disc space narrowing.

Diagnosis

Radiographic Appearances

The disease may affect the following main sites in the vertebrae: (1) the paradiscal region, (2) the center of the vertebral body, and (3) the anterior aspect of the vertebral body.[18] Involvement of the paradiscal region is most common. Paradiscal disease is usually present on either side of the intervertebral disc, leading to early narrowing of the disc (Fig. 2A,B). When the center of the vertebral body is involved, a concertina collapse occurs (Fig. 3), commonly associated with paraplegia. This type of change is more common in children. Involvement of the anterior aspect of the vertebral body is due to extension of a paravertebral abscess which strips the periosteum and ligaments away from the spine with the peripheral periosteal blood supply. The disease then attacks this devitalized bone and leads to anterior scalloping. This is sometimes referred to as an aneurysmal syndrome (Fig. 4). It is most

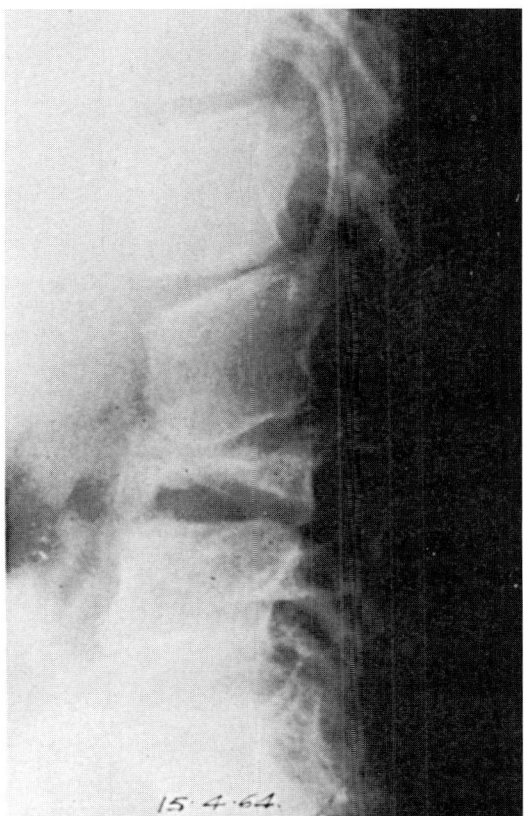

Figure 3. Concertina collapse of L3 vertebra in tuberculosis of the spine.

repeated microfatigue fracturing of the newly formed bone. Gradually, the latter becomes consolidated, but in the process, it is being slowly retropulsed posteriorly, forming an internal ridge. This causes pressure on the anterior aspect of the spinal cord.

Hsu and coworkers[21] confirmed that the pathologic process of active disease causes paraplegia of early onset. They also showed that, in paraplegia of late onset, a combination of active and healed disease or healed disease alone may be present. Hodgson and coworkers[20] found that anterior decompression and spinal fusion for Pott paraplegia due to active disease led to rapid recovery of the paraplegia in the majority of patients. Hsu and colleagues[21] showed that, in paraplegia of late onset, the prognosis is significantly worse in patients with healed disease compared with the case for those who have active disease. Surgical decompression of healed disease is technically difficult, and the outcome is also markedly less favorable.

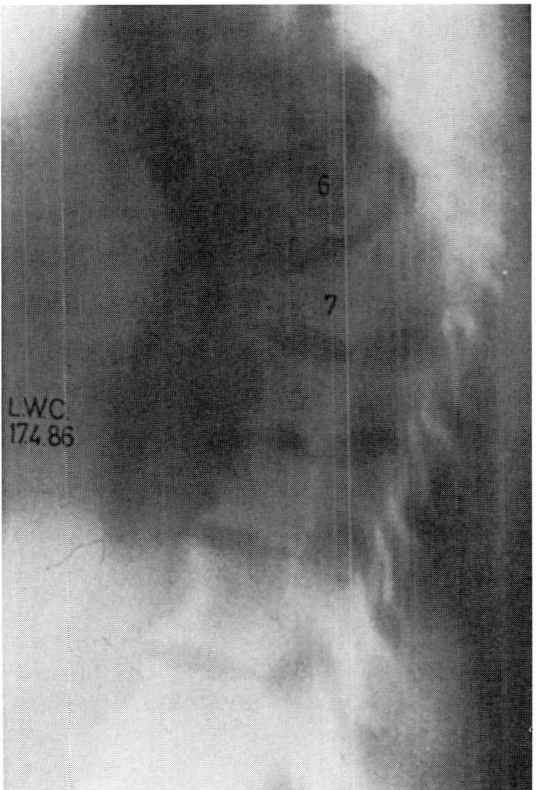

Figure 4. Aneurysmal syndrome affecting T6–T7 in tuberculosis of the spine.

common in the thoracic spine and in children.

Tuberculous infection rarely involves the transverse processes, the pedicles, the laminae, or the spinal processes. When it does, it falls into the group of patients with atypical presentation.

Malalignment of the spine may result from the disease, including scoliosis (sometimes mistaken for a hemivertebra [Fig. 5]), bayonet deformity (Fig. 6A,B), subluxation and dislocation (Fig. 7), and in the lower lumbar region, a reversed spondylolisthesis (Fig. 8). Subluxation or dislocation occurs when there is destruction of two or three vertebrae. In the dorsolumbar region, the anterior surface of the lowest thoracic vertebra or disc attached to it comes to lie on the upper surface of the first remaining lumbar vertebra or the disc. Reversed spondylolisthesis occurs because narrowing of the intervertebral disc causes the vertebral bodies to become closer together. The inclination of the facet joints dictates that the upper body moves backward on the lower ones.

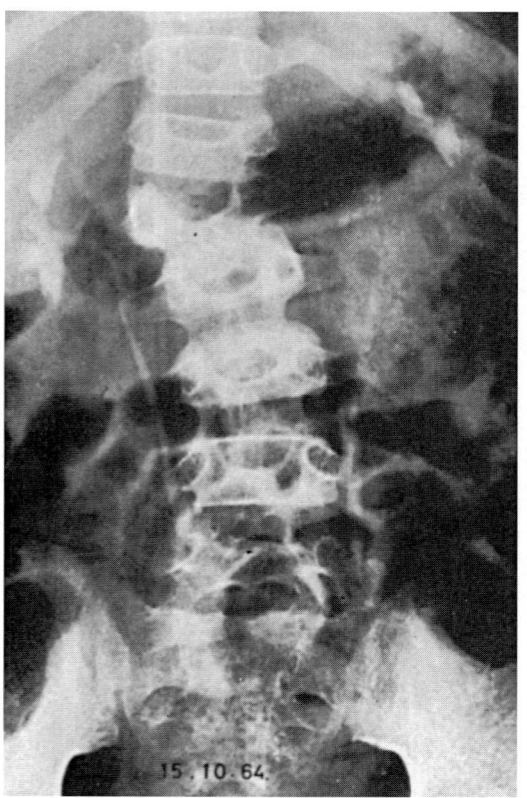

Figure 5. Tuberculosis of the spine mimicking a hemivertebra.

In the lumbar spine, another radiographic feature may be present. This is a bony bridging across the sides of two adjacent vertebrae. Masmonteil and Beclere[28] named it becs de perroquet. It is probably a true ossification of the paravertebral ligaments, possibly occurring as a response to infection.

A paravertebral abscess is commonly seen in the cervical, cervicodorsal, and thoracic regions. In the lumbar spine, however, because of the multiple origins of the psoas muscle arising from the vertebral bodies and intervertebral discs, the pus passes through a small opening to form an abscess in the psoas muscle. The psoas abscess does not show up well on plain x-ray films. If the disease affects the L5 vertebra or the sacrum, a presacral abscess forms, which again is difficult to detect by plain x-ray films, unless calcification has occurred.

Magnetic Resonance Imaging

Magnetic resonance imaging (MRI), although considerably more expensive than plain x-ray studies, is useful for the following reasons:

1. It has a higher sensitivity than do plain x-ray films in early lesions.
2. It can give some degree of differentiation between tuberculous and pyogenic spondylitis.
3. It is particularly useful in demonstrating paraspinal soft tissue abscesses and epidural extension as well as meningeal involvement.

Early in the disease process, T1-weighted images show decreased signal intensity from the affected vertebral marrow, and T2-weighted images show increased signal intensity (Fig. 9B). The cortical definition of involved vertebrae is invariably lost in tuberculous spondylitis[47] (Fig. 9A) in contradistinction to the case with pyogenic spondylitis. Enhanced MRI studies after intravenous injection of gadolinium are useful to categorize tuberculous spondylitis, especially to show epidural extension and meningeal involvement. There is evidence that rim enhancement around intraosseous and soft tissue abscesses is diagnostic of tuberculous infections (Fig. 9C).

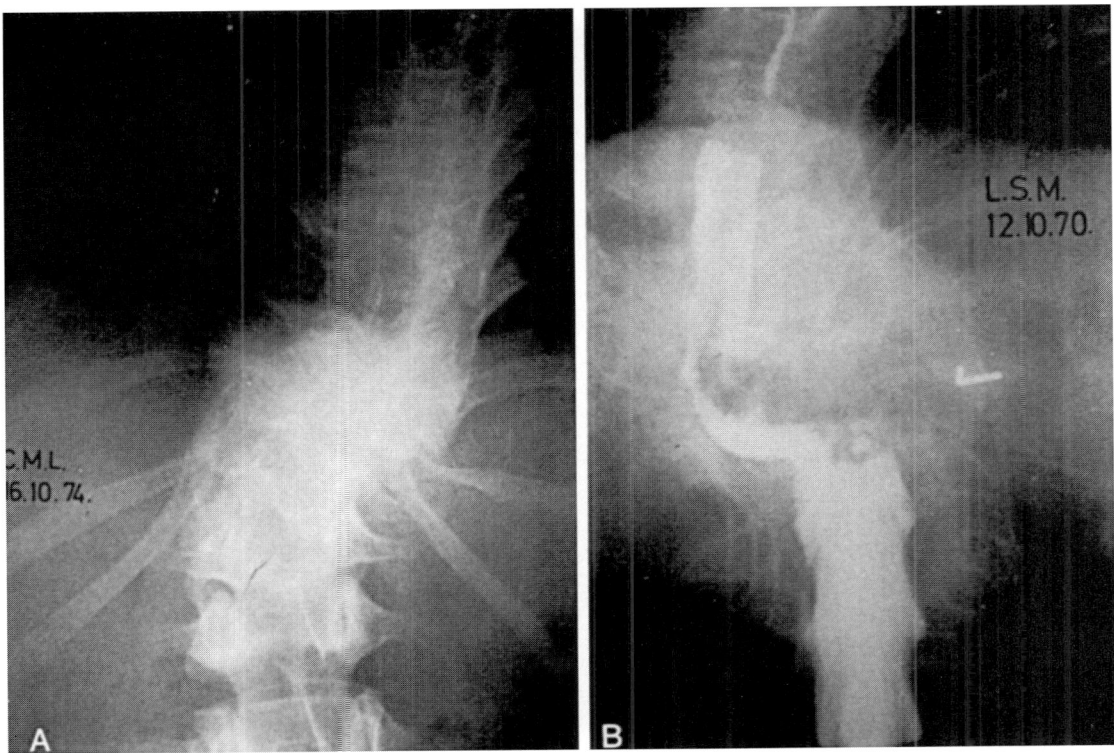

Figure 6. *A*, Bayonet deformity in tuberculosis of the spine. *B*, Myelogram of a different patient showing the same deformity.

Figure 7. Dorsolumbar subluxation in tuberculosis of the spine.

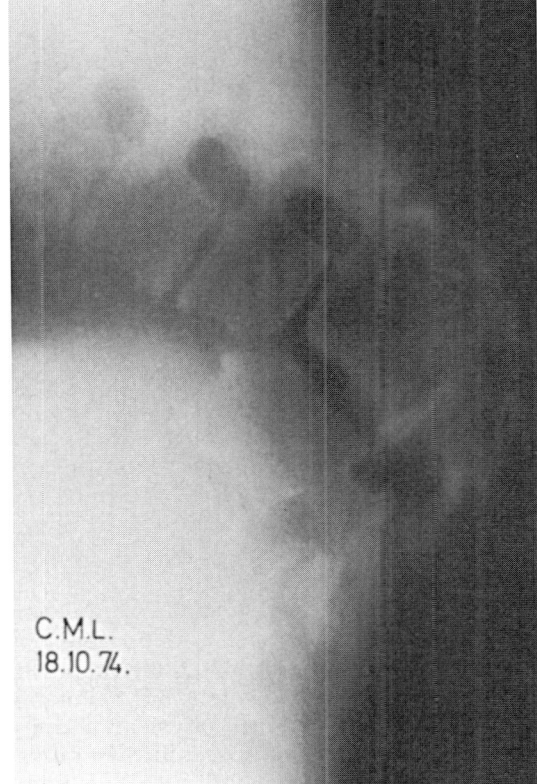

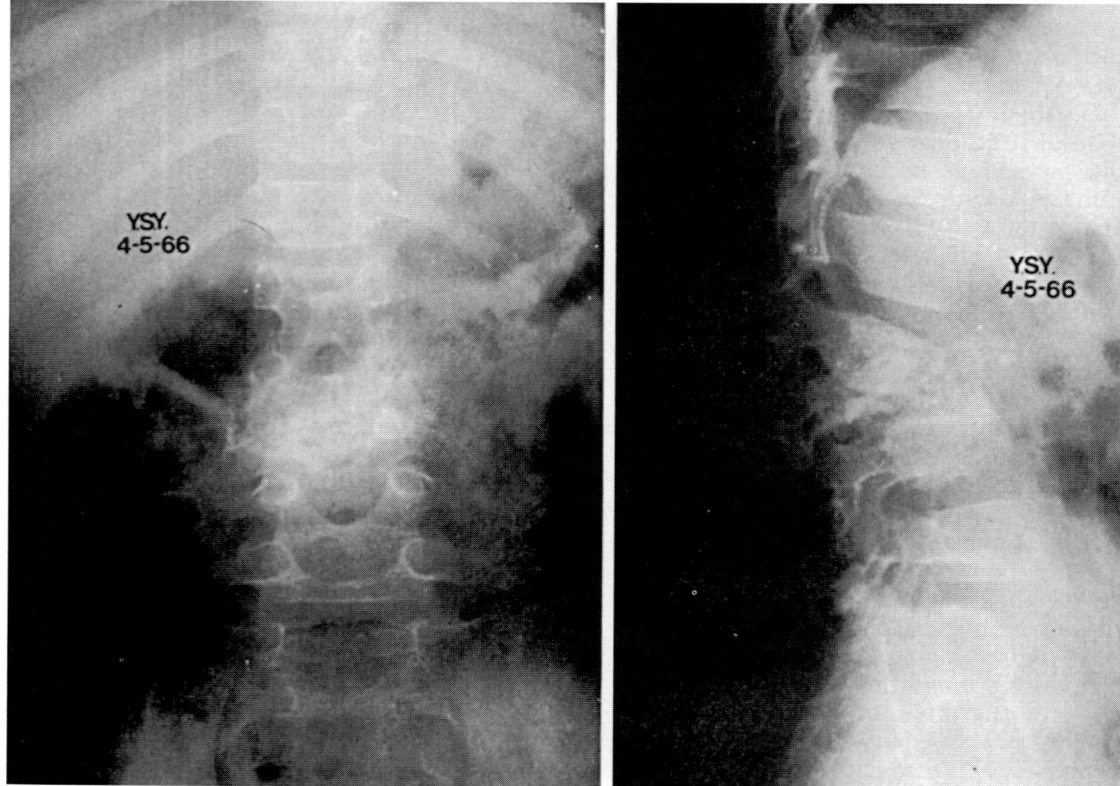

Figure 8. Reversed spondylolisthesis of L3 on L4 in tuberculosis of the spine.

Treatment

Conservative Treatment

The mainstay of treatment is antituberculous chemotherapy.[3] These drugs vary in (1) their bactericidal action, which is their ability to kill large numbers of actively metabolizing bacilli rapidly; (2) their sterilizing action, which is their capacity to kill slowly or intermittently by metabolizing semidormant bacilli; and (3) their ability to prevent emergence of acquired resistance by suppressing drug-resistant mutants. Isoniazid (INH) is the most potent bactericidal drug, and rifampicin is also an important one. On the other hand, rifampicin and pyrazinamide are the most important sterilizing drugs. INH, rifampicin, streptomycin, and ethambutol are effective in preventing the emergence of acquired resistance.

Short-course chemotherapy[3] is widely accepted as the treatment of choice for tuberculosis. The recommended regimen for patients with newly diagnosed disease is 2 months of pyrazinamide, INH, and rifampicin given daily, followed by 4 months of INH and rifampicin given daily. The dosage for INH is 5 mg/kg of body weight; for rifampicin, it is 10 mg/kg; and for pyrazinamide, 35 mg/kg. An alternative (and less potent) regimen is INH and rifampicin given daily for 9 months, with or without the addition of streptomycin or ethambutol daily for the first 2 months. (The dosage for streptomycin is 15 to 20 mg/kg of body weight.) The number of viable bacilli contained in bone and joint tuberculosis is small compared with the number in pulmonary lesions. A two-drug regimen, for example, 9 months of INH and rifampicin, is theoretically effective, provided that it is known that the level of initial resistance to INH in the population is low.

The Medical Research Council (MRC) of Britain conducted clinical trials comparing the effectiveness of ambulant chemotherapy alone with chemotherapy in combination with (1) bed rest for 6 months, (2) plaster jacket immobilization for 9 months, (3) sur-

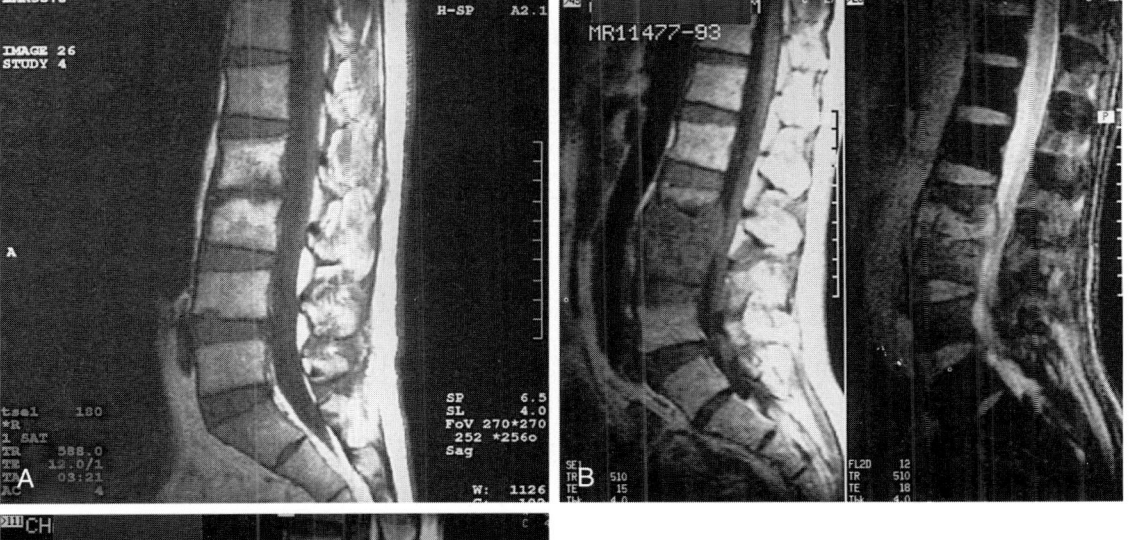
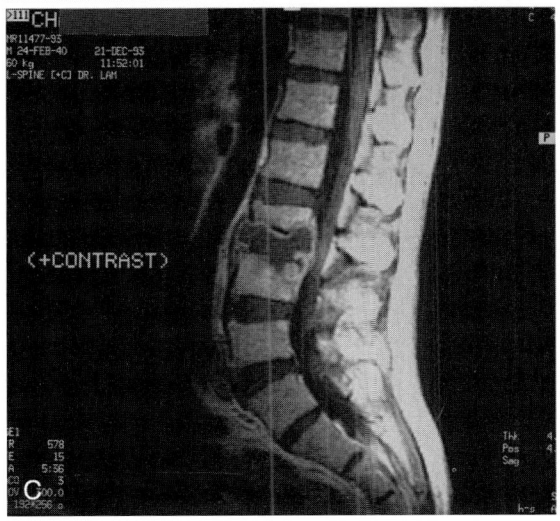

Figure 9. *A*, MRI scan of tuberculosis of the spine. Note the early loss of cortical definition of consecutive end plates of involved L2 and L3 vertebrae. *B*, In the T2-weighted image, note hyperintense signals in the superior half of L5 as well as in the entire vertebral bodies of L4 and L3. L5 involvement would have been undetectable by conventional x-ray films and computed tomographic (CT) scans. *C*, Gadolinium-enhanced image showing a large mass occupying the intervertebral disc space, in fact an abscess. The abscess has a nonenhanceable core with an enhanceable rim.

gical débridement (without fusion), and (4) anterior radical excision of disease focus and anterior spinal fusion. These are multicenter trials, some mainly studying children, and others mainly studying adults. The locations of centers include South Korea; Bulawayo, Zimbabwe; Hong Kong; and Madras.

They have compared the efficacy of different treatment regimens based on the percentages of patients achieving *favorable status* after 3, 5, and 10 years.[30-36] Favorable status is defined as full physical activity with clinically and radiographically quiescent disease, no sinuses or clinically evident abscesses, no myelopathy with functional impairment, and no modification of the allocated regimen. The first series, which was started in 1965, used a chemotherapy regimen consisting of 18 months of daily INH plus para-aminosalicylic acid, with or without streptomycin for the first 3 months. The percentage of patients with favorable status at 3 years was approximately 85% in all the groups. These results were maintained at 5 and 10 years. If the remaining patients who attained a favorable status after additional chemotherapy and/or operation were included, the proportion in all groups would rise to between 95% and 100%.

However, favorable status does *not* take into account symptomatic relief, fusion rate, or angle of kyphosis.

A second series of studies was begun in the 1980s, using short-course regimens of 6 or 9 months of INH and rifampicin with or without streptomycin. The 3-year results showed that favorable status was achieved in a slightly higher percentage of patients treated with the radical operation (plus chemotherapy) than in those ambulant chemotherapy alone, except in Madras.[37]

Anterior Radical Resection and Anterior Spine Fusion

The rationale for surgical treatment is based on the following findings:

1. The patient's general condition improves dramatically immediately after evacuation of the abscess.
2. Avascular material can be removed, and the insertion of an anterior strut graft under compression leads to early fusion.
3. Late recurrence is uncommon (after radical excision of the disease focus and solid fusion has been achieved).
4. Diseased material may be obtained for a definitive diagnosis.
5. Increasing deformity can be prevented.
6. Paraplegia can be prevented, or when it is established, anterior decompression with bone grafting leads to rapid recovery.

Tuberculosis of the spine mimics other conditions. Although diagnosis does not usually pose a problem in developing countries in which the disease is rife, it can be difficult in more affluent countries in which the condition is uncommon.

In the first 100 cases reported from the author's center in 1960, followed for an average of 3 years, the fusion rate was 94%.[17] The first 300 cases, published in 1964, had an overall radiologic fusion rate of 80%.[15] However, among those without radiologic union, 4.7% had died during the follow-up period, and 3% did not have bone grafts inserted because of technical reasons. The average time for fusion was 22.2 months, the shortest was 7 months, and the longest was 42 months. These included cases of extensive disease, including involvement of up to eight vertebral bodies.

In the same series of 300 cases, with 80% followed for longer than 5 years, there was a recurrence rate of 3.3%. Another series of 100 consecutive children from 18 months to 10 years old, after an average follow-up period of 8 years and 2 months (range from 1 to 15 years), again showed a low recurrence rate of 2%.[4] Although the true incidence of reactivation after healing as a result of conservative treatment is unknown, there is evidence from the MRC trials that a large proportion (50%) of children undergoing conservative treatment do not show evidence of bony fusion at up to 5 years of follow-up[33]; even at 10 years, 27% of cases still have *not* fused.[36] This compares with 90% fusion with the radical procedure at the 5-year follow-up,[34] and 97% at 10 years.[35]

The changes in the angle of kyphosis were compared at a 5-year follow-up among patients treated by the radical operation in Hong Kong, débridement in Bulawayo, and conservative measures in South Korea. The initial mean angles of kyphosis for the three groups were similar. Sixty patients in Hong Kong, 38 in Bulawayo, and 271 in Korea were assessed. The radically treated group had no change in the mean angle, whereas both those treated with débridement and those treated conservatively had a mean *increase* of 12 degrees in their kyphosis. More detailed analysis (Table 1) showed that 5% of patients in the conservative treatment group had an *increase* in their angle of kyphosis of 51 to 70 degrees. At 10 years of follow-up, although the number of patients assessed was smaller, those treated by the radical operation showed a mean *decrease* in kyphosis of 1.4 degrees in the thoracic and thoracolumbar regions and 0.5 degrees in the lumbar region, compared with an *increase* in the débridement group of 9.8 and 7.6 degrees, respectively, and in the conservative treatment group an *increase* of 17.8 and 5.2 degrees, respectively. Of 160 patients assessed for the conservative treatment, 52 patients had *increased* kyphosis between 11 and 30 degrees; 27 patients, between 31 and 50 degrees; and 9 patients, between 51 and 70 degrees. This poses a severe problem for the future (Table 2).

In a review of the outcome of deformity in children treated by radical resection and anterior spine fusion versus débridement only, the majority of children (56%) showed an improvement in deformity angle of 5 degrees or more after radical surgery, whereas 69% of children showed deterioration after débridement surgery, at the 6-month postoperative evaluation.[51] At the 17-year follow-up of patients with lumbar tuberculosis, 60% of those in the débridement group had 10 degrees or more (mean 24 degrees) kyphosis

Table 1

	Patients Assessed	Decrease 11 Degrees or More	Mean Increase (degrees)	Increase		
				11°–30°	31°–50°	51°–70°
Radical surgery (Hong Kong)	60	12	0	9	0	0
Débridement (Bulawayo)	38	0	12	11	3	0
Conservative treatment (Korea)	271	26	12	88	31	12

Changes in Angle of Kyphosis at 5-Year Follow-up

angle, whereas only one patient in the radical group had kyphosis due to graft failure.

Preferred Method of Treatment

The form of treatment offered should provide rapid relief from symptoms, especially pain and paraparesis or paraplegia. The end result should be firm evidence of eradication of the disease, as shown by a solid bony fusion with little or no deformity. This can be achieved predictably and in the majority of patients only by anterior radical resection of the diseased focus and anterior spine fusion. This requires good surgical expertise, good general anesthesia, and a high standard of postoperative care.

In the cervical spine, there is no place for conservative treatment alone. In the thoracic spine and the thoracolumbar junction, when there is early and limited disease without a large abscess causing pain, ambulant chemotherapy is justifiable. More extensive disease, significant pain, paraparesis, and presence of a kyphosis are strong indications for surgical treatment. It must be remembered that at 10 years of follow-up in the MRC trials, the average increase of kyphosis in the conservatively treated group amounted to 17.8 degrees. This is completely unacceptable in the thoracolumbar junction.

In the lumbar spine, the average increase in kyphosis for the conservatively treated group averaged only 5.2 degrees. Technically, radical resection and anterior spine fusion become more difficult with more caudal involvement. This is because the common iliac and segmental vessels may be involved in the abscess itself; sometimes, their walls become friable because of the inflammatory process, increasing the risk of damage that can lead to massive bleeding. The indication for ambulant chemotherapy is therefore stronger, unless there is extensive disease or significant deformity. At times, when surgical approach to the spine becomes too difficult, one can compromise by simply draining the abscess. Ideally, anterior radical resection and spine fusion still give the best end result (Fig. 10A,B).

Tuberculosis affecting the lumbosacral junction[42] is uncommon. Experience with 37 patients, 26 of whom had adequate records and follow-up (average of 20.2 years, range of 6 to 34.5 years) revealed that conservative and surgical treatment both resulted in firm

Table 2

Changes in Angle of Kyphosis at 10-Year Follow-up

	Site*	Patients Assessed	Mean Increase (degrees)†	Increase		
				11°–30°	31°–50°	51°–70°
Radical surgery	T&TL	27	−1.4	4	0	0
	Lumbar	4	−0.5			
Débridement	T&TL	21	9.8	9	3	0
	Lumbar	12	7.6			
Conservative	T&TL	125	17.8	52	27	9
	Lumbar	35	5.2			

*T, thoracic spine; TL, thoracolumbar spine.
†Mean increase. Negative values indicate a decrease in kyphosis.

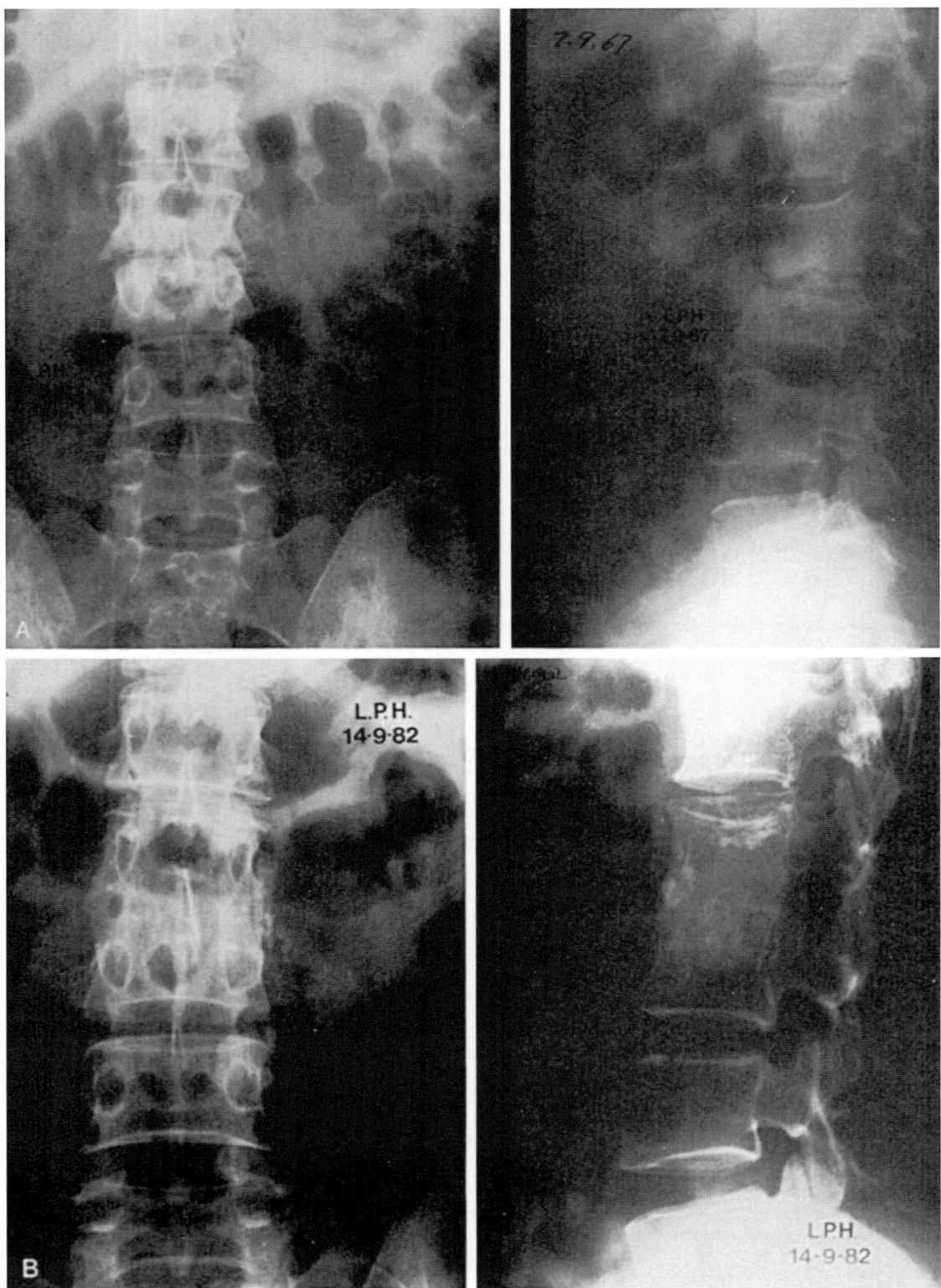

Figure 10. *A*, Tuberculosis affecting L2 and L3. *B*, Fifteen years after anterior excision and strut grafting, showing solid fusion.

fusion. However, only 25% of the group treated by anterior spine fusion had kyphosis (averaging 10.5 degrees) compared with 100% of the group treated conservatively (who had kyphosis averaging 60.4 degrees). Significant low back pain and a narrowed pelvic outlet necessitating cesarean section for pregnancy were correlated with the spinal deformity. The lumbosacral junction is technically highly demanding to operate on, but if the expertise is available, the outcome is superior to that achieved with conservative treatment (Fig. 11A to C). Conservative treatment cures the disease but results in significant deformity (Fig. 12A,B).

PYOGENIC INFECTIONS OF THE SPINE

Pyogenic infections have significant differences in clinical presentation, diagnostic criteria, treatment modalities, and outcome, as well as in causative organisms,[5, 7, 43] compared with those of tuberculosis of the spine. Three different groups of clinical entities have been described, although the relative frequency of occurrence of these groups vary from one geographic area to another. They are as follows:

1. Pyogenic spondylitis—The infection lies in the vertebral body and usually starts in the region of the end plates. Involvement of the neural arch is rare.
2. Septic intervertebral discitis.
3. Spinal epidural abscess.

Pyogenic Spondylitis

Pyogenic infections[43] of the spine constitute only about 1% of cases of osteomyelitis. The presentation may be acute or chronic. In the acute form, pain is the most constant symptom, whereas pyrexia, local tenderness, muscle spasm, constitutional upset, and neurologic involvement may or may not be present. The pain may radiate to the abdomen or legs. The presence of abdominal pain may confuse the diagnosis. The incidence of paraplegia or paraparesis varies from 3% to 15% in different series. Radiculopathy may also occur. It appears that advanced age, a more cephalad level of infection, and associated diseases of diabetes mellitus and rheumatoid arthritis predispose one to paraplegia.

In about half the cases, Staphylococcus is the causative organism, with Streptococcus, Proteus, and Escherichia coli involved in most of the remainder. Other organisms occasionally involved include Pseudomonas, Klebsiella, Salmonella typhi, Brucella, and Streptococcus pneumoniae.

The evidence is that the infection is hematogenous, with the urinary tract being the most common primary focus. Spinal infection has arisen after cardiac or urinary catheterization. Drug addicts and diabetics are also vulnerable.

INVESTIGATIONS

Erythrocyte sedimentation rate elevation is the most consistently abnormal finding. Elevation of the white blood cell count and a positive blood culture occur less consistently. Rising antibody titers, in response to specific organisms or antigens, when present, are valuable diagnostic aids.[8] These include anti-α and anti-γ staphylococcal hemolysin, antistreptolysin O, brucellin antibody, Widal tests for S. typhi, and gonococcal complement tests.

Needle biopsy is a useful procedure in obtaining material for both culture and pathologic study. However, the success rate of the procedure for diagnosis varies from 20% to 100%.

RADIOGRAPHIC APPEARANCES

Plain X-ray Films. No radiologic pattern is completely reliable in distinguishing a pyogenic infection from a tuberculous one. One or more of the following features may be present:[12]

1. Symmetric destruction of the adjacent surfaces of two vertebrae—this is not a specific feature (Fig. 13).
2. Loss of disc space—This may be variable in amount and is not a specific feature (Fig. 14).
3. New bone formation—This is much more common in pyogenic infections (Fig. 15) than in tuberculous ones. In a prospective study of 45 patients with spinal infection proved by bacteriologic and/or histologic findings, new bone formation occurred in 50% of white patients with pyogenic in-

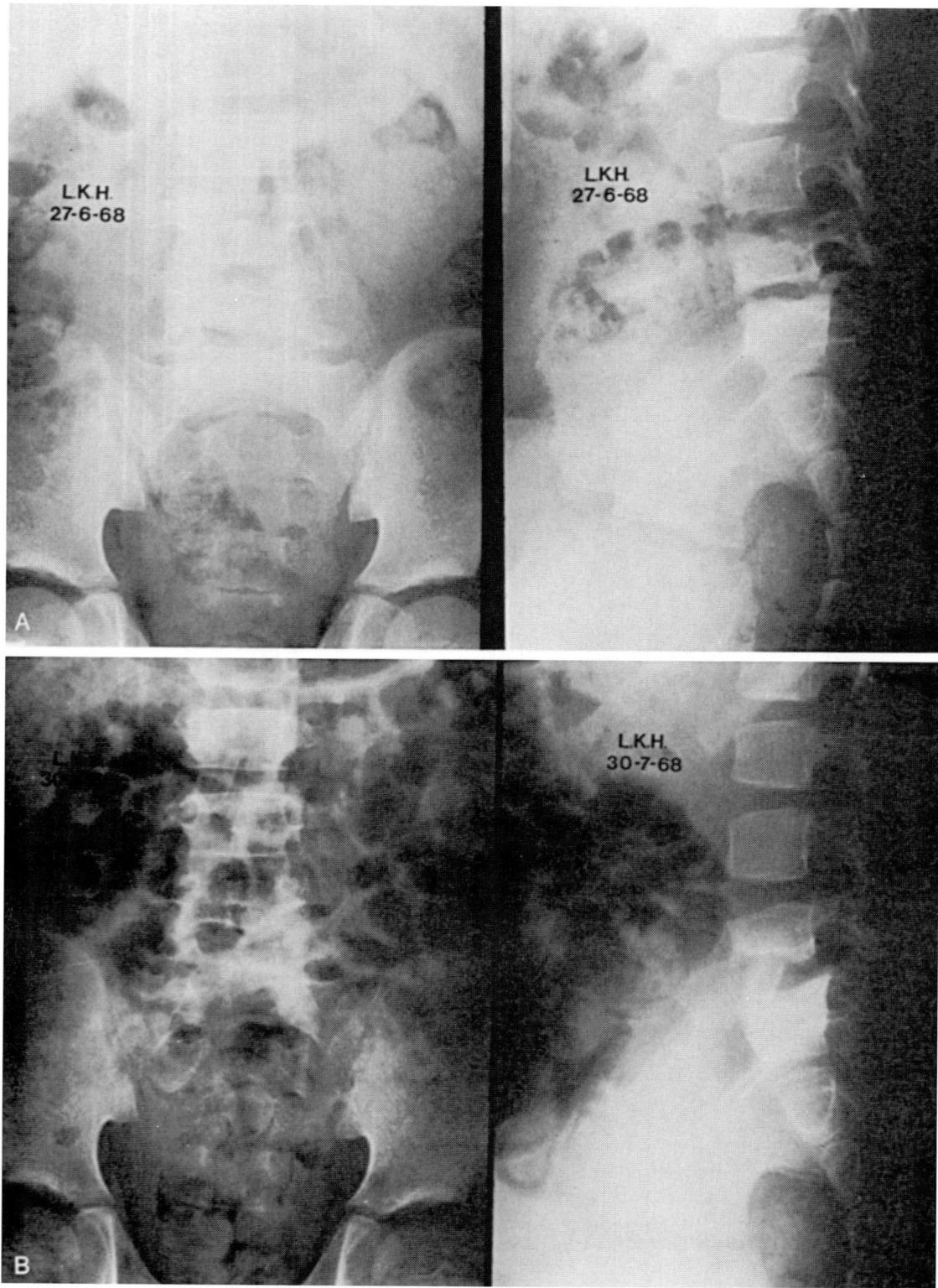

Figure 11. *A*, Tuberculosis affecting lumbosacral junction. *B*, After anterior excision and strut grafting.

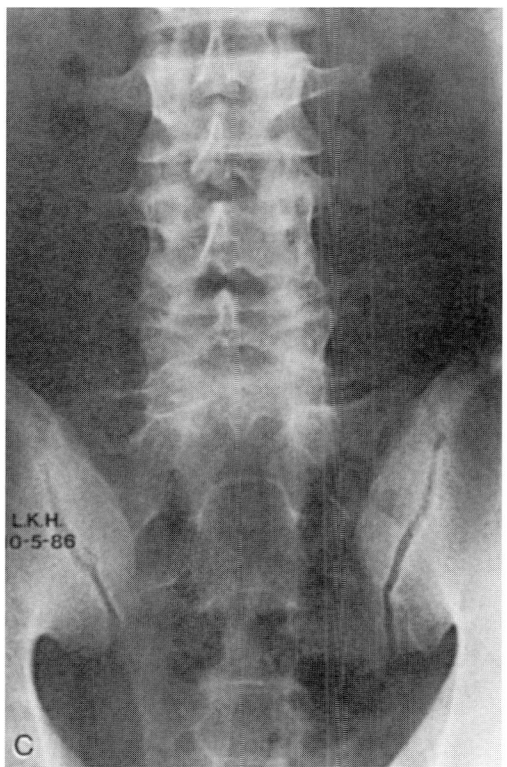
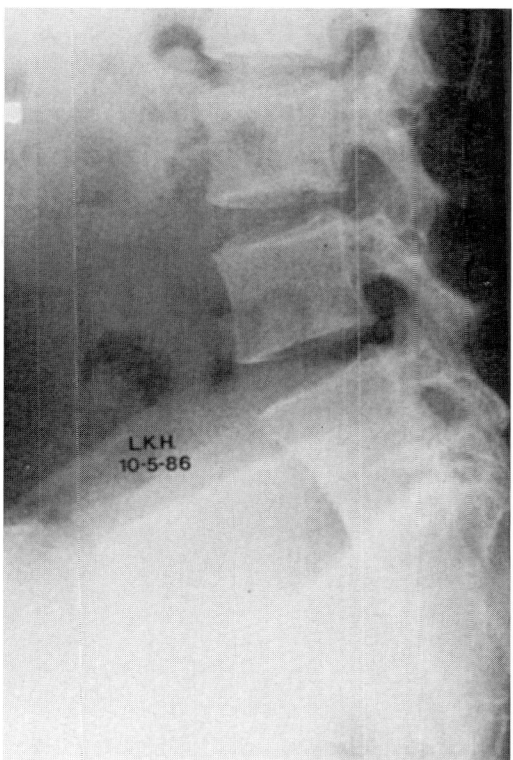

Figure 11 *Continued C,* Eighteen years later, showing solid anterior fusion.

fection, but none occurred in tuberculous infection.[2] However, in black patients, new bone formation occurred in 20% with tuberculous infection.

4. Sclerosis of bone, with or without marked destruction—This is more common in pyogenic infections (Fig. 15).

5. Paravertebral abscess—This is uncommon, and even when present, it is less prominent.

6. Kyphosis and subluxation—This is not a specific feature, and it tends to be less severe than in tuberculosis, because the number of vertebrae involved is usually smaller (Fig. 16).

Computed Tomography. There are certain advantages of this type of radiologic investigation.[6] These are as follows:

1. Multiplanar depictions of disturbances of bone integrity are possible by means of image reformation.
2. Precise definition of paraspinal soft tissue is possible. This is most useful in detecting paravertebral abscess formation, as well as extension of the disease process into the spinal canal. The combination of CT and small-volume, low-concentration metrizamide administration in the subarachnoid space also increases accuracy.
3. CT can also be used to guide percutaneous needle biopsy.

There is no evidence to show, however, that CT is more sensitive than conventional radiography in the earliest stages of spinal infection.

OTHER RADIOLOGIC INVESTIGATIONS

Radionuclide Bone Imaging.[1, 12] Technetium Tc 99m–labeled medronate discdium (^{99m}Tc MDP) imaging is the most sensitive screening test. An abnormal bone image increases the probability of the disease, even if findings of conventional x-ray films and CT scans are normal. A normal bone image virtually rules out suspected acute or chronic active osteomyelitis. The sensitivity of the three-phase bone scan varies from

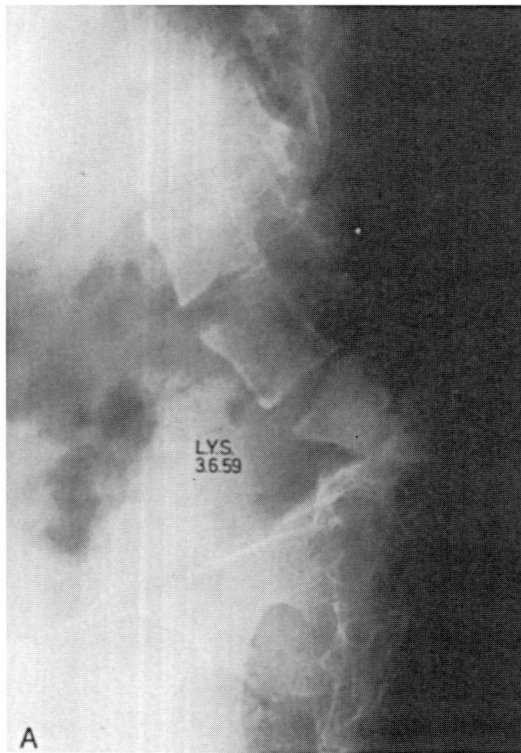
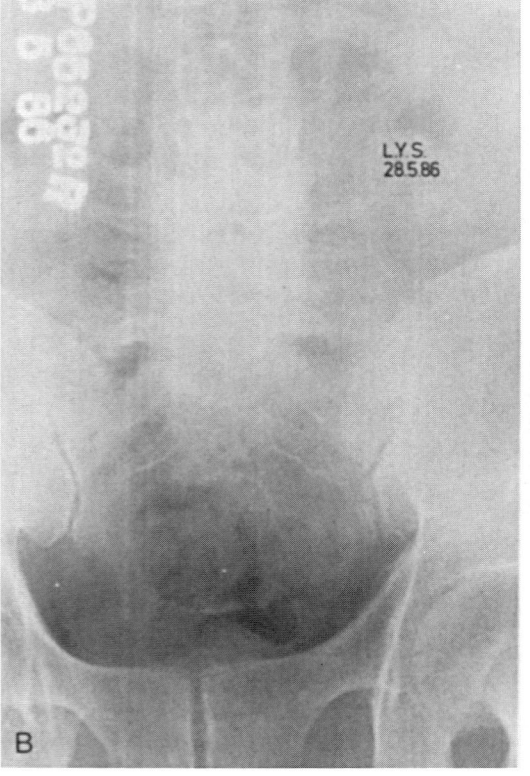
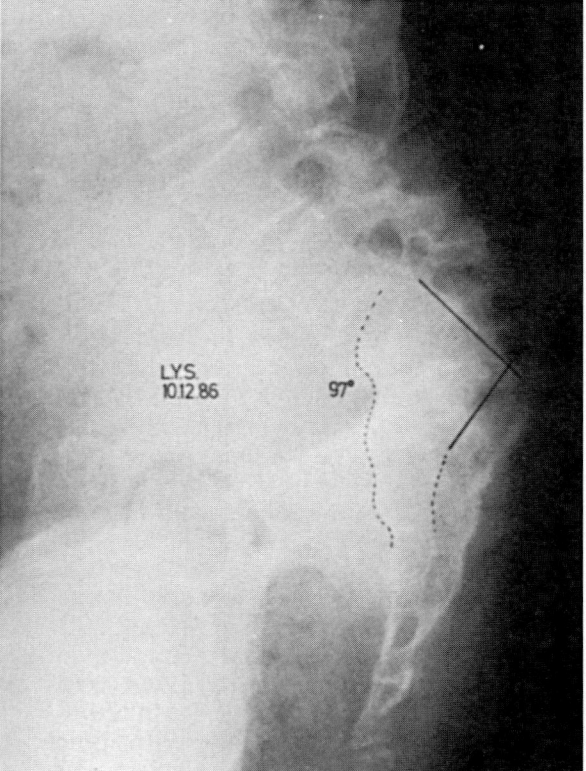

Figure 12. *A*, Tuberculosis affecting lumbosacral junction. *B*, Twenty-seven years after conservative treatment, showing solid fusion, but a kyphosis angle of 97 degrees, and exaggerated lumbar lordosis above.

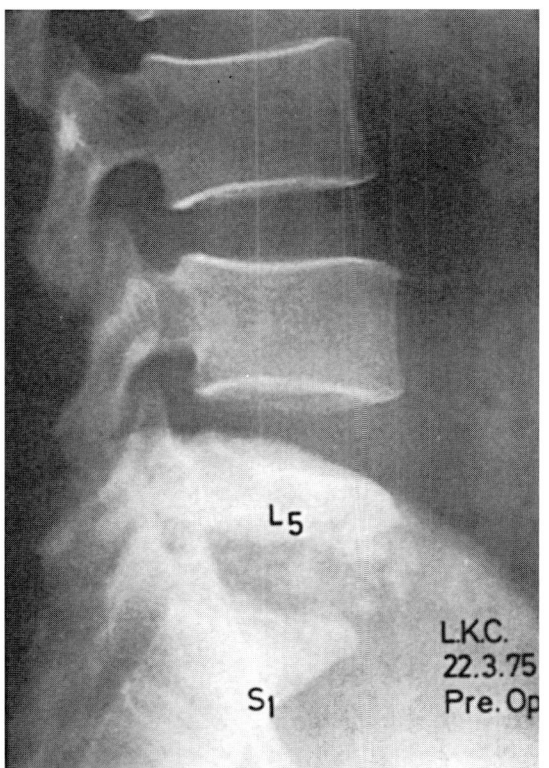

Figure 13. Pyogenic spondylitis showing symmetric destruction of the adjacent surfaces of L5 and S1.

89% in osteomyelitis to 100% in vertebral osteomyelitis.

Total-body gallium 67 (^{67}Ga) imaging is generally used sequentially after ^{99m}Tc MDP. An abnormal ^{67}Ga image following an abnormal technetium Tc 99m (^{99m}Tc) bone image increases the specificity of the diagnosis. Normal technetium and gallium bone images of the vertebra virtually exclude the diagnosis of pyogenic spondylitis.

In patients with paravertebral abscesses, abnormalities on both technetium and gallium scans may extend into the paravertebral region. The pattern of this uptake has been termed the butterfly sign.

Magnetic Resonance Imaging. MRI is at least as sensitive as radionuclide bone imaging and is therefore useful in early diagnosis. In pyogenic spondylitis, there is an increase in extracellular fluid within the vertebral marrow, because of the inflammatory reaction. This results in a reduced signal intensity on T1-weighted images and a high signal intensity on T2-weighted images. The affected vertebrae do not loose their cortical margin (Fig. 17A,B), as occurs in tuberculous infection. Involvement is mainly confined to the vertebral marrow with no significant extension into the paraspinal region.[47] Epidural extension is also infrequent. The soft tissue involvement can be demonstrated more confidently with enhancement by gadolinium. The intervertebral disc is usually affected and shows high signal intensity on T2-weighted images in the abscence of a nuclear cleft. The signal intensity is further enhanced by gadolinium.

Septic Intervertebral Discitis

This condition is believed to be a pyogenic infection arising primarily in the intervertebral disc. In children, as a rule, the disease is relatively benign with rapid resolution of symptoms.[46] Many patients respond well to bed rest or immobilization alone. Because of that, there is doubt as to whether it is a true bacterial infection. In

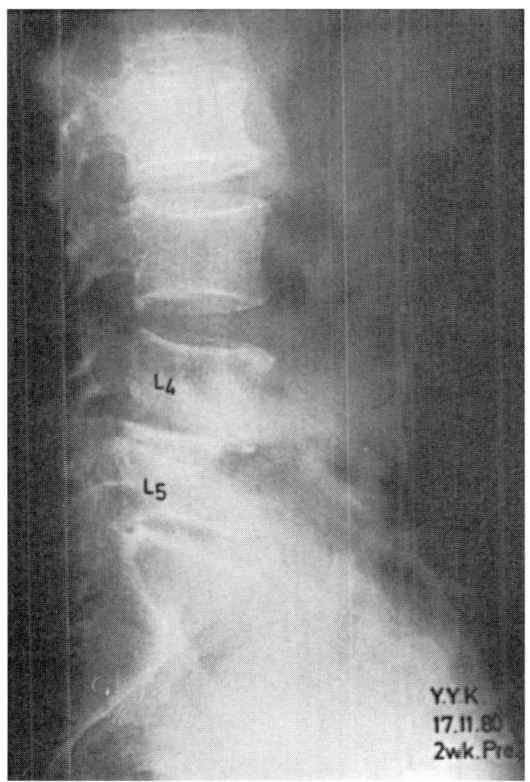

Figure 14. Pyogenic spondylitis showing early loss of joint space between L4 and L5.

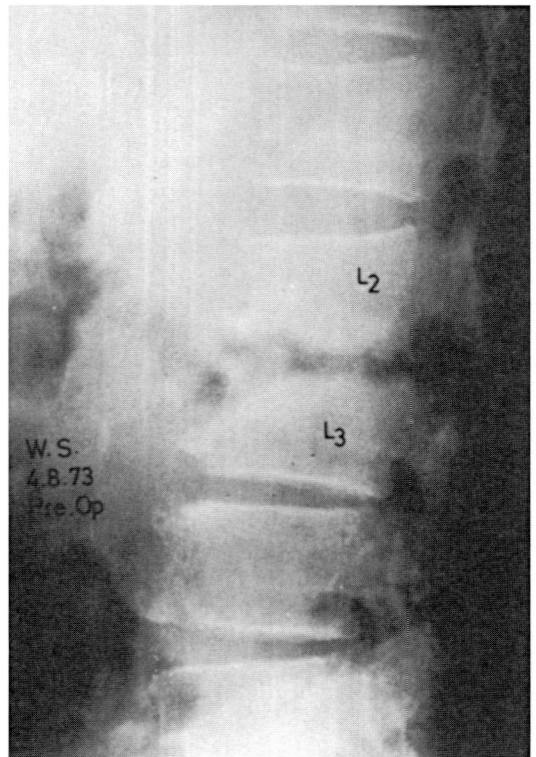

Figure 15. Pyogenic spondylitis showing subchondral and adjacent bone sclerosis and new bone formation anteriorly.

via the end plates, but that an adequate circumferential supply was maintained from the periphery, with vessels penetrating as far as the junction between the annulus fibrosus and the nucleus pulposus.

The clinical picture may include features of a prodromal infection before spinal involvement. Locally, there is back pain with or without referred pain of femoral or sciatic distribution, point tenderness, paravertebral muscle spasm, and limitation of movement. Paraparesis or paraplegia occurs in as many as 40% of patients. The level of involvement varies from one series to another, but is mainly thoracic and lumbar, with infrequent involvement of the neck, except in children.

BLOOD INVESTIGATIONS

Investigations similar to those used in pyogenic spondylitis may be helpful, although a normal value does not rule out the diagnosis.

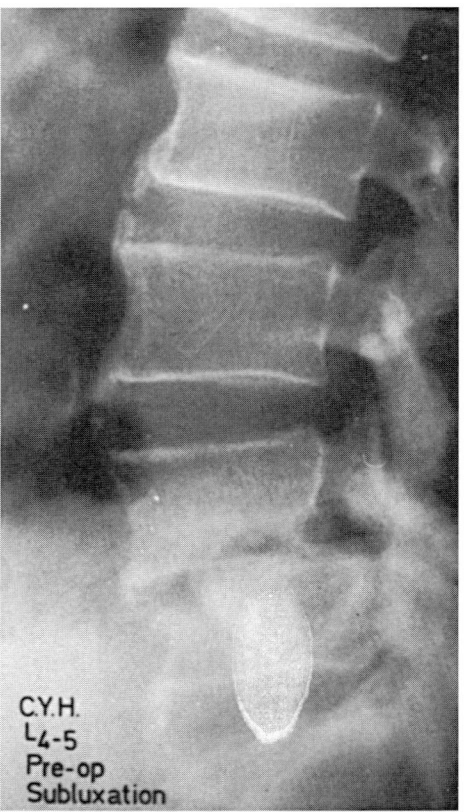

Figure 16. Lumbar pyogenic spondylitis showing mild anterior subluxation.

late adolescence and adulthood, intervertebral discitis is a more ominous disease.

A significant percentage of adult patients with intervertebral discitis present with prodromal infection, suggesting that, as is the case in pyogenic spondylitis, the bacteria reach the spine by a hematogenous route. There is controversy as to whether it is due to venous or arterial spread. Doyle[9] postulated that infections occurred via the vertebral venous plexus of Batson. However, Wiley and Trueta[50] demonstrated by vascular studies that it was extremely unlikely that the venous plexus was responsible for the spread of infection to the spine. They believed that arterial spread was the more likely route. Although it is generally stated that the intervertebral disc becomes avascular in adult life, Wiley and Trueta,[50] Mineiro,[38] and Hassler[13] showed that, although the blood supply to the intervertebral disc diminished with age, the main decrease was in the number of vessels that enter the nucleus pulposus from the adjacent vertebrae

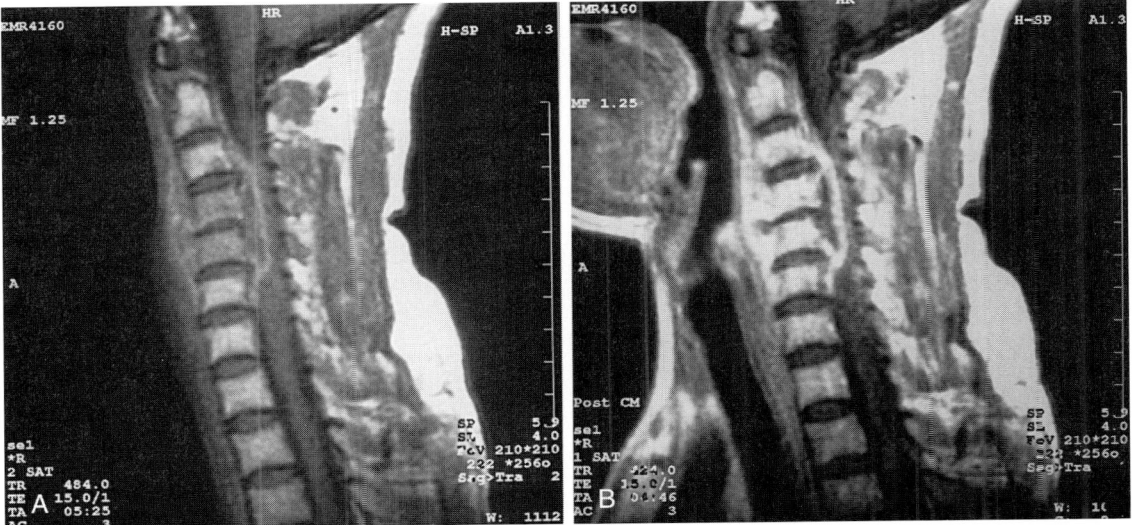

Figure 17. *A*, MRI scan of pyogenic spondylitis showing involved vertebrae with no loss of cortical margin, despite a significant epidural extension. *B*, Gadolinium-enhanced image showing hyperintense signal of epidural extension.

RADIOGRAPHIC APPEARANCES

The following features are observed in the plain films.[23] They tend to occur in sequence, although in individual cases the feature depends on the stage at which the patient presents (Fig. 18*A* to *D*).

1. Decrease in the vertical height of the affected intervertebral disc space—This feature is most constant and occurs during the first 3 months of the disease. The degree of narrowing is variable but does not relate to the subsequent progress of the disease (Fig. 18*A*).

2. Progressive sclerosis of the subchondral bone together with increase in radiodensity of the adjacent area of the vertebral bodies on either side of the affected disc—It usually follows disc space narrowing by 2 to 3 months. The density results from deposition of new bone on existing trabeculae, as

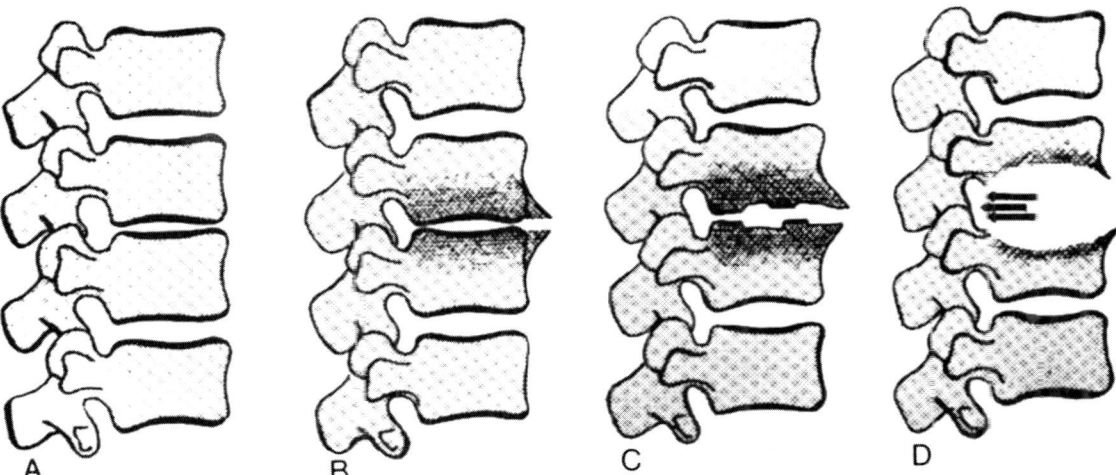

Figure 18. *A–D*, Septic intervertebral discitis showing different stages of radiographic presentation. (From Kemp, H. B. S., Jackson, J. W., Jeremiah, J. D., and Hall, A. J.: Pyogenic infections occurring primarily in intervertebral discs. J. Bone Joint Surg. 55B:701, 1973.)

well as associated subperiosteal new bone formation (Fig. 18B).

3. Progressive irregularity of the adjacent vertebral end plates—Kemp and coworkers[23] demonstrated that these changes were a local extension of the inflammatory process, which in turn evoked sclerosis of the margins of the vertebral body (Fig. 18C).

4. In 50% of the cases, the narrowing of disc space and adjacent sclerosis increased further. In the rest, there may be "ballooning" of the disc space as a result of erosion of the vertebral body (Fig. 18D).

5. Circumferential formation of bone around the annulus—This is attempted repair of the disease. Radiologically, it appears as a bony bridge.

In both tuberculous and pyogenic spondylitis, narrowing and subsequent loss of disc space are early and relatively common features. In tuberculous spondylitis, there is early destruction of bone, leading to loss of definition and collapse of the affected vertebral body. In pyogenic spondylitis, spontaneous intervertebral fusion occurs, which is not seen in septic discitis. Abscess formation is also extremely rare in septic discitis, although involvement of the spinal cord leading to paraplegia can occur by either pressure from inflammatory granulomatous tissue or septic thrombosis of spinal blood vessels.

OTHER RADIOLOGIC INVESTIGATIONS

Radionuclide Uptake Scanning. Both ^{99m}Tc MDP and ^{67}Ga imaging have been useful in the early diagnosis of this condition.

Magnetic Resonance Imaging. There is evidence that MRI is at least as sensitive as, and more specific than, radionuclide uptake scanning in disc space infection. In adults,[39] the use of a relatively long echo time (120-ms TE) and repetition time (3-second TR) shows a markedly increased signal intensity of the entire disc as well as the adjacent end plates. A 60-ms TE/1-second TR pulse sequence produces only an isointense signal of the body and disc space. In children,[14] an increase in signal intensity is not obtained, but an affected disc still shows up as being different from the adjacent normal structures.

Compared with radionuclide bone scanning, MRI specifically localizes the disease process to the disc space and has the added advantage of being completely noninvasive. Technetium scans have been found to be abnormal within 7 days of the onset of symptoms in cases of septic intervertebral discitis. This is much earlier than is the case for x-ray findings, in which usually 2 to 6 weeks must pass before changes are apparent. Whether MRI changes occur even earlier is not clear at present.

Spinal Epidural Abscesses

This condition is relatively uncommon,[22, 24] and patients are more frequently referred to neurosurgeons than to orthopedic surgeons.

CLINICAL FEATURES

Back pain is invariably present. Pyrexia may or may not be present. Root pain commonly follows. The incidence of paraparesis or paraplegia is high, ranging from 75% to 100%.

The presentation may be acute or chronic. The thoracic and lumbar spine are most commonly involved, and the disease is rarely seen in children younger than 12 years old.

INVESTIGATIONS

MRI is the most useful investigation for such lesions (Fig. 19A), especially when gadolinium enhancement is used in conjunction (Fig. 19B). MRI can also indicate whether there is intradural extensions involving the leptomeninges and the spinal cord.[47]

Treatment

Conservative Treatment

PYOGENIC SPONDYLITIS

A patient presenting with clinical features suggestive of this disease should be investigated with a blood culture or urine culture and plain x-ray studies of the spine. The findings lead to the following alternatives and the logical plan of management:[48]

1. Radiologic evidence and a positive blood culture—This group of patients

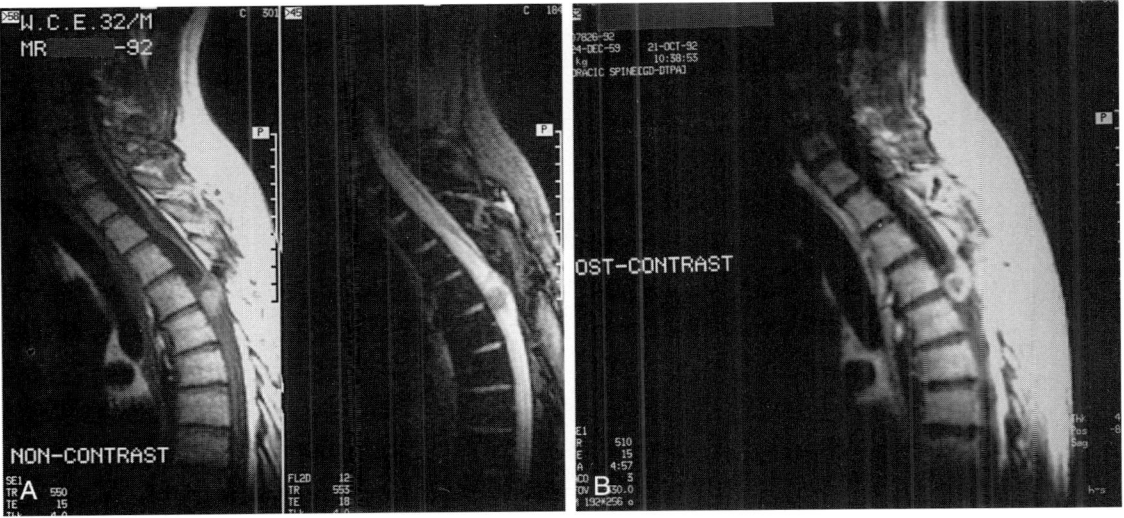

Figure 19. *A*, MRI scans showing gross cord atrophy plus a lump in the epidural space. The lump looks like a tumor, except that the T2 signal is more hypointense than would be expected for a tumor. *B*, After gadolinium injection, the typical appearance of an abscess is shown. This patient was subsequently operated on and the pathologic change confirmed.

should be treated by administration of the appropriate antibiotics intravenously for 6 weeks, then orally for a minimum of another 6 weeks. Bed rest is essential during the acute stage. When severe pain and muscle spasm have been alleviated, usually after 2 to 3 weeks of antibiotic administration, the patients can be mobilized with an external light spinal brace.

2. Abnormal radiologic evidence but negative blood and urine cultures—If there is a known prodromal infection, the organism is assumed to be the same. The appropriate antibiotic can then be selected. Specific antibodies to the more common organisms causing infections, such as *Staphylococcus* and *Streptococcus,* can be helpful if present. If the antibodies are absent and the disease is not responding to the chosen antibiotic, a needle biopsy is indicated to obtain material for culture.

3. No radiologic evidence—A radionuclide bone scan (^{m99}Tc MDP) is indicated to identify a lesion in the spine and the level of involvement. If it is followed by a ^{67}Ga scan, the specificity is increased. Abnormal bone scan findings, together with a positive blood culture, put the patient into the same plan of treatment as for the first group. If the bone scan is abnormal, but the blood culture is negative, the plan of treatment is the same as for the second group. Occasionally, a repeated needle biopsy may be necessary to obtain adequate material for culture.

Monitoring of the progress of the patient is essential. In addition to clinical features, the erythrocyte sedimentation rate obtained serially is extremely helpful. If the patient shows favorable progress on mobilization in a light spinal brace, he or she can be discharged to continue a regimen of antibiotics at home, after the initial 6 weeks of intravenous administration.

SEPTIC INTERVERTEBRAL DISCITIS

In adults, evidence is convincing that this condition results from a bacterial infection. The scheme of conservative treatment should closely follow that of pyogenic spondylitis. There is relatively little experience of this disease entity in the literature, and most series reported are small in numbers of patients studied.[29, 41] The following distinctive features need mentioning: (1) A positive blood culture is rarely encountered, so a needle biopsy (or open biopsy) is needed more frequently. Needle biopsy yields a positive culture in up to 70% of cases. (2) The incidence of paraplegia is up to 40%. Hence, some investigators advocate more liberal use of surgical débridement.

In children, the initial treatment should

consist of bed rest or immobilization in a plaster cast.[46] The majority respond to this treatment. Only if investigations show evidence of a systemic bacterial infection, with worsening of clinical features despite resting, is the use of antibiotics required.

SPINAL EPIDURAL ABSCESS

There is little or no place for conservative treatment alone.

Surgical Treatment

PYOGENIC SPONDYLITIS

The absolute indication for anterior débridement, with or without spine fusion, is paraparesis or paraplegia. Eismont and coworkers[10] identified the following factors that predispose one to paraplegia:

1. Higher age group
2. Cervical or thoracic involvement, which is more likely to cause paraplegia than is lumbar involvement
3. Staphylococcal infection (as opposed to, for example, *Pseudomonas* infection)
4. Coexisting diabetes mellitus or rheumatoid arthritis

Ryan and Taylor,[45] in a study of 49 patients, found that paraplegia occurred much more frequently in the acute form with a positive bacteriologic culture. The incidence was 21%, compared with 3% in the group with chronic disease and a negative bacteriologic culture. Furthermore, acute presentation occurred mainly in the cervical and thoracic regions, whereas chronic presentation was mainly in the lumbar region.

Eismont and coworkers[10] studied two patients with paraplegia, who subsequently died. Autopsies showed a moderate to severe degree of intrinsic damage with cystic degeneration of the spinal cord. They thought that this was an additional reason for urgent anterior decompression of the spinal cord when paraparesis is present.

Other more relative indications include severe back pain and muscle spasm that are not responding to intravenous antibiotic administration over a few weeks; uncertainly as to the infective organism; and extensive bone destruction with significant deformity, especially in the cervical spine.

The question of whether bone grafting should be performed, and whether the grafts will survive, in a site of the body involved by pyogenic infection is always raised. The author's center (in Hong Kong) has had experience in treating 43 patients with proven pyogenic spondylitis by anterior surgery, between 1957 and 1990.[11] The indications for surgery were (1) uncertain diagnosis, (2) neurologic involvement, (3) severe pain not responding to antibiotic administration after 2 to 3 weeks, (4) sepsis not controlled by conservative treatment, and (5) extensive involvement with deformity. The age of the patients ranged from 14 to 79 years. There were 13 cervical spine lesions, nine thoracic spine lesions, and 48 lumbosacral spine lesions. Thirty-eight patients had excision of the disease focus and anterior stable strut grafting (Fig. 20*A* to *D*).

Of these, 30 patients had an average follow-up of 5 years, with a range from 2 to 15 years. Radiologic fusion took an average of 6.8 months (range of 3 to 15 months). The fusion rate was 93%. Only two patients had pseudarthrosis; in one patient, it occurred at one level of a two-level fusion in the cervical spine. Two patients had an abnormally long fusion time. One patient had a disappearing graft in the initial few months after surgery, but this gradually reappeared on the subsequent radiographs, and radiologic fusion was seen at 28 months.

Two patients had recurrence. One had a chronic sinus and an acute abscess in the subcutaneous region of the scar 3 years after the surgery. This was treated by drainage of the abscess and excision of the sinus. The sinus was deep but did not involve the spine. The other patient had an adjacent (L1–L2) vertebral involvement by chronic spondylitis 2 years after the primary (D12–L1) surgery. This was treated similarly with excision and anterior spine fusion. A few months later, involvement of the L4–L5 vertebrae was noticed. This was treated by débridement without formal fusion. Chronic osteomyelitis was confirmed each time by histologic examination. At 14 years of follow-up, fusion was present in all the surgically treated levels. However, there was late onset of lower limb weakness (some years after third surgery), and a myelogram showed chronic adhesive arachnoiditis.

Fourteen patients had neurologic involvement. Nine had radiculopathy, and five had

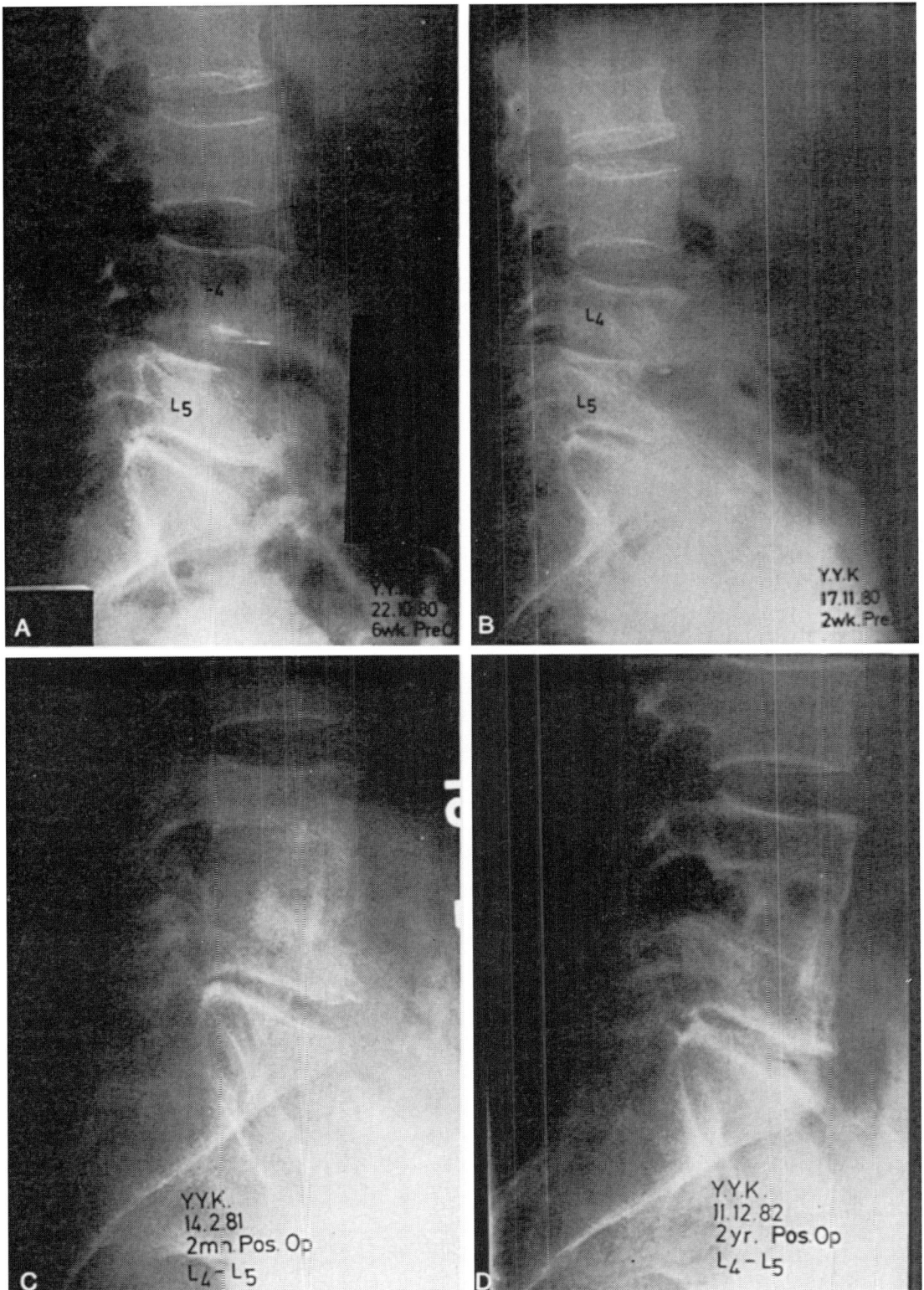

Figure 20. *A*, Pyogenic spondylitis affecting L4 and L5 6 weeks before operation, showing minimum changes on the x-ray film. *B*, Two weeks before operation showing marked narrowing of intervertebral disc L4–L5. *C*, X-ray film after anterior excision and interbody bone grafting. At 2 months after the operation, fusion is already progressing. *D*, Two years after operation, showing solid anterior spinal fusion, with preservation of disc height.

myelopathy. All those with radiculopathy improved after the operation. Of those patients with myelopathy, three cases were classified as Frankel grade C, and two grade D, preoperatively. Postoperatively, four patients recovered fully (grade E) and one improved from grade C to D. At long-term follow-up, one of the patients who improved from grade D preoperatively to grade E postoperatively subsequently had late deterioration to grade C (this is the patient with the multiple-level recurrence, referred to above).

Twenty-seven patients (90%) returned to the same work that they had before surgery, whereas three had to change their jobs (one owing to weakness, another owing to concomitant systemic lupus erythematosus, and the third because his job involved heavy manual labor). Of the 27 patients who returned to their original work, 15 patients were asymptomatic; six had occasional pain, one had a distinct limp, one had residual weakness, and four had mild deformity of the spine that did not bother them.

These results show that with adequate excision of the disease focus and administration of the appropriate antibiotic for an adequate period, bone graft survival is not a problem in pyogenic spondylitis. The fusion rate is greater than 93%. Neurologic involvement is generally well alleviated, which is the experience of other researchers as well.

Eismont and coworkers[10] reported a series of 31 patients affected by pyogenic spondylitis with paraparesis. Twenty-two were followed for longer than 2 years. These investigators showed that laminectomy for decompression did not achieve good results. Anterior débridement with or without grafting produced superior results. They thought that, if only minimum decompression with limited bone grafting was needed, the costotransversectomy approach is preferred. If extensive resection of necrotic bone with strut grafting is needed, the transthoracic or extraperitoneal approach is preferable. The costotransversectomy approach offers limited exposure and is useful only when a severe kyphosis is present, which rarely occurs in pyogenic spondylitis.

SEPTIC INTERVERTEBRAL DISCITIS

The absolute indication for surgical intervention is paraparesis or paraplegia. As noted above, the incidence is higher than in pyogenic spondylitis, by as much as 40%. Also, the onset is rapid and more frequently irreversible. Kemp and coworkers,[23] from operative findings, showed that paraplegia in this condition is mainly the result of direct extension of the inflammatory granulations posteriorly to involve the meninges and (occasionally) the cord. Septic thrombosis of spinal vessels may also be a cause.

Kemp and coworkers[23] advocated surgical clearance of diseased tissue in this condition, even in the absence of cord compression. Their reasons included preventing recurrence of the condition in some patients who had been treated conservatively, promoting rapid relief of symptoms, and obtaining material for culture of the infecting organism.

SPINAL EPIDURAL ABSCESS

The treatment of this condition constitutes an emergency, as permanent paraplegia or quadriplegia may otherwise result.[22, 24] The extent of the infection may span the length of many vertebrae and is most common at the thoracic and lumbar regions. Ventrally, the epidural space is practically nonexistent, but dorsally there is a larger amount of areolar tissue and a rich vascular plexus, where infection easily lodges. Therefore, a logical treatment is laminectomy over the entire extent of the infection, evacuation of abscess, and application of local as well as systemic antibiotics. Postoperative drains are recommended.

The results are worse if the patient has an acute presentation and if the infection has a subdural or intramedullary component. Mortality rate is still significant and varies from 3% to 30%. Morbidity in the form of residual weakness or sensory disturbance is also common (from 11% to 30%).

There is some suggestion that hyperbaric oxygen treatment may improve the outcome.[44] One center recommended one session per day, lasting 40 to 60 minutes at 1.7 to 2 units of atmospheric pressure. Ten to twenty sessions were needed.

OTHER UNCOMMON INFECTIONS

These infections may be bacterial or fungal. Most are insidious in onset, and a long interval may exist between onset of symptoms and diagnosis. Changes on x-ray films are slow to appear and are often nonspecific. Not infrequently, multiple levels of involvement may be present. The diagnosis is made possible only by awareness of such conditions, by the application of specific serologic tests, and by histologic examination of biopsy material.

Brucellosis Vertebral Osteomyelitis[26]

Brucellae are small nonmotile gram-negative capnophilic coccobacilli. There are three main species: *Brucella melitensis, B. abortus,* and *B. suis.* Brucellosis is an occupational disease found mainly in farmers, people working in meat-packing plants, veterinary surgeons, and livestock producers. Serologic studies include a brucelloslide test, which, if positive, is followed by a *Brucella* antibody tube dilution titer. The diagnosis depends on (1) a minimum *Brucella* antibody titer of 1:80, (2) radiographic evidence of spinal involvement, and (3) a clinical response to treatment. The lumbar spine, especially the lumbosacral region, is more commonly involved than other parts. The lesions may be single or multiple. Treatment consists of a combination of tetracycline and streptomycin, trimethoprim-sulfamethoxazole alone, or a combination of trimethoprim-sulfamethoxazole and rifampicin. Treatment should be for at least 3 months. Surgical decompression is required if there is neurologic involvement.

Actinobacillus actinomycetemcomitans Vertebral Osteomyelitis[40]

This is an extremely rare condition. The organism is part of the indigenous flora of the mouth. It is a gram-negative microaerophilic coccobacillus with fastidious growth requirements. There is no specific serologic test. Diagnosis depends on histologic findings and culture of the organism. Radiologically, the lesion may be osteoblastic. The bacteria are usually sensitive to streptomycin, tetracycline, and chloramphenicol.

Nocardial Vertebral Osteomyelitis[53]

Again, this is a rare infection. *Nocardia* organisms are true bacteria, gram positive and partially acid fast. The most frequent primary site of involvement by the disease is the pulmonary system. The x-ray findings in the spine are nonspecific, but multiple involvement sites are not uncommon. No specific serologic test is available. The mainstays of treatment are the sulfonamides. Minocycline is also effective.

Cryptococcal Vertebral Osteomyelitis[27]

This again is a rare condition. *Cryptococcus* infection is a true fungal infection. Diagnosis can be made by demonstrating rising serum cryptococcal titer (latex agglutination). Antifungal therapy, such as amphotericin B, may be useful.

REFERENCES

1. Adatepe, M. H., Powell, O. M., Isaacs, G. H., et al.: Hematogenous pyogenic vertebral osteomyelitis: Diagnostic value of radionuclide bone imaging. J. Nucl. Med. 27:1680–1685, 1986.
2. Allen, E. H., Cosgrove, D., and Millard, F. J. C.: The radiological changes in infections of the spine and their diagnostic value. Clin. Radiol. 29:31–40, 1978.
3. Antituberculosis Regimens of Chemotherapy. Bull. Int. Union Tuber. Lung Dis. 63:60–64, 1988.
4. Bailey, H. L., Gabriel, M., Hodgson, A. R., and Shin, J. S.: Tuberculosis of the spine in children. J. Bone Joint Surg. 54A:1633, 1972.
5. Bonfiglio, M., Lange, T. A., and Kim, Y. M.: Pyogenic vertebral osteomyelitis. Clin. Orthop. 96:234–247, 1973.
6. Brant-Zawadzki, M., Burke, V. D., and Jeffrey, R. B.: CT in the evaluation of spine infection. Spine 8:358–364, 1983.
7. Collert, S.: Osteomyelitis of the spine. Acta Orthop. Scand. 48:283–290, 1977.
8. Digby, J. M., and Kersley, J. B.: Pyogenic nontuberculous spinal infection. J. Bone Joint Surg. 61:47–55, 1979.
9. Doyle, J. R.: Narrowing of the intervertebral-disc space in children. Presumably an infectious lesion of the disc. J. Bone Joint Surg. 42A:1191–1200, 1960.
10. Eismont, F. J., Bohlman, H. H., Soni, P. L., et al.: Pyogenic and fungal vertebral osteomyelitis with paralysis. J. Bone Joint Surg. 65A:19–29, 1983.
11. Fang, D., Cheung, K. M. C., Remedios, I, et al.: Pyogenic vertebral osteomyelitis: Treatment by anterior spinal débridement and fusion. J. Spinal Disord. 7:173–180, 1994.
12. Fernandez-Ulloa, M., Vasavada, P. J., Hanslits, M. L., et al.: Diagnosis of vertebral osteomyelitis: Clinical, radiological and scintigraphic features. Orthopedics 8:1144–1150, 1985.
13. Hassler, O.: The human intervertebral disc. Acta Orthop. Scand. 40:765, 1970.
14. Heller, R. M., Szalay, E. A., Green, N. E., et al.: Disc space infection in children: Magnetic resonance imaging. Radiol. Clin. North Am. 26:207–209, 1988.

15. Hodgson, A. R.: Report on the findings and results in 300 cases of Pott's disease treated by anterior fusion of the spine. J. West. Pacific Orthop. Assoc. 1:3–7, 1964.
16. Hodgson, A. R., Skinsnes, O. K., and Leong, J. C. Y.: The pathogenesis of Pott's paraplegia. J. Bone Joint Surg. 49A:1147–1156, 1967.
17. Hodgson, A. R., and Stock, F. E.: Anterior spine fusion for the treatment of tuberculosis of the spine: The operative findings end results of treatment in the first 100 cases. J. Bone Joint Surg. 42A:295–310, 1960.
18. Hodgson, A. R., Wong, W., and Yau, A.: X-ray Appearances of Tuberculosis of the Spine. Springfield, IL, Charles C Thomas, 1969.
19. Hodgson, A. R., and Yau, A.: Pott's paraplegia: A classification based upon the living pathology. Paraplegia 5:1–16, 1967.
20. Hodgson, A. R., Yau, A., Kwon, J. S., and Kim, D.: A clinical study of 100 consecutive cases of Pott's paraplegia. Clin. Orthop. 36:128–149, 1964.
21. Hsu, L. C. S., Cheng, C. L., and Leong, J. C. Y.: Pott's paraplegia of late onset. The cause of compression and results after anterior decompression. J. Bone Joint Surg. 70B:534–538, 1988.
22. Kaufman, D. M., Kaplan, J. G., and Litman, N.: Infectious agents in spinal epidural abscesses. Neurology 30:844–850, 1980.
23. Kemp, H. B. S., Jackson, J. W., Jeremiah, J. D., and Hall, A. J.: Pyogenic infections occurring primarily in intervertebral discs. J. Bone Joint Surg. 55B:698–714, 1973.
24. Kumar, S., and Gulati, D. R.: Spinal abscesses. Neurol. India 26:193–195, 1978.
25. Leong, J. C. Y., and Hodgson, A. R.: Surgical treatment of tuberculosis of the spine. In Leach, R. E., Hoaglund, F. T., and Riseborough E. J. (eds.): Controversies in Orthopaedic Surgery. Philadelphia, W. B. Saunders, 1982, pp. 472–486.
26. Lifeso, R. M., Harder, E., and McCorkell, S. J.: Spinal brucellosis. J. Bone Joint Surg. 67B:345–351, 1985.
27. Litvinoff, J., and Nelson, M.: Extradural lumbar cryptococcosis. J. Neurosurg. 49:921–923, 1978.
28. Masmonteil, F., and Beclere, H.: Diagnostic radiographique des tuberculoses osteo-articulaires. J. Radiol. Electr. 7:259–266, 1923.
29. McCain, G. A., Harth, M., Bell, D. A., et al.: Septic discitis. J. Rheumatol. 8:100–109, 1981.
30. Medical Research Council Working Party on Tuberculosis of the Spine (First Report): A controlled trial of ambulant out-patient treatment and in-patient rest in bed in the management of tuberculosis of the spine in young Korean patients on standard chemotherapy. A study in Masan, Korea. J. Bone Joint Surg. 55B:678–697, 1973.
31. Medical Research Council Working Party on Tuberculosis of the Spine (Third Report): A controlled trial of débridement and ambulatory treatment in the management of tuberculosis of the spine in patients on standard chemotherapy. A study in Bulawayo, Rhodesia. J. Trop. Med. Hyg. 77:72–92, 1974.
32. Medical Research Council Working Party on Tuberculosis of the Spine (Fourth Report): A controlled trial of anterior spinal fusion and débridement in the surgical management of tuberculosis of the spine in patients on standard chemotherapy. A study in Hong Kong. Br. J. Surg. 61:853–866, 1974.
33. Medical Research Council Working Party on Tuberculosis of the Spine (Fifth Report): A five-year assessment of controlled trials of in-patient and out-patient treatment and of plaster-of-Paris jackets for tuberculosis of the spine in children on standard chemotherapy. Studies in Masan and Pusan, Korea. J. Bone Joint Surg. 58B:399–411, 1976.
34. Medical Research Council Working Party on Tuberculosis of the Spine (Sixth Report): A five-year assessments of controlled trials of ambulatory treatment, débridement and anterior spinal fusion in the management of tuberculosis of the spine. J. Bone Joint Surg. 60B:163–177, 1978.
35. Medical Research Council Working Party on Tuberculosis of the Spine (Eighth Report): A 10-year assessment of a controlled trial comparing débridement and anterior spinal fusion in the management of tuberculosis of the spine in patients on standard chemotherapy in Hong Kong. J. Bone Joint Surg. 64B:393–398, 1982.
36. Medical Research Council Working Party on Tuberculosis of the Spine (Ninth Report): A 10-year assessment of controlled trials of inpatient and outpatient treatment and of plaster-of-Paris jackets for tuberculosis of the spine in children on standard chemotherapy. J. Bone Joint Surg. 67B:103–110, 1985.
37. Medical Research Council Working Party on Tuberculosis of the Spine (Tenth Report): A controlled trial of 6-month and 9-month regimens of chemotherapy in patients undergoing radical surgery for tuberculosis of the spine in Hong Kong. Tubercle 67:243–259, 1986.
38. Mineiro, J. D.: Coluna Vertebral Humana: Alguns Aspectos da Sua Estrutura e Vascularizacao. Ph.D. Dissertation. Lisbon, Lisbon University, 1965.
39. Modic, M. T., Pavlicek, W., Weinstein, M. A., et al.: Magnetic resonance imaging of intervertebral disk disease. Radiology 152:103–111, 1984.
40. Muhle, I., Rau, J., and Ruskin, J.: Vertebral osteomyelitis due to Actinobacilius actinomycetemcomitans. JAMA 241:1824–1825, 1979.
41. Onofrio, B. M.: Intervertebral discitis: Incidence, diagnosis, and management. Clin. Neurosurg. 27:481–516, 1980.
42. Pun, W. K., Chow, S. P., Luk, K. D. K., et al.: Long-term follow-up on tuberculosis affecting the lumbosacral junction. J. Bone Joint Surg. 72B:675–678, 1990.
43. Pyogenic infections of the spine. Lancet 1:619–620, 1985.
44. Ravicovitch, M. A., and Spallone, A.: Spinal epidural abscesses. Eur. Neurol. 21:347–357, 1982.
45. Ryan, M. D., and Taylor, T. K. F.: The bacteriological diagnosis and antibiotic treatment of haematogenous vertebral osteomyelitis in adults. Aust. N. Z. J. Surg. 48:81–83, 1978.
46. Scoles, P. V., and Quinn, T. P.: Intervertebral discitis in children and adolescents. Clin. Orthop. 162:31–36, 1982.
47. Sharif, H. S.: Role of MR imaging in the management of spinal infections. AJR Am. J. Roentgenol. 158:1333–1345, 1992.
48. Silverthorn, K. G., and Gillespie, W. J.: Pyogenic spinal osteomyelitis: A review of 61 cases. N. Z. Med. J. 99:62–65, 1986.
49. Sorrel, E., and Sorrel-Dejerine, Y.: Recherches sur

Iatrogenic Discitis

ROBERT D. FRASER
BARRIE VERNON-ROBERTS
ORSO L. OSTI

Discitis is a potential complication of any procedure that involves entering the intervertebral disc. Contamination can occur during open or percutaneous surgical removal of the nucleus pulposus. Discitis may also result from the use of a contaminated needle during such procedures as discography, chemonucleolysis, lumbar puncture, myelography, and chemical sympathectomy.

Very few reports have described possible local complications of intradiscal injection. Discitis following discography with contrast material has been considered a rare complication,[4, 5, 19, 27-30, 45] with some investigators attributing it to a chemical or aseptic reaction.[4, 6, 28, 45] It has been suggested that discitis following discography is more common than previously recognized and may occur as often as once in 30 cases.[6, 12, 15]

The term discitis was more commonly associated with chemonucleolysis because of the exacerbation of back pain that frequently followed this procedure. Radiographic evidence of discitis following chemonucleolysis has been reported in as many as 2% of patients[32] and was generally attributed to a chemical or an aseptic process. Some studies described infective discitis following chemonucleolysis, but this seems to have been regarded as a separate entity.[1] In a review of 29,075 patients in the United States treated with chymopapain, Agre and colleagues[1] reported that 22 patients had developed discitis. The patients had severe back pain and spasm from a few days to many weeks following injection. In nine of them, bacterial infection had been confirmed by culture. A number of the remaining patients were considered to have aseptic discitis on the basis of negative cultures, and some had been treated with steroid therapy. These researchers did not state the time intervals between discography and needle biopsy. McCulloch and Macnab[31] reported no cases of infective discitis following chemonucleolysis in over 6000 patients. They believed that the incidence of "chemical" discitis was probably less than 1% and attributed the apparently low incidence of infective discitis to the bactericidal effect of chymopapain.

The evidence used to support the idea of a noninfective cause of discitis following discography and after chemonucleolysis was the following: the failure to isolate bacteria from biopsy material in most cases, the associated raised erythrocyte sedimentation rate (ESR) in the presence of a normal white blood cell count, the histopathologic findings of a chronic inflammatory process with lymphoid cell infiltration, and the tendency toward natural resolution. The same reasons have been advanced to support the idea of a noninfective cause for some cases of discitis after discectomy, although most investigators consider discitis following open procedures to be infective.[10, 25, 26, 36] In a review of the literature concerning postlaminectomy disc space infection, Fernand and Lee[10] stated that the route of infection was still not clear, as both hematogenous spread and local contamination may occur in a surgically traumatized area that has a poor blood supply.[25, 26, 44]

Discitis following discography was previously considered a rare occurrence, with a reported incidence of about 0.1%.[4, 5, 19, 27, 29, 40] Later studies have reported a higher incidence of discitis following both discography and treatment with chymopapain.[6, 7, 15, 30] However, because many individuals present with less severe symptoms and the disorder apparently resolves without treatment, the actual incidence of discitis following both discectomy and intradiscal injections is likely to be higher than the reported rates. The reported incidence of discitis following a standard discectomy varies from 0% to 2.8%,[10, 18] whereas the use of the operating microscope has been associated with a higher rate of discitis.[24, 30] Percutaneous discectomy complicated by discitis has also been reported.[8]

ETIOLOGY

Although there are claims of an aseptic causation,[11] there is compelling evidence to suggest that all cases of discitis with accompanying end-plate changes that result from an intradiscal procedure are due to bacterial contamination and are not due to a chemical, allergic, or some other aseptic process. The evidence for this is based on clinical and experimental studies:

In a clinical study,[15] the case records and radiographs of 432 patients who had undergone lumbar discography were reviewed. When an 18-gauge needle without a stylet had been used, discitis was diagnosed in 2.7% of 222 patients, but the use of needles with stylets in a two-needle technique at each level reduced the incidence to 0.7%. Seven patients with discitis after discography required anterior discectomy and fusion; their histopathologic findings were those of a chronic inflammatory response. Bacteria were isolated only from the discs of three of the four patients who had open biopsy less than 6 weeks from the time of discography. These findings suggest that bacteria were initiators rather than promoters of the response.

In an experimental study,[15] multiple-level lumbar discography was carried out in 11 mature sheep by injecting contrast material with or without various concentrations of bacteria. Radiographs were taken, and the discs and end plates were examined histologically and cultured for bacteria at intervals after injection. None of the controls showed any evidence of discitis, but all sheep injected with bacteria had typical radiographic and pathologic changes of discitis by 6 weeks, although cultures were almost all negative. The process did not seem to be dose related, and only a few bacteria were required to produce discitis. At 1 and 2 weeks after injection, bacteria could be isolated, but usually this could not be done after 3 weeks.

Despite the known bactericidal effect of chymopapain, similar results were obtained in a further experimental study.[13] Multiple-level lumbar intradiscal injections of chymopapain were carried out in eight mature sheep. Sixteen discs in four sheep were injected with a mixture of reconstituted chymopapain and a *Staphylococcus epidermidis* suspension, and 16 discs in another four sheep were injected with reconstituted chymopapain only. All sheep were sacrificed at 6 weeks. The discs and end plates were examined by means of radiologic and histopathologic procedures, and nuclear material was cultured for bacteria. None of the controls showed evidence of discitis, whereas all sheep injected with bacteria showed typical radiographic and pathologic changes of discitis, which occurred after the injection of very few bacteria. However, for most cases in which end-plate lesions were well established, there was no evidence of bacteria at sacrifice.

The intradiscal use of cephazolin sodium (Kefzol) in discography has caused the incidence of discitis to fall from 4.9% of 61 patients for one radiology practice[15] in a 12-month period to 0% of 127 patients during the first 12-month period when radiographic contrast material was mixed with cephazolin in a concentration of 1 mg/ml as a prophylactic measure against bacterial contamination.[35] The role of prophylactic antibiotics in the prevention of discitis following discography and chemonucleolysis was tested in another experimental study.[14] In 16 adult sheep lumbar intradiscal injections of bacteria were carried out at five adjacent levels. Eight of the animals were treated with intradiscal cephazolin, and the other eight were treated with a single intravenous injection of cephazolin. At the time of sacrifice at 6 weeks, all sheep showed no evidence of discitis at any level, and all cultures of disc material were negative. The results of this study indicated that either intradiscal or intravenous cephazolin was likely to substantially reduce the incidence of iatrogenic discitis resulting from intradiscal procedures. Varying doses of intravenous or intradiscal cephazolin as early as 1 day following inoculation of bacteria failed to arrest the sequence of changes typical of discitis.

Thus, the results of these studies strongly suggest that discitis is due to contamination of the intervertebral disc by bacteria and that antibiotics, while effective prophylactically, seem to have no effect on the development of the typical end-plate lesion after the condition is established.

PATHOLOGY

The histopathologic findings after discography of seven patients with discitis who required anterior discectomy and fusion are summarized in Table 1. Bacteria were recovered from three of four patients who had open biopsies carried out within 6 weeks of discography, but they were not isolated from any of the three patients who had open biopsies carried out more than 6 weeks after discography. The observation of disc vascularization, mature granulation tissue formation in both discs and vertebral bodies, the association of the more marked histologic changes with vertical disc protrusions, and the occasional presence of acute inflammatory cells in addition to chronic inflammation were features also common to the pathologic changes observed in experimental studies of discitis in sheep.[13, 15] In these studies, the histologic findings suggested that the earliest change was the disorganization of the end-plate region associated with granulation tissue and herniation of the nucleus pulposus. Although lesions were not visible at 1 week after injection, at 2 weeks macroscopic examination of the affected discs showed small herniations of nuclear material with an inflammatory reaction confined to the zone close to the end plate. Microscopically, the bony end plates and hyaline laminae had been breached in several places by granulation tissue (Fig. 1) and by the herniation of nuclear material. At 3 weeks, there was much more extensive loss of the end plates and hyaline laminae associated with larger protrusions of nuclear material into the vertebral bodies. The extruded nuclear material showed marked "capping" by neutrophil polymorphs in some places (Fig. 2), but the granulation tissue generally showed a paucity of acute inflammatory cells. A striking feature was the extensive replacement of vertebral bone by granulation tissue, even in regions where the end plate and nucleus were normal (Fig. 3). By 6 weeks, extruded and residual nuclear material had been extensively replaced by relatively avascular fibrous tissue and there was evidence of new bone forming at the periphery of the lesions in the vertebral bodies (Fig. 4). In most of the lesions, the granulation tissue contained moderate to few inflammatory cells, and these were mainly lymphocytes and plasma cells forming small aggregates. However, one or two microabscesses were found in the granulation tissue in a few discs (Fig. 5).

As has been seen in human specimens, the site of the lesion in experimental discitis corresponds to the needle-tip position (Fig. 6).

The following stages in the development of discitis after intradiscal procedures have been determined (Fig. 7):

1. Bacteria are introduced on the tip of a needle.
2. At the end of a week, the bacteria have multiplied, but there are no other abnormalities.
3. At 2 weeks, the end plate is thin but may still be intact. Immature granulation tissue has formed on the vertebral side of the end plate, and this is surrounded by a vascular response.
4. Three weeks after inoculation, the end plates have been ruptured with the herniation of nuclear material into the vertebral bodies. Granulation tissue lies against the herniated nucleus, and a more marked vas-

Text continued on page 907

Table 1

Summary and Grading of Histopathologic Features

		Disc Features					Vertebral Body Features					
					Inflammatory Cells						Inflammatory Cells	
Case	Disc	Vascular-ization	Granulation Tissue	Mature Fibrous Tissue	Acute	Chronic	End-Plate Defects	Nuclear Herniation	Granulation Tissue	Mature Fibrous Tissue	Acute	Chronic
1	L5–S1	++	+	−	−	−	++	−	++	++	+	++
2	L4–L5	+++	+++	++++	−	+	+++	++	++	+++	−	++
3	L4–L5	+++	+++	+++	−	+	++++	++	+	++	−	+++
4	L5–S1	++	−	−	++	−	+	−	++	++	++	+++
5	L4–L5	++	++++	++++	++	+++	++++	++	+++	++	++	+++
6	L4–L5	++	+	−	+	++	+	−	+	−	+	−
7	L4–L5	+++	+++	+++	−	+	+++	++	+++	++	−	+

Subjective assessment of the extent of the features listed is from minimal (+) to marked (++++).

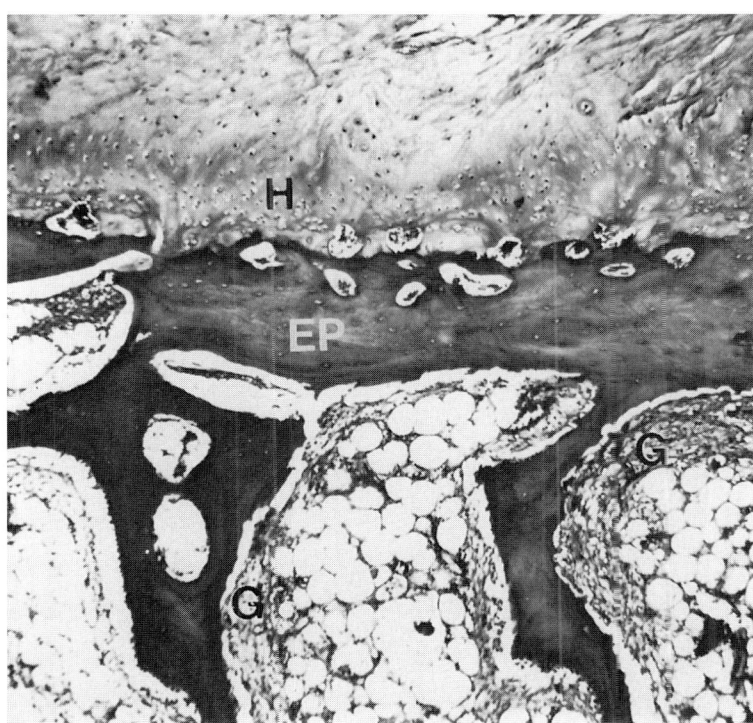

Figure 1. Low-power micrograph of L1–L2 disc in a sheep 2 weeks after injection of iothalamate meglumine 60% (Conray) and *S. epidermidis*. It shows intact regions of the end plate (EP) and prominent vascular channels extending into the hyaline lamina (H). The marrow spaces in the adjoining bone show young granulation tissue (G) extending along the trabecular surfaces, which are undergoing resorption. (Hematoxylin and eosin, × 50.) (From Fraser, R. D., Osti, O. L., and Vernon-Roberts, B.: Discitis after discography. J. Bone Joint Surg. 69B:26–35, 1987.)

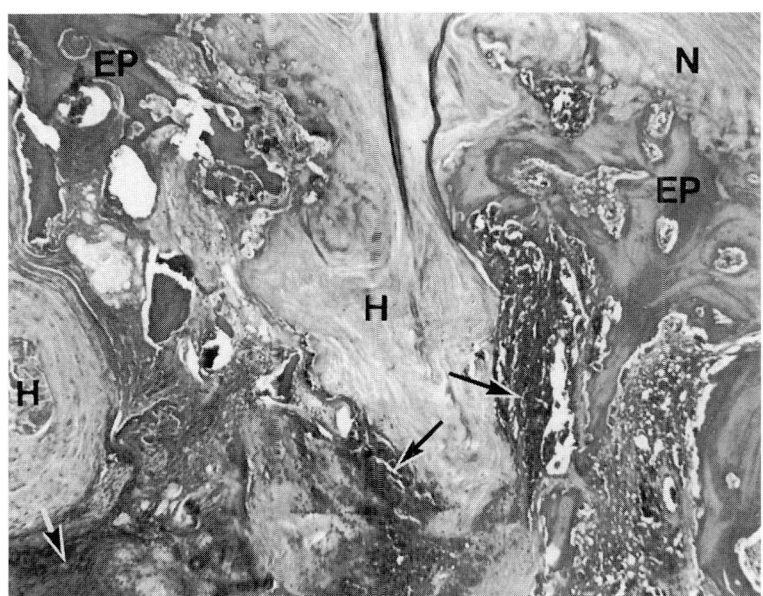

Figure 2. Low-power micrograph of L2–L3 disc in a sheep 3 weeks after injection of Conray and *S. epidermidis*. It shows herniations (H) of material from the nucleus pulposus (N) through the end plate (EP). The dark areas *(arrows)* capping the herniations represent an acute inflammatory reaction with numerous neutrophil polymorphs. (Hematoxylin and eosin, × 50.)

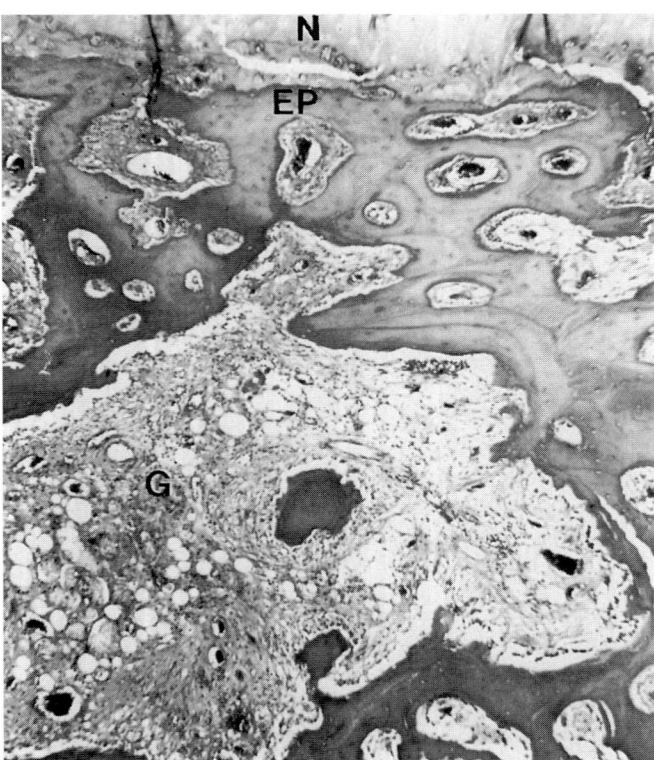

Figure 3. Low-power micrograph of L2–L3 disc in a sheep 3 weeks after injection of Conray and *S. epidermidis*. It shows extensive replacement of vertebral cancellous bone by granulation tissue (G) adjoining the intact end plate (EP) and normal nucleus pulposus (N). (Hematoxylin and eosin, × 50.) (From Fraser, R. D., Osti, O. L., and Vernon-Roberts, B.: Discitis after discography. J. Bone Joint Surg. 69B:26–35, 1987.)

Figure 4. Low-power micrograph of L3–L4 disc in a sheep 6 weeks after injection of Conray and *S. epidermidis*. It shows the disorganization of the nucleus with preservation of the outer annulus (A), disappearance of end plates and adjoining vertebral cancellous bone, herniation of nuclear material into both vertebral bodies, granulation tissue and fibrous tissue extending into the central region of the disc with (dark) intradiscal hemorrhages, and new bone forming at the junction of fibrous tissues with the residual cancellous bone of the vertebral bodies. (Hematoxylin and eosin, × 8.) (From Fraser, R. D., Osti, O. L., and Vernon-Roberts, B.: Discitis after discography. J. Bone Joint Surg. 69B:26–35, 1987.)

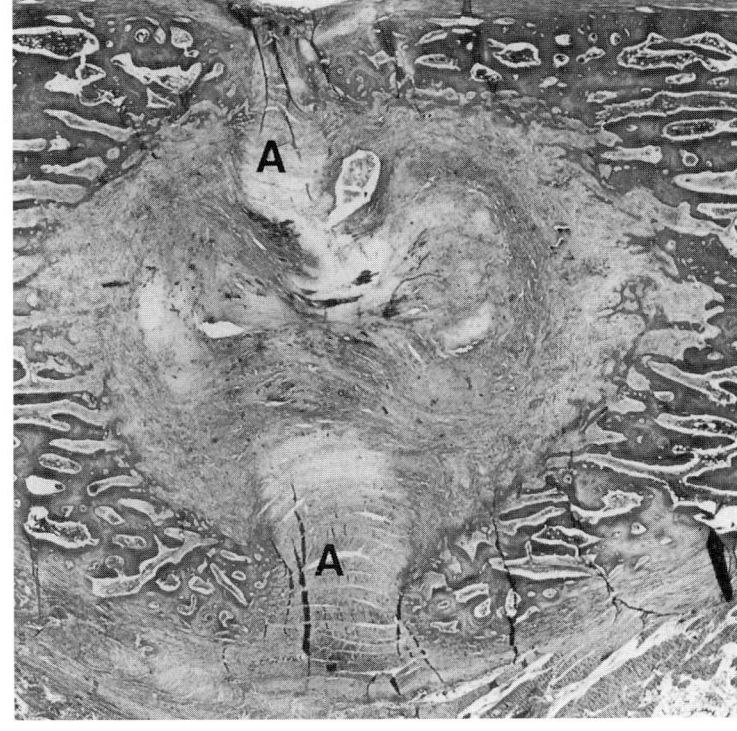

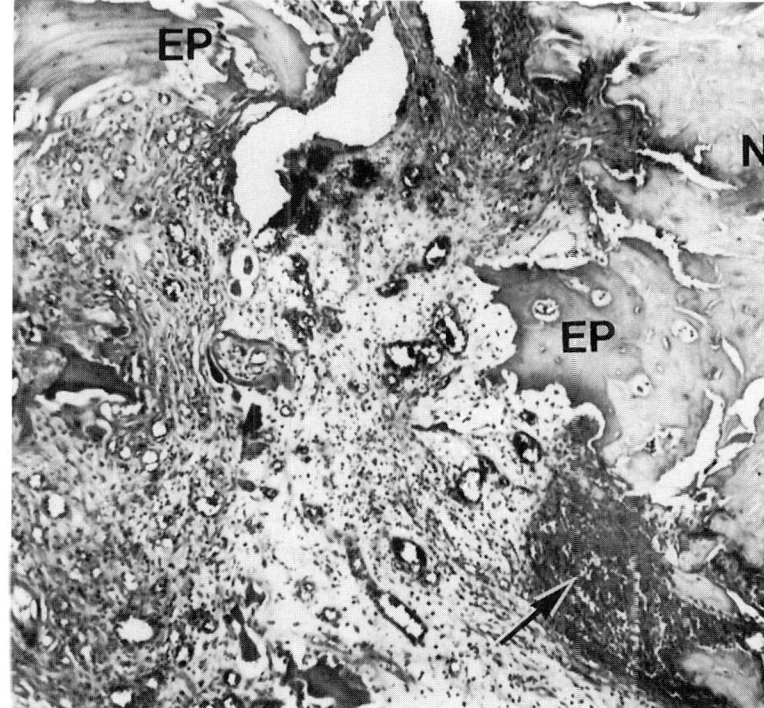

Figure 5. Low-power micrograph of L2–L3 in a sheep 6 weeks after injection of Conray and *S. epidermidis*. It shows that the end-plate (EP) has been breached by granulation tissue extending into the nucleus (N), and the presence of a microabscess *(arrow)*. (Hematoxylin and eosin, × 50.)

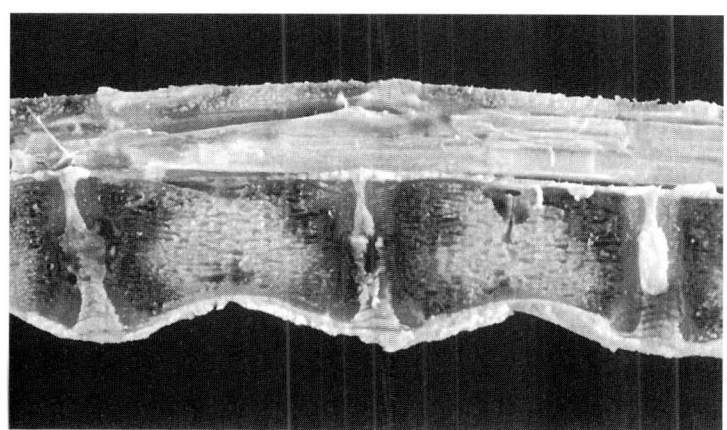

Figure 6. Macroscopic view of portion of spine in a sheep following injection of chymopapain and bacteria at all three levels illustrated. L3–L4 disc *(left)* shows largely central discitis; L2–L3 disc *(center)* shows combination of central and anterior discitis; and L1–L2 disk *(right)* shows anterior discitis alone. (From Fraser, R. D., Osti, O. L., and Vernon-Roberts, B.: Discitis following chemonucleolysis: An experimental study. Spine 11:34–43, 1986.)

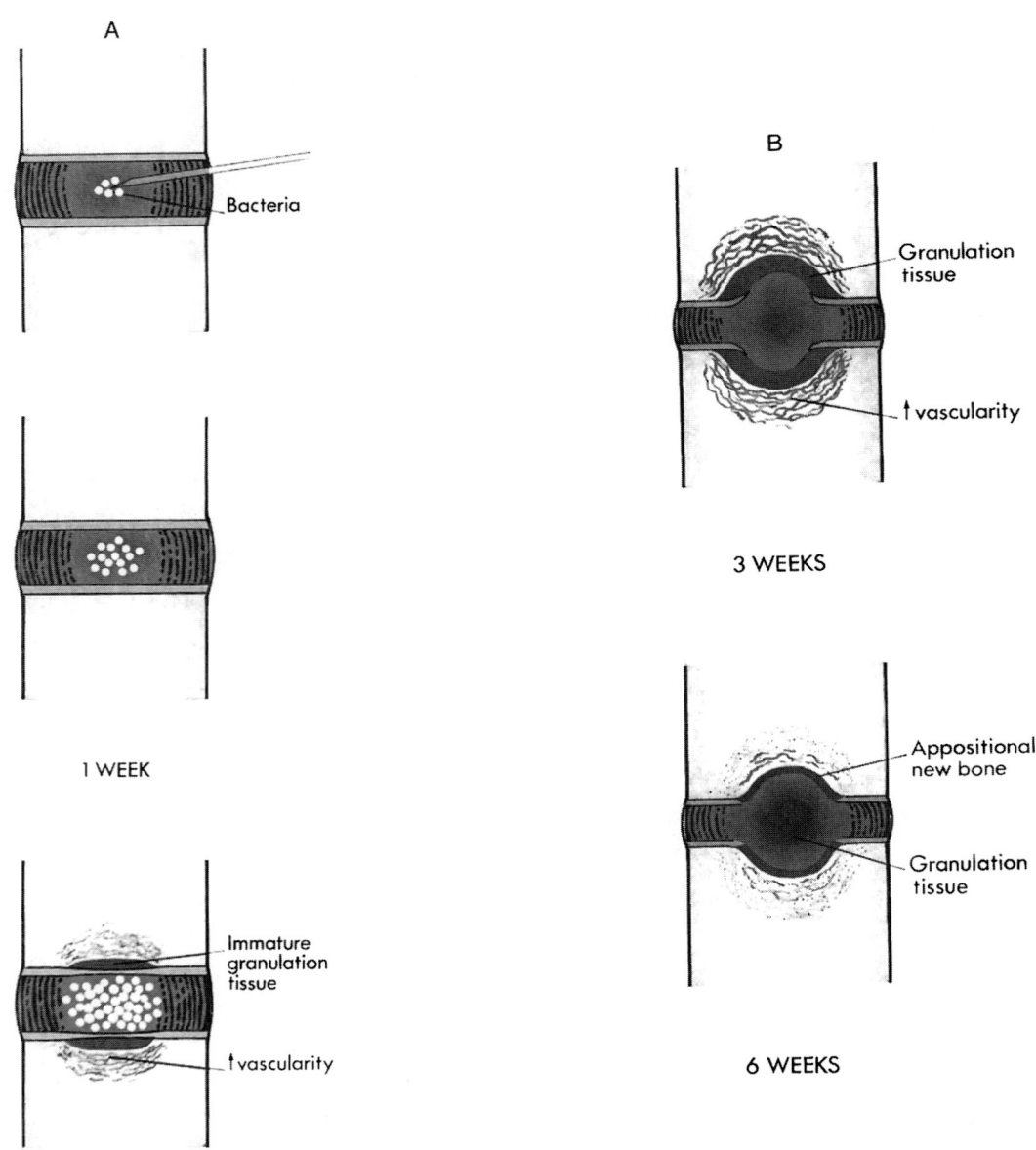

Figure 7. *A, B,* The stages in the development of discitis after discography.

cular response is present. At this stage, the bacteria are usually destroyed.

5. By 6 weeks, the lesion is approaching maturity with appositional new bone formation, and the nuclear material has been largely replaced by granulation tissue. In most cases, the bacteria have been eradicated. In a few instances, the lesion takes longer to reach maturity, and bacteria may persist, leading to osteomyelitis.

The pathologic response in postdiscectomy discitis is altered by the extent of the disc space clearance As with postinjection discitis at a level with gross degenerative changes, the end-plate lesion produced in postdiscectomy discitis tends to be more diffuse, as distinct from the classic discrete lesions of discitis following discography at a normal level.

PRESENTATION AND CLINICAL COURSE

Although the severity of symptoms of discitis varies widely, the clinical features are similar, irrespective of the cause. The clinical hallmark of discitis is back pain. Postoperative or postinjection pain may persist and then gradually increase in severity. In some individuals, the pain is excruciating, not relieved by rest, and poorly relieved by the administration of narcotic analgesics. The pain is aggravated by any attempt at movement and is accompanied by severe muscle spasm. Often, the spine is held rigidly in extension in a manner similar to that seen in childhood discitis. Not only does the patient resist moving the back, but straight leg raising is grossly limited on both sides by back pain. In this more severe form of postinjection discitis, fever may be present for 1 or 2 days, but in most cases the patient remains afebrile. An elevated temperature is more commonly associated with discitis after open procedures.[10, 26] Some patients have increased back pain, which develops insidiously following the procedure and may slowly subside over a period of several weeks or months.

The diagnosis of iatrogenic discitis may be overlooked because the clinical expression of the disease varies markedly and because the physical, laboratory, and radiologic findings may be masked by the recent intervention. Some patients are likely to be regarded as hyperreacting to operative or postinjection pain or their problems may be dismissed as "functional." Many patients experience an exacerbation of back pain following intradiscal injections, possibly owing to a mechanical or chemical effect, but the pain invariably resolves spontaneously within 1 to 2 weeks.

Although the clinical course of postinjection discitis varies considerably, there is a tendency for spontaneous resolution over a period of several weeks to 6 months or so, in which the patient's symptoms usually gradually subside. Sometimes, however, disabling back symptoms persist. Although the infective process is usually self-limited, individuals occasionally progress to a vertebral osteomyelitis and the possible extension of an abscess to the epidural space[7] with the risk of neural compression.

The prognosis of patients with postoperative discitis is poor.[20, 26] In a review of 33 patients with discitis following open discectomy, Lindholm and Pylkkanen[25] found the average duration of the disease was 7.4 months (range of 1.5 months to 2 years). At an average follow-up of 7.5 years, they found that most patients had disabling back symptoms and more than 60% had still not returned to work. Radiographic assessment revealed that bone bridging or spontaneous fusion had occurred in 42% of cases. They advised prophylaxis and early appropriate treatment to prevent a chronic disorder and protracted disability.

INVESTIGATIONS

The ESR is usually increased, but in postoperative cases this is partly attributable to the surgical procedure itself. Jonsson and colleagues[21] found that the ESR rapidly increases and then declines after lumbar spine surgery in patients without postoperative infection. The maximum mean peak value was seen 4 days after surgery (disc surgery, ESR of 75 mm/h; fusion surgery, ESR of 102 mm/h). After 2 weeks, the values were normal for the majority of patients. After contamination by an intradiscal needle, the ESR may not become elevated for 10 to 14 days, even in patients who have increased back pain with associated muscle spasms within a few days of the procedure. There is variation in

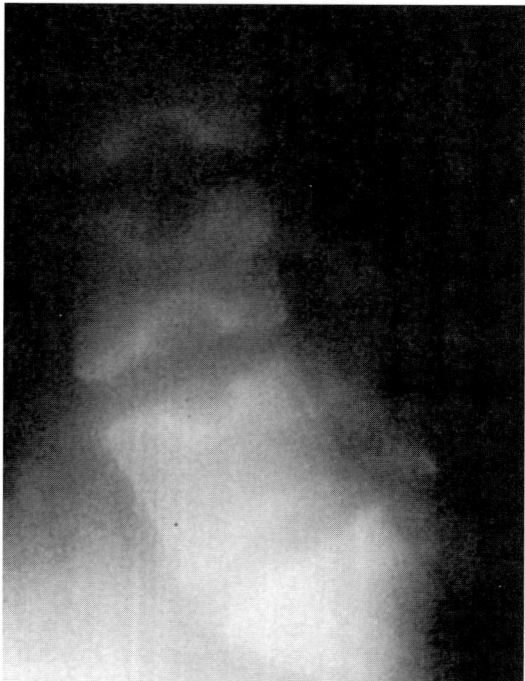

Figure 8. Lateral tomogram of lumbar spine 3 months after two-level discography shows the erosions of the end plates at both levels, a classic characteristic of postdiscography discitis. The sclerotic margins of the erosions are typical of late lesions.

erosions may be seen. These changes are better demonstrated by lateral tomography (Fig. 8) or by computed tomography, although generally 2 or 3 weeks must pass before they appear. This sequence of radiographic changes in the human is similar in timing and extent to that seen in experimental discitis in the sheep (Fig. 9).

A technetium bone scan often confirms the diagnosis of discitis following an intradiscal injection, but it is less useful in diagnosis following open surgery because of the increased amount of tracer around the surgically treated vertebral segment. A gallium scan appears to be more reliable in confirming the diagnosis of discitis.[34] Sometimes, the identification of the level or levels involved when multiple-level discography has been carried out can be difficult because bone scans may not be positive, particularly in the early acute phase of the disease. Magnetic resonance imaging is probably more sensitive in confirming the diagnosis early in the disease process[33, 41] by an alteration of

the effect on the ESR, which has ranged from normal levels to 90 mm/h in the authors' experience. An elevation of the C-reactive protein is a more consistent finding in these patients.

The white blood cell count nearly always remains normal, although it may be near the upper limit of normal values, and an associated neutrophilia is common. A leukocytosis is more frequently associated with postdiscectomy discitis and is partly attributable to the procedure itself. Blood cultures are usually negative, unless obtained early in the disease process. This is similar to the findings in childhood discitis; in one large series, blood cultures were positive only within the first 6 weeks of the onset of symptoms.[43]

The earliest radiographic change is narrowing of the height of the disc space, which may occur as early as 2 to 3 weeks after the procedure but in some cases may take some months to develop. As time passes, there is usually loss of definition of the bony end plate as seen on radiographs, and vertebral

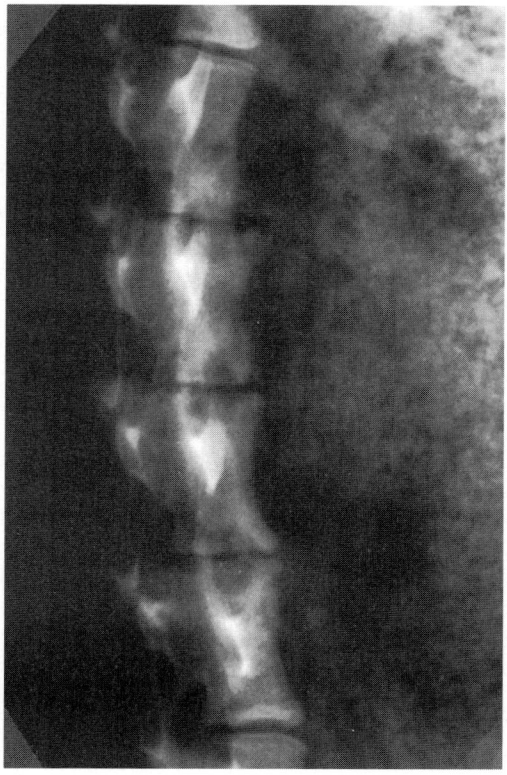

Figure 9. Three-level end-plate erosions in the sheep at 6 weeks after the intradiscal injection of Conray and *S. epidermidis*.

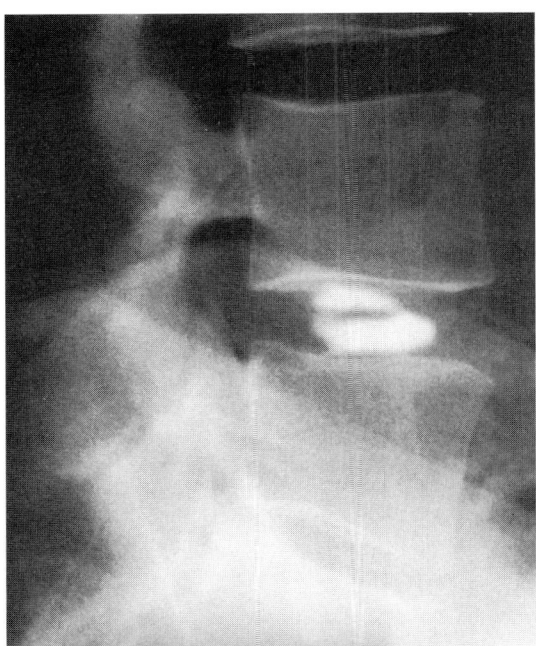

Figure 10. Normal L4–L5 discogram (case 1) is shown. (From Fraser, R. D., Osti, O. L., and Vernon-Roberts, B.: Discitis after discography J. Bone Joint Surg. 69B:26–35, 1987.)

the signal in the end-plate region. Furthermore, gadolinium-enhancement has heightened the sensitivity of this investigation, particularly in patients who develop postoperative discitis.[2, 37]

An aspiration or core biopsy of the affected disc space is likely to result in the identification of the bacteria, provided that this procedure is performed within a few weeks of inoculation Localization of the offending organism becomes less likely with the passage of time.

ILLUSTRATIVE CASES

From 1982 to 1984, seven patients with discitis after discography required anterior discectomy and fusion at the affected level. At operation, the disc and adjacent end plates were removed en bloc using dowel-cutting instruments.[3] Swabs were taken from the disc space and sent for microbiologic examination. The case histories of these patients are summarized in Table 2 and the histopathologic findings in Table 1. Two illustrative cases are reported in detail.

CASE ■ 1

A 28-year-old soldier presented with an 8-month history of increasing low back pain following repeated falls at work, where he was an army physical instructor. Examination revealed bilateral restriction of straight leg raising to 45 degrees by back pain, and there were no abnormal neurologic signs in the lower limbs. Discography at the L4–L5 level demonstrated a normal disc with no pain reproduction (Fig. 10). At the L5–S1 level, the injection was directed into a false cavity in the annulus and was reported to reproduce the patient's typical symptoms. Immediately following discography, the pain was more severe. Six weeks later, the patient's ESR was 24 mm/h. Under general anesthesia, discography was repeated, and a major extravasation of contrast material was observed through the upper and lower end plates of the L4–L5 level (Fig. 11). At the L5–S1 level, a more limited end-plate lesion was demonstrated posteriorly, corresponding to the position of the false cavity injection. The patient underwent anterior disc clearance and interbody fusion at L4–L5 and L5–S1, using a muscle-splitting retroperitoneal approach. Histologic examination of L5–S1 disc material showed heavily inflamed granulation tissue in both the hyaline laminae and the bone of the region of the end plate; acute inflammatory cells and chronic inflammation in disc material were observed (Fig. 12). A culture of this material demonstrated a light growth of *Pseudomonas aeruginosa*. The postoperative course was uneventful, and 9 months after the procedure the patient was assessed as being pain free. X-ray studies demonstrated consolidation at both levels.

CASE ■ 2

A 21-year-old naval rating presented with a 12-month history of disabling low back pain after lifting heavy drums along a gangway. He was unable to work, and his condition failed to respond to conservative treatment. Plain x-ray findings demonstrated a grade I spondylolisthesis. This was investigated by lumbar discography, which demonstrated minimal nuclear degeneration at the L4–L5 level and a degenerated disc at L5–S1 with reproduction of his typical back pain (Fig. 13). His symptoms became progressively more severe following discography, and arrangements were made to carry out an anterior interbody fusion at the L5–S1 level. A diagnosis of discitis was considered at the time but was thought to have been excluded by an ESR of only 22 mm/h and a plain lateral x-ray study 1 month after discography, which showed no evidence of disc space narrowing or erosion. Two weeks after anterior interbody fusion at L5–S1 (Fig. 14), he was still reporting severe pain and needed a par-

Table 2

Details of Seven Patients Having an Open Biopsy After Discography

Case	Age (years)	Original Diagnosis	ERS Between Discography and Surgery (mm/h)	Radiographs	Bone Scan	Interval Between Discography and Biopsy	Histologic Evidence of Discitis	Bacterial Culture
1	28	L5–S1 internal disc disruption	24	Large end-plate erosion	—	5 weeks	Yes	*Pseudomonas aeruginosa* (light growth)
2	21	Grade I isthmic spondylolisthesis of L5–S1	2	Large end-plate erosion at L4–L5	—	3 months	Yes	No growth
3	47	Discogenic back pain at L5–S1	50	End-plate erosion at L4–L5	Patchy nonspecific uptake	6 months	Yes	No growth
4	38	Back pain after compression fracture of L4	30	End-plate erosion at L5–S1	Abnormal at L5–S1	4 weeks	Yes	*S. epidermidis*
5	40	Grade II traumatic spondylolisthesis	99	—	Abnormal at L4–L5	3 weeks	Yes	No growth
6	18	Grade II isthmic spondylolisthesis	—	—	—	4 weeks	No	*Klebsiella pneumoniae*
7	46	Grade II degenerative spondylolisthesis	105	End-plate erosion at L4–L5	Abnormal at L4–L5	3 months	Yes	No growth

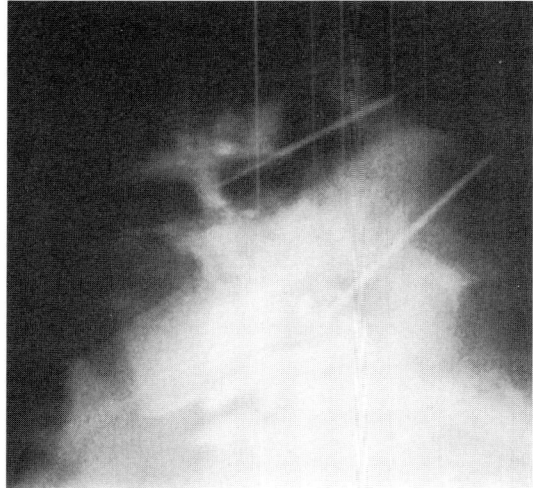

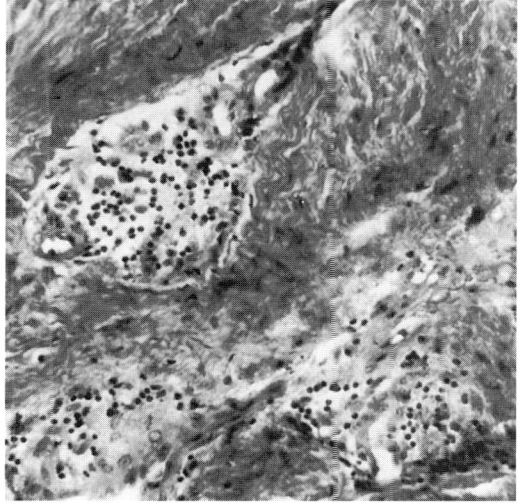

Figure 12. Chronic inflammation in the mature fibrous scar tissue within the disc shows clusters of lymphocytes grouped around small blood vessels (case 1). (Hematoxylin and eosin, × 100.) (From Fraser, R. D., Osti, O. L., and Vernon-Roberts, B.: Discitis after discography. J. Bone Joint Surg. 69B:26–35, 1987.)

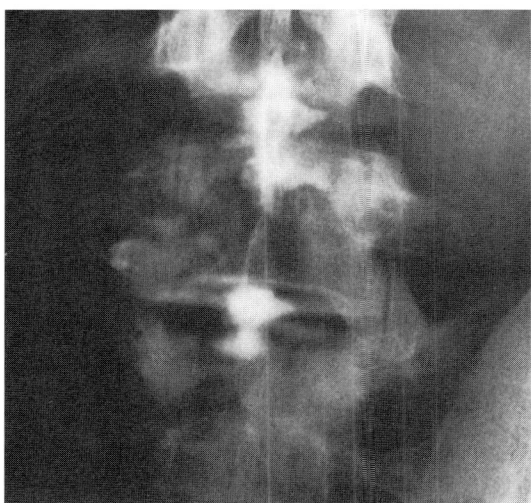

Figure 11. Lateral (top) and anteroposterior (bottom) discograms 5 weeks after the initial procedure show end-plate disruption at L4–L5 and L5–S1 (case 1).

enteral narcotic. He continued to require large amounts of analgesics, and 3 months after his interbody fusion plain x-ray films demonstrated that the disc space narrowing had occurred at the L4–L5 level together with a massive erosion in the L5 vertebral body (Fig. 15). Under general anesthesia, aspiration biopsy of the L4–L5 disc space was carried out, but a culture of this failed to reveal an organism. Contrast material was injected to outline the defect (Fig. 16), and he was treated with an intradiscal corticosteroid injection. This failed to result in the relief of his symptoms, and he had not improved after 6 weeks' immobilization in a brace. Seven months after the initial discogram had been carried out,

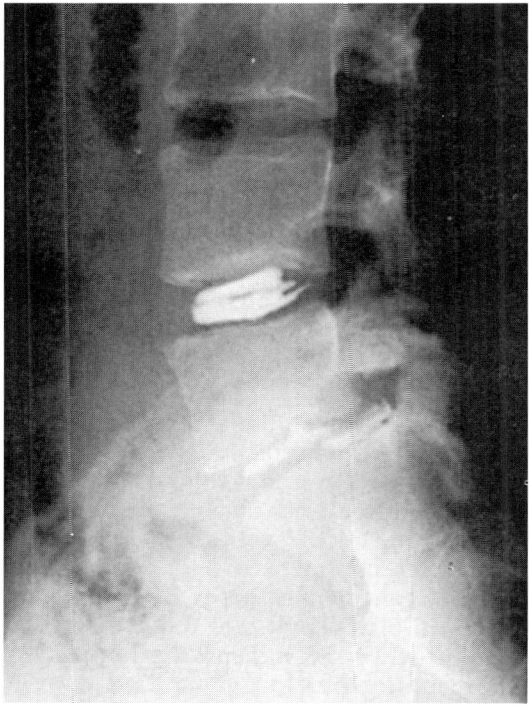

Figure 13. Lateral discograms demonstrate minimum nuclear degeneration at L4–L5 and a degenerated disc at L5–S1 (case 2). (From Fraser, R. D., Osti, O. L., and Vernon-Roberts, B.: Discitis after discography. J. Bone Joint Surg. 69B:26–35, 1987.)

he underwent anterior disc clearance and interbody fusion at the L4–L5 level, and this was followed by dramatic pain relief that has been sustained. Histologic examination of the L4–L5 intervertebral disc and adjacent end plates showed extensive destruction of the end-plate region (Fig. 17). There was abundant anterior granulation and fibrous tissue extending into the nucleus, but chronic inflammatory cells were few.

TREATMENT

Treatment should mainly be directed toward prevention. A strict aseptic technique is required for any intradiscal procedure. The skin should be prepared over a wide area and the drapes firmly fixed. The patient should be sedated to minimize movement for procedures carried out under local anesthesia. Care must be taken to avoid contamination of the drapes by x-ray equipment. Only needles with stylets should be used for intradiscal injection procedures, and a two-needle technique for each level is recommended. The operator should avoid touching the needle shaft, particularly near the tip, and a separate needle should be used for each skin puncture. Similar principles should be observed during percutaneous discectomy. Because of the increased inci-

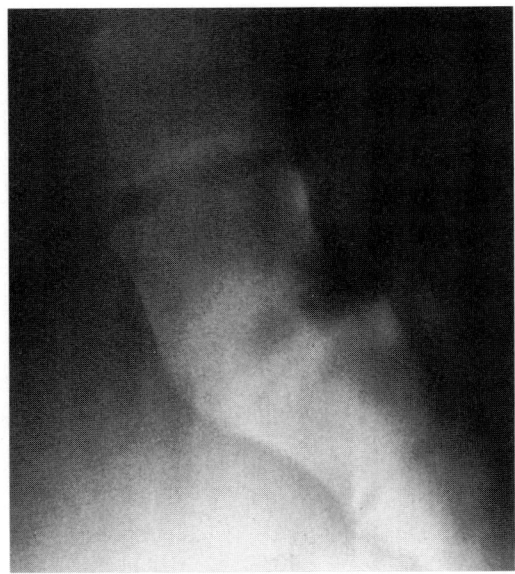

Figure 15. Lateral radiograph 3 months after interbody fusion demonstrates disc space narrowing at L4–L5 and a massive erosion of L5 vertebral body (case 2).

dence of discitis accompanying the use of the operative microscope, one should take great care when using this equipment to avoid contaminating the surgical gloves and the operative field.

Clinical and experimental evidence now supports the prophylactic use of a suitable antibiotic such as cephazolin administered either intradiscally or intravenously. For intradiscal injection procedures, the authors recommend that cephazolin be added to the contrast agent, when this is used, to a concentration of 1 mg/ml. For other intradiscal procedures, the intravenous administration of 1 to 2 g of cephazolin just before the commencement of the procedure is recommended. Boscardin and associates[3] demonstrated that the optimum level of intradiscal cephazolin is reached 15 to 18 minutes after the intravenous bolus is given.

Some doubt remains about the role of antibiotics in the treatment of established discitis. Although in most cases the bacterial response is self-limited, appropriate antibiotic administration may hasten recovery; however, this has yet to be proved. Pilgaard[36] found that antibiotics made no difference in the outcome of disc space infection following laminectomy. However, most investigators have advocated the use of antibiotics when a bacteriologic diagnosis has

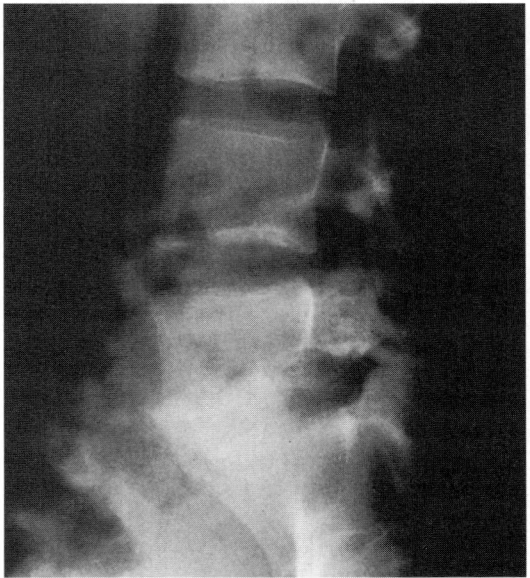

Figure 14. Lateral radiograph was taken 6 weeks after discography and 2 weeks after anterior interbody fusion at L5–S1 (case 2).

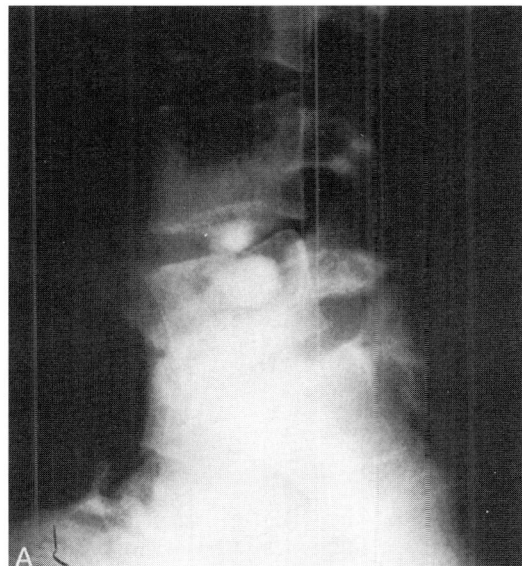

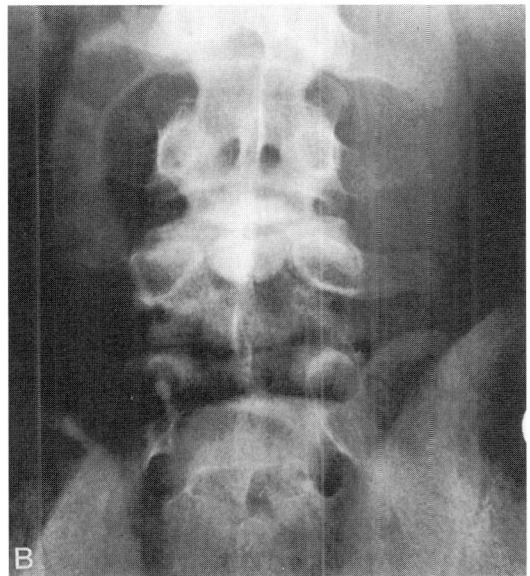

Figure 16. A, Lateral discogram demonstrates end-plate disruption 4 months after discography and 3 months after anterior interbody fusion at L5–S1 (case 2). B, Anteroposterior discogram demonstrates end-plate disruption (case 2). (From Fraser, R. D., Osti, O. L., and Vernon-Roberts, B.: Discitis after discography. J. Bone Joint Surg. 69B:26–35, 1987.)

been made.[10, 25, 26] Gibson and coworkers[17] were unable to assay antibiotics from disc material in humans after the intravenous injection of high doses of various preparations. Other studies in animals have since demonstrated by indirect means that antibiotics do cross the end plate[6, 14] and in sufficient amounts eradicate up to 2000 bacteria, but these studies have failed to demonstrate any therapeutic effect of antibiotics in the control of established discitis.[16] Antibiotics may, however, have a definite role in the few cases in which iatrogenic discitis proceeds to a vertebral osteomyelitis. Because of this small but important group of patients, a case can be made for an early attempt to isolate the bacteria by a needle biopsy of the affected disc followed by the intravenous administration of an appropriate antibiotic.

Some patients gain worthwhile symptomatic relief from the use of a brace or a spinal

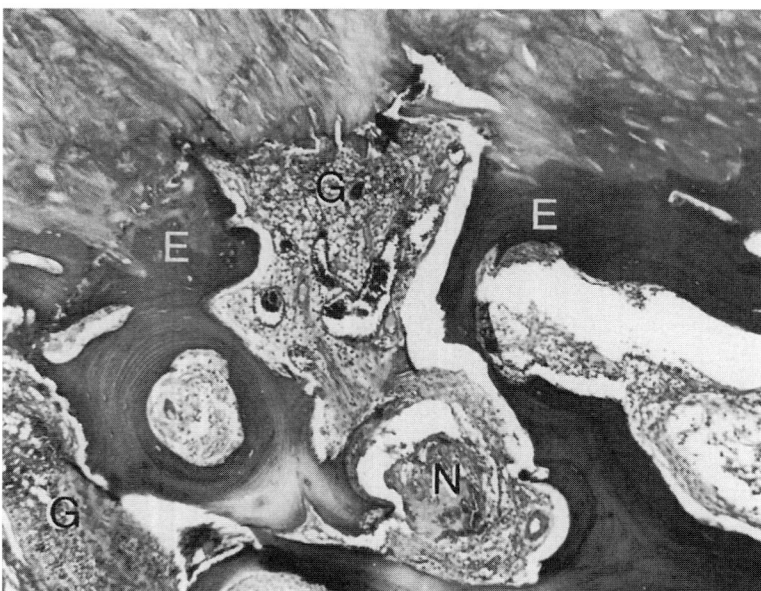

Figure 17. Low-power micrograph shows a breach in the end plate (E) with herniation of nuclear material (N) and granulation tissue (G) extending into the disc and marrow spaces (case 2). (Hematoxylin and eosin, × 50.) (From Fraser, R. D., Osti, O. L., and Vernon-Roberts, B.: Discitis after discography. J. Bone Joint Surg. 69B:26–35, 1987.)

jacket, which may need to be worn for 3 to 6 months. Successful treatment of postinjection discitis has been reported with both intradiscal[6] and systemic[16] steroids. In light of research,[13, 15] steroids should be considered only in the late phase when the radiographic lesion is quiescent, with a smooth sclerotic margin demonstrated by lateral tomography.

When a patient with disabling back symptoms develops discitis following preoperative discography at either the intended or an adjacent level of the spinal fusion, it seems appropriate to treat the patient by means of anterior disc clearance and interbody fusion after the diagnosis has been confirmed, rather than to wait for spontaneous resolution of the discitis, which would at best return the patient to the preinjection level of symptoms. In patients who have already undergone surgery prior to the development of postdiscographic discitis at an adjacent level, conservative measures as detailed above seem more appropriate for initial treatment. In cases of postinjection discitis in which the patient has persistent severe pain that does not respond to appropriate vigorous conservative measures, anterior disc clearance and interbody fusion should be considered, given the poor prognosis of patients with postoperative discitis managed conservatively.[20, 26] In light of the poor results of conservative measures, anterior disc clearance and interbody fusion should be considered also in this group of patients if there are few signs of response to early appropriate treatment.

NOMENCLATURE

The term discitis is logically reserved for a primary infection of the intervertebral disc. Spontaneously occurring discitis in the adult is undoubtedly an osteomyelitis of the vertebral body with secondary involvement of the intervertebral disc space. In most cases of iatrogenic discitis, the bacteria are removed after the vertebral end plate is breached. However, in a few cases a secondary vertebral osteomyelitis develops.

Apart from iatrogenic discitis, primary disc space infection occurs only in childhood. Some authorities consider discitis of childhood to be always secondary to osteomyelitis.[38, 43] Schmorl and Junghanns[39] described the sequence of the development of a small abscess in the end-plate region of the vertebral body with subsequent eruption into the adjacent disc rather than destruction of the vertebral bone. Childhood discitis is typified by radiographic disc space narrowing, and both end plates are usually involved. The observation that one end-plate lesion is larger than the other has been used as evidence to support the contention that discitis in childhood is a vertebral osteomyelitis with secondary involvement of the disc.[43] However, asymmetric adjacent end-plate lesions have commonly been encountered with iatrogenic discitis, and in some cases an end-plate lesion on one side only (usually the lower end plate) occurs.[16]

The clinical picture and clinical course of childhood discitis closely parallel those of discitis from needle contamination; both conditions are dissimilar to spontaneously occurring discitis in the adult, except for the development of spontaneous interbody fusion, which rarely occurs in the child. Frank purulence and paravertebral abscesses are extremely rare complications of childhood discitis[23, 38] and more commonly occur in iatrogenic discitis in association with a secondary vertebral osteomyelitis. The sheep studies have demonstrated that few bacteria are required to produce iatrogenic discitis, and it seems possible that a few bacteria could enter the inner annulus of a child's intervertebral disc from a vascular outer annulus.

CONCLUSION

All cases of iatrogenic discitis with accompanying end-plate changes resulting from an intradiscal procedure are attributable to bacterial contamination. In most cases, the bacterial infection resolves spontaneously, even though the patient may continue to have disabling back symptoms. It is likely that the incidence of discitis is higher than that reported in most series. The popularity of percutaneous disc excision[22] is likely to be associated with a significant incidence of discitis[8] unless appropriate preventive measures are taken, including the prophylactic use of a suitable antibiotic.

REFERENCES

1. Agre, K., Wilson, R. R., Brim, M. and McDermot, D. J.: Chymodiactin: Post marketing surveillance: Demographic and adverse experience data in 29,075 patients. Spine 9:479–485, 1984.
2. Boden, S. D., David, D. O., Dina, T. S., et al.: Postoperative diskitis: Distinguishing early MR imaging findings from normal postoperative disk space changes. Radiology 184:765–771, 1992.
3. Boscardin, J. B., Ringus, J. C., Feingold, D. J., and Ruda, S. C.: Human intradiscal levels with cefazolin. Spine 17:S145–S148, 1992.
4. Brodsky, A. E., and Binder, W. F.: Lumbar discography—its value in diagnosis and treatment of lumbar disc lesions. Spine 4:110–120, 1979.
5. Collis, J. S., and Gardner, W. J.: Lumbar discography: An analysis of one thousand cases. J. Neurosurg. 19:452–461, 1962.
6. Crock, H. V.: Practice of Spinal Surgery. Wien, Springer-Verlag, 1983.
7. Crock, H. V., and Patrikios, S. J.: Unpublished data, 1986.
8. Dendrinos, G. K., and Polyzoides, J. A.: Spondylodiscitis after percutaneous discectomy. A case diagnosed by M.R.I. Acta Orthop. Scand. 63:219–220, 1992.
9. Eismont, F. J., Wiesel, S. W., Brighton, C. T., and Rothman, R. H.: Antibiotic penetration into rabbit nucleus pulposus. Spine 12:254–256, 1987.
10. Fernand, R., and Lee, C. K.: Post laminectomy disc space infection: A review of the literature and a report of three cases. Clin. Orthop. 209:215–218, 1986.
11. Fouquet, B., Goupille, P., Jattiot, F., et al.: Discitis after lumbar disc surgery. Features of "aseptic" and "septic" forms. Spine 17:356–358, 1992.
12. Fraser, R. D.: Chymopapain for the treatment of intervertebral disc herniation: The final report of a double-blind study. Spine 9:815–818, 1984.
13. Fraser, R. D., Osti, O. L., and Vernon-Roberts, B.: Discitis following chemonucleolysis: An experimental study. Spine 11:34–43, 1986.
14. Fraser, R. D., Zhang, Y.-F., and Vernon-Roberts, B.: The role of prophylactic antibiotics in the prevention of discitis following chemonucleolysis: An experimental study. Presented to the International Society for the Study of the Lumbar Spine Meeting, Rome, 1986.
15. Fraser, R. D., Osti, O. L., and Vernon-Roberts, B.: Discitis after discography. J. Bone Joint Surg. 69B:26–35, 1987.
16. Fraser, R. D., Osti, O. L., and Vernon-Roberts, B.: Unpublished data, 1988.
17. Gibson, M. J., Karpinsky, M. R. K., Slack, R. C. B., et al.: The penetration of antibiotics into the normal intervertebral disc. J. Bone Joint Surg. 69B:784–786, 1987.
18. Graf, R., Reinhardt, H., and Gratzl, O.: Prolapses in adolescents of lumbar intervertebral discs: I—clinical observations. Neurochirurgia (Stuttg.) 27:12–15, 1984.
19. Gresham, J. L., and Miller, R.: Evaluation of the lumbar spine by discography and its use in selection of proper treatment of the herniated disc syndrome. Clin. Orthop. 67:29–41, 1969.
20. Iversen, E., Nielsen, V. A., and Hansen, L. G.: Prognosis in postoperative discitis. A retrospective study of 111 cases. Acta Orthop. Scand. 63:305–309 1992.
21. Jonsson, B., Soderholm, R., and Stromqvist, B.: Erythrocyte sedimentation rate after lumbar spine surgery. Spine 16:1049–1050, 1991.
22. Kambin, P., and Sampson, S.: Posterolateral percutaneous suction-excision of herniated lumbar intervertebral discs: Report of interim results. Clin. Orthop. 207:37–43, 1986.
23. Kemp, H. B. S., Jackson, J. W., Jeremiah, J. D., and Hall, A. J.: Pyogenic infections occurring primarily in intervertebral discs. J. Bone Joint Surg. 55B:698–714, 1973.
24. Kho, H. C. H., and Steudel, W. I.: Comparison be-

tween lumbar microdiscectomy and standard discectomy in lumbar disc herniations: A retrospective analysis of 267 cases. Neurochirurgia (Stuttg.) 29:181–185, 1986.
25. Kirkaldy-Willis, W. H.: Complications of disc surgery—discitis. Orthop. Trans. 7:110, 1983.
26. Lindholm, T. S., and Pylkkanen, P.: Discitis following removal of intervertebral disc. Spine 7:618–622, 1982.
27. Massie, W. K., and Stevens, D. B.: A critical evaluation of discography. J. Bone Joint Surg. 49A:1243–1244, 1967.
28. McCulloch, J. A.: Chemonucleolysis. J. Bone Joint Surg. 59B:45–52, 1977.
29. McCulloch, J. A., and Waddell, G.: Lateral lumbar discography. Br. J. Radiol. 51:498–502, 1978.
30. McCulloch, J. A.: Chemonucleolysis: Experience with 2,000 cases. Clin. Orthop. 146:128–135, 1980.
31. McCulloch, J. A., and Macnab, I.: Sciatica and Chymopapain. Baltimore, Williams & Wilkins, 1983, p. 203.
32. McCulloch, J. A.: Unpublished data, 1985.
33. Mulholland, R., Gibson, M., Buckley, J., and Worthington, B.: The changes in the intervertebral disc after chemonucleolysis shown by MRI. Presented at the International Society for the Study of the Lumbar Spine Meeting, Dallas, May 28–June 2, 1986.
34. Nolla-Sole, J. M., Mateo-Soria, L., Rozadilla-Sacanell, A., et al.: Role of technetium 99m diphosphonate and gallium 67 citrate bone scanning in the early diagnosis of infectious spondylodiscitis. A comparative study. Ann. Rheum. Dis. 51:665–667, 1992.
35. Osti, O. L., Fraser, R. D., and Vernon-Roberts, B.: Discitis after discography. The role of prophylactic antibiotics. J. Bone Joint Surg. 72B:271–274, 1990.
36. Pilgaard, S.: Discitis (closed space infection) following removal of intervertebral disc. J. Bone Joint Surg. 51A:713–716, 1969.
37. Post, M. J., Sze, G., Quencer, R. M., et al.: Gadolinium-enhanced M. R. in spinal infection. J. Comput. Assist. Tomogr. 14:721–729, 1990.
38. Ryan, M. D., and Taylor, T. K. F.: Septic discitis—a misnomer. Med. J. Aust. 147:415, 1987.
39. Schmorl, G., and Junghanns, H.: The Human Spine in Health and Disease, 2nd American Ed. (trans. by E. F. Besemann) New York, Grune & Stratton, 1971.
40. Simmon, E. H., and Segil, C. M.: An evaluation of discography in the localization of symptomatic levels in discogenic disease of the spine. Clin. Orthop. 108:57–69, 1975.
41. Smith, A. S., and Blaser, S. I.: Infectious and inflammatory processes of the spine. Radiol. Clin. North Am. 29:809–827, 1991.
42. Smith, R. F., and Taylor, T. K. F.: Inflammatory lesions of intervertebral discs in children. J. Bone Joint Surg. 49A:1508–1520, 1967.
43. Wenger, D. R., Bobechko, W. P., and Gilday, D. L.: The spectrum of intervertebral disc-space infection in children. J. Bone Joint Surg. 60A:100–108, 1978.
44. Wiley, A. M., and Trueta, J.: The vascular anatomy of the spine and its relationships to pyogenic vertebral osteomyelitis. J. Bone Joint Surg. 41B:796–809, 1959.
45. Wiltse, L. L., Widell, E. H., and Yuan, H. L.: Chymopapain chemonucleolysis in lumbar disc disease. JAMA 231:474–479, 1975.

14

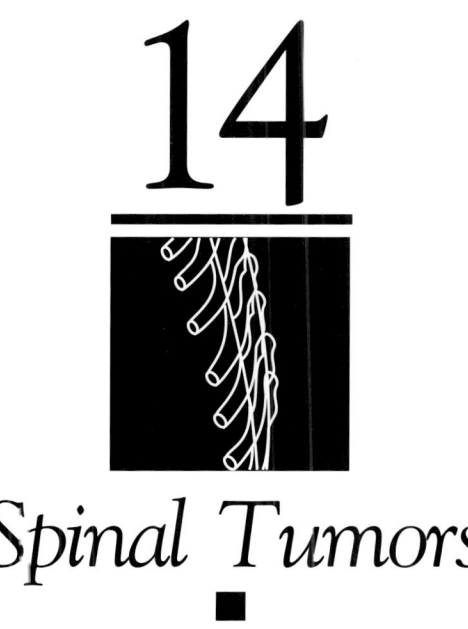

Spinal Tumors

JAMES N. WEINSTEIN

Primary tumors of bone are rare, accounting for approximately 0.4% of all tumors. Primary tumors of the spine account for less than 10% of all bone tumors.[10] Primary tumors are far less common than metastatic spine lesions, particularly in adults.[63] Other nonneoplastic conditions producing spinal symptoms are much more common. Nevertheless, primary tumors of the spine represent a diagnostic and therapeutic challenge to spine surgeons.[10, 13, 25, 65, 71, 80] A high index of suspicion is necessary if these lesions are to be accurately diagnosed and successfully treated, because the most common early symptom is back pain, which is an almost universal symptom among humans. These lesions are often found in compromising locations: specifically, around the spinal cord, the nerve roots, major organs, and blood vessels. Nevertheless, the results of treatment can positively affect survival and quality of life.

Improved therapies for systemic disease, more sophisticated preoperative evaluation and staging, the introduction of new surgical techniques and materials, and a trend toward a more aggressive surgical approach has led to improvements in both the short-term and long-term outcomes for patients with spinal tumors. Unfortunately, there is no uniform approach to treatment in these patients and little uniformity in reporting outcomes. This makes comparison of treatment protocols difficult and conclusions regarding definitive management somewhat tenuous. For appropriately selected patients, however, surgical treatment offers a reasonable likelihood of functional improvement, pain relief, and in some cases, cure of the disease.

Because of the opportunity to provide patients with such significant improvement, it is more imperative than ever that the treating physician appreciate the symptoms and characteristics of spinal neoplasm and that the principles of tumor staging and management be followed closely whenever such a lesion is suspected. Goals of treatment should be as follows: (1) to obtain a definitive diagnosis through biopsy or primary excision, (2) to institute appropriate surgical or medical treatment according to tumor type and the patient's condition at initial examination, (3) to preserve neurologic function, and (4) to maintain spinal column stability. Although the treatment of patients with spinal tumors must be individualized, specific principles should be observed in managing tumors in general and in managing specific tumor types to meet these goals.

SPINAL NEOPLASMS IN GENERAL

Neoplastic disease of the spine may arise from local lesions developing within or adjacent to the spinal column or from distant malignancies spreading to the spine or paraspinous tissues by hematogenous or lymphatic routes. Local involvement of the spine may result from primary tumors of bone, primary lesions arising in the spinal cord or its coverings, or contiguous spread of tumors of the paraspinous soft tissues and lymphatics. Regional or distant spread of metastatic disease to the spine may occur with almost any of the solid tumors of the body, with osseous malignancies of the appendicular skeleton, and with systemic lymphoreticular malignancies such as multiple myeloma and lymphoma. The likelihood that any one of these tumors accounts for any given lesion depends on intrinsic patient-related and tumor-related characteristics. Understanding these relationships allows the surgeon faced with an unknown spinal lesion to formulate a useful differential diagnosis and appropriately direct subsequent examinations. Such a directed approach allows the physician to establish a definitive diagnosis and treatment plan quickly.

Although both metastatic and primary tumors can be found in all age groups and at all levels of the spinal column, metastatic tumors are far more common than primary lesions. Metastatic carcinoma accounts for skeletal lesions in 40 times more patients than are affected by all other forms of bone cancer combined. An estimated 50% to 70% of patients with carcinoma develop skeletal metastases before death, and this number may be as high as 85% for women with breast carcinoma.[93] Primary tumors of the spine are rare, and for the most part, their relative incidence reflects that of tumors of the skeleton in general. Certain tumors (chordoma, osteoblastoma) show a predilection for the spinal column, but these still make up a small proportion of all spinal tumors.

Clinical Observations

The clinical presentation can vary considerably from patient to patient, but the primary symptom in most cases is back pain[94] (Table 1). Symptoms of back pain at night, pain at rest, or a neurologic deficit should prompt consideration of a spinal tumor. In one series, 84% of patients had some pain, either localized back pain (60%) or radicular pain (24%). There was no symptomatic distinction made between benign and malignant tumors.[94] In such cases, the pain is not usually relieved by rest or recumbency. It is usually of an insidious onset and is usually progressive over time (Table 2).

Despite these symptoms, diagnosis is often delayed.[55, 94] The delays are usually in terms of years. Unfortunately, delays affect adequate (optimum) treatment and survival. Patients often relate their pain to a fall or some other mishap, thus providing the unsuspecting physician with a likely but incorrect explanation of their pain. At the time of the initial neurologic examination, an objective deficit may be identified in 50% of patients.[71, 75, 80, 85, 94] This is directly related to the location and nature of the tumor mass. Herniated discs and various types of spinal stenoses have been confused with primary tumors.[75] A palpable detectable mass is uncommon.[94] The inter-

Table 1

Patterns of Presenting Symptoms		
Presenting Symptom	Number of Patients	Percentage of Patients
Back pain	25	30.50
Radicular pain	8	9.75
Weakness	7	8.50
Back pain and weakness	15	18.30
Radicular pain and weakness	8	9.75
Mass	4	4.90
Pain and mass	9	11.00
Pain, weakness, and bowel and bladder dysfunction	4	4.90
No symptoms	2	2.40
TOTAL	82	100

From Weinstein, J. N., and McLain, R.: Primary tumors of the spine. Spine 12:843–851, 1987.

Table 2

Incidence of Presenting Symptom	
Presenting Symptom	Percentage of Patients
Pain: localized or radicular	84.2
Weakness	41.5
Mass	15.9

From Weinstein, J. N., and McLain, R.: Primary tumors of the spine. Spine 12:843–851, 1987.

val from onset of symptoms to diagnosis is often prolonged, particularly in individuals with benign lesions.

Radiologic Studies

Judicious use of radiologic investigations is essential. Plain radiographs are satisfactory for diagnosing a majority of spinal tumors, with thoracic spinal lesions being the most difficult to detect.[25, 26, 63, 65, 75, 94] Evaluation for treatment planning, however, must include appropriate use of bone scans, computed tomography (CT), magnetic resonance imaging (MRI), tomography, and occasionally myelography and angiography. With these techniques and appropriate preoperative x-ray staging, a treatment algorithm can be instituted (Fig. 1). On plain radiographs, cortical disruptions and soft tissue masses are common for both benign and malignant spinal tumors. Fluoroscopy using C arm control or CT-scan–guided techniques are useful when closed percutaneous biopsies are indicated (Fig. 2). It is strongly recommended that spinal tumors undergo biopsy and be treated only by surgeons experienced

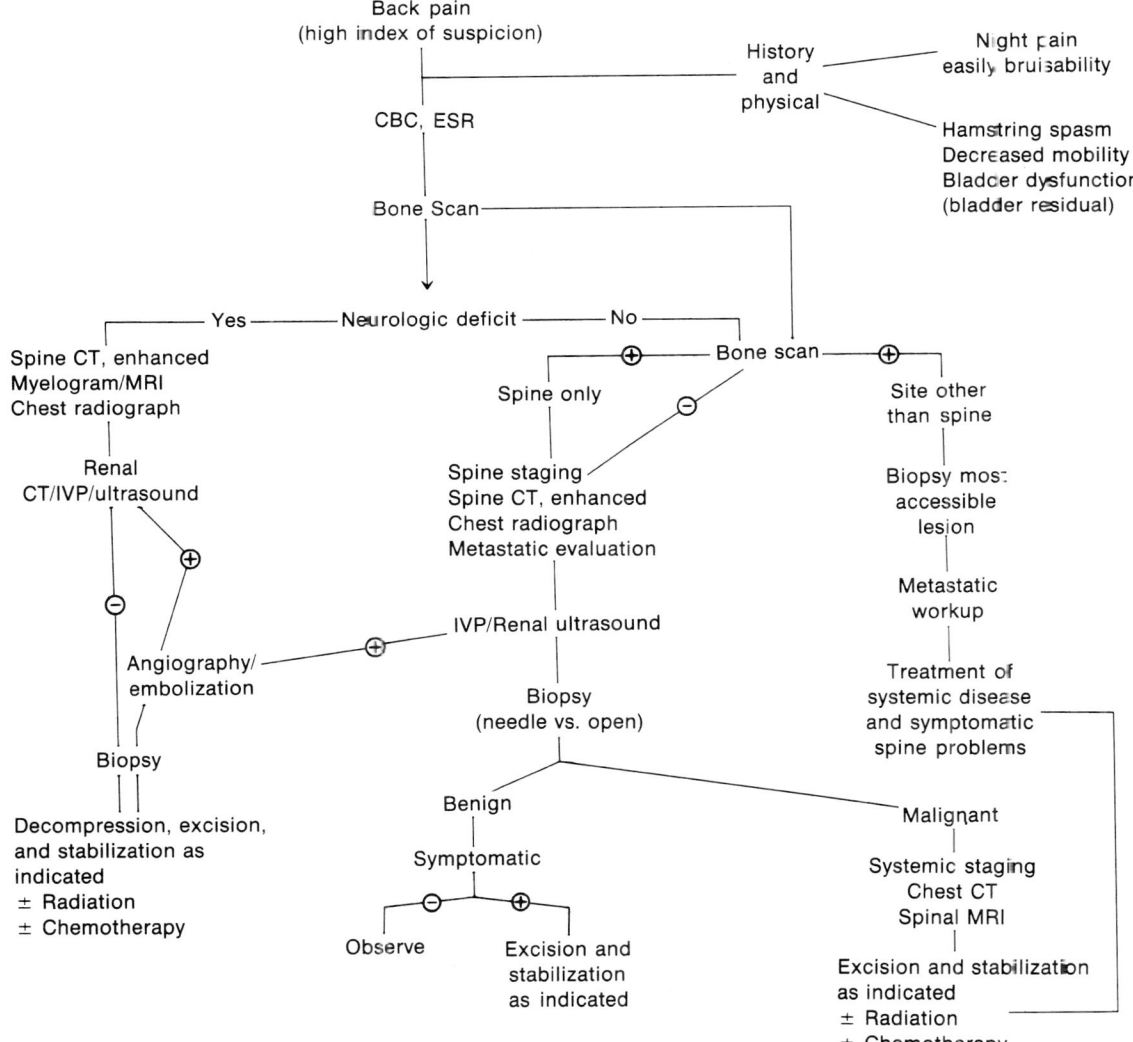

Figure 1. Algorithm for pediatric spinal tumors. (From Weinstein, J. N.: Spine neoplasms. *In* Weinstein, S. L. [ed.]: The Pediatric Spine: Principles and Practice. New York, Raven Press, 1994, pp. 887–916.)

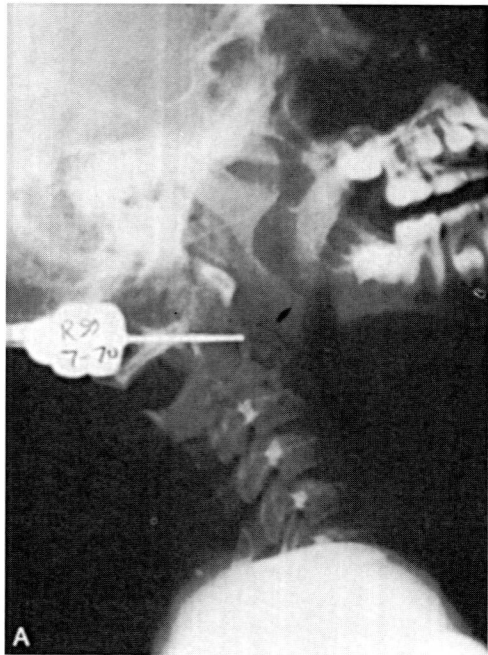
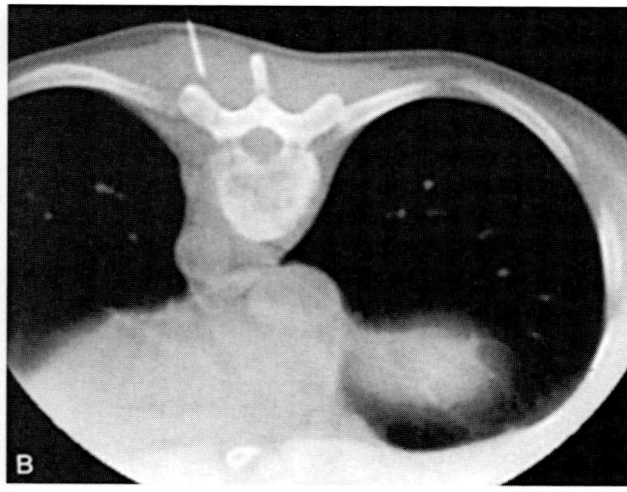

Figure 2. *A*, Percutaneous needle biopsy of C2 osteoblastoma. *B*, CT scan–directed needle biopsy of T6 metastatic breast cancer.

in the approach and management of these most difficult problems.[30, 35, 94]

Bone Scan

The technetiun Tc 99m bone scan is the most sensitive diagnostic tool for detecting spinal metastases. However, false-negative results occur if vascular response has been low because of the tumor. Primary tumors such as multiple myeloma and some sarcomas may produce negative results on bone scan. Also, the extent of technetium Tc 99m uptake does not necessarily correlate with the extent of tumor involvement.[31]

Computed Tomography and Myelography

CT may be the best diagnostic and surgical planning tool. It provides clear visualization of even minimum vertebral destruction and a good look at the surrounding soft tissues, allowing surgical decisions to be based on a clear visualization of the extent of invasion of the spinal canal.[94] A small amount of water-soluble dye in the subarachnoid space, used to enhance the CT scan, aids in distinguishing tumor from thecal sac. Myelography by itself is rarely indicated, although it can be useful in defining the extent of involvement or identifying multiple-site involvement.[31, 94] However, MRI has, in the author's opinion, replaced myelography in delineating multiple-site involvement and extent of disease. Myelographic or MRI blocks do not necessarily correlate with symptoms or outcome.[2] The progressive neurologic compromise, rather than the diagnostic studies, indicates the treatment course to be taken.

Magnetic Resonance Imaging

Although myelography has been the gold standard for evaluation of epidural metastases and cord compression, there are inherent risks involved in the test. MRI, on the other hand, has proved useful in evaluating a variety of spinal diseases, and it is well tolerated, noninvasive, and safe. The superior soft tissue detail provided by MRI and the ability to obtain multiplanar images enhance the diagnostic and treatment planning capabilities considerably. MRI often provides better delineation than does CT scanning of soft tissue tumor extension and adherence or invasion of paravertebral structures. Direct sagittal and coronal images are for some lesions superior to reconstructions available through CT scanning; unlike CT scanning, MRI is able to directly depict the spinal cord without the aid of intrathecal contrast material.[90, 92] The use of titanium and other MRI-compatible materials should be kept in mind during treatment to allow MRI to be used to monitor the patient for tumor recurrence.

Angiography

The effectiveness of spine surgery is sometimes compromised by excessive bleeding. Metastatic renal cell and thyroid carcinomas can be highly vascular, increasing morbidity and mortality. Aneurysmal bone cysts, hemangiosarcomas, and other primary tumors may also present a vascular challenge to spine surgeons. Angiography with selective embolization can be an effective way to manage such lesions.[76] Use of this technique can reduce intraoperative blood loss and perioperative morbidity and mortality. Identification of the origin of the artery of Adamkiewicz may also be helpful.[76]

PRIMARY TUMORS

Location

Primary spinal tumors involve all spinal segments. Cervical spinal tumors are, however, less common than thoracic, lumbar, and sacral lesions[94] (Fig. 3). The vertebral body is four times more likely to be involved with primary malignant tumors than are the posterior elements[24, 39, 63, 71, 94] (Fig. 4).

BENIGN TUMORS

Benign tumors of the spine, as with those elsewhere in the musculoskeletal system, generally carry a better prognosis than do malignant neoplasms. Surprisingly, with the exception of giant cell tumors, survival does not appear to correlate with treatment.[17, 35, 67, 94] Giant cell tumors of the spine, as with

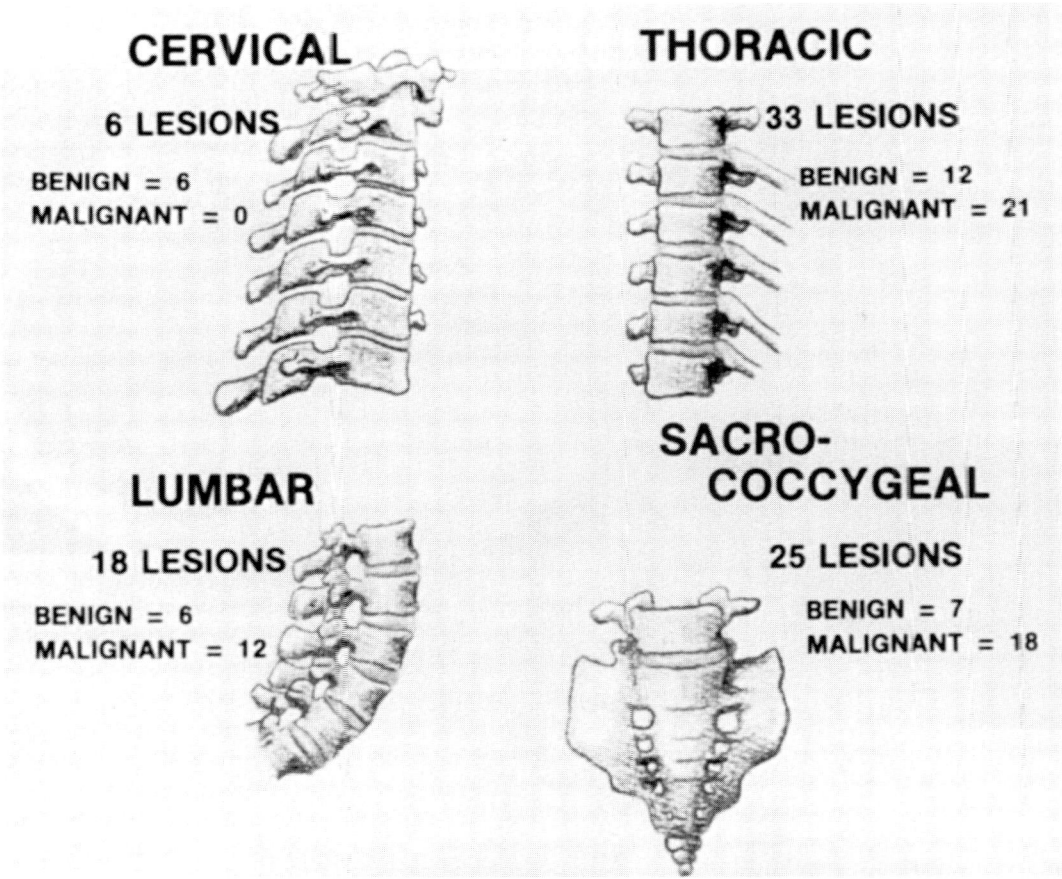

Figure 3. Primary spinal tumors by location.

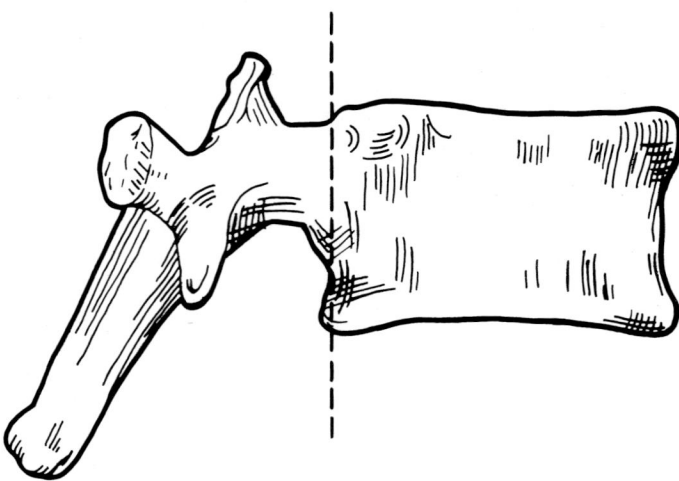

Figure 4. Location of tumor origin by tumor grade, benign versus malignant.

Posterior Elements
34%
10 malignant
18 benign

Vertebral Body
66%
41 malignant
13 benign

those in other locations, tend to have recurrences, and these are extremely difficult to treat.[17, 44, 45, 67, 82] Radiation therapy is almost never indicated in the treatment of benign spinal lesions. Appropriate primary treatment is essential.

The more common benign spinal lesions are hemangioma (Fig. 5), osteoid osteoma[40] (Fig. 6), and osteoblastoma[40] (Fig. 7). These are followed in frequency by osteochondroma (Fig. 8), giant cell tumor (Fig. 9), and aneurysmal bone cyst[80] (Fig. 10). Eosinophilic granuloma and other lesions such as angiolipoma are less common but must be part of the differential diagnosis. Eosinophilic granuloma (Fig. 11) is part of the histiocytosis X series, but is benign and can usually be treated by benign observation.[36]

Hemangioma is rarely symptomatic and is found in approximately 10% of all spines. It usually is located between T12 and L4. Women are affected three times more often than men. Usually, this lesion is an incidental x-ray finding or is found at autopsy without known clinical symptoms. Hemangiomas have the classic vertical reticular stripelike appearance on x-ray films. Rarely, hemangiomas expand to the adjacent pedicles and lamina or adjoining ribs. Soft tissue extension of hemangiomas causing neurologic deficit has been reported.[90] No treatment is required if the lesion is not symptomatic. However, if there is soft tissue extension or ballooning of the bone that causes symptoms of nerve root or spinal cord impingement, radiation therapy or surgical decompression should be considered.[88, 90]

Young patients with acute scoliosis who report back pain that is worse at night and during recumbency are suspected of having an osteoid osteoma. Their symptoms are usually relieved by aspirin administration.[69] Roentgenograms supplemented by CT or bone scan may be necessary to demonstrate and to guide treatment of these lesions. Treatment in symptomatic cases should be directed at marginal to wide excision of the lesion and appropriate stabilization if necessary (Fig. 12). The scoliosis and pain usually resolve with treatment of the tumor.

MALIGNANT TUMORS

The outcome for patients with malignant tumors of the spine varies with the specific

Text continued on page 927

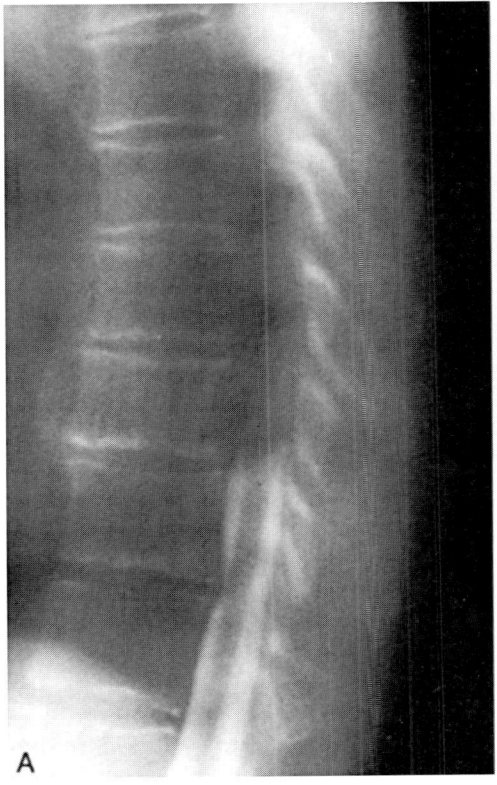
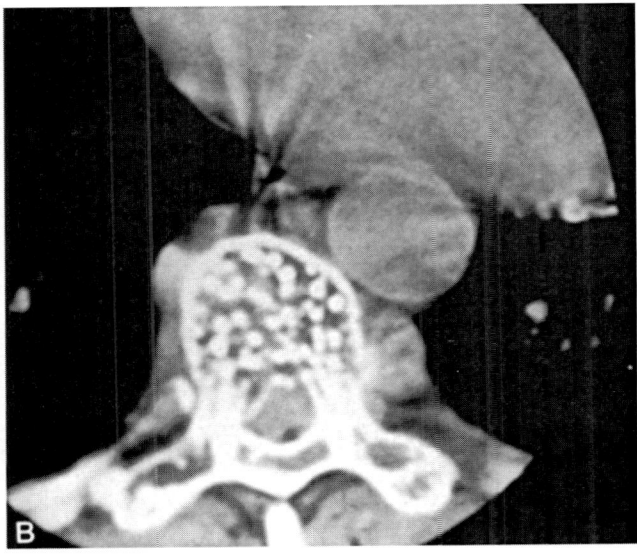

Figure 5. *A*, Lateral thoracic myelogram demonstrating obstruction of flow of contrast material. Diagnosis is hemangioma of T8 with soft tissue extension. *B*, CT scan of T8 hemangioma with extradural extension.

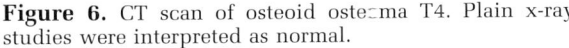
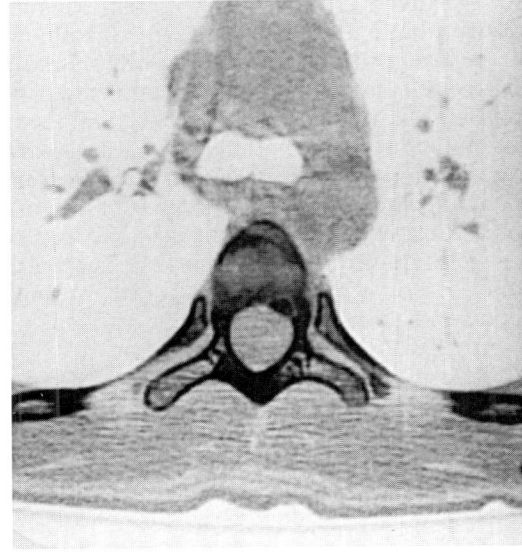

Figure 6. CT scan of osteoid osteoma T4. Plain x-ray studies were interpreted as normal.

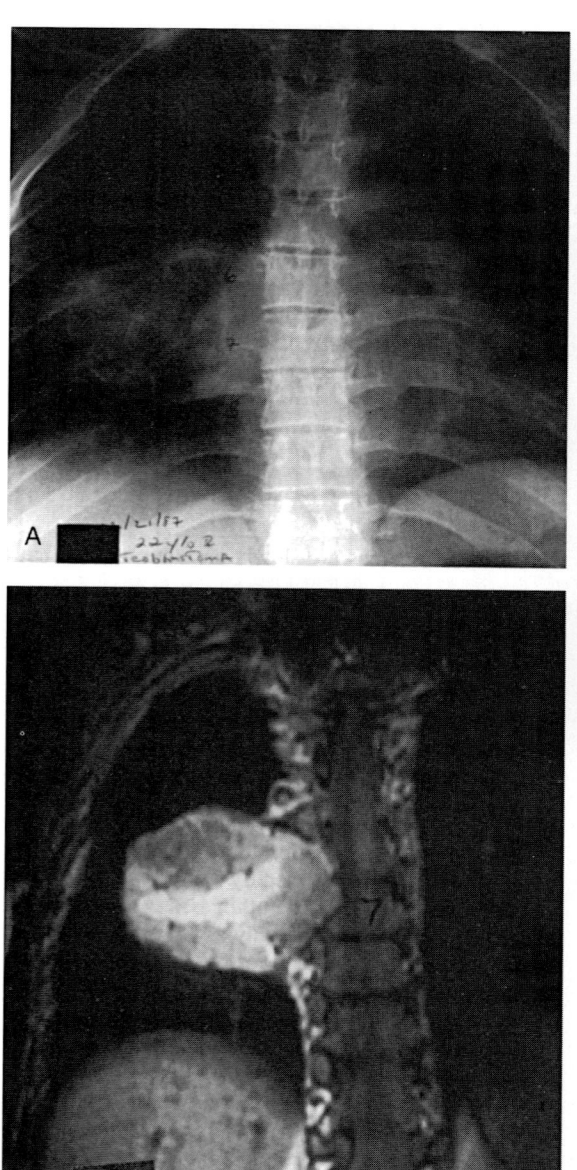
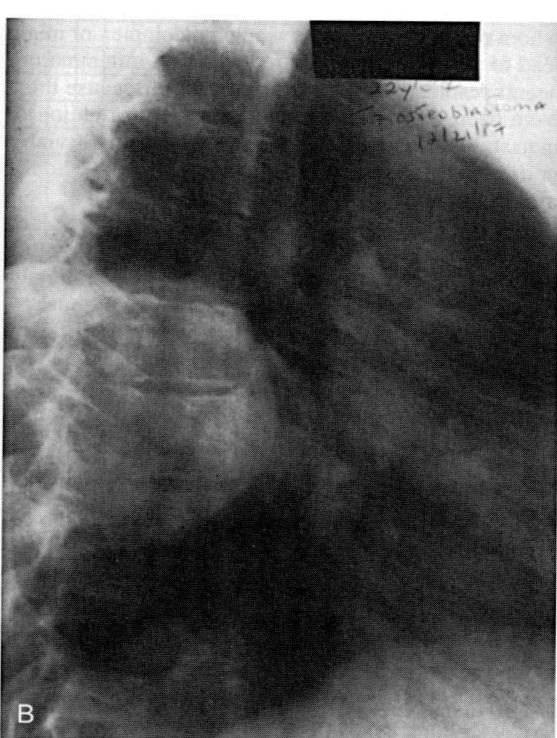

Figure 7. A T7 osteoblastoma. *A,* Anterior radiograph shows the expansile lesion from the body of T7 including and up to the body of T6; the ribs of T7 and T8 are clearly involved. Some calcification of the lesion is apparent. *B,* Lateral image shows a large expansile mass in the area of T6, T7, and T8, with some calcification. *C,* Coronal MRI scan shows growth of a large osteoblastoma off the vertebral bodies of T6 and T7 with some central calcification. (From Weinstein, J. N.: Spine neoplasms. *In* Weinstein, S. L. [ed.]: The Pediatric Spine: Principles and Practice. New York, Raven Press, 1994, p. 892.)

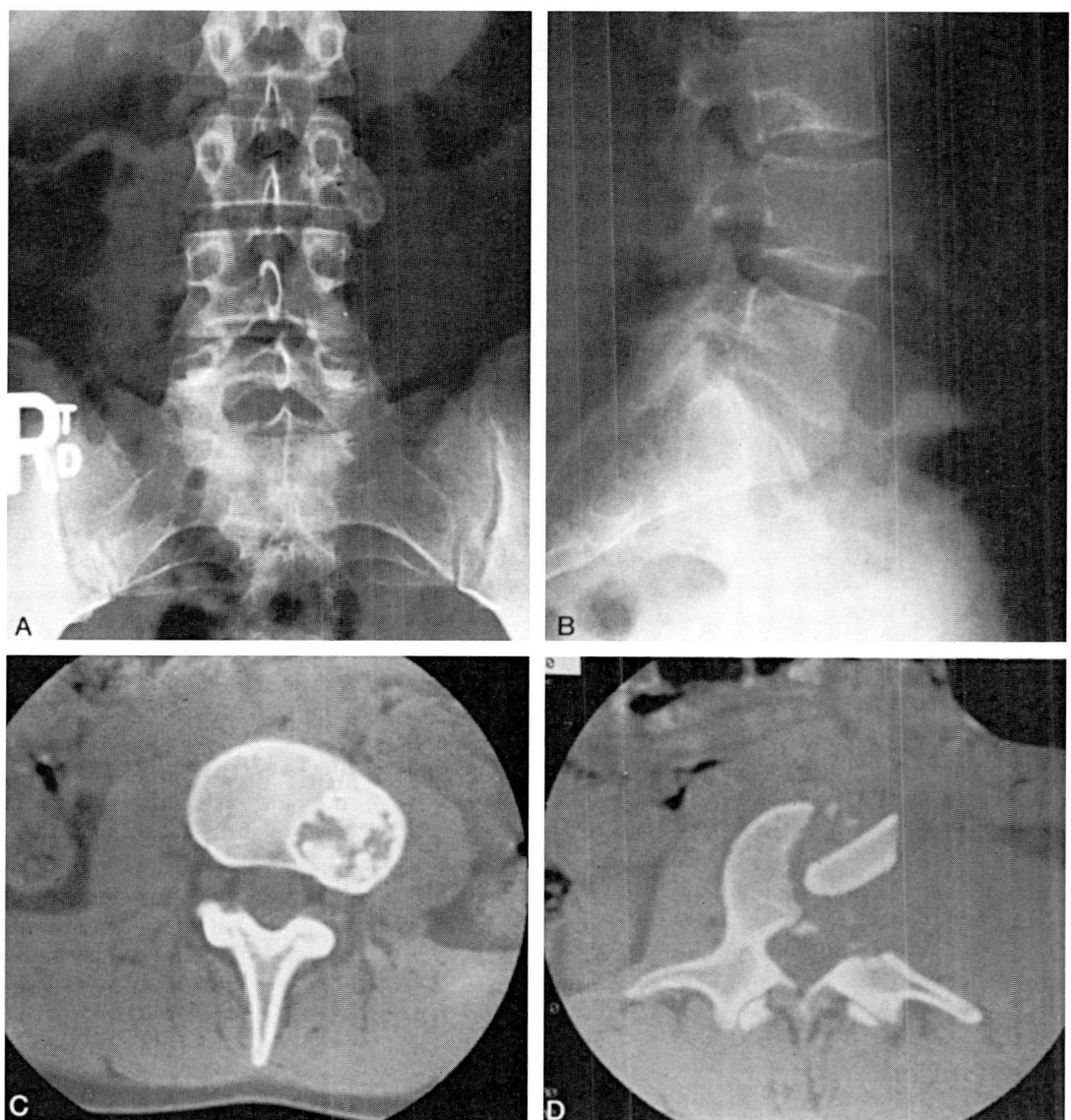

Figure 8. *A, B,* Osteochondroma at L3 (anteroposterior and lateral x-ray films). *C,* Osteochondroma at L3 (CT scan). *D,* Osteochondroma at L3 (CT scan 2 years postoperatively).

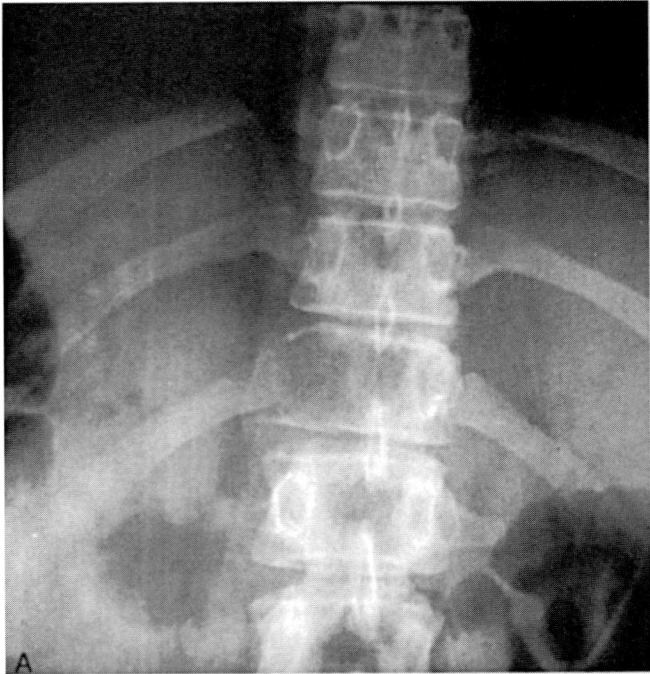

Figure 9. *A*, Giant cell tumor at T12. *B*, Lateral x-ray studies 5 years after total vertebrectomy show no recurrence.

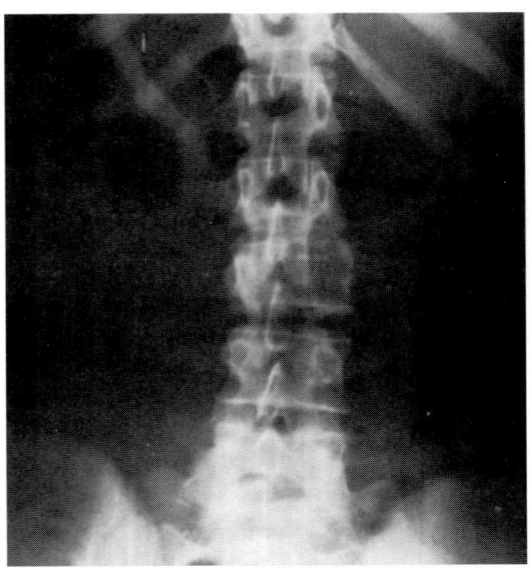

Figure 10. Aneurysmal bone cyst at L3.

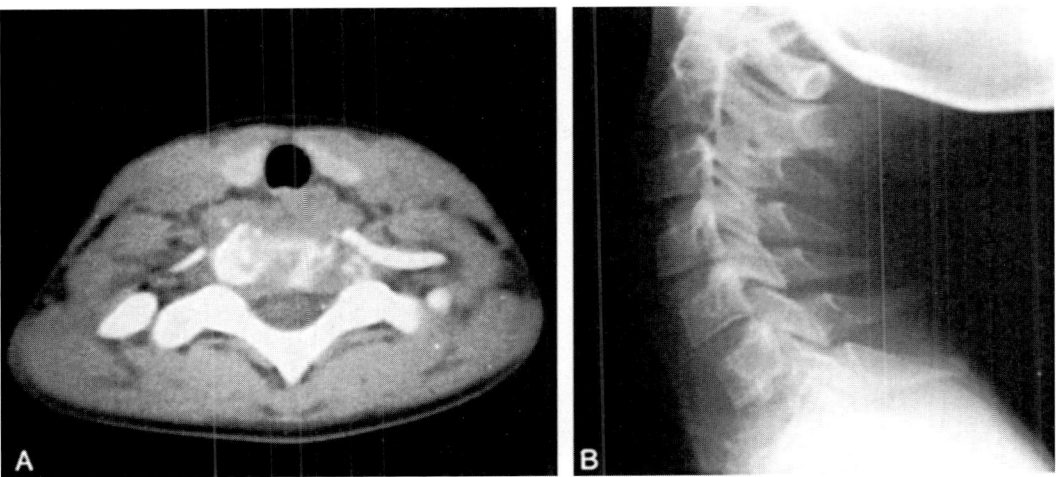

Figure 11. *A*, CT scan of eosinophilic granuloma at C7. *B*, Lateral x-ray film of C7 eosinophilic granuloma.

tumor type and the extent of the initial surgical excision.[17, 94]

Malignant neoplasms are much more likely to arise from the vertebral body than are benign lesions.[63, 71, 94] The correlation between age at diagnosis and tumor type is significant.[25, 65, 75, 94] The mean age at diagnosis is substantially higher for patients with malignant tumors than for those with benign tumors (49 years versus 21 years). In one series of 51 primary spinal tumors reported in patients older than 18 years of age, 80% had malignant neoplasms.[94] Patients with primary malignant tumors of the spine more commonly have associated neurologic findings, have a propensity for vertebral body involvement, and are older at the time of diagnosis[71, 75, 80, 94] (Table 3).

The most common malignant spinal lesion is plasmacytoma (myeloma). Other, less common, primary malignant tumors of the spine are chordoma, chondrosarcoma, lymphoma, Ewing sarcoma, and osteosarcoma.

Slow-growing, locally aggressive malignant tumors are associated with greater mean survival rates and overall survival rates compared with rapidly progressive and early metastasizing lesions. Multimodality therapy has allowed some long-term survivals in aggressive lesions.[64, 92, 94] Patients with solitary plasmacytoma and chondrosarcoma have greater overall survival rates than patients with osteosarcoma and lymphoma[94] (Table 4). Solitary plasmacytoma is sensitive to irradiation, and such treatment positively affects the survival of patients.[47, 36, 62, 35] However, if this bias for plasmacytoma is eliminated in the assessment of the long-term survival of patients with malignant spinal

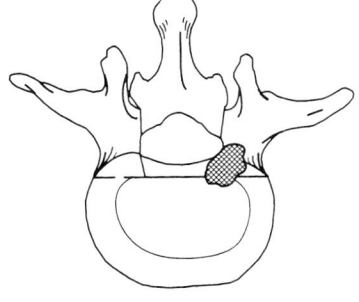
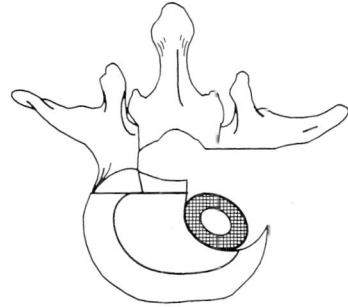

Figure 12. Illustration from CT scan of Figure 6, T4 osteoid osteoma, after resection and rib grafting.

Lesion

Resection with Rib Graft

Table 3

Clinical Features of Patients with Spinal Neoplasms

	Benign	Malignant	p Value
Mean age at diagnosis	20.9 y	48.7 y	.0001
Age greater than 18 years	32%	80%	.0001
Neurologic deficit	35%	55%	.09
Anterior location	42%	80%	.0005

From Weinstein, J. N., and McLain, R.: Primary tumors of the spine. Spine 12:843–851, 1987.

neoplasms, the relative outcome of surgically treated lesions was significantly affected only by complete surgical excision of the tumor when compared with other less aggressive treatments.[94] Thus, the best treatment results (i.e., survival) are affected by the most radical surgical extirpation of malignant spinal lesions* (Table 5).

METASTATIC TUMORS

Cancer in general is the second leading cause of death in the United States.[31] There are nearly 1 million new cases per year. Two thirds of these cases develop metastases, the skeletal system being the third most common site. Metastases are by far the most common skeletal tumors seen by orthopedists, and the spine is the most common site of skeletal involvement.[10] These metastatic foci are sometimes painful secondary to

*References 35, 52, 67, 71, 77, 79, and 94.

Table 4

Survival in Patients with Spinal Malignancy, by Tumor Type

Tumor Type	No.	Mean Survival (mo)*
Solitary plasmacytoma	15	38.27
Chondrosarcoma	4	28.00
Chordoma	11	27.73
Ewing sarcoma	4	27.50
Osteogenic sarcoma	3	18.33
Lymphoma	5	13.40
Others	4	36.25

*Survival scores truncated to 60 months.
From Weinstein, J. N., and McLain, R.: Primary tumors of the spine. Spine 12:843–851, 1987.

fracture, marrow disruption, and neural deficits. The most common primary tumors metastatic to bone are tumors of breast and prostate (84%), thyroid (50%), lung (44%), and kidney (37%). Breast cancer is the principal source of bony metastasis in women; in 65% to 85% of women with breast cancer, skeletal disease develops before death.[87] Among men, metastases from bronchogenic and prostatic carcinomas occur with the greatest frequency.

Lymphoma and myeloma are also commonly metastatic. The spine is the most common site of skeletal metastasis, irrespective of the primary tumor that is involved. It is followed by the ribs, the pelvis, the proximal long bones, the sternum, and the skull. However, vertebral metastases are often asymptomatic and are often discovered only by routine bone scans performed as part of a protocol to follow patients with tumors.

In the spine, the vertebral body is usually the first anatomic part to be involved, although pedicle destruction is often the first part involved on roentgenographic observation. This is easily explained by the fact that 30% to 50% of the vertebral body must be destroyed before these changes can be recognized on a roentgenogram. However, with only minimum involvement, the pedicle exhibits early roentgenographic cortical changes that can be seen when the pedicle in cross-section is inspected on an anteroposterior roentgenogram. Metastases to the posterior elements are seen in about 14% of cases.[37,81] Thoracic spinal metastases are usually from lung and breast, whereas lumbar spinal metastases are more commonly of prostatic origin. Spinal cord and nerve root compression occur only rarely (5%).[5,10] Spinal cord compression can occur at multiple levels in the same patient. This possibility, although rare, must be considered before treatment. If the symptoms are not consistent with the findings of routine roentgenographic studies, MRI or myelography should be performed to rule out the possibility of multiple-level involvement.

The prognosis for metastatic spinal disease is variable. The rapidity of neurologic deficit is extremely important and generally correlates with the ultimate prognosis. In general, a rapidly declining neurologic picture yields a poor prognosis, whereas persons with slowly progressive (days to

Table 5

Survival in Patients with Spinal Malignancy by Surgical Excision

Type of Surgical Treatment	No.	Mean Survival (mo)*	Percentage with 5-year Survival
None	5	17.00	15.0
Curettage	4	17.50	0.0
Incomplete resection	17	23.18	18.7
Biopsy only	10	33.50	33.0
Complete resection	10	48.40	75.0

*Survival scores truncated to 60 months.
From Weinstein, J. N., and McLain, R.: Primary tumors of the spine. Spine 12:843–851, 1987.

weeks) neurologic deficit have much more favorable outcomes.[51]

Treatment of metastatic spinal lesions falls into two general categories: surgical and nonsurgical.* Patients with roentgenographic evidence of spinal metastases or abnormal findings on bone scan but no bony vertebral collapse or neurologic impairment are candidates for irradiation, if their pain has been unresponsive to chemotherapy or hormonal manipulation. These patients may temporarily respond to the administration of epidural narcotics for pain management. Certain tumors (renal cell) with single metastatic foci without vertebral collapse are best treated by extirpation, when possible, and no irradiation, to allow the best long-term survival.[79, 94]

In patients without bony collapse or instability but with neurologic deficit or pain secondary to soft tissue involvement, the response to irradiation is usually good. However, depending on the tumor type and its particular prognosis, surgical extirpation followed by appropriate spine stabilization and irradiation may be the procedure of choice.[73] This view is contrary to the work by Gilbert and colleagues,[28] who reported that irradiation alone was as effective as decompressive laminectomy in the treatment of patients with epidural cord compression.

In patients with widespread metastases involving multiple levels, Fitzpatrick and Rider[22] advocated hemibody irradiation of 700 to 1000 rad. Fifty-three percent of those who received hemibody irradiation obtained complete or partial relief of their pain, despite disease progression.

Patients who have vertebral collapse and progressive pain are unlikely to be experience pain relief with irradiation alone. In these patients, the pain is caused by a mechanical problem of the bone, the disc, or other structures, and surgery with or without irradiation and chemotherapy may be the best course of treatment.

Pathophysiology

The distribution of metastatic disease in the skeleton is influenced by three factors. First, tumor emboli entering the blood stream tend to arrest in the natural filters of the vascular tree—the capillary beds of the liver, lungs, and bone marrow.[33, 94] To become established in the medullary canals of the spine, tumor emboli must first go through the capillary beds of the liver and lungs, often by establishing a metastasis at those locations, or alternatively circumvent these filters and reach the medullary sinusoids by an entirely different route. Tumors of the lung may seed the vertebral column directly through the segmental arteries, whereas carcinomas of the breast and prostate are thought to reach the vertebral system through communications with the paravertebral venous plexus originally described by Batson.[1] Venous drainage from the breast by the azygos veins communicates with the paravertebral venous plexus in the thoracic region, whereas the prostate drains through the pelvic plexus, which communicates in the lumbar region. Retrograde flow through the Batson plexus occurs during a Valsalva maneuver and may allow implantation of tumor cells in the vascular sinusoids of the vertebral body without passing through the usual capillary networks.

A second factor thought to be important

---

*References 2, 3, 5, 9, 13, 22, 28, 31, 32, 37, 38, 73, 81, 93, and 94.

in tumor distribution involves the tissue receptivity to embolic neoplasms. Certain tissues probably provide a more favorable environment for the survival of the tumor embolus. This "seed and soil" theory postulates that the red marrow of bone provides a biochemically and hemodynamically suitable environment for implantation and proliferation of tumor cells. Because the capillary network of the vertebral red marrow is particularly susceptible to tumor implantation and invasion, tumor cells find it easier to escape from the circulation and multiply within the fine network of cancellous bone.[31]

Finally, intrinsic factors inherent to the tumor cells may give one cell line a particular advantage in surviving and growing in the medullary space. Specifically, the elaboration of prostaglandins and the stimulation of osteoclast activating factors by breast cancer cells has been associated with the establishment of lytic metastases in bone.[27, 61] These cells may also produce a protective fibrin sheath that further isolates them within the marrow after a metastatic nidus is established.

Tumor Biology

The inherent nature of specific primary and metastatic neoplasms determines their biologic behavior, dictating which have slow or rapid growth, which are invasive, and which produce metastases. Although metastatic lesions usually demonstrate behavior similar to their parent lesions, this is not always true; some metastases may be far more invasive or rapidly growing than the primary lesion of origin. This biologic behavior of the primary or metastatic lesion determines the likelihood and rate of spinal cord compression. Rapid tumor expansion may produce vertebral erosion and fracture and may result in acute cord compression, with a poorer prognosis for improvement. Understanding the tumor type and its biology allows a surgeon to predict reasonably when, and if, a specific lesion will endanger neurologic structures.

The pathogenesis of a metastasis is controlled by several factors, some of which are contact inhibition, cell adhesiveness, and cell membrane mediation. Tumor cell survival depends on antigen-stimulated macrophage response, nonspecific immunologic response to fibrin clot, and permeability of endothelial and basement membranes, lymph vessels, and capillaries[27, 61] (Fig. 13).

Neurologic Status

The pretreatment neurologic status clearly correlates with posttreatment outcome as measured by the likelihood and extent of recovery, the ability to maintain or regain ambulation, and the preservation or loss of bowel and bladder function. Depending on the patient population surveyed, between 60% and 95% of the patients who can walk at the time of diagnosis retain that ability after treatment. Only 35% to 65% of the patients with paraparesis regain their ability to walk, and less than 30% of paraplegic patients regain ambulation.* The rate of progression of the neurologic deficit also has clear prognostic significance. If a patient progresses from the earliest onset of symptoms to a major deficit in less than 24 hours, the prognosis for recovery is poor, irrespective of treatment. Conversely, slow progression of neurologic involvement has a favorable prognosis for neurologic recovery after treatment.[31] All these factors, plus the surgical approach, determine the eventual return of neurologic function, which in favorable cases can be dramatic.

On the other hand, patients with a complete neurologic loss (i.e., complete paraplegia or quadriplegia), regardless of the cause, generally are not candidates for decompression. Patients with metastatic carcinoma of the lung, particularly those with oat cell carcinoma, who show widespread metastases must also be seriously considered as noncandidates for surgery because many of these patients have a survival of less than 2 to 3 months.

Radiation therapy has been the traditional standard of treatment for cord impingement, particularly in metastatic disease. Surgical decompression in the past has usually consisted of a laminectomy with removal of whatever tumor could be reached laterally in the spinal canal or through the pedicle. Laminectomy was sometimes combined with posterior stabilization and frequently combined with radiotherapy. Unfortunately,

---

*References 3, 20, 30, 33, 34, 42, 49, and 58.

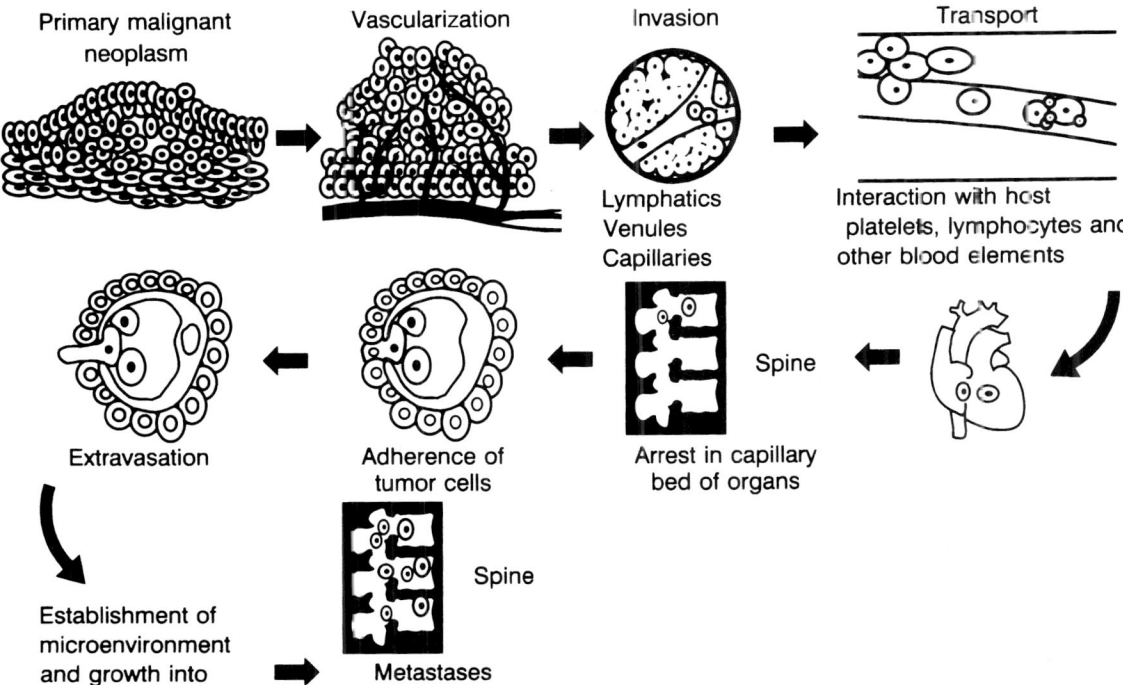

Figure 13. The pathogenesis of metastasis. (Data from Constans et al.[9] and Fidler et al.[19]) (From Weinstein, J. N.: Spine neoplasms. In Weinstein, S. L. [ed.]: The Pediatric Spine: Principles and Practice. New York, Raven Press, 1994, p. 905.)

the results of laminectomy were often no better than those of radiotherapy alone, and posterior decompression often resulted in a postoperatively acquired instability.[28, 31, 70]

Constans and associates[9] reported that 46% of their patients treated with decompressive laminectomy and radiotherapy had significant neurologic improvement compared with 39% of patients treated with radiotherapy. Similarly, Gilbert and coworkers[28] reported that satisfactory results were obtained in 46% of patients treated with laminectomy and radiotherapy, compared with 49% of patients treated with radiotherapy alone. Other investigators have noted that fewer than half of the patients treated by either radiotherapy or laminectomy obtained a satisfactory result in terms of retaining or regaining their neurologic function.[68]

Today, the results of surgical decompression through the anterior approach are more favorable and offer a genuine improvement over the results obtained with radiotherapy alone. Table 6 shows published data that compare recovery of neurologic function with anterior and posterior decompressions. How these tumors are approached is therefore determined by a number of the following factors.

TREATMENT OPTIONS

Surgery

O'Neil and associates[60] reviewed the treatment of 33 patients with metastatic lesions to the thoracic and lumbar spine. They found that 94% had good to excellent pain relief. Of 24 patients unable to walk preoperatively, 75% regained the ability to walk independently postoperatively.[60] Kostuik and colleagues[42] analyzed 71 metastatic lesions of the cervical, thoracic, and lumbar spine. Both anterior and posterior surgical approaches were used, and stabilization was augmented with methyl methacrylate. Good to excellent pain relief was obtained in 81% of cases. Significant improvement of neurologic deficits was obtained in 40% of patients with posterior decompression and 71% of patients with anterior decompression. Overall, survival averaged 11.3 months.[42] In a series reported by Harrington,[33, 34] 72 (94%) of 77 patients

Table 6

Maintenance and Recovery of Neurologic Function in Patients Treated Surgically for Cord Compression due to Metastatic or Primary Spinal Tumor

Investigator	Number of Patients	Percentage with Improvement	Percentage with Satisfactory Outcome
Anterior Decompression			
Sundaresan	160	80	78
Siegal[72]	75	80	80
Fidler[19]	17	73	78
Harrington[33]	77	84	73
Kostuik[41]	70	73	84
Manabe[49]	28	82	89
TOTAL	427	AVERAGE 78	AVERAGE 80
Posterior Decompression			
Wright[96]	86	35	33
White[95]	226	38	37
Hall[30]	123	30	29
Gilbert[28]	65	45	46
Nather[58]	42	13	29
Siegal[73]	25	39	39
Sherman[70]	149	27	48
Kostuik[42]	30	36	37
TOTAL	746	AVERAGE 33	AVERAGE 37

From Weinstein, J. N.: Differential diagnosis and surgical treatment of primary benign and malignant neoplasms. *In* Frymoyer, J. W. (ed.): The Adult Spine: Principles and Practice. New York, Raven Press, 1991, pp. 829–860.

treated by anterior decompression and stabilization experienced good to excellent pain relief. Sixty-two of these patients had a major neurologic impairment preoperatively, and 42 (68%) made significant improvement after surgery; 26 had a complete recovery and 16 others had a significant functional improvement after decompression.

Radiotherapy

Even though favorable results are obtained by surgical decompression, radiotherapy historically has been the treatment of choice for spinal osseous metastases and remains the most reasonable treatment option for many patients. In particular, patients with spinal pain and occasionally patients with neurologic compromise without vertebral collapse receive significant benefit from radiotherapy alone.

As with surgery, the preoperative neurologic status of the patient dictates the likely outcome. Although 70% of the patients who are ambulatory retain that functional ability after radiotherapy, rarely do patients who have lost this ability regain it after radiation alone.[83] The nature of the metastasis is also important to the outcome after radiotherapy because of the significant difference in radiosensitivity between tumor types and between different clones of the same tumor type. Prostatic and lymphoreticular tumors are usually radiosensitive, and excellent clinical results can be obtained by radiation alone in most patients.[7, 56, 83] Metastases from breast carcinoma are usually responsive to irradiation, but as many as 30% of the patients treated may be unresponsive to radiation alone.[32, 83, 93] Gastrointestinal and renal tumors usually are resistant to radiotherapy.

Braces

The halo vest is an important option for neurologically intact patients with cervical metastasis who have instability or pain. Used in conjunction with appropriate radiotherapy, symptomatic relief is reasonably good and bony healing of the lesion occurs in many cases. Most importantly, neurologic injury can be prevented by the halo vest while medical therapy is instituted. In patients with metastatic prostate carcinoma Danzig and associates[12] reported good maintenance of neurologic function and no morbidity using the halo vest. However, these patients wore the halo for roughly a third of their remaining lives.[12] Braces such as the thoracolumbo sacral orthosis (TLSO) are likewise viable and important tools in the management of thoracolumbar and sacral lesions, but their use is indicated only as an adjunct to treatment rather than as the primary treatment modality.

INDICATIONS FOR SURGICAL TREATMENT

The broad indications for surgical treatment, if the patient's overall status permits and there is a likelihood for survival, have been outlined by a number of researchers. Gilbert and coworkers[14, 28] suggested that decompressive laminectomy was indicated in metastatic disease when (1) the nature of the primary tumor was not known or the diagnosis was in doubt, (2) relapse of tumor occurred after maximum radiotherapy to that segment, and (3) symptoms progressed inexorably during radiotherapy. With the acceptance of more aggressive surgical treatments, these indications have been expanded. Surgical intervention has been recommended in instances of (1) an isolated primary and some isolated metastatic lesions or a solitary site of relapse, (2) pathologic fracture or deformity producing neurologic symptoms or pain, (3) radioresistant tumors—metastatic or primary, and (4) segmental instability following radiotherapy.[15, 23, 26, 31, 42, 49] These recommendations presume that the patient is healthy enough to survive surgery, but it is not incumbent to expect a long survival. Any patient with expectations of surviving 6 weeks or longer who is not hopelessly bedridden may be given consideration for surgery.

SURGICAL APPROACHES

A number of different surgical approaches are available to the spine surgeon, and variations to each have been described (Table 7). Choosing the correct approach for the given situation is perhaps the most important step in treating metastatic malignancies.

In situations in which conservative therapy is not feasible or has proved ineffective, surgical decompression is indicated In general, below the level of T2, anterior approaches may be used to restore stability, whereas above T2, posterior stabilization is usually indicated. Laminectomy should be restricted to those rare cases in which the site of compression has been shown to be strictly posterior.[20] In lesions of the cervical spine above the level of C3, a posterior approach is advocated, but if the dens is preserved and the body of C2 is destroyed, an anterior approach may be used, fixing the dens to C3 or C4 with metal-reinforced methyl methacrylate. In a series of 11 patients with high cervical metastases, posterior decompression and stabilization provided good to excellent pain relief in all patients but was not adequate to prevent collapse in one case with severe anterior vertebral destruction.[20] In metastatic lesions below C3, an anterior approach with decompression and methyl methacrylate stabiliza-

Table 7

Surgical Approaches to Spinal Neoplasms

Level	Anterior	Posterior
Cervical (C1–C2)	Transoral	Midline posterior
(C1–T2)	Anterolateral	Posterolateral
	Transsternal	
Thoracic	Thoracotomy	Midline posterior
		Costotransversectomy
Thoracolumbar (T11–L2)	Thoracoabdominal—10th–12th rib resection, detachment of diaphragm	Midline posterior
	Retroperitoneal	Posterolateral
Lumbar	Transabdominal	Midline posterior

From Weinstein, J. N.: Differential diagnosis and surgical treatment of primary benign and malignant neoplasms. In Frymoyer, J. W. (ed.): The Adult Spine: Principles and Practice. New York, Raven Press, 1991, pp. 829–860.

tion has been advocated. Some surgeons, however, prefer the posterolateral approach to lesions involving multiple adjacent cervical levels. Below C3, a single nerve root may need to be sacrificed to allow adequate anterior decompression by this approach. Stabilization after a posterolateral decompression may be accomplished by segmental fixation and sublaminar wiring augmented with methyl methacrylate as needed.[41, 42]

Anterior Versus Posterior Decompression

The selection of anterior decompression versus posterior decompression depends to some degree on the extent of involvement of the spine and the presence or absence of skip lesions and the degree of epidural tumor. A careful analysis of preoperative plain radiographs, CT scans combined with myelography, or MRI scans helps to define the extent of destruction and epidural spread. MRI sometimes has limits in defining the extent of the tumor. Therefore, myelography with CT scanning is necessary and may provide the best preoperative evaluation.

Anterior compression in the presence of epidural tumor over five or six levels usually does not respond well to anterior vertebrectomy alone. Generally, the selection of anterior decompression is restricted to patients with metastatic disease ideally limited to one or two adjacent vertebral segments or to patients with significant kyphosis in conjunction with vertebral body destruction. Skip lesions with single-level anterior destruction can be treated anteriorly, but the possible morbidity to the patient must be considered. Ideally, multiple-level lesions are best treated by a posterior approach.

The use of costotransversectomy for debulking of metastatic tumors combined with posterior segmental stabilization has been reported, but the results have not been as good as with the anterior approach. Only one of five patients regained the ability to walk with assistance, and survival was limited to a mean of 5 months.[14] Somewhat better results have been reported through a modified costotransversectomy approach with anterolateral decompression, but access to the tumor is always limited anteriorly and results are still inferior to those obtained by a formal anterior approach.

Posterior Laminectomy

In an uncontrolled, retrospective review of 38 patients treated by laminectomy, only 24% of patients demonstrated any improvement in neurologic function.[59] Whether laminectomy provides any significant benefit to patients with cord compression beyond that provided by radiotherapy is debatable. Although Constans and associates[9] showed some improvement in results using laminectomy with radiotherapy, the results of Gilbert and coworkers[28] showed little difference of results between patients treated with radiotherapy alone and those treated with both laminectomy and radiation. The proportion of satisfactory outcomes was less than 50% in each case.

Livingston and Perrin[48] in 1978 reviewed the results of 100 extensive laminectomies for neurologic deficits in metastatic disease. They defined satisfactory results as the ability to walk, retention of urinary continence, and survival of 6 months or longer. This was achieved in 40% of the patients; however, they did not differentiate between those who were ambulatory preoperatively and postoperatively. Doppman and Girton[16] in 1976 reported the results of laminectomies in anterior epidural masses in an angiographic study in 16 rhesus monkeys. They concluded that an anterior epidural mass of greater than 4 mm in diameter could not be adequately decompressed with posterior laminectomy.

A number of investigators have reported their results in cases of cord or cauda equina compression treated by posterior decompression, and most researchers graded deficits and outcome by the classification of Brice and McKissock.[6] This classification, based on mild, moderate, and severe neurologic deficits, defined satisfactory outcome as restoration and maintenance of ambulation and bowel and bladder function. It is not directly comparable with the most objective Frankel classification widely used today. This lack of continuity makes comparison of data for anterior and posterior approaches more difficult, but the trend seen in comparison is still clear (see Table 6). Of 746 reported cases treated by posterior decompression, only 37% of patients had a satisfactory neurologic outcome, and only 33% with neurologic deficit showed significant improvement.* Although the addition of stabilization substantially improved the pain relief and maintenance of neurologic function relative to laminectomy alone, the overall results were still somewhat disappointing. It therefore is evident that laminectomy does not provide adequate decompression in all lesions and may in fact increase instability.

The spinal cord is also endangered during laminectomy, especially in the thoracic region, because of the narrowness of the canal and the need to manipulate the cord to reach anterior or anterolateral tumor tissue.[51] In certain cases, laminectomy may be distinctly detrimental to neurologic outcome in patients with cord compression. Findlay[21] reviewed the results of laminectomy in patients with and without vertebral collapse and noted a poorer rate of recovery and twice the rate of postoperative paraplegia in patients with collapse. Laminectomy fails in these patients for two reasons. First, often inadequate decompression of the cord is obtained. Second, the resulting destabilization of the spinal column puts these patients at high risk for postoperative cord compression and paraplegia. Combining a destabilizing posterior decompression with an already unstable anterior column is clearly unwise.

If in metastatic disease the process is at more than two adjacent levels and is essentially posterior where there is extensive epidural spread as shown by MRI scanning, myelography, or enhanced CT scanning, decompression can be performed posterolaterally on the most affected side. In the thoracic spine one or more roots may be sacrificed. Stabilization is then achieved with segmental fixation and the liberal use of methyl methacrylate bone cement.

SURGICAL STABILIZATION

The specific types of stabilization depend on the specific tumor type and the anticipated response to treatment, as well as the extent of destruction of the anterior and posterior columns, the general condition of the patient, and the expected survival time.

---

*References 28, 30, 42, 58, 70–72, 95, and 96.

A Preferred Approach

Clearly, surgical extirpation for primary tumors of the spine can play a significant role in overall patient survival, recovery, and maintenance of neurologic function. Although true anatomic compartments as defined by Enneking[18] do not exist in the spinal column, anatomic structures do provide natural planes for dissection and wide excision.

Anatomic Extent of Spine Tumors: Level, Location, and Layer (Depth)

The spine is divided by vertebral level, with 12 locations and five layers[35, 92] (Fig. 14). Categorization of tumor by anatomic extent using this classification is possible. The level simply defines the vertebra or vertebrae that are involved. The 12 locations correspond to the numbers on a clock. Clockwise movement from left to right allows classification of tumor location and distinguishes left from right and anterior from posterior. More than one location is usually involved.

Layers define the depth of tumor involvement. Each location has five layers: A to E. Layer A is extraosseous and includes all soft tissues: skin, muscle, ligaments, blood vessels, nerves, discs, and other soft tissues, around each bony vertebra. Layer B is completely intraosseous: anterior, lateral (right and left), and posterior in the vertebrae. Layer C is also intraosseous but is deeper and involves only bone. Layer D indicates extraosseous spread within the vertebral canal (i.e., extradural tumor that has extended beyond the bone into the extradural space but has not invaded the dura). Layer E designates intradural tumor that has invaded the dura or has a purely intradural location. This classification allows the location and anatomic extent of a tumor of the spine to be defined and reported more clearly.

Zones for Surgical Resection

For surgical planning, the vertebral body is divided into four surgically resectable zones: I to IV. Tumor resection is designated as intraosseous (B and C), extraosseous (A, D, and E), and distant tumor metastasis (M)[82, 84] (Fig. 15A, B). Zone IB,C includes the spinous process, the pars interarticularis,

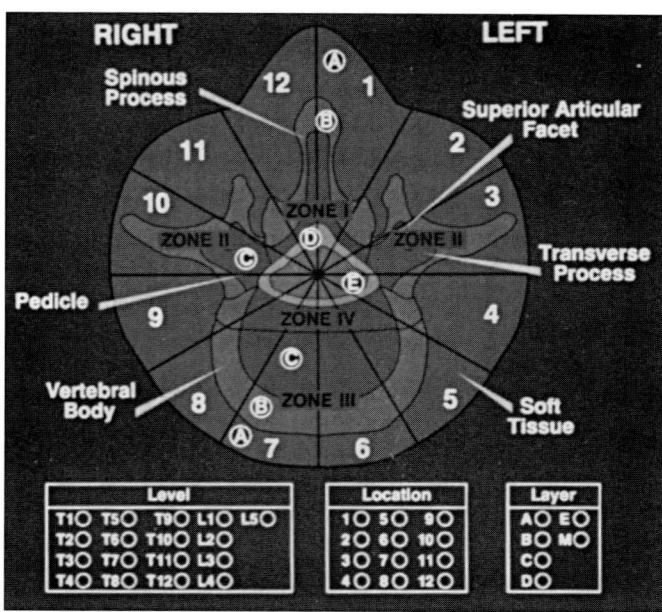

Figure 14. Schematic used by the international registry defining the level, location, and layer (depth) of the tumor. (From Weinstein, J. N.: Spine neoplasms. In Weinstein, S. L. [ed.]: The Pediatric Spine: Principles and Practice. New York, Raven Press, 1994, p. 909.)

and the inferior facets. Zone IIB,C includes the superior articular facet, the transverse process, and the pedicle from the level of the pars to its junction with the vertebral body. Zone IIIB,C includes the anterior three fourths of the vertebral body, and zone IVB,C designates involvement of the posterior one fourth of the body, that segment immediately anterior to the spinal cord. Zones IA to IVA are the extraosseous extensions of tumor beyond the boundaries of the cortical bone. Zones IM to IVM designate associated regional or distant metastatic involvement from the primary tumor. Surgical resection and outcome in many cases is determined by the zones involved and the extent of local or distant tumor spread, as well as the type of tumor and its grade.

Complete radiologic evaluation, including CT and MRI scanning, allows accurate tumor localization and extent, which in turn enables a more informed prediction of the tumor's grade and possibly the actual histologic type. Additional laboratory and screening studies obviously help to focus the differential diagnosis further, allowing the surgeon to plan the appropriate operation to treat the primary tumor adequately without exposing the patient to needless risks. Accurate determination of tumor type is essential in each case before surgical intervention because overtreatment of benign disease can be nearly as disastrous as undertreatment of malignancy. The algorithm shown in Figure 1 may be of help in evaluating a child seen for the first time with a spinal lesion.

Obtaining the widest surgical margin possible is essential for locally aggressive or malignant tumors, particularly those that do not respond well to adjuvant treatment. A wide margin can be obtained in most isolated lesions in zones IB,C to IVB,C because the tumor can usually be completely resected. An adequate margin can be extremely difficult to obtain in layer A tumors when they involve neurovascular structures. For lesions of the lumbosacral or cervical spine in zones IA to IVA and locations 1 to 12, resection may not be possible without producing serious neurologic deficits when associated neurovascular structures are involved, especially at locations 4 to 9. In these cases, the benefits of surgery may be marginal at best and, of necessity, surgery is most likely intralesional. The decision to attempt a wide or radical resection in these cases must weigh the benefit against the risk.

The appropriate surgical approach is selected on the basis of the ability to achieve sufficient access for both tumor extirpation and later stabilization of the spine. If both procedures cannot be performed adequately through the same incision, the surgeon must combine various approaches to achieve this

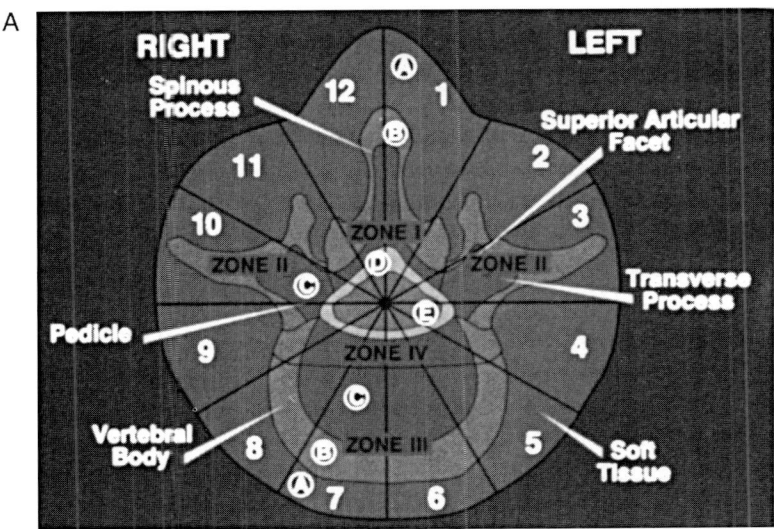

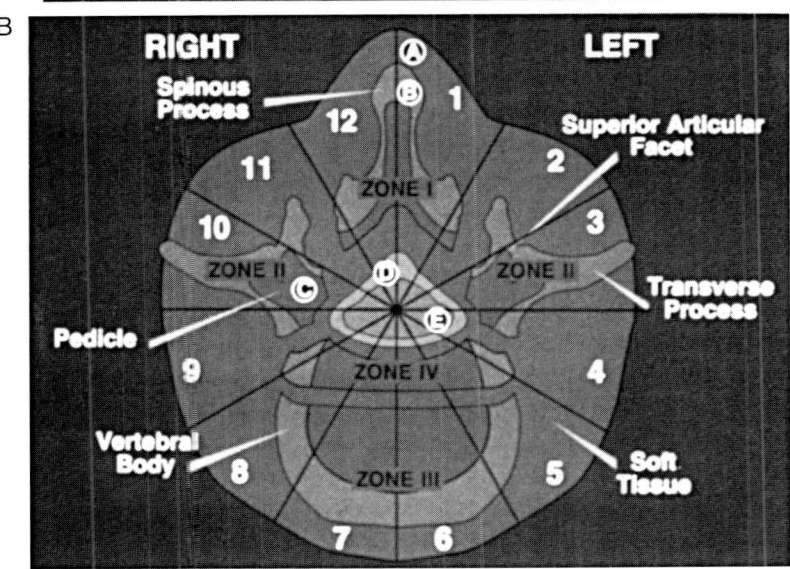

Figure 15. Anatomic extent (modified). *A,* Zones I to IV for surgical resection. *B,* Surgical resection by zone. These represent anatomically resectable zones according to tumor classification scheme. (From Weinstein, J. N.: Spine neoplasms. *In* Weinstein, S. L [ed.]: The Pediatric Spine: Principles and Practice. New York, Raven Press, 1994, p. 910.)

goal. An ill-planned approach may prevent the surgeon from completing extirpation of the tumor, which should be avoided if possible.

Zone I lesions in locations 12 and 1 are best approached posteriorly, and excision margin is based on any soft tissue (layer A) extent observed on preoperative studies. After posterior excision is performed, the resulting tensile loads are best minimized through posterior instrumentation. The type of instrumentation is left to the surgeon's experience and choice, but one must be well versed in all possible options. Zone II (locations 2 to 4 and 9 to 11) lesions are also more easily approached through a posterior or posterolateral approach.

Lesions in zone III (locations 5 to 8) should most often be approached anteriorly. Adequate resection of lesions in zone III involving layers B and C can usually be obtained throughout the spinal column, but layer A lesions must be carefully analyzed preoperatively, with anticipation of invasion or adherence to the great vessels or critical neurovascular elements, as well as other soft tissue structures. Reconstruction is then performed with or without internal fixation, depending on the extent of resection and the inherent stability of the remaining segments. In children, anterior fixation devices must be scaled down and should be avoided when possible.

Zone IV lesions in locations 4 to 9 require a combined anterior and posterior approach in most cases. These lesions involve the most inaccessible region of the vertebral body and are the most difficult lesions to reconstruct, providing technical challenges to the surgeon before, during, and after actual tumor resections. In many cases, zone I, II, or III must be crossed at some point to provide access to zone IV lesions, and frequently more than one zone is involved with tumor. Excision can be obtained through vertebrectomy or complete vertebral extirpation by essentially separating zones II and IV through combined approaches (Fig. 16A, B); in such cases, both anterior and posterior grafting are necessary. Failure to provide good fixation and adequate grafting is likely to result in loss of fixation and deformity, with potentially catastrophic complications.[46]

CASE ■ 1

A 25-year-old man had a history of back pain for 9 months, hamstring tightness, and bladder residual (Fig. 17A–C). His plain radiographs were interpreted as normal. Preoperative MRI scans and surgery clearly demonstrated a lesion solely within layer (depth) E (intradural), and locations 1 to 12 were involved but only in layer E (intradural). With this classification, this can be identified as a large intradural lesion with a level of top of L1 to near bottom of L2 involving locations 1 to 12 and layer E. Therefore, this tumor is classified by:

- Level: L1–L2
- Location: 1–12
- Layer: E

Treatment is now based on the anatomic extent of the tumor, and involves previously published but modified anatomic extent of resection classification[90–92] (see Figs. 14 and 15A, B):

- Level: L1–L2
- Zone: 1A

In this case, laminectomy was performed at L1 and L2, removing all of zone IB,C. The dura was entered but not removed, because the tumor, an ependymoma, was resected and the dura was closed. In cervical spine and sacrum, a similar system can be used (Figs. 18 and 19). The vertebral artery in the cervical spine is a separate layer F.

The vertebral body, the anterior and posterior longitudinal ligaments, the intervertebral disc, and the dura may all be resected to avoid leaving residual tumor. Neural, muscular, and vascular structures may, when indicated, all be sacrificed to obtain an adequate surgical margin. Such an aggressive approach may be justified, depending on tumor type and location. As in extremity surgery, extirpation often provides the best prognosis for local control and cure of the disease.

Appropriate treatment of spinal neoplasms requires an objective approach with significant preoperative planning. The anatomic extent of the lesion must be understood in three dimensions. Reconstruction and stabilization must be anticipated in planning the surgical approach. After the tumor is accurately localized by level, location, and layer, surgical reconstruction is planned.

Surgical intervention with metastatic disease must be considered in the face of all other options. It should not be considered as only a final alternative, however. In selected cases, surgery may offer the more conservative approach and may actually be less morbid to the patient than chemotherapy, radiation, or the administration of high-dose narcotics. A surgical oncologist specializing in the surgical treatment of tumors of the spine should be consulted early and often as decision-making proceeds in these difficult cases.

Complications

It is important to consider the complications in these most difficult cases, because management of complications sometimes is more difficult than management of the primary or metastatic tumor. Second chances are often too late. The first chance is not only the most important but may be the only chance. The ability to combine the best surgical and nonsurgical treatments can influence not only the immediate care of the patient but, more important, may also affect long-term survival.[53, 93, 94]

Several series have implicated acquired instability and deformity as reasons for lack

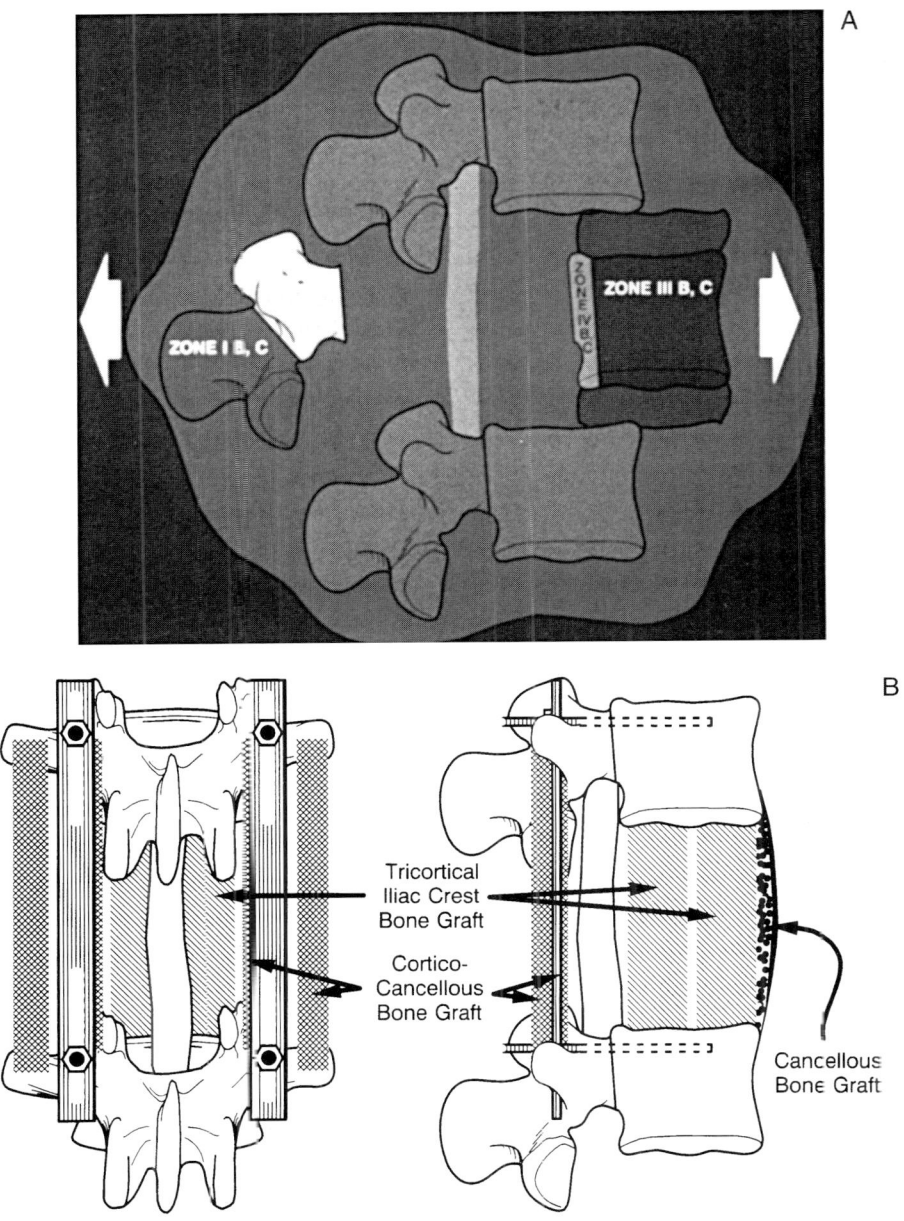

Figure 16. *A*, Zones I and II and III and IV can be resected together to perform a vertebrectomy. *B*, After resection, anterior and posterior bone grafting with posterior instrumentation is performed. (From Weinstein, J. N.: Spine neoplasms. *In* Weinstein, S. L. [ed.]: The Pediatric Spine: Principles and Practice. New York, Raven Press, 1994, p. 911.)

of neurologic improvement and occasionally for progression of neurologic dysfunction. Hypermobility or acquired instability may be the result of inadequate reconstruction or stabilization at the time of initial surgery or the result of late failure of fixation caused by disease progression or implant failure. Attention to the mechanics of reconstruction obviously is important.

In Harrington's[31] series of 77 patients treated with posterior stabilization and adjuvant methyl methacrylate, five patients had loss of fixation and required restabilization. In addition, in six patients, spinal hypermobility subsequently developed because of metastatic disease at adjacent levels of the spine.

Of the 24 complications reported by McAfee and colleagues,[52] only five occurred after anterior stabilization using methyl

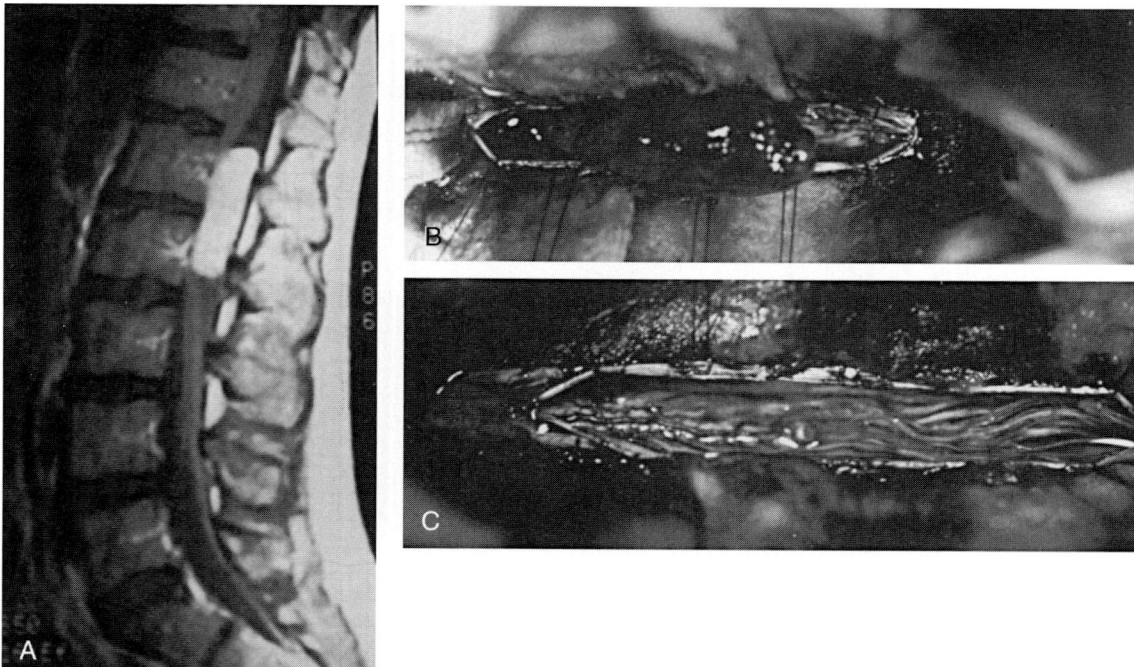

Figure 17. Ependymoma at L1–L2. *A,* MRI scan shows an intradural (E) tumor. *B,* Surgical extirpation of tumor. *C,* After surgical extirpation, cauda equina remains undisturbed (classified as level L1–L2, location 1–12, and layer E). (From Weinstein, J. N.: Spine neoplasms. *In* Weinstein, S. L. [ed.]: The Pediatric Spine: Principles and Practice. New York, Raven Press, 1994, p. 912.)

methacrylate. Of the 19 patients with posterior stabilization, 15 had loss of fixation and significant kyphosis subsequently developed in some patients. Six patients developed deep infections; three of them had associated significant neurologic deterioration.[52]

In the series of Kostuik and coworkers,[42] among 100 patients, there were three cases of instrumentation failure. One occurred in a patient who had anterior reinforced methyl methacrylate with metastatic disease in the cervical spine. Failure occurred because it was not recognized that the disease

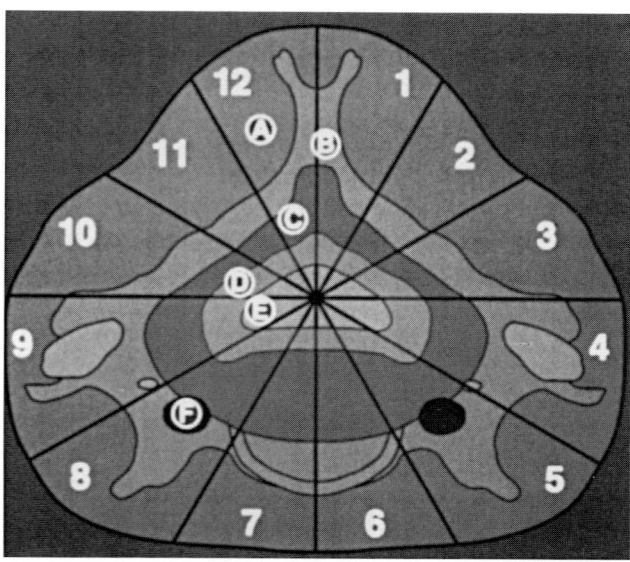

Figure 18. Schematic for international registry use for cervical spine, defining level, location, and layer of tumor. (From Weinstein, J. N.: Spine neoplasms. *In* Weinstein, S. L. [ed.]: The Pediatric Spine: Principles and Practice. New York, Raven Press, 1994, p. 913.)

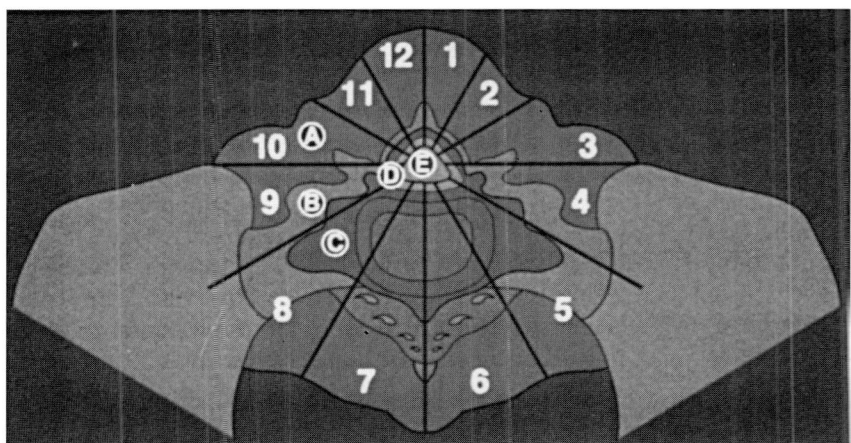

Figure 19. Schematic for international registry use for sacral tumors, defining level, location, and layer. (From Weinstein, J. N.: Spine neoplasms. *In* Weinstein, S. L. [ed.]: The Pediatric Spine: Principles and Practice. New York, Raven Press, 1994, p. 913.)

extended into the proximal vertebral body. A second procedure was successful. Two other major failures occurred; both were in the thoracic spine and both were associated with use of Harrington instrumentation without the use of sublaminar wires. A proximal hook pulled out in one patient, and both lower hooks pulled out in another. Both patients underwent reconstruction without sequelae.[42]

In patients for whom long-term survival may be possible, either autogenous bone grafting or autogenous bone grafting supplemented with various synthetic vertebral replacements, of which several are now available, rather than methyl methacrylate is recommended.

The complications of radiation have already been suggested: sarcomatous degeneration, neurologic dysfunction, and stunted growth. Before surgery, radiation has a significant effect. Radiation can increase the risk of infection at the time of surgery by 36%.

In a review of technical considerations and complications in tumor surgery by McLain and colleagues,[53] pedicle fixation was noted to have significant technical advantages in spinal reconstruction, with complications comparable with those of other methods of posterior segmental fixation, although operative times were slightly longer. With this system, fewer levels had to be fused compared with the case with systems using sublaminar hooks or wires. Preoperatively irradiated patients experienced 42% of all complications and had 70% of the major complications. Wound infections occurred in 18%, vascular injuries occurred in 18%, and transient neurologic deficits occurred in 36%. Clinical pseudarthrosis developed in two patients, and tumor progression produced late instability in two patients with renal carcinoma. Thecal compression and late collapse led to therapeutic failure in four patients at 1 year to 1 year 6 months after surgery. Fixation failure occurred in four patients, resulting in loosening of the hardware. Failure to address the anterior column disease adequately was the primary cause of treatment failure in these patients; had it been addressed, the fixation devices may have remained intact throughout the illness. Appropriate instrumentation, however, provided rigid fixation and allowed more extensive tumor resection with sparing of vertebral motion segments. Failure to address key technical and biomechanical principles, however, can lead to serious complications. Pedicle fixation may not be possible, but when it is, it appears to have the advantage of involving fewer motion segments.

SUMMARY

In the United States, approximately 2000 malignant tumors of bone are diagnosed each year.[74] Of these, between 4% and 20% are primary spinal tumors (80 to 400 tumors). Therefore, it would be unusual or impossible for any one institution to acquire the necessary understanding of the natural history of these tumors and their response to various forms of treatment. It would be helpful if an international registry was organized through which centers with special interest in these cases could work together. Only through a collaborative effort will enough information be obtained to enable rational surgical and nonsurgical decisions for patients.

Treatment of vertebral spinal tumors has evolved over years. More aggressive treatment has helped tremendously, as have improved diagnostic techniques. Diagnosis is the most important factor in treating tumors. The earlier the diagnosis occurs, the more beneficial treatment is. Although no single technique has emerged as superior, combinations of techniques for individual cases have given the best results. Many problems in treating cancer still exist, however. Many neoplasms are still not curable, and treatments of these tumors can in and of themselves lead to future problems (e.g., excision of tumors may result in spinal deformity and instability of the spine). The younger the patient is, the more susceptible to severe deformity that patient becomes. Complete excision is the best cure, although in the spine this can be difficult. Radiation therapy or chemotherapy may not only affect growth but can also be responsible for sarcomatous degeneration and secondary neoplasms.

In the future, the origin of human cancer as explained by molecular and cellular mechanisms in the various stages of carcinogenesis may provide the most effective clues to cancer prevention and treatment. The mechanisms by which normal cell growth fails and cells become malignant is believed to be related in part to the absence of tumor suppressor genes or an activated oncogene.[66, 89] The suppressor genes are involved in cell cycle control, signal transmission, angiogenesis, and development of tumor cells, indicating that they contribute to normal cell and tumor cell functions. These suppressor genes are believed to provide an untapped resource for treatment of cancer.[66] It is hoped that this technology will bring better understanding of the cellular mechanism of cancer and that currently crude methods will give way to a more basic and reasonable approach to these cancer patients. Clearly time will tell, but in the meantime, clinicians must not intervene without cause or delay without reason. Surgical intervention can at times be a valuable adjunct and occasionally the primary treatment for spinal neoplasms. Intervention can sometimes be worse than no intervention; at other times, aggressive intervention may be the best alternative.

REFERENCES

1. Batson, O. V.: The role of the vertebral veins in metastatic processes. Ann. Intern. Med. 16:38–45, 1942.
2. Bernat, J. L., Greenberg, E. R., and Barrett, J.: Suspected epidural compression of the spinal cord and cauda equina by metastatic carcinoma. Clin. Diagn. Surviv. Cancer 51:1953–1957, 1983.
3. Black, P.: Spinal metastasis: Current status and recommended guidelines for management. Neurosurgery 5:726–746, 1979.
4. Bohlman, H. H., Sachs, B. L., Carter, J. R., et al.: Primary neoplasms of the cervical spine. J. Bone Joint Surg. 68A:483–494, 1986.
5. Boland, P. J., Lane, J. M., and Sundaresan, N.: Metastatic disease of the spine. Clin. Orthop. 169:95–102, 1982.
6. Brice, J., and McKissock, W.: Surgical treatment of malignant extradural spinal tumors. Br. Med. J. [Clin. Res.] 1:1341–1344, 1965.
7. Bruckman, J. E., and Bloomer, W. D.: Management of spinal cord compression. Semin. Oncol. 5:135–140, 1978.
8. Coman, D. R., and deLong, R. P.: The role of the vertebral venous system in the metastasis of cancer to the spinal column: Experiments with tumor-cell suspensions in rats and rabbits. Cancer 4:610–618, 1951.
9. Constans, J. P., DeVitus, E., Donzelli, R., et al.: Spinal metastases with neurological manifestations. Review of 600 cases. J. Neurosurg. 59:111–118, 1983.
10. Dahlin, D. C.: Bone Tumors: General Aspects and Data on 6,221 Cases, 4th Ed. Springfield, IL, Charles C Thomas, 1986.
11. Dahlin, D. C.: Bone Tumors: General Aspects and Data on 6,221 Cases, 3rd Ed. Springfield, IL, Charles C Thomas, 1978.
12. Danzig, L. A., Resnick, D, and Akeson, W. H.: The treatment of cervical spine metastasis from the prostate with a halo cast. Spine 5:395–398, 1980.
13. Denis, F.: Spinal instability as defined by the three-column spine concept in acute spinal trauma. Clin. Orthop. 189:65–76, 1984.
14. DeWald, R. L., Bridwell, K. H., Prodromas, C., and Rodts, M. F.: Reconstructive spinal surgery as palliation for metastatic malignancies of the spine. Spine 10:21–26, 1985.
15. Dolin, M. G.: Acute massive dural compression secondary to methylmethacrylate replacement of a tumorous lumbar vertebral body. Spine 14:108–110, 1989.
16. Doppman, J. L., and Girton, M.: Angiographic study of the effect of laminectomy in the presence of acute anterior epidural masses. J. Neurosurg. 45:195–202, 1976.
17. Enneking, W. F.: Musculoskeletal Tumor Surgery. New York, Churchill Livingstone, 1983.

18. Enneking, W. F., Spanier, S. S., and Goodmann, M.: A system for surgical staging of musculoskeletal sarcoma. Clin. Orthop. 153:106–120, 1980.
19. Fidler, I. J., Gersten, D., and Hart, I.: The biology of cancer invasion and metastasis. Adv. Cancer Res. 28:149–250, 1978.
20. Fidler, M. W.: Pathological fractures of the cervical spine. J. Bone Joint Surg. 67B:352–357, 1985.
21. Findlay, G. F.: The role of vertebral body collapse in the management of malignant spinal cord compression. J. Neurol. Neurosurg. Psychiatry 50:151–154, 1987.
22. Fitzpatrick, P. J., and Rider, W. D.: Half body radiotherapy. Int. J. Radiol. Oncol. Biol. Phys. 1:197–207, 1976.
23. Flatley, T. J., Anderson, M. N., and Anast, G. T.: Spinal instability due to malignant disease. Treatment by segmental spinal stabilization. J. Bone Joint Surg. 66A:47–52, 1984.
24. Floman, Y., Milgrom, C., Kenan, S., et al.: Spongious and cortical osteoblastoma of the axial skeleton. Orthopaedics 8:1478–1484, 1985.
25. Francis, K. C., and Hutter, R. V. P.: Neoplasms of the spine in the aged. Clin Orthop. 26:54–66, 1963.
26. Fraser, R. D., Paterson, D. C., and Simpson, D. A.: Orthopaedic aspects of spinal tumors in children. J. Bone Joint Surg. 59B:143–151, 1977.
27. Galasko, G. S. B.: The development of skeletal metastases. In Weiss, L., and Gilbert, H. A. (eds.): Bone Metastases. Boston, G. K. Hall Medical, 1981.
28. Gilbert, R. W., Kim, J. H., and Posner, J. B.: Epidural spinal cord compression from metastatic tumor: Diagnosis and treatment. Ann. Neurol. 3:40–51, 1978.
29. Greenberg, H. S., Kim, J. H., and Posner, J. B.: Epidural spinal cord compression from metastatic tumor. Ann. Neurol. 8:361–366, 1980.
30. Hall, A. J., and MacKay, N. N.: The results of laminectomy for compression of the cord or cauda equina by extradural malignant tumour. J. Bone Joint Surg. 55B:497–505, 1973.
31. Harrington, K. D.: Metastatic disease of the spine, current concepts. J. Bone Joint Surg. 68A:1110–1115, 1986.
32. Harrington, K. D.: Anterior cord decompression and spinal stabilization for patients with metastatic lesions of the spine. J. Neurosurg. 61:107–117, 1984.
33. Harrington, K. D.: Anterior decompression and stabilization of the spine as a treatment for vertebral collapse and spinal cord compression from metastatic malignancy. Clin. Orthop. 233:177–194, 1988.
34. Harrington K. D.: Metastatic disease of the spine. In Harrington K. D. (ed.): Orthopaedic Management of Metastatic Bone Disease. St. Louis, C. V. Mosby, 1988, pp. 309–383.
35. Hart, R., Boriani, S., Weinstein, J. N., et al.: Spine tumors: Surgical staging and clinical outcome. Application to giant cell tumors of the spine. Presented at the International Society for the Study of the Lumbar Spine Meeting, Seattle, WA, June 21–25, 1994.
36. Ippolito, E., Farsetti, P., and Tudisco, C.: Vertebral plana. J. Bone Joint Surg. 66A:1364–1368, 1984.
37. Jaffee, W. F.: Tumors and Tumorous Conditions of the Bones and Joints. Philadelphia, Lea & Febiger, 1958.
38. Johnson, J. R., Leatherman, K. D., and Holt, R. T.: Anterior decompression of the spinal cord for neurological deficit. Spine 8:396–405, 1983.
39. Keim, H. A., and Reina, E. G.: Osteoid osteoma as a cause of scoliosis. J. Bone Joint Surg. 57A:159–163, 1975.
40. Kirwan, E. O., Hutton, P. A. N., Pozo, J. L., and Ransford, A. O.: Osteoid osteoma and benign osteoblastoma of the spine. J. Bone Joint Surg. 66B:21–26, 1984.
41. Kostuik, J. P.: Anterior spinal cord decompression for lesions of the thoracic and lumbar spine: Techniques, new methods of internal fixation, results. Spine 8:513–531, 1983.
42. Kostuik, J. P., Errico, T. J., Gleason, T. F., and Errico, C. C.: Spinal stabilization of vertebral column tumors. Spine 13:250–256, 1988.
43. Kostuik, J. P., and Weinstein, J. N.: Differential diagnosis and surgical treatment of metastatic spine tumors. In Frymoyer, J. W. (ed.): The Adult Spine: Principles and Practice. New York, Raven Press, 1991, pp. 861–888.
44. Larsson, S. E., Lorentzon, R., and Boquist, L.: Giant cell tumors of the spine and sacrum causing neurologic symptoms. Clin. Orthop. 111:201–211, 1975.
45. Larsson, S. E., Lorentzon, R., and Boquist, L.: Giant cell tumor of bone. J. Bone Joint Surg. 57A:167–173, 1975.
46. Leeson, M. C., Makley, J. T., and Carter, J. R.: Metastatic skeletal disease in the pediatric population. J. Pediatr. Orthop. 5:261–267, 1985.
47. Lichtenstein, L.: Bone Tumors. St. Louis, C. V. Mosby, 1965.
48. Livingston, K. E., and Perrin, R. G.: The neurosurgical management of spinal metastases causing cord and cauda equina compression. J. Neurosurg. 49:839–843, 1978.
49. Manabe, S., Tateishi, A., Abe, M., and Ohno, T.: Surgical treatment of metastatic tumors of the spine. Spine 14:41–57, 1989.
50. Mankin, H. J., Lange, T. A., and Spainer, S. S.: The hazards of biopsy in patients with malignant primary bone and soft-tissue tumors. J. Bone Joint Surg. 64A:1121–1127, 1982.
51. Martin, N. S., and Williamson, J.: The role of surgery in the treatment of malignant tumours of the spine. J. Bone Joint Surg. 52B:227–237, 1970.
52. McAfee, P., Bohlman, H., Ducker, T., and Eismont, F.: Failure of stabilization of the spine with methylmethacrylate. A retrospective analysis of twenty-four cases. J. Bone Joint Surg. 68A:1145–1157, 1986.
53. McLain, R., Kabins, M., and Weinstein, J.: VSP stabilization of lumbar neoplasms: Technical considerations and complications. J. Spinal Disord. 4:359–365, 1991.
54. McLain, R. F., and Weinstein, J. N.: Solitary plasmacytomas of the spine: A review of 84 cases. J. Spinal Disord. 2:69–74, 1989.
55. McLain, R., and Weinstein, J. N.: Primary tumors of the spine. Spine 12:843–851, 1987.
56. Millburn, L., Hibbs, G. C., and Hendrickson, F. R.: Treatment of spinal cord compression from metastatic carcinoma. Cancer 21:447–452, 1968.
57. Mindell, E. R.: Chordoma: Current concepts review. J. Bone Joint Surg. 63A:501–505, 1981.
58. Nather, A., and Bose, K.: The results of decompression of cord or cauda equina compression from

metastatic extradural tumors. Clin. Orthop. 169:103–108, 1982.
59. Nicholls, P. J., and Jarecky, T. W.: The value of posterior decompression by laminectomy for malignant tumors of the spine. Clin. Orthop. 201:210–213, 1985.
60. O'Neil, J., Gardner, V., and Armstrong, G.: Treatment of tumors of the thoracic and lumbar spinal column. Clin. Orthop. 227:103–112, 1988.
61. Powles, T. J., Dowsett, M., Easty, G. C., et al.: Breast-cancer osteolysis, bone metastases, and the anti-osteolytic effect of aspirin. Lancet 1:608–610, 1976.
62. Raven, R. W., and Willis, R. A.: Solitary plasmacytoma of the spine. J. Bone Joint Surg. 31B:369–375, 1949.
63. Rothman, R. H., and Simeone, F. A.: The Spine, 2nd Ed. Philadelphia, W. B. Saunders, 1982.
64. Russin, L. A., Robinson, M. J., Engle, H. A., and Sonni, A.: Ewing's sarcoma of the lumbar spine. Clin. Orthop. 164:126–129, 1982.
65. Sachs, B. L., Makley, J. T., Carter, J. R., et al.: Primary osseous neoplasms of the thoracic and lumbar spine. Orthop. Trans. 8:422–423, 1984.
66. Sager, R.: Tumor supressor genes: The puzzle and the promise. Science 246:1406–1412, 1989.
67. Schajowicz, F.: Solitary plasmacytomas. In Schajowicz, F. (ed.): Tumors and Tumor-Like Lesions of Bone and Joints. New York, Springer-Verlag, 1981, pp. 296–298.
68. Shaw, M. D., Rose, J. E., and Paterson, A.: Metastatic extradural malignancy of the spine. Acta Neurochir. (Wien) 52:113–120, 1980.
69. Sherman, M. S., and McFarland, G., Jr.: Mechanism of pain in osteoid osteoma. South. Med. J. 58:163–166, 1965.
70. Sherman, R. M., and Waddell, J. P.: Laminectomy for metastatic epidural spinal cord tumors. Clin. Orthop. 207:55–63, 1986.
71. Shives, T. C., Dahlin, D. C., Sim, F. H., et al.: Osteosarcoma of the spine. J. Bone Joint Surg. 68A:660–668, 1986.
72. Siegal, T., and Siegal, T.: Surgical decompression of anterior and posterior malignant epidural tumors compressing the spinal cord. Neurosurgery 17:424–430, 1985.
73. Siegal, T., Tiqva, P., and Siegal, T.: Vertebral body resection for epidural compression by malignant tumors. J. Bone Joint Surg. 67A:375–382, 1985.
74. Silverberg, B., and Lubera, J.: Cancer statistics. CA 37:12, 1987.
75. Sim, F. H., Dahlin, D. C., Stauffer, R. N., and Laws, E. R., Jr.: Primary bone tumors simulating lumbar disc syndrome. Spine 2:65–74, 1977.
76. Smith, T. P., and Cragg, A. H.: Angiography of the spine. In Frymoyer, J. W. (ed.): The Adult Spine: Principles and Practice. New York, Raven Press, 1991, pp. 511–525.
77. Stener, B.: Total spondylectomy in chondrosarcoma arising from the seventh thoracic vertebra. J. Bone Joint Surg. 53B:288–295, 1971.
78. Stener, B.: Total spondylectomy for removal of a giant-cell tumor in the eleventh thoracic vertebra. Spine 2:197–201, 1977.
79. Stener, B., Henriksson, C., Johansson, S., et al.: Surgical removal of bone and muscle metastases of renal cancer. Acta Orthop. Scand. 55:491–500, 1984.
80. Thommesen, P., and Poulsen, J. O.: Primary tumors in the spine and pelvis in adolescents: Clinical and radiological features. Acta Orthop. Scand. 47:170–174, 1976.
81. Thompson, J. E., and Keiller, V. H.: Multiple skeletal metastases from cancer of the breast. Surg. Gynecol. Obstet. 38:367–375, 1924.
82. Tillman, B. P., Dahlin, D. C., Lipscomb, P. R., et al.: Aneurysmal bone cyst: An analysis of ninety-five cases. Mayo Clin. Proc. 93:478–495, 1968.
83. Tomita, T., Galicich, J. H., and Sundaresan, N.: Radiation therapy for spinal epidural metastases with complete block. Acta Radiol. 22:135–143, 1983.
84. Uribe-Botero, G., Russell, W. D., and Sutow, W. W.: Primary osteocarcoma of bone. A clinical pathological investigation of 243 cases, and the necroscopy studies in 54. Am. J. Clin. Pathol. 67:427–435, 1977.
85. Valderama, J. A. F., and Bullough, P. G.: Solitary myeloma of the spine. J. Bone Joint Surg. 50B:82–90, 1968.
86. Verbiest, H.: Giant cell tumors and aneurysmal bone cysts of the spine. J. Bone Joint Surg. 47B:699–713, 1965.
87. Verbiest, H.: Lesions of the cervical spine: A critical review. In Carrea, R. (ed.): Neurological Surgery, International Congress Series 433. Amsterdam-Oxford, Excerpta Medica, 1978, pp. 374–383.
88. Virinder, M., Gupta, S. K., Tuli, S. M., and Sanyal, B.: Symptomatic vertebral hemangiomas. Clin. Radiol. 31:575–579, 1980.
89. Weinstein, B.: The origins of human cancer: Molecular mechanisms of carcinogenesis and their implications for cancer prevention and treatment. Cancer Res. 48:4135–4143, 1988.
90. Weinstein, J. N.: Differential diagnosis and surgical treatment of primary benign and malignant neoplasms. In Frymoyer, J. W. (ed.): The Adult Spine: Principles and Practice. New York, Raven Press, 1991, pp. 829–860.
91. Weinstein, J. N.: Surgical approach to spine tumors. Orthopedics 12:897–905, 1989.
92. Weinstein, J. N.: Spine neoplasms. In Weinstein, S. L. (ed.): The Pediatric Spine: Principles and Practice. New York, Raven Press, 1994, pp. 887–916.
93. Weinstein, J. N., Collalto, P., and Lehmann, T. R.: Long-term follow-up of nonoperatively treated thoracolumbar spine fractures. J. Orthop. Trauma 3:152–159, 1988.
94. Weinstein, J. N., and McLain, R. F.: Primary tumors of the spine. Spine 12:843–851, 1987.
95. White, A. A., III, and Panjabi, M. M.: Surgical constructs employing methylmethacrylate. In White, A. A., III, and Panjabi, M. M. (eds.): Clinical Biomechanics of the Spine. Philadelphia, J. B. Lippincott, 1978, pp. 423–431.
96. Wright, R. L.: Malignant tumors in the spinal extradural space: Results of surgical treatment. Ann. Surg. 157:227–231, 1963.

15

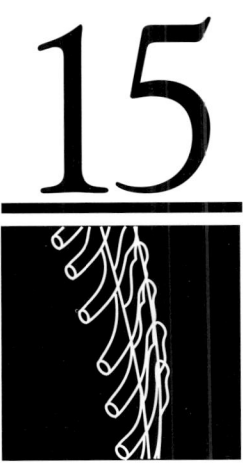

Complications of Lumbar Spine Surgery

GORDON R. BELL

Complications of lumbar spine surgery can be either general types of complications, which are common to any type of spine surgery, or complications related to particular types of surgery or to certain surgical approaches. The latter include complications of posterior approaches for neural decompression, of anterior approaches, and of bone graft harvesting for spinal arthrodesis. This chapter examines each of these areas with the hope that an understanding of potential pitfalls will enable the surgeon to avoid them or will at least permit their prompt recognition and therefore minimize both morbidity and impact on surgical outcome.

GENERAL COMPLICATIONS

All lumbar spine surgery, and indeed all surgeries generally, share certain broad groups of potential complications that occur preoperatively, intraoperatively, or postoperatively.

Preoperative Complications

Preoperative factors that are important determinants of surgical outcome involve primarily surgical decision-making. Therefore, complications of this process can be thought of as being judgment errors in patient selection. The most common indication for lumbar spine surgery is pain palliation. Numerous researchers have emphasized that surgery is more likely to produce symptomatic relief of radicular leg pain (sciatica) than low back pain.[27, 28, 55] This is primarily because the cause of the leg pain can usually be determined accurately and precisely so that surgery can be directed to the source of the leg pain.

Spangfort[113] showed that, for disc herniation, the surgical success rate is directly proportional to the magnitude of neural compression noted at surgery, which is reflected by the size of the disc herniation. The ability to predict accurately the size of the disc herniation is based on the preoperative correlation of an objective neurologic deficit with a positive straight leg raising sign and a confirmatory objective radiographic imaging test. When all three of these preoperative factors are present, the chance of finding a definite disc herniation at surgery approaches 95%.[60]

The difficulty with surgery for low back pain lies not so much with the technical aspects of the surgical procedure but with localization of the source of low back pain. Discography has been advocated as a diagnostic test for determining the origin of back pain.[20, 80, 109, 119] The role of discography is still controversial, and it may not accurately predict the painful level, even when the pain might be coming from the disc.[62, 95] Discography comprises three components: the radiographic image, concordant pain reproduction, and resistance to injection. The incidence of abnormal radiographic discograms in asymptomatic persons has been reported to be as high as 79%.[20] Therefore, the presence of an abnormal image as the primary determinant of an abnormal discogram is fraught with error.

The anatomic basis for the controversy surrounding the concept of concordant pain reproduction as the discriminator for discographic results is that sensory innervation of the outer layer of the annulus fibrosus is from a sinuvertebral nerve, which not only supplies the annulus at the same level but arborizes superiorly and inferiorly to supply adjacent discs as well. Therefore, the assumption that concordant pain reproduction after a disc injection indicates that the pain is coming from the injected disc is not necessarily true. The pain could theoretically come from a different level innervated by a sinuvertebral nerve either above or below the injected disc.

Finally, a normal disc exhibits some resistance to injection of dye because of its turgidity and high water content. A degenerated or herniated disc exhibits less resistance to injection and a larger volume of dye can be injected more easily than in a normal disc.

Intraoperative Complications

In general, the complications related to anesthesia for spine surgery are comparable to those associated with other nonspine surgical procedures. These include airway complications related to intubation or aspiration; fluid management problems, including shock, fluid overload, and transfusion reactions; pulmonary conditions such as atelectasis and postoperative pneumonia; cardiac risks related to intraoperative or postoperative myocardial infarction, cardiogenic shock, or congestive heart failure; and vascular complications related to blood loss, hypertension, hypotension, and thrombotic or embolic phenomena. The latter category includes conditions associated with hypoperfusion of vital organs such as the kidney and the brain. This chapter deals primarily with anesthesia-associated complications related to spine surgery.

For anterior thoracic or thoracolumbar spine surgery in which the diaphragm must be detached from its origin, there are additional potential complications that can affect pulmonary function. In addition, there are risks associated with potential damage to major blood vessels, the spinal cord, and spinal nerves. These are dealt with separately below.

Posterior spine surgery poses problems related to prone positioning of the patient, which is the least physiologic position for a patient under general anesthesia.[120, 122] These include potential problems with maintaining ventilation and in managing the airway. In addition, there is the risk of pressure to structures such as the eyes, which can cause central retinal artery occlusion and result in blindness. To maintain the patient in the prone position required for posterior spine surgery, pressure must be exerted on the patient by either the operation table itself or various positioning devices. This can produce compression of various neural structures, which may result in temporary or permanent nerve palsies.[13] These include compression of the sciatic nerve or its branches from prolonged pressure of the buttocks against a buttress while in the kneeling position,[13, 31] pressure on the ulnar nerve at the elbow,[18] injury to the anterior interosseous nerve in the cubital tunnel,[3] axillary nerve injury,[53, 96] brachial plexus injuries from excessive shoulder abduction,[21] and cervical radiculopathy from prolonged neck rotation.

Some of these position-associated complications can be obviated by the use of spinal rather than general anesthesia. The advantage of spinal anesthesia in posterior surgery is that the patient is awake and can therefore control the head and upper extremities. This minimizes the risk of pressure on the eyes, compression to the ulnar nerve at the elbow, and brachial plexus palsies. Spinal anesthesia, however, is not without its own particular complications. Problems related to spinal anesthesia include persistent cerebrospinal fluid leak and hypotension from venous pooling of blood in the lower extremities.

The syndrome of inappropriate antidiuretic hormone secretion (SIADH) is characterized by the release of antidiuretic hormone from the posterior pituitary gland in the absence of the usual osmometric or volumetric stimuli of dehydration or hypovolemia.[5] This results in failure to excrete free water, producing dilutional hyponatremia. SIADH occurs in many circumstances, including surgery, and has been reported during and after spine surgery in particular.[6] It is thought that secretion of antidiuretic hormone reaches its maximum level during surgery and that the syndrome gradually resolves by approximately the third postoperative day. It is imperative to distinguish between SIADH and hypovolemia as a cause of low urine output, because the former demands treatment by fluid restriction, whereas the latter requires fluid administration. SIADH should always be considered as a cause of low urine output and dilutional hyponatremia during and immediately after spine surgery.

Postoperative Complications

Some postoperative complications are common to many surgical procedures, including spine surgery. These include conditions such as *urinary retention*. Some uncommon spinal conditions, such as cauda equina syndrome, however, may predispose to urinary retention owing to impairment in function of the nervous supply to the bladder. It is important to distinguish benign postoperative urinary retention from retention due to a spinal cause, such as cauda equina syndrome from epidural hematoma, because the treatment of these two conditions may be radically different. When urinary retention is the result of cauda equina syndrome, prompt surgical decompression is imperative. Urinary retention, regardless of its etiology, may require either intermittent straight catheterization or indwelling catheterization. A urinary catheter, particularly when used for a lengthy period, may predispose the patient to urinary tract infection, necessitating treatment with antibiotics.

Ileus can also follow any surgical procedure but is common after some spine procedures, particularly anterior lumbar or thoracolumbar surgery. In addition, it is more likely to follow lengthy or complicated posterior procedures, such as instrumented lumbar fusions. When the intertransverse membrane is violated during transverse process recipient site preparation for bilateral lateral (posterolateral) fusion, entry to the retroperitoneal space occurs, making ileus more likely.

Deep venous thrombosis (DVT) and *pulmonary embolism (PE)* are serious complications of any type of surgery. DVT is thought to be the precursor to PE in approximately 90% of cases.[100] The risk of DVT after general surgery ranges between 5% and 63%, but it is particularly common with certain orthopedic surgeries. Such procedures include repair of hip fracture and total hip and total knee arthroplasty, in which the incidence of DVT after unprotected joint replacement is as high as 60% to 80%.[51] DVT after routine spine decompressions, however, was thought to be rare. Bell and associates[7] reported that the incidence of DVT in unprotected lumbar decompression for disc herniation or spinal stenosis performed under spinal anesthesia was 27.5%. Prophylaxis with pneumatic compression stockings reduced the incidence to 4.5% in patients receiving spinal anesthesia. Pneumatic compression stockings seemed to provide no significant protection from DVT in patients receiving general anesthesia, in which cases the incidence of DVT was 13.6% without pneumatic compression stockings and 8.1% with pneumatic compression stockings. DVT and PE are discussed in more detail later.

Scar Tissue

Postoperative scar tissue may be classified by anatomic location as being either within the dura (arachnoiditis) or external to the dura (epidural fibrosis). Arachnoiditis is an inflammation of the pia-arachnoid membrane that surrounds the cauda equina or spinal cord.[17] It is one of the more serious complications of spine surgery, which can result in surgical failure and continued pain. The etiology of arachnoiditis is often unclear, but has been associated with many conditions including the use of oil-based contrast agents for myelography and surgery.[104] The exact mechanism of arachnoiditis that occurs after surgery is not completely understood, but arachnoiditis is thought to be more likely to follow dural laceration in which blood gains entry to the dural sac and mixes with neural elements.[22] It is also associated with intraoperative trauma to neural structures.

Arachnoiditis has a spectrum of severity, from mild pia-arachnoid thickening to severe scarring with complete blockage of the flow of contrast agents or cerebrospinal fluid. In milder cases, radiographic diagnosis can be subtle, but in more obvious cases, the condition is characterized by a clumping together of the cauda equina such that individual nerve roots are not visualized. In such cases, a myelogram with water-soluble contrast medium presents the radiographic appearance of a myelogram with oil-based contrast medium, with poor definition of individual nerve roots. Magnetic resonance imaging (MRI) or contrast medium–enhanced computed tomography (CT) may also show individual elements of the cauda equina clumped together. Surgical treatment of true arachnoiditis rarely produces any significant pain relief and may be complicated by further damage to the neural structures and more scarring.[17, 22]

Epidural fibrosis is extradural, rather than intradural, scar tissue in which adhesive constrictions can form around neural tissue. It commonly arises from contact with the paraspinal musculature and is probably a relatively frequent event after spine surgery.[77] Although constricting extradural scar tissue can result in postoperative pain, symptoms are relatively infrequent. When postoperative pain exists, the primary differential diagnostic possibilities are scar and recurrent disc herniation. Radiographic distinction between these two conditions is best made with gadolinium-enhanced MRI scanning or contrast-enhanced (CT) scanning.[105, 106]

Efforts to prevent postoperative scar formation include delicate surgical technique, adequate illumination and magnification, meticulous hemostasis and drainage, and the use of some form of an interposition membrane as a barrier to scar formation.[72, 76, 77] The latter includes a thin layer of fat or synthetic agents such as absorbable gelatin sponge (Gelfoam). A free fat graft has been considered the gold standard for interposition membranes, although the use of large grafts has been associated with postoperative cauda equina syndrome.[103]

Deep Venous Thrombosis and Pulmonary Embolism

PE is the third most common cause of death in the United States, accounting for up to 200,000 deaths annually. In hospitalized patients, PE is the most frequent preventable cause of hospital death, detectable in more than one quarter of all routine autopsy examinations. DVT, the precursor to PE in 90% of cases, is common in hospitalized patients.[100] The etiology of PE includes immobilization associated with hospitalization, as well as factors related to surgery itself. The incidence of DVT in patients undergoing general surgery has been reported to be between 5% and 63% but is even more common in other types of surgery, particularly orthopedic surgery. The frequency of DVT in patients undergoing surgery for fracture of the hip without DVT prophylaxis ranges between 36% and 60%. The incidence of DVT after unprotected elective hip surgery ranges between 40% and 60%; after unprotected total knee replacement arthroplasty, the incidence is between 60% and 80%.[51]

DVT following routine spine surgery has been thought to be a rare event, although it has been reported after scoliosis surgery. Ferree and associates[37, 38] reported only a 6% incidence of DVT in 86 patients undergoing routine lumbar decompressive surgeries using compression ultrasonography as the method of diagnosis. This low rate probably represents an underestimation of the true incidence of DVT, because compression ultrasonography is considered a less accurate method of diagnosis than venography, particularly for the detection of distal (calf) thrombi. Bell and colleagues[7] examined 31 patients undergoing unprotected laminectomy for spinal stenosis or hemilaminotomy and discectomy for disc herniation and found a 25.8% incidence of venographically proven DVT. This incidence is similar to that reported in general surgery patients.

Traditional prophylaxis against DVT by the use of medications such as aspirin, heparin, and sodium warfarin (Coumadin) is thought to pose an increased risk of bleeding with the potential for postoperative epidural hematoma and cauda equina syndrome. The use of mechanical methods of DVT prophylaxis, such as pneumatic compression stockings, offers the advantage of decreased morbidity from bleeding.

Bell and associates[7] examined 194 patients undergoing routine decompressive lumbar surgery under either spinal or general anesthesia who were randomized to receive either no DVT prophylaxis or pneumatic compression stockings. The method of DVT diagnosis was venography. For patients receiving spinal anesthesia, none of the 51 patients with pneumatic compression stocking prophylaxis developed DVT, whereas 14 (27.5%) of 51 patients without prophylaxis developed DVT ($p < .001$). For patients undergoing general anesthesia, 7 (14.6%) of 48 patients with pneumatic compression stocking prophylaxis and 6 (13.6%) of 44 patients without prophylaxis had DVT, a statistically insignificant difference. Because this study involved randomization only for DVT prophylaxis or no prophylaxis, but was not randomized for type of anesthesia (general versus spinal), the investigators attempted to explore further the potential relationship between type of anesthesia and DVT by controlling for prophylaxis and adding another 112 nonrandomized patients receiving only pneumatic compression stocking prophylaxis, bringing the total number of patients to 306. The overall rate of DVT in this group was 10.8% but varied by type of anesthesia. Patients receiving spinal anesthesia and prophylaxis had a 4.5% DVT rate; without prophylaxis, the DVT rate was 27.5% ($p < .001$). For patients undergoing general anesthesia with and without prophylaxis, the DVT rate was 8.1% and 13.6%, respectively ($p = .363$). Although pulmonary emboli were not specifically looked for by means of ventilation/perfusion scans, no clinically detectable PE was noted. This study suggested that the best combination of type of anesthesia and DVT prophylaxis for prevention of DVT was spinal anesthesia with pneumatic compression stocking prophylaxis. The worst was spinal anesthesia without pneumatic compression stockings. General anesthesia, regardless of prophylaxis, was intermediate between these two.

Wound Infection

Postoperative spine infections may be divided into superficial and deep infections. Although the treatment of both types of infections is often similar (i.e., débridement and antibiotic therapy), it is useful to make this distinction because the duration of treatment (e.g., short-term antibiotic administration for superficial infections versus long-term intravenous antibiotic use for deep infections), morbidity, and long-term outcome are often different between the two.

SUPERFICIAL WOUND INFECTION

Superficial wound infections are located beneath the dermis and subcutaneous tissue but superficial to the deep thoracolumbar fascia and are characterized by tenderness and localized erythema. They usually have associated drainage and fluctuance, although in milder cases consisting of only cellulitis, these may be absent. Patients may be febrile but usually show no systemic signs of illness. Laboratory data usually show elevated concentrations of acute phase reactants, particularly increased erythrocyte sedimentation rate (ESR) and elevated C-reactive protein (CRP) levels, although the white blood cell count is usually within normal limits.

Treatment of superficial wound infections consists of aggressive surgical débridement of all necrotic tissue and short-term parenteral antibiotic administration. In most cases, the wound can be closed primarily even if débridement involves removal of a moderate amount of tissue from the wound margins, because the edges can be mobilized by undermining the subcutaneous tissues, thereby permitting closure without excessive tension on the edges of the wound. The short-term placement of suction-irrigation tubes is left to the discretion of the surgeon, although their use is usually not required. In cases of a small, well-localized area of superficial wound dehiscence with infection, treatment may consist of only localized conservative wound care and oral antibiotic administration without the need for formal surgical débridement.

DEEP WOUND INFECTIONS

As opposed to superficial infections, in which the diagnosis is usually readily apparent, deep infections may be difficult to identify and a high index of suspicion is often required.[47] Delay in diagnosis is often encountered, and the amount of tissue necrosis is therefore frequently more extensive than with superficial infection. Symptoms include back pain or referred leg pain that is more severe than the pain usually encountered postoperatively. This may follow a relatively painless immediate postoperative period. The patient may feel ill and may exhibit generalized malaise. Fever is often present but may be deceptively low grade. If an epidural abscess is also present, radicular leg pain may occur and may be accompanied by a neurologic deficit. Although the patient may exhibit a leukocytosis, elevation of the white blood cell count may be absent. Acute phase reactant concentrations, such as manifested by ESR and CRP levels, are usually elevated.

If there is a strong suspicion of a deep abscess, the diagnosis may be confirmed by sterile aspiration with subsequent culture and sensitivity testing of the fluid obtained.[69] More commonly, additional confirmation must first be obtained by radiographic imaging studies. MRI scanning provides the best and most useful information by revealing both the presence and the extent of the deep abscess.[92] This often aids in delineating the site for subsequent aspiration. Typically, an abscess is demonstrated by the presence of a well-demarcated area of increased signal intensity on the T2-weighted image. When MRI scanning is not available, the diagnosis may be confirmed radiographically by the presence of a circumscribed area of fluid density on the CT scan.

Treatment of a deep wound infection, particularly one associated with spinal instrumentation, should be aggressive. Surgical débridement of all necrotic tissues should be followed by appropriate administration of parenteral antibiotics.[82] Surgical exposure should begin with careful débridement and irrigation or lavage of each layer sequentially, to avoid inadvertent contamination of potentially uninfected deeper layers. If the infection extends deeply into the laminectomy site, care should be taken to remove any fat graft or absorbable gelatin sponge (Gelfoam). After the removal of tissues with gross infection or suspected infection, the wound should be thoroughly irrigated with pulsatile lavage. If an instrumented spine fusion was performed and the fixation appears rigid and well fixed to the bone, the hardware and bone graft should probably be left in place, as this may minimize the risk of subsequent pseudarthrosis.

Wound closure should be meticulous, and the wound should be drained. The deep fascia should be tightly closed by interrupted absorbable suture, which may be oversewn with a continuous running stitch. The wound should be closed primarily unless there is extensive loss of tissue by a particularly virulent organism. Because recently performed postoperative incisions are friable and because wound edges may have been débrided and subcutaneous tissue undermined, resulting in wound edges that are under some tension, it is usually advisable to close the wound using large throws of a sturdy, nonabsorbable suture rather than staples. The use of suction-irrigation tubes for a few days may be considered, although this is usually not necessary.

Postoperative Discitis

Postoperative discitis is infection of the disc space after surgical discectomy that usually results from direct inoculation of the disc at the time of surgery. It is to be distinguished from pyogenic vertebral osteomyelitis, in which the disc is secondarily infected after hematogenous spread from an infective focus to the vertebral body. The clinical presentation is fairly typical, with the patient experiencing a period of relief of preoperative leg, and sometimes back, symptoms.[78, 102] This period of relief may vary from a few days to several weeks, but it is ultimately followed by increasing back pain. Often, the pain appears out of proportion to the magnitude of the surgery. The patient typically has marked lumbar paravertebral muscle spasm and persistent lumbar lordosis on attempted flexion and may even have scoliosis due to muscle spasm. A positive straight leg raising sign may be present, but other neurologic findings are typically absent.

Fever is nearly always absent and routine laboratory tests such as the white blood cell count are usually within normal limits. Concentrations of acute phase reactants, such as manifested by the ESR, are typically elevated but their significance may be difficult to determine in the immediate postoperative period because they are nonspecific and are usually elevated after any surgical procedure. Progressive serial increases of the ESR, however, are highly significant and strongly suggest the presence of some type of postoperative infection.[10] CRP levels are thought to be a more sensitive and specific indicator of infection and may therefore be a better test than the ESR in the immediate postoperative period.

Routine radiographic diagnosis is notoriously difficult in the early stages of disc space infection because, except for loss of typical lumbar lordosis, early plain x-ray findings are usually absent for the first few weeks after surgery. Early radiographic findings include progressive narrowing of the disc space and blurring of the vertebral end plates. Subsequently, reactive bone formation may occur and bony sclerosis may be evident. Fusion of adjacent vertebrae may occur, although in some cases the infection may progress with further loss of bone and collapse of the vertebrae. Technetium Tc 99m bone scan may suggest infection before such changes are evident on plain x-ray studies, although such changes are not expected until bone involvement occurs. MRI scanning is the most accurate imaging test to detect the early presence of infection within the disc before bone involvement is evident on plain x-ray films or bone scans. Both the morphologic features and the signal characteristics of the disc are readily demonstrated by MRI scanning and should be compared with those on the preoperative scan to detect any differences.[92] Typically, the changes on MRI scan are similar to those found with early pyogenic vertebral osteomyelitis, particularly before more significant bone changes occur in the latter (Fig. 1). On the T2-weighted image, the disc has an abnormal configuration and an increased signal intensity. In addition, there is usually a similar increased signal within the adjacent vertebral bodies. On the T1-weighted image, there is decreased signal intensity within the disc and a similar signal intensity within the adjacent vertebral bodies.

Treatment consists of a regimen appropriate antibiotics, an initial period of bed rest if warranted by the pain, and usually a period of bracing. Although the most common infectious organism is *Staphylococcus aureus*, which is often methicillin resistant, an attempt should usually be made to confirm the diagnosis by obtaining appropriate tissue for bacteriologic examination. This can most easily be done by CT-guided biopsy of the disc space. If this does not yield a diagnosis, percutaneous Craig needle biopsy, which employs a larger-bore needle than that used for CT-guided biopsy, can be attempted.[24, 101] Alternatively, an open biopsy can be attempted. The latter procedure has the advantage of permitting removal of some of the infected disc and phlegmatic material, thereby decreasing the bacterial load and theoretically allowing more effective penetration of the infected area by the antibiotics. After bacteriologic diagnosis has been confirmed, either an infectious disease consultation can be obtained or appropriate parenteral antibiotic administration can be initiated and continued for approximately 6 weeks.[34] Additional surgery for postoperative discitis is indicated if there is a progressive neurologic deficit, such as cauda equina syndrome; a documented epidural abscess; or frank sepsis from spinal infection that is unresponsive to parenteral antibiotics.[34] The patient's course should be followed by clinical examination and by serial determination of acute phase reactants. The prognosis of aggressively treated disc space infection is generally favorable, although reported success rates are variable, ranging between 39% and 88%.[81, 102]

Pyogenic Vertebral Osteomyelitis

As opposed to postoperative discitis, in which the disc space is primarily infected and the adjacent vertebral bodies are secondarily involved, pyogenic vertebral osteomyelitis results from primary involvement of the vertebral body, most commonly from hematogenous spread from a remote infectious focus. Vertebral osteomyelitis most commonly occurs not postoperatively as a complication of spine surgery, but rather as a sequela of infection elsewhere. Commonly, this may occur as a complication of genitourinary infection or instrumentation, but it may result from any infection or intravenous drug abuse. One may theorize that an increase in reactive blood flow to recently operated tissue, together with the presence of a fresh postoperative wound hematoma, might render the postoperative spine vulnerable to secondary involvement with infection from either a remote infection or even a simple bacteremia.

Symptoms may be similar to those found

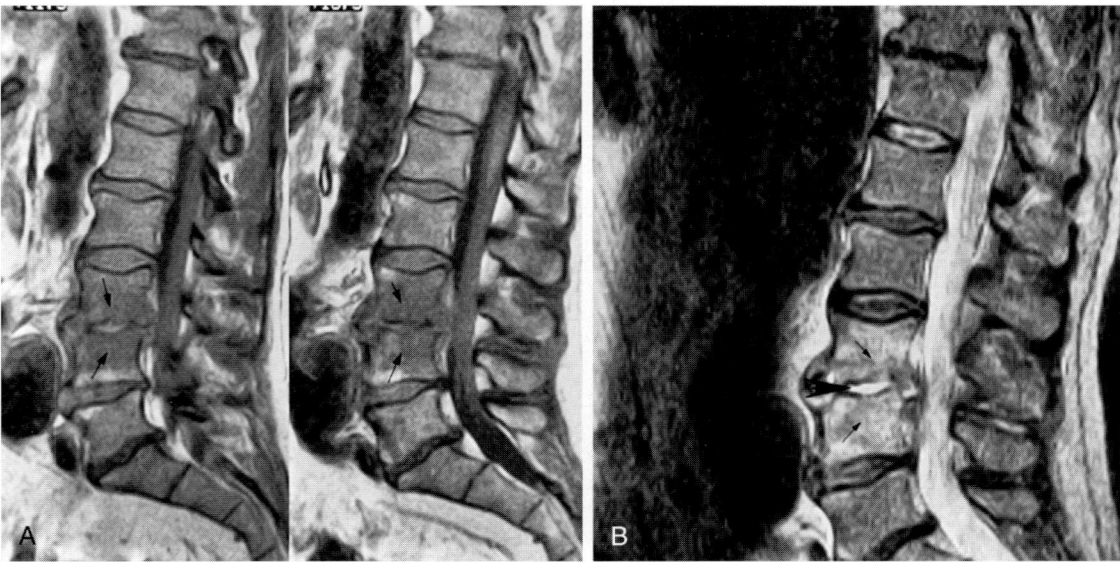

Figure 1. Sagittal lumbar MRI of patient with postoperative disc space infection at L3–L4. *A*, Sagittal T1-weighted image showing decreased signal intensity involving the inferior aspect of L3 and the superior aspect of L4 adjacent to the L3–L4 disc *(arrows)*. *B*, Sagittal T2-weighted image showing increased signal of L3 and L4 vertebrae adjacent to the affected L3–L4 disc *(arrows)*. Note the increased signal and abnormal configuration of the L3–L4 disc *(arrowhead)*.

with postoperative discitis, but the presence of bone involvement subjects the spine to potentially more deformity and therefore renders the neural elements more liable to mechanical compression from spine instability or deformity, with a potential for either paresis or paralysis.[47] Paralysis may also result from septic thrombi to the blood vessels of the spinal cord. Paralysis is therefore more of a risk in this instance than in discitis, and it varies with the level of spine involvement and the nature of the infecting organism.[33]

Diagnosis of vertebral osteomyelitis is based on signs and symptoms similar to those of postoperative discitis and requires a high index of suspicion. True sepsis is usually absent, and therefore temperature and results of routine blood tests such as complete blood count are often normal. Measurements of acute phase reactants such as the ESR and CRP levels, however, are nearly always elevated. Definitive radiographic diagnosis is by MRI scan, with findings similar to those of postoperative discitis, except that bone involvement may be more extensive and may show collapse or other deformity.[92] As is the case with postoperative discitis, the diagnosis should be confirmed bacteriologically by CT-guided biopsy or open biopsy. Treatment is similar to that of postoperative discitis, with bed rest as needed, 6 weeks of parenteral antibiotic administration, and usually the use of bracing to provide comfort and to minimize the risk of late deformity. Additional surgery is reserved for the treatment of a complicating epidural abscess, neurologic deterioration, or significant deformity.[34, 47] Follow-up entails primarily clinical examination, serial acute phase reactant determination, and serial x-ray studies to detect early deformity.

Epidural Abscess

Epidural abscess, because of its risk of paresis or frank paralysis, is one of the most feared complications of spine surgery. Fortunately, it is rare after surgery of the spine, with only 16% of epidural abscesses resulting from postoperative infection.[4] The signs and symptoms are obvious and constitute a typical presentation.[4, 56] Patients nearly always have significant back pain and often have neurologic findings such as nuchal rigidity or weakness and paralysis of the lower extremities. The patient appears much sicker than with either postoperative discitis or vertebral osteomyelitis and therefore typically exhibits fever and elevation of both the white blood cell count and acute phase reactant concentrations. MRI scanning is the diagnostic imaging modality of choice, and it clearly visualizes the abscess as a discrete, well-circumscribed entity within the subarachnoid space[92] (Fig. 2). MRI, like conventional myelography, delineates the upper and the lower extent of the abscess and is therefore invaluable in preoperative planning.

Treatment must be prompt. Evacuation of the abscess should be followed by parenteral antibiotic administration. The preferred surgical approach is generally posterior laminectomy when possible. An anterior approach, however, may be required for a well-circumscribed loculated anterior abscess, particularly in the cervical and the thoracic spine, where retraction of the spinal cord is contraindicated. In addition, an anterior approach may be necessary if there is significant deformity, such as severe kyphosis, in which bony collapse may compromise the neural structures and in which reconstruction and bone grafting may be required.

COMPLICATIONS RELATED TO POSTERIOR APPROACH

Although each of the various posterior surgical procedures involves complications

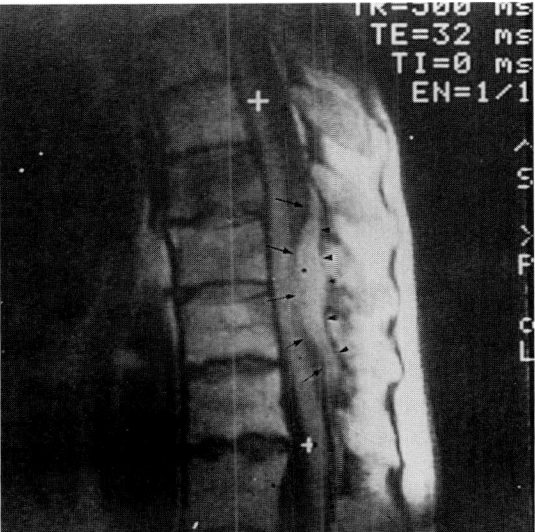

Figure 2. Thoracic MRI of patient with epidural abscess *(arrows* and *arrowheads)* posterior to the spinal cord secondary to tuberculosis.

specific to the particular type of procedure being performed, most such procedures share some complications related to surgical anatomy and exposure. Complications of spinal instrumentation are not considered in this chapter but are presented elsewhere in the text. Furthermore, this section is not intended to encompass all aspects of surgical complications, as discussions in other chapters of the various surgical techniques also provide information on specific complications.

Laminectomy and Discectomy

Both laminectomy and discectomy, whether radical, limited, or microsurgical, share common bony, soft tissue, and neural anatomy and, therefore, have common potential complications (see below). For complications of a particular surgical procedure, the reader is referred to the discussion of that procedure in other chapters.

Inadequate Neural Decompression

Failure to obtain symptomatic relief of radicular leg pain, in the absence of an error in surgical decision-making, must be considered a complication of surgery. Avoidance of this complication requires precise correlation of the preoperative imaging study with the surgical anatomy and necessitates that the surgeon continue to search for the cause of the neural compression until it is found. It also requires a thorough knowledge of surgical anatomy and the potential sources and sites of neural compression as described by Macnab.[83] In addition, it is imperative that the surgeon have a precise understanding of potential anatomic variations in the location of disc herniations and know precisely where to look for neural compression, particularly when predicted pathologic change is not found.[115, 116]

It is important for the surgeon to recognize and to look for additional sites of neural compression, which may account for inadequate relief after decompression of only one site. This condition, sometimes referred to as a double-crush phenomenon, is thought to be at least partially due to venous congestion of the neural segment located between the two sites of compression, resulting in a compartmentlike syndrome of the intervening segment.[71] This may involve central compression of the cauda equina at two or more sites, or it may entail some element of concomitant lateral compression, within the lateral recess, within the neural foramen, or at an extraforaminal site. It is important to identify all potential sites of neural compression that may explain the clinical picture and to achieve adequate decompression at those levels.

Recurrent Disc Herniation

Distinguishing recurrent disc herniation from scar formation is a complex decision-making process that requires a precise history and high-quality radiographic imaging.[64, 125, 126] Failure to obtain even temporary pain relief after decompressive lumbar surgery suggests either that there was additional neural compression at the operated level or at another level that was not adequately addressed at the time of surgery, or that there is a nonspinal cause of the pain. A pain-free interval of less than 6 months suggests the onset of scar formation as the cause of recurrent pain. Recurrence of pain after a pain-free interval of longer than 6 to 12 months suggests a new process such as a recurrent disc herniation.[39, 125, 126]

The incidence of recurrent disc herniation has been reported as approximately 3%.[46] Although many surgeons do not consider a remote recurrence a true complication of spine surgery, most surgeons believe that a recurrent herniation within a few months of surgery represents a complication of the surgical procedure. Experimental work in animal models has shown that the risk of instability, and the theoretic risk of recurrence, is greater with both a box annulotomy and a cruciate incision of the annulus fibrosus than it is with merely a slit made through the annulus.[2, 36] The first two surgical options, particularly the former, cause more disruption of the annulus than does a slit, which theoretically separates the fibers of the annulus fibrosus and therefore comes closer to maintaining its integrity.

Durotomy

Incidental violation of the dura (durotomy) most commonly occurs when the edge of a biting instrument, such as a Kerrison rongeur, inadvertently grabs the dura and produces either a punctate hole in the dura or a frank laceration.[125] Usually, the injury is noted immediately by the sudden appearance of cerebrospinal fluid within the wound. Occasionally, however, the tear is not noted until later by the clinical appearance of persistent spinal headache or by the onset of obvious swelling in the back, suggesting a pseudomeningocele.[88] The incidence of the latter complication has been estimated at between 0.07% and 2%.[54]

When the durotomy is noted intraoperatively, the dura should be repaired primarily.[88] It is imperative that there be adequate exposure to visualize the full extent of the laceration. If an operating microscope is not used, the surgeon should employ a headlight and loupe magnification. Closure of the defect is facilitated by placing the patient in a slightly head-down (Trendelenburg) position to minimize the amount of cerebrospinal fluid in the operative field. This provides the dual advantage of providing a drier operative field and minimizing the tendency for the individual roots of the cauda equina to float to the surface, which can result in inadvertent injury to the roots during dural repair. For larger tears, a small cottonoid patty can be placed over the exposed nerve roots for the initial portion of the repair to protect the roots.[32] Just before the final portion of the dural closure, the cottonoid can be removed and the final dural sutures placed. For tears associated with loss of tissue, or for tears in locations that are difficult to repair, a fat graft or a piece of fascia (thoracolumbar fascia, fascia lata, or freeze-dried fascia) may be used to facilitate closure of the defect.[32] A watertight closure is performed with a running 6–0 silk or nylon suture. After meticulous closure, the patient is returned to a neutral or slightly head-up (reverse Trendelenburg) position and a Valsalva maneuver is performed to assess the integrity of the closure. The use of a fibrin glue may also be considered for additional strength and integrity of the repair. The remainder of the surgical wound closure proceeds as usual, except that a drain is generally not employed; the interrupted fascial closure is oversewn with a running stitch and a routine skin closure is performed. Theoretically, if the closure is watertight, the patient may be ambulatory the day after surgery. If there is any doubt about the integrity of the closure, the patient should be restricted to bed rest for 3 to 5 days.[32]

If a dural leak is not noticed intraoperatively and becomes clinically evident postoperatively owing to persistent spinal headache or pseudomeningocele, an attempt should be made to confirm the diagnosis by myelogram or MRI scan, and the patient should generally be returned to the operating room for dural closure.[88] Alternatively, particularly with smaller leaks, a subarachnoid drain can be inserted at the bedside and the patient restricted to bed rest until the leak subsides. This generally involves removal of approximately 300 ml of cerebrospinal fluid per 24 hours in a sterile blood collection bag, which is titrated by adjusting the height of the bag to produce this rate of cerebrospinal fluid flow.[70]

Nerve Root Injury

Peripheral nerve injuries related to improper positioning of the patient during surgery have been discussed previously. Neural injury may also occur owing to direct trauma to the nerve root during surgery. Such injury may result from excessive neural retraction, contusion, laceration, or electrocauterization.[118] The incidence of neurologic complications after lumbar spine surgery has been estimated at 0.2%.[89] Such injury may be suspected postoperatively by the presence of a new or increased objective neurologic deficit or subjective parasthesias of new onset. This condition, sometimes referred to as the battered root, may occur either as an unavoidable consequence of severe neural compression or as a result of indelicate surgery.[12]

Meticulous surgical technique, therefore, is paramount to minimize such complications. Adequate surgical exposure is imperative to minimize excessive neural retraction. In cases of a large central disc herniation or a large midline bulging disc in the presence of concomitant spinal stenosis, for example, a bilateral laminectomy rather than a keyhole laminotomy may be required to remove the disc fragment safely.

It is important to obtain an anteroposterior x-ray film of the lumbar spine to identify anatomic variants that might be of surgical significance. The presence of spina bifida occulta, for example, should be noted because cautious surgical exposure of a level with this defect is imperative to minimize the risk of damage to the underlying dura and nerve roots. Similarly, the presence of a laminectomy defect from prior surgery should be noted to reduce blunt or sharp injury to neural elements during surgical exposure. Other preoperative studies should also be carefully examined to identify other potentially significant anatomic variants, such as an anomalous nerve root, which could be injured during surgical decompression.[115, 116]

During surgical exposure of neural elements during laminotomy or laminectomy, particularly for surgical discectomy, it is always important to visualize the lateral edge of the nerve root to be sure that exposure is not inadvertently being performed in the axilla of the nerve root, where accidental dural laceration and neural injury could occur and where repair of such injuries is particularly difficult. This is especially important during revision lumbar surgery, during which dissection should usually be performed by staying lateral to the root, thereby avoiding a potentially dangerous midline scar. When performing lateral nerve root decompressions, it is essential to work parallel, rather than perpendicular, to the long axis of the nerve root to limit the risk of inadvertently cutting across a root.

Epidural Hematoma

Epidural hematoma causing symptomatic neurologic compression or cauda equina syndrome is one of the most feared complications of spine surgery. Fortunately, the risk of this complication can be minimized by meticulous attention to preoperative, intraoperative, and postoperative detail.

Preoperatively, it is advisable that the patient stop the administration of all nonsteroidal antiinflammatory drugs approximately 1 week before surgery. In addition, it is important that the patient is not hypocoagulable and that the prothrombin time, partial thromboplastin time, and platelet counts are within normal limits.

Intraoperatively, the patient should be positioned with the abdomen hanging free to minimize bleeding from epidural venous congestion. The blood pressure should be kept below 100 mmHg systolic, if possible, to decrease bleeding. Electrocautery should be used to restrict bleeding during the surgical exposure. Raw bone surfaces should be dried with bone wax to decrease the amount of bleeding on bone surfaces. Epidural bleeding should be controlled with bipolar electrocoagulation. At the end of the surgical procedure when the paraspinal muscle retractors are removed, the muscle walls should be checked for bleeders, because prolonged muscle retraction may temporarily occlude potentially significant muscle bleeders, which could begin bleeding after muscle layer closure. In general, the author prefers to use a drain postoperatively to minimize the amount of postoperative hematoma formation.

Postoperatively, the drain should be left in place for 24 to 48 hours, or until the amount of collected blood is less than approximately 30 ml/8 hours. Nonsteroidal antiinflammatory drugs are generally not used in the immediate postoperative period because of the risk of bleeding from the fresh wound.

A characteristic clinical feature of epidural hematoma is the presence of severe pain, which appears to be out of proportion to what is normally expected.[87] This is usually accompanied by, or rapidly followed by, an obvious and sometimes rapidly progressive neurologic deficit. Depending on the extent and location of surgical exposure and the magnitude of the hematoma, the neurologic deficit may be focal and unilateral or widespread, involving multiple muscle groups in both legs.

The key to diagnosis of this condition is having a high index of suspicion. When possible, and when time permits, radiographic confirmation should be attempted by MRI scan, myelogram, or CT scan. After the diagnosis is suspected, treatment should be immediate. This situation mandates an emergent return to the operating room and drainage of the hematoma or other compressing structures.

Compression by Fat Grafts or Absorbable Gelatin Sponge

Postoperative neurologic compression may be due to structures other than blood. The use of free fat grafts as a barrier to scar formation has been associated with symptomatic neurologic compression mimicking epidural hematoma (Fig. 3).[103] This has prompted some surgeons to abandon fat grafts in favor of other substances such as absorbable gelatin sponge. Even these substitutes, however, may cause neural compression if proper care is not exercised (Fig. 4). The use of a thin 3- to 5-mm piece of fat, rather than a large thick piece, is recommended. For multilevel laminectomy requiring the use of a lengthy piece of scar barrier material, the author prefers absorbable gelatin sponge rather than fat, because the latter could theoretically become balled up and exert focal compression on the dura, with resulting cauda equina syndrome.

Vascular Complications

Vascular injuries associated with posterior lumbar spine procedures are nearly always due to surgical discectomy in which the major abdominal vessels are injured by passage of an instrument through the anterior annulus (Fig. 5).[44, 117] Such injuries may be recognized early by brisk bleeding, hypotension, and abdominal distention, or they may manifest late by formation of an arteriovenous fistula.[65] The latter most commonly presents with high-output cardiac failure or abdominal bruits. Early injury from laceration of a major abdominal vessel is associated with a high mortality. The mortality rate from acute arterial injuries has been reported at 78%, whereas the mortality of venous injuries is 89%. Late formation of arteriovenous fistula is more compatible with long-term survival than are acute injuries, with mortality reported between 9% and 11%.[30]

Vascular injury occurs most commonly at L4–L5, followed by L5–S1.[8, 30] This reflects, to some extent, the incidence of symptomatic herniations of the lumbar spine, although regional differences in the vascular anatomy of the lower lumbar spine play a role. The most common vascular injury is arteriovenous fistula formation. This occurs most frequently between the right common iliac artery and vein (29.1%), between the left common iliac artery and vein (25.5%), the right common iliac artery and the inferior vena cava (21.8%), and the right common iliac artery and the left common iliac vein (12.7%).[93]

The true incidence of vascular complications after posterior spine surgery is unknown, but their occurrence is, to some extent, directly proportional to the amount of

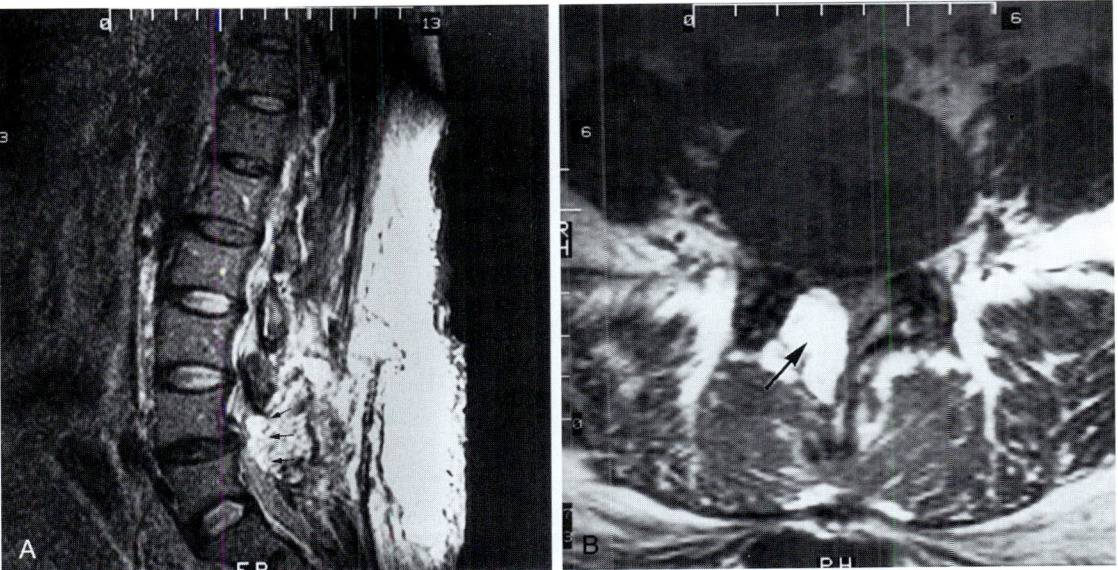

Figure 3. MRI of a patient with cauda equina syndrome from postoperative compression by fat graft. *A*, Right parasagittal T2-weighted image showing darkened L4–L5 disc with high-signal-intensity epidural fat graft *(arrows)*. *B*, Axial MRI showing mass effect of high-signal-intensity right-sided epidural fat graft *(arrow)*.

disc removed surgically, because aggressive attempts at disc removal are more likely to involve perforations of the anterior annulus. The instrument most commonly implicated is the pituitary rongeur.[44] If care is taken to avoid excessive penetration of the rongeur into the disc, this devastating complication can be avoided. Limiting the depth of penetration to less than 2.5 cm provides a safe margin for error. This depth can be ensured by measuring and marking the instrument before surgery. With current emphasis on more limited disc removal techniques, rather than radical discectomy, in which a more aggressive extirpation of the disc is advocated, the incidence of such vascular complications will undoubtedly be less than previously reported.[114]

Postoperative Instability

Instability after surgical decompression can be considered an iatrogenic complication of spine surgery. Such instability can occur in the anteroposterior plane (spondylolisthesis), the mediolateral plane (lateral listhesis or scoliosis), or both planes simultaneously. In general, the risk of postoperative anteroposterior instability can be minimized by maintaining the integrity of a total of at least one facet joint at the level decompressed. In other words, if a unilateral complete facetectomy is performed on one side, the integrity of the entire opposite facet must be maintained. Similarly, if half of one facet is removed during surgical decompression, at least half of the contralateral facet joint should be spared. If a total of more than one facet at a single level is removed during decompression, consideration should be given to prophylactic fusion at that level.

When decompression of a spinal stenotic level associated with degenerative spondylolisthesis is undertaken, concomitant fusion should generally be performed because the surgical outcome has been shown to be better than that with decompression alone.[58] This is thought to result at least partially from minimizing the risk of a subsequent increase in the slip, although a direct relationship between increase in magnitude of subsequent slip and poorer surgical outcome has not been demonstrated.[58]

Isthmic spondylolisthesis with frank fracture of the pars interarticularis may also occur in the absence of prior slip as a result of surgical decompression. In such cases, the patient has evidence of a de novo spondylolisthesis occurring either at one of the levels decompressed or at a level above the level of decompression. The presumed mechanism is either a mechanical stress fracture

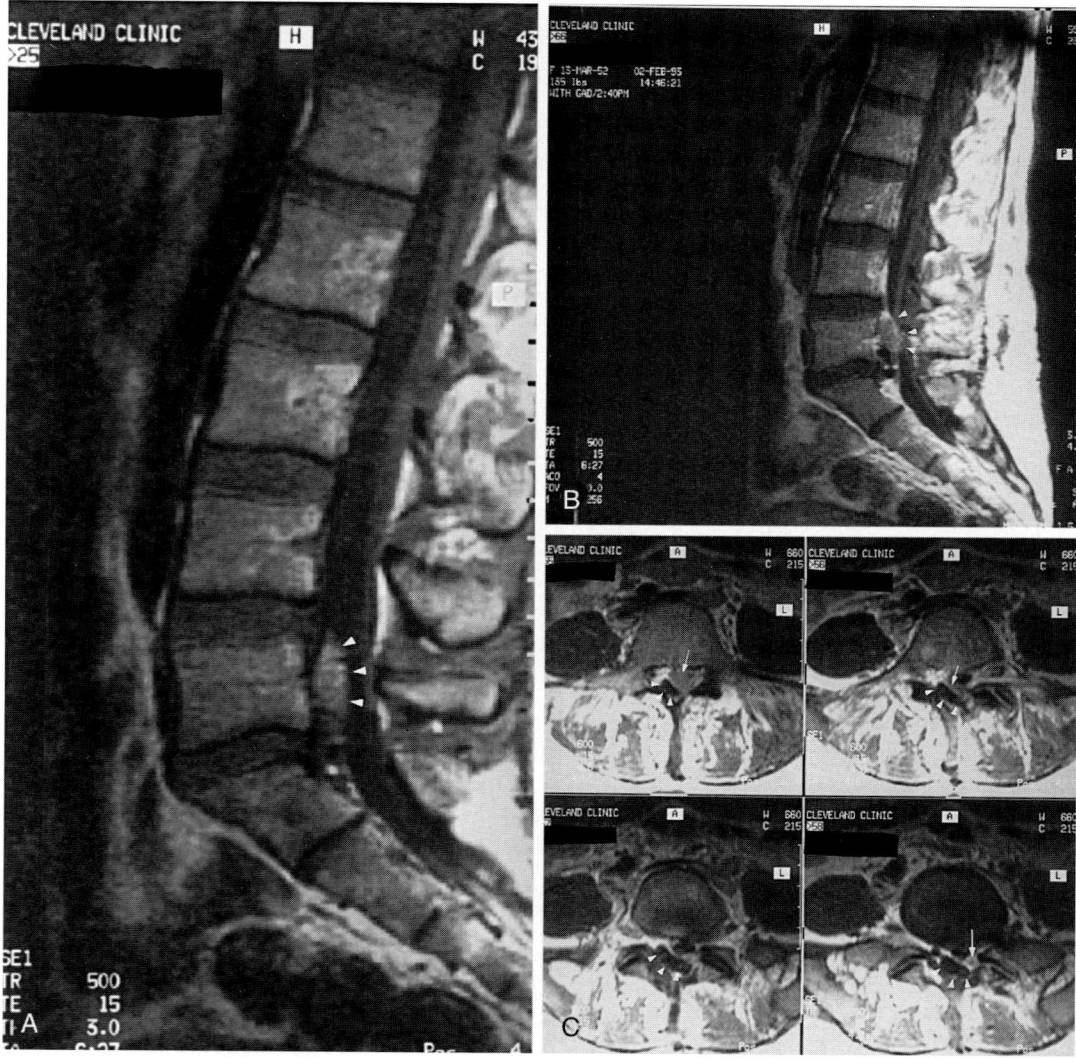

Figure 4. Patient with postoperative left footdrop due to compression of left L5 nerve from absorbable gelatin sponge (Gelfoam) mass. *A,* T1-weighted sagittal MRI showing epidural Gelfoam mass *(arrowheads)* posterior to L5 vertebral body. *B,* Post-gadolinium T1-weighted MRI showing nonenhancing Gelfoam mass *(arrowheads).* *C,* Axial T1-weighted MRI showing Gelfoam mass *(arrows)* exhibiting mass effect with compression and distortion of cauda equina *(arrowheads).*

or impairment of the blood supply to the affected level.

Alternatives to Traditional Discectomy

Microdiscectomy, chemonucleolysis, percutaneous discectomy, and laser discectomy are surgical alternatives to traditional discectomy for relief of radicular leg pain. As such, the indications for these procedures should be viewed in the same critical manner as those for discectomy: primarily leg pain, objective neurologic findings such as neurologic deficit or positive tension sign, and a correlative imaging test finding. In addition, the compressive pathologic change should be due to a contained disc herniation without any significant concomitant bony stenosis. Indications for these procedures should not be be less stringent than those for traditional discectomy merely because these procedures may be perceived as less invasive. Each of these procedures has potential complications and poses a potential

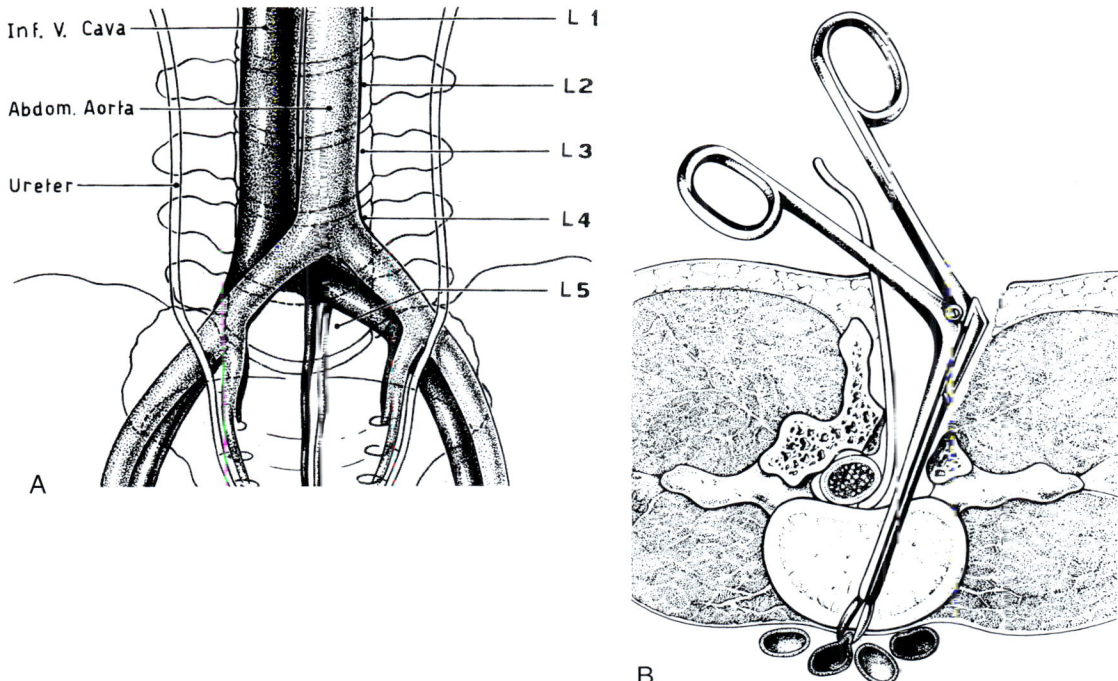

Figure 5. *A*, Relationship of the abdominal vessels and the ureters to the lumbar vertebrae and disc spaces. Note that the aorta bifurcates at approximately the lower border of the L4 vertebral body or the L4–L5 disc. The inferior vena cava is formed by the confluence of the right and left common iliac veins dorsal to the aorta and slightly to the right of the midline. *B*, Potential for injury to the abdominal vessels by penetration of the anterior annulus fibrosus by a pituitary rongeur during surgical discectomy. (From Montorsi, W., and Ghiringhelli, C.: Genesis, diagnosis and treatment of vascular complications after intervertebral disk surgery. Int. Surg. 58:233–235, 1973.)

economic liability to the patient and to society if good results are not achieved.

Microdiscectomy

Microdiscectomy is an alternative to radical or limited discectomy that uses illumination and magnification. It has the theoretic advantage of a smaller skin incision, less exposure of neural elements and less dural scarring, minimum tissue disruption, and more rapid wound healing.[90] It also has the advantage of better visualization for the first surgical assistant and is therefore useful as a teaching tool. First advocated by Williams[127] in 1978, microdiscectomy, as originally described, involved a purely interlaminar approach without bone removal. Subsequent modification of the procedure by Hudgins[63] and Wilson and Harbaugh[129] involved removal of enough bone and ligamentum flavum to visualize the nerve root. Early studies reported an 85% to 98% success rate, with a reoperation rate of 4% to 9.1%.[50, 63, 127, 129]

Complications of microdiscectomy are similar to those of standard discectomy. These include inadequate pain relief, infection, nerve injury, and bleeding. McCulloch[90] reported 24 complications (10.8% complication rate) in 223 patients undergoing microsurgery for disc herniation and lateral zone stenosis. These included minor dural tears (2.7%), exploration of the wrong level recognized during surgery (2.7%), hemorrhage requiring transfusion (1.35%), superficial wound infection (0.9%), disc space infection (0.9%), transient increase in neural deficit (0.9%) and hematoma (0.45%).

Inadequate relief of leg pain may be at least partially due to inadequate visualization, including failure to visualize the lateral edge of the nerve root. It may also be due to failure to address the main compressive pathologic change, which may include a significant lateral recess stenosis or other bony pathologic alteration and which may occur in as many as 30% of patients with symptomatic disc herniation.[114] Surgically adequate microdiscectomy technique must therefore include removal of bone if necessary.

A higher rate of infection after microdiscectomy than after standard discectomy has been reported by Wilson and associates,[128, 129] probably owing to contamination from the microscope. Later work by Dauch,[25] however, reported an infection rate of only 0.4%, comparable with or lower than that for standard discectomy. Major bleeding during microdiscectomy, as during standard discectomy, is possible. Indeed, even in McCulloch's[90] series, three patients required transfusion owing to hemorrhage. However, because even a small amount of blood within the field of the operating microscope makes adequate visualization extremely difficult, hemostasis is more important during microdiscectomy than during standard discectomy and bleeding complications therefore tend to be less common.[90] Neurologic injury during microdiscectomy is uncommon, with a reported incidence of approximately 1% to 2%.[90]

Chemonucleolysis

Chemonucleolysis, an intradiscal therapeutic procedure whereby an enzyme is introduced into the intervertebral disc, has traditionally used two types of enzymatic injection: chymopapain and collagenase.[15] Chymopapain is an extract of the tropical fruit papaya that when injected into the intervertebral disc, acts on the proteoglycan aggregates of the nucleus pulposus to split off the glycosaminoglycan side chains, thereby interfering with the ability of the proteoglycan to imbibe and hold water.[91] This effect is thought to result in reduced pressure of the disc on the adjacent inflamed nerve root and therefore less pain from the root.

Chymopapain has been shown to have an efficacy of approximately 70% to 80% in double-blind studies and is therefore is somewhat less effective than results reported for traditional discectomy.[14, 41, 66] Chymopapain was widely used in Canada and Europe before it was released for general use in the United States in 1982. By 1985, its widespread use in the United States resulted in 37 major neurologic catastrophes and six deaths among the initial 80,000 patients injected.[110] By 1987, postmarketing surveillance of the first 110,000 patients revealed 58 severe neurologic complications.[40] These complications included anaphylaxis, transverse myelitis, subarachnoid hemorrhage, cerebral hemorrhage, Brown-Séquard syndrome, and paraplegia. Most of these complications seemed to be related to technique and therefore were potentially avoidable. The occurrence of transverse myelitis, however, was particularly disturbing, because these patients typically exhibited a benign postoperative course for the initial 3 to 5 weeks. Severe back and leg pain then developed, followed by paraplegia and bowel and bladder dysfunction. It was thought that this might be due to a delayed antigen-antibody reaction from intrathecal injection of the enzyme. Although subsequent surveillance information reported only a 0.02% mortality rate,[110] much of the enthusiasm for this procedure has waned to the extent that it is no longer commonly used in the United States.

Chymopapain is neurotoxic when injected into the subarachnoid space because it causes microvascular damage to the basement membrane of the pia-arachnoid vessels, with resulting subarachnoid hemorrhage and paraplegia.[15] This complication has a reported incidence of 0.0003% and is technique related.[1] It is therefore imperative that intrathecal injection of the enzyme be avoided. A saline acceptance test or injection of contrast material into the disc before chymopapain injection can help to ensure proper needle placement, although some data suggest that the latter should be avoided because the combination of chymopapain and dye may predispose to subarachnoid hemorrhage and serious neurologic complications.[111]

Anaphylaxis, which may occur after chymopapain injection, is thought to result from an antigen-antibody reaction to chymopapain or one of its degradation products. Its overall incidence is approximately 0.5%, but it is less common in patients who are prescreened with a chymopapain skin test.[1, 91] In addition, the use of local rather than general anesthesia permits earlier recognition and treatment of this complication and thereby ameliorates its potential danger to the patient.[91]

In addition to the serious neurologic complications described, other sequelae include low back pain, inadequate relief of leg pain, and discitis. Initial studies reported approximately a 2.7% incidence of discitis. This was subsequently reduced to approximately 0.7% by the use of a two-needle technique in which the initial 18-gauge needle is advanced to the posterolateral corner of the annulus and a smaller 22-gauge needle is then inserted into the larger needle and passed into the center of the disc.[42] Postinjection low back pain has been reported to occur in as many as 50% of patients, with severe back spasm occurring in approximately 30%.[111] Inadequate relief of leg pain is commonly due to the presence of a noncontained disc fragment or to the presence of concomitant bony stenosis such as lateral recess stenosis. It is therefore imperative that concise preoperative imaging studies be performed and examined closely to identify these potential contraindications to chymopapain injection.

Percutaneous Discectomy

Percutaneous discectomy is an alternative to traditional discectomy or microdiscectomy and has a success rate of approximately 70% to 80%.[99] Initially described by Hijikata[59] in 1975, the technique has since been modified by numerous investigators.[45, 68, 108] It involves the percutaneous introduction of a cannula into the lateral annulus and removal of disc fragments. Subsequent modifications have included an automated technique whereby a reciprocating suction cutting device automatically removes disc material.[99] Later modifications have also included the use of the laser to vaporize nuclear material. Like chemonucleolysis, percutaneous discectomy is indicated primarily for relief of radicular leg pain due to a contained disc herniation. Leg pain from other causes, such as noncontained disc herniation or bony stenosis, is generally not relieved by this procedure.

The most common complication of percutaneous procedures is a small risk of discitis, estimated at approximately 0.2%.[84] Less common complications include cauda equina syndrome and nerve root injury, retroperitoneal bleeding, and bowel injury due to a retrorenal colon.[11, 43, 57]

ANTERIOR SURGERY COMPLICATIONS

Complications related to anterior lumbar spine surgery are considered in the categories of vascular, neurologic, genitourinary, and abdominal complications. Specific complications related to particular procedures are not dealt with here but instead in the chapters dealing with them.

Vascular Complications

The two major vessels encountered in anterior approaches to the lumbar spine are the abdominal aorta and the inferior vena cava and their branches[93] (see Fig. 5A). The abdominal aorta bifurcates at the lower border of the L4 vertebral body or the L4–L5 disc to become the right and left common iliac arteries. Similarly, the vena cava is formed by the confluence of the right and left common iliac veins, which lie dorsal to their arterial counterparts and slightly to the right of midline at the level of the L5 vertebral body.

The right common iliac artery crosses the bifurcation of the vena cava and the left common iliac artery. The common iliac arteries bifurcate to become the internal and external iliac arteries, usually at the upper border of the sacrum. Similarly, the common iliac veins are formed by the confluence of the external and internal iliac veins. The internal iliac artery and vein pass lateral to the sacral promontory to enter the pelvis, whereas the external iliac artery and vein pass ventrally over the sacroiliac joint.

The iliolumbar artery and vein are generally recurrent branches of the internal iliac artery and vein, respectively, and pass cephalad at the level of the sacral ala. The middle sacral artery, generally formed at the bifurcation of the aorta, lies along the anterior sacrum. The middle sacral vein, joining the left common iliac vein, lies slightly to the right of the middle sacral artery.

Anterior approaches to the lumbar spine may be accomplished either retroperitoneally or transperitoneally. The retroperitoneal approach to the lumbar spine is a modified sympathectomy approach originally described by Fey.[94] Although vascular injuries are potentially devastating, they are relatively uncommon.[30, 43, 44, 61] Any vascular structure is potentially at risk during anterior surgical approaches, but the iliolumbar vein, a branch of the vena cava or the left iliac vein, is most frequently jeopardized by anterior retroperitoneal approaches to the lumbar spine.[123] Because retraction of this vessel may result in its avulsion from the vena cava, the surgical approach is generally made from the left side, as it is easier and safer to retract the aorta than the vena cava. The use of some anterior spine fixation devices, notably the Dunn device, has been associated with delayed aortic erosion and retroperitoneal hemorrhage,[16] prompting some concern that a right-sided approach might be safer when implantable devices are being considered.

The middle sacral vessels can be injured during anterior approaches to the lower lumbar spine. They are often deliberately sacrificed during the approach to the L5–S1 disc and are therefore of no particular significance. When these vessels are sacrificed, care should be taken to avoid electrocautery because of the risk of damage to the superior hypogastric plexus.

The left iliac artery is at risk with anterior exposures at L4–L5 owing to retraction of this vessel. This can result in either temporary spasm or frank occlusion of the artery. Other vessels may be at risk when associated conditions such as prior anterior surgery, spinal or retroperitoneal infection, aneurysm, or tumor produce scarring. Careful preoperative history and physical examination should alert the physician to these possibilities so that additional care can be exercised at surgery.

Transperitoneal approach to the anterior lumbar spine affords access to the lumbosacral junction but necessitates exposure of, and working at or below, the bifurcation of the abdominal aorta and vena cava.[75, 103] The left common iliac vein and iliolumbar vein are in jeopardy with this exposure, and the middle sacral vessels must be ligated to expose the L5–S1 disc. A risk of surgery with this approach to L5–S1, or with a retroperitoneal approach to this level, is damage to the preaortic sympathetic plexus that lies along the anterior surface of the aorta at the level of its bifurcation.[123]

Neurologic Complications

Most of the neurologic complications of the anterior approaches to the lumbar spine are related to injury to the sympathetic plexus, with potential implications regarding sexual function.[67] Although penile erection is primarily a parasympathetic function, ejaculation is predominantly sympathetically innervated. The parasympathetic nerve supply is via the pelvic splanchnic nerves (S2, S3, and S4)—the nervi erigentes.[67] The parasympathetic nerve supply innervates the prostate, the corpora cavernosa, and the bladder detrusor muscle. The sympathetic nerve supply to the urogenital system is from the thoracolumbar spinal cord (T11 to L2) and it innervates the seminal vesicles, the vas deferens, the urethra, and penile blood vessels. Anterior L5–S1 approaches jeopardize the superior hypogastric plexus, which contains the sympathetic innervation to the urogenital system.[123] In particular, electrocautery should be avoided, because it can result in damage to the superior hypogastric plexus. When hemostasis is required, vascular clips should be used.

Damage to the superior hypogastric plexus can result in impairment of bladder neck closure and retrograde ejaculation with subsequent sterility, although it has no effect on erection, which is a parasympathetically controlled function. Indeed, injury to the parasympathetic nervous system should not occur if the surgical approach is confined above the pelvic brim. Therefore, impairment of erection should never occur in approaches to the mid and upper lumbar spine and should not occur in approaches to the L5–S1 junction if proper care is exercised and the approach is limited. Stauffer and Coventry[119] reported on the Mayo Clinic experience with anterior lumbar interbody fusion and described only one case of impotence in 83 cases. Similarly, Sacks[107] noted no instances of impotence and only two cases of sterility in 200 patients undergoing anterior lumbar interbody fusion.

The lumbar sympathetic chain (T12 to L4) may be injured in anterior approaches to the lumbar spine.[123] This can result in a sympathetic effect with vasodilatation and a feeling of increased warmth in the ipsilateral foot and therefore a feeling of coolness in the opposite foot. This complication is rarely of any significance, although the patient should be warned of its possibility in advance.

Damage to lumbar neural innervation to the lower extremities may occur from two potential sources. The cauda equina itself could be damaged directly by penetration through the disc space during attempted anterior interbody fusion. The risk of this complication can be eliminated, or at least minimized, by careful technique in performing disc curettage and in sizing and introducing the graft. Damage to the lumbosacral plexus may occur by vigorous retraction or penetration of the psoas muscles. Care should be taken to avoid unnecessary retraction of the psoas and to minimize the risk of hematoma formation by sweeping the muscle off the disc by proceeding from the midline laterally.[123] Care should also be exercised when dealing with the psoas muscle to avoid damage to the genitofemoral nerve that lies on its surface.

Damage to Intraperitoneal and Retroperitoneal Structures

Retroperitoneal approaches to the anterior lumbar spine may result in inadvertent perforation of the peritoneum. If this is repaired promptly and carefully, it is usually of no significance, although it may result in the development of later adhesions. After the peritoneum is entered, either inadvertently during retroperitoneal exposure or during a transperitoneal approach, damage to intraperitoneal structures may occur, including injury to the large bowel. Injury to the ureter may also occur during anterior exposures to the lumbar spine, particularly with retroperitoneal approaches.[97] With transperitoneal exposures, the ureter is usually laterally located and therefore not routinely visualized.[123] With the retroperitoneal approach, the ureter is reflected anteriorly with the peritoneal sac but can be damaged, particularly when dense adhesions are present from prior surgery or infection.

BONE GRAFTING COMPLICATIONS

In lumbar spine surgery requiring autologous bone, pain from the donor site is often more debilitating, and sometimes has a higher morbidity, than that associated with the primary spine procedure itself. These findings have been summarized by Kurz and associates[73, 74] in an extensive review of the complications of iliac bone grafting. Some of these complications occur with either anterior or posterior grafting procedures, whereas other complications are more common with only one of these approaches.

Although the incidence of pain from posterior grafting procedures is reportedly similar to that from anterior iliac grafting, morbidity from the former seems to be greater. Up to 15% of patients may have significant pain lasting longer than 3 months.[26, 29] Attempts to ameliorate the pain from posterior iliac grafting include meticulous hemostasis and suction drainage to minimize hematoma formation, careful closure of the gluteal musculature after periosteal stripping, and blocking of periosteal pain with alcohol.[79]

Infection of a bone graft site can occur as in any other surgical procedure. When it occurs in conjunction with instrumented posterior spine fusion, however, spread of infection to the primary surgical site can occur. This is more common when the primary site and bone graft site share a common longitudinal skin incision, which promotes easy access between the two sites. The use of a separate iliac graft skin incision minimizes this risk. The chance of infection can also be reduced by minimizing hematoma formation through proper hemostasis, including the use of bone wax, absorbable gelatin sponge, and suction drainage.

Stress fracture through the ilium after bone grafting has been reported[52] (Fig. 6). This is more common in patients with pre-existing metabolic bone disease, such as rheumatoid arthritis, that renders the bone osteoporotic. Fracture after anterior iliac grafting results from pull of the rectus femoris and sartorius muscles on the anterior superior iliac spine with its ultimate avulsion. Treatment is usually symptomatic, although primary repair of a large avulsion with screw fixation can be attempted. Fracture through the posterior ilium can also occur if a generous bicortical graft is taken that results in only a small bridge of remaining bone between the osteotomy site and the sciatic notch. This can result in shifting of the entire hemipelvis by its attachment with the other side of the pelvis through the symphysis pubis (Fig. 7). A similar phenomenon may occur after posterior sacroiliac ligament injury, when pelvic instability may occur with subluxation of the ipsilateral hemipelvis.

The most common arterial injury during

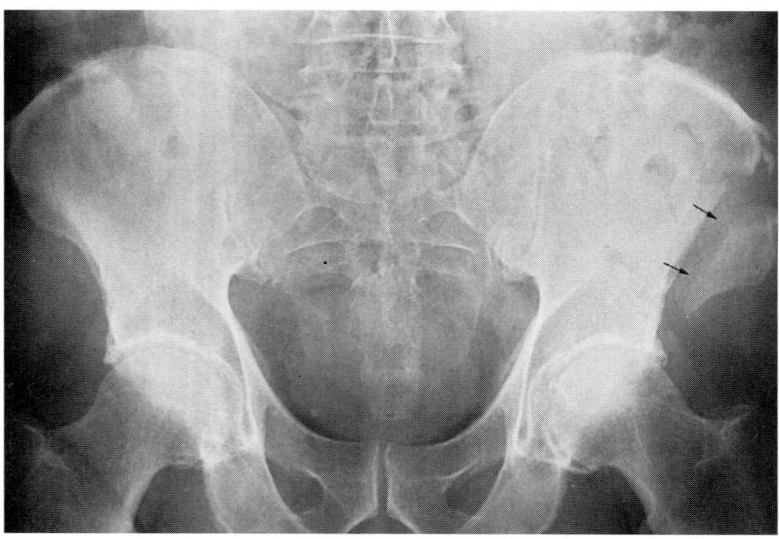

Figure 6. Avulsion of anterior left ilium *(arrows)* after harvesting of tricortical iliac graft.

posterior iliac grafting is to the superior gluteal artery as it exits the pelvis through the sciatic notch. This may occur from its penetration by the tip of a Taylor retractor or from its injury by a chisel, an osteotome, or a saw. After division of the superior gluteal artery, it may retract into the pelvis, making control of bleeding difficult. When this happens, the bleeding may sometimes be controlled by hooking a finger around the sciatic notch to compress the artery. Grasping the artery with a long hemostat may also be successful, although direct exposure of the artery by either a retroperitoneal approach or removal of bone from the sciatic notch may be necessary.[73, 74] Attempts at blind grabbing of the artery may result in inadvertent injury to the sciatic nerve, which courses with the superior gluteal artery through the sciatic notch.

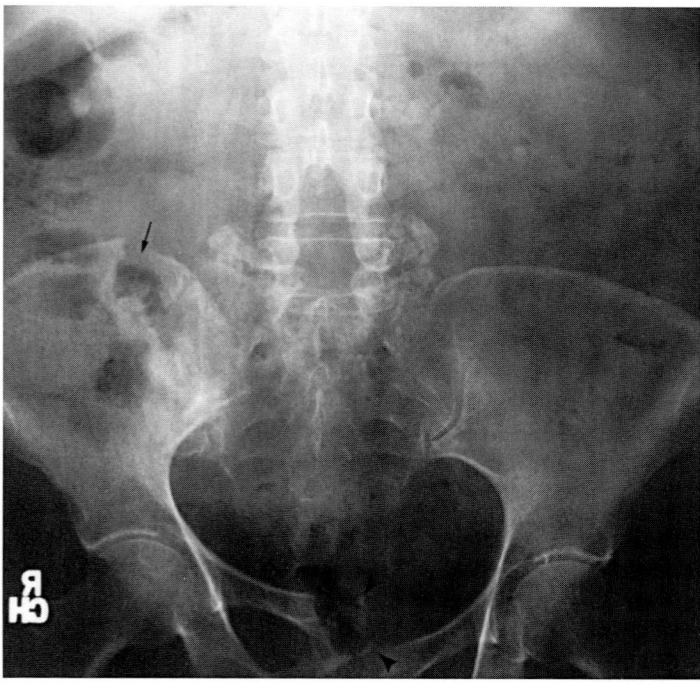

Figure 7. Fracture through right posterior iliac wing *(arrow)* and disruption of symphysis pubis *(arrowheads)* with resulting superior migration of the entire right hemipelvis *(arrowheads)* after harvesting of posterior iliac bone graft in rheumatoid patient.

Exposure of the inner table of the ilium may result in injury to the anastomotic network of vessels from the deep circumflex iliac artery, the iliolumbar artery, and the fourth lumbar artery, vessels that traverse the iliacus muscle to supply the iliacus, psoas, and quadratus lumborum muscles.[73, 74]

Nerve injury to three nerves may potentially occur during posterior iliac bone grafting procedures: the superior cluneal nerves, the sciatic nerve, and the superior gluteal nerve.[73, 74] The superior cluneal nerves are cutaneous branches from L1, L2, and L3, which cross the posterior iliac crest approximately 8 cm lateral to the posterior superior iliac spine. Injury to these nerves may result in an area of numbness over the buttocks and occasionally in a painful neuroma. The sciatic nerve exits the pelvis with the superior gluteal nerve through the sciatic notch. Injury to the sciatic nerve may mimic an individual lumbosacral root injury if the formation of the nerve from its individual branches occurs distal to the site of injury at the sciatic notch. The superior gluteal nerve passes through the sciatic notch with the superior gluteal artery and can therefore be injured by the same mechanism as injury to the artery. Because of its innervation of the gluteus medius and minimus, injury to the nerve results in weakness of hip abduction.

Anterior iliac bone grafting is more commonly performed in conjunction with cervical procedures, but this is also done for reconstruction after anterior lumbar vertebral corpectomy. Injury to four nerves may occur with anterior iliac bone techniques: the lateral femoral cutaneous nerve, the ilioinguinal nerve, the iliohypogastric nerve, and the femoral nerve.[73, 74]

Meralgia paresthetica is a complication of anterior iliac grafting due to injury to the lateral femoral cutaneous nerve.[86, 124] It results in paresthesias or pain along the lateral aspect of the thigh. The lateral femoral cutaneous nerve generally passes beneath the sartorius muscle and the inguinal ligament, both of which attach to the anterior superior iliac spine. The nerve therefore usually passes medial to the anterior superior iliac spine; it can be protected during surgery by an approach that stays lateral to it.[48] However, this nerve may be located up to 2 cm lateral to the anterior superior iliac spine in up to 10% of cases and thus may be at risk for injury during anterior bone harvesting.[48]

The ilioinguinal and iliohypogastric nerves enter the inguinal canal and may be injured by traction on the nerves during harvesting of bone from the inner wall of the ilium.[112] The former supplies sensation to an area of skin beneath the medial half of the inguinal ligament along the proximal and medial thigh, to portions of the scrotum, and to the penis. The latter provides sensation to the anterior two thirds of the iliac crest. Injury to these two nerves may result in either pain or paresthesias in the involved areas.

Injury to the femoral nerve is uncommon, but it is theoretically vulnerable to injury during bone harvesting from the inner table of the ilium.[74]

Other injuries from bone grafting that are less common include injury to the ureter owing to its proximity to the sciatic notch and to the superior gluteal vessels.[35] Injury to these vessels may also result in damage to the ureter directly, or it may be injured indirectly during blind attempts to control bleeding from the superior gluteal artery. Herniation of abdominal contents through a full-thickness defect in the wall of the ilium has also been reported and results from failure of the iliacus muscle to restrain these structures after its detachment from the inner wall of the ilium.[12, 19, 23, 98]

REFERENCES

1. Agre, K., Wilson, R., Brim, M., et al.: Chymodiactin post-marketing surveillance. Spine 9:479–485, 1984.
2. Ahlgren, B., Lydon, C., Brower, E., et al.: Strength of healing lumbar discs after surgical incisions. Presented at the International Society for the Study of the Lumbar Spine Meeting, Marseilles, France, June 1993.
3. Albanese, S., Buterbaugh, G., Palmer, A. K., et al.: Incomplete anterior interosseous nerve palsy following spinal surgery. A report of two cases. Spine 11:1037–1038, 1986.
4. Baker, A. S., Ojemann, R. G., Swartz, M. N., et al.: Spinal epidural abscess. N. Engl. J. Med. 293:463–468, 1975.
5. Bartter, F. C., and Schwartz, W. E.: The syndrome of inappropriate secretion of antidiuretic hormone. Am. J. Med. 42:790–806, 1967.
6. Bell, G. R., Gurd, A. R., Orlowski, J. P., et al.: The syndrome of inappropriate antidiuretic hormone secretion following spinal fusion. J. Bone Joint Surg. 68A:720–724, 1986.
7. Bell, G. R., Boumphrey, F. R., Piedmont, M. A., et al.: The incidence and prophylaxis of deep ve-

nous thrombosis (DVT) following spinal surgery. Spine (in press).
8. Berkeland, I. W., and Taylor, T. K. F.: Major vascular injuries in lumbar disc surgery. J. Bone Joint Surg. 51B:41–19, 1969.
9. Bertrans, G.: The battered root problem. Orthop. Clin. North Am. 6:305–310, 1975.
10. Bircher, M. D., Tasker, T., Crawshaw, C., et al.: Discitis following lumbar surgery. Spine 13:98–102, 1988.
11. Blankstein, A., Rubinstein, E., Ezra, E., et al.: Disc space infection and vertebral osteomyelitis as a complication of percutaneous lateral discectomy. Clin. Orthop. 242:311–312, 1989.
12. Bosworth, D.: Repair of herniae through iliac crest defects. J. Bone Joint Surg. 37A:1069–1073, 1955.
13. Britt, B. A., and Gordon, R. A.: Peripheral nerve injuries associated with anesthesia. Can. Anaesth. Soc. J. 11:514–537, 1964.
14. Brown, M. D., and Daroff, R. B.: The double blind study comparing disease to placebo: An editorial comment. Spine 2:233, 1977.
15. Brown, M. D.: Intradiscal therapy: Chymopapain or collagenase, Chicago, Year Book Medical Publishers, 1983, pp. 77–93.
16. Brown, L. P., Bridwell, K. H., Holt, R. H., and Jennings, J.: Aortic erosions and lacerations associated with the Dunn anterior spinal instrumentation. Abstract presented at the 20th Annual Scoliosis Research Society, San Diego, 1985.
17. Burton, C.: Lumbar arachnoiditis. Spine 3:24–30, 1978.
18. Cameron, M. G. P., and Stewart, O. J.: Ulnar nerve injury associated with anaesthesia. Can. J. Anaesth. 22:253–264, 1975.
19. Challis, J. H., Lyttle, J. A., and Stuart, A. E.: Strangulated lumbar hernia and volvulus following removal of iliac crest bone graft. Acta Orthop. Scand. 46:230–233, 1975.
20. Collis, J. S., and Gardner, W. J.: Lumbar discography—an analysis of one thousand cases. J. Neurosurg. 19:452–461, 1962.
21. Cooper, D. E., Jenkins, R. S., Bready, L., et al.: The prevention of injuries of the brachial plexus secondary to malposition of the patient during surgery. Clin. Orthop. 228:31–41, 1988.
22. Coventry, M. B., and Stauffer, R. N.: The multiply operative back. In American Academy of Orthopaedic Surgeons: Symposium on the Spine. St. Louis, C. V. Mosby, 1969, pp. 132–142.
23. Cowley, S. P. and Anderson, L. D.: Hernias through donor sites for iliac bone grafts. J. Bone Joint Surg. 65A:1023–1026, 1983.
24. Craig, F. S.: Vertebral-body biopsy. J. Bone Joint Surg. 38A:93–102, 1956.
25. Dauch, W. A.: Infection of the intervertebral space following conventional and microsurgical operation on the herniated lumbar intervertebral disc. Acta Neurochir. (Wien) 82:43, 1986.
26. Dawson, E. G., Lotysch, M., III, and Urist, M. R.: Intertransverse process lumbar arthrodesis with autogenous bone graft. Clin. Orthop. 154:90–96, 1981.
27. DePalma, A. F., and Rothman, R. H.: Surgery of the lumbar spine. Clin. Orthop. 63:162–170, 1969.
28. DePalma, A. F., and Rothman, R. H.: The Intervertebral Disc. Philadelphia, W. B. Saunders, 1970.
29. DePalma, A., Rothman, R., Lewinnek G., and Canale, S.: Anterior interbody fusion for severe cervical disc degeneration. Surg. Gynecol. Obstet. 134:755–758, 1972.
30. DeSaussure, R. L.: Vascular injury coincidence to disc surgery. J. Neurosurg. 16:222–229, 1959.
31. Dornette, W. H. L.: Compression neuropathies: Medical aspects and legal implications. Int. Anesth. Clin. 24:201–229, 1986.
32. Eismont, F. J., Wiesel, S. W., and Rothman, R. H.: Treatment of dural tears associated with spinal surgery. J. Bone Joint Surg. 63A:1132–1136, 1981.
33. Eismont, F. J., Bohlman, H. H., Soni P. L., et al.: Pyogenic and fungal vertebral osteomyelitis with paralysis. J. Bone Joint Surg. 65A:19–29, 1983.
34. Eismont, F. J., and Kitchel, S. H.: Pyogenic infections of the spine. In Evarts, C. M. (ed.): Surgery of the Musculoskeletal System, 2nd Ed. New York, Churchill Livingstone, 1990, pp. 2277–2297.
35. Escalas, F., and De Wald R. L.: Combined traumatic arteriovenous fistula and ureteral injury: A complication of iliac bone-grafting. J. Bone Joint Surg. 59A:270–271, 1977.
36. Ethier, D. B., Cain, J. E., Yaszemski, M. J., et al.: The influence of annulotomy selection in disc competence: A biomechanical, radiographic, and histologic analysis. Presented at the International Society for the Study of the Lumbar Spine Meeting, Marseilles, France, June 1993.
37. Ferree, B., Stern, P., Jolson, R., et al.: Deep venous thrombosis after spinal surgery. Spine 18:315–319, 1993.
38. Ferree, B. A., and Wright, A. M.: Deep venous thrombosis following posterior lumbar spinal surgery. Spine 18:1079–1082, 1993.
39. Finnegan, W. J., Tenlin, J. M., Marvel, J. P., et al.: Results of surgical intervention in the multiply operated back patient. J. Bone Joint Surg. 61A:1077–1082, 1979.
40. Flint Laboratories, Spinal Therapies Group: Chemonucleolysis Update. Northbrook, IL, Flint Laboratories, January 1987.
41. Fraser, R. D.: Chymopapain for the treatment of intervertebral disc herniation: Preliminary report of a double blind study. Spine 7:275–279, 1982.
42. Fraser, R. D., Osti, O. L., and Vernon-Roberts, B.: Discitis following chemonucleolysis. Spine 11:679–687, 1986.
43. Freebody, D., Bendal, R., and Taylor, R.: Anterior transperitoneal lumbar fusion. J. Bone Joint Surg. 53B:617–627, 1971.
44. Freeman, D. G.: Major vascular complications of lumbar disc surgery. West. J. Surg. Gynecol. Obstet. 69:175–177, 1961.
45. Friedman, W. A.: Percutaneous discectomy: An alternative to chemonucleolysis? Neurosurgery 13:542–547, 1983.
46. Garfin, S. R., Glover, M., Booth, R. E., et al.: Laminectomy: A review of the Pennsylvania hospital experience. J. Spinal Disord. 1:116–133, 1988.
47. Gepstein, R., and Eismont, F. J.: Postoperative spine infections. In Garfin, S. R. (ed.): Complications of Spine Surgery. Baltimore, Williams & Wilkins, 1989, pp. 302–322.
48. Ghent, W. R.: Further studies on meralgia paresthetica. Can. Med. Assoc. J. 85:871–875, 1961.
49. Gill, K.: Retroperitoneal bleeding after automated percutaneous discectomy. Spine 15:1376–1377, 1990.

50. Goald, J. H.: Microlumbar discectomy: Follow-up of 477 patients. J. Microsurg. 2:95–100, 1980.
51. Goldhaber, S. Z.: Prevention of venous thromboembolism. In Goldhaber, S. Z . (ed.): Pulmonary Embolism and Deep Venous Thrombosis. Philadelphia, W. B. Saunders, 1985, pp. 135–157.
52. Guha, S. C., and Poole, M. D.: Stress fracture of the iliac bone with subfascial femoral neuropathy: Unusual complications at a bone graft donor site: Case report. Br. J. Plast. Surg. 36:305–306, 1983.
53. Gwinnutt, C. L.: Injury to the axillary nerve. Anaesthesia 43:205–206, 1988.
54. Hadani, F. G., Knoler, N., Tadmor, R., et al.: Entrapped lumbar nerve root in pseudomeningocele after laminectomy: Report of three cases. Neurosurgery 19:405–407, 1986.
55. Hakelius, A.: Progress in sciatica: A clinical follow-up of surgical and non-surgical treatment. Acta Orthop. Scand. (Suppl.) 129:6–76, 1970.
56. Hancock, D. O.: A study of 49 patients with acute spinal extradural abscesses. Paraplegia 10:285–288, 1973.
57. Helms, C. A., Munk, P. L., Witt, W. S., et al.: Retrorenal colon: Implications for percutaneous diskectomy. Radiology 171:864–865, 1989.
58. Herkowitz, H. N., and Jurz, L. T.: Degenerative lumbar spondylolisthesis with spinal stenosis. A prospective study comparing decompression with decompression and intertransverse process arthrodesis. J. Bone Joint Surg. 73A:802–808, 1991.
59. Hijikata, S., Yamagishi, M., Nakayama, T., et al.: Percutaneous discectomy: A new treatment method for lumbar disc herniation. J. Toden. Hosp. 5:5, 1975.
60. Hirsch, C., and Nachemson, A.: The reliability of lumbar disk surgery. Clin. Orthop. 29:189–195, 1963.
61. Holf, R. P.: Arterial injuries occurring during orthopaedic operations. Clin. Orthop. 28:21–37, 1963.
62. Holt, E. P.: The question of lumbar discography. J. Bone Joint Surg. 50A:720–725, 1968.
63. Hudgins, W. R.: The role of microdiscectomy. Orthop. Clin. North Am. 14:589–603, 1983.
64. Hueftle, M. G., Modic, M. T., Ross, J. S., et al.: Lumbar spine: Postoperative MR imaging with Gd-DTPA. Radiology 167:817–824, 1988.
65. Jarster, B. S., and Rich, N. M.: The challenge of the arteriovenous fistula formation following disc surgery: A collective review. J. Trauma 16:726–733, 1976.
66. Javid, M. J.: Treatment of herniated lumbar disc syndrome with chymopapain. JAMA 243:2043–2048, 1980.
67. Johnson, R. M., and McGuire, E. J.: Urogenital complications of anterior approaches to the lumbar spine. Clin. Orthop. 154:114–118, 1981.
68. Kambin, P., and Schaffer, J. L.: Percutaneous lumbar discectomy: Review of 100 patients and current practice. Clin. Orthop. 238:24, 1989.
69. Keller, R. B., and Pappas, A. M.: Infections after spinal fusion using internal fixation instrumentation. Orthop. Clin. North Am. 3:99–111, 1972.
70. Kitchel, S. H., Eismont, F. J., and Green, B. A.: Closed subarachnoid drainage for management of cerebrospinal fluid leakage after an operation on the spine. J. Bone Joint Surg. 71A:984–987, 1989.
71. Konno, S., Olmarker, K., Byrod G., et al.: Intermittent cauda equina compression. Presented at the International Society for the Study of the Lumbar Spine Meeting, Seattle, June 1994.
72. Kuivila, T., Steffe, A., Bell, G. R., et al.: Controlling the formation of the laminectomy membrane. Clin. Orthop. 236:166–170, 1988.
73. Kurz, L. T., Garfin, S. R. and Booth, R. E.: Harvesting autogenous iliac bone grafts: A review of complications and techniques. Spine 14:1324–1332, 1989.
74. Kurz, L. T., and Herkowitz, H. N.: Complications of bone graft harvest. Semin. Spine Surg. 5:145–152, 1993.
75. Lane, J. D., and Moore, E. S.: Transperitoneal approach to the intervertebral disc in the lumbar area. Ann. Surg. 127:537–551, 1948.
76. Langenskjold, A., and Kiviluoto, O: Prevention of epidural scar formation after operating on the lumbar spine by means of free fat transplants. Clin. Orthop. 115:92–95, 1976.
77. LaRocca, H., and Macnab, I.: The laminectomy membrane. J. Bone Joint Surg. 56B:545–550, 1974.
78. Lestini, W. F., and Bell, G. R.: Spinal infections: Patient evaluation. Semin. Spine Surg. 2:244–256, 1990.
79. Levy, J. W.: Personal communication.
80. Lindblom, K.: Diagnostic puncture of intervertebral disks in sciatica. Acta Orthop. Scand. 17:231–239, 1948.
81. Lindholm, T. S., and Pylkkanen, P.: Discitis following removal of intervertebral disc. Spine 7:618–622, 1982.
82. Lonstein, J., Winter, R., Moe, J., et al.: Wound infection with Harrington instrumentation and spine fusion for scoliosis. Clin Orthop. 96:222–223, 1973.
83. Macnab, I.: Backache. Baltimore Williams & Wilkins, 1977.
84. Maroon, J. C., and Onik, G.: Percutaneous automated discectomy. In Rothman, R. H., and Simeone, F. A. (Eds.): The Spine, 3rd. Ed. Philadelphia, W. B. Saunders, 1992.
85. Massey, E. W., and Plee, A. E.: Compression injury of the sciatic nerve during a prolonged surgical procedure on a diabetic patient. J. Am Geriatr. Soc. 28:188–189, 1980.
86. Massey, E. W.: Meralgia paresthetica secondary to trauma of bone graft. J. Trauma 20:342–343, 1980.
87. Marshall, L. F.: Complications of surgery for degenerative cervical and lumbar disc disease. In Garfin, S. R. (ed.): Complications of Spine Surgery. Baltimore, Williams & Wilkins, 1989.
88. Marshall, L. F.: Cerebrospinal fluid leaks: Etiology and repair. In Rothman, R. H., and Simeone, F. A. (eds.) The Spine, 3rd Ed. Philadelphia, W. B. Saunders, 1992.
89. Mayfield, F.: Complications of laminectomy. Clin. Neurosurg. 23:435–439, 1975.
90. McCulloch, J. A.: Microdiscectomy. In Rothman, R. H., and Simeone, F. A. (eds.): The Spine, 3rd Ed. Philadelphia, W. B. Saunders 1992.
91. McCulloch, J. A.: Alternative forms of disc excision: Chemonucleolysis. In Rothman, R. H., and Simeone, F. A. (eds.): The Spine, 3rd Ed. Philadelphia, W. B. Saunders, 1992.
92. Modic, M. T., Feiglin, D. H., Piraino, D. W., et al.: Vertebral osteomyelitis: Assessment using MR. Radiology 157:157–166, 1985.

93. Montorsi, W., and Ghiringhelli, C.: Genesis, diagnosis and treatment of vascular complications after intervertebral disc surgery. Int. Surg. 58:233–235, 1973.
94. Mouat, T. B.: The operative approach to the kidney of Bernard Fey. Br. J. Urol. 2:126–132, 1939.
95. Nachemson, A.: Lumbar discography—where are we today? Spine 14:555–556, 1989.
96. Nambisan, R. N., and Karakousis, C. P.: Axillary compression syndrome with neurapraxia due to operative positioning. Surgery 105:449–454, 1989.
97. Noyes, D. T., and Morrisseau, P. M.: Ureteral transection secondary to lumbar disc surgery. Urology. 19:651–652, 1982.
98. Oldfield, M. C.: Iliac hernia after bone grafting. Lancet 248:810–812, 1945.
99. Onik, G., Mooney, V., Maroon, J. C., et al.: Automated percutaneous discectomy: A prospective multi-institutional study. Neurosurgery 2:228–233, 1990.
100. Oster, G., Tuden, R. L., and Colditz, G. A.: A cost-effectiveness analysis of prophylaxis against deep-vein thrombosis in major orthopedic surgery. JAMA 257:203–208, 1987.
101. Ottolenghi, C. E.: Aspiration biopsy of the spine: Technique for the thoracic spine and results of twenty-eight biopsies in this region and over-all results of 1050 biopsies of other spinal segments. J. Bone Joint Surg. 51A:1531–1544, 1969.
102. Pilgaard, S.: Discitis (closed space infection) following removal of lumbar intervertebral disc. J. Bone Joint Surg. 51A:713–716, 1969.
103. Prusick, V. R., Lint, D. S., and Bruder, W. J.: Cauda equina syndrome as a complication of free epidural fat grafting. J. Bone Joint Surg. 70A:1256–1258, 1988.
104. Quiles, M., Marchisello, P. S., and Tsairis, P.: Lumbar adhesive arachnoiditis: Etiologic and pathologic aspects. Spine 3:45–50, 1978.
105. Ross, J. S., Masaryk, T. J., Modic, M. T., et al.: Lumbar spine: Postoperative assessment with surface-coil MR imaging. Radiology 164:857–860, 1987.
106. Ross, J. S., Masaryk, T. J., and Modic, M. T.: MR imaging of lumbar arachnoiditis. AJNR 8:885–892, 1987.
107. Sacks, S.: Anterior interbody fusion of the lumbar spine. J. Bone Joint Surg. 47B:211–223, 1965.
108. Schreiber, A., Suezawa, M. D., and Leu, H.: Does percutaneous nucleotomy with discoscopy replace conventional discectomy? Eight years of experience and results in treatment of herniated lumbar disc. Clin. Orthop. 238:35, 1989.
109. Simmons, J. W., Aprill, C. N., Dwyer, A. D., et al.: A reassessment of Holt's data on: "The question of lumbar discography." Clin. Orthop. 237:120–124, 1988.
110. Smith Laboratories: Data from Postmarketing Surveillance. Northbrook, IL, Smith Laboratories, 1985.
111. Smith Laboratories: Package Insert. Northbrook, IL, Smith Laboratories, July 1986.
112. Smith, S. E., De Lee, J. C., and Ramamurthy, S.: Ilioinguinal neuralgia following iliac bone-grafting. Report of two cases and review of the literature. J. Bone Joint Surg. 66A:1306–1308, 1984.
113. Spangfort, E. V.: The lumbar disc herniation. Acta Orthop. Scand. (Suppl.) 142:1–95, 1972.
114. Spengler, D. M.: Lumbar discectomy—results with limited disc excision and selective foraminotomy. Spine 7:604–607, 1982.
115. Stambough, J. L., and Booth, R. E.: Complication in spine surgery as a consequence of anatomic variations. In Garfin, S. R. (ed.): Complications of Spine Surgery. Baltimore, Williams & Wilkins, 1989.
116. Stambough, J. L.: Surgical technique for lumbar discectomy. Semin. Spine Surg. 1:47–53, 1989.
117. Stambough, J. L., and Simeone, F. A.: Vascular complications in spine surgery. In Garfin, S. R. (ed.): Complications of Spine Surgery. Baltimore, Williams & Wilkins, 1989.
118. Stambough, J. L., and Simeone, F. A.: Neurogenic complications in spine surgery. In Rothman, R. H., and Simeone, F. A. (eds.): The Spine, 3rd Ed. Philadelphia, W. B. Saunders, 1992.
119. Stauffer, R. N., and Coventry, M. B.: Anterior interbody lumbar spine fusion. Analysis of Mayo Clinic series. J. Bone Joint Surg. 54A:756–768, 1972.
120. Tetzlaff, J. E.: Personal communication.
121. Walsh, R. R., Weinstein, J. N., Spratt, K. F., et al.: Lumbar discography in normal subjects—a controlled, prospective study. J. Bone Joint Surg. 72A:1081–1088, 1990.
122. Ward, C. F.: Complications of positioning for spine surgery. In Garfin, S. R. (ed.): Complications of Spine Surgery. Baltimore, Williams & Wilkins, 1989.
123. Watkins, R. G.: Cervical, thoracic, and lumbar complications—anterior approach. In Garfin, S. R. (ed.): Complications of Spine Surgery. Baltimore Williams & Wilkins, 1989.
124. Weikel, A. M., and Habal, M. B.: Meralgia paresthetica: A complication of iliac bone procurement. Plast. Reconstr. Surg. 60:572–574, 1977.
125. Wiesel, S. W.: Neurologic complications and lumbar laminectomy: A standardized approach to the multiply operated lumbar spine. In Garfin, S. R. (ed.): Complications of Spine Surgery. Baltimore, Williams & Wilkins, 1989.
126. Wiesel, S. W., Feffer, H. L., and Rothman, R. H.: A lumbar spine algorithm. In Weinstein, J. N., and Wiesel, S. W. (eds.): The Lumbar Spine. Philadelphia, W. B. Saunders, 1990.
127. Williams, R. W.: Microlumbar discectomy. Spine 3:175–182, 1978.
128. Wilson, D. H., and Kenning, J.: Microsurgical lumbar discectomy: Preliminary report of 83 consecutive cases. Neurosurgery 4:137, 1979.
129. Wilson, D. H., and Harbaugh, R.: Lumbar discectomy: A comparative study of microsurgical and standard technique. In Hardy, R. W. (ed.): Seminars in neurosurgery—lumbar disc disease. New York, Raven Press, 1982, pp. 147–156.

16

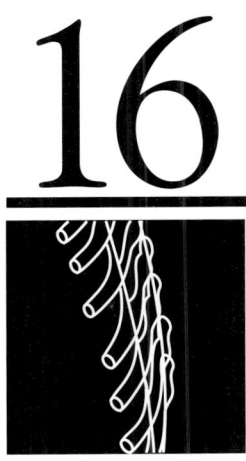

Osteoporosis of the Spine

TOMMY HANSSON
TONY S. KELLER

Osteoporosis, which is characterized by a reduction in skeletal bone mass and concomitant change in skeletal structure, produces an increased risk of fracture and thus has a devastating effect in terms of morbidity, mortality, and the cost of health care in an increasing senile population. Osteoporosis affects both the appendicular and the axial skeleton of adults and is a well-recognized public health problem of increasing proportions. More than 1.2 million fractures occur in the United States each year, including more than 500,000 cases of vertebral fracture and 200,000 cases of hip fractures, one third to one half of which occur in women older than 65 years.[102] In the United States, the personal and medical costs associated with osteoporotic fractures are expected to increase dramatically in the next 2 decades, because the number of persons older than age 65 years is predicted to double by the year 2010 (1985 United States Census).[125a]

A close association between bone mineral loss due to osteoporosis and the risk of fracture has been clearly established. Skeletal structures such as the vertebral bodies and the proximal femur, which are composed primarily of trabecular bone, appear to be particularly at risk. Thus, the development of clinical diagnostic tools sensitive enough to identify imminent fracture or collapse of vertebral bodies and other weight-bearing tissues is essential. Until these tools are developed, the ability of a clinician to evaluate a patient's bone status clearly, to prevent osteoporosis, or to determine the effect of therapeutic treatments is severely limited. This chapter discusses the prevalence of vertebral osteoporosis, provides an overview of skeletal physiology and mechanics, and reviews the basic biomechanical, radiographic, and clinical aspects of assessment of vertebral strength and fracture risk.

EPIDEMIOLOGY

The aging skeleton is characterized by a gradual loss of bone mass, which decreases bone strength (force or stress at failure), increases bone fragility associated with mechanical trauma, and increases fracture risk. A more rapid loss of bone mass occurs in postmenopausal women. Collectively, these processes are referred to as primary osteoporosis. At present, the precise cause of primary osteoporosis is unknown.

Because of increased morbidity and immobility produced by hip fractures, many epidemiologic studies of osteoporosis have focused on hip fractures. Until recently, vertebral fractures were deemed to be of lower incidence and less concern than hip fractures. There are, however, no reasons why increases in the incidence of hip fractures should not reflect a similar increasing incidence of osteoporotic spine fractures.[9] A Swedish study found that 43% of the subjects who had a hip fracture also had one or more vertebral fractures of an osteoporotic type.[136] Osteoporosis seems to have become more and more common, particularly in industrialized countries. This increase is partly explained by the fact that the populations in most industrialized countries are growing older, but it is also an indication of increased risk associated with more industrialized countries.[96, 137] Osteoporotic vertebral fracture is probably the most frequent of all fragility fractures, particularly if every vertebral fracture in the spine is considered.

Vertebral fracture is about four times more common in women than in men, and the risk of a vertebral fracture has been found to increase almost exponentially with age. The frequency of osteoporotic vertebral fracture also increases during menopause in women. After menopause, there is a steady increase in the frequency of vertebral fracture throughout life. In this respect, the vertebral fragility fractures differ from fractures of the distal radius. The prevalence of the latter increases with age but levels out after age 60 to 65 years. An interesting finding is that the increase in risk of a fragility fracture between 1985 and 1991 in Sweden was almost twice as high for men as for women.[137] Depending on the age groups studied (40 to >80 years), the prevalence of osteoporotic vertebral fractures varies from about 5% to somewhat more than 50%.[48, 71, 90, 136]

Radiographically detectable compression fractures of the spine verify the presence of osteoporosis or bone fragility. Without any known pathomorphologic aberrations distinguishing osteoporotic bone from nonosteoporotic bone tissue, the fracture itself defines a pathologic process. Because a fracture is not only the result of the mechanical properties of the bone but also a function of the fracturing trauma, both factors must be considered in the definition of osteoporosis. If a patient has a recent fracture and nothing or little is known about the patient's bone quality or the forces involved in the trauma, the most practical way of clarifying whether a fracture is osteoporotic is to apply Frost's[43] criteria of everyday trauma. Frost stated that a fracture that occurs as a consequence of an everyday trauma indicates the presence of osteoporosis or bone fragility. Even if available technology allows the determination of the amount of bone mineral in different parts of the human skeleton, practical techniques for measuring the fracture-generating forces are still lacking. Therefore, the everyday trauma definition is still useful for identifying bone fragility.

Although there are no distinct differences between the bone tissue in osteoporotic versus normal subjects, there are apparent difficulties in assessing the limits of normality. Because demineralization of the human skeleton is usually a more or less continuous process from relatively early in life, weakening of the skeleton is a part of normal aging.[102] An osteoporotic type of fragility fracture occurs in subjects in whom demineralization progresses to a level at which the spine or other parts of the skeleton no longer can resist an everyday trauma. In many subjects with spinal osteoporosis, the vertebrae may become so demineralized that they cannot resist the spinal loads accompanying everyday life. Because the amount of bone mineral in combination with the loading conditions determines the occurrence of a fracture, a subject with a low amount of bone mineral, but no fracture, has osteopenia. A subject with a low amount of bone mineral and a fracture sustained during a minor everyday trauma is likely to have osteoporosis.

BASIC BONE PHYSIOLOGY

Bone is a two-phase, porous, directional composite material, composed of hydroxyapatite (inorganic or mineral phase) and collagen (organic phase). In the normal adult skeleton, hydroxyapatite constitutes approximately two thirds of the weight or about 50% of the volume of dry bone tissue. Bone composition can be described by several histologic variables, including mineral content, porosity, and density. The density (mass/volume) may refer to either the wet or dry tissue density (mass/unit volume of solids) or the wet or dry bulk density (mass per unit volume of a region of bulk bone). Bone devoid of pores has a tissue density, or specific gravity, of approximately 2 g/cm³. Bulk density, or apparent density (ρ_a), however, is a measure of both the porosity and the mineral content of bone. Bulk density ranges from less than 0.1 g/cm³ to approximately 2 g/cm³. All of these histologic variables have been used to describe the composition of bone.

From a morphologic point of view, two principal types of bone are recognized, cortical and cancellous. In the adult skeleton, both cortical and cancellous bone have roughly the same amount of mineral, except in metabolic diseases such as osteogenesis imperfecta in which the mineral content is significantly reduced. Cortical, or compact, bone is generally distinguished from cancellous, or trabecular, bone by its lower porosity (<30% pores by volume) and higher apparent density (>1.7 g/cm³). It is most prevalent in the shafts of long bones. The ends of long bones and the axial skeleton (spine) are composed primarily of trabecular bone, which in the case of the axial skeleton has a porosity greater than 70% or an apparent density less than 0.6 g/cm³. By virtue of its inherent porosity, trabecular bone has an extremely complex structure, or architecture. Decreases in bone mass associated with aging, inactivity, and menopause have profound effects on the architecture of trabecular bone. Collectively, the changes, or adaptations, in skeletal mass and architecture are referred to as modeling and remodeling processes.

Modeling and Remodeling

Modeling and remodeling are the two different biologic activities that can affect the architecture of cortical and trabecular bone. The work of Frost,[37, 38, 43] spanning more than 3 decades and ingeniously synthesizing developments in bone research, has defined the modern concepts of modeling and remodeling skeletal tissues.

Modeling, or structural adaptation, can change the shape and size of the surfaces of the bone via resorption and formation processes. Adaptation can take place as large-scale change in the shape or size of an entire skeletal part, small-scale change in the shape and size of an individual trabecula, or mini modeling (a change that determines the type of bone formed). Modeling is postulated to have an aging component as well as a loading component, and in terms of the latter, structural adaptation seems to be the response to the strain history experienced by the tissue. Frost[42, 43] stated that modeling can increase bone mass, but it cannot decrease bone mass.

Remodeling takes place through basic multicellular units (BMUs). Each unit remodels a microscopic quantum, or packet, of bone.[43] The remodeling sequence is an orderly cascade of activation, resorption, and formation. Activation involves the initiation of the resorptive ability of the BMU. Resorption by osteoclast cells creates cavities when bone and matrix are removed. Formation is the repair phase by which the resorption cavities are filled with new tissue via osteoblast cells. The end result of the activation-resorption-formation BMU sequence is a new packet of bone, or a so-called basic structural unit.

The amount of bone replaced in one remodeling sequence (about 4 months) is roughly 0.05 mm³. There are three possible outcomes for the basic structural unit during one remodeling sequence: a net increase in the amount of bone, a net decrease in the amount of bone, or an equal amount of bone. Remodeling takes place on all surfaces of the bone—periosteal, cortical endosteal, haversian, and trabecular. Without pharmacologic help, however, a net gain of bone can appear only on the periosteal surface. On the trabecular and cortical endosteal surfaces, the remodeling sequences generally result in bone loss. The loss of trabecular and cortical endosteal surface bone during one activation-resorption-formation sequence is estimated to be about 0.003 mm³. Bone remodeling is a lifelong process and is considered somewhat faster in children than in adults. Remodeling events explain skeletal changes, such as the expansion of the marrow cavities in long bones, the widening of these bones (increased outer diameter), and the concomitant thinning of the cortices with increasing age. Bone remodeling also explains why skeletal structures proportionally rich in spongy bone (vertebrae, hip region, proximal humerus, distal radius, pelvic bones, and knee region) are more likely to lose bone mass throughout life.

Microfracturing, or fatigue fracture formation, can also affect modeling and remodeling. Fatigue fracture formation is considered a normal occurrence in the human skeleton.[8, 39] Indeed, healing microfractures have been found in many locations within the skeleton, including the spine and the hip.[36, 58, 123, 126] Hence, one must assume that both modeling and remodeling respond to microfracturing to prevent the accumulation of microtrauma, which if unchecked, produces gross fracture. Remodeling processes replace the damaged bone with new bone, whereas modeling processes modify bone structure in a manner that may make it more resistant to failure during periods of overloading.

Stimulus for Skeletal Adaptation

Although numerous theories regarding the stimuli for skeletal adaptation have been proposed, tissue strain (ϵ), or deformation per unit length, is considered by many investigators to be of central importance to this process.[18, 75, 109] A normal bone fractures at strains corresponding to about 25,000 $\mu\epsilon$ (10^{+6} mm/mm). During normal daily activity, bone strains do not usually exceed about 1500 $\mu\epsilon$. Strains above this magnitude are likely to initiate modeling processes: woven bone formation in the immature skeleton, and lamellar bone formation in the mature skeleton. Continuous exposure to strains lower than 1500 $\mu\epsilon$ presumably does not elicit a modeling response. However, during exposure of the skeleton to strains below 50 $\mu\epsilon$, such as during episodes of acute disuse, skeletal remodeling is initiated through the activation of more BMUs than normal. Consequently, the trabecular and endosteal surfaces experience a deficit in the formation of new bone during the activation-resorption-formation sequence.[132] Because no compensatory mechanisms (modeling and microfracturing) are present during the period of disuse, the result is a net loss of bone.

During normal activity, strains in the range 50 to 1500 $\mu\epsilon$ are hypothesized to keep resorption and formation at a similar magnitude. This implies that, over a long period, bone is lost because the activation-resorption-formation remodeling sequence tends to maintain a negative balance between resorption and formation. Physical exercise producing strains of sufficient magnitude and/or changes in skeletal loading that alter the distribution of strains within a skeletal structure can activate modeling processes to form new lamellar bone and thereby preserve or even increase skeletal mass, which in turn limits the range of strain in the skeleton.[19] The overall result of a strain-limiting strategy, therefore, is to preserve or to maintain a safety factor (strength > physiologic loads) within the bone material. Given the complexity of the skeleton's functional loading environment, it is not obvious how remodeling and modeling, which are cellular processes, determine how strain levels in the skeleton become deleterious during activity and adjust mass accordingly. Consequently, some researchers have proposed that bone cells are predominantly sensitive to strains within specific frequency bands and react to increases or decreases in the strain energy within that band.[109] Another possibility is simply that the stimulus threshold at which bone cells respond in a positive, or osteogenic, manner is mediated by the stimulus frequency. Thus, certain frequencies elicit a lower stimulus threshold in the process of bone cell transduction.

VERTEBRAL STRENGTH

The spine is a weight-bearing structure, which besides protecting the spinal cord and offering exceptional flexibility and range of motion, must continually support the weight of the torso and the head. During everyday activities, the spine must to a significant degree, support axial compressive forces on the vertebrae and intervening disc tissues. In the L1 to L4 lumbar spine, the compressive forces are approximately 50% to 60% of the subject's body weight.[111] Consequently, numerous investigators have examined the axial compressive strength properties of cadaveric human thoracolumbar vertebrae.* Ultimate strength values ranging from about 1 to 15 kN have been recorded in these experimental studies, most of which have examined tissues from older subjects (e.g., >40 years). To what extent the inability to obtain specimens representative of the entire population has influenced these strength values is hard to estimate. However, it is reasonable to assume that the compressive strength of vertebrae is grossly underestimated for ages below 50 years. Experimentally, as well as clinically, large variations in bone strength have made it difficult to de-

---

*References 2, 7, 8, 14, 30–32, 34, 44, 53, 54, 63, 73, 85, 97, 99, 100, 103, 105, 107, and 129.

fine a specific threshold or even a range with which to differentiate normal bone from osteoporotic bone. The latter also requires knowledge of the physiologic forces and stresses that act on the vertebral structures.

Vertebral Fracture Threshold

In vivo measurements of disc pressure are still the most realistic reference values for estimating the actual physiologic loads acting on the human lumbar spine.[93] By simply extrapolating the lumbar disc pressure results corresponding to everyday activities, one can predict that ultimate compressive stress values for the L3–L4 spine should range from 150 to 175 N/cm². Presumably, this might represent the threshold at or below which the risk of a vertebral fracture is increased during everyday activities.[56] Because of the small number of clinical studies in which the magnitude of fracture trauma has been considered, however, it seems likely that these values are much too narrow in range to represent realistic physiologic values with which to define vertebral fracture risk.[56] As a result, considerable effort has been devoted to establishing reliable experimental and clinical measures of skeletal strength and fracture risk.

Experimental Assessment of Skeletal Strength and Fracture Risk

In vitro studies of cadaver spines long ago revealed close relations between measures of the amount of bone (ash weight, wet and dry weight, apparent density, and so on) and the compressive strength of vertebrae.[7, 8, 44, 104, 129] Initially, interest in characterizing the mechanical and physical properties of vertebrae and other skeletal structures originated in the need to evaluate fracture risk associated with aging and disease. This interest has intensified owing to the need to understand implant-bone interactions and biologic fixation. Thus, numerous in vitro studies of the physical and mechanical behavior of bony tissues can be found in the literature, most of which has been reviewed by Evans,[32] Currey,[22a] Gibson,[50] Goldstein,[51] and Rice.[101] Some of these studies have established significant mathematic relationships between clinical, noninvasive measures of bone density and bone mechanical properties.[26, 59, 70, 74, 88, 116] One of the most striking features of both the in vitro and in vivo data is the large variation in density, modulus, and strength reported.

Relationship Between Bone Density and Compressive Strength

Both linear and nonlinear mathematic relationships have been used to characterize the dependence of modulus and strength on trabecular bone density, with current sentiment among investigators tending to favor the power law formulations originally described for human and bovine trabecular and cortical bone tested in compression and tension.[17] In describing trabecular bone compressive mechanical behavior most investigators have found skeletal strength to be proportional to apparent density squared, but significant variations of data are commonly found among different studies. Variations in mineral content (ash fraction, calcium and phosphorus fractions), such as those that are evident during growth, also influence bone mechanical properties.[22, 23] In the normal adult skeleton, however, variations in mineral content are generally small and contribute little to the mechanical response of cortical and trabecular bone, except in metabolic diseases such as osteogenesis imperfecta.

In a comprehensive study[79] of human vertebral trabecular and femoral cortical bone, the apparent dry density of 496 specimens ranged from 0.05 to 1.89 g/cm³, resulting in a greater than 3000-fold difference in bone strength over this range.[79] Bone strength was closely correlated with tissue apparent dry density (ρ_a), mineral fraction (α), and apparent ash density (ρ_α = mineral fraction × apparent dry density). The variation in bone strength was best described by power functions ($y = ax^b$) of bone apparent ash density. Bone strength (S) in megapascals was approximately proportional to the square of the apparent ash density (in grams per cubic centimeter) in the case of the vertebral bone specimens ($n = 200$; $\rho_\alpha < 0.1$ g/cm³):

$$S = 284 \, \rho_\alpha^{2.27 \pm 0.09} \quad (R^2 = .79) \quad (1)$$

and to the square of the apparent ash density in the case of the femoral bone specimens ($n = 296$; $0.1 < \rho_\alpha < 1.22$ g/cm³):

$$S = 116 \rho_\alpha^{2.03 \pm 0.03} \quad (R^2 = .93) \quad (2)$$

Each model explains roughly 80% to 90% of the variation in bone strength. Theoretic analyses of the mechanisms of cell wall deformations of idealized open- and closed-cell porous engineering materials support the use of a squared power law to describe the relationship of bone strength to apparent density.[49, 50]

More than 90% of the variance in skeletal strength was explained by apparent density when the vertebral and femoral bone data were combined ($n = 496$; $0.03 < \rho_\alpha < 1.22$ g/cm^3):

$$S = 117 \rho_\alpha^{1.93 \pm 0.02} \quad (R^2 = .97) \quad (3)$$

On the basis of the 97.5% confidence intervals associated with these models of bone strength, predictions obtained by extrapolating equation 1 high-density values ($\rho_\alpha = 1.22$ g/cm^3) resulted in gross underestimation of bone strength (by approximately threefold) in comparison with the values obtained from the appropriate regression equation. Closer agreement between femoral model extrapolations of strength to the lowest-density specimens was obtained. These findings are consistent with the statistical analysis of pooled trabecular bone data performed by Rice and coworkers.[101] Similar predictions based on the values obtained from the combined data (equation 3), however, resulted in close agreement to the 97.5% confidence intervals for strength computed separately from the vertebral (equation 1) and femoral (equation 2) bone data. These results support the notions that extrapolations do not yield valid results and that reliable predictions can be obtained only over the data range evaluated.

This remarkable difference in mechanical properties reflects, at least in part, the skeleton's adaptive response to its mechanical environment. In addition to environmental and testing conditions, much of this variation can also be attributed to the anatomic origin and age of the specimens.

Clinical Estimates of Skeletal Strength and Fracture Risk

Recognition that there is a close association between bone apparent density and bone mechanical properties has prompted numerous in vivo investigations focusing on establishing mathematic relationships between bone strength and clinical measures of skeletal density.

The advent of noninvasive techniques for determining the amount of bone mineral in the spine (e.g., dual- and triple-photon energy absorptiometry, quantitative computed tomography [CT], and double- and triple-energy x-ray absorptiometry) have made nondestructive bone quantifications possible in vitro as well as in vivo. Each of these techniques provides a precision of about 1% to 4%[27, 46, 84] and is accurate to about 3% to 10%[46, 128] in comparison with a precision of $\leq 0.1\%$ for direct measurements of bone ash content (inorganic weight). These techniques also allow quantitative measurement of bone density in relationship to average density for both age-matched and younger persons and can be used as a criterion for the definition of osteoporosis. The definition of osteoporosis has varied but generally ranges from 2 to 2.5 standard deviations below the mean density for an average 30-year-old adult of the same sex. Because all of these measurement approaches can be used both in vitro and in vivo, they have provided great advantages in spinal research.

In general, noninvasive measurements of bone density—bone mineral content (grams per centimeter), bone mineral density (grams per square centimeter), and trabecular density (grams per cubic centimeter)*—have explained roughly 25% to 80% of the variation in trabecular bone axial compressive strength of the thoracolumbar vertebrae when expressed as linear ($y = bx + a$) relationships[12, 31, 54-56, 98] or power ($y = ax^b$) relationships.[74] Predictions of vertebral trabecular bone strength (S) in megapascals based on bone mineral content (BMC) obtained from the latter study.[74]

$$S = 0.13 \text{BMC}^{2.25} \quad (R^2 = .76) \quad (4)$$

are more consistent with predictions from the aforementioned in vitro studies[74, 79] in which similar squared relationships between trabecular strength and apparent density or apparent ash density were reported.

---

*Trabecular density can be derived only from radiographic measures of bone mineral content using in vitro bone mineral content–bone mineral density correlations or in vivo calibration phantoms.

However, as is the case for other clinical estimates, they do not yield the same high correlations found using histologic measures of bone quality.

Significant positive correlations between ultimate strength and bone mineral content have also been found when the vertebral specimens have been tested in flexion-compression, distraction, and distraction-extension nodes.[53, 94] Testing of vertebral specimens in flexion-compression did not reveal any unique relations between the amount of bone and strength or stress in comparison with results achieved with testing under axial compression. In addition, except for the general fragility of the osteopenic spine, there are no indications that osteopenia increases the spine's susceptibility to fail with loading in any specific direction.[53, 94] Studies comparing trabecular bone failure patterns in osteopenic specimens with failure patterns in specimens with normal amounts of bone mineral have not identified any unique differences.[53] In contrast to most other fragility fractures, osteoporotic vertebral fracture is less frequently related to a distinct trauma, such as a fall.[48] More often, trauma causing vertebral fracture seems to be associated with normal activities (e.g., a moderate or light lift when bending forward, a change of position, a sudden twist of the trunk, and even coughing).

Nonlinear relationships between vertebral strength and density such as those noted above imply that, in already osteopenic vertebrae, a further reduction of the amount of bone brings about a proportionally greater strength reduction. For example, a 50% reduction in bone density (analogous to bone losses associated with long-term bed rest, paralysis, and senile osteoporosis) corresponds to a fourfold decrease in bone strength.

Influence of Vertebral Level on Mechanical and Physical Properties

The compressive mechanical strength (stress at failure) of vertebral trabecular bone specimens does not appear to vary significantly at different levels within the lumbar spine.[55, 74] The vertebral levels T12 and L1 have the highest risk of an osteoporotic fracture of any region of the human spine; one hypothetic explanation for this observation is that these levels are intrinsically more susceptible to fracture.[112] A more plausible explanation for an increased fracture risk at these two levels may be that the intervertebral joint between T12 and L1 is the fulcrum for motions between the relatively stiff thoracic cage and the more freely movable lumbar spine. Therefore, stress concentrations, especially in flexion, predispose these vertebrae to a higher risk of fracture in an osteopenic person.

Rate of Bone Loss in Aging Trabecular and Cortical Bone

Age-related bone losses are purported to occur earliest in trabecular bone. The earliest changes observed in the spine are a decrease in the amount of osseous tissue, a loss of the horizontal trabeculae, and a thickening of the vertical trabeculae.[6] Of note is the finding that bone losses are eightfold to 10-fold greater in the trabecular skeleton (2% to 3% per year) than in the cortical skeleton (0.3% to 0.5% per year).[92] This has been hypothesized to be related to functional differences in the time course of the remodeling process.[39] Another explanation, which deserves further attention, is the hypothesis that measured differences in the rate of trabecular and cortical bone loss reflect the greater surface (S)/volume (V) ratio of trabecular bone ($S/V \cong 4$) in comparison with whole cortical bone ($S/V \cong 0.4$).[76] Assuming a constant rate of remodeling for both cortical and trabecular bone, a 10-fold greater amount of exposed trabecular bone surface would result in a 10-fold greater loss of trabecular bone in comparison with that of cortical bone. This observation correlates well with the reported differences in the pattern of bone loss for these tissues. Hence, skeletal structures, such as the vertebral bodies, which have trabecular bone as the primary constituent, are particularly susceptible to fracture.

Because trabecular bone is a highly porous material, changes in the internal architecture of vertebrae in age- and disease-related bone loss also have a profound effect on vertebral mechanical strength. Thus, accurate assessment of fracture risk in patients must include, in addition to traditional estimates of density, considerations of skeletal architecture. At present, however, clinical considerations of skeletal architecture are limited to radiographic signs such as loss of horizontal trabeculae and concomitant accentuation of vertically oriented trabeculae, which may ultimately produce a pattern of biconcavity, or "codfish" vertebrae, in elderly persons.

VERTEBRAL MORPHOLOGY

Although noninvasive measures of bone density are now considered the most effective method known for predicting fracture risk, these techniques appear to be only about 70% accurate. Presumably, other material features of bone and supporting structures are needed to explain the additional 30% of causes of fracture. On the basis of work of Mazess,[86] it appears that these additional factors play a greater role in the spine, making bone density less predictable in the spine than in other regions of the skeleton that are composed of higher density bone. Trabecular bone researchers currently attribute the unexplained variation in mechanical properties to differences in the morphologic features of this tissue.

In vertebrae, large variations in trabecular density and mechanical properties have been noted within adjacent regions separated by only a few millimeters.[74–76] Five morphologically distinct regions of trabecular bone are found in the vertebral centrum: superior, first transitional, center, second transitional, and inferior levels (Fig. 1). The superior and inferior sections each occupy approximately 30% to 35% of the total segment height and exhibit patterns of orientation distinct from those of the center and transitional sections. The transitional and middle portions of the centrum consist primarily of platelike trabeculae forming a closed-cell structure, in contrast to the superior and inferior sections of the centrum, which consist primarily of rodlike trabeculae forming an open-cell structure. Trabecular bone structure is more dense in the inferior and superior sections than in the central sections of the lumbar centrum. Platelike trabeculae are associated with the central regions of lesser density bone. This observation is consistent with that of earlier investigators, who in describing vertebral architecture, noted that ". . . even in the more porous areas . . . the basic structure consists

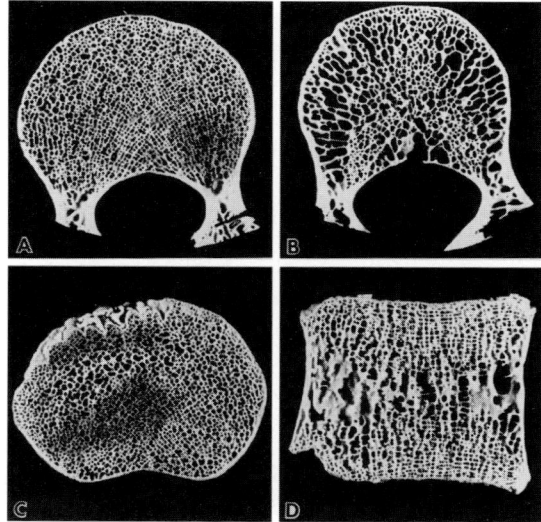

Figure 1. Photomicrographs of transverse and sagittal sections of the lumbar vertebral centrum obtained from an 18-year-old male patient. *A*, *B*, and *C* correspond to superior, central, and inferior levels, respectively, of the second lumbar vertebra. *D* corresponds to the midsagittal section of the third lumbar vertebra. Note that the proximal and distal regions of the spine are composed of an open-cell, rodlike structure in contrast to the central region of the vertebra, which is characterized by the presence of closed-cell, platelike bone (*D*). (From Keller, T. S., Hansson, T. H., Abram, A. C., et al.: Regional variations in the compressive properties of lumbar vertebral trabeculae: Effects of disc degeneration. Spine 14:1012–1019, 1989.)

of perforated plates rather than true trabeculae in the sense of struts or bars."[3] This observation differs from that of Gibson,[50] who after evaluating structure-density relationships for a variety of bone types, indicated that open-cell structures dominate for relatively low-density trabecular bone, whereas closed-cell structures dominate in higher-density trabecular bone. The central, platelike regions of the lumbar spine, therefore, appear to be unique in terms of their trabecular architecture. The functional significance of this finding remains to be determined.

The complex organization and distribution of vertebral trabeculae and trabeculae in other regions of the skeleton support the generally accepted hypothesis that function directly influences the structure and strength of bone, a relationship known as Wolff's law.[135] From a mechanical engineering standpoint, trabecular bone behaves similarly to porous engineering materials because of its cellular structure and large energy absorption capabilities. The distribution of trabecular bone density and mechanical properties within vertebrae vary along the axis and within the cross section of vertebrae. Some investigators have reported a variable or heterogeneous distribution of trabecular bone tissue physical and mechanical properties for the vertebral centrum.* Most of these studies have noted that anterior regions of the vertebral centrum are generally less dense and less strong than posterior regions. Keller and associates[76] noted that the superior and inferior regions of lumbar vertebrae are denser than the central and transitional regions. This observation is consistent with the observation of wedging and compressed vertebrae in elderly persons.[114]

Structural Indices of Trabecular Bone

In anisotropic materials such as bone, the organization of individual material components may be more important than the actual amount of material present. Indeed, the dependence of mechanical properties on the structure of trabecular bone has been noted by numerous investigators, but difficulties in adequately characterizing the two-dimensional and three-dimensional structure of trabecular bone have severely limited the development of predictive models relating structure to mechanical properties. Beginning with the work of von Meyer,[127] many anatomic studies have provided general descriptions of trabecular bone architecture, and it is commonly accepted that variations in trabecular architecture can be attributed to the magnitude and distribution of functional stresses or strains.[106] In some skeletal structures such as the vertebral body, trabecular bone is the primary load-bearing constituent,[87, 105] and it is surrounded by only a thin layer of cortical bone. Schmorl and Junghanns[113] noted that the number and directions of trabeculae within the spine varied with spinal curvature, which they also attributed to adaptations to functional stresses. Other researchers have reported a decrease in vertebral trabecular plate thickness and tissue volume with increasing age.† Variations in trabecular morphologic features have important clinical implications in terms of the type and severity of injuries to the spine and the sites where functional disturbances are potentially most harmful.[82, 89]

One of the first detailed studies of vertebral structure was conducted by Amstutz and Sissons,[3] who created stacked celluloid models from serial transverse histologic sections of the third lumbar vertebra of a young woman. On the basis of an analysis of four $6 \times 7 \times 1$-mm thick models from the superior, central (neural arch), and inferior sections, they reported an increased density of bone in superior and inferior surfaces of the vertebra. Trabeculae were preferentially oriented in the vertical and horizontal planes and, at the level of the vertebral arch, exhibited an anterior radial orientation that condensed toward the vertebral arch. Using a scanning electron microscope, Whitehouse and coworkers[132] studied the general three-dimensional arrangement of trabeculae and the distribution of trabecular bone within the lumbar vertebral body of a young man. Their analysis of relative bone area, volume, and trabecular boundary estimates from 12 areas of a transverse and a sagittal section of the vertebral centrum indicated a relatively high degree of tissue heterogeneity, most notably in the superior and inferior sections near the intervertebral discs. These and other similar studies, while providing quantitative data on the distribution of bone, have been primarily descriptive in terms of the orientation of trabecular bone.[28, 91, 132, 133]

During the past 2 decades, investigators have used quantitative imaging techniques, based on stereologic theory,[111, 125, 130] to characterize structural anisotropy in trabecular bone.* Using histologic sections and high-resolution micro CT imaging techniques, stereologic analyses can provide planar mathematic indices of skeletal structure, including trabecular number (TN), trabecular width (TW), trabecular orientation (θ), trabecular anisotropy (MIL_{ratio}), and bone volume fraction (V_f). Each of these structural variables has been shown, to a certain degree, to predict the mechanical behavior of trabecular bone, but none has proved to be more effective than apparent density and mineral content. Some of the ambiguities associated with these variables may be related to the fact that these are two-dimen-

---
*References 26, 29, 74, 76, 78, 88, and 122.
†References 4–6, 16, 25, 39, 72, 92, and 99.

*References 20, 35, 61, 68, 81, 83, 117, 121, and 134.

sional descriptions of a complex three-dimensional structure.

In a morphologic study, Zhu and associates[138] described the multiplanar structural variations of vertebral trabecular bone. These investigators examined a series of more than 200 high-resolution (20-μm voxels [volume pixels]) serial images of lumbar vertebral trabeculae. The results of this study indicated that the surface planar structural properties of the vertebral specimens could not adequately describe the complex and heterogeneous distribution of bone present; an accurate description of the bulk structural properties of vertebral trabecular bone required multiple serial plane sections distributed at least every 100 μm along a given axis. They also found that the vertebral bone specimens were characterized by smooth and repetitive transitions of plane structural indices (TW, TN, MIL_{ratio}, and θ) along the superior-inferior axis of the specimens, suggesting a high degree of connectivity within the vertebral trabecular bone. In addition, these researchers noted that the trabecular bone area centers within the vertebral specimens exhibited a helical variation. This helical variation in the bone area centers was hypothesized to reflect the intrinsic springlike structure of vertebral trabecular bone that provides an efficient means to absorb energy and withstand external impact during loading.

Quantitative information from these and other studies has provided insight into the effect of structural variables on mechanical properties. It has been used to characterize changes in skeletal architecture associated with bone remodeling, implant loosening, and pathologic changes to the skeleton.

Relationship Between Bone Structural Indices and Mechanical Properties

Researchers often attribute the unexplained variance in bone mechanical properties to bone structure, but few studies have performed detailed analysis of trabecular bone structure in comparison with mechanical properties. Indices of surface planar structure have been used, together with traditional measures of apparent density or porosity, to improve predictions of the mechanical properties of trabecular bone. Using a high-resolution micro CT scan imaging technique, Goulet and colleagues[52] noted that surface planar structural indices could reliably predict the bulk mechanical properties of trabecular bone as long as the bone specimens were relatively homogeneous in structure. Snyder and associates[118] reported a close correlation between trabecular structural indices (TN and TW) and calculated strengths of trabecular bone specimens from L1 vertebral bodies, which were within 20% of values predicted by previous experimental studies for similar density specimens. Hodgskinson and Currey[66, 67] reported that approximately 93% of the variance in the Young's modulus of human tibial and femoral cancellous bone and nonhuman tibial and femoral cancellous bone could be explained using mineral volume fraction, apparent density, and two structural variables. However, given that the architecture of vertebral trabecular bone is highly heterogeneous,[138] such high correlations are not expected for human vertebral trabecular bone. Other investigators have established relationships that explain roughly 60% to 90% of the variance in the elastic modulus of trabecular bone using both apparent density and three-dimensional descriptions of trabecular bone fabric.[24, 124] Three-dimensional connectivity measures, such as the Euler number (EN), are hypothesized to be good indicators of osteopenia.[35] Additional quantitative structural analyses of trabecular bone are needed and may provide insight into mechanical behavior not explained by tissue physical properties and gross structure alone.

Simulations of Osteoporosis in Human Vertebrae

With progressive demineralization, the vertical trabeculae become thinner and the horizontal cross-linkings become fewer.[6] Because the buckling strength of a slender column is largely dependent on its diameter, its length, and the distance between cross-linkings (Euler buckling), a loss of bone in some regions reduces the total number of cross-linkings. Consequently, a small reduction in bone mineral content, at these points, produces a proportionally much greater decrease in strength.

Simulations of osteoporosis have been reported in which planar and multiplanar structural indices were quantified using three-dimensional binary image arrays obtained from high-resolution serial histologic sections of lumbar vertebral trabecular bone.[77] In this study, structural measurements of the image arrays were repeated several times after sequential removal of layers of bone pixels from the surfaces of the trabeculae at 20-μm increments (Fig. 2). Here, the sequential removal of bone pixels simulates age-related bone loss associated with osteoporosis (assuming a uniform loss of bone in both space and time). After three iterations of the computer simulation of aging (removal of 60 μm), there was a 60% loss in bone volume fraction (V_f) accompanied by significant fragmentation of the horizontal trabeculae. In terms of the structural indices computed after each iteration, the connectivity (EN) decreased in direct proportion to V_f, whereas the structural indices (TN and TW) decreased at a slightly lower rate than V_f and EN.

The biomechanical implications of these variations in trabecular structure and relative density (V_f) can be estimated from this analysis. After 50% of the bone has been resorbed (comparable with losses associated with severe osteoporosis or long-term bed rest), there is an estimated fourfold decrease in bone strength (assuming $S \propto \rho_a^2 \propto V_f^2$). At this point, there is also a concomitant 50% and 30% decrease in EN and TW, respectively (see dashed line in Figure 3). If the trabeculae have a constant length, the decrease in TW is equivalent to an approximately 50% (0.7^2) decrease in the critical elastic buckling load, indicating that there is a markedly greater risk of fracture (e.g., twofold) associated with bone loss than one would predict from density or mineral content changes alone. One would also expect that the trabecular fragmentation seen in Figure 2 would further decrease the ability of the trabecular network to resist loading. This highly simplified analysis does not consider bone stress-adaptive changes, which could be used to model local rather than global changes in the remodeling process.

BIOMECHANICAL ADAPTATION OF THE SPINE

A link between degenerative changes in the intervertebral disc (IVD) and those in spinal ligaments was originally suggested by Harris and Macnab.[62] Keller and colleagues[74, 78] noted that there is a similar link

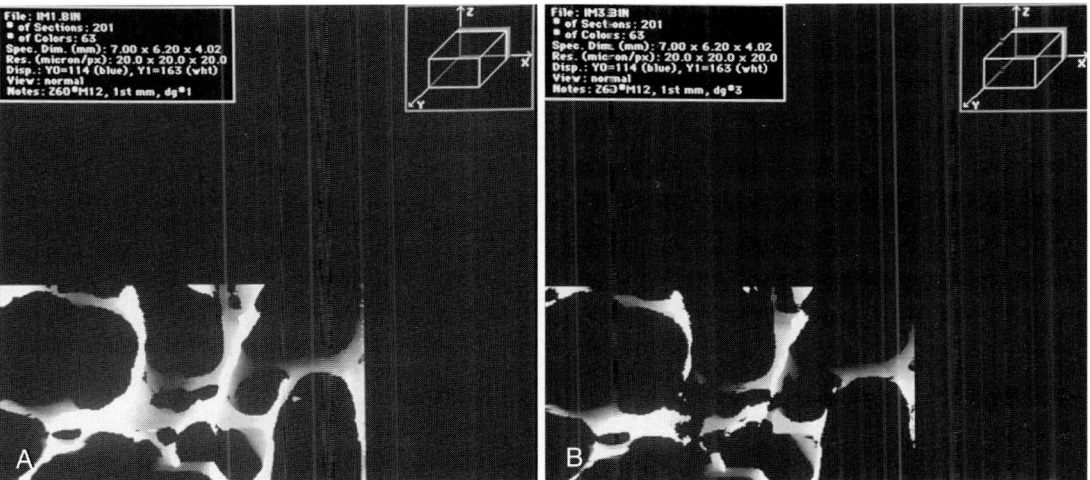

Figure 2. Reconstructed, three-dimensional image arrays for a 7 × 1 × 4.02 mm region (x, y, z, respectively) of L4 vertebral trabecular bone from a 60-year-old man. A, The original trabecular bone structure. B, The same specimen following the third iteration of the osteoporosis simulation by bone demineralization, at which point 60 μm of bone has been removed from the surfaces of the trabeculae. The top portion of each image corresponds to the superior axis (z coordinate) of the vertebral specimen. Note that there is significant trabecular fragmentation and loss of trabecular connectivity after bone demineralization—simulated osteoporosis. These 20-μm voxel (volume pixel) images were reconstructed from a histologic specimen using a destructive, quantitative serial sectioning and surface image capture procedure.[138]

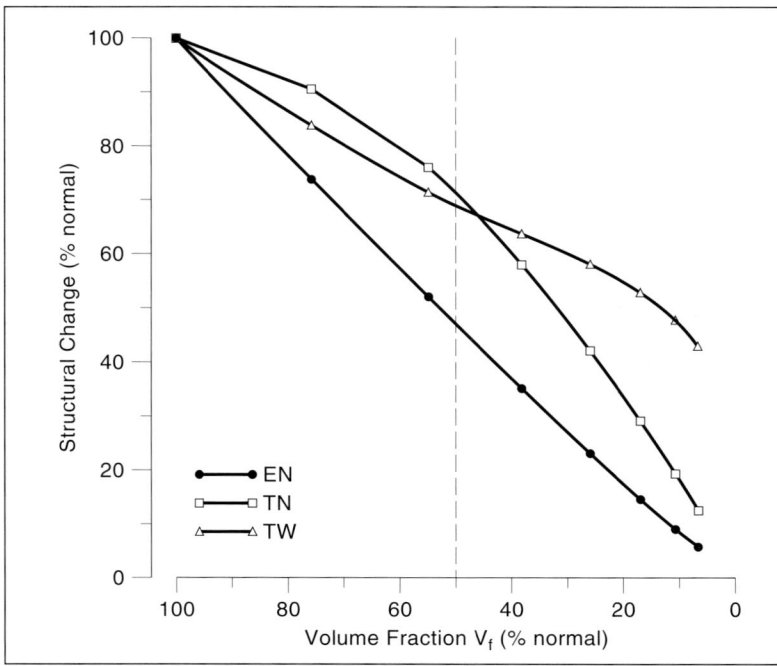

Figure 3. Change in vertebral trabecular bone structure as a function of V_f (relative density). The structural indices—TN, TW, EN—are expressed as a percentage of the values obtained before computer-simulated removal of bone from the trabecular surfaces. EN is a measure of the trabecular connectivity in the vertebral trabeculae, and it decreases in a linear manner with V_f. Each data point shown represents removal of 20 μm of bone from the trabecular surfaces (see Fig. 2).

between the IVD and the underlying trabecular bone. This hypothesis reflects the fact that the properties of ligaments, discs, and bone in the spine are interrelated and stems from biomechanical considerations of load sharing by these structures.

During aging, degenerative changes in the IVD that reduce the water content of the nucleus also lower the nucleus pressure.[1, 139] Ordinarily, this pressure creates higher compressive stresses in the nucleus region in comparison with those in peripheral regions of the IVD and allows the IVD to retain flexibility and resilience during extreme loading conditions. Hence, additional density and strength are needed for trabecular bone underlying high-stress regions in the normal disc if the stress-adaptive properties of bone (Wolff's law) are to be observed. This implies that a heterogeneous distribution of physical and mechanical properties in trabecular bone tissue underlying the disc should be present. Indeed, heterogeneous distributions of trabecular structural and physical properties have been described for the young lumbar vertebral centrum.[74–78] In contrast, a more uniform pressure or stress distribution across the IVD and adjacent end plates and subdiscal bone is predicted for the severely degenerated IVD, in which case the subdiscal variations in mechanical and physical properties should be more homogeneous. This notion has been previously validated using mathematic models.[117] Findings by Keller and associates[78] provided further support for this view. In the latter study, physicochemical properties of the disc were well correlated with subdiscal bone mechanical properties. Age-related changes in the physicochemical properties of the disc also closely paralleled age-related changes in subdiscal bone mechanical properties.

The notion that IVD, spinal ligaments, and vertebral bone properties are interdependent has important implications for degenerative processes in the spine as well as for the etiology of vertebral osteoporosis. Alterations in disc function that somehow change disc properties propagate changes in bone properties via disturbances in spine mechanical function, which in turn produces further alterations in disc function. A similar scenario for alterations in bone properties arises, creating a vicious circle of events that facilitates degeneration of the spine (Fig. 4). The consequences of alterations in disc properties, however, are probably more damaging than those of alterations in bone properties, because adult IVD lacks a direct blood supply and hence has limited regenerative capabilities. The amount of bone mineral in the spine determined with dual-pho-

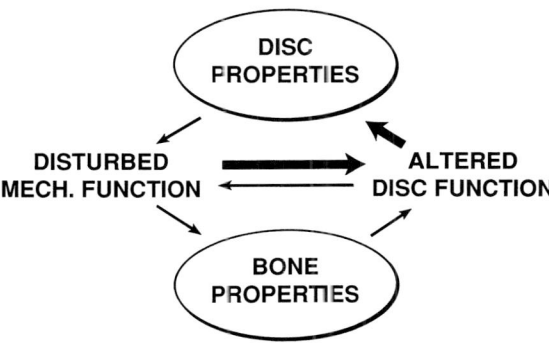

Figure 4. The biomechanically controlled regulation of IVD and subdiscal bone properties. Changes in disc properties (e.g., degeneration) are hypothesized to produce changes in trabecular bone properties, and vice versa. The bold arrows emphasize the consequences of altered disc and mechanical function. An analogous functional interdependence has also been hypothesized for lumbar spinal ligaments and vertebral bone. (From Keller, T. S., Ziv, I., Moeljanto, E., and Spengler, D. M.: Interdependence of lumbar disc and subdiscal bone properties: A report of the normal and degenerated spine. J. Spinal Disord. 6:106–113 1993.)

ton absorptiometry has also been found to be an accurate predictor of tensile properties of the spinal ligaments.[95] This also seems to confirm that the spine is a functional entity composed of interdependent structures that respond to remodeling stimuli in a similar manner.

Each of these studies demonstrates how the properties of the vertebral disc and/or spinal ligaments determine the load-sharing conditions between two neighboring vertebrae, which in turn also control the remodeling of the trabecular bone beneath the disc. Although there is little knowledge of how disc or ligament degeneration is related to the long-term development of osteopenia and osteoporosis, one can speculate that the relation of the properties of the disc, the ligaments, and/or the adjacent bone in some way determines the failure pattern in spinal osteoporosis. Consequently, it is reasonable to assume that discrepancies between the properties of the discs and those of the vertebral bodies (the end plates and the adjacent trabecular bone) may contribute to the formation of a central compression fracture.

FAILURE PATTERNS IN OSTEOPOROSIS

Perey[99] was perhaps the first to report that the weakest part of a compressed thoracolumbar vertebra was the central end plate and the underlying trabecular bone. Numerous studies have confirmed these results, and there is some evidence that the amount of bone mineral does not alter this failure pattern.[57] Under combined compression-flexion, quasistatic loading (<10 mm/s) of lumbar vertebrae produces a typical central end-plate fracture, together with an anterior wedge type of fracture.[53] Axial compression testing at high strain rates (200 mm/s), which more closely resemble the body motions that occur during normal activities, also produced central end-plate failures (Neumann, P., personal communication, 1994). These higher but more physiologic strain rates, however, nearly doubled the ultimate compressive strength of the spine in comparison with the corresponding values obtained during quasistatic compression conditions.

Central end-plate fractures are also often the first sign of failure during in vitro repetitive loading experiments conducted on normal and osteopenic human lumbar vertebral motion segments.[11, 59, 60] Hansson and associates[60] also noted that the type of end-plate fracture formed (Schmorl node or central end plate) was correlated with the age and degree of disc degeneration of the specimens. Schmorl nodes were predominantly associated with younger, less degenerated discs, whereas central end-plate fractures were predominantly associated with older, more degenerated specimens (Fig. 5). This study also demonstrated how remarkably close to failure the human spine is when it is subjected to repetitive loading; compressive stresses as low as 50% of the failure strength of the vertebrae produce fatigue fractures after fewer than 1000 cycles.

RADIOGRAPHIC ASSESSMENT OF SPINAL OSTEOPOROSIS

Radiographically, at least three different types of vertebral fractures are related to osteoporosis:[69]

1. Osteoporotic compression collapse, or crush fractures, which involve the entire vertebral body, including the anterior as well as the posterior cortices.
2. Wedge-type fractures in which the

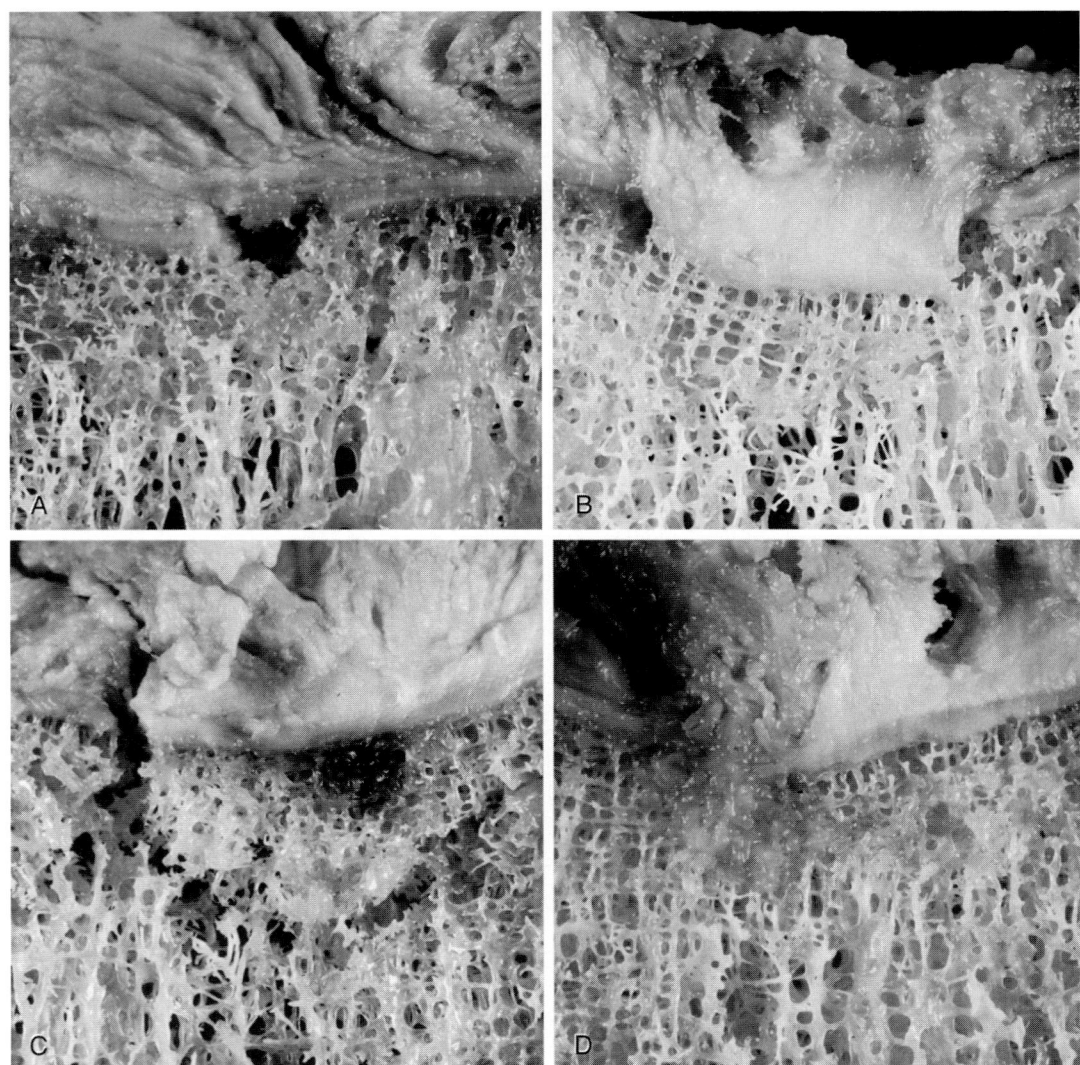

Figure 5. Typical vertebral end-plate fractures resulting from dynamic axial compressive fatigue loading experiments. *A* and *B* illustrate Schmorl node fractures, which occurred more frequently in specimens from young persons with nondegenerated IVDs. *C* and *D* illustrate the central end-plate type of fractures, which were predominantly found in specimens from older subjects with degenerated IVDs. Located centrally in the vertebral bodies, the minimally dislocated fractures can be difficult to detect even in vitro. (Adapted from Hansson, T., Keller, T., and Jonson, R.: Fatigue fracture morphology in human lumbar motion segments. J. Spinal Disord. 1:33–38, 1988.)

height of the posterior aspect of the vertebral body remains relatively intact.

3. Central compression type with a ballooning, concave disc, which gives the spine a codfishlike appearance. The deformity can occur on one or both sides of the same vertebra. The anterior and posterior cortices are relatively unaffected.

Both central end-plate fractures and the anterior wedge type of fractures observed during in vitro testing of ultimate strength were difficult to visualize radiographically, even when all the surrounding soft tissues were excised.[53, 57] Thus, it is likely that a conventional radiographic examination of the spine in an osteoporotic patient may overlook fractures such as those caused by in vitro strength testing. Typically, fractures that are readily detectable on anteroposterior or lateral radiographs are actually gross fractures involving major wedging, biconcavity, or collapse (crush) of the entire vertebral body.[47, 69] Considerable controversy remains concerning (1) the precise relationship between vertebral fracture type and the quality of bone and (2) the precise amount of reduction of the anterior cortex that should be classified as a fracture. Radiologic criteria, such as translucency, sparse trabecular pattern, and thickness of the vertebral cortices, are difficult to quantify reliably, at least using conventional radiographic techniques. For this reason, much interest has focused on the possibilities of finding accurate and reproducible radiographic measures to describe the shape of the human vertebrae.*

Digital x-ray studies, CT scans, and MRI scan analysis offer promise in terms of improved definition of vertebral structure and/or trabecular structure, and they may ultimately improve the chances of detecting minor vertebral fractures, such as the central end-plate fracture. Quantitative analysis of these images may also assist in the clinical assessment of vertebral fracture risk. With regard to quantitative CT, Chevalier and coworkers[21] used a spatial filter to obtain enhanced two-dimensional CT images of lumbar vertebral trabecular networks. From the resulting digital images, they computed a so-called trabecular fragmentation index, defined as the ratio of the number of network discontinuities to the total length of the network. This index distinguished normal and osteoporotic female subjects regardless of age, and it was significantly correlated ($R = -.60$) with bone mineral density values obtained for the same subjects. High-resolution multiplanar models of trabecular structures derived from micro CT scans have also been used to describe the connectivity of trabecular bone.[35] Reliable radiographic techniques may also improve the ability to assess the effects of various pharmacologic and physical treatment regimens on prevention and treatment of osteoporosis.

CLINICAL ASPECTS IN OSTEOPOROSIS

In some patients, the first clinical sign of osteoporosis is a sudden pain in the back after an exertion. Typically, the fracture-evoking forces are by definition light to moderate. Some patients remark that their fracture was preceded by a period of more strenuous physical exertion involving activities such as lifting, bending, and climbing stairs. The pain is usually located in the lower thoracic or upper lumbar spines and may be referred to the lower lumbar or lumbosacral spines. In some cases the pain is segmental, whereas in other cases the pain may be completely incapacitating. The period of severe pain always subsides spontaneously, but it can last for weeks in some patients. When severe, the pain can cause an ileuslike condition. Neurologic complications or deficits, however, are rare. The presence of other more severe problems, including metastasis, must be considered. The pain eventually decreases with the healing of the fracture and gradually disappears. In a minority of patients, back problems may develop after the fracture episode.

Although a more or less distinct episode often marks the occurrence of an osteoporotic vertebral fracture, the majority of patients with spinal osteoporosis are unaware of such an episode. Their diagnosis is made through an incidental radiographic examination. Patients with the silent type of vertebral fracture are typically older than 75 years, whereas patients with a well-defined fracture episode and severe pain are generally younger than 70 years.[119] Silent fracturing is also four times more likely to be associated with mild or moderately severe wedge or concave-biconcave fracture.[71] A strong indication of a compressed vertebra is body height loss, irrespective of the presence or absence of pain. In many cases, these patients have been aware of an increasing kyphosis of their upper thoracic spine, sometimes for several years preceding the first clinical examination. When asked why they did not seek medical help at an earlier time, many women explain that they were reluctant to seek medical advice for their increasing kyphosis because their mother or grandmother had a similar problem for many years. Some of these patients also report having long periods of nonspecific backache.

The risk of a recurrent fracture episode seems to be lower among patients whose first fracture occurred through a distinct trauma. Among patients without such a well-defined episode, the risk of more or less continual fracturing is greatly increased. Reports of up to a five times in-

---

*References 13, 45, 64, 65, 80, 103, and 120.

creased risk for new vertebral fractures have been noted in women who currently have severe spinal fracture deformities.[10, 15] From a biomechanical perspective, it seems reasonable that patients who experience fractures only during heavier loading of the spine, as a group, have a stronger spine than patient with fragile spines who have more or less axially insufficient vertebral strength and who experience fractures with less severe trauma. As long as the first type of patient can avoid a trauma of similar or greater magnitude, the risks are relatively small that they will have additional vertebral fractures. On the other hand, subjects with inherently weaker vertebrae typically continue to have fractures, often in a stepwise manner. This process is characterized by a reduced body height and an advancing kyphosis, or humpback. If compression and kyphosis continue, other clinical symptoms occur, including collision of the ribs and the iliac crest, and pronounced protrusion of the belly.

The initial evaluation of a patient with a suspected vertebral fracture should include anteroposterior and lateral radiographs. Fractures in the thoracic spine might result in an increased kyphosis, whereas lumbar fractures can increase lordosis. Osteoporotic fractures above the T6–T7 level are rare, and the differential diagnosis in such a case includes multiple myeloma, metastasis, chondromalacia, hyperthyroidism, hypercalcemia, and infectious disorders. Scintigraphy might be helpful when differential diagnostic possibilities cannot be ruled out.

Bed rest for few days might be necessary to alleviate severe pain. Bed rest should be as brief as possible, because prolonged bed rest enhances bone loss in the already demineralized spine. Symptomatic treatments may include the administration of analgesics, but medication should not include any substance that can exacerbate the obstipation in some patients due to a pain-induced ileus or subileus. However, this usually resolves within a couple of days. Mobilization can start as soon as the worst period of discomfort has subsided. Some patients receive some relief with the use of a soft corset during early mobilization. Most patients appreciate self-training instructions on a modified back exercise program, although patients should be informed that virtually all osteoporotic fractures will heal and that the pain prognosis is also optimistic.

REFERENCES

1. Adams, P., and Muir, H. M.: Qualitative changes with age of proteoglycans of human lumbar discs. Ann. Rheum. Dis. 35:289–295, 1976.
2. Adams, M. A., Hutton, W. C., and Stott, J. R. R.: The resistance to flexion of the lumbar intervertebral joint. Spine 5:245–253, 1980.
3. Amstutz, H. C., and Sisson, H. A.: The structure of the vertebral spongiosa. J. Bone Joint Surg. 51B:540–550, 1969.
4. Arnold, J. S., and Wei, L. T.: Quantitative morphology of vertebral trabecular bone. In Stover, B., and Jee, W. S. S. (eds.): Radiobiology of Plutonium. UT, Salt Lake City, J. W. Press, 1972, pp. 333–354.
5. Arnold, J. S.: Trabecular pattern and shapes in aging and osteoporosis. In Jee, W. S. S., and Parfitt, A. M. (eds.): Bone Histomorphometry, Third International Workshop. Paris, Armour Montagu, 1981, pp. 297–308.
6. Atknison, P. J.: Variations in trabecular structure of vertebrae with age. Calcif. Tissue Res. 1:24–32, 1967.
7. Bartley, M. H., Arnold, J. S., Haslam, R. K., and Jee, W. S. S.: The relationship of bone strength and bone quantity in health, disease and aging. J. Gerontol. 21:517–521, 1966.
8. Bell, G. H., Dunbar, O., and Beck, J. S.: Variations in strength of vertebrae with age and their relation to osteoporosis. Calcif. Tissue Res. 1:75–86, 1967.
9. Bengnér, U., Johnell, O., and Redlund-Johnell, I.: Changes in incidence and prevalence of vertebral fractures during 30 years. Calcif. Tissue Int. 42:293–296, 1988.
10. Black, D. M., Nevitt, M. C., Palermo, L., et al.: The study of osteoporotic fractures research group. Prediction of new vertebral deformities. J. Bone Miner. Res. 8(suppl. 1):S135, 1993.
11. Brinckmann, P., Biggemann, M., and Hilweg, D.: Fatigue fracture of human lumbar vertebrae. Clin. Biomech. Suppl. 1:1–23, 1988.
12. Brinckmann, P., Biggemann, M., and Hilweg, D.: Prediction of the compressive strength of human lumbar vertebrae. Spine 14:606–610, 1989.
13. Brinckmann, P., Frobin, W., Biggemann, M., et al.: Quantification of overload injuries to thoracolumbar vertebrae and discs in persons exposed to heavy physical exertions or vibration at the workplace. Part I. The shape of vertebrae and intervertebral discs—study of a young, healthy population and a middle-aged control group. Clin. Biomech. 9(suppl. 1), 1994.
14. Brown, T., Hansen, R. J., and Yorra, A. J.: Some mechanical tests on the lumbosacral spine with particular reference to the intervertebral discs. J. Bone Joint Surg. 5A:1135–1164, 1957.
15. Burger, H., van Daele, P. L. A., Algra, D., et al.: Vertebral fractures as a risk factor for developing future non-vertebral fractures. J. Bone Miner. Res. 8(suppl. 1): S326, 1993.
16. Caldwell, R. A.: Observations on the incidence, aetiology and pathology of senile osteoporosis. J. Clin. Pathol. 15:421–431, 1962.
17. Carter, D. R., and Hayes, W. C.: Bone compressive strength: The influence of density and strain rate. Science 194:1174–1176, 1976.
18. Carter, D. R.: Mechanical loading history and skeletal biology. J. Biomech. 20:1095–1109, 1987.

19. Carter, D. R., Orr, T. E., and Fyrhie, D. P.: Relationships between loading history and femoral cancellous bone architecture. J. Biomech. 22:231–244, 1989.
20. Cheal, E. J., Snyder, B. D., Nunamaker, D. M., and Hayes, W. C.: Trabecular bone remodeling around smooth and porous implants in the equine patellar model. J. Biomech. 20:1121–1134, 1987.
21. Chevalier, F., Laval-Jeantet, A. M., Laval-Jeantet, M., and Bergot, C.: CT image analysis of the vertebral trabecular network in vivo. Calcif. Tissue Int. 51:8–13, 1992.
22. Currey, J. D.: Effects of differences in mineralization on the mechanical properties of bone. Philos. Trans. R. Soc. Lond. [Biol.] 13:509–518, 1984.
22a. Currey, J. D.: Power law models for the mechanical properties of cancellous bone. Eng. Med. 15:153–154, 1986.
23. Currey, J. D.: The effects of porosity and mineral content on the Young's modulus of elasticity of compact bone. J. Biomech. 21:131–139, 1988.
24. Dalstra, M., Huiskes, R., Odgaard, A., and van Erning, L.: Mechanical and textural properties of pelvic trabecular bone. J. Biomech. 26:523–535, 1993.
25. Delling, G.: Age-related bone changes. Pathology 58:117–147, 1978.
26. Dickie, D. L., Goldstein, S. A., Flynn, M. J., et al.: Vertebral rBMD distributions and fracture characteristics: In vitro and in vivo results. Trans. Orthop. Res. Soc. 13:368, 1988.
27. Dunn, W. L., Wahner, H. W., and Riggs, B. L.: Measurement of bone mineral content in human vertebrae and hip by dual photon absorptiometry. Radiology 136:485–487, 1980.
28. Dyson, E. D., Jackson, C. K., and Whitehouse, W. J.: Scanning electron microscope studies of human trabecular bone. Nature 225:957–959, 1970.
29. Edwards, W. T., McBroom, R. C., and Hayes, W. C.: Variation of density in the vertebral body measured by quantitative computed tomography. Trans. Orthop. Res. Soc. 11:205, 1986.
30. Eie, N.: Load capacity of the low back. J. Oslo City Hosp. 4:75–98, 1966.
31. Eriksson, S. A., Isberg, B. O., and Lindgren, J. U.: Prediction of vertebral strength by dual photon absorptiometry and quantitative computed tomography. Calcif. Tissue Int. 44:243–250, 1989.
32. Evans, F. G., and Lissner, H. R.: Biomechanical studies on the lumbar spine and pelvis. J. Bone Joint Surg. 2A:278–290, 1959.
33. Evans, F. G.: Mechanical Properties of Bone. Springfield, IL, Charles C Thomas, 1973.
34. Farfan, J.: Mechanical Disorders of the Low Back. Philadelphia, Lea & Febiger, 1973.
35. Feldkamp, L. A., Goldstein, S. A., Parfitt, M. A., et al.: The direct examination of three-dimensional bone architecture in vitro by computed tomography. J. Bone Miner. Res. 4:3–11, 1989.
36. Freeman, M. A. R., Todd, R. C., and Pirie, C. J.: The role of fatigue in the pathogenesis of senile femoral neck fractures. J. Bone Joint Surg. 56B:698–702, 1974.
37. Frost, H. M.: Laws and Bone Structure, Springfield, IL, Charles C Thomas, 1964.
38. Frost, H. M.: Mathematical Elements of Lamellar Bone Remodelling. Springfield, IL, Charles C Thomas, 1964.
39. Frost, H. M.: The pathomechanics of osteoporosis. Clin. Orthop. 200:198–225, 1985.
40. Frost, H. M.: Structural adaptations to mechanical usage (SATMU): 1. Redefining Wolff's law: The bone modelling problem. Anat. Rec. 226:403–413, 1990.
41. Frost, H. M.: Structural adaptations to mechanical usage (SATMU): 2. Redefining Wolff's law: The bone remodelling problem. Anat. Rec. 226:414–422, 1990.
42. Frost, H. M.: Perspective: The role of changes in mechanical usage setpoints in the pathogenesis of osteoporosis. J. Bone Miner. Res. 7:253–261, 1992.
43. Frost, H. M.: Suggested fundamental concepts in skeletal physiology. Calcif. Tissue Int. 52:1–4, 1993.
44. Galante, J., Rostoker, W., and Ray, R. D.: Physical properties of trabecular bone. Calcif. Tissue Res. 5:236–246, 1970.
45. Gallagher, J. C., Hedlund, L. R., Stoner, S., and Meeger, C.: Vertebral morphometry: Normative data. Bone Miner. 4:189–196, 1988.
46. Genant, H. K., Cann, C. E., Ettinger, B., et al.: Quantitative computed tomography for spinal mineral measurement. Current status. J. Comput. Assist. Tomogr. 9:602–604, 1985.
47. Genant, H. K., Wu, C. Y., van Kuijk, C., et al.: Vertebral fracture assessment using a semiquantitative technique. J. Bone Miner. Res. 8:1137–1148, 1993.
48. Gershon-Cohen, J., Rechtman, A. M., and Schraer, H.: Asymptomatic fractures in osteoporotic spines of the aged. JAMA 153:625–627, 1953.
49. Gibson, L. J., and Ashby, M. F.: The mechanics of three-dimensional cellular materials. Proc. R. Soc. Lond. A382:43–59, 1982.
50. Gibson, L. J.: The mechanical behaviour of cancellous bone. J. Biomech. 18:317–328, 1985.
51. Goldstein, S. A.: The mechanical properties of trabecular bone: Dependence on anatomic location and function. J. Biomech. 20 1055–1061, 1987.
52. Goulet, R. W., Feldkamp, L. A., Kubinski, D. J., and Goldstein, S. A.: Predicting the architectural orientation of trabecular bone. Trans. Orthop. Res. Soc. 14:263, 1989.
53. Granhed, H., Hansson, T., and Jonson, R.: Mineral content and ultimate compressive strength of lumbar vertebrae. A cadaver study. Acta Orthop. Scand. 60:105–109, 1989.
54. Hansson, T.: Bone Mineral Content and Biomechanical Properties of Lumbar Vertebrae. Thesis. Gothenburg, Sweden, Gothenburg University, 1977.
55. Hansson, T., and Roos, B.: The bone mineral content of the lumbar spine at the time of the first vertebral crush fracture. Trans. Orthop. Res. Soc. 5:195, 1980.
56. Hansson, T., Roos, B., and Nachemson, A.: The bone mineral content and ultimate compressive strength in lumbar vertebrae. Spine 1:46–55, 1980.
57. Hansson, T., and Roos, B.: The relation between bone mineral content, experimental compression fractures and disc degeneration in lumbar vertebrae. Spine 2:147–153, 1981.
58. Hansson, T., and Roos, B.: Microcalluses of the trabeculae in lumbar vertebrae and their relation to the bone mineral content. Spine 4:375–380, 1981.

59. Hansson, T., Keller, T., and Panjabi, M. M.: A study of the compressive properties of lumbar vertebral trabeculae: Effects of tissue characteristics. Spine 12:56–62, 1987.
60. Hansson, T., Keller, T., and Jonson, R.: Fatigue fracture morphology in human lumbar motion segments. J. Spinal Disord. 1:33–38, 1988.
61. Harrigan, T. P., and Mann, R. W.: Characterization of microstructural anisotropy in orthotropic materials using a second rank tensor. J. Mater. Sci. 19:761–767, 1984.
62. Harris, R. I., and Macnab, I.: Structural changes in the lumbar intervertebral discs: Their relationship to low back pain and sciatica. J. Bone Joint Surg. 36:304–322, 1954.
63. Hartman, W. F.: Deformation and failure of spinal materials. Exp. Mech. 3:98–103, 1974.
64. Hedlund, L. R., and Gallagher, J. C.: Vertebral morphometry in diagnosis of spinal fractures. Bone Miner. 5:59–67, 1988.
65. Hedlund, L. R., Gallagher, J. C., Meeger, C., et al.: Change in vertebral shape in spinal osteoporosis. Calcif. Tissue Int. 44:168–172, 1989.
66. Hodgskinson, R., and Currey, J. D.: Effects of structural variation on the Young's modulus of non-human cancellous bone. Proc. Inst. Mech. Eng. [H] 204:43–52, 1990.
67. Hodgskinson, R., and Currey, J. D.: The effect of variation in structure on the Young's modulus of cancellous bone: A comparison of human and non-human material. Proc. Inst. Mech. Eng. [H] 204:43–52, 1990.
68. Hollister, S. J., Goldstein, S. A., Jepsen, K. J., and Goulet, R. W.: Continuum and microstructural stress morphology relationships for trabecular bone subject to controlled implant loads. Trans. Orthop. Res. Soc. 15:74, 1990.
69. Hurxthal, L. M.: Measurement of anterior vertebral compressions and biconcave vertebrae. Am. J. Roentgenol. 3:635–644, 1968.
70. Husby, T., Heiseth, A., Ronningen, H., and Alho, A.: Computed tomographic density of the femur related to rotating loading—a cadaver study. Trans. Orthop. Res. Soc. 14:107, 1989.
71. Jensen, G. F., Christiansen, C., Boesen, J., et al.: Epidemiology of postmenopausal spinal and long bone fractures: A unifying approach to postmenopausal osteoporosis. Clin. Orthop. 166:75–81, 1982.
72. Jowsey, J., Phil, D., Kelly, P. J., et al.: Quantitative microradiographic studies of normal and osteoporotic bone. J. Bone Joint Surg. 47A:785–806, 1965.
73. Kazarian, L., and Graves, G. A.: Compressive strength characteristics of the human vertebral centrum. Spine 1:1–14, 1977.
74. Keller, T. S., Hansson, T. H., Abram, A. C., et al.: Regional variations in the compressive properties of lumbar vertebral trabeculae: Effects of disc degeneration. Spine 14:1012–1019, 1989.
75. Keller, T. S., and Spengler, D. M.: Regulation of bone stress and strain in the immature and mature rat femur. J. Biomech. 22:1115–1128, 1989.
76. Keller, T. S., Moeljanto, E., Main, J. A., and Spengler, D. M.: Distribution and orientation of bone in the human lumbar vertebral centrum. J. Spinal Disord. 5:60–74, 1992.
77. Keller, T. S., Zhu, M., and Pope, M. H.: Fracture risk associated with changes in vertebral architecture: Implications for the aging spine. International Society for the Study of the Lumbar Spine, Chicago, IL, 1992, pp. 114–115.
78. Keller, T. S., Ziv, I., Moeljanto, E., and Spengler, D. M.: Interdependence of lumbar disc and subdiscal bone properties: A report of the normal and degenerated spine. J. Spinal Disord. 6:106–113, 1993.
79. Keller, T.: Predicting the compressive mechanical behavior of bone. J. Biomech. 27:1159–1168, 1994.
80. Kleerekoper, M., Parfitt, A. M., and Ellis, B. I.: Measurement of vertebral fracture rates in osteoporosis. In Christiansen, C., Arnaud, C. D., Nordin, B. E. C., et al. (eds.): Osteoporosis. Glostrup, Denmark, Aalborg Stiftsborgtrykkeri, 1984, pp. 103–109.
81. Kuo, A. D., and Carter, D. R.: Computational methods for analyzing the structure of cancellous bone in planar sections. J. Orthop. Res. 9:918–931, 1991.
82. Lane, J. M., and Vigorita, V. J.: Current Concepts Review. Osteoporosis. J. Bone Joint Surg. 65A:274–278, 1983.
83. Layton, M. W., Goldstein, S. A., Goulet, R. W., et al.: Examination of subchondral bone in experimental osteoarthritis by microscopic computed axial tomography. Arthritis Rheum. 31:1400–1405, 1988.
84. LeBlanc, A. D., Evans, H. J., March, C., et al.: Precision of dual photon absorptiometry measurements. J. Nucl. Med. 27:1362–1365, 1986.
85. Lindahl, O.: Mechanical properties of dried defatted spongy bone. Acta Orthop. Scand. 47:11–19, 1976.
86. Mazess, R. B.: Bone densitometry for clinical diagnosis and monitoring. In DeLuca, H. G., and Mazess, R. B. (eds.): Osteoporosis: Physiological Basis, Assessment, and Treatment. New York, Elsevier Science, 1990.
87. McBroom, R. J., Hayes, W. C., Edwards, W. T., et al.: Prediction of vertebral body compressive fracture using quantitative computed tomography. J. Bone Joint Surg. 67A:1206–1214, 1985.
88. McCubbrey, D. A., Cody, D. D., Kuhn, J. L., et al.: Static and fatigue failure properties of thoracic and lumbar vertebral bodies and their relation to regional density. Trans. Orthop. Res. Soc. 15:178, 1990.
89. Melton, L. J., and Riggs, B. J.: Epidemiology of age-related fractures. In Avioli, L. V. (ed.): The Osteoporotic Syndrome. Orlando, FL, Grune & Stratton, 1983, p. 45.
90. Melton, L. J.: Epidemiology of vertebral fractures. Proceedings of the International Symposium on Osteoporosis, Aalborg, Denmark, September 27-October 2, 1987.
91. Mertz, W. A., and Schenk, R. K.: Quantitative structural analysis of human cancellous bone. Acta Anat. 75:54–66, 1970.
92. Meunier, P. J.: Bone histomorphometry in osteoporotic states. In Barzel, U. S. (ed.): Osteoporosis II. New York, Grune & Stratton, 1979, p. 27.
93. Nachemson, A., and Elfström, G.: Intravital dynamic pressure measurements in lumbar discs. Scand. J. Rehabil. Med. Suppl 1:1–40, 1970.
94. Neumann, P., Osvalder, A. L., Nordwall, A., et al.: The ultimate flexural strength of the lumbar spine and vertebral bone mineral content. J. Spinal Disord. 6:314–323, 1993.

95. Neumann, P., Ekström, L., Keller, T., et al.: Aging, vertebral density, and disc degeneration alter the human anterior longitudinal ligament. J. Orthop. Res. 12:103–112, 1994.
96. Obrandt, K. J., Bengner, U., Johnell, O., et al.: Is there a secular change in the incidence of hip fractures? Calcif. Tissue Int. 44:175–178, 1988.
97. Örtoft, G., Mosekilde, L., Hasling, C., et al.: Estimation of vertebral body strength by dual photon absorptiometry in elderly individuals: Comparison between measurements of total vertebral and vertebral body bone mineral. Bone 14:667–673, 1993.
98. Parfitt, A. M., Mathews, C. H. E., Villanueva, A. R., and Kleerekoper, M.: Relationship between surface, volume, and thickness of iliac trabecular bone in aging and osteoporosis. Implications for the microanatomic and cellular mechanism of bone loss. J. Clin. Invest. 72:1396–1409, 1983.
99. Perey, O.: Fracture of the vertebral end-plate in the lumbar spine; an experimental biomechanical investigation. Acta Orthop. Scand. Suppl. 25:1–101, 1957.
100. Plaue, R.: Das frakturverhalten von Brust—und Lendenwirbelkörpern. Z. Orthop. 110:357–362, 1972.
101. Rice, J. C., Cowin, S. C., and Bowman, J. A.: On the dependence of the elasticity and strength of cancellous bone on apparent density. J. Biomech. 21:155–168, 1988.
102. Riggs, B. L., and Melton, L. J., III: Medical progress: Involutional osteoporosis. N. Engl. J. Med. 314:1676–1684, 1986.
103. Roaf, R.: A study of the mechanics of spinal injuries. J. Bone Joint Surg. 4B:810–823, 1960.
104. Rockoff, S. D., Zettner, A., and Albright, J.: Radiographic trabecular quantitation of human lumbar vertebrae in situ. Invest. Radiol. 2:339–352, 1967.
105. Rockoff, S. D., Sweet, E., and Bleustein, J.: The relative contribution of trabecular, and cortical bone to the strength of human lumbar vertebrae. Calcif. Tissue Res. 3:163–175, 1969.
106. Roesler, H.: Some historical remarks on the theory of cancellous bone structure (Wolff's law). In Cowin, S. C. (ed.): Mechanical Properties of Bone, Vol. 45. New York, American Society of Mechanical Engineers, 1981, pp. 27–42.
107. Rolander, S. D., and Blair, W. E.: Deformation and fracture of the lumbar vertebral end-plate. Orthop. Clin. North Am. 1:75–81, 1975.
108. Ross, P. D., Davis, J. W., Epstein, R. S., et al.: Ability of vertebral dimensions from a single radiograph to identify fractures. Calcif. Tissue Int. 51:95–99, 1992.
109. Rubin, C. T., Mcloed, K. J., and Bain, S. D.: Functional strains and cortical adaptation: Epigenetic assurance of skeletal integrity. J. Biomech. 23:43–54, 1990.
110. Ruff, S.: Brief acceleration: Less than one second. German Aviat. Med. World War II, 1:584–597, 1950.
111. Saltykov, S. A.: Stereometric Metallography, 2nd Ed., Metallurgizdat, Moscow, 1958.
112. Saville, P. D.: The syndrome of spinal osteoporosis. Clin. Endocrin. Metabol. 2:177–185, 1973.
113. Schmorl, G., and Junghanns, H.: The Human Spine in Health and Disease. New York, Grune & Stratton, 1959.
114. Shane, E.: Osteoporosis In Manolagas, S. C., and Olefsky, J. M. (eds.): Metabolic Bone and Mineral Disorders. New York, Churchill Livingstone, 1988, pp. 151–192.
115. Shirazi-Adl, Shrivastava, S. C., and Ahmed, A. M.: Stress analysis of the lumbar disc-body unit in compression. A three-dimensional nonlinear finite element study. Spine 9:120–134, 1984.
116. Smith, M. D., Cody, D. D., Emery, S. E., and Meyers, S.: Prediction of bone graft mechanical properties using computed tomography. Trans. Orthop. Res. Soc. 16:642, 1991.
117. Snyder, B. D., Hayes, W. C., and Saltzman, W. M.: A general purpose, automated system for the quantitative description of anisotropic structures. Trans. Eur. Soc. of Biomech. 5:250, 1986.
118. Snyder, B. D., Cheal, E. J., Hipp, J. A., and Hayes, W. C.: Anisotropic structure property relation for trabecular bone. Trans. Orthop. Res. Soc. 14:262, 1989.
119. Spector, T. D., McCloskey, E. V., Doyle, D. V., et al.: Prevalence of vertebral fracture in women and the relationship with bone density and symptoms: The Chingford study. J. Bone Miner. Res. 8:817–822, 1993.
120. Spencer, N. E., Steiger, P., Cummings, S. R., et al.: Placement of points for digitizing spine films. J. Bone Miner. Res. 5(suppl. 2): S247, 1990.
121. Stone, J. L., Snyder, B. D., Hayes, W. C., and Strang, G. L.: Three-dimensional stress-morphology analysis of trabecular bone. Trans. Orthop. Res. Soc. 9:199, 1984.
122. Struhl, S., Goldstein, S. A., Dickie, D. L., et al.: The distribution of mechanical properties of trabecular bone within vertebral bodies and iliac crests: Correlation with computed tomography. Trans. Orthop. Res. Soc. 12:262, 1987.
123. Todd, R. C., Freeman, M. A. R., and Pirie, C. J.: Isolated trabecular fatigue fractures in the femoral head. J. Bone Joint Surg. 4B:723–728, 1972.
124. Turner, C. H., Cowin, S. C., Rho, J. Y., et al.: The fabric dependence of the orthotropic elastic constants of cancellous bone. J. Biomech. 23:549–561, 1990.
125. Underwood, E. E.: Quantitative Stereology, 2nd Ed. Moscow, Metallurgizdat, 1970.
125a. United States Department of Commerce: Statistical Abstract of the United States, Ed. 106. Washington, DC, Bureau of the Census, 1986.
126. Vernon-Roberts, B., and Pirie, C. J.: Healing trabecular microfractures in the bodies of lumbar vertebrae. Ann. Rheum. Dis. 32:406–412, 1973.
127. von Meyer, G. H.: Die architectur der spongiosa. Arach. Anat. Physiol. Wiss. (Med. Reich. DuBois-Reymonds Arch.) 34:615–628, 1867.
128. Wahner, W. H., Dunn, W. L., Mazess, R. B., et al.: Dual-photon Gd-153 absorptiometry of bone. Radiology 156:203–206, 1985.
129. Weaver, J. K., and Chalmers, J.: Cancellous bone: Its strength and changes with aging and an evaluation of some methods for measuring its mineral content. J. Bone Joint Surg. 2A:289–299, 1966.
130. Weibel, E. R., and Elias, H. E.: Quantitative Methods in Morphology. Berlin, Springer-Verlag, 1967.
131. Weinreb, M., Rodan, G. A., and Thompson, D. D.: Osteopenia in the immobilized rat hind limb is associated with increased bone resorption and

decreased bone formation. Bone 10:187–194, 1989.
132. Whitehouse, W. J., Dyson, E. D., and Jackson, C. K.: The scanning electron microscope in studies of trabecular bone from the human vertebral body. J. Anat. 108:481–496, 1974.
133. Whitehouse, W. J.: The quantitative morphology of anisotropic trabecular bone. J. Microsc. 101:153–168, 1974.
134. Whitehouse, W. J.: Cancellous bone in the anterior part of the iliac crest. Calcif. Tissue Res. 23:67–76, 1977.
135. Wolff, J.: Das Gesetz der Transformation der Knochen. Berlin, Hirschwald, 1892.
136. Zetterberg, C., Mannius, S., Mellström, D., et al.: Osteoporosis and back pain in the elderly. A controlled epidemiologic and radiographic study. Spine 15:783–786, 1990.
137. Zetterberg, C., Sjöstedt, Å, Zidén, L., et al.: Epidemiology of hip fractures in Göteborg, Sweden 1940–1991. Scandinavian Orthopaedic Association. Proceedings of the 47th Assembly, Reykjavik, Iceland, June 8–11. Acta Orthop. Scand. 65(suppl. 260):30, 1994.
138. Zhu, M., Keller, T. S., Moeljanto, E., and Spengler, D. M.: Multiplanar variations in the structural characteristics of cancellous bone. Bone 15:251–259, 1994.
139. Ziv, I.: The Changes in the Properties of the Intervertebral Disc and Facet Cartilage in Ageing and Degeneration. Doctoral thesis. Haifa, Israel, Technion, Israel Institute of Technology, 1989.

17

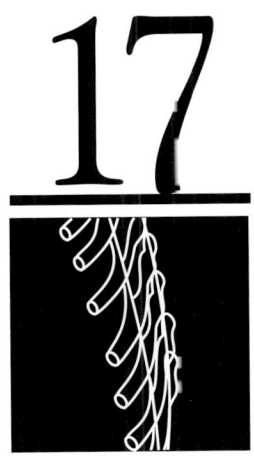

Rehabilitation

Education and Training

MICHELE CRITES BATTIÉ
MARGARETA NORDIN

No clear consensus exists on the conditions underlying most cases of back symptoms, their causes, or their treatment.[18] Thus, one could question the value of patient education given the current state of knowledge. However, what is known about nonspecific low back problems may help patients to control their symptoms and reduce associated anxieties and may provide a basis for more informed decisions about health care. In addition, patient satisfaction[10, 11, 14] and even speed of recovery[5, 44] depend in part on the information that the patient receives and the style in which it is given.

Nonspecific low back pain cases constitute the vast majority of low back problems among patients seeking health care and include ailments of the back in the lumbar region with or without radiating pain. The natural history of nonspecific low back pain is encouraging, with about 75% of patients recovering within 4 weeks of the onset of pain.[41] The symptoms are considered acute during the first week and subacute in the period from 7 days to 7 weeks. Spitzer and colleagues[41] offered these classifications as operational guidelines. They are also useful as time indicators related to patient care, which should include the prevention of chronicity as a primary focus.

The classic theory of illness implies that interaction between a person and a disease leads to illness.[50] In the case of nonspecific low back pain, the interaction is complex, and a biopsychosocial model is necessary to understand the problem more fully and to prevent long-term disability.[45] Behaviors related to health and pain are deeply rooted, and an effective clinician-patient relationship is needed that allows an effective exchange of information, including education of the patient.

This discussion focuses on education for patients with acute or subacute nonspecific low back pain. Patient information can include verbal advice and information from health care providers, printed material, and/or information in an audiovisual format. This approach to education is less formal than a back school, a structured program of group sessions that is usually conducted in a classroom setting, includes handouts, and is taught by a health care provider with special interest in low back pain.

THE LEARNING PROCESS

A person given new information tends to select what is personally relevant to incorporate into prior knowledge. If the information goes far beyond the person's level of education, it is either dismissed or changed according to what is understood.[35] This process is called adaptation.[37] The adaptation process is an equilibrium between assimilation and accommodation that is idiosyncratic. The patient modifies the information and constructs personal theories.

Providing information to the patient with back pain is a two-way process that involves both the patient's and the health care provider's concepts of and theories about the symptoms.[24] A patient seeing several health care providers for his or her low back symptoms may receive several explanations and diagnoses. This often creates chaos for the patient and increases the fear that something is seriously wrong. The educator must thus be sensitive to the patient's health-related beliefs, level of understanding, and prior experience with the health care system. If education is provided by a health care team, its members must have a common goal and provide and reinforce the same message to the patient. If a consistent message is not delivered to the patient, confusion arises, fear about a serious condition increases, and the patient may seek additional health care evaluations or treatments.

EDUCATION AND CLINICIAN-PATIENT INTERACTION

The first contact between the patient and the health care provider is crucial,[45] because it is the point at which trust is established. At the initial encounter, knowledge can be transferred and the fear of a serious condition decreased for the patient. Studies suggest that, for ill-defined symptomatic conditions, communication between the clinician and the patient may have more impact on patient outcomes than does the specific treatment choice. In particular, agreement about the nature of the problem and the provider's confidence in his or her diagnosis and optimism about recovery can affect patient outcomes.[5, 10, 21, 26, 42, 44]

Providing information that addresses several basic patient expectations and concerns can increase the chances that the consultation will be satisfying and effective. These expectations include an adequate explanation of the problem, a sense of the prognosis (which in the case of nonspecific acute or subacute back symptoms should be generally positive), recommendations for controlling symptoms, and activity guidelines that take into account the patient's work and leisure activities.

Provide an Adequate Explanation of the Condition

Persons with symptoms often visit clinicians more for information than for treatment. As Barksy[4] noted, patients "seek not so much palliation or cure but rather knowledge and education: a diagnostic label for their condition, an etiologic explanation, a pathophysiologic model or a prognostic estimate." He went on to cite evidence that many patients with pain want information about etiology even more than they want analgesics. Although it may not be possible to provide a specific diagnosis for the majority of patients with back pain, they can be reassured that serious disease is not present in most cases and that rapid improvement is likely. The clinician can also offer an explanation of the types of anatomic structures and injury or illness mechanisms that may be involved.[14]

Deyo and Diehl[14] found that the most frequently cited source of dissatisfaction among patients with low back pain was failure to receive an adequate explanation of the problem. These patients were less satisfied with their medical office visit, less likely to want to consult the same physician again, and likely to want more diagnostic tests than were patients who received an adequate explanation of their problem. Meeting this patient expectation was not associated with more physician time or diagnostic testing. In contrast, patients who thought that they did not receive a satisfactory explanation desired more tests and were more concerned about the possibility of serious illness.

Bass and colleagues[5] conducted a study to

determine which actions of family practice physicians influence the outcome of symptoms, including back and neck pain. The factor that was most strongly associated with early resolution of symptoms was agreement between the patient and the physician about the nature of the underlying problem. Other important prognostic factors were patient reports of stress, the presence of other psychosocial factors, and the duration of symptoms and medical history. Remarkably, there was no relationship between resolution of the patient's symptoms and the adequacy of history taking or physical examination, although the criteria for assessing these factors were not well described. The use of diagnostic tests or the prescription of drugs also had no significant effect on the resolution of symptoms. This finding is consistent with a British study[42] in which the prescription of medication for nonspecific problems had no effect on symptom resolution.

Abenhaim and colleagues[1] found that among approximately 2000 back-related workers' compensation cases in the province of Quebec, patients who were given a specific diagnosis incurred more time loss from work. The reasons for this could be that (1) the pathophysiologic progression for some specific diagnoses may be slower (e.g., sciatica) than for nonspecific back pain; (2) specific diagnoses may have been dealt with differently administratively; (3) a specific diagnosis may be associated with more diagnostic tests and consultations that delay return to work; or (4) labeling of a patient with a specific diagnosis can carry the message that the condition is serious and warrants more work loss. For example, a diagnosis of degenerative changes of the spine was classified as a disease. Thus, reassuring the patient that serious disease is not present in the case of nonspecific low back pain may be a critical component of discussions of likely diagnoses.

Set Positive, Realistic Expectations

Is there any point in a clinician's projecting confidence and positive expectations for recovery? The answer would appear to be a resounding yes. Thomas[44] asked this question in a randomized clinical trial examining the effects of providing a firm diagnosis and positive expectations of recovery, as opposed to expressing honest uncertainty about the diagnosis and recovery expectations. Two weeks after the consultation, patient satisfaction was significantly greater among patients who received a positive, confident consultation. Similarly, of those receiving positive expectations regarding prognosis, 64% recovered, as compared with 39% of those whose physicians expressed uncertainty. Prescribing versus not prescribing a medication (administering placebo) did not have a significant effect on satisfaction with care or length of time to recovery. The findings of this investigation demonstrate that patients with nonspecific pain symptoms associated with minor illness are more satisfied with care and more likely to recover from their illness within 2 weeks if they receive a positive, confident consultation rather than one that highlights uncertainty.

Another study by Fordyce and colleagues[21] lends further credence to the value of providing a plausible explanation of symptoms and positive expectations about recovery time to patients with nonspecific low back pain symptoms. They examined the effects of using a behavioral approach with medication and treatment activities based on the suspected structures involved and expected healing time, as contrasted with a more traditional treatment approach that responds to symptoms presented over time. Patients with the onset of back pain in the preceding 10 days were randomly assigned to either traditional or behavioral treatment methods and later compared on a set of outcome measures. Patients treated with the behavioral approach, using a diagnostic model with positive expectations of healing and time-contingent interventions, had significantly less claimed impairment at 9 to 12 months after treatment. The investigators concluded that the clinician "who would rely on patient definitions of pain or illness is at peril to promote chronicity."[21]

Furthermore, Bush and colleagues[10] found that patient satisfaction was related to physicians' confidence in their abilities to manage low back pain effectively. The patients of providers reporting more confidence were significantly more satisfied with the information they received than patients of less confident providers. These differences could not be explained by the physicians' years in practice, the length of the visit, the severity and duration of symptoms, or patient demographic factors. In particular, provider confidence was significantly related to patient satisfaction with the information received, but not to patient satisfaction with the caring nature of the provider or with the effectiveness of the treatment approach. These findings support other research demonstrating that patient satisfaction is influenced by how effectively clinicians communicate information.[14] Variations in the confidence with which information is conveyed may also explain, in part, why patients of chiropractors have reported more satisfaction with the information they received about their back problems than have patients of family practice physicians. The patients seeing chiropractors were more likely to affirm strongly that their provider seemed confident and comfortable in diagnosing and effectively treating their low back pain than were patients of family physicians (60% versus < 25%, respectively).[11]

Setting positive expectations and conveying such information in a confident manner appears to increase patient satisfaction and hasten recovery. Fortunately, for nonspecific back pain, there is every reason to be optimistic about the resolution of symptoms and return to normal activities. Recurrent bouts of back symptoms, however, are common and should be acknowledged. Although patients should be aware of the possibility of a recurrent episode, they can be reassured that these episodes are typically self-limited and may be easier to deal with given the patient's experiences in managing their present symptoms. There is also evidence to suggest that the risk of recurrences and their frequency may decrease with the passage of time since the last episode.[7]

Advise on Symptom Control

Over-the-counter medications, such as acetaminophen and aspirin, may benefit patients with nonspecific back symptoms, and they generally have fewer side effects than do prescription medications. In general, there is little evidence that prescription medications are more effective at alleviating back symptoms or returning patients to activity.[9] In addition, several studies have shown no increase in patient satisfaction when medication was prescribed for ill-defined symptomatic conditions, including back pain.[5, 44]

The greatest symptom relief may come simply with frequent changes of position and experimentation with different standing, sitting, and lying positions to find those that are most comfortable. Some suggestions for resting or work positions can also be offered on the basis of decreased spinal loads as determined by intradiscal pressure measurement studies and other biomechanical studies,[33, 48] as well as from clinical experience. Patients can be advised that heat or cold packs may offer some short-term symptom relief and that they can be applied conveniently at home while patients are resting in a comfortable position.

On the basis of national surveys in the United States, Deyo and Tsui-Wu[17] reported in 1987 that bed rest was the most frequently used treatment for low back pain. However, attitudes and practices regarding the prescription of bed rest have changed dramatically. This may be due, in part, to the results of two well-publicized, randomized clinical trials conducted in primary care medical practice.[15, 22] One study examined the effects of prescribing 2 versus 7 days of bed rest for patients with acute back pain without neurologic deficits. Patients who were prescribed 2 days of bed rest returned to work significantly sooner (3.1 versus 5.6 days) than did those prescribed 7 days. There were no significant between-group differences with respect to time until pain resolution and return of other functions. A similar study comparing recommendations of 4 days of bed rest versus none in patients without neurologic deficits who were seen in family practice clinics found that patients in the group that was not prescribed bed rest reported returning to their normal level of activities 42% sooner than those for whom bed rest was recommended. Again, there were no other significant differences in pain resolution.[22] These studies suggest that bed rest is not helpful in the resolution of back symptoms in patients without neurologic deficits and may serve only to delay return to work and other usual activities.

The reluctance to recommend bed rest was seen in a study in which 293 physical therapists were queried about how they would treat three hypothetic patients with back symptoms.[6a] None of the therapists recommended bed rest for the patient depicted as having chronic back pain or acute-recurrent symptoms, and only 35% of therapists recommended bed rest (mean of 1.8 days) for the patient with acute sciatica and neurologic deficit.[6a] Support for bed rest appears to have substantially decreased among other health care providers as well.[9]

Provide Recommendation for Work and Leisure Activities

Instead of being encouraged to be inactive, patients are more likely to be advised to stay active and to use discretion when engaging in specific activities that substantially increase the load on the spine, which may exacerbate symptoms.[8, 41] Physical activities such as walking, cycling, and swimming are commonly recommended, as is a gradual return to normal activities.[8, 41] If prolonged sitting exacerbates symptoms, as is the case in some patients, they can try changing positions at frequent intervals and, when possible, reclining slightly and using a small pillow or towel roll at the base of the lumbar spine.[2, 48] Some patients may also be able to adapt their work areas temporarily so that they can do some of their activities in more comfortable positions (e.g., standing).

In the early stages of recovery, minimizing heavy lifting, or at the very least avoiding lifting that involves twisting and bending, particularly in combination, is recommended.[3] The manner in which an object is lifted can influence the forces across the spine to a greater extent than the weight of the object. Although controversies still exist about the preferred lifting method, few clinicians would argue that getting the object as close to the body as possible and avoiding twisting while lifting are advisable to reduce the forces on the back, the intervertebral discs in particular.

By recognizing physical activity and return to work as important parts of the rehabilitation process, health care providers can play an important role in minimizing the negative consequences of work loss. General activity guidelines, as opposed to statements that patients can work or cannot work, give patients a clearer idea of activities to avoid or to engage in with caution, whatever their environment. Such guidelines also give the employer an opportunity to accommodate an employee's restrictions.

Provide Information for Better Health Care Consumerism

It has been argued that an effective relationship between the physician and the patient must include patient participation in medical decision-making.[40, 47] These studies note that communication rated as satisfactory is not necessarily effective communication. Encouraging patients to take an active role in their treatment may transform a satisfying relationship between the physician and the patient into an effective one.[10]

With greater public awareness of new diagnostic tools and medical innovations, clinicians may have to face some unrealistic patient expectations regarding diagnosis and symptom relief. At the same time, clinicians are under increasing pressure to use diagnostic tools and treatment interventions judiciously because of growing concerns about health care financing. It may become essential to provide adequate information to patients to alter their expectations about diagnosis and treatment while maintaining their satisfaction with care.

Deyo and colleagues[16] examined whether patient expectations about diagnostic tests could be altered by spending less than 5 minutes discussing information about the likely causes of back pain, the low yield of useful findings on roentgenograms, and the radiation involved. The study findings supported the effectiveness of this strategy for decreasing the use of diagnostic tests in the early management of low-risk patients while maintaining patient satisfaction. Other studies also provide evidence that the use of diagnostic tests and the prescription of medications are not important factors influencing satisfaction with care or length of recovery time among patients in whom severe disease is not suspected.[5, 44]

Consider Written Material as Adjunct to Education

Several studies suggest that providing written educational materials in the clinical setting can be an effective adjunct to verbal patient instruction and education.[23, 38] Written instructions in the therapy setting have been associated with higher compliance with exercise recommendations.[23] In the primary care setting, providing educational materials on back pain management, including how to control symptoms and when to seek medical advice, has been linked to reduced health care utilization during the subsequent year.[38] Conversely, unsolicited self-care brochures provided to the general population have yet to demonstrate an effect on subsequent health care utilization for back problems, although they have been successful in curbing utilization for some other conditions.[43]

A practical consideration in planning or selecting written materials is deciding which information is most important for patients to remember. Patients who are overburdened with too much written information may forget the most salient points.[25] Therefore, it may be advisable to be judicious with handouts or at least to highlight the more relevant facts and recommendations.

As computer technologies continue to develop and become a familiar means of accessing information, they will also begin to appear more frequently as educational tools in clinical settings.[34] Such technologies also allow interactive sessions that can be tailored to the patient's condition and specific interests. Deyo and others in the Back Pain Outcome Assessment Team are currently involved in efforts to determine whether the availability and use of interactive videodiscs can ease the educational burden for clinicians seeing patients with back symptoms and create more informed consumers of back care. The impact of the videodisc program on patient satisfaction, knowledge relevant to medical decision-making, and health care utilization are under investigation (Deyo, R.A., personal communication, 1994).

BACK SCHOOLS

Back schools are typically composed of a series of structured group sessions with the objective of transferring knowledge to help participants change their behavior and increase function. A back school has a defined content (e.g., information on anatomy, physiology, and the natural history of nonspecific or specific lower back pain). The goals often include teaching the group simple principles of nonpainful postures, relaxation techniques, ergonomic principles to apply to sport and work activities, and simple exercises. More than 50 articles have been published on the topic of back schools. These educational programs offer diverse messages and styles of presentation, resulting in obvious limitations in grouping all educational programs together to evaluate their efficacy. Nevertheless, several studies have attempted to examine the efficacy of group back education programs.[13, 27, 28, 31, 39] These reviews analyzed approximately 20 separate controlled trials of back schools, a half dozen of which included randomization.

The randomized controlled study by Berquist-Ullman and Larsson[7] performed in an occupational setting provides some evidence of the efficacy of back school with respect to promoting earlier return to work. At a 1-year follow-up, they found shorter duration of sick leave for patients attending a back school that included a work site visit compared with the duration of sick leave for patients receiving manipulation and shortwave diathermy treatment.

The efficacy of back schools for patients with subacute nonspecific low back pain in nonoccupational settings, however, is inconclusive. As stated by Klingenstierna,[28] "In treating LBP the main challenge is to beat the good natural prognosis. It seems unlikely that permanent behavioral changes would take place after a short time of education, as of a few back school sessions." The metaanalysis by Linton and Kamwendo[31] and Keijsers and associates[27] found that back school by itself appears to be, at most, marginally successful, although insufficient evidence was available. Studies on the efficacy of back school have encountered several problems, such as lack of an adequate control group, absence of blinded evaluation, and other design flaws.

In a review, Cohen and colleagues[13] uncovered 89 articles but only 13 met the inclusion criteria, based in part on quality of study design and the inclusion of a control group, for evaluating the effects of group education. It is interesting to note that they found poor agreement when raters were asked to score the quality of the educational content, which was characterized as good or very good by both raters in only two cases.

Although limited information provided in the articles may have biased the raters, this underscores the need to define what constitutes good educational curricula for patients with back pain. Cohen and colleagues[13] also brought up several points of importance for planning and evaluating future educational programs. These included setting reasonable goals with respect to the expected effects of the educational approach, such as the outcomes to be evaluated, and providing sufficient descriptions of objectives, content, and educational methods used in the interventions. These are required to repeat the work and to allow readers to interpret study results adequately.

COMBINED PROGRAMS, INCLUDING BACK SCHOOLS

In several notable studies, the back school has been used as an adjunct to extensive interventions to prevent long-term disability. Chöler[12] and Lindström and associates[29, 30] performed early intervention studies in the city of Gothenburg, Sweden. Chöler[12] performed a controlled trial of two urban populations. Persons off from work for 4 to 6 weeks owing to nonspecific low back pain participated in a program emphasizing return to work, which included a careful evaluation, the Swedish back school, fitness training, a site visit at work by a physical therapist trained in ergonomics, and when indicated, judicious use of surgery. This approach, using a multidisciplinary team that included an orthopedic surgeon, a physical therapist, and a nurse, was associated with 90% less disability than with the approach used for patients with back pain in another area of the city where the program was not provided. Lindström and colleagues[29, 30] used a similar approach in a randomized clinical trial with Volvo company employees, with similarly good results.

These programs point out the importance of a structured approach to nonspecific low back pain for symptoms and disability lasting 4 to 6 weeks.[21] They also emphasize the benefits of using a multidisciplinary team approach with return to activity and work as the primary objective. It should be noted, however, that both studies were conducted in Sweden, and the results may vary in other health care systems and cultures.

EDUCATION AND TRAINING IN THE WORKPLACE

Prevention of back pain in the workplace remains an elusive goal, but there is encouraging evidence suggesting that workplace-based programs focusing on preventing long-term disability may be effective.[6, 19, 20, 49] A key component of these programs has been educating management personnel in appropriate ways of responding to employees who report back problems.

Prolonged disability from back problems is often associated with a lack of follow-up and absence of concern from workplace personnel, the development of adversarial situations, and litigation. It appears that employers may be able to prevent many of these situations by appropriate training of supervisors, workplace medical personnel, and upper-level management.

Immediate supervisors, in particular, are in key positions to support return-to-work initiatives, to create a welcoming work environment, and to identify potential problems at the worksite that may influence the patient's return to normal activities. There is evidence that supervisor training on how to deal appropriately with musculoskeletal symptoms in the workplace can be effective in positively influencing both attitudes and behaviors.[32]

An example of a program focusing on changing the attitudes of management toward back problems was reported by Fitzler and Berger.[20] In this program, management personnel were trained in the positive acceptance of low back pain. An atmosphere was created in which workers were encouraged to report episodes of low back pain to the company clinic. Conservative, in-house treatment, including worker education, was provided by the company nurse. Attempts were made to keep the worker on the job, often with modified duties that were consistent with the worker's condition. If necessary, referrals were made to the company physician, and treatment and progress were closely monitored. During a 3-year period, workers' compensation costs for low back claims were reduced from more than $200,000 per year to less than $20,000 per year, a 10-fold decrease. The results are impressive, even though the study was uncontrolled.

Wood[50] also reported on the effects of a personnel program directed at minimizing the impact of back problems among hospital workers. He encouraged changes in managers' attitudes toward reports of low back pain and improvement of the quality and quantity of communications among all parties involved in the employee's care, particularly between the employee and workplace personnel. Gradual return to work was also organized if needed, for example, by part-time work, light duty, or other solutions. After adoption of the program, the proportion of high time loss claims demonstrated a significant decrease compared with the prior period (7.1% versus 1.7%). Another program designed to reduce back pain disability in a long-term health care facility involved informal training sessions of managers and supervisors in appropriately responding to reports of back pain.[6] The emphasis was on maintaining helpful, regular contact with the employee, beginning immediately after the report of symptoms and continuing throughout recovery, and providing temporary work modifications when necessary. The results suggest a significant effect, with a reduction in medical and indemnity costs of 77% in the year after the onset of the program, as compared with the mean costs of the prior 3 years. Similar decreases were not seen in other facilities during the year.

Although it is unlikely that any single approach can resolve all the problems surrounding back pain in the workplace, education and training of management and supervisors in dealing appropriately with reports of symptoms appears to be a fruitful area for further development and investigation. Interventions of this type are likely to be successful only through a commitment by management at the highest levels.

CONCLUSIONS

The information that the patient receives and the style in which it is given can improve patient satisfaction with care and can assist patients with nonspecific low back problems in controlling their symptoms and reducing associated anxieties. Education also provides a basis for more informed decisions about health care. As concluded in the low back problem guidelines, funded by the United States Agency for Health Care Policy and Research,[9] "evidence indicates that educating patients about back problems may reduce use of medical resources, decrease patient apprehension, and speed recovery."

Education given in the form of a structured back school, as the sole treatment, seems to be only marginally successful on the basis of evidence of efficacy in patients with subacute back symptoms. Back schools used as adjuncts to other multimodal approaches, in which return to activity and work is the primary objective, may enhance the success of the program, although further evaluation is necessary.

REFERENCES

1. Abenhaim, L., Rossignol, M., Gobeille, D., et al.: Prognostic consequences in the making of initial medical diagnosis of work-related back injuries. Spine 20:791–795, 1995.
2. Andersson, G. B. J., Ortengren, R., Nachemson, A., and Elfstrom, G.: Lumbar disc pressure and myoelectric back muscle activity during sitting: Studies on an experimental chair. Scand. J. Rehabil. Med. 6:104–114, 1974.
3. Andersson, G. B. J., Ortengren, R., and Nachemson, A.: Intradiscal pressure, intraabdominal pressure, and myoelectric back muscle activity related to posture and loading. Clin. Orthop. 129:156–164, 1977.
4. Barsky, A. J.: Hidden reasons some patients visit doctors. Ann. Intern. Med. 94:492–498, 1981.
5. Bass, M. J., Buck, C., Turner, L., et al.: The physicians actions and the outcome of illness in family practice. J. Fam. Pract. 23:43–47, 1986.
6. Battié, M. C.: The effect of improved communication and work accommodations on back injury claims. Presented at the International Society for the Study of the Lumbar Spine Meeting, Seattle, June 22–25, 1994.
6a. Battié, M. C., Cherkin, D. C., Dunn, R., and Wheeler, K.: Managing low back pain: Attitudes and treatment preferences of physical therapists. Phys. Ther. 74:219–226, 1994.
7. Berquist-Ullman, M., and Larsson, U.: Acute low back pain in industry. A controlled prospective study with special reference to therapy and confounding factors. Acta Orthop. Scand. 170:117, 1977.
8. Bigos, S. J., and Andary, M. T.: The practitioner's guide to the industrial back problem: Part 1. Helping the patient with the symptoms and pathology. Semin. Spine Surg. 4:42–54, 1992.
9. Bigos, S., Bower, O., Braen, G., et al.: Acute Low Back Problems in Adults. Clinical Practice Guideline no. 14. AHCPR Publication no. 95–0642. Rockville, MD, Agency for Health Care Policy and Re-

search, Public Health Service, U.S. Department of Health and Human Services, December 1994.
10. Bush, T., Cherkin, D., and Barlow, W.: The impact of physician attitudes on patient satisfaction with care for low back pain. Arch. Fam. Med. 2:301–305, 1993.
11. Cherkin, D., and MacCornack, F. A.: Patient evaluations of low back pain care from family physicians and chiropractors. West. J. Med. 150:351–355, 1989.
12. Chöler, U.: Back-pain attempt at a structured treatment program for patients with low-back pain (in Swedish). Stockholm, SPRI Report 188, Social Planeringsoch Rationaliserings Institutet Rapport, 1985.
13. Cohen, J. E., Goel, V., Frank, J. W., et al.: Group education interventions for people with low-back pain: An overview of the literature. Spine 19:1214–1222, 1994.
14. Deyo, R. A., and Diehl, A. K.: Patient satisfaction with medical care for low-back pain. Spine 11:28–30, 1986.
15. Deyo, R. A., Diehl, A. K., and Rosenthal, M.: How many days of bedrest for acute low back pain? A randomized clinical trial. N. Engl. J. Med. 315:1064–1070, 1986.
16. Deyo, R. A., Diehl, A. K., and Rosenthal, M.: Reducing roentgenography use: Can patient expectations be altered? Arch. Intern. Med. 147:141–145, 1987.
17. Deyo, R. A., and Tsui-Wu, Y.: Descriptive epidemiology of low back pain and its related medical care in the United States. Spine 12:264–268, 1987.
18. Deyo, R. A., Cherkin, D., Conrad, D., and Volinn, E.: Cost, controversy, crisis: Low back pain and the health of the public. Annu. Rev. Public Health 12:141–156, 1991.
19. Fitzler, S. L., and Berger, R. A.: Attitudinal change: The Chelsea back program. Occup. Health Saf. 51:24–26, 1982.
20. Fitzler, S. L., and Berger, R. A.: Chelsea back program: One year later. Occup. Health Saf. 52:52–54, 1983.
21. Fordyce, W. E., Brockway, J. A., Bergman, J. A., and Spengler, D.: Acute back pain: A control-group comparison of behavioral vs. traditional management methods. J. Behav. Med. 9:127–140, 1986.
22. Gilbert, J. R., Taylor, D. W. and Hildebrand, A.: Clinical trial of common treatments for low back pain in family practice. Br. J. Med. 291:791–794, 1985.
23. Glossop, E. S., Goldenberg, E., Smith, D. S., and Williams, M.: Patient compliance in back and neck pain. Physiotherapy 68:225–226, 1982.
24. Helman, C. G.: Feed a cold, starve a fever—folk model of infection in an English suburban community and their relation to medical treatment. Cult. Med. Psychiatry 3:107–137, 1978.
25. Joyce, C. R., Caple, G., Mason, M., et al.: Quantitative study of doctor-patient communication. Q. J. Med. 38:183–194, 1969.
26. Kaplan, S. H., Greenfield, S., and Ware, J. E.: Assessing the effects of physician-patient interactions on the outcomes of chronic disease. Med. Care 27(suppl.):S110–S127, 1989.
27. Keijsers, J., Bouter, L. M., and Meertens, R. M.: Validity and comparability of studies on the effects of back schools. Physiother. Theory Pract. 7:177–184, 1991.
28. Klingenstierna, U.: Back schools: A review. Crit. Rev. Phys. Rehab. Med. 3:155–171, 1991.
29. Lindström, I.: Mobility, strength, and fitness after a graded activity program for patients with subacute low back pain: A randomized prospective clinical study with a behavioral therapy approach. Spine 17:641–652, 1992.
30. Lindström, I., Öhlund, C., Eek, C., et al.: The effect of graded activity on patients with subacute low-back pain: A randomized prospective clinical study with an operant-conditioning behavioral approach. Phys. Ther. 72:279–293, 1992.
31. Linton, S. J., and Kamwendo, K.: Low back schools: A critical review. Phys. Ther. 67:1375–1383, 1987.
32. Linton, S. J.: A behavioral workshop for training immediate supervisors: The key to neck and back injuries? Percept. Motor Skills 73:1159–1170, 1991.
33. Nachemson, A.: The lumbar spine: An orthopaedic challenge. Spine 1:59, 1976.
34. Nelson, C. W.: Helping patients decide: From Hippocrates to videodiscs—an application for patients with low-back pain. J. Med. Sys. 12:1–10, 1988.
35. Nordin, M.: Back schools in the prevention of chronicity. Baillieres Clin. Rheumatol. 6:685–703, 1992.
36. Nordin, M., and Vischer, T. L.: Common low-back pain: Prevention of chronicity Baillieres Clin. Rheumatol. 6:685–704, 1992.
37. Piaget, J.: The Origin of Intelligence in the Child. Harmonds Worth, Penguin, 1977
38. Roland, M., and Dixon, M.: Randomized controlled trial of an educational booklet for patients presenting with back pain in general practice. J. R. Coll. Gen. Pract. 39:244–246, 1989.
39. Schlapbach, P.: Backschool. In Schlapbach, P., and Gerber, N. J. (eds.): Physiotherapy: Controlled Trials and Facts. Basel, Karger, 1991, pp. 25–46.
40. Speedling, E. J., and Rose, D. N.: Building an effective doctor-patient relationship: From patient satisfaction to patient participation Soc. Sci. Med. 21:115–120, 1985.
41. Spitzer, W. O., LeBlanc, F. E., and Dupuis, M.: Scientific approach to the assessment and management of activity-related spinal disorders. A monograph for clinicians. Report of the Quebec Task Force on Spinal Disorders. Spine 12(suppl.):S1–S59, 1987.
42. Starfield, B., Wray, C., Hess, K., et al.: The influence of patient-practitioner agreement on outcome of care. Am. J. Public Health 71:127–131, 1981.
43. Terry, P. E., and Pheley, A. The effect of self-care brochures on use of medical services. J. Occup. Med. 35:422–426, 1993.
44. Thomas, K. B.: General practice consultations: Is there any point in being positive? Br. Med. J. 294:1200–1202, 1987.
45. Waddell, G.: A new clinical mode for the treatment of low back pain. 1987 Volvo Award in Clinical Sciences. Spine 12:632–644, 1987.
46. Waddell, G.: Biopsychosocial analysis of low back pain. Baillieres Clin. Rheumatol. 6:523–557, 1992.
47. Wartman, S. A., Morlock, L. L., Malitz, F. E., and Palm, E. A.: Patient understanding and satisfaction as predictors of compliance. Med. Care 21:886–891, 1983.
48. Williams, M. M., Hawley, J. A., McKenzie, R. A., and van Wijmen, P. M.: A comparison of the effects

of two sitting postures on back and referred pain. Spine 16:1185–1191, 1991.
49. Wood, P. W. N.: The basis of rheumatologic practice, including nomenclature and classification. In Scott, J. T., (ed.): Copeman's Textbook of the Rheumatic Diseases, 6th Ed. London, Churchill Livingstone, 1986, pp. 59–142.
50. Wood, D. J.: Design and evaluation of a back injury prevention program within a geriatric hospital. Spine 12:77–82, 1987.

Mechanical Diagnosis and Therapy for Low Back Pain: Toward a Better Understanding

ROBIN McKENZIE
RONALD DONELSON

In the past, little was known about the likely causes of low back pain. Every health care specialty attempted to obtain for itself the responsibility for care of the back by administering the skills of that particular specialty.

This same situation persists today to a lesser degree. Some physicians propose that the answers to most back problems lie in the dispensing of medicines, pills, and embrocations, despite evidence that most cases of low back pain have mechanical and not inflammatory causes. Surgeons attempt to provide solutions by removing, replacing, or modifying various parts of the spinal column. Osteopaths and chiropractors have for almost 100 years applied spinal manipulative therapy (SMT) to the painful back, albeit for different reasons. Physiotherapists have traditionally used heat, massage, exercises, and electrotherapeutic modalities, which are still used in some clinics today. Only in the past 40 years have physiotherapists adopted manipulative procedures for spinal therapy.

Since Hippocrates first described methods of treatment of low back pain more than 2000 years ago, mechanical therapy has played a dominant role in the conservative care of patients with the disorder. Especially in the early stages of the problem, patients who seek treatment today usually receive some form of conservative care from a physiotherapist, a chiropractor, or an osteopath. These professionals dominate the field of health care providers who dispense mechanical therapies. The most common mechanical therapies used are exercise, traction, massage, mobilization, and spinal manipulation.

Health care consumers and providers will eventually recognize and choose the system of conservative care for low back pain that provides cost-effective therapies with the potential for long-term benefit. No treatment has yet been found to provide a reliable long-term positive outcome for people with low back pain.

Physicians can be bewildered by the claims and counterclaims from proponents of mechanical therapies. The authors attempt here to present an organized and rational approach to the mechanical treatment of spinal pain, one that is available and growing in use worldwide.

Increasing numbers of chiropractors have adopted some of the orthodox elements of medical practice and have attempted to moderate the extravagant claims of effectiveness in treating spinal and visceral disorders that persist from the past. Chiropractors are now employing modalities commonly seen in physiotherapy clinics. A patient with back pain will almost certainly receive SMT from the chiropractor. However, it is unnecessary and unacceptable to deliver manipulative therapy to every patient with back pain so that the few patients who really need it are treated appropriately. The chiropractic concept that an alteration of the pathologic state or modulation of the neurophysiologic structure is best achieved by the delivery of mechanical forces applied from without remains controversial and unproved.

The advantages of physiotherapy and its practice should encourage physicians to work interdependently with physiotherapists. Most physicians have neither the time nor the skills to deliver mechanical therapy in its current form. If patients are to receive appropriate current mechanical therapy, they must avail themselves of the services of a mechanical therapist.

Chiropractors, physiotherapists, and physicians, with new concepts in mechanical spinal pathology, can deliver a complete spectrum of mechanical forces (including SMT). These mechanical therapies, when applied with appropriate guidelines, can identify outcome predictors, remove clinical guesswork, and thereby prevent the waste of time through application of treatment modalities of dubious value.

During the next few years, clinicians who can provide the techniques of modern mechanical spinal therapy will have an opportunity to be the key medical professionals in the delivery of conservative care for mechanical disorders of the spine. They will earn that responsibility only by working within the medical profession and thereby subjecting themselves to stringent criticism necessary for scientific evolution.

To better understand the present predicament, it is necessary to review some aspects of the pathologic processes of low back pain, the treatments delivered, and the philosophies underlying various approaches.

PATHOLOGY

The pathologic processes or the micromechanical disorders that give rise to low back pain are still rather obscure, just as they were when Hippocrates first described his methods of treatment for "hyboma" or acute lumbar kyphosis.[26] Hippocrates believed the cause to be a backward dislocation of one vertebra onto another. Although the understanding of mechanical disorders has improved immensely, especially in the past 20 years, it is still not possible to identify with certainty or precision the offending structure causing pain in many cases.[42, 53]

Since the search for exact causes of low back pain began, every structure in the lower back has been suspect at one time or another. The reasons proposed for onset of pain have been innumerable. They have ranged from a witch's curse inflaming the nerves to the proverbial chill in the kidneys acquired by sitting in a draft. The search within the medical field for the causes of low back pain has narrowed to two structures likely to be involved in the production of most cases of mechanical back pain—the intervertebral disc and the zygapophyseal joint.[42]

The intervertebral disc, with its strong annulus fibrosus retaining the gel-like nucleus, probably attracts the most attention. Since its appearance in 1974, the journal *Spine* has published the results of innumerable studies aimed at the examination of intervertebral disc structure, function, pathologic changes, and treatment. Growing sophistication of and experience with magnetic resonance imaging and discographic interpretation are providing increasing understanding of the pain-producing mechanisms of the intervertebral disc.

The other mobile structure to capture the attention of those investigating back pain is the zygapophyseal joint. Although this joint is a probable source of pain, the precise pathologic conditions causing the pain have been difficult to identify.

The intervertebral disc changes that occur with the aging process are now well described, but disagreement remains about certain fundamental aspects.[7, 8, 58, 60] For example, it has been proposed that the intervertebral disc actually thickens, rather than thins, with aging.[58] This would inevitably lead to reappraisal of the hypothetic basis of some therapies.

Until more sophisticated technology provides an answer, the conceptualization regarding the reasons for treatment effectiveness must continue to remain flexible and open to change. However, there are certain established findings within orthopedics that many health care professionals either remain unaware of or choose to ignore.

Most disorders of the sacroiliac joint are inflammatory in origin. That true mechanical lesions occur is also recognized. They are uncommon and usually occur only after pregnancy.[14] Especially in North America and wherever therapists are receiving instruction from osteopaths, physiotherapists are "discovering" sacroiliac disorders in many of their patients.[49] It is likely that either these proponents are wrong or the literature is in error.

The historical obsession of physiotherapists with the musculature as the main source of backache has already been exposed.[10] Although orthopedic opinion does not support the proposal,[57] muscle imbalance and muscle strain are still considered by some physiotherapists to be common causes of persistent back pain and to influence the degree of lordosis.

It appears to be generally accepted medical opinion that the origin of most cases of low back pain is mechanical, probably arising in the intervertebral disc early in life and in the zygapophyseal joints much later.[7, 8, 40, 58, 60] The treatment of these particular problems, therefore, should mainly be mechanical. This fact has been recognized through 2500 years of recorded history, and most treatments provided today for the alleviation of back pain contain mechanical components.[51]

However, even with the most sophisticated and detailed investigations, the precise pathologic process responsible for back pain remains a mystery. In their attempts to fill this void, some therapists develop a system of pathology, and a consequent terminology, separate from and contradictory to that existing within the medical field as a whole, and orthopedics in particular. The medical profession has always been able to exert control over and put pressure on its wayward practitioners to protect the public from outrageous claims and methods of treatment. It is time that similar controls were applied to other practitioners treating disorders of the low back, especially when fringe concepts such as cranial suture mobilization, craniosacral techniques, and myofascial release techniques are being taught to physiotherapists without the slightest scientific evidence to support their therapeutic value for spinal pathologic conditions. If physiotherapists fail to curb the development of unscientific cultism, they deserve to lose what should be their rightful place in the medical team approach to back pain.

MEDICAL DIAGNOSIS

Although it is frustrating to accept that a complete or even a partial diagnosis is lacking at the start of therapies, mechanical low back pain has one important advantage over other disorders: a successful outcome of treatment does not depend on positive identification of the site of the lesion. Not until invasive treatment interventions are considered is the precise identification of the affected structure and its location critical.

A patient should be screened by the family medical practitioner before commencing mechanical spinal assessment and treatment. This is to identify nonmechanical and more serious pathologic processes. The mechanical practitioner is then able to define the mechanical problem.

MECHANICAL DIAGNOSIS

There is almost universal agreement that it is necessary to obtain detailed history from the patient. However, confusion reigns about the relevance of various questions posed by the examiner and answers provided by the patient and the best method of establishing a mechanical diagnosis.

Some clinicians attach much importance to a particular response; other clinicians disregard a given response as irrelevant. Some practitioners obtain large amounts of detailed information. This is idealistically appropriate but may not be practically useful. The clinician has a simple choice. If he or she obtains a large range of detailed information, much of it will be irrelevant or unreliable.[44] If the clinician is prepared to limit the information to mechanically relevant data, he or she will increase its reliability and relevance.

Some clinicians decide the nature of the mechanical problem principally by palpation. Some even claim to be able to determine by palpation alone the extent of the existing disorders. Many practitioners have found that rather gross losses of movement are detectable by palpation. However, intertherapist reliability, especially regarding palpatory skills, has been extremely poor.[24, 34, 43] A study comparing intertester reliability in the examination of sacroiliac dysfunction also showed extremely poor correlation: in 11 of 13 tests, agreement was 50% or less. Palpatory skills were fundamental to each of those 11 tests. All the therapists involved were experienced and trained in orthopedic manual therapy.[49] One study that indicates that palpation is reliable is flawed because no objective and independent assessors were involved.[28]

Clinicians who base their diagnosis mainly on palpatory findings tend to confuse whether the information they receive is derived from tactile sources alone—a claim that is frequently made—and whether the information is imparted to them by stressing the offending structure during the process of palpation, thus reproducing the patient's symptoms. Pain provoked by localized movement or pressure from palpation itself has been found to be more reliable in diagnosis.[39, 49] Therefore, practitioners who claim to have developed finely tuned palpation skills should recognize that only the ability to detect the patient's painful response is required to identify affected levels.

Chiropractors rely on a combination of diagnostic criteria, but mainly on information obtained from palpatory and radiographic findings. Both tools are of dubious value. Not only do many studies demonstrate palpatory assessment to be unreliable, but radiographs analyzed by either a chiropractor or a radiologist have been of little value in detecting the presence or absence of back pain.[22] As for the lavish claims made by chiropractors about the validity of radiographic findings in producing symptoms, no study of posttreatment radiographs has ever demonstrated that improvement or correction of the radiographic abnormalities parallels the recovery of the patient.

Physiotherapists in various parts of the world exhibit differing attitudes toward mechanical diagnosis. These have been influenced by the theories of three people in particular:

1. The osteopathic concepts and subsequent modifications developed by Freddy Kaltenborn, a Norwegian physiotherapist
2. The more orthopedically oriented approach of James Cyriax, an English physician
3. An Australian, Geoffrey Maitland, also a physiotherapist, who blended an orthopedic system with his own, using palpatory examination and treatment.

In the long run, however, regardless of the amount of data obtained from the patient's history, physical examination, and laboratory tests, the final decision as to the mechanical approach to be adopted is determined by the patient's response to the mechanical forces applied. The clinician's conception of the appropriate treatment is frequently, and must always be, overruled by the emergence of an adverse painful reaction to the initiation of that treatment.

After serious disorders not suited to mechanical therapy are excluded, the remaining nonspecific back problems (which affect the great majority of patients) are best evaluated by an organized, dynamic, mechanical assessment. This assessment can determine, usually at the initial evaluation, the status of the structures and their potential to react to certain maneuvers.

Pain Patterns

Intensity and Location

Persons familiar with this assessment approach realize that serious pathologic processes should already have been eliminated by medical screening. Radiologic assessment, when indicated, rules out most disorders unsuited to the mechanical approach. However, radiologic assessment is otherwise not helpful in determining patient suitability for mechanical treatment. Palpatory diagnosis is rejected because of the widespread incidence of tropism[11, 64] and an inability to demonstrate intertester reliability.

The search for diagnostic information can be based on mechanical principles. Increasing mechanical deformation of a structure results in increasing pain. It also causes radiating and referred pain. Reducing mechanical deformation obviously decreases the intensity and radiation of pain. The effects of mechanical forces on existing pain patterns are therefore likely to be more reliable in determining the nature of the mechanical disorder than any palpatory, radiologic, or other laboratory investigations.

Thus, a dynamic mechanical evaluation, using repetitive end-range motion with simultaneous monitoring of pain location and intensity, is recommended for examination and assessment. The consequent expression of pain, whether it is peripheral or central, determines the mechanical diagnosis. No longer is it sufficient to ask the patient during the physical examination if a single movement performed in each direction produces pain. It is paramount to assess the effects of repeating end-range movement in each direction. One movement may well increase peripheral symptoms, but what if repetition of that movement were to abolish those same symptoms? Judgment made on the performance of one movement may deprive the patient of appropriate therapy.

Usually, information derived from the initial assessment identifies patients with pathologic conditions unsuitable for the mechanical approach. This information may not identify the pathologic process itself but, under certain circumstances, can frequently indicate the nature of the problem.

Pain provocation and increase of referred symptoms while using all mechanical variables during the initial assessment is almost certain to expose discogenic disorders unsuited to mechanical treatment at the current stage of the disorder. A study has found that the ability of certain directions of spinal end-range test movements to centralize pain in patients with chronic disorders is highly reliable at predicting painful annular and nuclear morphologic changes as visualized by discography followed by axial imaging.[4] This study strongly suggested that reported changes in the location of pain may well be related to mechanical changes or shifts of nuclear content within the intervertebral disc.[4]

Information emerging from the use of repetitive end-range motion also identifies rapid responders to mechanical therapy and separates slow responders from nonresponders. The process enables the health care provider to determine at the initial visit the directions in which patients should and should not be moved (their directional preference).[16,17] Repeated movements that cause symptoms to diminish progressively or that cause pain to change from a peripheral to a more central location (centralization) (see Fig. 2) are considered desirable and should be encouraged and used as a basis for self-treatment. Movements that cause symptoms to become increasingly painful or to radiate to more distal sites are considered undesirable and, once identified, should be avoided. Likewise, positions that produce pain should be avoided and substituted by positions that abolish pain.

Conclusions from this evaluation process are based almost entirely on the effects produced on the patients' symptoms by repeating well-defined movements performed with the patient in the standing and recumbent positions (Fig. 1). Special importance is placed on the centralization of pain, which the authors regard as absolutely reliable in predicting successful outcome in the treatment of mechanical disorders of the low back (Fig. 2). The intertester reliability in interpreting both pain location[35,53] and changes in intensity, the effects of repeated test movements,[45,54] and the value of these findings in the selection of effective treatment interventions,[12,15] is increasingly supported in the literature.

Classification of Nonspecific Pain Syndromes

The effects of repetitive end-range motion on the patient's pain pattern identify three main categories in the spectrum of nonspecific pain: postural, dysfunction, and derangement. Each group is characterized by differing pain responses to the application of similar mechanical forces. Persons in each group describe similar pain responses to the application of similar mechanical forces. After assessment by repetitive motion, a classification of patients with nonspecific back pain is possible. The categories are the postural, dysfunction, and derangement syndromes. The derangement syndrome category is further subdivided into seven clinically identifiable entities.[38,39]

The precise means of identification and the concepts and methods of treatment of these syndromes are described in detail elsewhere.[38,39] Only a brief summary is provided here.

POSTURAL SYNDROME

Patients with the postural syndrome are usually younger than 30 years of age, have sedentary occupations, and frequently do not engage in regular exercise. Pain appears locally, usually adjacent to the midline of the spinal column. The affected person fre-

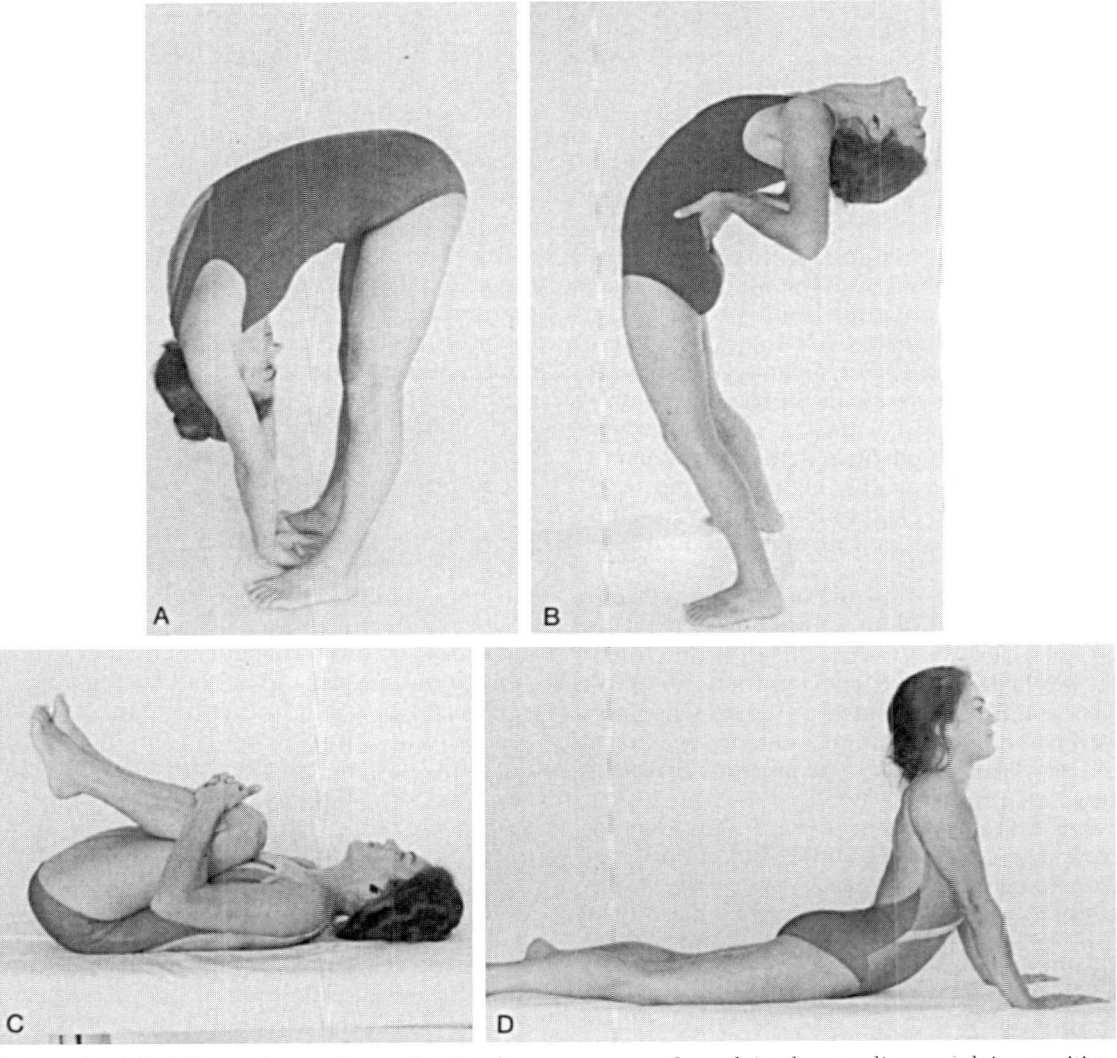

Figure 1. *A–D*, Effects of repeating well-defined movements performed in the standing and lying positions are observed.

quently reports pain felt either separately or simultaneously in the cervical, thoracic, and lumbar areas.

Pain from the postural syndrome is never induced by movement, is never referred, and is never constant. No pathologic process, no loss of movement, and no signs are found during the assessment with this syndrome. There is nothing to see.

Movements are normal, and patients are sometimes described as being hypermobile. The only objective information is discovered on examination of posture at the time of onset of pain, when the patient adopts a slouched posture and "hangs" at the end range of ligamentous and capsular tension.

The pain seems to be provoked by mechanical deformation of normal soft tissues occurring only when spinal segments are subjected to prolonged static loading with joints held at end range. This occurs most commonly when poor sitting or standing postures are adopted and when the person is required to maintain a prolonged bending or stooping position.

Pain from the postural syndrome probably arises from any part of the mobile segment or from the adjacent soft tissues. It is probably ligamentous, annular, or periarticular in origin. Described simply, postural pain eventually appears by, or arises from, prolonged overstretching of normal tissue.

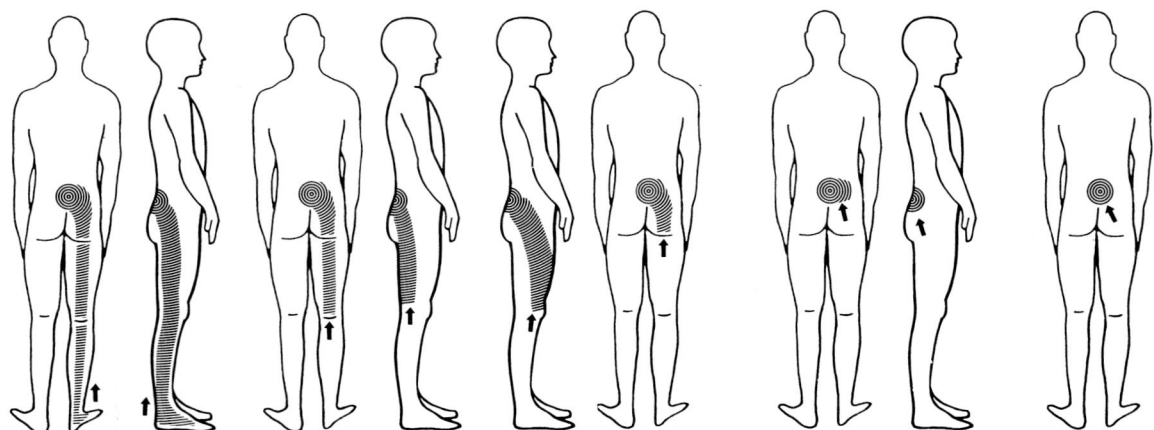

Figure 2. Progressive centralization of pain indicates the suitability of the exercise program.

DYSFUNCTION SYNDROME

Patients with the dysfunction syndrome are usually older than 30 years of age, except for those in whom trauma can be identified as the original cause. They commonly exhibit poor posture and are frequently sedentary.

Their pain usually remains after the initial acute symptoms resolve and may subsequently increase insidiously over a long period. Pain is provoked when they attempt full movement. Motion is restricted by mechanically deforming shortened, sensitive soft tissues in segments that have reduced elasticity and movement. The pain is always felt at end range, never during movement. With the exception of that due to an adherent nerve root, pain from dysfunction is never referred.

The loss of movement evident in the dysfunction syndrome arises from two common causes. The first and most frequent cause of reduced spinal mobility is the maintenance of poor postural habits during the first few decades of life. This is especially likely if the person does not exercise regularly. Poor postural habits allow adaptive shortening of certain structures. The result is a gradual reduction of mobility with aging. The movements reduced are usually the extension movements essential for maintenance of an erect posture.

The second cause of reduced spinal mobility is contracture of fibrous scar tissue resulting from repair after trauma. Thus, an inextensible scar can form within or adjacent to otherwise healthy structures and cause reduced mobility. The pain resulting from stretching of this inextensible scar appears only on attempts at full end-range movement. The pain does not occur during the movement or before the structure is placed under tension. Surrounding healthy structures are capable of further extensibility, but those ranges of movement are restricted by the scar.

It is not possible to identify the structure causing the pain of dysfunction, but any of the soft tissues related to or adjacent to the vertebral column may adaptively shorten or may be damaged. Thus, the pain may result from adaptive shortening of, or injury to, any of the ligamentous structures in the segment, including those pertaining to the intervertebral disc, the zygapophyseal joints, or the superficial or deep muscles or their attachments. The pain may also result from adherence of the spinal nerve root or dura after severe intervertebral disc bulging or rupture, but this is more easily identified.

Described simply, the pain of dysfunction is produced immediately by the overstretching of shortened tissues.

DERANGEMENT SYNDROME

Patients with the derangement syndrome are usually between 20 and 55 years of age. They invariably have a poor sitting posture. Pain usually develops suddenly, over a few hours or 1 or 2 days. During this time, patients change from completely normal to significantly disabled individuals. Often, this syndrome appears for no apparent reason.

The symptoms may be felt locally, adjacent to the spinal midline, and may radiate and be referred distally in the form of pain, paresthesia, or numbness. The symptoms historically are produced, abolished, increased, or reduced by the performance of certain movements or the maintenance of certain positions.[63]

Pain from the derangement syndrome may alter and change in regard to both the site of the pain and the extent of the affected area. Pain from the derangement syndrome may cross the midline and move, for example, from the right side of the low back to the left side.

Embryonic discogenic pathologic processes must always be suspected when the patient describes the pain as changing position and radiating when he or she changes position or performs certain movements. In cases in which referred pain changes its distribution or location, some evidence supports the conceptual model signifying the development of nuclear displacement through incomplete annular cracks or tears within the intervertebral disc. The displacement occurs as the disc changes its shape or position during movement or sustained postures.[2, 30, 60]

Pain from the derangement syndrome is frequently constant. There may be no position in which the patient can find relief. Therefore, the pain may be present regardless of whether movement is performed. It is usually described as an ache that at times can be severe. The ache is then made more severe by movement in certain directions and is reduced by movement in other directions.

In patients with the derangement syndrome, especially those with severe cases, gross obstruction of movement may occur. Postural deformities, such as kyphosis and scoliosis, are also seen frequently. Sudden obstruction of movement with loss of spine mobility and the sudden appearance of postural deformity in acute cases of low back and neck pain may be likened to the sudden locking that may occur in the knee joint, commonly caused by internal derangement of the meniscus.

The mechanism of internal derangement of the intervertebral disc is not fully understood. That the nucleus pulposus can be displaced toward and escape through a damaged annular wall is inarguable.[1, 2] It is highly likely that this is a consequence of sudden or violent movement or a result of poor postures sustained by younger patients. Older patients have a stiffer, less fluid nucleus, which is less likely to be displaced from within its annular envelope.[1, 2, 19] Another hypothesis is that, prior to a frank annular lesion with nuclear herniation, there are incomplete tears into which nuclear material may be displaced. This condition alters joint biomechanics and may be responsible for temporary postural deformities (e.g., localized scoliosis and kyphosis).

Creep of the fluid nucleus-annulus complex disturbs the normal alignment of adjacent vertebrae and changes the resting shape of the disc.[19, 47] This change of shape also affects the ability of the joint surface to move in its normal pathway. Deviation to the right or the left of the sagittal plane results when flexion or extension is attempted.[47] Laboratory and cadaveric observations carried out by Stahl[55] and Vogel[61] in 1977 and described in a monograph by Kramer[30] exactly duplicated the conceptual model that one of the authors (R.M.) presented in 1980.[37] This model proposed a simple mechanism of displacement that could account for the production of acute low back problems, especially those conditions causing acute lumbar list and acute kyphosis.[30, 36, 38]

Described simply, the pain of derangement is consequent to a change in disc shape, with related malalignment of the mobile segment and its associated abnormal stresses.

Identification of Nonspecific Pain Syndromes

Identification of the different syndromes is based on the following:

- The effects that repeated end-range spinal movements have on the initiation of pain
- The point in the movement pathway at which pain is first perceived
- The anatomic site of the pain and subsequent change of location of the pain (centralization)
- The increasing or decreasing intensity of the pain
- The abolition of the pain
- Any corresponding changes in range of

motion, or the presence of postural deformity.

Mechanical pain can arise from only a limited number of events or combination of events causing force to be applied to innervated soft tissues. Those soft tissues may be in a normal state, a shortened state, or an anatomically altered state with a change in the shape or distribution of the disc and its fluids. Any of these soft tissue states can be identified by the response of the patient's pain to the deliberate application of certain mechanical forces.

Patients with inflammatory disorders, with spondylolisthesis or other undetected minor fractures, or with pathologic conditions unsuited to mechanical therapies do not respond in a predictable fashion. These persons are quickly recognized when tested appropriately.[38]

MECHANICAL TREATMENTS

Methods

Spinal Manipulative Therapy and Self-Treatment

All over the world, enthusiastic physiotherapists, disillusioned by the use of ineffectual methods of physical therapy, are rediscovering mobilization and manipulation and providing it as the treatment of choice for many patients with spinal pain. No one experienced in the use of such therapy has failed to be excited on the many occasions when a spectacular improvement is obtained. Undoubtedly, many patients benefit from SMT. Several studies support the finding of short-term relief of pain.[5, 18, 20, 25, 27, 52]

From within the ranks of physiotherapists, and especially from chiropractors and osteopaths, there emerge claims expounding the advantages of one form of SMT over another. Although one cannot with any hope of resolution enter the arguments for or against the concepts underlying the various systems, it is comparatively simple to demystify the manipulative procedures used to achieve the same result. No study demonstrates that any one form of SMT is superior to another. One report established that osteopathic manipulation at the end of 4 weeks was no better than a placebo (detuned short-wave diathermy).[23] Schiotz and Cyriax[51] described these situations well: "It is not the elegance or alleged specificity of some maneuver that matters, it is its therapeutic effectiveness." The effectiveness of patient-performed repetitive motion is frequently superior to the most elegant SMT technique.

Physiotherapists should avoid the tendency of those schooled in one particular method of mobilization to denigrate other systems. Devotees of Kaltenborn, Maitland, Cyriax, and Paris enthusiastically support their particular gurus. They fail to recognize that each group of practitioners is probably dispensing the same maneuver and effect using a different title, philosophy, and variation.

Once one is familiar with the various techniques of SMT, it becomes clear that the basic maneuvers in common use today are essentially the same. Although differences may exist in the manner of treatment delivery, these differences have not yet been shown to affect the final outcome. This statement will be strenuously challenged by the purists. This is the way it should be, of course, and the definitive study that demonstrates the superiority of one form of SMT over another is eagerly awaited.

Manipulative treatments are now dispensed by physiotherapists with extensive training in modern mechanical concepts. The current mechanical physiotherapist has the advantage of being able to use the entire spectrum of mechanical concepts and tools. So in considering the form of mechanical therapy most appropriate for the patient, whether it be exercise, traction, mobilization, or manipulation, the well-trained mechanical therapist can provide this treatment.

Several problems and concerns arise from the current wave of enthusiasm for SMT and its related techniques. These problems exist because, in many parts of the world, manipulation by physiotherapists is only now being developed. The initial enthusiasm, although understandable, must be tempered and brought into perspective. Inexperienced physical therapists see manipulation as the cure for back pain and a panacea for whatever ails the patient.

Professionals who have longer experience with the benefits and limitations of SMT must make that experience available to moderate the enthusiasm of persons entering the field. Until therapists have learned to distinguish between a patient's responsiveness to treatment and a natural resolution of symptoms with the passage of time, their credibility is at risk. When patients improve over 3 to 4 months, can their recovery be attributed to the manipulative or mechanical treatments delivered during this period? Failure to recognize and to understand the natural history and self-limited characteristics of low back problems perpetuates an inability to review treatment methods and results critically.

To dispense SMT, it has always been necessary for the therapist to do something passively to the patient. Thus, whether the patient's improvement results from the passage of time or is attributable to the techniques of therapy, the patient, correctly or incorrectly, attributes the recovery to the treatment. The patient may become dependent on the therapy and, in the event of recurrence, hurry back to the therapist. In the mind of the patient, and often in the mind of the therapist, the patient must receive more of the same treatment to recover.

SMT provides short-term benefit.[5, 18, 20, 25, 27, 52] There are no known long-term benefits.[41] If physiotherapists acting as part of a medical team are to become the professionals responsible for conservative treatment and management of mechanical spinal problems, treatments with the potential to provide long-term advantages must be provided.

In 1956, the author (R. M.) witnessed several patients who experienced rapid and inexplicable improvement from the performance of casual movements or positions. The observations clearly demonstrated a cause-and-effect relationship between these movements or positions and the presence or intensity of symptoms. One patient who had been in pain for 3 weeks lay inadvertently in a certain position on a treatment table. After about 10 minutes, he arose, completely relieved of leg pain. He returned the following day almost totally symptom free. Another patient, after a change of position, experienced a complete transfer of his pain from the right to the left side. Another patient with a neck problem abolished all symptoms by repeatedly combing his hair with the head laterally flexed to one side. The pain did not return. These and other clinical observations allowed the development of several rather different avenues of diagnosis and therapy.[36, 37]

The main conclusions arising from these observations were that patients, with the use of self-treatment principles and without manipulation by a therapist, could significantly affect the courses of their own disorders. For patients with nonspecific back pain, it is estimated that more than 70% of patients can be taught these principles and can achieve a good result with greater safety, with greater speed and efficiency, with less expense, and with lasting benefit.[37] The routine use of SMT cannot be justified for the treatment of low back pain if the same result can be obtained using forces applied by the patient independently.

The time to apply special techniques of mobilization and manipulation arrives only after the patient has exhausted all self-treatment options without success. Temporary improvement for only a few hours after self-treatment suggests that the applied forces, although appropriate directionally, were inadequate in degree. The introduction of mobilization at this time is indicated. Failing improvement with the use of mobilization, then and only then is manipulation indicated.

The author (R.M.) has further proposed that mobilization and manipulation should be postponed until it has been determined that resolution of the problem is impossible using the patient's own movements and positions. Patients unable to apply self-treatment procedures with lasting benefit and those with any lumbar or sciatic list always require the special skills of the physiotherapist versed in correction of this problem.[36] Other patients need therapy in the form of mobilization techniques, and a few of those additionally require manipulative thrust procedures.[35, 39]

Thus, the gradual development of increasing force to bring about change is a logical and safe method of applying mechanical therapies, assuming that vertebral and vascular pathologic processes have been excluded. The ultimate weapon is the manipulative thrust technique. Why immediately use that technique when the patient may well be capable of causing change without the help of the therapist, at the same time learning an important self-management lesson?

The authors are not proposing that mobilization and manipulation are no longer necessary. SMT has a particular and important part to play in the treatment of mechanical spinal pain. However, it is greatly misused and overused. It is now possible to determine, usually within the first 24-hour period after assessment, whether manipulative therapy is needed. It should no longer be necessary to apply SMT to find out retrospectively whether the procedure was of value or even indicated. Spinal mobilization and manipulation should not be dispensed to the entire population of patients with back pain to ensure that the few persons who really need it actually receive it. It is conceivable that in the not too distant future, mechanical spinal disorders (apart from the obvious exceptions) will be so well understood that few problems affecting the spinal segments will require manipulation. Most patients will then be able to treat their own mechanical disorders.

Traction

As with studies of the efficacy of SMT,[5] most investigations of clinical efficacy of traction are flawed. However, some evidence remains to suggest that it is premature to discard the treatment as entirely ineffectual. An addition to the various types of traction is the autotraction table, which was devised by Lind but studied by Larsson.[32]

Originally designed for the treatment of frank disc herniation causing sciatic syndromes, autotraction has been recommended by some practitioners in the United States as a panacea for back pain in general. Its worth may be misjudged accordingly. No such claims were made by its innovator, and it is hoped that it will be further investigated by independent assessors. One study indicated that the response to autotraction was no different from that to manual traction at 2 weeks and 3 months.[33] Another study noted that, during autotraction, pressures within the disc increased considerably.[3] No negative pressures were recorded.

Gravity traction and inversion traction are also currently in vogue in the United States. There are no reliable data or objective assessments that indicate that these treatments are beneficial. As is true of other therapies, improvement with traction must be seen to result from the treatment and not from the passage of 3 or 4 weeks as the natural history of the condition runs its course.

In the authors' experience,[38, 39] patients with sciatica with list and neurologic disorder appear to improve with the passage of time rather than with traction itself. All other patients benefit more rapidly by using self-treatment procedures than by undergoing traction.

Massage

Massage is still used for the treatment of low back pain, and it can certainly have a mechanical effect on superficial structures. When it is applied with sufficient pressure, there must also be a mechanical effect on the articulations of the spine. Under certain circumstances, it is likely that firm massage is as beneficial as gentle mobilization.

Exercise

Exercise has been the mainstay of the physiotherapy profession, especially since the development of Swedish Remedial Exercises in the early part of the 20th century.[50] In the treatment of spinal disorders, conflict has always existed between therapists who have advocated flexion exercises, on the basis of the rationale proposed by Williams,[62] and practitioners who have advocated extension to treat low back pain.[10, 26, 39] Williams' philosophy is most strongly established in the United States and Canada, where almost anyone with low back pain or sciatica receives the standard flexion procedure from physiotherapists.

Extension, on the other hand, having been graphically described by Hippocrates,[26] has been used throughout the rest of the world, it seems, since the earliest records were kept.[51]

Of course, it is not possible to impose one treatment arbitrarily on the entire spectrum of mechanical disorders of the low back, deciding that all patients must undergo flexion or all patients must undergo extension. Several studies indicate that exercises tailored to suit individual needs are of benefit.* Most but not all patients benefit from extension. Flexion and lateral flexion, when necessary to centralize referred pain during assessment, are also then necessary for treatment. Repetitive end-range movements[38, 39] and the study of centralizing pain phenomena make it possible to determine the direc-

---

*References 11, 15, 29, 37, 46, 48, and 58.

tion in which any particular patient must be moved to bring about resolution of a particular problem.

Some patients must flex in a particular way to abolish pain. Other patients must extend in a particular way to achieve that state. Still other patients must first flex and then immediately extend to become free of symptoms.

Mechanical Treatment of Nonspecific Pain Syndromes

Three clinically identifiable syndromes exist in the nonspecific spectrum of low back pain.[38, 39] Identification of any one of these syndromes is not dependent on the identification of the structures responsible for the presenting symptoms. Soft tissues are affected by mechanical forces that result in the production of pain under only three particular conditions: (1) normal, (2) shortened, and (3) anatomically disrupted and displaced tissues.

POSTURAL SYNDROME

Normal tissues can become painful in daily life by the application of prolonged stresses commonly appearing during static postural loading conditions, such as prolonged sitting, standing, or bending. Correction of faulty postural habits removes causative stresses. No other treatment is required. SMT mobilization and traction are of no use. To remove the cause of pain, the therapist must instruct the patient as to the correct position and the patient, and only the patient, must carry out the corrective changes in postural habit.

DYSFUNCTION SYNDROME

Shortened structures limit movement and simultaneously cause pain when placed on stretch. Essentially, treatment is a remodeling process. Short structures are lengthened by the regular application of stretching exercises. Dysfunction is not rapidly reversible; weeks are required to remodel and lengthen. SMT is of no use. Structures that have adaptively shortened over weeks and months cannot suddenly lengthen by the application of high-velocity thrusts without incurring damage.

DERANGEMENT SYNDROME

An example of the derangement syndrome is the presence of frank tears of the annulus fibrosus with nuclear displacement or annular bulging. The patient experiences aching without movement, increased pain with movement in certain directions as displacement increases, and reduced pain in other directions as displacement decreases. This syndrome is subject to mostly rapid reversal. The derangement is reduced by applying appropriate movements; the reduction is maintained by correcting posture and avoiding wrong positions. Function is restored before adaptive changes are established.

CONCLUSIONS

It is not yet possible to identify precisely the structures involved in the production of common low back problems, with one exception—the intervertebral disc.[42] Treatment has been by trial and error, and no reliable predictors of outcome have been available. Although further research is required, the centralization of pain phenomena appears to offer promise as a reliable prognostic indicator.[15]

Physiotherapists, by virtue of their training, their relationship with the medical profession, and their improved public esteem, appear to be the professionals most appropriately equipped to assume responsibility to dispense conservative spinal therapy for mechanical disorders. Therapists must ensure, however, that this opportunity is not lost by allowing less discriminating colleagues to perpetuate the deceptive use of invalidated treatments. Eliminating outmoded, ineffective therapies is an urgent priority. It is appropriate to quote Nachemson:

In the therapeutic field today, it is virtually impossible to introduce a new drug without clinical and laboratory tests to prove its effectiveness, and we are increasingly alert to and critical of different types of pharmacological side effects. The same approach should be used for the different forms of treatment of low back pain and we should critically re-assess our present methods.[35]

Mechanical forces used to treat mechanical disorders of the low back should be applied in a graduated form, first by using the repeated movements of self-treatment, then progressing through mobilization, and finally applying manipulative procedures. If there is no resolution of symptoms, the use of other mechanical devices such as traction should follow. The only patients to receive electrotherapeutic modalities should be those failing to respond to the mechanical approach. Electrotherapeutic modes, such as transcutaneous electrical nerve stimulation, interferential therapy, and microwave therapy, should be used to modulate pain only when mechanical methods have failed. Physiotherapy professionals, however, must ask themselves whether modulating pain by using expensive modalities is of greater benefit to the patient and society than dispensing rather inexpensive medications.

REFERENCES

1. Adams, M. A., and Hutton, W. C.: Prolapsed intervertebral disc: A hyperflexion injury. Spine 7:3, 1982.
2. Adams, M. A., and Hutton, W. C.: Gradual disc prolapse. Spine 10:6, 1985.
3. Andersson, B. J. G., Schulz, A. B., and Nachemson, A: Intervertebral disc pressures during traction. J. Rehabil. Med. 9(suppl.):88, 1983.
4. Aprill, C. A., Medcalf, R., Donelson, R. G., et al.: Discographic outcomes predicted by the centralization of pain and directional preference: A prospective, blinded study. Presented at the North American Spine Society Meeting, Washington, D.C., October 1995.
5. Brunarski, D. J.: Clinical trials of spinal manipulation. J. Manip. Physiol. Ther. 7:4, 1984.
6. Carron, H., DeGood, D. E., and Tait, R.: A comparison of low back pain patients in the United States and New Zealand: Psychosocial and economic factors affecting severity of disability. Pain 21:77–89, 1985.
7. Coventry, M. B., Ghormley, R. K., and Kernohan, J. W.: The intervertebral disc: Part II. Changes in the intervertebral disc concomitant with age. J. Bone Joint Surg. 27:233, 1945.
8. Coventry, M. B., Ghormley, R. K., and Kernohan, J. W.: The intervertebral disc: Part III. Pathological changes in the intervertebral disc. J. Bone Joint Surg. 27:460, 1945.
9. Cyriax, J.: Textbook of Orthopaedic Medicine, Vol. 1. London, Bailliere Tindall, 1954.
10. Cyriax, J.: Textbook of Orthopaedic Medicine, 5th Ed., Vol. I. London, Bailliere Tindall, 1980.
11. Cyron, B. M., and Hutton, W. C.: Articular tropism and instability of the lumbar spine. Spine 5:168, 1980.
12. Delitto, A. A., Cibulka, M. T., Erhard, R. E., et al.: Evidence for an extension-mobilization category in acute low back syndrome: A prescriptive validation pilot study. Phys. Ther. 73:216–228, 1993.
13. DiMaggio, A., and Mooney, V.: Conservative care for low back pain: What works? J. Musculoskel. Med. 4:27–34, 1987.
14. Dixon, A.: Diagnosis of low back pain. In Jayson, M. (ed.): The Lumbar Spine and Back Pain. Tunbridge Wells, Great Britain, Pitman Medical, 1980.
15. Donelson, R., Silva, G., and Murphy, K.: Centralization phenomenon: Its usefulness in evaluating and treating referred pain. Spine 15:211–213, 1990.
16. Donelson, R., Grant, W., Kamps, C., and Medcalf, R.: Pain response to sagittal end-range spinal motion: A prospective, randomized, multicentered trial. Spine 16:S206–S212, 1991.
17. Donelson, R., Grant, W., Medcalf, R., et al.: Pain response to end-range spinal motion in the frontal plane: A multi-centered, prospective trial. Presented at the International Society for the Study of the Lumbar Spine Meeting, Heidelberg, Germany, May, 1991.
18. Doran, M. L., and Newell, D. J.: Manipulation in treatment of low back pain: A multicentre study. Br. Med. J. 2:161, 1975.
19. Farfan, H. F.: Mechanical disorders of the low back. Philadelphia, Lea & Febiger, 1973.
20. Farrell, J. B., and Twomey, L. T.: Acute low back pain. Comparison of two conservative treatment approaches. Proceedings of the Manipulative Therapists Association of Australia, Perth, Western Australia, 1983, p. 162.
21. Fredrickson, B., Murphy, K., Donelson, R., and Yuan, H.: McKenzie treatment of low back pain: A correlation of significant factors in determining prognosis. International Society for the Study of the Lumbar Spine Meeting, Dallas, 1986.
22. Frymoyer, J. W., Phillips, R. B., Newbert, A. H., and MacPherson, B. V.: A comparative analysis of the interpretations of lumbar spinal radiographs by chiropractors and medical doctors. Spine 11:10, 1986.
23. Gibson, T., Blagrave, P., and Harkness, J.: Low back pain treated by an osteopath. Br. J. Rheumatol. 24:92, 1985.
24. Gonella, C., Paris, S., and Kutner, M.: Reliability in evaluating passive intervertebral motion. Phys. Ther. 62:437, 1982.
25. Hadler, N. M., Curtis, P., Gillings, D. B., and Stinnett, S.: A benefit of spinal manipulation as adjunctive therapy for acute low-back pain. A stratified controlled trial. Spine 12:7, 1987.
26. Hippocrates: Corpus Hippocrateum. Peri Arthron. 400 BC. Cited by Cyriax, J.: Textbook of Orthopaedic Medicine, 5th Ed., Vol. 1. London, Bailliere Tindall, 1980.
27. Hoehler, F. K., Tobis, J. S., and Buerger, A. A.: Spinal Manipulation for low back pain. JAMA 245:1835, 1981.
28. Jull, G.: The reliability of manual palpation. Proceedings of the Manipulative Therapists Association of Australia Conference, Brisbane, Australia, 1985.
29. Kopp, J. R., Alexander, A. H., and Turocy, R. H.: The use of lumbar extension in the evaluation and treatment of patients with acute herniated nucleus pulposus. Clin. Orthop. 202:211–218, 1986.
30. Kramer, J.: Intervertebral Disk Diseases, 1st Ed. Chicago, Year Book, 1981.
31. Kuslich, S., and Ulstrom, C.: The tissue origin of low back pain and sciatica: A report of pain response to tissue stimulation during operations on the lumbar spine using local anesthesia. Orthop. Clin. North Am. 22:181–187, 1991.

32. Larsson, U., Choler, U., and Lidstrom, A.: Auto traction for treatment of lumbago-sciatica. Acta Orthop. Scand. 51:791, 1980.
33. Ljunggren, A. E., Webber, H., and Larson, S.: Auto traction v. manual traction in patients with prolapsed lumbar intervertebral discs. Scand. J. Rehabil. Med. 16:17, 1984.
34. Matyas, T. A., and Bach, T. M.: The reliability of selected techniques in clinical arthrometrics. Aust. J. Physiother. 1:175, 1985.
35. McCombe, P. F., Fairbank, I. C. T., Cockersole, B. C., et al.: Reproducibility of physical signs in low-back pain. Spine 14:908–913, 1989.
36. McKenzie, R. A.: Manual correction of sciatic scoliosis. N. Z. Med. J. 76:484, 1972.
37. McKenzie, R. A.: Prophylaxis in recurrent low back pain. N. Z. Med. J. 89:627, 1979.
38. McKenzie, R. A.: The Lumbar Spine. Waikanae, New Zealand, Spinal Publications, 1980.
39. McKenzie, R. A.: The cervical and thoracic spine: Mechanical diagnosis and therapy. Waikanae, New Zealand, Spinal Publications, 1991.
40. Mooney, V.: Presidential address. Spine 12:8, 1987.
41. Moritz, U.: Evaluation of manipulation and other manual therapy. Criteria for measuring the effect of treatment. Scand. J. Rehabil Med. 11:173, 1979.
42. Nachemson, A.: A critical look at conservative treatment of low back pain. In Jayson, M. (ed.): The Lumbar Spine and Back Pain. Tunbridge Wells, Great Britain, Pitman Medical, 1980, p. 355.
43. Nachemson, A.: Lumbar spine instability. Spine 10:3, 1985.
44. Nelson, M. A., Allen, P., and Clamp, S.: Reliability and reproducibility of clinical findings in low-back pain. Spine 4:2, 1979.
45. Nelson, R. M., and Nester, D. E.: Standardized assessment of industrialized low-back injuries: Development of NIOSH low-back atlas. Top. Acute Care Trauma Rehabil. 2:16–30, 1988.
46. Nwuga, G., and Nwuga, V.: Relative therapeutic efficacy of the Williams and McKenzie protocols in back pain management. Physiother. Pract. 1:99–106, 1985.
47. Panjabi, M., Krag, M. H., and Chung, T. Q.: Effects of disc injury on mechanical behaviour of the human spine. Spine 9:7, 1984.
48. Ponte, D. J., Jensen, G. J., and Kent, B. E.: A preliminary report on the use of the McKenzie protocol versus Williams protocol in the treatment of low back pain. J. Orthop. Sports Phys. Ther. 6:2, 1984.
49. Potter, N. A., and Rothstein, J. M.: Intertester reliability for selected clinical tests of the sacroiliac joint. Phys. Ther. 65:1671, 1985.
50. Prosser, E.: Manual of Massage and Movements. London, Faber & Faber, 1945.
51. Schiotz, E. H., and Cyriax, J.: Manipulation, Past and Present. London, Heinmann, 1975.
52. Sims-Williams, H., Jayson, M. I. V., and Young, S. M. S.: Controlled trial of mobilisation and manipulation for patients with low back pain in general practice. Br. Med. J. 2:1338, 1978.
53. Spitzer, W. O., LeBlanc F. E., Dupuis, M., et al.: Scientific approach to the assessment and management of activity-related spinal disorders. Spine 12:7S, 1987.
54. Spratt, K. F., Lehmann, T. R., Weinstein, J. N., and Sayre, H. A.: A new approach to the low back physical examination, behavioral assessment of mechanical signs. Spine 15:2, 1990.
55. Stahl, C.: Experimentelle Untersuchungen zur Biomechanik der Halswirbelsaule. Medical Dissertation. Dusseldorf, University of Bochum, 1977.
56. Stankovic, R., and Johnell, O.: Conservative treatment of acute low back pain: A prospective randomized trial: McKenzie method of treatment versus patient education in "mini back school." Spine 15:120–123, 1990.
57. Suzuki, N., and Seiichi, E.: A quantitative study of trunk muscle strength and fatigability in the low back pain syndrome. Spine 8:1, 1983.
58. Twomey, L., and Taylor, J.: Age changes in the lumbar intervertebral discs. Acta Orhop. Scand. 56:496, 1985.
59. Vanharanta, H., Videman, T., and Mooney, V.: A comparison of McKenzie exercises, Back Trac and back school in lumbar syndrome; preliminary results. International Society for the Study of the Lumbar Spine, Dallas, 1986.
60. Vernon-Roberts, B.: Pathology and interrelation of intervertebral disc lesions. In Jayson, M. (ed.): The Lumbar Spine and Back Pain, 2nd Ed. Tunbridge Wells, Great Britain, Pitman Medical, 1980.
61. Vogel, G.: Experimentelle Untersuchungen zur Mobilitat des Nucleus Pulposus in Lumbalen Bandscheiben. Medical Dissertation. Dusseldorf, University of Bochum, 1977.
62. Williams, C. P.: The Lumbosacral Spine. New York, McGraw-Hill, 1965.
63. Williams, M. M., Hawley, J. A., McKenzie, R. A., et al.: A comparison of the effects of two sitting postures on back and referred pain. Spine 16:1185–1191, 1991.
64. Willis, T. A.: The lumbo-sacral anomalies. J. Bone Joint Surg. 41A:935, 1959.

Manipulation of the Lumbar Spine

STANLEY V. PARIS

Spinal manipulation is perhaps the most controversial of conservative spinal management techniques. The controversy is no doubt attributable to the fact that the origin and development of the technique have been outside the sphere of orthodox medical influence. More recent times have given rise to the bone setters of England and Europe and the osteopaths and chiropractors of North America. Although it incurs the healthy skepticism of the medical profession, spinal manipulation enjoys ever-increasing acceptance by physical therapists and, indirectly, by their referring medical colleagues. The methods by which manipulation is practiced differ greatly among the various professional groups, and even within those groups. However, there is a trend toward conformity as some of the more cultlike methods give way to those based, at least to some extent, on science.

Until recently, little was known of the mechanism underlying the reported benefits from manipulation of the spine. With the development of information on collagen synthesis and on the mechanisms for the formation of capsular restrictions, a mechanical basis for stretching joints to improve motion has emerged. Again, the neurophysiologic responses of articular mechanoreceptors have been identified[26] as possibly underlying the relief from pain provided by manipulative techniques, especially those that incorporate repeated motions or oscillations.

Both mechanical and neurophysiologic effects can be added to the already recognized psychologic or placebo effect of the intensive manipulation and, of course, to the occasional audible crack or snap of the joint, to which many patients and some practitioners attach great importance.

There have been attempts at clinical investigations into the possible benefits of manipulation. These investigations attempt to compare manipulation with other modalities, such as the administration of medication or placebo, the use of bed rest, and physiotherapy. The studies illustrate that manipulation is most effective in acute back pain states. However, there is still no study of manipulation as it is practiced by most practitioners (physical therapists) in North America. They use manipulation not as the sole treatment but along with preparatory modalities, such as heat application and massage, and supportive modalities, such as exercises, posture modifications, and back school. Just as back surgery is not practiced without explanation, anesthesia, medication, and supportive care (e.g., physical therapy), neither is manipulation practiced without preparation and supportive treatments. Thus, to assess it as an isolated treatment is meaningless and will have little effect on its acceptance or rejection.

DEFINITION OF JOINT MANIPULATION

Joint manipulation has been defined as "the skilled, passive movement of a joint (or spinal segment), either within or beyond its active range of motion."[23] The definition contains no mention of the term thrust or force. It uses the word skilled, and it does not distinguish between the words mobilization and manipulation, which the author holds to be synonymous. Therefore, the techniques of manipulation may be gentle oscillations within the existing range, stretches at the end of range, or thrusts either within or at the end of range. One joint sound commonly heard, especially when joints are moved passively, is a pop, which is probably caused by the release of gas from the joint fluid. This results, no doubt, in an increase in the intraarticular volume and thus produces a temporary increase in range of motion. The pop and its resultant swelling are also thought to have an effect on the muscle tone inhibitors of the type III mechanoreceptors in the joint capsule and/

or the Golgi tendon end organs in the overlying multifidus muscle, which also attaches to the capsule. In either case, there is a temporary increase in range of motion, along with a sensation of pain relief. This is the common experience of persons who crack their own backs. The pain relief could be explained by the gate control mechanisms postulated by Melzack[15] and the muscle relaxation response from the Golgi tendon end organs in the multifidus muscle.

A multitude of techniques are available, each with different objectives and adherents, which are usually divided along professional lines. Furthermore, most practitioners who have taken graduate education in manipulation rarely use it as the sole modality. Preparatory treatment, such as heat application and massage, followed by a manipulation, such as gentle oscillations for pain relief or stretch techniques to increase range, is essential to obtain the best results. The treatments are followed by rest, exercises, and of course, education in the use and care of the back. Unfortunately, most of the research on manipulation fails to take into account these factors and renders on an unprepared individual either a rotary thrust to the lumbar spine or a passive hip flexion. The former is considered a test of manipulation and the latter a test of mobilization.[8] This is an outdated approach that may represent the medical practitioner's idea of manipulation, but it is not practiced by most physical therapists and chiropractors who have specialized in manipulative techniques. Manipulation without appropriate preparatory and supportive treatments does not fairly represent the current state of practice.

Thrust techniques are still common in chiropractic practice but are becoming less so since it has been recognized that the gentler techniques of progressive stretch produce similar results that are less likely to aggravate the underlying symptom. When practiced by chiropractors, thrust techniques may be either specific, in which case the force is directed to a vertebra, or nonspecific, in which case the force is applied to an area. Thrust techniques, and indeed most techniques in physical therapy, are not directed against vertebrae but rather against the joint to increase its range. Far more common in physical therapy is a stretch technique directed primarily toward one facet joint or segment for the purpose of increasing range.

Manipulation is used, therefore, for its mechanical effects to increase range, its neurophysiologic effects to abate pain, and of course, the placebo effect, which no doubt is enhanced by the hands on nature of both the examination and the treatment.

Table 1 delineates the classification of manipulative techniques for the lumbar spine.

HISTORY

First described by Hippocrates,[25] spinal manipulation has been practiced by distinguished forefathers of orthopedics, including Galen,[19] Sir James Paget,[20] Hugh Owen Thomas (whose father was a bone setter [lay manipulator]),[14] Hood,[10] Mennell[5,16] and Cyriax.[3] In the United States, osteopathy, beginning in the 1870s, and chiropractic, beginning in the 1890s, generated more practitioners of manipulation.

By the 1920s, physical therapists in Scandinavia, England, and the United States had taken an interest in manipulation.[7] Since the 1960s the technique has become well established in their practices; articles and texts

Table 1

Classification of Lumbar Manipulative Techniques

Nonthrust
Oscillations—principal effect is neurophysiologic; several grades, classification depending on range and force
Stretches—principal effect is mechanical on the capsule and adjacent myofascia
  Sustained, which are done within comfort
  Repeated, which are more comfortable
  Progressive, in which repeated maneuvers go progressively further

Thrust
Specific—usually used to correct a vertebral position (chiropractic) or to correct a movement restriction (physical therapy)
Nonspecific—usually directed toward a region of the spine and usually involves a torque; commonly the method practiced by physicians who have not had formal training in manipulative techniques

Distraction (a more precise term for traction)—may be intermittent or sustained in combination with positioning for the involved segment and side of the segment, or without positioning.

have been written by the author[21-23] and other physical therapists.[5, 12]

PURPOSE

The principal purpose of manipulation is to increase the range of motion in a spinal segment, which in turn is believed to help improve nutrition, gate pain, increase tolerance to insult, and improve function.

Manipulation has two primary effects: the first is on pain, and the second is on mechanics. In the relief from pain, particularly acute pain, manipulation appears to fare better than all other modalities and procedures. One study showed manipulation in the treatment of acute low back pain with or without leg pain to be superior to drug therapy, physiotherapy, bed rest, and placebo.[24] However, for chronic back and leg pain, manipulation slipped to third place, behind physiotherapy and back school. In fact, this is the combination used by most therapists practicing manipulation (i.e., with physical therapy and back school).

These data point to the effects of manipulation on pain. The effect of the technique seems to resemble that of Codman's exercises on the shoulder[2]; that is, the gentle oscillatory motions appear to control the onward transmission of nociceptive impulses[15, 26] and thus close the gate to pain. Not only is the pain relieved, but the involuntary muscle holding is also abated and function is improved. Although oscillations are usually performed manually, some manipulation tables permit patients to oscillate their own lumbar spine (Fig. 1)

Mechanically, manipulation may stretch

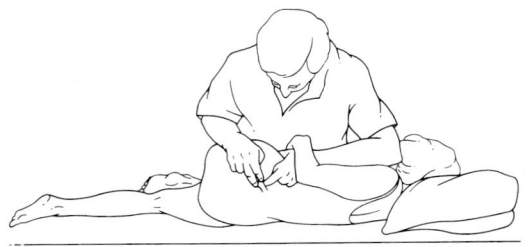

Figure 2. Midlumbar rotation stretching the left capsule at L4–L5 is used to regain range of motion or to release a mechanical locking or an incarcerated capsule. The forces are localized by placing the subject in a forward bending position and then by rotating to the desired level. The position is held by pressure on the shoulder and pelvis and further localized with pressure on the adjacent spinous processes. (From Payton, O. D. [ed.]: Manual of Physical Therapy. New York, Churchill Livingstone, 1989.)

tightened capsular adhesions[1] of the facet joints and help restore shortened muscles to normal length (Fig. 2). On occasion, manipulation may correct the alignment of a joint, such as the sacroiliac joint, which owing to hypermobility may have overridden its normal restraints and become locked in a faulty position.

Neither manipulation nor the closely related distraction (traction) has been shown to have long-term effect on the intervertebral disc.[13] When relief of pain follows manipulation in patients diagnosed as having disc lesions, one can assume that the disc was not the primary or sole cause of the pain.

Likewise, the use of manipulation to correct (adjust) vertebral misalignments has not been shown to be a valid concept. The principal protagonists of its use for this purpose are chiropractors, and they are currently showing an increasing interest in manipulation for correcting movement dysfunctions rather than vertebral misalignments.

INDICATIONS

The indications for manipulation vary, depending on the stage of the condition. Clinically, low back pain can be divided into immediate, acute, subacute, settled, and chronic stages. The treatment at each of these stages is somewhat different.

Immediate and Acute Stages

In the immediate and acute stages, it is sometimes observed that a patient has a pos-

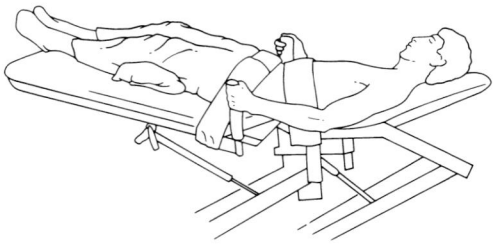

Figure 1. Automanipulation is an effective means of introducing motion into the acute spine. The patient controls the movement and can use the low back muscles to assist in motion. The use and effect is akin to that of Codman's exercises for the shoulder. (From Payton, O. D. [ed.]: Manual of Physical Therapy. New York, Churchill Livingstone, 1989.)

ture characterized by a combination of forward bending and side bending. In the absence of a current history and neurologic signs, the most likely cause of this posture is either a mechanical lock of the facets or the voluntary adoption of a posture that unburdens the side of the back that is in pain as a result of, perhaps, a painful capsular entrapment.

If the examination of the passive movements detects a locked facet, the treatment of choice is a facet distraction technique, actually rotation to the segment (Fig. 2). However, if the posture has been maintained for any length of time, backward bending as both a passive and an active exercise may also need to be added after the facet mechanical lock or painful entrapment has been released (Fig. 3). Of course, one could argue about whether facets are capable of becoming locked. Given that they—like the knee, the wrist, or the temporomandibular joint—possess menisci and that these latter joints can lock spontaneously, it seems plausible that the same mechanism may occasionally affect the spine.

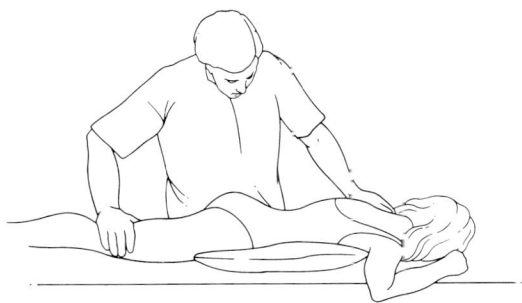

Figure 4. Using isometric multifidus contraction to pull on the capsule of a suspected facet capsular impingement. The shoulder on the affected side and the pelvis on the opposite side are held firm while a leg raise is requested. Note that the lumbar spine should be supported with one or more firm pillows. (From Payton, O. D. [ed.]: Manual of Physical Therapy. New York, Churchill Livingstone, 1989.)

If the examination suggests a possible acute facet capsule entrapment as evidenced by a restriction (by pain) of movements that increase the load of the involved facet (i.e., posture of backward bending or side bending to the painful side and rotation to the opposite side), an exercise or a manipulation technique that calls on a strong isometric contraction of the multifidus muscle may be successful. The mechanism at work here is the use of the multifidus attachment to the facet capsule to pull out the entrapped capsule; in the clinical picture just described, it is highly effective (Fig. 4). The principle of this procedure is not unlike using the capsular attachment of the rectus femoris to avoid painful passive hip flexion. If this is not successful, the distraction technique illustrated in Figure 2 modified by using more side bending (e.g., over a pillow) may be effective.

Subacute Stage

In the subacute stage, once any postural malalignment has been corrected, the emphasis is on maintaining range of motion and facilitating healing. Forceful manipulations have no place, but oscillatory and active exercises are valuable.

Settled Stage

In the settled stage, usually at about the 10th day after the injury, manipulation, par-

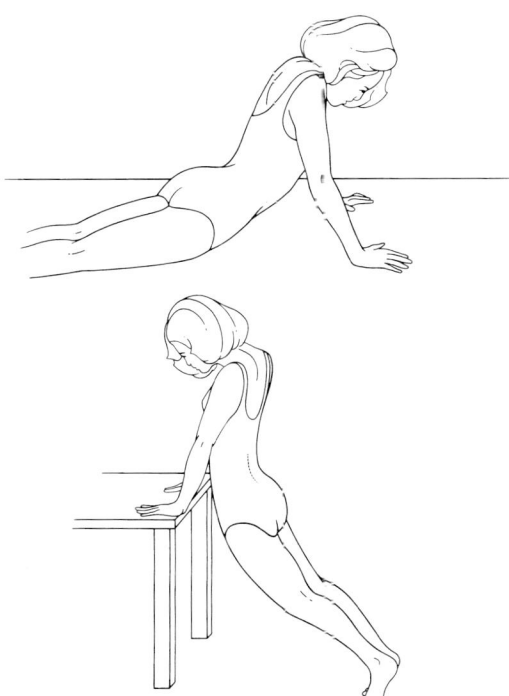

Figure 3. *A, B,* Backward bending to provide motion and to gate pain may be accomplished in a number of ways, as depicted in these illustrations. (From Payton, O. D. [ed.]: Manual of Physical Therapy. New York, Churchill Livingstone, 1989.)

ticularly that of a mechanical nature, is most effective. Tired and cramped muscles may be assisted by heat application, massage, and manipulative stretching, and any adhesions that may be forming within either the facet joints or the soft tissues surrounding them can also be stretched at this stage, with little risk of causing an exacerbation of symptoms.

Likewise, back school concepts will have already been introduced along with whatever exercises the patient's condition indicates may be of assistance. Furthermore, the therapist will have looked at not only the lumbar spine but also at such factors as a pronated foot, which would functionally shorten the leg and result in lateral curvature. Likewise, a hip restriction or a tight iliopsoas might well influence spinal function and thus either cause or prolong the patient's symptoms.

Chronic Stage

In the chronic stage, which begins about 3 months after the injury, manipulation as the sole treatment does not fare as well as the combination of physical therapy, heat application, massage, and back school. In addition, the emphasis is placed on improving physical fitness, increasing work activity, and if necessary, using some behavioral techniques.

LIMITATIONS

Manipulation is not successful in all cases of low back pain, but when combined with education in the form of back school and general physical therapy, it offers the best possible approach to low back pain conditions in patients for whom surgery is not indicated.

There are contraindications to some forms of manipulation. However, even in the presence of nearby fracture or disease, gentle oscillations may provide a significant degree of relief from pain.

Some practitioners have stated that pain below the buttock[11] or pain below the knee[9] is a contraindication to manipulation, no doubt because of the assumption that such pains are discogenic in origin and thus indicate considerable severity. However, Mooney and Robertson[19] showed that such pains can come from facet joints. In addition, the nerves of the lumbar spine also receive nociception from the muscles and ligaments of the lumbar spine as well as from the facets and discs. Furthermore, the sacroiliac joint is likewise innervated by the lumbar nerves, notably the medial branch of the postprimary rami from L4 and L5 and from S1 to S3. These nerves also have the ability of forwarding noxious stimuli, which could be interpreted as back and leg pains. Thus, leg pain does not seem to be a contraindication to manipulation. Nevertheless, most practitioners agree that, when the procedure reproduces the patient's intensity of pain and especially when it increases its radiation, the procedure should be abandoned because it will probably aggravate the condition.

Many practitioners consider that manipulation has little, if any, beneficial effect on intervertebral disc dysfunction. The movement of manipulation may help to relieve the patient's discomfort and encourage a return to activity. However, there is very little evidence that a pathologic process in the disc can be reversed by manipulation or, for that matter, by lumbar traction.

Most practitioners are careful to avoid placing a rotary or torque stress on an intervertebral disc when signs of imminent disc disease are present. Instead, a distraction or side bending technique designed to open up the foramen and to flatten the natural disc convexity is preferred. The effect of such maneuvers may be to relieve pressure on a nerve root, thus reducing its sensitivity. These techniques are termed positional distraction and are illustrated in Figure 5.

When a proven disc herniation is thought to be the cause of the patient's pain, manipu-

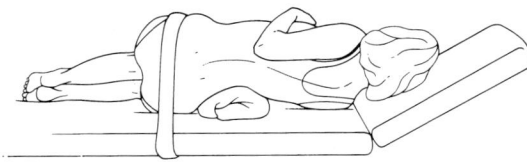

Figure 5. When neurologic signs suggest nerve root pressure, this form of distraction (traction), in which the patient is placed over a bolster during side bending and forward bending to the involved level, is effective in gaining a wide opening of the intervertebral foramen. It should not be used during the acute stage, in which case there may be a danger of increasing the disc injury. (From Payton, O. D., [ed.]: Manual of Physical Therapy. New York, Churchill Livingstone, 1989.)

lation is probably not indicated[21] and should be replaced by positional distraction techniques during the settled stage. However, in several studies, manipulation has been performed in the presence of demonstrated myelographic defects and has resulted in good or excellent pain relief, although no discernible difference was observed in the myelogram.[4] It must be concluded that its use in the presence of a known or suspected disc lesion must be carefully graded and monitored and is at best controversial.

CONCLUSION

In a number of studies spinal manipulation has been shown to be the superior treatment modality for the relief of low back pain in the acute phase. In the chronic stages of low back and leg pain, spinal manipulation as a treatment by itself has not been shown to produce any advantage over other conservative treatment. However, manipulation combined with physical therapy and back school techniques provides the most favorable clinical results. This is the manner in which increasing numbers of physical therapists practice manipulation.

REFERENCES

1. Akeson, W. H., Amiel, D., and Woo, S.: Immobility effects of synovial joints: The pathomechanics of joint contracture. Biorheology 17:95, 1980.
2. Codman, E. A.: The Shoulder. Boston, Thomas Todd, 1934.
3. Cyriax, J. H.: Textbook of Orthopaedic Medicine, 8th Ed., Vol. I. Diagnosis of Soft Tissue Lesions. London, Bailliere and Tindall, 1982.
4. Doran, P. M. L., and Newall, P. J.: Manipulation in the treatment of low back pain: A multicenter study. Br. J. Med. 2:161, 1975.
5. Edwards, B. C.: Low back pain and pain resulting from lumbar spine conditions: A comparison of treatment results. Aust. J. Physiother. 15:104, 1969.
6. Glover, J. R., Morris, J. G., and Knosla, T.: Back pain: A randomized clinical trial of rotational manipulation of the trunk. Br. J. Indust. Med. 31:39, 1974.
7. Grunewald, L. R.: A study of physiotherapy as a vocation. Physiother. Rev. 8:38–39, 1928.
8. Hadler, N. M., Curtis, P., Gillings, D. B., and Stinnett, S.: A benefit of spinal manipulation as adjunctive therapy for acute low-back pain: A stratified controlled trial. Spine 12:702–706, 1987.
9. Hay, M. C.: Incidence of low back pain in Busselton. Proceedings of Conference on Low Back Pain, West Australia Institute of Technology, September 7–13, 1974.
10. Hood, W.: A Treatise on Bone-Setting. London, 1871.
11. Hooper, J.: Low back pain and manipulation: Paraparesis after treatment of low back pain by physical methods. Med. J. Aust. 1:549, 1973.
12. Maitland, G. D.: Vertebral Manipulation. Stoneham, Butterworth, 1964.
13. Mathews, J. A., and Yates, D. A.: Reduction of lumbar disc prolapse by manipulation. Br. Med. J. 3:696, 1969.
14. McMurray, T. P.: Life of Hugh Owen Thomas. Centenary Lecture, Liverpool Medical Institution, Feb. 7, 1935. Liverpool Med. Chir. J. 43:3, 1935.
15. Melzack, R.: The Puzzle of Pain. London, Penguin, 1973.
16. Menell, J.: Back Pain. Boston, Little, Brown, 1960.
17. Mennell, J.: Physical Treatment by Movement, Manipulation and Massage. London, Churchill, 1934.
18. Mensor, M. C.: Non-operative treatment including manipulation for lumbar intervertebral disc syndrome. J. Bone Joint Surg. 17A:925, 1955.
19. Mooney, V. T., and Robertson, J.: The facet syndrome. Clin. Orthop. 115:149, 1976.
20. Paget, J.: Cases that bonesetters cure. Br. Med. J. 1867, p. 1.
21. Paris, S. V.: The theory and technique of specific spinal manipulation. N. Z. Med. J. 62:320, 1963.
22. Paris, S. V.: The Spinal Lesion. San Diego, Pegasus Press, 1965.
23. Paris, S. V.: Spinal manipulative therapy. Clin. Orthop. 179:55–61, 1983.
24. Posstacchini, F., Facchini, M., and Palieri, P.: Efficacy of various forms of conservative treatment in low back pain. A comparative study. Paper presented at International society for the Study, Rome, 1987.
25. Withington, E. T.: Hippocrates with an English Translation, Vol. 3. Cambridge, Harvard University Press, 1959, pp. 278–307.
26. Wyke, B. D.: The neurology of low back pain in the lumbar spine. In Jayson, I. V. (ed.) Back Pain. London, Pitman Medical, 1980, pp. 265–339.

Psychologic Approaches to the Management and Treatment of Chronic Low Back Pain

■

SHAUL SCHREIBER
DANIEL STEIN
YIZHAR FLOMAN

Chronic low back pain is defined as pain in the lumbosacral region that occurs daily for a period of at least 6 months.[153, 154] Some studies, however, have required that the definition specify a longer period, emphasizing the association of the duration of the illness with various dimensions of chronic low back pain.[162] At the time of this writing, chronic low back pain is regarded as one of the most common chronic pain disorders that interfere with patients' lifestyles[162] worldwide, as demonstrated by cross-cultural studies.[159] Traditional approaches to chronic pain have been characterized by a somatosensory model.[178] Pain has been seen as a purely sensory event, and the pain experience has been assumed to be directly proportional to the peripheral damage.[122, 178] Although the model may be appropriate for acute pain,[160] it may be misleading and inadequate with regard to chronic pain.[16, 178] This assumption stems from the many instances of chronic pain that have no discernible peripheral damage,[121] from the cases of emotional conditions that can lead to the development of chronic pain,[21] and from the clinical reports on the absence of pain expression despite severe injury.[178] In addition, many studies have demonstrated that various psychosocial variables may be closely related to chronic low back pain[44, 77] and that chronic low back pain may have a significant influence on a patient's psychosocial adaptation.[75, 150]

Melzack and Wall[114] were the first to incorporate such observations into a multidimensional model of chronic pain. Their gate control theory emphasized the link between neurophysiology and psychology and defined three principal dimensions of pain perception. The sensory-discriminative dimension provides a neutral description of the nociceptive input, and the motivational-affective and cognitive-evaluative dimensions modulate the perception of the input according to the affective state and the interpretation of the input, respectively. It is thus suggested that complex biopsychosocial models may be applicable for understanding chronic low back pain.[16, 63] This highlights the role of the psychiatrist as part of a multidisciplinary team evaluating and treating patients with chronic low back pain.[160]

This discussion focuses on the following dimensions: psychologic and social factors associated with chronic low back pain; the risk of the progression from acute to chronic low back pain; the controversial issue of organic versus psychogenic chronic low back pain; the indications for psychiatric assessment in chronic low back pain; the role of the psychiatrist in a team evaluating and treating patients with chronic low back pain; and the most important drug and psychologic treatments of chronic low back pain.

PSYCHOLOGIC AND SOCIAL FACTORS ASSOCIATED WITH CHRONIC LOW BACK PAIN

Depression and Chronic Low Back Pain

A close link between the experience of chronic pain and the state of depression has been described in many studies.[15, 75] Several findings strongly support the association between chronic low back pain and depression, although the exact nature of this relationship remains unclear.[30, 38] The findings are as follows:

- Patients with chronic low back pain are often depressed.[75, 91] Between 60% and 100% of these patients have demonstrable symptoms of a depressive disorder.[7, 145]
- Patients with chronic low back pain often demonstrate neurovegetative symptoms of depression.[1, 168]
- Many patients with a depressive disorder (between 60% and 100%) report considerable somatic pain.[165, 188]
- Patients with chronic low back pain have been shown to have significantly increased rates of affective disorders (particularly unipolar depression) and alcoholism among first-degree relatives.[1, 39] These results are similar to the findings in depression.[131] Interestingly, a significantly higher incidence of major depression has been found in first-degree relatives of depressed patients with chronic low back pain, compared with those of nondepressed patients with chronic low back pain.[39]
- In a manner resembling that of depressed patients,[156] persons with chronic low back pain demonstrate increased rate of neuroendocrine abnormalities, including nonsuppression on the dexamethasone suppression test[1, 18] and a blunted thyrotropin response to the administration of thyrotropin-releasing hormone.[55] They also demonstrate shortened rapid eye movement latency on the polysomnogram.[1, 16] Moreover, patients with chronic low back pain and major depression have been differentiated from patients with chronic low back pain without depression on the basis of dexamethasone nonsuppression.[56]
- Many patients with chronic pain improve significantly with either the administration of antidepressive medications[72, 150, 191] or electroconvulsive therapy.[23, 107]

Various suggestions have been offered to explain the associations between chronic low back pain and depression, reflecting the ambiguity and inconsistencies regarding these relationships. The suggestions are as follows:

- Chronic low back pain leads to the development of depression.[15, 89] Ranga Rama Krishnan and colleagues,[145] for example, found in a study of 71 patients with chronic low back pain that in the majority the depression developed after the onset of pain. Hendler[75] regarded depression as a normal reaction in chronic low back pain. Blumer[16] suggested that "the depressive symptomatology of the chronic pain patients tends to be viewed as the consequence of physical suffering from which there appears to be no relief."
- A depressive disorder may lead to the development of chronic low back pain.[7] This hypothesis probably stems from the well-known finding that depression is often manifested in somatic symptoms, including pain.[15, 89] Although Hendler[75] claimed that "depression is rarely manifested by chronic pain" other studies have found that depressive symptoms usually precede the pain[118] and that relief from pain is concomitant with relief from the depression.[23, 123, 189]
- Chronic low back pain is regarded as "masked" depression[100, 179] or as a specific variant of the depressive disease.[17] This suggestion probably reflects the well-known finding that patients with chronic low back pain tend to deny or to have difficulty in expressing feelings.[63, 101] Thus, when depression develops in such patients, it is not expressed directly as an emotional state but rather indirectly as a somatic disorder, including pain.[63, 89]
- Some investigators suggest that chronic pain may be neither primary nor secondary to depression,[1, 16] but that similar mechanisms may be involved in the development of chronic pain and depression.[89] The aforementioned findings of an increased incidence of depression in first-degree relatives of patients with chronic low back pain may be related to a genetic vulnerability to depression in these patients.[39] In addition, similar biologic abnormalities, mainly depletion of serotonin in critical central nervous system synapses[73] and the previously mentioned neuroendocrine abnormalities, reported in both conditions, may suggest some common underlying biologic basis.
- Another possibility is that chronic low back pain may be a physical variant of or may have many common symptoms and clinical signs with the entity of posttraumatic stress disorder.[68, 106, 108, 135, 163] In fact,

pain has been recognized to be a strong enough psychologic stressor in traumatic circumstances to be the core trauma of posttraumatic stress disorder,[161] and some patients with chronic low back pain may have "an intrusive recollection of pain," not actual pain. Posttraumatic stress disorder is characterized by three categories of symptoms: (1) persistent reexperiencing of the traumatic event (either recurrent intrusive recollections and dreams or flashbacks), (2) persistent avoidance of cues reminiscent of the event or numbing of general responsiveness; and (3) persistent symptoms of increased arousal (difficulty in falling or staying asleep, irritability, difficulty in concentrating, and hypervigilance or exaggerated startle response). Like patients with posttraumatic stress disorder, patients with chronic low back pain frequently have major depressive episodes concomitantly; withdrawal from work, social, and family activities; and a tendency to self-medication, which may lead to drug and substance abuse. Moreover, both groups are frequently suspected of malingering. In both cases, the chronicity of the symptoms and the poor response to a simple treatment modality necessitates a multidimensional approach, a multiprofessional team, and a comprehensive rehabilitation approach.

- Macnab,[103] writing of whiplash (but the discussion is just as valid for chronic low back pain), made an important point. The clinician often does not recognize a patient's pain as legitimate. By failing to do so, the clinician may provoke iatrogenic psychologic problems. Whether the patient receives adequate treatment may depend on the clinician's preconceived notions about the type of injury involved. By failing to treat the injury adequately, the physician may be responsible for producing the so-called litigation neurosis. This viewpoint is reinforced by the report of a National Academy of Sciences committee.[81]

Most depressed patients with chronic low back pain apparently do not demonstrate a major (endogenous) depressive disorder, according to standardized psychiatric diagnostic criteria.[3] The rate of major depression in these patients is between 20% and 45%.[7, 38, 101, 145] Thus, it seems that most depressed patients with chronic low back pain demonstrate an atypical depressive picture.[165] Studies employing standardized diagnostic criteria have identified subgroups of depressed patients in those with chronic low back pain.[7, 145] These studies emphasized that the depression seen in chronic low back pain represents a continuum, ranging from no depression to major depression. Interestingly, 20% of persons with chronic low back pain have no depression at all.[38, 145] Some controversy seems to exist regarding the association between depression and the organicity of the chronic low back pain. Although Magni[104] and Crisson and associates[37] reported similar rates of depression in chronic low back pain of organic or functional origin, Ranga Rama Krishnan and colleagues[145] found the incidence of major depression to be twice as high among patients without organic findings.

Social Factors

Keefe and coworkers[87, 88] identified variables that can predict which individuals are susceptible to chronic low back pain. They distinguished between primary predictors (which uninjured workers are likely to develop chronic low back pain) and secondary predictors (which workers with acute episodes develop chronic pain). The study addressed the issue of what psychosociomedical variables are predictive of success or failure in response to a comprehensive functional restoration treatment program by workers who are chronically disabled with low back pain. This was done by identifying an array of 42 variables, from a larger pool of quantified physical, psychosocial, and medical factors rated to be important with this patient population.

Specific social factors affecting back pain can be divided into three distinct categories. Primary factors are predictive of who, in an uninjured population, might have a low back pain episode, whereas secondary and tertiary factors are predictive of how individuals respond after a low back injury is present: secondary factors identify persons with an acute low back pain incident who are likely to develop chronic difficulties (5% to 10% of the injured population), and tertiary factors identify those patients, who, after chronic symptoms have developed, are likely to resolve their difficulties and return to a productive lifestyle.

The social factors that have been related to low back pain are

I. Primary social factors
   A. Direct occupational factors
      1. Physical job demands (lifting, twisting, and bending activities; vibration; and so on)
      2. Work environment (noisy versus quiet, the quality of lighting, and the presence or absence of safety features)
   B. Indirect occupational factors
      1. Level of job satisfaction
      2. Supervisor ratings of job performance
      3. Employee's relationship with co-workers
II. Secondary social factors
   A. Occupational variables
      1. Level of job satisfaction
      2. Job type and physical demands
      3. Work history
   B. Family response to injury or pain behaviors
   C. Attorney involvement in a disability case
   D. Education level
III. Tertiary social factors
   A. Occupational variables
      1. Availability for a job after treatment
      2. Job type and physical demands
      3. Job performance and satisfaction
   B. Family response to the injured member
   C. Past surgical history
   D. Attorney involvement in a disability case

Primary Factors. Bigos and coworkers,[13] in a retrospective review of 900 back injury cases from Boeing Company employees during a 15-month period, reported that back injury claims were related to specific types of jobs, particularly those that involve lifting, and to previous industrial back injuries. This is consistent with previous findings that have linked jobs involving lifting, twisting, and bending to back injuries.[124] Length of time on the job was a significant factor in the Boeing study, with those with less time on the job having a higher incidence of injuries. Furthermore, previous supervisors' ratings were found to be important as well: a disproportionate number of injured employees had the lowest appraisal rating from their supervisor in the 6 months prior to their injury. Biering-Sorensen and Thomsen[12] reported that longer travel distances from home to work were found to be risk indicators for first-time episodes of back injury in a Danish population. Eastrand[43] reported low education (<6 years) and low occupational status as indicative of a higher incidence of low back pain among a group of Swedish men.

A variety of other social factors have been identified as possibly playing a role in the causation of low back pain. Cigarette smoking is one such variable that has been thoroughly examined, and the link between smoking and increased incidence of low back pain is well documented.[60, 90] According to some researchers, habitual cigarette smoking relates to physical and psychologic indices of chronic pain.[84] Most smoking patients (91%), however, believed that smoking had no effect on their pain intensity. When smoking and nonsmoking patients with back pain were compared, the smokers showed significantly higher levels of emotional distress, they tended to remain inactive, and they relied on medication more often than did the nonsmoking patients.[84]

Poor general physical fitness, gender differences, and overall social satisfaction are other factors that have been linked with low back pain.[19, 105]

Secondary Factors. Simply stated, secondary predictive factors relative to back pain determine those acute episodes that are likely to become chronic. Occupational and psychosocial factors were the two categories weighted highest (accounting for 40% of the total weight) within the model developed by Frymoyer and Cats-Bril,[58, 59] at the Vermont Rehabilitation Engineering Center, to identify and assess whether low back disability can be predicted. Specific factors identified included numerous job-related variables (e.g., lack of job satisfaction, physical demands, and instability of work history), injury-related variables (e.g., perception of fault, compensability, and attorney involvement) and other social variables (e.g., low level of education, previous history of disability, and major life events).

Many other studies have focused on the identification of social factors that affect the course of a pain episode or low back injury. The role of the family of the patient with low back pain is probably the most important social factor considered in this regard.[47, 136] Along with family variables, many occupational factors that were identified as primary predictors also influence response to a low back pain episode. A low supervisor's rating during the previous 6-month period, job dissatisfaction, perception of job-related tasks as repetitive and boring, and a noisy, unpleasant work environment were identified not only as primary predictors of a low back pain episode but also as secondary predictors of episodes that were likely to become chronic.[14, 58]

Tertiary Factors. Comparatively little effort has focused on the discovery of tertiary predictors (i.e., social factors that predict successful resolution after a chronic low back pain syndrome is present).[47, 59] The evidence that does exist relative to tertiary predictive factors is more anecdotal but qualitatively not dissimilar from that identified for primary and secondary factors. Because by definition a chronic low back pain episode indicates longer periods of disability, the availability of a job to return to and attitudes of employers related to taking back injured workers become significant tertiary predictors.[14, 109] The perception of the injured worker as susceptible to recurrence or reinjury further retards the successful resolution of low back pain disability. Additional complicating factors include habituation to benzodiazepines and narcotic pain relievers (a too-frequent iatrogenic consequence of the medical treatment) and social isolation resulting from decreased social contact subsequent to an industrial injury. Certainly, one major factor that is a significant tertiary predictor is the status of the injured worker's compensation. Financial compensation to injured workers during periods of work injury–related disability can become a disincentive to return to work as disability extends well into a chronic phase. However, empirical evidence of the effects of compensation and litigation on resolution of low back pain disability remains equivocal.[42]

Other Psychodynamic Factors

Many different psychodynamic factors have been found to be associated with chronic low back pain. The following list seems to point out the most consistent and significant ones:

1. The development and persistence of chronic low back pain as a fulfillment of unmet and unacknowledged passive-dependent wishes,[16] as well as wishes to receive affection.[17]
2. Inhibition and repression of aggressive impulses that may lead to muscle activation and increased muscle tone, and thus to the development of chronic low back pain.[45, 51]
3. A sustained cycle of anxiety and muscle tension causing pain, which produces more anxiety.[122] Although anxiety has primarily been associated with the reaction to acute pain,[70, 162] it is nevertheless often found in chronic low back pain.[146, 162] An association has also been demonstrated between chronic pain and various anxiety disorders.[121]
4. The somatic expression of unresolved psychic pain.[16, 178]
5. Imitation of or identification with a significant person with a crippling disease or chronic pain.[17]
6. The finding, by projective psychologic tests, that patients with chronic low back pain derive little pleasure from life, have considerable tension,[96] are overly adapted,[148] and demonstrate self-criticism and guilt.[21]
7. The finding, by the Oswestry Low Back Pain Disability Questionnaire, that patients with chronic low back pain derive little pleasure from work and that the best predictor for the outcome of the treatment and for spontaneous recovery was work satisfaction.[60, 80]
8. Some evidence suggests that patients with chronic pain who receive workers' compensation benefits have a tendency to exaggerate their symptoms and not to benefit from treatment.[51] Some studies indicate that time-limited compensation may not affect treatment outcome or interfere with return to work, whereas unlimited compensation may adversely influence overall treatment outcome and the probability that patients will return to work.[57, 83]

INDICATIONS FOR PSYCHIATRIC ASSESSMENT

Chronic low back pain has often been associated with various forms of the somatoform disorders,[2] known in the past as hysterical neuroses.[122] These include the conversion disorders,[120] somatization disorders,[157] psychogenic pain disorders,[157] and hypochondriasis.[120] These definitions all imply that the painful physical symptoms or irrational anxiety and conviction about physical illness exist in the absence of organic findings or known physiologic mechanisms[64] and suggest the existence of some basic underlying repressed psychologic conflict as the cause of the disorder.[16] Some controversy seems to exist, however, regarding the association between chronic low back pain and hysteria. Merskey,[121] summarizing the results of many of his studies, suggested that in many patients with chronic pain, a conversive or hysterical mechanism represents a leading cause and that these patients often demonstrate a histrionic personality. On the other hand, Blumer[16] claimed that suggesting a connection between chronic pain and hysteria is highly inappropriate. Most patients with chronic pain lack the colorful and highly dramatic presentation and the "belle indifference" of a classic hysteric, and histrionic personality traits tend to be noticeably absent.

Moreover, some studies suggest that much chronic pain is myofascial in origin. Myofascial trigger points were the culprits in 31% of patients with pain (10% of all patients) in an internal medicine group study.[49, 166] Most significantly, in a comprehensive pain center study, 85% of 283 patients were assigned a diagnosis of primary myofascial pain syndrome.[152] One report claimed that 28% of patients with chronic low back pain have no organic findings when examined.[127] This is so common in clinical practice that a special diagnostic label was created for these patients—chronic intractable benign pain.[38] In the pain center study cited above,[166] clinicians examined patients with chronic intractable benign pain. Myofascial trigger points in the low back muscles were found in almost 97% of patients with chronic low back pain. Many of these patients had decreased ranges of motion, nondermatomal sensory abnormalities, and hypertonic muscles—all common features of myofascial pain syndromes. This study raised the possibility that chronic pain that may be blamed on psychogenic mechanisms may be due to myofascial lesions. There is a high interrater reliability between palpators who are trained and experienced at diagnosing myofascial trigger points.[158] Moreover, features of these lesions can be reliably demonstrated with both algometry[138] and thermography.[49]

The extensive employment of the Minnesota Multiphasic Personality Inventory (MMPI) in the study of chronic low back pain has also demonstrated an apparent association between chronic pain, somatization, and hypochondriasis. This instrument is a broad-based, self-administered inventory, consisting of 566 true or false questions and yielding data on 10 clinical scales.[65] A frequent finding in chronic low back pain patients is the conversion V[63] or somatization[169] profile of the MMPI. This constellation is characterized by significant elevations of hysteria (scale 3) and hypochondriasis (scale 5) and, to a lesser degree, an elevation of depression (scale 4). Many studies have consistently described this profile in chronic low back pain.[1, 163, 194]

A controversy seems to exist, however, regarding the interpretation of these findings. Goldstein[63] suggested the conversion V pattern to reflect a conversion reaction in which the chronic low back pain substitutes for depression. Similarly, Dhanens and Jarrett[40] claimed that this pattern is indicative of the defensive style of the patient with a psychogenic disorder, who exhibits a denial of awareness of psychologic conflict and a subsequent expression of this conflict through somatic concerns. On the other hand, Sternbach and colleagues[168] saw this pattern as an example of a psychophysiologic disorder with depression. Keel[89] also suggested that these patients can be characterized as typical psychosomatic patients, that is, demonstrating a physical condition affected by psychologic factors.

Interestingly, some researchers have argued that the conversion V pattern of the MMPI is representative of a general group characteristic that actually disguises important subgroup differences in the psychologic adjustment to chronic low back pain.[1, 102] The introduction of multivariate statistical techniques has yielded strong support for the contention that several distinct subtypes of psychologic response to chronic low back pain can be identified with the use of the MMPI.[1, 102] Several studies have reported such results,[1, 25, 95, 169] casting considerable doubt regarding the apparent psychologic homogeneity of patients with chronic low back pain.[16, 142]

Hazard and colleagues[66] tested the assumption that disability exaggeration affects treatment outcomes. They concluded that there were no significant associations between any individual factor and days lost from work over a 2-year period. Only two of the 12 disability exaggeration models tested distinguished between rehabilitation program graduates and dropouts, and none of the models accurately predicted return to work after treatment.

Attempts have been made to provide support for some of the outlined psychodynamic assumptions. Employing various electromyographic (EMG) techniques, some studies have found EMG changes, reflecting muscle hyperactivity, associated with various psychologic conflicts or stressors.[35, 41] Unfortunately, most of these studies, except those of Collins and coworkers[35] and Turk and Flor[178] are uncontrolled, and they have various methodological problems.[178] Other studies have demonstrated a correlation between decreased mobility in chronic low back pain and various psychodynamic factors.[51, 126]

Alexithymia—the Psychophysiologic Model

Many studies have consistently reported that patients with chronic low back pain tend to have difficulty with recognizing and expressing their feelings, particularly those of hostility and anger.[16, 142, 168, 184] Sifneos[164] coined the term alexithymia to refer to this condition; it has been suggested that alexithymia is common not only in chronic pain, but also in psychosomatic (or psychophysiologic) disorders in general.[16, 89] In this context, pain is viewed as a kind of body language expressing feelings that these patients cannot otherwise show.[16, 89] Approximately 45% of patients with chronic low back pain demonstrate significant alexithymia.[5, 117] It has been found that patients who report preoccupation with their symptoms and difficulty in expressing emotional distress are more significantly impaired by persistent pain than patients who do not report such responses.[92, 142]

Personality Type

Many researchers have attempted to correlate the development of chronic low back pain with specific personality types. The most frequent personality disorders associated with chronic low back pain were dependent personality[70] and histrionic (hysterical) personality.[70, 120] Keel[89] suggested that some patients may be more vulnerable and prone to develop chronic pain than others in similar conditions. Engel[45] and Blumer and Heilbronn[17] coined the term pain-prone personality (or disorder) in agreement with such a hypothesis. In his retrospective studies of a large number of patients with chronic pain, Blumer[16] noticed a remarkable psychologic homogeneity. Prior to the development of pain, these patients tended to demonstrate excessive work performance, industriousness, overactivity, and a general denial of interpersonal difficulties and hostile aggressive trends. After a significant loss or disappointment and often with the advent of an injury, these patients tended to develop intractable pain and a complete alteration in lifestyle, changing from responsible, overly active, and industrious individuals to passive-dependent invalids. Blumer suggested that, in these patients, basic passive-dependent needs are concealed and denied as unacceptable from an early age, only to reappear when pain ensues. However, the multiplicity of personality subtypes found by using the MMPI seems to contradict the tendency to associate chronic pain with only one specific or a few specific personality types.[1, 102, 126]

Keefe and associates[88] used a hierarchic cluster analysis procedure to identify homogeneous subgroups of patients with low back pain who show similar pain behavior patterns during a videotaped behavior sample. One hundred six patients with chronic low back pain were divided into two groups. The cluster analysis procedure identified four similar subgroups in both groups. The first subgroup showed a low or moderate level of guarding and a low level of other pain behaviors. The second subgroup showed a high level of guarding and a moderate level of rubbing of the painful area. The third subgroup showed high levels of guarding and moderate levels of bracing and rubbing. The fourth subgroup exhibited a high level of rubbing and moderate levels of bracing. Keefe and associates[88] concluded that the subgroups identified may require somewhat different approaches to pain assessment and treatment.

It is generally agreed that chronic pain as a major symptom is rare among patients with schizophrenia.[122] It is not common among those with major (endogenous) depression,[101, 122] and is often associated with other types of depression[38, 120] and anxiety.[120, 146] Although one investigator claimed that "chronic pain due to neurotic illness (mainly somatoform disorders or hysteria) and personality disorder is probably the most common variant,"[122] other researchers suggested that the patient with chronic low back pain has basically a psychosomatic (psychophysiologic) disorder.[16, 168] The difference between the two definitions is obvious. Whereas hysteria relates to pain in the absence of organic findings, the psychophysiologic model suggests some organic dysfunction attributable to emotional causes. It should be noted that at least some patients with chronic low back pain (as many as 20% to 30% in some studies[1, 7]) do not demonstrate evidence of psychopathologic changes.[70, 120]

Another important, and still controversial, issue is whether the psychodynamic and personality factors mentioned precede or result from chronic low back pain. It is obviously difficult to reach a definite conclusion, owing to difficulties in performing prospective studies in this case. Several studies have suggested that the patient's emotional condition not only precedes the pain[70] but is actually associated with its development.[111, 122] Pilowski and Spence[143] found that the illness behavior of patients with chronic pain (i.e., how they perceive, evaluate, and act on their symptoms[112]) is significantly associated with preexisting personality factors. Similarly, although patients with clearly physical lesions and good premorbid adjustment do not demonstrate significant emotional and personality changes,[70, 120] those with chronic pain thought to reflect a psychogenic cause tend to report at least some premorbid disturbance.[70, 120] In addition, the pretreatment psychologic condition of patients with chronic low back pain as evaluated by the MMPI[102] and other tests[70] has been found to be significantly related to the results of treatment, including surgery; poor pretreatment adjustment has been consistently linked with a poor response.

On the other hand, some investigators have suggested that chronic low back pain may lead to the development of emotional and even personality changes.[120, 150] For example, Pelz and Merskey[138] found that chronic pain due to organic causes results in emotional responses and disturbances in the patient's personal and social life (e.g., a significant degree of disturbance of work, sleep, and social activities and of sexual relationships). Other researchers have emphasized that patients with chronic low back pain develop a variety of psychologic, cognitive, and behavioral coping strategies to adjust to and to manage their pain.[75, 151] In addition, it has been demonstrated that the relief of chronic pain may result in some amelioration of personality change and psychologic disturbance.[170, 193]

Interpersonal (Environmental) Stressors

There has been a growing body of research suggesting an association between various environmental (psychosocial) stressors and the development, maintenance, and exacerbation of chronic low back pain.[63, 89, 178] Increased pain has thus been related to increased psychosocial stress.[47, 51] It has been demonstrated that a number of variables indicating family-related distress (e.g., family conflict and marital dissatisfaction) may be increased in patients with chronic low back pain compared with a control group.[47, 125] Factors reflecting familial maladjustment have also been associated with increased pain perception in patients with chronic low back pain.[47] In addition, it has been suggested that pain may occur more frequently in certain families, and specifically, that relatives of patients with chronic low back pain demonstrate substantially more reports of pain than do control subjects.[17] Although attempts have been made to identify specific family models of patients with chronic low back pain[98, 192] and to associate them with families with psychosomatic disorders in general,[178] specific characteristics of the families of patients with chronic pain have been delineated only rarely.[47]

It has been suggested that the patient's pain may fulfill the emotional needs of other family members. Thus, although acute pain appears at random, it may evolve into a chronic pain problem if it fulfills the object-related needs of a family.[98, 192] Similarly, the immediate precipitation of the symptom may be caused, according to these assumptions, by a threat to the family homeostasis.[98] In addition to the contribution of the family to the development and maintenance of chronic low back pain, chronic pain may exert a significant influence on the family.[17, 123] Extrafamilial stressors have also been associated with chronic low back pain. These include mainly factors related to work, such as type of occupation,[120] increased vocational stress,[125] reduced work satisfaction,[174] and decreased peer cohesion at work.[47] Interestingly, patients with chronic low back pain judged to have an organic cause have been found to demonstrate an increased rate of overall psychosocial distress.[67]

PROGRESSION FROM ACUTE TO CHRONIC LOW BACK PAIN

Acute low back pain is generally defined as pain of a duration not exceeding 6 months.[145, 162] This dichotomy between acute low back pain and chronic low back pain is somewhat arbitrary,[168] as changes in pain experience may be gradual[74] and are highly associated with the duration of the illness.[74, 162] In general, it seems that patients with chronic low back pain demonstrate significantly more psychopathology than do patients with acute low back pain.[75, 162, 168] Whereas acute low back pain may not be associated with significant emotional disturbance (with the exception of anxiety),[184] the development of chronicity has been found to lead to increased depression,[70, 168] anxiety,[162] and somatic preoccupation[75, 168] and to decreased coping ability.[75] The development of chronic pain has been also associated with alterations in pain perception and tolerance.[162] Fordyce[52] and Schofferman[160] claimed that acute pain tends to persist if it is treated solely as the result of a local lesion, while important psychologic considerations are ignored.

Keel[89] identified the following biopsychosocial factors that may lead to the development of chronic low back pain: (1) repeated investigations that fail to identify a clear course or explanation for the illness, and repeated treatment failures; (2) persistent disability and prolonged absence from work; (3) increasing physical inactivity; (4) secondary gains presumably associated with the illness, for example, improvement in family relations, the chance of being freed from an unpleasant duty, and financial compensation; (5) the development of medication abuse; and (6) negative side effects of surgery or drugs that may increase the patient's pain and hypochondriasis.

ORGANIC VERSUS PSYCHOGENIC (FUNCTIONAL) CHRONIC LOW BACK PAIN

The concept of psychogeneity has often been applied to the problem of chronic low back pain because many patients report greater pain and disability than their organic lesions apparently warrant.[67, 113, 154] Many studies have attempted to differentiate between demonstrable organic causation and a nonorganic, presumably psychogenic (functional) disorder. This dichotomy is currently regarded as a complex and controversial issue.[30, 102, 113] The differentiation would be valid if consistent and replicable findings would appear in various centers using different assessment techniques, and if these findings would demonstrate predictive validity regarding differences in prognosis or in the effects of various treatment modalities.[70, 110] Some studies have found, for example, that patients with chronic low back pain of organic causes demonstrate a favorable response to conservative,[75, 95] as well as surgical,[70, 132] treatment. Other studies regard the organic-psychogenic dichotomy as being confusing and misleading[27, 63, 64, 102, 176] and as having limited value in regard to prognosis and treatment decisions.[102, 176] They suggest that an integrated approach, emphasizing complex interactions among biologic, psychologic, and social correlates is more applicable for understanding chronic low back pain[16, 63, 89, 178]; they also recommend the formation of valid and reliable subgroups of patients, according to their psychosocial adjustment and ability to cope with chronic low back pain.[102, 176]

Ransford and colleagues[147] developed the concept of the pain drawing as a screening device to assess the psychologic status of patients with pain. They used a scoring system for pain drawings and assumed that only certain anatomic distributions of back pain and sciatica could be accepted as of organic origin. The patient's score was then compared with results of the MMPI. They concluded that "the pain drawing may allow the physician to screen out most (93%) of the patients who are likely to have poor psychometrics and allow him to obtain a full psychologic assessment before proceeding with the necessary treatment."[147] Udén and associates[182, 183] assessed pain drawings by categorizing the pain as organic, possibly organic, possibly nonorganic, and nonorganic. They also stated that correlation of the pain drawing with the MMPI or other psychologic assessments should not be regarded as a prerequisite for validating the pain drawing. They evaluated the precision and reliability of this system and concluded that "pain drawing thus appears to be as efficient and reliable as many other commonly used clinical routines despite its simplicity and the fact that no complicated machinery is involved."[9, 32]

Waddell and coworkers[186] suggested the Waddell score to describe a set of nonorganic physical signs (tenderness, simulation, distraction, regionalization, and overreaction) that are independent of those commonly used to detect organic disease, but that correlate with treatment failure, with long-standing symptoms, with elevated hypochondriasis and hysteria scores of the MMPI, and with various other psychologic factors. The Waddell score was validated as a useful tool to distinguish between nonorganic physical signs and physical disorders in low back pain. Chan and colleagues[32] examined the reliability of the pain drawing test using experienced and inexperienced evaluators and found an interevaluator reliability of between 73% and 78%. A correlation between pain drawings and Waddell's nonorganic physical signs demonstrated that a large proportion of patients with high Waddell scores had pain drawings indicating nonorganic pain. Moreover, no significant differences were noted in the distribution of Waddell scores and pain drawings on the basis of patient gender or payment status (e.g., medicolegal or workers' compensation involvement).

The differentiation between organic and psychogenic chronic low back pain is still established according to physical examination, x-ray study, computed tomography, myelography, electromyography, and nerve conduction studies, as well as by magnetic resonance imaging. The entire approach emphasizes the definition of psychogenic chronic low back pain as nonorganic; that is, the disorder is presumably functional when there is no evidence of objective organic findings.[176] As do other investigators[7, 30, 76, 157] the authors suggest that an organic disease and a psychiatric disorder may coexist independently; thus, the definition of functional causation should be based on the existence of positive psychologic findings. The rate of presumably psychogenic pain in various populations with chronic low back pain is between 20% and 50%.* Most studies suggest that patients with functional disorders demonstrate a significantly higher level of psychosocial disturbance compared with those who have organic disorders.[78, 89, 121, 145, 154] This relates, for example, to increased premorbid personality disturbance[70] and psychosocial maladjustment[75, 154] or to increased depression[70, 145] and anxiety.[70] Other studies, however, have found either no difference between the organic and nonorganic groups[146, 168] or increased psychopathologic changes among patients with organic conditions.[67]

Various psychologic assessment procedures have been used to differentiate between organic and functional chronic low back pain. Hackett and Bouckoms[64] identified some clinical characteristics that correlate with the psychogenicity of pain: the pain is in more than one place or is of more than one variety; the patient seems more interested in convincing others that the pain is genuine than in receiving a cure for it; the presence of emotional problems is denied; the pain is reported to be insensitive to any emotional state; the pain varies according to the interpersonal setting; the patient is convinced about the uniqueness and singularity of the pain; the patient projects to the physician the attitude that "only you can save me"; the pain either does not fluctuate over time or consistently becomes more severe, and nothing alleviates it.

Some studies found the MMPI to be useful in differentiating organic and psychogenic chronic low back pain.[29, 61, 110] Patients with psychogenic pain were thought to demonstrate the conversion V pattern of the MMPI

---

*References 44, 95, 145, 154, 157, 168, and 176.

to a greater degree.[61, 110] In addition, specific scales,[29] consisting of selected MMPI items, were constructed to distinguish between the two populations. Many studies, however, found a considerable similarity and overlap between the MMPI profiles of patients with functional and organic chronic low back pain.[7, 76, 95, 102, 168] Some investigators suggested that this overlap is a valid finding.[1, 7, 168] Other researchers claimed that this state actually reflects the inadequacy of the MMPI scale in the assessment of chronic low back pain and that other procedures could be more effective in distinguishing between organic and functional disorders.[76, 95] The following instruments have been used:

Pain Drawing Test. The pain drawing test[147] consists of an outline drawing of the human body on which patients map the nature and distribution of their pain. The patients are asked to describe four categories of pain: pins and needles, burning, stabbing, and deep ache. In chronic low back pain of organic origin, the patient should describe only one of the categories and the pain should follow an anatomic distribution matching the organic diagnosis. In psychogenic chronic low back pain, the pain drawings tend to be bizarre, patients describe multiple pain sensations, and the pain spreads to an unrelated area of the body in a nonanatomic distribution.[63, 147, 154] Various scoring systems have been developed to standardize the results. Although some studies have found this instrument to discriminate significantly between organic and functional pain,[147, 154] other reports have failed to replicate these findings.[9]

McGill Pain Questionnaire. This instrument, developed by Melzack,[115] consists of 20 sets of adjectives from which the patient is asked to choose the words best describing his or her pain. It also includes a pain drawing test, a rating of present pain intensity, and a selection of words that describe the temporal quality of the pain. Although some studies have found that patients with organic chronic low back pain use characteristic wordings and descriptions,[121] other reports have found a considerable overlap with nonorganic (functional) chronic low back pain.[120] All the words employed in the McGill Pain Questionnaire imply some physical change in the body.[120] Although the McGill Pain Questionnaire can identify patients with chronic low back pain with certain patterns of psychologic disturbances, it is not considered effective in distinguishing organic from functional pain.[89]

Back Pain Classification Scale. This instrument, developed by Leavitt and Garron[93] consists of various pain-related terms. The patient is instructed to choose the terms best describing his or her pain. By means of discriminant analysis, Leavitt and Garron[93] identified 13 items reliably differentiating organic from functional chronic low back pain. Replication of these results,[94, 95] however, was not reported independently.

Mensana Clinic Back Pain Test. This 15-question test,[76] which is essentially a structured medical interview, records the patient's physical and psychologic response to chronic low back pain. It has been found to differentiate between organic and functional pain in some studies.[70, 76] Other specific pain questionnaires have also attempted to tackle this issue,[133, 154] although so far their use has been limited.

Waddell's Nonorganic Physical Signs in Chronic Low Back Pain. This is a set of nonorganic physical signs that are independent of those commonly used to detect organic disease, but that correlate with treatment failures, long-standing symptoms, elevated hypochondriasis and hysteria scores of the MMPI, and various other psychologic factors.[186]

Pain and Impairment Relationship Scale. Few validated instruments are available to assess beliefs and attitudes that patients have regarding pain or ability to function despite discomfort. The Pain and Impairment Relationship Scale (PAIRS)[167] was developed to tap these important beliefs and attitudes in patients with chronic pain. Validation of the PAIRS to a general sample of patients with chronic benign low back pain supported the discriminant, convergent, and divergent validity, as well as the reliability and relative independence from favorable self-report response bias of the PAIRS by demonstrating, respectively, that (1) the impairment beliefs assessed with the PAIRS were more prominent in patients with chronic low back pain than in matched healthy control subjects without pain; (2) scores on the PAIRS were significantly related to measures of physical impairment, but not to physicians' ratings of disease severity; (3) the impairment beliefs assessed with the PAIRS are readily distinguishable from cognitive distortions and emotional distress; (4) PAIRS scores for patients with chronic low back pain are relatively consistent over time; and (5) PAIRS scores are not significantly associated with measures of favorable self-report response bias.

In summary, despite the many controversies and inconsistencies associated with the distinction between organic and functional chronic low back pain, treatment is still often recommended (or not recommended) on this basis.[70, 176] This may lead to serious errors in the treatment of patients with either disorder.[176] The authors suggest that, in each case, the organic and psychologic conditions have to be carefully scrutinized. Decisions as to treatment should be based simultaneously on the orthopedic evaluation and the patient's ability to benefit from the treatment.

ROLE OF PSYCHIATRIST IN TEAM EVALUATION AND TREATMENT APPROACH

The discussion above emphasizes the highly complex interactions between physical and emotional dimensions in chronic low back pain. Psychologic factors have a great influence on the development of chronicity,[7, 89] and different personality profiles[102] or coping styles[151] are found to be associated with the prognosis and different responses to treatment. Such a view seems to call for a radical change in the role of the psychiatric consultant. Traditionally, psychiatrists have been employed when pain has continued for a long time and has become resistant to conventional therapies and when pain behaviors appear inappropriate to the organic condition (e.g., to solve issues of organicity versus psychologic overlay.[63, 89, 184]). Thus, the psychiatrist has been called relatively late in the treatment, when the patient and the physician are already highly frustrated and equally mistrustful.[64]

It has been suggested that the psychiatric consultant should be brought into the case early.[64] All patients have to be routinely assessed by a psychiatrist if the pain does not respond to conventional treatment within a few weeks, because only such early screening can prevent chronicity.[89] Moreover, the psychiatrist should be an integral part of a multidisciplinary team employing a biopsychosocial approach[64, 160] and should be introduced to patients as such.[64] One role of the psychiatrist is to evaluate and identify the psychiatric condition, the emotional adjustment, and the success in coping with pain according to standardized interviews, including those with family members, and accepted psychologic batteries.[64] In addition, the psychiatrist should serve as a consultant to the other professionals and as a full-fledged member in an integrated team.[64, 160] According to Schofferman,[160] a chronic low back pain management program "that uses a multidisciplinary team approach and a biopsychosocial treatment model, may have the highest likelihood of success." This team includes the following professionals: an orthopedic surgeon, a psychiatrist or a psychologist, a physical therapist, an occupational therapist, an anesthesiologist, and occasionally, a neurosurgeon.[160]

DRUG TREATMENT OF CHRONIC LOW BACK PAIN

The typical patient with chronic low back pain has backache for longer than 6 months. Although the individual usually has a defined disorder in the lumbar spine, the pain is out of proportion to the organic lesion and is not amenable to standard treatment modalities, including surgical intervention. These patients are not working, are increasingly incapacitated, and consume improper medications such as narcotic analgesics and tranquilizers. These drugs usually provide little, if any, help. Pain plays a major role in the lives of these patients and their families.[6]

About 50% of patients admitted to chronic pain programs are routinely using narcotic analgesics, tranquilizers, hypnotic sedatives, and muscle relaxants.[149] These medications not only provide little relief from pain but also possess a strong potential for exacerbating the pain and the related symptoms. Narcotic analgesics lose their effectiveness in reducing chronic back pain because tolerance develops.[26] In addition, the use of narcotic analgesics leads to dependence and depression. The administration of benzodiazepines as tranquilizers for treating chronic low back pain (e.g., diazepam [Valium]) is inappropriate and contraindicated. By virtue of the ability of these agents to deplete serotonin levels in the central nervous system, they decrease the pain threshold and induce depression, habituation, and sleep disturbances.[73] Unfortunately, these are the drugs most commonly prescribed by many practitioners managing chronic low back pain.[72]

Therefore, the essential first step in any chronic low back pain program is to discontinue the use of these harmful agents. After the medication use is successfully discontinued, patients may even notice some alleviation of pain.[145] (For a description of a detoxification program, see under Operant Behavioral Treatment Programs below.) Sleep disturbances that were present before detoxification or were brought about by the process are managed by the administration of tricyclic antidepressants[2] (TCAs) or the newer heterocyclic antidepressants[197] (HCAs), with relatively few side effects and safe profile for use in elderly or physically ill patients,[46, 48, 97] in increasing dosages.

Sympathetic overactivity is an important feature of acute pain. In chronic pain, on the other hand, the sympathetic activity subsides, and appetite and sleep disturbances, irritability, and somatic preoccupation increase.[150] Therefore, the pharmacologic management of acute pain is completely different from that of chronic pain. For treating acute pain, analgesics are in order. For treating chronic pain, narcotics, and tranquilizers may be harmful, whereas tricyclic[2, 8, 187] and heterocyclic antidepressants, and low doses of butyrophenone, thioxanthenes, and phenothiazines are in order. The analgesic efficacy of TCAs in treating chronic pain has been documented in peripheral neuropathies, postherpetic neuralgia, and tic douloureux.[39, 139, 195, 196] The analgesic efficacy of the newer HCAs in treating pain is under research, and preliminary reports are encouraging.[140] Because pain and depression coexist in patients with chronic low back pain, it is reasonable to administer TCAs or HCAs. Sternbach[171] hypothesized that chronic pain is associated with the depletion of brain serotonin levels. This depletion accounts for the frequent occurrence of depression in chronic pain. Sternbach and colleagues[172] also speculated that serotoninergic TCAs (e.g., clomipramine), by virtue of correcting the serotonin deficit, successfully ameliorate depression and chronic pain. Indeed, a single dose of 40 mg of fenfluramine, a selective releaser of serotonin, reduces both pain and depression in some patients with chronic low back pain.[190] Other researchers have hypothesized that TCAs may relieve pain by affecting endogenous opiates[64] or by reducing anxiety or muscle tension.[73]

Ward[191] conducted a double-blind study testing the effects of desipramine or doxepin on patients with chronic low back pain and depression. Sixty percent of the patients had significant pain relief as well as relief of the depression with either drug. Patients who had pain relief after an acute challenge with fenfluramine were significantly more likely to have pain relief with either antidepressant.[191] Neither drug changed cerebrospinal fluid endorphin levels, acute pain tolerance, or EMG findings. Ward[191] suggested that his data may support the idea of a sertoninergic mechanism of action for TCAs in chronic pain. Although desipramine is usually regarded as a noradrenergic antidepressant and the exact mechanism of action of doxepin is uncertain, both drugs may exert serotoninergic uptake blocking effects.[191] Amitriptyline, doxepin, or clomipramine may be administered to fight chronic low back pain, anxiety, depression, and insomnia. Because TCAs have anticholinergic side effects on the cardiovascular, gastrointestinal, and genitourinary systems, care should be exercised in elderly patients[175] and in those with cardiac disease, prostatism, and glaucoma.

In instituting treatment with antidepressant medication, it is often advantageous to administer the drug in divided doses throughout the day. This is done so that the patient can gradually accommodate to unwanted side effects, and there is an opportunity to titrate the dosage upward until the desired clinical effect is achieved. After the optimum therapeutic dosage is achieved, any of the currently available TCAs or HCAs (except fluoxetine, which should be given in the morning) can be given as a single bedtime dose with equal therapeutic efficacy. However, a single bedtime dose is not recommended in elderly patients, who are likely to be sensitive to the anticholinergic effects of the antidepressant, and in patients who have a moderate or high degree of anxiety. These patients may tolerate the drug better if it is administered in three or four smaller doses divided throughout the day.[11] The dosage is increased gradually, starting with 25 to 50 mg at bedtime.[72] Usual adult daily dosage are listed in Table 1, and blood level monitoring is available if the desired effect is not achieved at those dosages.[62] Moreover, one study has supported a possible therapeutic window for amitriptyline,[22] but at this time there are inadequate data to support reliable statements regarding correlation of therapeutic response and plasma levels for the newer antidepressants.[62] The full effect may not be noticed for 2 to 4 weeks.

One of the continuing problems in achieving a prompt and therapeutically satisfactory response to antidepressant drugs is the inability to predict which patient will respond optimally to which type of antidepressant. Attempts to use blood, cerebrospinal fluid, and urine tests of neurotransmitter metabolites to predict responsiveness to specific antidepressant drugs have been unsuccessful. Most often, the process of arriving at an optimum response involves considerable trial and error, employing different antidepressant drugs until a satisfactory therapeutic response is established with a tolerable level of side effects. The association between the effect of TCAs on amelioration of pain and improvement of depression in patients with chronic pain is equivocal. Some studies found simultaneous improvement in both aspects on the administration of TCAs.[23, 189] They also found that the duration of treatment (about 4 weeks) and the dosage of TCAs (150 to 250 mg daily) are similar for chronic pain and depressive disorders.[85, 189] Other reports suggest that TCAs may have a differential effect on chronic low back pain and depression.[198]

Pain amelioration may be attained with smaller dosages[198] and in a shorter duration,[72] as compared with the time and dosage required to affect depression. This means that antidepressants should be administered to patients with chronic low back pain, regardless of whether they have concomitant depression. If therapy is successful, it should be maintained for 3 to 6 months. The success rate of TCAs has been documented, by several investigators, to be about 60% to 70%.[17, 99] Anxiety commonly complicates chronic low back pain. The usual antianxiety agents, such as diazepam, are contraindicated in chronic pain syndromes because they deplete brain serotonin levels. On the other hand, phenothiazine tranquilizers, which are potent anxiolytics,[72] are also effective in the management of chronic low back pain.[72, 150] Chlorpromazine, a standard phenothiazine, blocks dopamine

Table 1
■

Daily Dosages of Antidepressant Medication for Adults		
	Daily Dosage (mg)*	Range (mg)
Tertiary amine—tricyclic		
Amitriptyline	125–200	50–300
Imipramine	125–200	50–300
Clomipramine	125–200	50–300
Secondary amine—tricyclic		
Desipramine	150–250	50–300
Nortriptyline	75–100	30–100
Bridged tricyclic		
Maprotiline	125–200	50–225
Tetracyclic		
Mianserin	60–90	30–120
Triazolopyridine derivate		
Trazodone	100–250	50–400
Nefazodone	20–40	10–60
SSRIs	20–40	5–80
Fluoxetine	10–20	10–40
Paroxetine	20–40	10–50
Fluvoxamine	100–200	50–300

*Elderly patients should generally be treated with one half of the usual adult dosage of any of these antidepressants
SSRIs, serotonin selective reuptake inhibitors.

postsynaptically and has blockade effects; in addition, haloperidol has been shown to bind to opiate receptors as an agonist. The combination of TCAs and phenothiazines may be more efficacious than either drug alone.[75, 150]

In summary, the goals of drug therapy in chronic low back pain are (1) cessation of inappropriate drug administration; (2) management of pain, depression, and anxiety; (3) management of sleep disturbances; and (4) appropriate use of analgesics.[72]

PSYCHOLOGIC TREATMENT OF CHRONIC LOW BACK PAIN

General Principles

Mental health care professionals are playing an increasingly important part in the management of chronic low back pain. Although they are still concerned with the various psychosocial aspects of pain,[64] psychologists and psychiatrists are also currently involved in the treatment of chronic pain. In this regard, some important psychologic principles have been established, which are considered by many mental health care practitioners to be an integral part of the treatment of chronic low back pain.

Patients with chronic pain must be treated in a manner different from that for patients with acute pain.[160] The treatment goal often becomes not eliminating the pain[160] but learning how to live with it.[31, 89, 160] Thus, the continuation or resumption of work and other regular activities becomes a paramount goal in the treatment of chronic low back pain.[16, 160] Characteristically, most psychologic treatments stress the importance of the patient's taking an active role in treatment and the establishment of a cooperative relationship with the therapists.[31, 178] Patients must experience their own actions as influencing the pain, thus gaining a sense of control and mastery over their situations.[31, 89] In addition, patients must receive clearly presented information about their illness and its treatment.[89] This orientation should also include the spouse or significant other and other family members who may otherwise continue to reinforce pain behaviors, because such behaviors are associated with conflicts in the family.[16, 89] If the cause of chronic low back pain is presumably mainly psychogenic, therapists should respond to it as they would to organic pain.[16] Patients have to be told that pain of an uncertain origin or that resulting from mental stress may exist and can be treated.[16, 89] This must be conveyed to the patient with an empathic and accepting attitude.[89] Although the exact nature of a psychogenic origin (e.g., depression and anxiety) has to be elucidated and treated,[16, 160] invasive somatic investigations must be avoided in these cases, unless they are absolutely indicated.[16, 89]

The available psychologic treatments are reviewed below. Regardless of the treatment, however, the best results are achieved when psychologists and psychiatrists are an integral part of a multidisciplinary team, including professionals from several specialities.[160, 178] This has been established in various studies,[20, 177] emphasizing the importance of treating chronic low back pain as a multifunctional problem that requires attention to the physical as well as psychologic and social aspects of pain.[178]

Behavioral Intervention Procedures

Operant Behavioral Treatment Programs

Operant approaches do not deal with the pain experience per se but rather with its behavioral consequences.[89, 178] The goals of operant treatment are the extinction of maladaptive pain behaviors (e.g., verbally reporting pain, taking medications, and avoiding activities associated with pain) and the promotion of healthy behaviors (e.g., participating in exercise and work).[31, 150, 178] To increase the rate of the desired behaviors, they should systematically be followed by effective positive reinforcement. Unwanted pain behaviors are usually reduced by extinction (i.e., by withdrawal of attention and reinforcements for these behaviors).[31, 89, 150, 178] As Reuler and associates[150] described, "if a chronic low back pain patient lies in bed excessively, one can either withdraw the reinforcers for remaining in bed, such as withdrawing housecleaning services, or give reinforcement to walking as mechanisms to increase up time."

Another goal of operant treatment is to increase physical activity.[89, 150, 178] This is achieved through step-by-step training programs,[89] in which activity is associated with various positive reinforcers, but not with pain.[16, 150, 178] A third goal of such programs is the elimination or reduction of medication use.[16, 31, 89, 150, 178] After the establishment of the required dosage, medications are not prescribed as needed, but are provided at regular time intervals. Thus, medication administration and the attention associated with it are no longer contingent on pain. Because the medication is in liquid form, masked by color and taste, and is given in the same volume for each dose, the total amount of medication may be gradually reduced.[16, 89, 150, 178]

Operant programs must usually be conducted on an inpatient basis[16, 150, 178] and are costly, time consuming, and complex.[31] Some uncontrolled studies have reported significant increases in activity and employability and marked medication dosage reduction, both after treatment and at follow-up.[4, 27] However, with the exception of the study of Cairns and Pasino,[28] no control group studies have been conducted to test the efficacy of the operant approach in treating chronic low back pain.[31, 178] Although they are considered promising, operant treatments have several limitations.[178] Reinforcements seem to fail to generalize to activities that are not directly treated, and the results may be not maintained when the reinforcers are removed.[28, 178] Another issue to be considered is the importance of family involvement and the patient's natural environment (in terms of stress versus tranquility) in the maintenance of treatment effects.[51]

Respondent Treatment Approaches

The respondent treatment approaches include distraction, relaxation, imagery techniques, and biofeedback. The goal of these treatments is to influence the assumed psychologic basis of chronic low back pain.[178] The theoretic basis of this approach is the assumption of a pain-tension-pain circle. Accordingly, treatment should interrupt this vicious circle by replacing the increased muscle tension with an adequate and tension-incompatible reaction such as relaxation.[94, 178] These techniques all aim to assist the patients in controlling and regulating the sensory input and thus in experiencing mastery over the pain experience.[89]

Distraction (Attention Diversion). The rationale of this technique is concentration on thoughts to divert the patient's attention from the pain.[178] Attention diversion can be also achieved through a variety of activities, such as walking, talking, or exercising.[89] These activities should require enough attention to make the patient forget the pain. The efficacy of this technique has been demonstrated in patients with chronic low back pain.[89, 160]

Relaxation. A variety of procedures can be used to induce profound muscle relaxation. The most prevalent method, progressive muscle relaxation,[82] consists of having the patient tense and then relax the major muscle groups of the body in a fixed order and symmetric manner.[24] The rationale is that the patient's negative expectations about pain can increase anxiety; this, in turn, fosters muscle tension, which leads to more pain and consequently more anxiety.[89, 178] This cycle can be interrupted by relaxation.[89, 178] In addition, improvement may also be related to changes in the sympathetic nervous system.[79] Studies evaluating the efficacy of relaxation techniques in chronic low back pain, with concomitant biofeedback[10, 86] or without it,[89, 160, 180] including those with controlled designs,[180] have reported this modality to be useful. In addition, relaxation is relatively inexpensive and easy to manage, in both outpatient and group settings.[89, 180]

Imagery Techniques. In imagery procedures, the patient focuses attention on a comfortable picture that is incompatible with pain or tries to transform the pain perception or the situation (context) in which the pain is perceived. Examples of imaginative pain perception transformation are reinterpreting the chronic low back pain as mildly disturbing, instead of extremely painful, or imagining comfortable warmth spreading into the painful areas. Changing the context may be accomplished by imagining, for example, the chronic low back pain to be the result of strenuous work, while realizing that one is now resting in a comfortable chair.[89]

Biofeedback. Biofeedback is the process of providing visual or auditory information feedback to a subject of the status of some somatic or autonomic function.[71, 150] With biofeedback-measuring devices sensitive to responses in the body beneath the threshold of usual awareness (e.g., visceral responses and muscle tension), it is possible to provide moment-to-moment information about these responses and thus to help the patient to control and modify them.[173] Two types of biofeedback application may be distinguished. One is a specific type in which the patient is provided feedback about the actual condition that needs to be controlled. The other, more applicable to chronic low back pain, is the nonspecific type. The patient is taught a more general skill—such as controlling the amplitude of a component in the electroencephalogram or achieving EMG reduction in various muscles—that has been found to be associated with pain reduction.[71, 173] EMG biofeedback, for example, may use a clanging signal, the rate of which increases as the EMG level rises and decreases as the EMG level falls. The patient's task is to learn to relax with the biofeedback's assistance.

Most studies on biofeedback treatment in chronic low back pain are anecdotal or systematic case studies[10, 129] or group outcome or comparison studies.[69, 86, 137] Only a few controlled studies have been performed.[50, 130] In general, the biofeedback studies are difficult to evaluate. According to Truk and Flor,[178] "different methodological procedures, different patient group, variation in the number and length of treatment sessions and numerous design studies, including the combination of biofeedback with relaxation training in some studies but not in others, make conclusions tentative." The evaluation of biofeedback effects in chronic low back pain, in general, permits no clear conclusions.[31] When pain reduction is used as the relevant criterion, some studies report significant reduction in pain intensity and/or frequency after treatment,[10, 50, 129, 130] whereas other reports have not found significant change.[69, 86, 137] When EMG values are used as the criterion, the results are still not clear. Some studies have demonstrated significant posttreatment EMG reductions,[50] whereas other investigations have not shown significant changes.[69, 137] However, the two controlled studies that have assessed the influence of biofeedback alone in chronic low back pain[50, 130] demonstrate strong effects of EMG biofeedback on pain and tension levels. Thus, it is suggested that, although the research on the efficacy of biofeedback in chronic low back pain is preliminary,[50] it appears to be a promising treatment modality for such patients.[71, 178] Some researchers emphasize, however, that because biofeedback is a costly and complex procedure, it should be reserved for patients who have no success with other behavioral techniques.[89, 181] In addition, it has been demonstrated that the nonspecific type of biofeedback application often requires continued and frequent practice. This raises such issues as how to transfer the training to the real world from a quiet, clinical setting.[173]

The mechanisms presumed to underlie EMG biofeedback's effectiveness in chronic low back pain are the reduction of both muscle hyperreaction and anxiety.[178] Although some studies have demonstrated a significant association between muscle tension and/or anxiety reduction and a decrease in pain,[50] other reports have not.[69, 130] Thus, the following other mechanisms have been proposed: distraction,[116] suggestion,[116] increase of the patient's sense of control and mastery over the pain,[71, 116] the mental calm experienced by patients receiving EMG biofeedback,[199] and the effect of biofeedback on modifying maladaptive cognitive evaluations and responses associated with the experience of pain.[50, 130]

Cognitive Approaches

The cognitive approaches are closely related to the gate control model of pain of Melzack and Wall.[114] As mentioned earlier, this model emphasizes that motivational-affective and cognitive-evaluative dimensions may modulate the perception of the sensory input. The basic assumption underlying the cognitive perception is that the behavior of individuals is determined not only by how patients perceive sensory phenomena (e.g., pain), but also by the way in which they construe their world and apply meaning to it.[178] The goal of these approaches is to alter maladaptive thoughts, feelings, or behaviors related to pain and thereby to modify the experience of pain.[178] The treatment involves educating the patient about the identification of pain-eliciting and pain-aggravating situations, thoughts, and behaviors, as well as the identification and modification of maladaptive pain-related cognition.[177] The cognitive approach has successfully been employed in various pain syndromes, including chronic low back pain.[180] A significant reduction in pain intensity and general suffering and a concomitant decrease in the use of the health care system have been reported. Cognitive treatment also has the advantage of being applicable in group and outpatient settings.[178, 180]

Hypnosis

When employing hypnosis in the management of chronic pain syndromes, various induction and deepening procedures are typically used and followed by specific analgesia-inducing techniques. These may include the direct suggestion of analgesia (e.g., loss or decrease of sensation in the affected body part), transformation of the pain experience (e.g., movement of the pain from one part of the body to another where it is more manageable), and various forms of attention diversion.[78, 155]

Most studies evaluating the effects of hypnosis in pain control are uncontrolled clinical case studies, in which the subjective report of pain reduction is often the sole criterion of success.[178] Usually, these studies report impressive pain reduction.[36, 155] However, the total lack of controlled clinical research precludes confident conclusions about the efficacy of hypnosis in chronic low back pain.[178] Interestingly, some leading authorities in the field of pain have considerable reservations regarding the employment of hypnosis in chronic pain. Hacket and Bouckoms[64] found that "only about one in four subjects is able to achieve (in hypnosis) a state of concentration of sufficient magnitude for lasting pain control." Merskey[119] emphasized that relief of pain with hypnotic techniques is "rarely complete where there is an important physical cause of pain, and frequently it is of only modest proportions." In Orne's[134] experience, on the other hand, although hypnotherapy has been efficacious in managing chronic organic pain, it is frequently ineffective in relieving functional pain. Hendler and Fernandez[71] suggested that, although hypnosis is an effective treatment for acute pain problems, there is only limited evidence of its efficacy in treating patients with chronic pain, with the exception of chronic muscle tension and its resulting pain.

Psychodynamic Psychotherapy

Psychodynamic psychotherapy, when offered as the sole treatment, has had limited success in alleviating chronic low back pain.[64] Psychotherapy may, however, produce significant benefit if used in conjunction with other treatment modalities, such as behavioral therapy.[64, 160] Its role then is to gain the patient's cooperation in the treatment program and to promote realistic expectations to help the person adjust to chronic pain and to achieve insight into the psychosocial problems associated with pain. Merskey[119] suggested that psychotherapy may be useful, particularly for pain of assumed psychogenic origin, although it may also assist the patient with organic pain to maintain a more useful and affective adjustment. In his experience, relatively brief psychotherapy (10 to 12 sessions) is usually sufficient. If it does not work within this time schedule, the chances for any significant change are minimum. When intensive psychotherapy is not appropriate, patients may nevertheless be helped by supportive psychotherapy[119] or counseling.[160] Keel[89] suggested that, because many patients with chronic low back pain are alexithymic, methods that help to activate feelings or that focus on body awareness seem more suitable than psychodynamic psychotherapy.

Group Treatment and Eclectic Approaches

Group programs have become popular in the treatment of chronic low back pain.[168] Various models exist. The main principles of group treatment may be elucidated through one model, pain control classes.[77] These involve patients with chronic pain in various stages of treatment and therapists experienced both in group treatment and in the various mechanisms of chronic low back pain. The goals of these classes are to correct misconceptions and to reduce fears about illness, to replace self-defeating patterns of thinking with more constructive ones, and to provide a forum for mastery experience. Each meeting consists of the following parts: (1) educating patients about their attitudes toward pain and ways to modify them, (2) conducting group interactions and discussions related to pain, and (3) conducting group experiences of various behavioral techniques.

The efficacy of pain control classes has been associated with several factors. The group experience involves exposure to others and thus involves peer pressure that forces the individual to change pain-related thinking and behavior.[77] The group may instill hope through processes such as imparting information and providing encouragement, group support, and constant feedback.[77, 200] During group interaction, patients may explore and vent their pain-related feelings and perceive the commonality of their problem (i.e., others also have chronic low back pain).[77, 200] In addition, good role models are provided by inviting successful graduates of preceding groups to each new group.[77, 169] Employing this model in chronic low back pain, Herman and Baptiste[77] demonstrated a considerable reduction in depression, pain perception, and analgesic intake and a significant increase in employment rates after treatment. Other models of group programs, combining several different treatment methods, have also been successful.[30, 188] Obvious advantages of group treatment in chronic low back pain are that it is inexpensive and may be employed on an outpatient basis.

Another relatively recent development in the treatment of chronic low back pain includes the eclectic (or comprehensive) approaches.[89, 160, 178] These simultaneously employ a range of techniques that draw from various theoretic perspectives, such as operant behavioral procedures, physical rehabilitation, family participation, group discussions, biofeedback and relaxation, and supportive treatment.[188] Most studies of eclectic approaches,[33, 188] although not all of them,[34] provide some evidence of the usefulness of such programs; the combinations are probably more efficient than each treatment alone.[89, 159] For example, there are marked reduction in pain and the use of medication, an increase in activity, and significant extent of vocational rehabilitation in a large number of patients. However, the lack of control groups and comprehensive pain assessment in these studies, and the uncertainty about the effective components, prevent definite conclusions.[178]

REFERENCES

1. Adams, K. M., Heilbronn, M., and Blumer, D.: A multimethod evaluation of the MMPI in a chronic pain patient sample. J. Clin. Psychol. 42:878–886, 1986.
2. Alcoff, J., Jones, E., Rust, P., and Newman, R.: Controlled trial of imipramine for chronic low back pain. J. Fam. Pract. 14:841–846, 1982.
3. American Psychiatric Association: Diagnostic and Statistical Manual of Mental Disorders, 4th Ed. Washington, DC, American Psychiatric Association, 1994.
4. Anderson, T. P., Cole, T. M., Gullickson, G., et al.: Behavior modification of chronic pain: A treatment program by multidisciplinary team. Clin. Orthop. 129:96–100, 1977.
5. Antczak-Bouckoms, A., and Bouckoms, A. J.: Affective disturbance and the denial of problems in dental patients with pain. Int. J. Psychosom. 32:9–11, 1985.
6. Aronoff, G. M., and Evans, W. O.: Evaluation and treatment of chronic pain at the Boston Pain Center. J. Clin. Psychiatry 4(suppl.):4–9, 1982.
7. Atkinson, J. H., Jr., Ingram, R. E., Kremer, E. F., and Saccuzzo, D. P.: MMPI subgroups and affective disorder in chronic pain patients. J. Nerv. Ment. Dis. 174:408–413, 1986.
8. Baldessarini, R. J.: Drugs and the treatment of psychiatric disorders In Gilman, A. G., Rall, T. W., Nies, A. S., Taylor, P., et al. (eds.): Goodman and Gilman's The Pharmacological Basis of Therapeutics, 8th Ed. New York, Macmillan, 1985.
9. Bayer, C. L. von: Invalid use of pain drawings in psychological screening of back pain patients. Pain 16:103–107, 1983.
10. Belar, C. D., and Cohen, T. L.: The use of EMG feedback and progressive muscle relaxation in the treatment of a woman with chronic back pain. Biofeedback Self Regul. 4:349–352, 1979.
11. Bernstein, J. G.: Drug interactions. In Hacket, T. P., and Cassam, N. H. (eds.): Massachusetts General Hospital Handbook of General Hospital Psychiatry, 2nd Ed. Littleton, MA, PSG Publishing, 1987, pp. 538–571.
12. Biering-Sorensen, F., and Thomsen, C.: Medical, social and occupational history as risk indicators for low-back trouble in a general population. Spine 11:720–725, 1986.
13. Bigos, S., Spengler, D. M., Martin, N. A., et al.: Back injuries in industry: A retrospective study: II. Injury factors. Spine 11:246–251, 1986.
14. Bigos, S., Spengler, D. M., Martin, N. A., et al.: Back injuries in industry: A retrospective study: III. Employee-related factors. Spine 11:252–256, 1986.
15. Blumer, D., Roth, T., and Heilbronn, B.: Biological markers for depression in chronic pain. Presented at the Annual Meeting of the American Psychiatric Association, New Orleans, May 1981.
16. Blumer, D.: Psychiatric aspects of chronic pain: Nature identification and treatment of the pain-prone disorder. In Rothman, R. H., and Simeone,

F. A. (eds.): The Spine, 2nd Ed. Philadelphia, W. B. Saunders, 1982, pp. 1090–1117.
17. Blumer, D., and Heilbronn, B.: Chronic pain as a variant of depressive disease. The pain-prone disorder. J. Nerv. Ment. Dis. 170:381–406, 1982.
18. Blumer, D., Zorick, F., and Heilbronn, B.: Biological markers for depression in chronic pain. J. Nerv. Ment. Dis. 170:425–428, 1982.
19. Boden, S. D., Lestini, W. F., and Wiesel, S. W.: Compensation low back pain. Semin. Spine Surg. 1:68–75, 1989.
20. Bonica, J. J.: Basic principles in managing chronic pain. Arch. Surg. 112:783–788, 1977.
21. Bouras, N.: Psychological aspects of patients having multiple operations for low back pain. Br. J. Med. Psychol. 57:147–151, 1984.
22. Boyer, W. F., Lake, C. R.: Initial severity and diagnosis influence the relationship of tricyclic plasma levels to response: A statistical review. J. Clin. Psychopharmacol. 7:67–71, 1987.
23. Bradley, J. J.: Severe localized pain associated with the depressive syndrome. Br. J. Psychiatry 109:741–745, 1963.
24. Bradey, J. P.: Behavior therapy. In Kaplan, H. I., and Sadock, B. J. (eds.): Comprehensive Textbook of Psychiatry, 4th Ed. Baltimore, Williams & Wilkins, 1985, pp. 1365–1373.
25. Bradley, L. A., and Van der Heide, L. H.: Pain-related correlates of MMPI profile subgroups among back pain patients. Health Psychol. 3:157–174, 1984.
26. Brodner, R. A., and Taub, A.: Chronic pain exacerbated by long term narcotic use in patients with nonmalignant disease: Clinical syndrome and treatment. Mt. Sinai J. Med. 45:233–237, 1978.
27. Cairns, D., Thomas, L., Mooney, V., and Pace, J. B.: A comprehensive treatment approach to chronic low back pain. Pain 2:301–308, 1976.
28. Cairns, D., and Pasino, J. A.: Comparison of verbal reinforcement of feedback in the operant treatment of disability due to chronic low back pain. Behav. Ther. 8:621–630, 1977.
29. Calsyn, D. A., Louks, J., and Freeman, C. W.: The use of the MMPI with chronic low back pain patients with mixed diagnosis. J. Clin. Psychol. 32:532–536, 1976.
30. Cameron, A. J. R., and Shepel, L. F.: Psychological assessment. In Kirkaldy-Willis, W. H. (ed.): Managing Low Back Pain. New York, Churchill Livingstone, 1983, pp. 63–73.
31. Cameron, A. J. R., Shepel, L. F., and Bowen, R. C.: Psychological treatment of back pain and associated problems. In Kirkaldy-Willis, W. H.: Managing Low Back Pain. New York, Churchill Livingstone, 1983, pp. 229–239.
32. Chan, C. W., Goldman, S., Ilstrup, D. M., et al.: The pain drawing and Waddell's nonorganic physical signs in chronic low back pain. Spine 18:1717–1722, 1993.
33. Chapman, S. L., Brena, S. F., and Bradford, L. A.: Treatment outcome in a chronic pain rehabilitation program. Pain 11:255–268, 1981.
34. Cohen, M. J., Heinrich, R. L., Collins, G. A., and Bonebakker, A. D.: Group outpatient physical or behavioral therapy for chronic low back pain. Paper presented at the Annual Meeting of the American Pain Society, New York, September 1980.
35. Collins, G. A., Cohen, M. J., Naliboff, B. D., and Schandler, S. L.: Comparative analysis of paraspinal and frontalis EMG, heart rate, and skin conductance in chronic low back pain patients and normals in various postures and stress. Scand. J. Rehabil. Med. 14:39–46, 1982.
36. Crasilneck, H. B.: Hypnosis in the control of chronic low back pain. Am. J. Clin. Hypn. 22:71–78, 1979.
37. Crisson, J., Keele, F. J., Wilkins, R. H., et al.: Self-report of depressive symptoms in low back pain patients. J. Clin. Psychol. 42:425–430, 1986.
38. Crue, B. L., and Pinsky, J. J.: An approach to chronic pain of non-malignant origin. Postgrad. Med. J. 60:858–864, 1984.
39. Davis, J. L., Lewis, S. B., Gerlich, J. E., et al.: Peripheral diabetic neuropathy treated with amitriptyline and fluphenazine. JAMA 238:2291–2293, 1977.
40. Dhanens, T. P., and Jarrett, S. R.: MMPI assessment index. Predictive and concurrent validity. Int. J. Clin. Neuropsychol. 6:46–49, 1984.
41. Dorpat, T. L., and Holmes, T. H.: Backache and muscle tension origin. In Kroger, W. S. (ed.): Psychosomatic Obstetrics, Gynecology, and Endocrinology. Springfield, IL, Charles C. Thomas, 1962.
42. Dworkin, R. H., Handlin, D. S., Richlin, D. M., et al.: Unraveling the effects of compensation, litigation, and employment on treatment response in chronic pain. Pain 23:49–59, 1985.
43. Eastrand, N.: Medical, psychological, and social factors associated with back abnormalities and self reported back pain: A cross sectional study of male employees in a Swedish pulp and paper industry. Br. J. Ind. Med. 44:327–336, 1987.
44. Edelstein, E. L.: Experience and mastery of pain. Is. Ann. Psychiatry 12:216–226, 1974.
45. Engel, G.: "Psychogenic" pain and the pain-prone patient. Am. J. Med. 26:899–918, 1959.
46. Feighner, J. P., Boyer, W. F., Meredith, C. H., and Hendrickson, G.: An overview of fluoxetine in geriatric depression. Br. J. Psychiatry 153(suppl. 3):105–108, 1988.
47. Feurstein, M., Sult, S., and Houle, M.: Environmental stressors and chronic low back pain: Life events, family and work environment. Pain 22:295–307, 1985.
48. Fisch, C.: Effect of fluoxetine on the electrocardiogram. J. Clin. Psychiatry 46:42–44, 1985.
49. Fischer, A. A., and Chang, C. H.: Temperature and pressure threshold measurements in trigger points. Thermology 1:212–215, 1986.
50. Flor, H., Haag, G., Turk, D. C., and Koehler, H.: Efficacy of EMG biofeedback pseudotherapy and conventional medical treatment for chronic rheumatic back pain. Pain 17:21–31, 1983.
51. Fordyce, W. E.: Behavioral Methods for Chronic Pain and Illness. St. Louis, C. V. Mosby, 1976.
52. Fordyce, W. E.: Learning processes in pain. In Sternbach, R. A.: The Psychology of Pain. New York, Raven Press, 1978, pp. 49–72.
53. France, R. D., Houpt, J. L., Skott, A., et al.: Depression as a psychopathological disorder in chronic low back pain patients. J. Psychosom. Res. 30:127–133, 1986.
54. France, R. D., Ranga Rama Krishnan, K., and Trainor, M.: Chronic pain and depression. III. Family history study of depression and alcoholism in chronic low back pain patients. Pain 24:185–190, 1986.

55. France, R. D., Ranga Rama Krishnan, K., Galli, V., et al.: Preliminary study of thyrotropin-releasing hormone stimulation test in chronic low back pain patients. Pain 27:51–55, 1986.
56. France, R. D., Ranga Rama Krishnan, K., Trainor, M., and Pelton, S.: Chronic pain and depression. IV. DST as a discriminator between chronic pain and depression. Pain 28:39–44, 1987.
57. Fredrickson, B. E., Trief, P. M., VanBeveren, P., et al.: Rehabilitation of the patient with chronic back pain. A search for outcome predictors. Spine 13:351–353, 1988.
58. Frymoyer, J., and Cats-Bril, W.: Predictors of low back pain disability. Clin. Orthop. 221:89–98, 1987.
59. Frymoyer, J.: Helping your patients avoid low back pain. J. Musculoskel. Med. 5:83–101, 1989.
60. Gallagher, R. M., Rauh, V., Haugh, L. D., et al.: Determinants of return-to-work among low back pain patients. Pain 39:55–67, 1989.
61. Gentry, W. D., Shows, W. D., and Thomas, M.: Chronic low back pain: A psychological profile. Psychosomatics 15:174–177, 1974.
62. Glassman, A. H., Perel, J. M., Shostak, M., et al.: Clinical implications of imipramine plasma levels for depressive illness. Arch. Gen. Psychiatry 34:197–204, 1977.
63. Goldstein, R.: Psychological evaluation of low back pain. In White, A. H. (ed.): Failed Back Surgery Syndrome, Evaluation and Treatment, Vol. 1. Spine: State of the Art Reviews. Philadelphia, Hanley & Belfus, 1986, pp. 103–114.
64. Hackett, T. P., and Bouckoms, A.: The pain patient: Evaluation and treatment. In Hackett, T. P., and Cassem, N. M. (eds.): Massachusetts General Hospital Handbook of General Hospital Psychiatry. Littleton, MS, PSG Publishing, 1987, pp. 42–68.
65. Hathaway, S. R., and McKinley, J. C.: Minnesota Multiphasic Personality Inventory Manual, Rev. Ed. New York, Psychological Corporation, 1951.
66. Hazard, R. G., Bendix, A., and Fenwick, J. W.: Disability exaggeration as a predictor of functional restoration outcomes for patients with chronic low-back pain. Spine 16:1062–1067, 1991.
67. Heaton, R. K., Getto, C. J., and Lehman, R. A. W.: A standardized evaluation of psychosocial factors in chronic pain. Pain 12:165–174, 1982.
68. Helzer, J. E., Robins, L. N., and McEnvoi, L.: Posttraumatic stress disorder in the general population. N. Engl. J. Med. 317:1630–1634, 1987.
69. Hendler, N., Derogatis, L., Avella, J., and Long, D.: EMG biofeedback in patients with chronic pain. Dis. Nerv. Sys. 38:505–514, 1977.
70. Hendler, N., Viernstein, M., Gucer, P., and Long, D.: A preoperative screening test for chronic back pain patients. Psychosomatics 20:801–808, 1979.
71. Hendler, N., and Fernandez, P.: Alternative treatments for patients with chronic pain. Psychiatr. Ann. 10:25–30, 1980.
72. Hendler, N.: Use of analgesic and psychotropic drugs for chronic pain of benign origin. Contemp. Neurosurg. 1:1–5, 1981.
73. Hendler, N.: The anatomy and psychopharmacology of chronic pain. J. Clin. Psychiatry 43:15–20, 1982.
74. Hendler, N.: The four stages of pain. In Hendler, N., Long, D., and Wise, T. N. (eds.): Diagnosis and Treatment of Chronic Pain. Littleton, MS, PSG Publishing, 1983.
75. Hendler, N.: Depression caused by chronic pain. J. Clin. Psychiatry 45:30–36, 1984.
76. Hendler, N., Mallett, A., Vierotein, M., et al.: A comparison between the MMPI and the "Mensana Clinic Back Pain Test" for validating the complaint of chronic back pain in women. Pain 23:243–251, 1985.
77. Herman, E., and Baptiste, S.: Pain control: Mastery through experience. Pain 10:79–86, 1981.
78. Hilgard, E. R.: The alleviation of pain by hypnosis. Pain 1:213–231, 1975.
79. Hoffman, J. W., Benson, H., and Arns, P. A.: Reduced sympathetic nervous system responsivity associated with the relaxation response. Science 215:190–192, 1982.
80. Hurri, H.: The Swedish back school in chronic low back pain. Part II. Factors predicting the outcome. Scand. J. Rehabil. Med. 21:41–44, 1989.
81. Institute of Medicine: Pain and Disability: Clinical, Behavioral and Public Policy Perspectives. Washington DC, National Academy Press, 1987.
82. Jacobson, E.: Progressive Relaxation. Chicago, University of Chicago Press, 1938.
83. Jamison, R. N., Matt, D. A., and Parris, W. C.: Effects of time-limited vs. unlimited compensation on pain behavior and treatment outcome in low back pain patients. J. Psychosom. Res. 32:277–283, 1988.
84. Jamison, R. N., Stetson, B. A., and Parris, W. C.: The relationship between cigarette smoking and chronic low back pain. Addict. Behav. 16:103–110, 1991.
85. Johansson, D., and von-Knorring, L.: A double blind controlled study of a serotonin uptake inhibitor (zimelidine) versus placebo in chronic pain patients. Pain 7:69–78, 1979.
86. Keefe, F. J., Black, A. F., Williams, R. B., and Surwit, R. S.: Behavioral treatment of chronic back pain. Clinical outcome and individual difference in pain relief. Pain 11:221–231, 1981.
87. Keefe, F. J., Crisson, J. E., Maltbie, A., et al.: Illness behavior as a predictor of pain and overt behavior patterns in chronic low back pain patients. J. Psychosom. Res. 30:543–551, 1986.
88. Keefe, F. J., Bradley, L. A., and Crisson, J. E.: Behavioral assessment of low back pain: Identification of pain behavior subgroups. Pain 40:153–160, 1990.
89. Keel, P. J.: Psychological evaluation and management of low back pain. In Floman, Y. (ed.): Disorders of the Lumbar Spine. Rockville, MD, Aspen, 1989.
90. Kelsey, J. L., Githens, P. B., O'Conner, T., et al.: Acute prolapsed lumbar intervertebral disc: An epidemiological study with special reference to driving automobiles and cigarette smoking. Spine 9:608–613, 1984.
91. Kraemlinger, K. G., Swanson, D. W., and Maruta, T.: Are patients with chronic pain depressed? Am. J. Psychiatry 140:747–749, 1983.
92. Large, R. G., and Mullins, P. R.: Illness behavior profiles in chronic pain: The Auckland experience. Pain 10:231–239, 1981.
93. Leavitt, F., and Garron, D. C.: The detection of psychological disturbance in patients with low back pain. J. Psychosom. Res. 23:149–154, 1979.

94. Leavitt, F., and Garron, D C.: Validity of a back pain classification scale among patients with low back pain not associated with demonstrable organic disease. J. Psychosom. Res. 23:301–306, 1979.
95. Leavitt, F.: Comparison of three measures for detecting psychological disturbance in patients with low back pain. Pain 13L:299–305, 1982.
96. Leavitt, F., and Garron, D. C.: Rorschach and pain characteristics of patients with low back pain and "conversion V" MMPI profiles. J. Pers. Assess. 46:18–25, 1982.
97. Lemberger, L., Bergstorm, R. F., Wolen, R. L., et al.: Fluoxetine: Clinical pharmacology and physiologic disposition. J. Clin Psychiatry 46:14–19, 1985.
98. Liebman, R., Honig, P., and Berger, H.: An integrated treatment program for psychogenic pain. Fam. Process 15:307–406, 1976.
99. Lindsay, P., and Wyckoff, M.: The depression-pain syndrome and its response to antidepressants. Psychosomatics 22:571–577, 1981.
100. Lopez-Ibor, T. J.: Masked depression. Br. J. Psychiatry 120:245–258, 1972.
101. Love, A. W.: Depression in chronic low back pain patients. Diagnostic efficiency of three self-report questionnaires. J. Clin. Psychol. 43:85–89, 1987.
102. Love, A. W., and Peck, C. L.: The MMPI and psychological factors in chronic low back pain: A review. Pain 28:1–12, 1987.
103. Macnab, I.: The whiplash syndrome. Clin. Neurosurg. 20:232–241, 1972.
104. Magni, G.: Chronic low-back pain and depression: An epidemiological survey. Acta Psychiatr. Scand. 70:614–617, 1984.
105. Magora, A.: Investigation of the relation between low back pain and occupation: V. Psychological aspects. Scand. J. Rehabil. Med. 5:191–196, 1973.
106. Malt, U. F., Blirka, G., and Hoivic, B.: The three-year biopsychosocial outcome of 551 hospitalized accidentally injured adults. Acta Psychiatr. Scand. Suppl. 355:84–93, 1989.
107. Mandel, M. R.: Electroconvulsive therapy for chronic pain associated with depression. Am. J. Psychiatry 132:632–636, 1975.
108. Martini, D. R., Ryan, C., Nakayama, D., and Ramenofsky, M.: Psychiatric sequelae after traumatic injury: The Pittsburgh Regatta accident. J. Am. Acad. Child. Adolesc. Psychiatry 29:70–75, 1990.
109. Mayer, T. G., and Gatchel, R. J.: Functional restoration for spinal disorders: The sports medicine approach. Philadelphia, Lea & Febiger, 1988.
110. McCreary, C. P., Turner, J., and Dawson, E.: Emotional disturbance and chronic low back pain. J. Clin. Psychol. 36:700–715, 1979.
111. McNeill, T. W., Sinkora, G., and Leavitt, F.: Psychologic classification of low-back pain patients: A progressive tool. Spine 11:955–959, 1986.
112. Mechanic D.: The concept of illness behavior. J. Chronic Dis. 15:189–194, 1962.
113. Mechanic D., and Angel, R. J.: Some factors associated with the report and evaluation of back pain. J. Health Soc. Behav. 28:131–139, 1987.
114. Melzack, R., and Wall, P. D.: Pain mechanisms: A new theory. Science 150:971–979, 1965.
115. Melzack, R.: The McGill Pain Questionnaire: Major properties and scoring methods. Pain 1:277–299, 1975.
116. Melzak, R.: The promise of biofeedback: Don't hold the party yet. Psychol. Today July:18–23, 1975.
117. Mendelson, G.: Alexithymia and chronic pain: Prevalence, correlates and treatment results. Psychother. Psychosom. 37:154–164, 1982.
118. Merskey, H., and Spear, F. G.: Pain: Psychological and psychiatric aspects. London, Bailliere-Tindall and Cassell, 1967.
119. Merskey, H.: Psychological aspects, hypnotherapy and psychotropic drugs. In Swerlow, M. (ed.): Relief of Intractable Pain. Amsterdam, Excerta Medica, 1974, pp. 90–115.
120. Merskey, H.: Pain and personality. In Sternback, R. A. (ed.): The Psychology of Pain. New York, Raven Press, 1978, pp. 111–127.
121. Merskey, H., and Boyd, D. B. Emotional adjustment and chronic pain. Pain 5:173–178, 1978.
122. Merskey, H.: Psychiatry and the treatment of pain. Br. J. Psychiatry 136:600–602, 1980.
123. Mohamed, S. N., Weisz, G. M., and Waring, E. N.: The relationship of chronic pain to depression, marital adjustment, and family dynamics. Pain 5:285–292, 1978.
124. Nachemson, A.: The lumbar spine: An orthopaedic challenge. Spine 1:59–71, 1976.
125. Nagi, S. Z., Riley, L. E., and Newby, L G.: A social epidemiology of back pain in a general population. J. Chronic Dis. 27:769–779, 1973.
126. Naliboff, B. D., Cohen, M. J., and Yellen, A. N.: Does the MMPI differentiate chronic illness from chronic pain? Pain 13:333–341, 1982
127. Naliboff, B. D., Cohen, M. J., Swanson, G. A., et al.: Comprehensive assessment of chronic low back pain patients and controls: Physical abilities, level and activity, psychological adjustment and pain perception. Pain 23:121–134, 1985.
128. Newman, R. I., Seres, J. L., and Yospe, L. P.: Multidisciplinary treatment of chronic pain: Long-term follow-up of low-back pain patients. Pain 4:283–292, 1978.
129. Nigl, A. J., and Fisher-Williams, M.: Treatment of low back strain with electromyographic biofeedback and relaxation training. Psychosomatics 21:495–499, 1980.
130. Nouwen, A., and Solinger, J. W.: The effectiveness of EMG biofeedback training in low back pain. Biofeedback Self Regul. 4:103–111, 1979.
131. Nurnberger, F. I., and Gershon, E. S.: Genetics. In Raykel, E. S. (ed.): Handbook of Affective Disorders. New York, Guilford Press 1982, pp. 126–145.
132. O'Brien, J. P.: The role of fusion for chronic low back pain. Orthop. Clin. North Am. 14:639–647, 1983.
133. Oostdam, E. M. M., and Duivenvoorden, H. J.: Description of pain and the degree to which the complaints fit the organic diagnosis of low back pain. Pain 18:71–82, 1984.
134. Orne, M. T.: Pain suppression by hypnosis and related phenomena. Adv. Neurol. 4:563–572, 1974.
135. Patterson, D. R. Carrigan, L., Questad, K. A., and Robinson, R.: Post-traumatic stress disorder in hospitalized patients with burn injuries. J. Burn Care Rehabil. 11:181–184, 1990.
136. Payne, B., and Norfleet, M. A.: Chronic pain and the family: A review. Pain 26:1–22, 1986.

137. Peck, C., and Kraft, G.: Electromyographic biofeedback for pain related to muscle tension. Arch. Surg. 112:889–895, 1977.
138. Pelz, M., and Merskey, H.: A description of the psychological effects of chronic painful lesions. Pain 14:293–301, 1982.
139. Pheasant, H., Bursk, A., Goldfarb, J., et al.: Amitriptyline and chronic low-back pain—a randomized double-blind crossover study. Spine 8:552–557, 1983.
140. Pick, C. G., Paul, D., Eison, M. S., and Pasternak, G. W.: Potentiation of opioid analgesia by the antidepressant nefazodone. Eur. J. Pharmacol. 211:375–381, 1992.
141. Pilling, L. F., Bronnick, T. L., and Swenson, W. M.: Psychologic characteristics of psychiatric patients having pain as a presenting symptom. Can. Med. Assoc. J. 97:387–394, 1967.
142. Pilowsky, I., and Spence, N. D.: Pain and illness behavior: A comparative study. J. Psychosom. Res. 20:131–134, 1976.
143. Pilowsky, I., and Spence, N. D.: Illness behavior syndromes associated with intractable pain. Pain 2:61–71, 1976.
144. Polatin, P. B., Gatchel, R. J., Barnes, D., et al.: A psychosociomedical prediction model of response to treatment by chronically disabled workers with low-back pain. Spine 14:956–961, 1989.
145. Ranga Rama Krishnan, K., France, R. D., Pelton, S., et al.: Chronic pain and depression. I. Classification of depression in chronic low back pain patients. Pain 22:279–287, 1985.
146. Ranga Rama Krishnan, K., France, R. D., Pelton, S., et al.: Chronic pain and depression. II. Symptoms of anxiety in chronic low back pain patients and their relationship to subtypes of depression. Pain 22:289–294, 1985.
147. Ransford, A. O., Cairns, D., and Mooney, V.: The pain drawing as an aid to the psychologic evaluation of patients with low-back pain. Spine 1:127–134, 1976.
148. Rauchfleisch, U.: Handbruch zum Rosenzweig Picture Frustration Test (PFT). Bern, Huber, 1979.
149. Ready, L. B., Sarkis, E., and Turner, J. A.: Self-reported vs. actual use of medications in chronic pain patients. Pain 12:285–294, 1982.
150. Reuler, J. B., Girard, D. E., and Nardone, D. A.: The chronic pain syndrome: Misconceptions and management. Ann. Intern. Med. 93:588–596, 1980.
151. Rosenstiel, A. K., and Keefe, F. J.: The use of coping strategies in chronic low back pain patients: Relationship to patient characteristics and current adjustment. Pain 17:33–44, 1983.
152. Rosomoff, H. L., Fishbein, D. A., Goldberg, M., et al.: Physical findings in patients with chronic intractable benign pain of the neck and/or back. Pain 37:279–282, 1989.
153. Roy, R.: Measurement of chronic pain in pain-depression literature during the 1980s: A review. Int. J. Psychiatry Med. 16:179–188, 1986–1987.
154. Ryden, O., Lindal, E., Udén, A., and Hansson, S. B.: Differentiation of back pain patients using a pain questionnaire. Scand. J. Rehabil. Med. 17:155–161, 1985.
155. Sacerdote, P.: Teaching self-hypnosis to patients with chronic pain. J. Human Stress 4:18–21, 1978.
156. Sachar, E. F.: Endocrine abnormalities in depression. In Paykel, E. S. (ed.): Handbook of Affective Disorders. New York, Guilford Press, 1982, pp. 191–201.
157. Sanders, S. H.: Cross-validation of the back pain classification scale with chronic, intractable pain patients. Pain 22:271–277, 1985.
158. Sanders, S. H., Brena, S. F., Spier, C. J., et al.: Chronic low back pain patients around the world: Cross-cultural similarities and differences. Clin. J. Pain 8:317–323, 1992.
159. Schiffman, E., Friction, J., Haley, D., and Tylka, D.: A pressure algometer for myofascial pain syndrome: Reliability and validity testing. In Dubner, R., Gebhart, G. F., and Bond, M. R. (eds.): Proceedings of the 5th World Congress on Pain. New York, Elsevier Science, 1988, pp. 408–413.
160. Schofferman, J.: Management of chronic pain. In White, A. H. (ed.): Failed Back Surgery Syndrome, Evaluation and Treatment, Vol. 1. Spine: State of the Art Reviews. Philadelphia, Hanley & Belfus, 1986, pp. 115–127.
161. Schreiber, S., and Galai-Gat, T.: Uncontrolled pain following physical injury as the core-trauma in post traumatic stress disorder. Pain 54:107–110, 1993.
162. Sedlak, K.: Low-back pain: Perception and tolerance. Spine 10:440–443, 1985.
163. Shalev, A. Y., Schreiber, S., Galai, T., and Melmed, R. N.: Post traumatic stress disorder following medical events. Br. J. Clin. Psychol. 32:247–253, 1993.
164. Sifneos, P. E.: Clinical observations on some patients suffering from a variety of psychosomatic diseases. Proceedings of the Seventh European Conference on Psychosomatic Research. Basel, Karger, 1967.
165. Skevington, S. M.: Chronic pain and depression: Universal or personal helplessness. Pain 15:309–317, 1983.
166. Skootsky, S.: Incidence of myofascial pain in an internal medicine group practice. Presented at the American Pain Society, Washington, DC, November 6–7, 1986.
167. Slater, M. A., Hall, H. F., Atkinson, J. H., and Garfin, S. R.: Pain and impairment beliefs in chronic low back pain: Validation of the Pain and Impairment Relationship Scale (PAIRS). Pain 44:51–56, 1991.
168. Sternbach, R. A., Wolf, S. R., Murphy, R. W., and Akeson, W. H.: Traits of pain patients: The low-back "loser." Psychosomatics 14:226–229, 1973.
169. Sternbach, R. A.: Pain patients, traits, and treatment. New York, Academic Press, 1974.
170. Sternbach, R. A., and Timmermans, G.: Personality changes associated with reduction of pain. Pain 1:177–181, 1975.
171. Sternbach, R. A.: The need for an animal model of chronic pain. Pain 2:2–4, 1976.
172. Sternbach, R. A., Janowsky, D. S., Huey, L. Y., and Segal, D. S.: Effects of altering brain serotonin activity on human chronic pain. In Bonica, J. J., and Albee-Fessard, D. (ed.): Advances in Pain Research and Therapy, Vol. 1. New York, Raven Press, 1976, pp. 601–606.
173. Stroebel, C. F.: Biofeedback and behavioral medicine. In Kaplan, H. I., and Sadock, B. J. (eds.): Comprehensive Textbook of Psychiatry, 4th Ed. Baltimore, Williams & Wilkins, 1985, pp. 1467–1473.

174. Svenson, H. O., and Anderson, G. J.: Low back pain in 40–47 year old men: Work history and work environment factors. Spine 8:272–276, 1983.
175. Thomson, T. L., Moran, M. G., and Nies, A. S.: Psychotropic drug use in the elderly, N. Engl. J. Med. 308:194–238, 1983.
176. Trief, P. M., Elliott, D. J., Stein, N., and Frederickson, B. E.: Functional vs. organic pain: A meaningful distinction? J. Clin. Psychol. 43:219–226, 1987.
177. Turk, D. C., and Kerns, R. D.: Conceptual issues in the assessment of clinical pain. Int. J. Psychiatr. Med. 113:57–68, 1983.
178. Truk, D. C., and Flor, H.: Etiological theories and treatments for chronic back pain. II. Psychological models and interventions. Pain 19:209–230, 1984.
179. Turkington R. W.: Depression masquerading as diabetic neuropathy. JAMA 243:1147–1150, 1980.
180. Turner, J. A.: Comparison of group progressive-relaxant training and cognitive-behavioral therapy for chronic low back pain. J. Consult. Clin. Psychol. 50:757–765, 1982.
181. Turner, J. A., and Chapman, C. R.: Psychological interventions for chronic pain: A critical review. I. Relaxation training and biofeedback. Pain 12:1–21, 1982.
182. Udén, A., Åström, M., and Bergenudd, H.: Pain drawings in chronic back pain. Spine 13:389–392, 1988.
183. Udén, A., and Landin, L. A.: Pain drawing and myelography in sciatic pain. Clin. Orthop. 216:124–130, 1987.
184. Villard, H. P., Imbeault, J., and Duguay, M.: Low back pain: A psychosomatic clinical study. Psychother. Psychosom. 45:78–83, 1983.
185. Von Knorring, L.: The experience of pain in depressed patients. Neuropsychobiology 1:155–165, 1975.
186. Waddell, G., McCulloch, J. A., Kummel, E. D., and Venner, R. M.: Nonorganic physical signs in low back pain. Spine, 5:117–125, 1980.
187. Walsh, T. D.: Antidepressants in chronic pain. Clin. Neuropharmacol. 6:271–295, 1983.
188. Wanson, D., Floreen, A., and Swenson, W.: Program for managing chronic pain. II. Short-term results. Mayo Clin. Proc. 51:409–411, 1976.
189. Ward, N. G., Bloom, V. L., and Friedel, R. O.: The effectiveness of tricyclic antidepressants in the treatment of coexisting pain and depression. Pain 7:331–341, 1979.
190. Ward, N. G., Bokon, J. A., Ang J., and Butler, S. H.: Differential effects of fenfluramine and dextroamphetamine on acute and chronic pain. In Fields, H. L., Dunber, R., and Cervero, F. (eds.): Advances in Pain Research and Therapy. New York, Raven Press, 1985, pp. 753–760.
191. Ward, N. G.: Tricyclic antidepressants for chronic low back pain. Spine 11:661–665, 1986.
192. Waring, E. M.: The role of the family in symptom selection and perception in psychosomatic illness. Psychother. Psychosom. 28:253–259, 1977.
193. Watkins, R. G., O'Brien, J. P., Draugelis, R., and Jones, D.: Comparisons of preoperative and postoperative MMPI data in chronic back patients. Spine 11:385–390, 1986.
194. Watson, D.: Neurotic tendencies among chronic pain patients: An MMPI item analysis. Pain 14:365–385, 1982.
195. Watson, C. P., Evans, R. J., Reed, K., et al.: Amitriptyline versus placebo in postherpetic neuralgia. Neurology 32:671–673, 1982.
196. Watson, C. P. N., and Evans, R. J.: A comparative trial of amitriptyline and zimelidine in post-herpetic neuralgia. Pain 23:387–394, 1985.
197. Wernicke, J. F.: The side effect profile and safety of fluoxetine. J. Clin. Psychiatry 46:59–67, 1985.
198. Whitlock, F. A.: Hypoalgesia in depressive illness. Br. J. Psychiatry 140:549–550, 1982.
199. Williams, R., and Rhoads, J.: Biofeedback: An adjunct for psychiatric treatment. Paper presented at the Annual Meeting of the American Psychiatric Association, Anaheim, CA, 1975.
200. Yalom, I. D.: The Theory and Practice of Group Psychotherapy, 2nd Ed. New York, Basic Books, 1975.

Functional Restoration for the Patient with Chronic Low Back Pain

ROWLAND G. HAZARD
TOM G. MAYER
HEIKKI VANHARANTA

NEED FOR MULTIDISCIPLINARY FUNCTIONAL RESTORATION

Despite phenomenal advances in diagnostic and therapeutic technologies, back pain continues to plague industrialized societies throughout the world. Earlier in this book, the point is clearly made that far beyond the direct medical costs of pain relief, modern societies bear a growing socioeconomic burden generated by disability from spinal disorders. How can this apparent incongruence between improving technology and increasing disability be explained?

For the vast majority of patients with spinal pain, there is no clear pathoanatomic diagnosis at the end of the clinical search through currently available imaging and electrodiagnostic tests.[24, 92, 96] A given patient may receive diagnoses of facet syndrome, muscle imbalance, degenerative disc disease, or fibrositis depending on the backgrounds of the health care practitioners involved. However, a diagnosis leading to tissue-specific intervention with significantly better results than with natural recovery is relatively rare.[16, 92]

The lack of an operational diagnosis may be inconsequential for the 90% of people who recover spontaneously from acute episodes of spinal pain. But people who continue to experience pain for longer than the expected several weeks of tissue repair face a series of confounding theoretic and practical problems. First, their pain is not measurable by any objective standard. Second, spinal pain is often disproportionate to extant pathologic change. This is most evident in the cases of asymptomatic disc herniations and radicular pain with normal results of diagnostic studies.[7, 24, 98] Third, self-assessments of pain and disability may not correlate well with observed physical capacity.[27, 93] Therefore, a significant minority of patients remain without diagnosis or cure a few months after spinal injury, their disability prevents recreation and gainful employment, and there are confusing mismatches of pain reports, physical impairments, and biopsychosocial disabilities.

These patients with chronic, disabling spinal pain are commonly beset with secondary problems, including depression, anxiety, economic stress, family discord, fear of reinjury, and low self-esteem. As the months and even years of disability accrue, the likelihood of functional and socioeconomic recovery gradually decreases. A quick and simple medical fix is frequently not available for these patients.

In the past decade, clinical and research efforts to help these patients have shifted somewhat from symptom palliation toward functional and socioeconomic recovery. This discussion presents the essential elements and outcomes of a therapeutic approach to disabling spinal pain: functional restoration. Because functional restoration depends heavily on objective physical capacity measurement, some of the theoretic and physiologic principles of spinal function are discussed initially. An outline of a specific functional restoration program is followed by presentation of published outcomes. Finally, political and health policy issues related to spinal rehabilitation are reviewed.

FUNDAMENTALS OF SPINE FUNCTION

Clinicians dealing with musculoskeletal conditions are occasionally overprivileged by visual access to most parts of the relevant organ system. However, in the spinal anatomy, the small, inaccessible, three-joint complexes stacked one on another do not lend themselves to easy inspection. Intersegmental spine movement is difficult to measure even with biplanar x-ray devices. Multiple small muscles interdigitate over variable numbers of segments, and ligamentous structures may share surprising amounts of load in certain joint positions. Moreover, bilateral comparisons are impossible. Until recently, there were no valid indirect measurement methods to assess spine function. Although the absence of direct dynamic visualization methodology persists, novel technology for assessing spine function has become part of the clinical routine. Controversy attends various aspects of spine functional analysis; however, ignorance and neglect of functional quantification can lead to inappropriate management.

In spinal disorders, lack of recognition of the deconditioning syndrome has adversely affected therapeutics. Eclectic therapies applied uniformly to all patients are not as effective as treatment programs individualized on the basis of functional testing. As many as 30% to 40% of patients with chronic spinal pain show some evidence of disuse and deconditioning, which makes them candidates for physical retraining after the functional deficits are identified. Without quantification, the deficits are simply not recognizable, leading to inevitable overutilization or underutilization of therapeutic services. Medicare requires periodic testing to document progress in other areas of rehabilitation. It is likely that similar rules will ultimately apply to treatment of spinal problems, once their necessity becomes more generally perceived.

The deconditioning associated with knee meniscal injuries and surgery was recognized during World War II and popularized by reporting of the injuries of highly visible football players 2 decades later. This led to a therapeutic revolution in combined surgery and rehabilitation for knee injuries that continues today. Despite differences in visual access, the experience with knee rehabilitation translates to that with the treatment of spinal disorders. Inactivity leads to loss of general whole-body task performance ability, which is appreciated by any athlete as uniform loss of functional capacity. More specifically, the injured area sustains greater loss of paraarticular soft tissue function, which becomes progressively more profound as disuse and immobilization continue. These changes create a weak link in the localized extremity joint or spinal region, the physical capacity of which must be measured separately.

How can an understanding of tissue reactions to stress and disuse elucidate the rehabilitation process? A brief consideration of the spinal components involved is in order.

Cartilaginous Tissues

There is ample evidence that back pain can originate from cartilaginous structures.[88, 89] Since 1980, the innervation of the intervertebral disc has been mapped.[8, 99] The nuclear material of the disc has chemically induced inflammatory effects outside its normal anatomic site, notably in the epidural space.[56] This inflammatory process is regarded as one of the mechanisms of nerve dysfunction and pain in disc herniations.[63] Even though these tissues can be painful, the relative focus of rehabilitation is to facilitate recuperation of a tissue's loading capacity.

To appreciate how rehabilitation facilitates this recovery, it is necessary to understand what the structure of cartilaginous tissues is and how they maintain their unique properties throughout the lives of human beings. In the lumbar motion segment, there is cartilaginous tissue in the disc, in the disc end plates, and in the apophyseal joints. These tissues are hydrated, fiber-reinforced composites that provide structural stability and strength. They are composed of collagen fibers embedded in a proteoglycan and water gel. The mechanical needs of different types of cartilaginous tissues actually influence their composition. The annulus of the disc has more type I collagen fibers than do the disc nucleus, the end plates, or the facet joints because type I collagen fibers offer greater tensile strength, which is needed in the annulus. Type I collagen is the main type of collagen found in tendons, ligaments, and bone. Type II collagen predominates in tissues exposed to compressive loads (e.g., disc nuclei and the cartilaginous surface of the joints).[17]

The other dominant matrix macromolecules are proteoglycans, which are entrapped in the collagen network. These macromolecules are composed of glycosaminoglycan polyanions that, with their counterions, exert an osmotic pressure of several atmospheres so that the cartilaginous tissue can remain exceptionally hydrated. This gives these tissues the characteristics of a hydraulic buffer.[17] The more quickly these tissues are compressed, the firmer their resistance is. When unloaded, the cartilage of a joint returns immediately to the shape and height it had before imposition of the load. Discs with thick hydraulic nuclear tissue regain their height after compression more slowly than does cartilage in peripheral joints. This tissue recuperation occurs only after a long rest.

The way that tissues maintain their mechanical properties across a lifetime is not completely understood; however, there is currently a great deal of research on this topic. Cells in these tissues constantly renew the cartilaginous matrix. The normal synthesis rate is slow. Collagen turnover proceeds over decades; proteoglycan turnover is faster, requiring only a couple of years.[17] However, when injury occurs, that renewal rate of collagen changes dramatically.[31] The rate and quality of the cell synthesis and cell degradation are influenced by many other factors as well.

In vitro and in vivo studies in animals have shown that the speed of both collagen and proteoglycan synthesis is partly controlled by the type of compressive impulses that the tissues receive.[61] If compressive stimuli are missing, the rate of synthesis decreases, the rate of deterioration increases, and the cartilaginous tissues atrophy.[64, 65, 75, 78] If there is constant or long-lasting (for hours) pressure on these tissues, the rate of synthesis of the matrix, likewise, decreases and degradation increases.[87] On the other hand, if compression lasts from a couple of seconds to tens of seconds, synthesis by the chondrocytes increases, sometimes even doubling.[66] The positive effect of repeated compressive stimuli on these tissues has been demonstrated best in continuous passive motion studies.[79] An explanation for this effect is that compressive stimuli are needed to keep the pH of the tissue in the optimum range for the cells producing matrix material. Acid products of cell energy metabolism accumulate as lactic acid in these anaerobic tissues without repetitive compression.[87] Nutrition of these cells is also dependent on motion.[29, 30] Discs are the largest avascular tissues in the body, and their nutrition depends on diffusion. Short, vibrating stimuli have also been found to be injurious to cartilaginous tissues.[90]

Many studies have shown that the orientation of macromolecules in scar tissue during healing depends on the direction of the mechanical stimuli received.[35, 83] This is also likely to prove true for the spine. The spine is multidimensional in its movements. To restore this multidimensionality, the spine should be trained so that formatted scar tissue can function without new injury during the usual twists and compressions that patients generate in their daily activities.

In fact, cartilaginous tissues allow only movements that they are accustomed to performing without irritation and without initial degenerative changes.[83] This inertia is one reason why the change in patient activity level at the beginning of rehabilitation can cause additional pain. Pain during early rehabilitation can be reduced with gradually progressive exercise, preceding and building up to intensive rehabilitation. Immediately after an injury, repeated loading increases damage to the cartilage.[21] Likewise, an immediate return to normal activities after a significant disc injury can exacerbate the injury and lengthen the pain episode. In the case of an acute back injury, initial rest can be beneficial.[97] Considerable clinical judgment is required to find a balance between protective rest and continued mechanical stress when patients with chronic spinal pain have acute flare-ups during rehabilitation. Such situations demand careful distinction between hurt and harm. Staff and patient dialogue over this issue can become the turning point in recovery, when it leads to more active and productive self-care behaviors.

Much of the information currently available about matrix synthesis has been obtained from in vitro studies and from animal experiments; these results cannot be applied directly to humans. However, epidemiologic data support the in vitro experimental results. Static sitting, for example, especially by truck drivers who spend long hours experiencing vibration, is related to disc degeneration, disc prolapse, and back symptoms. In persons with jobs that incorporate a lot of free motion, fewer symptoms, less disc degeneration, and fewer herniations develop.[28, 91] Performing physically demanding work and participating in sports contribute to the disc's ability to endure high loads.[72] However, the activities in many forms of physically demanding work and sports are so violent to the spine that, despite the increasing strength of the tissue, injury is likely to occur.[77] The available evidence is limited such that therapists must use extensive judgment in prescribing exercise and activity.

Tendons and Ligaments

The rehabilitation of tendons and ligaments of the back involves many of the same principles that apply to cartilaginous tissue. The macromolecules of all these tissues are alike, but the amount of different macromolecules varies. Even tendons have cartilaginous matrix and chondrocytes in areas in which compressive loads must be tolerated (i.e., close to the attachment of tendons to bones and in different bony canals).[22] Annular tissue in the disc that is designed to withstand tensile force resembles ligament or tendon tissue; its matrix is rich with type I collagen fibers.

In these ligaments, the load, its nature, and its direction affect the type of matrix that is produced after injury. In the absence of compressive stimuli, the cartilaginous matrix of the tendons deteriorates, and in the absence of tensile forces, so do other parts of the tendon. Tissue function determines what types of cells and matrix are generated.[22] Tensile strength and the loading ability of tendons is restored slowly.[20] This restoration is actually dependent on the production of macromolecules, which is slow. To regain the same tensile strength that existed before an injury, a patient must exercise for many months, and perhaps for as long as a year. Many types of active braces or continuous passive motion devices have been used to decrease the deterioration experienced while a patient is immobilized after tendon surgery. However, these are not widely available in back care today.

Muscles

When muscles are not used, they weaken. This observation is also true in the case of patients with chronic low back pain. Yet, there is little evidence to support a theory that weak muscles are the cause of back pain or that the muscles themselves might be the primary site of injury in cases of low back pain. There is also no evidence that, if muscles are strengthened, back pain disappears. Measurable trunk torque in patients with chronic back pain is weak. However, there is evidence that these measures relate more to general psychosocial problems than to pure muscle function. Back muscles atrophy, and biopsies have demonstrated atrophy, especially in type 2 muscle fibers.[74] This finding suggests that these muscles are underused because of pain or axonal injury. Part of the clumsiness that patients evidence after back injury can be explained by muscle atrophy. Atrophy also affects body coordination and balance (e.g., in lifting). Atrophied back muscles are more common in women older than age 40 years and in men and women after multiple back operations.[46]

Programs of rehabilitation exercise are planned to encourage patients to reuse atrophied muscles. That is why these programs are designed to include many lifting, carrying, and bending movements. Within a couple of weeks, a patient's measurable trunk torque may increase as much as 2000%, which suggests that these measurements are evaluating something other than muscle force. However, torque measurements can be used to indicate the success of the rehabilitation program. Muscle tissue itself is generally adaptive to new stimuli. The effect of exercises for muscle hypertrophy is apparent after several weeks. Coordination skills and body balance in lifting improve sooner, reflecting improved neuromuscular function. In a 5-year follow-up study, the structural changes in the muscles were well correlated with the clinical outcome. The muscle atrophic changes were reversible and could be diminished by adequate therapy.[8]

MEASUREMENT OF SPINE FUNCTION

Experience with evaluation of the extremities enables the identification of elements of performance that have functional value and that can be applied to spine function assessment. Trunk range of motion, strength, neurologic status, endurance combined with whole-body aerobic capacity, and ability to perform activities of daily living are some of the major factors traditionally assessed. Evaluation of extremity neurologic function (straight leg raising ability, lower extremity strength, and sensation and reflexes in dermatomal or myotomal patterns) is still viewed by the majority of clinicians as the ideal objective spine function evaluation. However, these neurologic characteristics may be irrelevant for several reasons. First, they are a measure of acute change, when noted in relation to surgical pathologic findings. In the chronic situation, persistence of neurologic changes generally reflects epidural fibrosis or other permanent, uncorrectable anatomic abnormalities. In addition, the neurologic deficits, although they may emanate from spinal structures, are perceived by the patient as extremity abnormalities that produce pain, sensory changes, and weakness of the arms or the legs. In summary, what the clinician currently views as standard objective functional tests may not be useful in efforts to overcome spinal deconditioning.

A critical principle of measurement is that the tests and methods should be accurate, reliable, and discriminating. They must also be relevant to the physiology being measured. As an example of the latter, an isometric leg lift strength test performed with the back straight, in a squatting position, probably reveals little about the strength of injured or deconditioned lumbar musculature. Moreover, physics-based principles must be used to evaluate quantitative measurement devices, much as they would be used to evaluate the performance of a scale or a speedometer. Terms such as accuracy and precision must be clarified. It is not sufficient to identify a device's measurement as reliable, because accurate devices may provide unreliable data because of normal human variability (which can be accounted for by appropriate normative data bases). Similarly, accurate devices may provide data that are clinically useless because of wide fluctuations in human performance due to a variety of sources of error. These sources of error may include the human-device interface, the training and skill of test administrators, or a low signal output by the device relative to the noise in the system. Because of a variety of issues involving secondary gain or fear, which may impede the performance of an injured person, an effort assessment capability is a desirable component of a device to be used in patients with low back pain. The physicians, therapists, and technicians using devices for indirect, objective measurement of spine function should have a basic understanding of the science of quantitative assessment to evaluate the merit of each device.

When patients have disability due to low back pain, the various psychosocial and socioeconomic concomitants of the physical symptoms are likely to make self-reports of pain symptoms an unreliable gauge of treatment progression. In addition, the clinician cannot obtain visual feedback regarding the complex trunk joints and musculature of the lower back. Thus, indirect objective assessment of function is necessary. Such quantitative measures are a necessity for deriving any objective information about the lumbar spine, as compared with extremity rehabilitation assessment, in which functional tests may be an adjunct luxury only. Objective, quantitative measurements of function provide the clinician with a definition of the patient's physical capacity, and succeeding tests document changes in performance with treatment. Suboptimal effort suggests psychosocial barriers to recovery, and identification of insufficient progress can lead to changes in psychosocial treatment interventions. Finally, when maximum medical recovery is achieved, the quantitative tests outline the patient's work capacity and the functional elements often required as part of an impairment or disability evaluation. The following discussion outlines the essentials of the quantitative functional evaluation in the standardized functional restoration program implemented at the Productive Rehabilitation Institute of Dallas for Ergonomics (PRIDE). These are the specific physical capacity and functional capacity tests used to assess the injured region and the individual, respectively.

Physical Capacity Testing

Range of Motion Measurements

Lumbar range of motion measurements involve an inclinometer or a gravity or bubble goniometer to provide angular motion measurements.* An inclinometer is placed over L1 to measure maximum lumbar flexion or extension, and a second inclinometer is placed over the sacrum to measure hip motion. Simultaneous readings are obtained. True lumbar motion is derived by subtracting the sacral reading from the L1 reading. Although this technique is somewhat cumbersome initially, the clinician's proficiency develops rapidly, and several computerized inclinometers are available. This technique has minimum variability and good interrater reliability. True lumbar motion is derived from the compound motion of the hips and spine, effort is delineated, and the spinal motion pattern is assessable as normal or abnormal.

Isolated Trunk Strength Measurements

Emerging technology has provided a number of accurate devices to assess trunk strength. These devices must actually measure the functional capacity of the lumbopelvic unit, and therefore, appropriate isolation of the segment is necessary.

Isometric Technology. These protocols measure the maximum force that a muscle can generate in contraction. (Some investigators believe these protocols to be more accurate than other technologies.) Trunk extensor strength, with good pelvic stabilization, is assessed by the MedX device (MedX, Ocala, FL). Training may also be done on this unit.

Isokinetic Technology. This testing measures dynamic performance by locking in the speed and acceleration variables. This makes calculation of both interindividual and intraindividual differences relatively easy. Other dependent variables, such as work and power, can be derived. Additionally, an approximate effort factor can be obtained from the average points variance, and fatigue and recovery ratios indicative of endurance and recovery after a completion of a specific task can be determined. Available devices providing these types of measurements include the Cybex trunk extension/flexion unit, the Cybex torso rotation unit, and the TMC attachment to the Cybex 6000 (Lumex, Ronkonkoma, NY); the Kin-Com device (Chatteck Corp., Chattanooga, TN); the Biodex Back attachment (Biodex Co., Shirley, NY); and the Lido Back unit (Loredan, Inc., Davis, CA).*

Functional Capacity Testing

Lift Testing

Isoinertial Testing. In isoinertial testing, the velocity is not controlled but the mass is held constant or is progressed. The end point of the test is determined by the subject's self-report of maximum capability, discomfort, or perception of pending injury (psychophysical test), or by the subject's attainment of a target heart rate (aerobic test). The progressive isoinertial lifting evaluation (PILE) offers a standardized protocol with a normative database to assess this capability in an individual.[43, 44, 47]

Isometric Testing. In this testing, distance is kept constant, so that force is measured directly, with no actual movement of the lever arm, so that velocity is zero. Several manufacturers produce equipment that employs this technology.[11, 12, 67]

Isokinetic Testing. In isokinetic testing, velocity is kept constant while distance is limited to a range, so that force may be studied dynamically. Ergonomic and anthropometric protocols are available. Effort is assessable through average points variance, as in isokinetic strength testing. Assessment devices include the Cybex Liftask and the Lido Lift. Both of these units are also capable of alternative protocols (isometric or isoinertial).[13, 34, 37, 45, 54, 73]

Aerobic Capacity Testing

Aerobic capacity testing is used in a typical bicycle ergometry protocol to measure a person's cardiovascular capacity. Protocols generally involve a progressively increasing workload, easily calibrated in watts or kilograms per meter. Nomograms based on body weight and age are available, in which maximum oxygen consumption can be derived from the workload with an accuracy of about ±10%.

---

*References 1, 2, 32, 37, 38, 48, 49, 51, 52, 76, and 94.

*References 9, 14, 15, 26, 40, 41, 50, 53, 59, 60, 80, 81, 84, and 85.

Obstacle Course

An obstacle course is used to measure other functional abilities relevant to activities of daily living. These whole-body tasks can be measured with equipment that is available for purchase, which usually permit testing of arm strength and manipulative activities (BTE, Baltimore Therapeutics, Baltimore, MD). Certain devices allow the use of both arms (e.g., to rotate heavy wheels or to push and pull), although most of these movements are either slowly dynamic or are completely isometric (i.e., static). Creative development of devices for testing bending, twisting, crawling, pushing and pulling, and so on, is common in secondary and tertiary treatment environments.

Effort Assessment

Effort assessment remains controversial. The various isokinetic devices use measurements that essentially capture a coefficient of variation that is generally believed to give some indication of patient effort.[26, 59, 60] The consistency factor definitely has its limitations and can be overridden by persons who are carefully pacing themselves. The patient's performance relative to anticipated normal levels must also be taken into consideration. Normalizing factors, such as age, sex, weight, and activity level appear important but remain controversial.[48, 50, 52–54, 59] Further work is needed to establish the accuracy of effort and normalization factors in individual cases.

PSYCHOSOCIAL ASSESSMENT

Early efforts to distinguish between functional (nonorganic) and organic low back pain did not meet with success. The complex nature of chronic pain makes it difficult to categorize component factors clearly as purely physical or purely psychologic. Instead, chronic pain must be understood as an interactive, psychophysiologic behavior pattern wherein the physical aspects and the psychological aspects constantly overlap and intertwine. The focus of psychologic evaluation of the patient with low back pain therefore must shift away from functional versus organic distinctions to the identification of important psychologic characteristics of each patient. These characteristics obviously affect a patient's disability and his or her response to treatment interventions. Identification of such characteristics facilitates treatment planning and assists in the prediction of treatment outcome. Although an extensive review of the various instruments used for psychologic assessment is not possible here, an analysis of some basic instruments commonly used within a functional restoration program may be useful.

Quantified Pain Drawing

The pain drawing provides a nonverbal assessment tool of pain location, severity, and subjective characteristics.[57] Patients are encouraged to display the locations of their pain and rate its intensity on a 10-cm line. Scoring uses an overlay that reliably quantifies pain by dividing the human drawing into a series of boxes, yielding a score for pain in the trunk, in the extremities, and outside the body. This latter dimension is useful for identifying pain magnifiers and also suggests the possibility of somatic delusions in rare cases. The pain drawing provides an easy and reliable method for documentation of changing pain perception in response to treatment.

Million Visual Analog Scale

The Million Visual Analog Scale consists of 15 questions relating to perceptions of pain and disability. Responses are recorded by placing a mark on a 10-cm line that represents an index of severity. Scores are easily obtained using a ruler or grid. This scale is particularly useful because of its nonverbal form of expression. Its ease of administration and reproducibility make it ideal for monitoring progress on repeated administrations. Extremely exaggerated responses that do not correlate with clinical assessment may also indicate the need for further, in-depth psychologic evaluation.

Depression Scales

The Beck Depression Inventory (BDI) consists of 21 items pertaining to symptoms of depression, such as sleep disturbance, sexual dysfunction, weight change, and anhedonia. It is brief and easy to complete and has a cumulative scoring system that takes less than 1 minute to complete. The BDI is designed to identify cognitive factors of depression, and along with the Hamilton Depression Rating Scale, can provide the clinician with valuable information about the existence and the severity of depression in patients with low back pain.[3, 68, 69, 95] The ease of administration of the BDI makes it easy to use on repeated visits, offering the clinician a relatively simple means of following depressive symptoms and treatment progress.

Minnesota Multiphasic Personality Inventory

The Minnesota Multiphasic Personality Inventory (MMPI) is one of the oldest and most frequently used indices of psychologic functioning. Its first three clinical scales, hypochondriasis, depression, and hysteria, provide valuable information in the evaluation of patients with chronic low back pain. Relative elevations of these three clinical scales can alert the clinician to the possibility of important problems, such as symptom magnification, poor insight into emotions, and defenses based on denial and somatization tendencies. Many ancillary scales have been developed within the MMPI, which also provide specific information pertinent to the treatment of chronic low back pain. Notable among these are the McAndrews and ego strength scales. The McAndrews scale helps to identify patients with alcoholic or drug-dependent personality types, which may assist the treatment team in preventing drug abuse before habituation actually occurs. The ego strength scale is designed to identify persons with limited emotional resources who might lack the motivation and personal responsibility to benefit adequately from an intensive treatment regimen.

Other Psychological Assessment

The structured clinical interview for *Diagnostic and Statistical Manual of Mental Disorders,* fourth edition (DSM-IV) diagnosis is an interview test designed to help a trained mental health provider to establish a DSM-IV psychiatric diagnosis. The most important scales are the axis I and II diagnoses, which occur commonly in chronic spinal disorders.[33, 70] The Hamilton Depression Rating Scale is a clinician-administered test that supplements the self-report of the BDI. A clinical interview by psychologists helps to focus on the various critical issues that constitute the essential barriers to recovery that must be addressed. These barriers may be social problems (e.g., child care or transportation problems) that specifically affect the patient's ability to participate in rehabilitation or may involve financial, psychologic, legal, and employer-related issues. Similar interviews performed by professional disability managers are useful in evaluating the specific occupational aspects of ongoing disability. This role is currently being assumed by occupational therapists, social workers, vocational rehabilitation specialists, or rehabilitation nurses. Tests that evaluate a person's level of education, training potential, and skills, such as the Wechsler Adult Intelligence Scale (WAIS-R), are also commonly used in assessments designed to achieve an outcome of returning the chronically disabled worker to a productive life style.

FUNCTIONAL RESTORATION

The functional restoration program described is that of the PRIDE program. Tertiary treatment uses the physical and functional capacity and psychosocial assessments described previously to organize a physician-directed, interdisciplinary team treatment approach to restoring patients to productivity. Multiple disciplines are available on site, so that all patients have the benefit of access to each specialized group of health care providers in an intensive program individualized according to the initial assessments.* An additional feature of functional restoration programs involves attention to outcome monitoring for all patients, with structured clinical interviews at a minimum follow-up of 1 year. These interviews focus on specific objective factors of cost and disability.[19, 42, 45, 48, 58]

After the initial assessment, a preprogram

---

*References 10, 23, 32, 34, 36, 40, 41, 71, 81, and 84.

phase of treatment is planned once or twice weekly. The duration and the frequency are determined by the patient's degree of deconditioning and psychosocial barriers that would interfere with participation in the subsequent 3-week intensive phase. In the preprogram phase, the physical and occupational therapists are involved primarily in confidence building to overcome the patient's inhibition and fear of injury that limits physical performance. Therapists use mobilization and stretching to prepare the patient for the intensive muscle-training phase of the physical program. Psychologists and disability managers, respectively, deal with psychologic (e.g., depression and substance dependence) and social (e.g., financial or transportation difficulties and family responsibilities) barriers to program participation. The preprogram cannot exceed 6 weeks and ranges from 2 to 6 weeks; it is followed by the intensive phase.

During the intensive portion of the program, the patient participates in a 3-week, 10-hour-a-day program consisting of reconditioning, work simulation, disability management, and a cognitive-behavioral program.[39, 42, 45] The reconditioning and work simulation aspects of the intensive phase particularly involve physical and occupational therapists using active treatment modalities. This approach may be difficult to promote. The traditional reimbursement schedules in much of the industrialized world encourage outdated, passive treatments, which produce temporary comfort and discourage exercise and education. Quantification is necessary for these aspects of the program, because they provide the initial levels of exercise from which a progressive resistive program emerges. The indirect assessments confirm functional deficits and psychosocial barriers to effort. This assessment leads to a combination of education and exercise training to resolve the deconditioning syndrome. Initial treatment is directed toward mobilizing and strengthening the weak link in the biomechanical chain, while whole-body work simulation integrates the performance of this link with other parts of the body deconditioned simply by inactivity (Table 1).

The cognitive-behavioral multimodal disability management program focuses initially on the identification of psychosocioeconomic barriers to functional recovery in

Table 1

Critical Elements of a Tertiary Functional Restoration Program

1. Quantification of physical and functional capacity
2. Psychosocioeconomic assessment
3. Physical reconditioning of the injured functional unit
4. Work simulation and whole-body retraining
5. Cognitive-behavioral multimodal disability management program
6. Education and training in work and fitness maintenance
7. Ongoing outcome assessment utilizing objective criteria

a given individual through the assessments mentioned previously and then on specific treatments of these problems. The initial treatment may be pharmacologic, involving detoxification from habituating opiate and tranquilizer medications, the use of antidepressants and antiinflammatory medications, and occasionally the use of major tranquilizers. Remaining treatments include a cognitive-behavioral program of education and counseling, including stress management, which is time limited and aggressively oriented toward sequential goal setting. Failure to meet mutually prearranged goals may result in dismissal from the program, an event currently occurring in about 5% of comprehensive program admissions. In practice, education and counseling account for approximately one half of total program time, with the remainder being spent in physical training.

Finally, just as the quantification of physical function and self-report provides feedback to the staff and the patient on individual performance, so follow-up outcome measures provide objective statistical confirmation of the patient's success in achieving program goals. The PRIDE comprehensive program performs routine 1- and 2-year structured follow-up telephone interviews. The interview includes information on employment status, additional surgical, medical or chiropractic treatment; resolution of compensation issues (long-term disability, Social Security Disability Income, permanent partial or total disability, and so on); and injury recurrence.[55] The interviews must be performed in the context of possible remaining barriers to full disclosure by the patient; this may necessitate further investigation through staff contacts with employers, attorneys, family members, or third-party payers in some cases. Combining the follow-up interview information with preprogram demographic data on the same subjects provides valid statistical comparisons of the ability of a comprehensive functional restoration program to deal with disability and cost. Because cases of chronic low back pain ultimately account for 80% of the cost of low back pain problems through a combination of medical treatment, lost productivity, indemnity, and government support, program evaluation, including involvement of other members of the disability system, provides a major resource to clinicians, employers, health care planners, and legislators.

FUNCTIONAL RESTORATION OUTCOMES

Progressive Rehabilitation Institute of Dallas for Ergonomics

In 1985, Mayer and associates[39] reported the first results of functional restoration in patients with chronic spinal pain from industrial injuries. They compared a group of patients graduating from the PRIDE program described earlier with patients who dropped out before completing the program and with an initially similar comparison group who pursued other treatments after authorization for functional restoration was denied by their insurance carriers. All patients met the entry criteria of at least 4 months' disability, willingness to participate in rehabilitation, and lack of a surgically correctable cause of pain. There were 38 patients in the control group. Of the 73 patients beginning the PRIDE program, seven dropped out and 66 graduated. Quantitative functional evaluations repeated on completion of the 3-week intensive program reflected significant improvements in pain, disability, and depression questionnaire scores. Major mean gains were also noted in lifting capacity, isokinetic trunk strength, and trunk flexibility.

One year after treatment, contact rates for the three patient groups exceeded 85%. Although only 45% of the comparison cohort and 20% of the dropouts had returned to work, 86% of the functional restoration graduates were working or were involved in vocational training programs. Expanding this study to a 2-year follow-up, Mayer and coworkers[42] reported results for more than 85% of 116 program graduates and 72 comparison patients. Of the graduates, 87% were working, whereas only 41% of the comparison group were employed. The graduates required less than half the spinal surgery and health care visits needed by the comparison group.

SPINE Institute of New England

In 1986, Hazard and colleagues[25] at the University of Vermont established a functional restoration program modeled after the PRIDE program. Using the same study design and patient criteria and groupings, they retested the efficacy of this treatment approach. Of the original 90 patients, 59 graduated from the program, five dropped out, and there were 17 comparison patients. Again, the treatment groups were essentially similar according to multivariate pretreatment analysis.

Pain, disability, and depression scores had significantly improved for the graduates at the time of program completion. Physical capacities had increased as well. At 1-year follow-up, return-to-work rates were 81% for graduates, 41% for dropouts, and 29% for comparison patients. Six patients initially denied treatment access for 6 months eventually completed the program, and all had returned to work 6 months later.

Partial discrepancies among pain, impairment, and disability outcomes in this study raised the question of which outcomes were most important to the patients themselves. A 5-year follow-up study compared patient treatment satisfaction according to these outcome categories. Program graduates' treatment satisfaction 5 years later was only weakly correlated with simultaneous pain and disability self-assessments. People who had returned to work 1 year after treatment had higher 5-year satisfaction than those who had not returned to work, although this difference was not evident when workers and nonworkers were compared at the 5-year follow-up.

Functional Restoration Variations

A somewhat similar program to those described above, supplemented by nerve blocks, was reported by Tollison and colleagues[86] in 1989. Using the same three-group study design, 88% of the program participants and 90% of the comparison patients were contacted 18 months after treatment. Of those in the contacted treatment group, 56% were working, and of the comparison contacts, only 27% were working. As in the original study by Mayer and colleagues,[39] patients who had functional restoration required far less subsequent medical and surgical care.

In 1991, Oland and Tveiten[62] reported the results of a Norwegian modern active rehabilitation program loosely patterned after the PRIDE approach. This program differed from the original in that functional testing and integrated counseling were deemphasized in favor of more passive interventions for some patients. Six and 18 months after treatment, the patients had no significant improvements in pain or disability scores. Only 23% had returned to work at 18 months. Although the investigators attributed some of their outcome failures to ambient differences between Norway and the United States, treatment factors, such as inadequate behavioral support and functional capacity monitoring, may better explain their results, particularly in view of the dismal self-assessment outcomes.

At the 1993 International Society for Study of the Lumbar Spine meeting, Bendix and associates[4] reported results from their program, which was based on the approach used at the SpINE Institute of New England. They randomized 118 chronically disabled patients with back pain to interdisciplinary functional restoration, physical training, or counseling with warm-up exercises. Four months after treatment, the group return-to-work rates were 66%, 47%, and 36%, respectively. Recognizing the adverse reemployment situation existing in Scandinavia, they reported work readiness rates of 76%, 56%, and 39%, respectively. The employment advantages in the treatment group were accompanied by superior self-reports of pain reduction.

POLITICS AND POLICIES

Unfortunately, although functional restoration of the patient with chronic pain is the most cost-effective approach to work-incurred spinal disability, employers and government agencies are often unmotivated to effect change in their policies. Although a Boeing Company study[5, 6, 82] clearly demonstrated that job dissatisfaction and personnel relations may be the best (or only) predictor of back injury, use of the medical system to avoid responsibility for good personnel relations has become endemic in some industries. These employers and government agencies may find it easier to ascribe back injury to the cost of doing business and pass these expenses on to the consumer or the taxpayer. An adversarial relationship, filled with rancor more often than not, alters the status of the patient from an employee to a claimant. Before too quickly falling into the trap of labeling the injured worker who seeks redress from perceived punitive employer actions as a faker or malingerer, one must consider the multitude of factors in the evolution of the workers' compensation and personal injury systems themselves.

Although a full discussion of nonmedical legal and administrative issues is a critical adjunct to the rehabilitation of the chronically disabled patient, for the purposes of this discussion, the reader should be slow to judge negatively the motivation of the injured worker. If in some cases manipulativeness, opportunism, and financial secondary gain characterize such patients' behaviors, their actions are often conditioned by perceived injustice in the essentially adversarial workers' compensation system. Employer-employee conflict is often played out through their respective representatives (the insurance carrier and the plaintiff attorney) in a contest over medical benefits, job retention rights, and disability-related indemnity benefits tied to perceived permanent impairment. The other players in the disability system may have a variety of personal and business interests that can diverge in certain critical areas from the best interest of the injured worker. As such, the interdisciplinary team's education on the particular rules of the workers' compensation venue can be an important aspect of treatment to assist the patient in escaping the maze of chronic disability.

In this regard, the tertiary care provider is probably the only relatively disinterested party capable of assisting the patient in formulating a problem-solving solution, thus accomplishing the specific socioeconomic benefits of interest to the injured worker and society. In so doing, the assessment and the treatment of the chronically disabled worker lead to tertiary prevention, in which the most dismal consequence of permanent disability of the young and potentially productive worker is avoided. Because spinal disorders are the greatest cause of disability for persons younger than age 45 years in all industrialized countries, an average of 25 to 30 years of taxpayer-supported welfare benefits (e.g., Social Security Disability Income, long-term disability, unemployment insurance, social welfare, and food stamps) can be avoided by judicious application of tertiary care to the identified chronically disabled worker.

In selected cases, tertiary care may be appropriate even before completion of a maximum period of normal soft tissue healing (4 to 6 months postinjury). Although secondary treatment is usually preferable for patients before 4 months of disability, the availability of effective tertiary care with cost- and duration-limited programs may make them desirable for selected cases even before 4 months have passed. In particular, with more aggressive employer involvement through transitional work return programs, with the recognition of early psychosocial stressors potentially leading to enhancement of disability, and with the advent of treatment guidelines to inform health care providers and administrative agencies of demonstrated ways to achieve treatment goals, tertiary treatment, at least in a limited form, may be instituted within 6 to 8 weeks of injury or disability in selected cases. A variety of criteria can be used to distinguish the suitability of secondary or tertiary care in these cases. These criteria include the match between physical capacity and job demands, recent prior injury, age, other medical conditions, preexisting psychosocial barriers, and job availability. Progressive education of health care providers to the more advanced concepts of rehabilitating injured workers is the best method to advance program effectiveness, ensuring quality of care.

In conclusion, the future lies in finding solutions that involve communication and cooperation among members of the disability system. The injured patient must be given the same opportunity for appropriate medical care, reemployment, and compensation for injury as is provided for patients with other industrial or personal injuries. If objective structural documentation cannot provide adequate means for assessing impairment, functional assessment–based awards must be considered. At this time, judicious combinations of surgical treatment, if appropriate, and tertiary rehabilitation are becoming more readily available and should help to prevent permanent total disability. Quantification may also lead the way to prevention through worker selection and placement and greater options for returning to work through the Americans with Disabilities Act. Prevention programs should be combined with job analysis and redesign after risk assessment, as well as enlightened education of high-risk workers and their personnel managers and supervisors. Multidisciplinary teams of occupational health care professionals, providing optimum early and late care for the gamut of industrial injuries in a cost-effective manner, is the ultimate goal. It can be accomplished with the increase in knowledge available through improved psychosocial and physical or functional capacity assessment technology, and through tertiary treatment of workers with chronic spinal disorders.

REFERENCES

1. Adams, M., Dolan, P., Marks, C., et al.: An electroinclinometer technique for measuring lumbar curvature. Clin. Biomech. 1:130–134, 1986.
2. American Medical Association Guides to the Evaluation of Permanent Impairment, 3rd Ed., Revised. American Medical Association, Chicago, 1990.
3. Beck, A., Steer, R., and Garbin, W.: Psychometric properties of the Beck Depression Inventory: Twenty-five years of evaluation. Clin. Psychol. Rev. 8:77–100, 1988.
4. Bendix, A. F., Bendix, T., Busch, E., et al.: Comparison of different active treatment programs for patients with chronic low back pain (abstract). Presented at the International Society for the Study of the Lumbar Spine Meeting, Marseilles, France, June 1993.
5. Bigos, S., Spengler, D., Martin, N., et al.: Back injuries in industry: A retrospective study. II. Injury factors. Spine 11:246–251, 1986.
6. Bigos, S., Spengler, D., Martin, N., et al.: Back injuries in industry: A retrospective study. III. Employee-related factors. Spine 11:252–256, 1986.
7. Boden, S. D., Davis, D. O., Dina, T. S., et al.: Abnormal magnetic-resonance scans of the lumbar spine in asymptomatic subjects. J. Bone Joint Surg. 72A:403–408, 1990.
8. Bogduk, N., Tynan, W., and Wilson, A. S.: The nerve supply to the human lumbar intervertebral discs. J. Anat. 132:39–56, 1981.

9. Brady, S., Mayer, T., and Gatchel, R.: Physical progress and residual impairment quantification after functional restoration, part II: Isokinetic trunk strength. Spine 19:395–400, 1994.
10. Cady, L., Bischoff, D., O'Connel, E., et al.: Strength and fitness and subsequent back injuries in firefighters. J. Occup. Med. 21:269–272, 1979.
11. Chaffin, D.: Human strength capability and low back pain. J. Occup. Med. 16:248–254, 1974.
12. Chaffin, D., Herrin, G., and Keyserling, W.: Pre-employment strength testing: An updated position. J. Occup. Med. 20:403–408, 1978.
13. Curtis, L., Mayer, T., and Gatchel, R.: Physical progress and residual impairment quantification after functional restoration, part III: Isokinetic and isoinertial lifting capacity. Spine 19:401–405, 1994.
14. Davies, G., and Gould, J.: Trunk testing using a prototype Cybex II isokinetic stabilization system. J. Orthop. Sports Phys. Ther. 3:164–170, 1982.
15. Delitto, A., Crandell, C., and Rose, S.: Peak torque to body weight ratios in the trunk: A critical analysis. Phys. Ther. 69:138–143, 1989.
16. Deyo, R. A.: Conservative therapy for low back pain: Distinguishing useful from useless therapy. JAMA 250:1057–1062, 1983.
17. Eyre, D. R., Benya, P., Buckwalter, J., et al.: Basic science perspectives. In Frymoyer, J. W., and Gordon, S. L. (eds.): New Perspectives on Low Back Pain. Park Ridge, IL, American Academy of Orthopaedic Surgeons, 1988, pp. 147–207.
18. Gatchel, R., Mayer, T., Capra, P., et al.: Quantification of lumbar function, part 6: The use of psychological measures in guiding physical functional restoration. Spine 11:36–42, 1986.
19. Gatchel, R., Mayer, T., Hazard, R., et al.: Editorial. Functional restoration: Pitfalls in evaluating efficacy. Spine 17:988–995, 1992.
20. Gelberman, R., Goldberg, V., An, K.-N., et al.: In Woo, S. L.-Y., and Buckwalter, J. A. (eds.): Injury and Repair of Musculoskeletal Soft Tissues. Park Ridge, IL, American Academy of Orthopaedic Surgeons, 1988, pp. 5–40.
21. Gill, K., Videman, T., Shimizu, T., et al.: Experimental intervertebral disc degeneration (abstract). Presented at the International Society for the Study of the Lumbar Spine Meeting, Rome, 1987.
22. Giori, N. J., Beaupre, G. S., and Carter, D. R.: Cellular shape and pressure may mediate mechanical control of tissue composition in tendons. J. Orthop. Res. 11:581–591, 1993.
23. Gould, J., and Davies, G. (eds.): Orthopedic and Sports Physical Therapy. St. Louis, C. V. Mosby, 1985.
24. Haldeman, S.: Presidential address, North American Spine Society: Failure of the pathology model to predict back pain. Spine 15:718–724, 1990.
25. Hazard, R. G., Fenwick, J. W., Kalisch, S. M., et al.: Functional restoration with behavioral support: A one-year prospective study of patients with chronic low-back pain. Spine 14:157–161, 1989.
26. Hazard, R., Reid, S., Fenwick, J., et al.: Isokinetic trunk and lifting strength measurements: Variability as an indicator of effort. Spine 13:54–57, 1988.
27. Hazard, R. G., Haugh, L. D., Green, P. A., et al.: Chronic low-back pain: The relationship between patient satisfaction and pain, impairment, and disability outcomes. Spine 19:881–887, 1994.
28. Heliövaara, M.: Epidemiology of Sciatica and Herniated Lumbar Intervertebral Disc. Helsinki, Finland, Social Insurance Institution, ML:76, 1988.
29. Holm, S., and Nachemson, A.: Nutritional changes in the canine intervertebral disc after spinal fusion. Clin. Orthop. 169:243–258, 1982.
30. Holm, S., and Nachemson, A.: Variations in the nutrition of the canine intervertebral disc induced by motion. Spine 8:866–874, 1983.
31. Kääpä, E., Holm, S., Han, X., et al.: Collagens in the injured porcine intervertebral disc. J. Orthop. Res. (in press).
32. Keeley, J., Mayer, T., Cox, R., et al.: Quantification of lumbar function, part 5: Reliability of range of motion measures in the sagittal plane and an in vivo torso rotation measurement technique. Spine 11:31–35, 1986.
33. Kinney, R., Gatchel, R., Polatin, P., et al.: Prevalence of psychopathology in acute and chronic low back pain patients. J. Occup. Rehabil. 3:95–103, 1993.
34. Kishino, N., Mayer, T., Gatchel, R., et al.: Quantification of lumbar function, part 4: Isometric and isokinetic lifting simulation in normal subjects and low back dysfunction patients. Spine 10:921–927, 1985.
35. Klebe, R. J., Caldwell, H., and Miam, S.: Cells transmit spatial information by orienting collagen fibers. Matrix 9:451–458, 1989.
36. Langrana, N., and Lee, C.: Isokinetic evaluation of trunk muscles. Spine 9:171–175, 1984.
37. Loebl, W.: Measurement of spinal posture and range of spinal movements. Ann. Phys. Med. 9:103–110, 1967.
38. Mayer, T., Tencer, A., Kristoferson, S., et al.: Use of noninvasive techniques for quantification of spinal range-of-motion in normal subjects and chronic low back dysfunction patients. Spine 9:588–595, 1984.
39. Mayer, T., Gatchel, R., Mayer, H., et al.: Objective assessment of spine function following industrial accident: A prospective study with comparison group and one-year follow-up. Volvo Award in Clinical Sciences, 1985. Spine 10:482–493, 1985.
40. Mayer, T., Smith, S., Keeley, J., et al.: Quantification of lumbar function, part 2: Sagittal plane trunk strength in chronic low back pain patients. Spine 10:765–772, 1985.
41. Mayer, T., Smith, S., Kondraske, G., et al.: Quantification of lumbar function, part 3: Preliminary data on isokinetic torso rotation testing with myoelectric spectral analysis in normal and low back pain subjects. Spine 10:912–920, 1985.
42. Mayer, T., Gatchel, R., Mayer, H., et al.: A prospective two-year study of functional restoration in industrial low back injury: An objective assessment procedure. JAMA 258:1763–1767, 1987.
43. Mayer, T., Barnes, D., Nichols, G., et al.: Progressive isoinertial lifting evaluation, part I: A standardized protocol and normative database. Spine 13:993–997, 1988.
44. Mayer, T., Barnes, D., Nichols, G., et al.: Progressive isoinertial lifting evaluation, part II: A comparison with isokinetic in a disabled chronic low back pain industrial population. Spine 13:998–1002, 1988.
45. Mayer, T., and Gatchel, R.: Functional Restoration for Spinal Disorders: The Sports Medicine Approach. Philadelphia, Lea & Febiger, 1988.
46. Mayer, T. G., Vanharanta, H., Gatchel, R., et al.:

47. Mayer, T., Barnes, D., Kishino, N., et al.: Progressive isoinertial lifting evaluation. An erratum. Spine 15:5, 1990.
48. Mayer, T., Mooney, V., and Gatchel, R.: Contemporary Care for Painful Disorders: Concepts, Diagnosis and Treatment. Philadelphia, Lea & Febiger, 1991.
49. Mayer, T., Brady, S., Bovasso, E., et al.: Noninvasive measurement of cervical tri-planar motion in normal subjects. Spine 18:2191–2195, 1993.
50. Mayer, T., Gatchel, R., Keeley, J., et al.: Optimal spinal strength normalization factor among male railroad workers. Spine 18:239–244, 1993.
51. Mayer, T., Tabor, J., Bovasso, E., et al.: Physical progress and residual impairment quantification after functional restoration, part I: Lumbar mobility. Spine 19:389–394, 1994.
52. Mayer, T., Gatchel, R., Keeley, J., et al.: A male incumbent worker industrial database, part I: Lumbar spinal physical capacity. Spine (in press).
53. Mayer, T., Gatchel, R., Keeley, J., et al.: A male incumbent worker industrial database, part II: Cervical spinal physical capacity. Spine (in press).
54. Mayer, T., Gatchel, R., Keeley, J., et al.: A male incumbent worker industrial database, part III: Lumbar/cervical functional testing. Spine (in press).
55. Mayer, T., Gatchel, R., and Prescott, M.: Functional restoration socioeconomics outcomes: The PRIDE outcome tracking system. Spine (in press).
56. McCarron, R. F., Wimpee, M. W., Hudkins, P., et al.: The inflammatory effect of nucleus pulposus. A possible element in the pathogenesis of low back pain. Spine 12:760–764, 1987.
57. Mooney, V., Cairns, D., and Robertson, J.: A system for evaluating and treating chronic back disability. West. J. Med. 124:370–376, 1976.
58. Nachemson, A.: Work for all. Clin. Orthop. 179:77–82, 1983.
59. Newton, M., and Waddell, G.: Trunk strength testing with iso-machines, part 1: Review of a decade of scientific evidence. Spine 7:801–811, 1993.
60. Newton, M., Thow, N., Somerville, D., et al.: Trunk strength testing with iso-machines, part 2: Experimental evaluation of the Cybex II Back Testing System in normal subjects and patients with chronic low back pain. Spine 7:812–824, 1993.
61. Ohshima, H., and Urban, J. P. G.: The effect of lactate and pH on proteoglycan and protein synthesis rates in the intervertebral discs. Spine 17:1079–1082, 1992.
62. Oland, G., and Tveiten, G.: A trial of modern rehabilitation for chronic low-back pain and disability: Vocational outcome and effect of pain modulation. Spine 16:457–459, 1991.
63. Olmarker, K., Rydevik, B., and Nordborg, C.: Autologous nucleus pulposus induces neurophysiologic and histologic changes in porcine cauda equina nerve roots. Spine 18:1425–1432, 1993.
64. Palmoski, M. J., Coyler, R. A., and Brandt, K. D.: Joint motion in the absence of normal loading does not maintain normal articular cartilage. Arthritis Rheum. 23:325–334, 1980.
65. Palmoski, M. J., and Brandt, K. D.: Effects of static and cyclic compressive loading on articular cartilage plugs in vitro. Arthritis Rheum. 27:675–681, 1984.
66. Parkkinen, J. J., Lammi, M. J., Helminen, H. J., et al.: Local stimulation of proteoglycan synthesis in articular cartilage explants by dynamic compression in vitro. J. Orthop. Res. 10:610–620, 1992.
67. Pederson, O., Peterson, R., and Staffeldt, F.: Back pain and isometric back muscle strength of workers in a Danish factory. Scand. J. Rehabil. Med. 7:125–128, 1975.
68. Polatin, P., Gatchel, R., Barnes, D., et al.: A psychosociomedical prediction model of response to treatment by chronically disabled workers with back pain. Spine 14:956–961, 1989.
69. Polatin, P.: Functional restoration for the chronically disabled low back pain patient. J. Musculoskel. Med. 7:17–39, 1990.
70. Polatin, P., Kinney, R., Gatchel, R., et al.: Psychiatric illness and chronic low back pain: The mind and the spine—which goes first? Spine 18:66–71, 1993.
71. Pope, M., Frymoyer, J., and Andersson, G.: Occupational Low Back Pain. New York, Praeger Publications, 1984.
72. Porter, R. W., Adams, M. A., and Hutton, W. C.: Physical activity and the strength of the lumbar spine. Spine 14:201–203, 1989.
73. Porterfield, J., Mostardi, R., King, S., et al.: Simulated lift testing using computerized isokinetics. Spine 12:683–687, 1987.
74. Rantanen, J., Hurme, M., Falck, B., et al.: The lumbar multifidus muscle five years after surgery for a lumbar intervertebral disc herniation. Spine 18:568–574, 1993.
75. Retterer, E.: De l'influence de la suractivité fonctionelle sur la structure du cartilage diarthrodial. C. R. Soc. Biol. (Paris) 64:117–120, 1908.
76. Reynolds, P.: Measurement of spinal mobility: A comparison of three methods. Rheum. Rehabil. 14:180–185, 1975.
77. Riihimaki, H.: Back pain and heavy physical work: A comparative study of concrete reinforcement workers and maintenance house painters. Br. J. Ind. Med. 42:226–232, 1985.
78. Saaf, J.: Effects of exercise on adult articular cartilage. Acta Orthop. Scand. (Suppl) 7:1–86, 1950.
79. Salter, R. B., Simmonds, D. F., Malcolm, B. W., et al.: The biological effect of continuous passive motion on the healing of full-thickness defects in articular cartilage. An experimental investigation. J. Bone Joint Surg. 62A:1232–1251, 1980.
80. Smidt, G., and Blantied, F.: Analysis of strength tests and resistive exercises commonly used for low-back disorders. Spine 12:1025–1034, 1987.
81. Smith, S., Mayer, T., Gatchel, R., et al.: Quantification of lumbar function, part 1: Isometric and multi-speed isokinetic trunk strength measures in sagittal and axial planes in normal subject patients. Spine 10:757–764, 1985.
82. Spengler, D., Bigos, S., Martin, N., et al.: Back injuries in industry: A retrospective study I. Overview and cost analysis. Spine 11:241–245, 1986.
83. Tammi, M., Paukkonen, K., Kiviranta, I., et al.: Joint loading-induced alterations in articular cartilage. In Helminen, H. J., et al. (eds.): Joint Loading. Wright 1987, pp. 64–88.
84. Thompson, N., Gould, J., Davies, G., et al.: Descriptive measures of isokinetic trunk testing. J. Orthop. Sports Phys. Ther. 7:43–49, 1985.

85. Thorstensson, A., and Nilsson, J.: Trunk muscle strength during constant and velocity movement. Scand. J. Rehabil. Med. 14:61–68, 1982.
86. Tollison, C. D., Kriegel, M. L., Satterthwaite, J. R., et al.: Comprehensive pain center treatment of low back workers' compensation injuries: An industrial medicine clinical outcome follow-up comparison. Orthop. Rev. 18:1115–1126, 1989.
87. Urban, J., and Hall, A.: Physical modifiers of cartilage metabolism. In Kuettner, K. E., (ed.): Articular Cartilage and Osteoarthritis, New York, Raven Press, 1992, pp. 393–406.
88. Vanharanta, H., Sachs, B. L., Spivey, M. A., et al.: The relationship of pain provocation to lumbar disc deterioration as seen by CT/discography. Spine 3:295–298, 1987.
89. Vanharanta, H., Guyer, R. D., Ohnmeiss, D. D., et al.: Disc deterioration in low-back syndromes: A prospective, multi-center CT/discography study. Spine 13:1349–1351, 1988.
90. Vanharanta, H., Nykanen, M., Eronen, I., et al.: Experimental study on the effect of vibration on rabbit joints. J. Orthop. Rheumatol. 1:109–112, 1988.
91. Videman, T., Nurminen, M., and Troup, J. D. G.: Lumbar spine pathology in cadaveric material in relation to history of back pain, occupation, and physical loading. Spine 15:728–740, 1990.
92. Waddell, G.: A new clinical model for the treatment of low-back pain. Spine 12:632–644, 1987.
93. Waddell, G.: Clinical assessment of lumbar impairment. Clin. Orthop. 221:110–120, 1987.
94. Waddell, G., Somerville, D., Henderson, I., et al.: Objective clinical evaluation of physical impairment in chronic low back pain. Spine 17:617–628, 1992.
95. Ward, N.: Tricyclic antidepressants for chronic low back pain: Mechanisms of action and predictors of response, 1986 Volvo Award in Clinical Sciences. Spine 11:661–665, 1986.
96. White, A. A.: Synopsis: Workshop on idiopathic low back pain. Spine 7:141–149, 1982.
97. Wiesel, S. W., Cuckler, J. M., DeLuca, F., et al.: Acute low back pain: An objective analysis of conservative therapy. Spine 5:324–330, 1980.
98. Wiesel, S. W., Tsourmas, N., Feffer, H. L., et al.: A study of computer-assisted tomography. 1. The incidence of positive CAT scans in asymptomatic group of patients. Spine 9:549–551, 1984.
99. Yoshizawa, H., O'Brien, J., Smith, W. T., et al.: The neuropathology of intervertebral discs removed for low back pain. J. Pathol. 132:95–104, 1980.

18

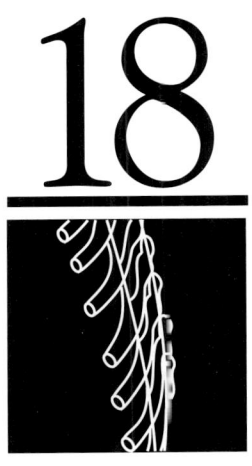

Low Back Pain in Pregnancy

GUNNAR B. J. ANDERSSON

Low back pain often develops in pregnant women. Women with ongoing or previous back pain are often afraid of pregnancy, which they believe will increase their pain or cause it to recur. The association of pregnancy and back pain, therefore, is a topic with which all persons involved in back care and those involved in maternity care should be familiar. Many orthopedic surgeons are apprehensive about treating pregnant women with back pain, because many standard examinations cannot be done and several treatment methods are contraindicated. This chapter begins by discussing the epidemiologic aspects of the problem and then proceeds to a discussion of its clinical presentation, pathogenesis, diagnosis, treatment, and prevention, as well as of postpartum back pain.

EPIDEMIOLOGIC ASPECTS

Back pain is common during pregnancy. Mantle and associates[19] reported that, in a consecutive, retrospective sample of 180 pregnant women, 48% experienced backache during pregnancy. Pain was severe in one third of these women. Fast and colleagues,[7] in a similar retrospective study of 200 women, estimated the 9-month prevalence to be 56% and stated that pain usually developed between the fifth and the seventh month.

A prospective Swedish study reported a prevalence of back pain during pregnancy of 49%.[11] Of the women in that study, 9% had back pain of sufficient severity that they were referred for orthopedic evaluation, and 19% were at some time unable to work because of their problem. In another prospective Swedish study, Ostgaard and colleagues[26] followed 917 women and found the 9-month prevalence to be 49%, with a point prevalence of between 22% and 28% from the 12th week until delivery. Because 22% of the women had back pain at the beginning of the study, the true prevalence of back pain was 27%. Previous back problems increased the risk of back pain, as did young age, multiparity, and several physical and psychologic work factors.[25, 26]

Other studies have shown that women experiencing backache often have the first episode of low back pain during pregnancy. In a study by Svensson and colleagues,[33] 10% of the women studied reported that back pain first occurred during pregnancy, whereas Biering-Sorensen[3] reported that

1057

20% of women with back pain related its onset to pregnancy and delivery. Because these studies are retrospective, the recall factor can easily explain the 10% difference between them. Other epidemiologic studies have found that women with a high number of live births have an increased risk of back pain.[9, 19, 33, 34]

Disc herniations occurring during pregnancy are rare. An incidence of 1:10,000 has been calculated, but the diagnosis is more difficult in pregnant women, and therefore, the true incidence may be different.[17] Pregnancy may or may not be a risk factor for future herniations. Both O'Connell[23] and Kelsey and associates[14, 15] found that previous pregnancies increased the risk of subsequent disc herniations. Kelsey and associates' studies indicated that the risk of herniation is even greater among women who have had many pregnancies. Heliovaara,[13] on the other hand, did not find any association between the prevalence of disc herniations and the number of births in a large cross-sectional study of Finnish women.

The risk of developing back pain during pregnancy when such pain has been a previous problem was studied prospectively by Ostgaard and Andersson.[25] Women with a history of back pain experienced back pain during pregnancy twice as often as women who never had back pain. Furthermore, the pain experienced by these women was more intense. The risk of pregnancy-related back pain increased with greater numbers of previous episodes of back pain and with longer previous episodes of back pain. In spite of these findings, none of the women thought that the back pain was so severe that they regretted the pregnancy.

CLINICAL PRESENTATION

Low back pain during pregnancy does not differ significantly in its clinical presentation from low back pain occurring at other times in life. The only major difference is that a larger proportion of the pregnant women have pain over the sacroiliac joints than is usually the case in other populations with back pain.[30] Using pain drawings, Ostgaard and associates[26] were able to differentiate three groups of pregnant women with different distributions of pain. The first group, and the smallest, included women with pain in the thoracic region only. A second group consisted of women who had pain in the lumbar regions with or without radiation into one or both legs. The third group were women with pain occurring primarily over the sacroiliac joint areas and sometimes radiating to the thighs (Fig. 1). Interestingly, the relative proportion of patients with pain near the sacroiliac joint increased as pregnancy progressed, whereas in the group with low back pain the proportion of those with back symptoms decreased (Fig. 2). Generally, the point prevalence of back pain remained the same at various times during pregnancy, ranging from 22% to 28%.

Most women have troublesome but not severe pain. However, in a Swedish study, about 19% of the women had disability sufficient to result in their being listed as sick for significant periods during their pregnancies.[11] Women with pain localized to the sacroiliac joint areas in that study seemed to present for treatment with more severe symptoms. Pain when walking was typical. Thus, almost 50% of these women had difficulties in walking with a normal stride length, compared with only about 20% of women with pain in the lumbar or the thoracic region. Furthermore, these women had difficulty in walking on stairs and inclines.

Typically, pregnancy-related back problems increase toward the end of the day. Back pain is usually aggravated by physical fatigue and by bending, lifting, and twisting activities. Some women have greater pain during sitting, but most women have pain that is troublesome during standing and walking. Mantle and colleagues[19] found that sexual intercourse was an aggravating factor for only a few women. Fast and coworkers[7] noted that as many as 36% of women with pain during pregnancy reported night pain. This proportion is higher than that usually found with mechanical back pain, indicating that the underlying mechanisms may be different.

Unfortunately, back pain during pregnancy does not disappear after delivery. Some women actually experience greater pain in the early postpartum period. In a Norwegian study,[11] the prevalence of back pain immediately after delivery was about 20%, and at 3 and 12 months postpartum it was 26.5% and 20%, respectively. As during

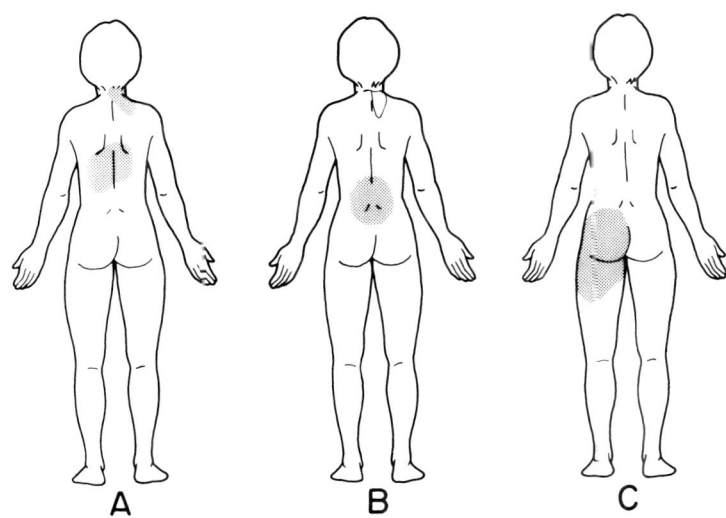

Figure 1. Three groups of women with different distributions of pain were identified by Ostgaard and colleagues.[26] *A*, Women with pain above the lumbar region. *B*, Women with pain in the lumbar region (and sometimes down one or both legs). *C*, Women with pain in the sacroiliac areas. (Modified from Ostgaard, H. C., Andersson, G. B. J., and Karlsson, K.: Prevalence of back pain in pregnancy. Spine 16:549–552, 1991.)

pregnancy, the pain was usually troublesome but not severe. Ostgaard and Andersson[28] followed 817 of the original cohort of 917 women for 18 months postpartum. Only 7% considered their pain "not better or worse." Thirty percent of the women with back pain recovered completely, usually within 6 months. Sick leave during pregnancy because of back pain and physically heavy work was associated with increased risk of persistent back pain, as were back pain during earlier pregnancies and multiple pregnancies, with or without back pain.

Melzack and Schaffelberg[21] recorded pain experienced by women during labor. They concluded that 33% of the women had continuous, severe low back pain that was qualitatively different from the pain associated with uterine contractions. It was believed to be attributable to distention and pressure on visceral and neural structures in the peritoneum. No attempt was made to follow the course of pain after labor. Ostgaard and associates[27] specifically studied the effect of back pain and pelvic pain on pregnancy outcome. No negative effects were observed.

A separate group consists of women with rheumatoid arthritis and associated low back problems. Approximately 75% of women with known rheumatoid arthritis have a pregnancy-induced remission. Of those women, however, 75% show improvement during the first trimester, another 20% improve during the second trimester, and

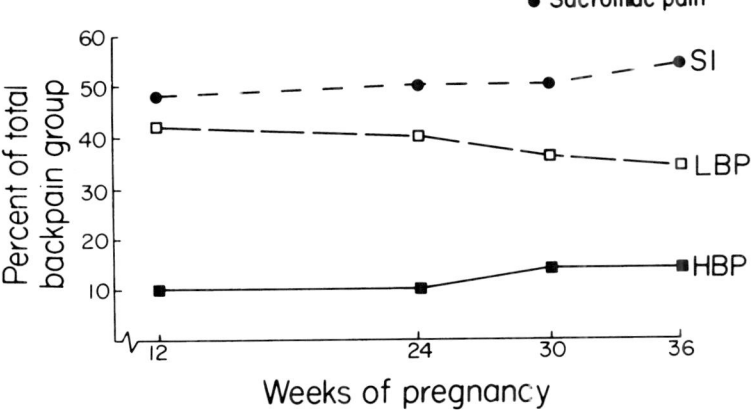

Figure 2. The proportion of women with sacroiliac (SI) area pain increased as pregnancy progressed, whereas the proportion of women with lumbar pain (LBP) decreased. The point prevalence of back pain was similar at each time during the pregnancy. (Modified from Ostgaard, H. C., Andersson, G. B. J., and Karlsson, K.: Prevalence of back pain in pregnancy. Spine 16:549–552, 1991.)

about 5% improve during the third trimester (Fig. 3). About 90% of patients experience a flare-up of arthritis after delivery, including women whose disease activity was unchanged during pregnancy. Most commonly, this flare-up occurs in the second and third months postpartum. It is unrelated to the return of menses or to breast-feeding.[24]

PATHOGENESIS

The reason why pregnancy influences the natural history of back pain is not completely known. However, several hypotheses can be made, including mechanical, hormonal, and vascular theories. Pregnancy causes an increase in the biomechanical load on the spine with an increased forward bending moment that varies somewhat among women and increases as pregnancy progresses. Ostgaard and associates[29] calculated that the additional load imposed on the lumbar spine by the near-term fetal material was similar to that caused by a forward lean of the trunk of about 22 degrees. The shape of the spine changes as a consequence of pregnancy. The effects on the anteroposterior curve (lumbar lordosis) and on the lumbar tilt are variable. Different studies have come to different conclusions. Snijders and colleagues[31] found that the lumbar spine straightened during pregnancy, and they postulated that this was due to equilibrium requirements of moments about the hip joint. This alone does not explain the straightening of lumbar lordosis, because equilibrium could be accomplished by a backward leaning of the trunk. Bullock and associates[5] measured the progression of kyphosis, lordosis, and pelvic tilt. Thoracic kyphosis was found to increase by an average of 6.6 degrees; the lordosis, by 7.2 degrees; and the pelvic tilt, by 1.9 degrees. Ostgaard and coworkers,[29] however, found no difference in lumbar lordosis from week 12 to week 36. Weight gain alone does not seem to increase the risk of back pain during pregnancy. Mantle and colleagues[19] concluded that weight, obesity, index weight gain, and the baby's weight were not associated with an increased risk of backache during pregnancy. Furthermore, it seems from most of the studies that there is no continuous increase in pain as pregnancy progresses, which would be expected if weight gain were a major factor.

An alternative hypothesis is that an increased laxity in collagen tissue occurs during pregnancy and that this makes the spine and the pelvic joints less stiff, altering their response to mechanical loading. It is known that the relaxin content in serum increases up to 10-fold during pregnancy.[6, 35] These levels seem to reach a maximum between the 38th and 42nd weeks and to decline rapidly after birth. The natural history of back pain during pregnancy does not seem to be directly related to the changes in relaxin levels. The combined effects of increased mechanical load and decreased collagen tissue stiffness may, however, be the cause of back pain in many pregnant women.

Ostgaard and colleagues[29] evaluated several biomechanical risk factors, including

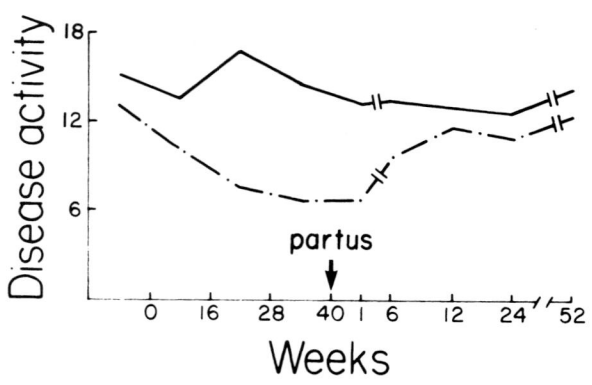

Figure 3. Of women with rheumatoid arthritis (RA), 75% have pregnancy-induced remission. After delivery, the disease activity increases to prepregnancy levels. (Modified from Östensen, M., and Husby, G.: Ensuring a healthy pregnancy for the woman with severe RA. J. Musculoskel. Med. 5:13–25, 1988).

weight gain, abdominal circumference, sagittal and transverse abdominal diameters, the amount of lumbar lordosis, finger laxity, and striae atrophicae in the skin of the abdomen, thighs, and breasts.[29] This information was gathered prospectively for 855 consecutive pregnant women at weeks 12, 20, 24, 30, and 36 of their pregnancies and was related to the occurrence of back pain. The primary biomechanical risk factor identified was the change in abdominal sagittal diameter, which on average increased by 55% from the 12th to the 36th week. An initially deep lumbar lordosis was also a risk factor. Peripheral joint laxity was important in women who were pregnant for the first time, because this population with back pain had decreased laxity (i.e., stiffer joints at the beginning of the pregnancy).

A vascular hypothesis has also been advanced and is based on the fact that many pregnant women with back pain have night pain.[8] The fluid increase over the course of pregnancy (average of 6.5 L) can result in dependent edema during the upright hours and increased venous return during recumbency. This could cause a stagnant hypoxia of neural tissue and vertebral bodies. This mechanism, while it may explain night pain, does not account for other features of pregnancy-related back pain.

In patients with rheumatoid arthritis, changes in steroid hormone levels and pregnancy-associated proteins have been thought to be important. Placenta-eluted γ-globulins have also been suggested as causes of pregnancy-induced remission. Nevertheless, the role of any of these factors remains unclear.

DIAGNOSIS

In any patient with low back problems, the physical examination is the cornerstone. Indeed, in the pregnant patient the clinical examination is even more important because the use of structural examinations (radiography and scans) is limited by the need to avoid irradiation. As mentioned above, a pain drawing is helpful in outlining the specific distribution of pain, which may provide clues to its origin. The patient history should include questions about previous back problems, the work situation, and any factors associated with relief or aggravation of the pain. In the physical examination of pregnant women, two specific areas need particular attention, the symphysis and the sacroiliac areas. Symphysiolysis (diastasis of the symphysis pubis) is detected as pain induced by pressure over the symphysis pubis as well as anterior pain induced when the pelvis is compressed and when the patient stands on one leg. These women also present with painful restriction of abduction and rotation of both hips. Symphysiolysis generally becomes a problem post partum rather than during pregnancy. Normally, the pubic symphysis widens maximally by the sixth month of pregnancy, returning to normal status within 3 to 5 months of delivery.[1] The problem appears to develop when this return to normal does not occur.

A multitude of tests are believed to be specific to the sacroiliac region.[13, 18, 32] These include the Patrick test, the knee-shoulder test, the hyperextended hip test, the sacral compression test, the pelvis separation test (ventral gapping), the pelvic compression test (dorsal gapping), and the Gaenslen test. In the author's opinion, none of these tests is entirely specific. However, increased pain during the performance of any of these tests seems to be more likely to originate from the sacroiliac joints than from the lumbar spine. Positive results of several tests at the same time strengthen this diagnosis.

Neither radiographs nor bone scans should be obtained during pregnancy. The only exception is if a tumor or infection is suspected. Lead shielding and collimated beams can reduce the fetal exposure. The effect of magnetic resonance imaging on the fetus is not sufficiently clarified to warrant recommending this method of investigation. Thus, structural examinations are usually out of the question. This is not a great loss because structural examinations usually add little to treatment decisions. Furthermore, the back problem is rarely so severe as to require these examinations with great urgency. Electromyography can be safely used to screen for herniated discs.

TREATMENT

The treatment of back pain in pregnancy is influenced by the fact that pregnancy precludes the use of some treatment modalities and the use of some types of medication.

Consequently, prevention is the best treatment method.

Information is an indispensable part of treatment. Women should be informed (reassured) that, although the back problem may be annoying, it is not in any way dangerous either to them or to their child and that usually the course is benign. They should also be taught proper body mechanics adapted to pregnancy and appropriate methods of relaxation.

Only patients with significant pain and discomfort should be given medication. They should first be advised about the possible risks. Physicians practicing in the United States should strongly consider having the patients sign a consent form documenting that this information has been transmitted. Drugs with short half-lives are preferred, and of course, the smallest possible dosage should be used for the shortest possible period. Simple analgesics such as acetaminophen are not believed to be teratogenic and therefore can be used safely during both pregnancy and lactation. Salicylates have not been shown to have teratogenic effects. However, prolonged gestation and labor, as well as maternal and neonatal bleeding and respiratory distress in the neonate, have been reported as side effects.[24] For that reason, if salicylates are necessary, only low doses should be given and treatment should be terminated 4 to 6 weeks before delivery. The same is true for other nonsteroidal antiinflammatory drugs such as indomethacin,[22] naproxen (Naprosyn), ibuprofen, and diflunisal, which should not be given during the third trimester of pregnancy. Further, salicylates and indomethacin should not be given to lactating women because they are excreted in breast milk and have significant side effects on nursing infants. Naproxen is considered compatible for nursing mothers and can be used to manage postpartum pain.[4]

Corsets may be used during pregnancy. Indeed, specific corsets, called maternity corsets, have been designed to allow for the increasing change in abdominal width as pregnancy progresses.[12] These corsets can provide significant support, particularly at the end of the day when fatigue often causes additional pain. Manipulation is not recommended. However, physical therapy adapted to pregnancy may prove beneficial. Abdominal muscle and pelvic floor muscle exercises are most commonly employed. Using a small cushion behind the back during sitting and resting in the early afternoon can also be helpful.

Almost all back pain in pregnant women can easily be managed with proper advice, appropriately reduced physical activities, the administration of mild analgesics, and perhaps the use of a supporting corset.

Surgery, obviously, should always be avoided in a pregnant woman. Even in patients with muscle weakness due to a disc herniation, the prognosis without surgery is good. Although O'Connell[23] found significant weakness and sometimes paresis in a few patients with disc herniations, the pain was later relieved and strength either recovered or improved without a surgical intervention. The only indication for disc surgery during pregnancy is severe neurologic dysfunction, as in cauda equina syndrome.

Backache and sciatica during pregnancy are not an indication for abortion. Previous spine fusion for scoliosis does not increase the risk for back pain during pregnancy.[2]

POSTPARTUM BACK PAIN

Usually, the low back pain that sometimes follows delivery is a continuing pain from the latter part of pregnancy. Occasionally, however, back pain occurs during delivery and remains for some time. Kogstad,[16] when examining a group of women post partum, found that low back pain in the preceding year, low back pain immediately after delivery, and smoking were negative factors with respect to continuous back pain during the first year after delivery. About one third of the women examined by Kogstad[16] were believed to have a relaxation of the pelvic girdle affecting primarily the sacroiliac joints and the symphysis pubis. Ostgaard and Andersson[28] reported that 67% of 817 women studied experienced pain directly after delivery. At follow-up examination about 12 months later, 37% still had some back symptoms. Those who recovered typically did so within 6 months. Physically heavy work was the main factor associated with persistent back pain at 12 months.

PREVENTION

Prevention of backache in pregnancy can be accomplished by any of three main approaches. The first is to change the life style and work environment to reduce the load on the spine. This is particularly helpful for women who have a history of back pain and who have had many previous pregnancies, some of which have been complicated by back pain. In these women, a modification of heavy physical work can be beneficial.

The second approach involves education. This includes prophylactic back education with an emphasis on posture, working positions, lifting technique, and methods of avoiding or alleviating backache. A pregnancy back school should preferably be combined with some abdominal muscle contraction and pelvic floor contraction exercises to enhance the muscle support. Instruction both in methods of coping with stress and discomfort and in methods of relaxation can be added. The effect of a pregnancy low back school was tested by Mantle and colleagues,[20] and it was found that women who were educated had less troublesome and severe backache than did a control group not placed in the program.

The third method of prevention is to place pregnant women in a prophylactic corset or brace. Because this has significant negative effects on the trunk muscles and is cumbersome, it cannot be recommended at this time. This is particularly true because there is no study supporting the beneficial effect of such prophylactic efforts.

CONCLUSIONS

Back pain is common in pregnancy, and the risk of back pain is greater in women who have had a previous back problem. Usually, however, pain is not severe and unremitting, but rather it is moderate, although annoying. A separate group of women tend to have problems that are more localized to the sacroiliac region. For this group, the prognosis is not as good as for those with pain in the lower back and the upper back. Prophylactic pregnancy back care programs should, ideally, be provided for all pregnant women. Should back pain occur, information and the judicious use of medication may be necessary. In more severe cases, it may be necessary to use pregnancy corsets. Unfortunately, the back pain does not seem to disappear immediately after pregnancy, and it may cause a problem for the patient, particularly during the first year postpartum. Women need not be fearful of the occurrence of back pain during pregnancy. Rather, they should become informed about the benign nature of these problems and ways of coping with them, should they occur.

REFERENCES

1. Abramson, D., Roberts, S., and Wilson, P.: Relaxation of the pelvic joints in pregnancy. Surg. Gynecol. Obstet. 58:595–613, 1934.
2. Betz, R. R., Bunnell, W. P., Lambrecht-Mulier, E., and MacEwen, D.: Scoliosis and pregnancy. J. Bone Joint Surg. 69A:90–96, 1987.
3. Biering-Sorensen, F.: A prospective study of low back pain in a general population. I. Occurrence, recurrence and aetiology. Scand. J. Rehabil. Med. 15:71–79, 1983.
4. Briggs, G. G., Freeman, R. K., and Yaffe, S. J.: Drugs in Pregnancy and Lactation. Los Angeles, Williams & Wilkins, 1986.
5. Bullock, J., Juli, G. A., and Bullock, M.: The relationship of low back pain to postural changes during pregnancy. Austr. J. Physiother. 33:10–17, 1987.
6. Calgunieri, M., Bird, H. A., and Wright, V.: Changes in joint laxity occurring during pregnancy. Ann. Rheum. Dis. 41:126–128, 1982.
7. Fast, A., Shapiro, D., Ducommun, E. J., et al.: Low back pain in pregnancy. Spine 12:368–371, 1987.
8. Fast, A., Weiss, L., Parich, S., and Hertz, G.: Night backache in pregnancy—hypothetical pathophysiological mechanisms. Am. J. Phys. Med. Rehabil. 68:227–229, 1989.
9. Frymoyer, J. W., Pope, M. H., Costanza, M. C., et al.: Epidemiologic studies of low-back pain. Spine 5:419–423, 1980.
10. Grieve, G. P.: The sacro-iliac joint. Physiotherapy 62:384–400, 1976.
11. Hammar, M., Berg, G., Lillieskold, U., et al.: Low-back pain and pregnancy—incidence, diagnostics and background factors. J. Swedish Med. Assoc. 83:1960–1962, 1983.
12. Heckman, J. D.: Managing musculoskeletal problems in pregnant patients. J. Musculoskel. Med. 7:29–41, 1990.
13. Heliovaara, M.: Epidemiology of Sciatica and Herniated Lumbar Intervertebral Disc. Helsinki, Finland, Social Insurance Institution, 1988.
14. Kelsey, J. L., Greenberg, R. A., Hardy, R. J., and Johnson, M. F.: Pregnancy and the syndrome of herniated lumbar intervertebral disc; an epidemiological study. Yale J. Biol. Med. 48:361–368, 1975.
15. Kelsey, J. L., and White, A. A., II: Epidemiology and impact of low-back pain. Spine 2:133–142, 1980.
16. Kogstad, O.: Low back pain. Post partum. Spine (submitted).
17. LaBan, M. M., Perrin, J. C. S., and Latimer, F. R.: Pregnancy and the herniated lumbar disc. Arch. Phys. Med. Rehabil. 64:319–321, 1983.
18. Lewit, K.: Manuelle Medizin in Rahmen des medizinischen rehabilitierung. Leipzig, Johan Ambrousius Barth, 1977.
19. Mantle, M. J., Greenwood, R. M., and Currey, H.

L. F.: Backache in pregnancy. Rheumatol. Rehabil. 16:95–101, 1977.
20. Mantle, M. J., Holmers, J., and Currey, H. L. F.: Backache in pregnancy. II. Prophylactic influence of back care classes. Rheumatol. Rehabil. 20:227–232, 1981.
21. Melzack, R., and Schaeffelberg, D.: Low back pain during labor. Am. J. Obstet. Gynecol. 156:901–905, 1987.
22. Moise, K. J., Hohta, J. C., Sharif, D. S., et al.: Indomethacin in the treatment of premature labor—effects on the fetal ductus arteriosus. N. Engl. J. Med. 319:327–331, 1988.
23. O'Connell, J. E. A.: Lumbar disc protrusion in pregnancy. J. Neurol. Neurosurg. Psychiatry 23:138–141, 1960.
24. Östensen, M., and Husby, G.: Ensuring a healthy pregnancy for the woman with severe RA. J. Musculoskel. Med. 5:13–25, 1988.)
25. Ostgaard, H. C., and Andersson, G. B. J.: Previous back pain and risk of developing back pain in a future pregnancy. Spine 16:432–436, 1991.
26. Ostgaard, H. C., Andersson, G. B. J., and Karlsson, K.: Prevalence of back pain in pregnancy. Spine 16:549–552, 1991.
27. Ostgaard, H. C., Andersson, G. B. J., and Wennergren, M.: The impact of low back pain and pelvic pain on the pregnancy outcome. Acta Obstet. Gynecol. Scand. 70:21–24, 1991.
28. Ostgaard, H. C., and Andersson, G. B. J.: Postpartum low back pain. Spine 17:53–55, 1992.
29. Ostgaard, H. C., Andersson, G. B. J., Schultz, A. B., and Miller, J. A. A.: The influence of biomechanical factors on low back pain during pregnancy. Spine 18:61–65, 1993.
30. Rungee, J. L.: Low back pain during pregnancy. Orthopedics 16:1339–1344, 1993.
31. Snijders, C. J., Scroo, J. M., Snijder, J. G., and Hoedt, H. T.: Change in form of the spine as a consequence of pregnancy. *In* Digest of the 11th International Conference on Medical and Biological Engineering, Abstract No. 49.4, Ottawa, 1976.
32. Stoddard, A.: Manual of Osteopathic Technique. London, Hutchinson Medical Publications, 1964.
33. Svensson, H.-O., Andersson, G. B. J., Johansson, S., and Wilhelmsson, V. A.: A retrospective study of low-back pain in 38–40 year old women. Spine 13:548–552, 1988.
34. Videman, T., Nurminen, T., Tola, S., et al.: Low-back pain in nurses and some loading factors of work. Spine 9:400–404, 1984.
35. Zarrow, M., Holmstrom, E. G., and Salhanich, H. A.: The concentration of relaxin in the blood serum and other tissues of women during pregnancy. J. Clin. Endocrinol. 15:22–27, 1955.

19

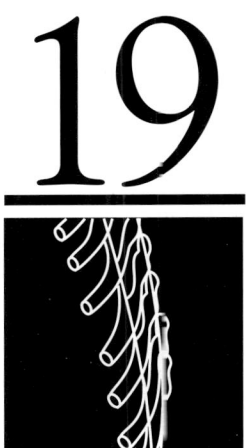

Industrial Low Back Pain

Risk Factors

STANLEY J. BIGOS
MICHELE CRITES BATTIÉ

Risk factors related to back problems have been a topic of interest in the literature since the 1920s.[19] Since then, back problems have become the most expensive musculoskeletal malady in the industrialized nations of the world. A major reason for the enormous cost is that back problems have also become the most common cause of disability in persons younger than age 45 years and are an extremely expensive health care problem in the working age group.[31, 38, 40, 67] The impact goes far beyond the pain and diminished quality of life experienced by workers and their families; back problems are an increasing burden for society as industry incorporates higher insurance costs into the costs of goods and services or as tax revenues are allocated to care for those declared disabled and their families.[65, 67]

Prevention has long been the goal of investigators studying risk factors for industrial back problems. Radiographs were introduced as preemployment screening tools in the 1920s,[19, 23] followed by preemployment medical history and physical examination. Testing of physical capacities has received a great deal of attention. These tests, even those using expensive technology, have not as yet clearly established any associations with future back problems and related work incapacity.*

Efforts to prevent industrial back problems by establishing and enforcing safety and health regulations to decrease suspected physical hazards at the workplace also produced equivocal results.[19] Although such techniques led to a substantial decrease in objectively verifiable industrial injuries, the reporting of more subjective injuries such as back strain increased. The inadequacy of prevention efforts is indicated by the almost 2700% increase in disability awards in the United States and the 3300% increase in Sweden during similar 20-year periods.[51, 67] Many of the ineffective attempts at prevention and intervention have been based on flawed assumptions about factors thought to be associated with increased risk of back pain.

---

*References 3–6, 11, 12, 28, 56, 61, and 71.

ETIOLOGY AND INCITING CAUSES

Epidemiologists state that 85% of older adults, irrespective of occupation, report having experienced back problems that interfere with work or recreational activity,[1, 34, 36, 37, 50] and up to 25% of people between the ages of 30 and 50 years report the presence of back symptoms at the time when they are surveyed.[1, 2, 34, 69, 73] The common and usually transitory nature of back pain has led some observers to question whether it can be called a disease, let alone fit into an injury model.[37]

Additional questions about the injury model arise during the study of the onset of back problems. Onset is commonly gradual and is frequently not related to an accidental cause.[29, 35, 59, 61, 78] In a study of patients with acute, subacute, and chronic back pain at the authors' institution, 77% of a patient population could not relate the onset of symptoms to a time within 24 hours of an accident or unusual activity.[29]

The failure of the injury model to explain industrial back problems led to the cumulative trauma model, which is now proposed to explain musculoskeletal problems of gradual onset among workers. Unfortunately, the difficulties in monitoring off-work activities make it virtually impossible to control all the factors needed to verify scientifically the cumulative model as an explanation of industrial back problems.

Medical technology allows a determination of a pathoanatomic diagnosis in only 12% to 15% of persons.[11, 24] Thus, there does not need to be an objective diagnosable condition to explain back symptoms or to file a back injury claim. Commonly used diagnostic terms such as back sprain or strain, myofascitis, disc syndrome, facet syndrome, and subluxations are not verified objectively and, for scientific purposes, must be considered synonyms for idiopathic back pain. Thus, the basis for studying back problems is less objective than that for studying more easily diagnosable problems such as fractures and lacerations.

In summary, both the injury model and the cumulative trauma model are clouded by numerous problems. The documentation of either is difficult, and medical science is unable to provide a specific diagnosis in the majority of cases. More important, both models may distort the perceptions of researchers attempting to find solutions to industrial back problems as well as the perceptions of patients experiencing symptoms.

PERCEPTIONS AFFECTING THE CLAIM-FILING PROCESS

Because medical technology usually cannot provide a verifiable diagnosis of back injury,[11, 24] often none is needed for a back injury claim to be filed or accepted. Therefore, the claim-filing process is somewhat subjective, and the perceptions of the employee seem especially significant. Although back symptoms may be the basis of a claim, the employee's perceptions about the *safety* of continuing to work and about the *impact* of a back injury claim on his or her personal situation may determine whether a claim is filed. Programs involving the presentation and interpretation of information about symptoms, safety, and personal environment affect a person's perceptions and thus the back injury claim process, for better or for worse.[25, 26, 58, 79]

Symptoms

Reports of back symptoms are so common that there is little reason to question whether a person has symptoms when a back injury claim is made.* The presence of symptoms alone may lead to a back injury claim, especially if they are severe or if the claimant believes that the problem is unusual, is caused by an accident, or is the fault of another person. However, comparing the high incidence of back problems (reported by more than 85% of adults) and point prevalence (as high as 30% in the 30- to 50-year age group) to the actual number of expected injury claims (2% to 5% of workers in the United States per year)[20, 43, 52, 74] indicates that all workers with symptoms do not file a claim.[65] In addition, 10% of those who file do not miss work because of their problem.[68]

Perceptions of Safety

Many workers with back symptoms are apparently confident that they can safely

---

*References 1, 2, 24, 33, 34, 36, 37, 62, 69, and 73.

perform tasks without jeopardizing their future health. Seemingly, if symptoms are minor, they continue working despite some back discomfort.

The physical requirements of a job can have a major impact on the decision to file a back injury claim.[65] Back symptoms that would lay up a furniture mover or heavy laborer may not interfere with the work of an administrator, a supervisor, or a clerk. If a worker perceives that performing certain tasks will actually cause physical harm, it is unlikely that the person will continue to work, if the industrial environment is insured. Changing only the perceptions about a job also can affect the claim-filing process. Ironically, there is evidence that increasing the employee's awareness of back-related work hazards, in an attempt to improve job safety, increases both the number reported and the cost of back injuries.[61]

Perceptions of Impact

For some persons with back symptoms, the desire to continue working overcomes difficulties with tasks or the fear of further injury. Common examples are the farmer who wears a footdrop brace so he or she can harvest crops before taking time for a surgical evaluation; the independent house framer who continues to work and thus avoids leaving the crew unsupervised during the busy season; or the parent with small children and inadequate social support who continues to carry out activities for the family. These cases illustrate that, in certain situations, concerns about back symptoms may be overcome by the need to continue activities that are essential to or that positively affect a personal situation.

Indirect evidence also suggests that similar scenarios occur in the industrial setting. Some jobs are stressful to the back but rarely generate back injury claims. In some instances, camaraderie and financial or personal status make the positions desirable for some workers. Surely, a number of these workers have back discomfort, but perhaps not sufficient to warrant filing a back injury claim and risking transfer to a less desirable position.

Conversely, suppose that the task at hand is not so coveted or is even dreaded. A back injury claim may lead to an escape or time out from the pressures of daily living or an unsatisfactory job or task. A back injury claim may also provide an opportunity to prove a point about a certain task that is perceived as dangerous. Filing a back injury claim could even become a more socially acceptable alternative to quitting a job.[14]

Perceptions about the potential personal impact of a back injury claim commonly raise questions about malingering. However, most employees filing injury claims under the above conditions seem to be reacting to misconceptions about back pain, back injury claims, or safety, which can be fueled by personal problems in the work or off-hours environment. The process rarely seems conscious or deliberate,[35, 66] and the authors caution against the use of the term malingering in regard to these situations. Furthermore, malingering is virtually impossible to document, and such accusations can jeopardize a successful resolution of the person's medical, insurance, and livelihood problems.

STUDY DESIGN

Retrospective Data. Data from scientific prospective studies have not always been available. Retrospective data, predominately from insurance records, generated controversy and contributed little to progress in curbing the industrial back problem.[1, 65]

Numerous retrospective studies of multiple factors related to industrial back problems have produced many conflicting associations.[15] Andersson[1] reported that findings were misleading because data derived from insurance company reports and absenteeism reports were incomplete and categorized for purposes other than back research. Another factor is inadequate study design. Snook[65] pointed out that "most studies of low back pain are of small-sample, short-term, and retrospective studies done without a control group." Thus, clear insights and solutions to the industrial back problem have been slow in coming.

Prospective Studies. Snook[65] emphasized that "the greatest need . . . is for a long-term, controlled longitudinal study that controls the many variables involved in low back pain. . . . Nevertheless we can approach the ideal experiment with a large sample, control groups, good experimental design, adequate statistical treatment, and sufficient funds and time to complete the study." Owing to the cost and effort required to meet these ideals, few prospective studies have been conducted to date of work-related back pain problems and most have been of limited scope, focusing on individual physical capacities among workers in occupations with high physical demands.

The specific definition of back problems and thus of predictors varies in longitudinal studies. Some investigations are about predictors of back symptoms as revealed on questionnaires.* Other studies concern predictors of industrial back incident reports or "injury" claims filed in the workplace.† These are distinctly different back-related outcomes, as indicated by an approximately 10-fold variation in the reported incidence.

PREDICTORS OF INDUSTRIAL BACK INCIDENT REPORTS OR INJURY CLAIMS

Industrial back incident reports and injury claims are specific definitions of back problems to be distinguished from reports of symptoms solicited on surveys. Most developed countries have systems for filing reports of work-related injuries and illnesses, and these systems may have effects of their own. Perhaps because of differences in reporting and compensation systems between countries, most of the prospective studies in this area have been conducted in the United States.† There have been few prospective, longitudinal studies investigating industrial back pain incident reports or claims, and most investigations have focused primarily on individual physical factors (Table 1).

Chaffin and Park,[22] in 1973, conducted a study of back incident reports in 411 men and women who engaged in manual lifting in their work at an electronics manufacturing company. The study focused on the effects of occupational lifting and mismatches between individual strength and job requirements. They noted an association between low back pain reports and jobs with higher lifting strength requirements in terms of position and magnitude of the weight lifted. They also found a higher incidence of back pain reporting in persons who demonstrated less strength on isometric strength testing than that deemed necessary to meet job demands. Strength in excess of job requirements did not appear to have an additional protective effect. However, only 25 low back incidents were reported among the study group and the result did not reach statistical significance and awaits verification.

In 1980, Keyserling and coworkers[41, 42] expanded on Chaffin and Park's earlier work and reported two studies examining the association between lifting strength with respect to job requirements and industrial injury and illness reports. These investigators found a greater tendency toward reports of medical problems during the following year among employees who were not matched to the job on the basis of meeting strength requirements (required to lift >75% of their maximum capacity, as determined by maximum isometric strength testing). However, neither study differentiated between back problems and other musculoskeletal problems. There was no indication that strength exceeding job requirements provided any extra protection from back problems. In addition, the relationship between inadequate strength to meet job demands and increased injury reports did not hold true for all strength testing positions. Employees with strength that matched job requirements in the arm lift position actually had the highest incidence of injury reports in one investigation.[42]

Isokinetic lifting strength was investigated as a predictor of low back injury claims among nurses.[7] It was concluded that it was a poor predictor of subsequent back symptoms and injury reports. Another prospective study of back injury reports in nurses reached similar conclusions about isometric lifting strength and other general fitness variables.[53] The factors that discriminated most between the nurses who did and did not report subsequent back injuries in the latter study were prior compensation pay, smoking status, and poorer job satisfaction. A history of compensation has been associated with work loss due to back problems in other studies as well.

Cady and associates[21] reported on physical fitness as an indicator of risk in 1652 firefighters over a 3-year period. Fitness was defined by a composite score based on aerobic capacity, strength, and flexibility measures. They found that firefighters with high

---

*References 11, 12, 21, 37, 42–45, 54, 69, and 73.
†References 3, 4, 6–8, 13, 15, 20, 21, 47, and 53.

Table 1

Summary of Prospective Studies of Predictors of Industrial Back Pain Reports or Injury Claims*

Study Subjects (No. Volunteers/ No. Solicited), Follow-up Duration Factors Considered	Aircraft Mfgr. Employees (3020/4027), 4 Years[18]	Electronics Mfgr. Employees (411/?), 1 Year[22]	Firefighters (1652/1900), 3 Years[21]	Nurses (171/?), 2 Years[49]	Nurses (131/255), 1.5 Years[55]
Demographic					
Gender	0	0			
Age	↓	0			
Education	0				
Anthropometric					
Standing height	↑, men only	0			0
Weight or obesity	↑, women only	0			↑
Lifestyle					
Smoking	↑				↑↑
Physical Capacities					
Lifting strength	0	↓		0	0
Aerobic capacity or fitness	0		↓		0
Trunk strength					0
Flexion or side bending	0				
Prereporting Back Examination					
Decreased patellar reflex	↑				
Decreased Achilles reflex	0				
Symptoms on SLR	↑↑				
Psychosocial					
Psychologic distress	↑↑				
Health locus of control	0				
Family social support	0				
Stress level					0
Work-Related					
Social support or job satisfaction	↓↓				↓↓
Perceived physical demands	0				
Frequency of heavy lifting		↑, >150 lifts/day			
Medical History					
Back pain history	↑↑	↑		↑	
Prior back-related compensation claim					↑↑
Prior MVA					↑
Health care utilization (for pain)	↑↑				

*All studies were conducted in the United States.
↑, positive association; ↑↑, strong positive association; ↓, negative association; ↓↓, strong negative association; 0, not a predictor; SLR, straight leg raising; MVA, moving vehicle accident.

fitness levels were about nine times less likely to report a back injury than those in the least fit group. However, the few injuries reported among the highly fit were the most serious in terms of costs. The effects of age and other potentially confounding factors were not reported, making interpretation of results difficult.

Since Porter[53] introduced the idea of using ultrasonography to detect a relatively narrow canal diameter, and reported significant differences in the canal diameters of patients with radicular symptoms as compared with those of control subjects, there has been interest in such measurements as screening tools.[46, 52] A study of ultrasound measurements of the lumbar spinal canals of 204 mine workers investigated their association with back problems. Previous medical and work attendance records were reviewed, and the subjects were followed for 3 years to observe absence from work and changes of employment. Workers who remained on the job had spinal canal measurements significantly larger than those of workers who retired. However, the evaluation was complicated because of the high retirement rate and a reduction in the size of the work force because of economic difficulties in the industry; thus, some of the information that led to the final conclusions had to be dealt with retrospectively.

A study examined D-scan ultrasonic measurements of the spinal canal as predictors of industrial back pain reports and extended work loss in aircraft manufacturing workers.[9] The investigators found that the mean canal measurements were smaller at all spinal levels in persons reporting industrial back pain than in persons without reports of symptoms. The differences, however, were extremely small and no association was found between canal measurements and extended work loss claims. The imprecision of

B-scan ultrasonography measurements and their poor predictive ability renders them of dubious screening value.

In a prospective, longitudinal study of industrial back pain reports in 3020 aircraft manufacturing (Boeing Company) workers, isometric lifting strength, maximum aerobic capacity, and range of motion in side bending and flexion were among the factors that were not associated with subsequent symptoms.[18] The strongest predictors of future back pain reports, other than current or recent back problems at the onset of the study, were negative perceptions of the workplace, including low job task enjoyment and social support, and emotional distress[18] (Fig. 1). The only factor from the baseline physical examination that was strongly associated with future reporting was back pain elicited on straight leg raising testing,[7] which probably represents another aspect of recent or current back problems, which are known to influence future risk. These findings underline the multifaceted nature of back pain reporting in industry.

Although some factors have been identified as risk indicators, their practical value in predicting specifically who will or will not experience or report symptoms is poor. For example, a positive straight leg raising test result in the study mentioned above more than doubled the risk of reporting, but less than 3% of subjects had this finding and only one in five of those reported subsequent back pain.[7] This result illustrates the inadequacy of such tests as preemployment or preplacement tools. It was similarly difficult to predict extended disability. In the Boeing Company study,[17] the factors that contributed to the prediction of extended time loss, and that differed significantly between claims of short- and long-term time loss, were a low scale 10 on the Minnesota Multiphasic Personality Inventory, indicating extroversion, and back pain elicited on straight leg raising testing as identified prior to the filing of the back injury claim. Physical capacity measures and psychologic findings commonly seen in chronically disabled patients did not contribute significantly to predicting extended back pain disability in this group of claimants.[13]

In summary, one study suggested an association between industrial back pain reports and insufficient isometric strength relative to job demands, but general strength testing failed to predict the filing of industrial back pain reports. A negative correlation between back incident reports and overall fitness in terms of strength, flexibility, and cardiovascular fitness factors may exist in firefighters.[21] However, similar associations between physical factors and back pain reporting were not corroborated in other occupational groups whose peak physical job demands were less extreme. A study of aircraft manufacturing workers found that perceptions of work and other psychosocial factors played a greater role in whether industrial back pain reports were filed than did the wide array of physical measures studied. These findings emphasize the importance of adopting a broader approach to understanding and dealing with the multifaceted problems of back pain symptoms that interfere with work, and offer an explanation as to why efforts focusing on purely physical or injury factors have met with little success.

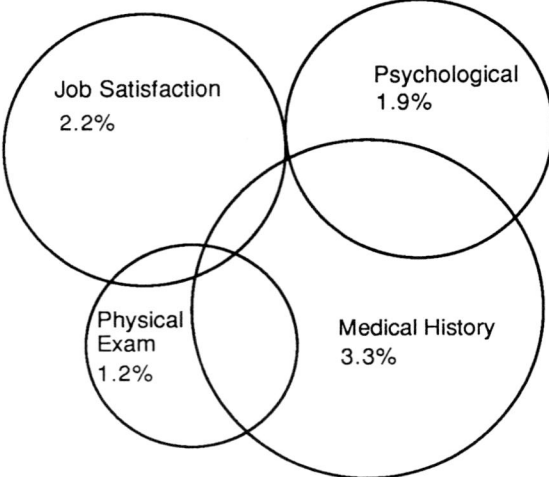

Figure 1. Venn diagram of final multivariate model for predicting industrial back pain reports. Medical history explains 3.3% of the uncertainty in predicting a subject's making or not making an industrial back pain report, as compared with 1.2% explained by physical examination (straight leg raising), 1.9% explained by psychologic findings (Minnesota Multiphasic Personality Inventory and HLOC), and 2.2% explained by job satisfaction (modified work adaptability, partnership, growth, affection, and resolve [WORK-APGAR]). The predictive value of medical history and physical examination together is 4%, of medical history and psychologic findings together is 4.5%, and of medical history and job satisfaction together is 5.4%. The predictive value of psychologic findings and physical examination considered together is 3.3%. The predictive value of job satisfaction and physical examination considered together is 3.3%. (From Bigos, S. J.: Industrial low back pain. Semin. Spine 4:8–9, 1992.)

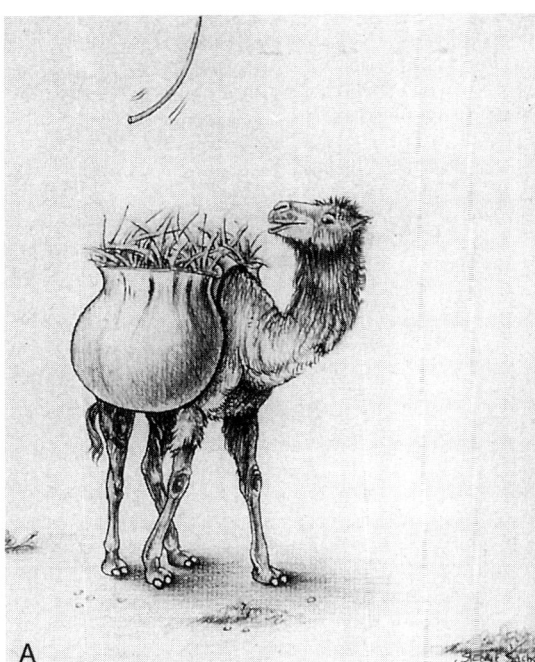
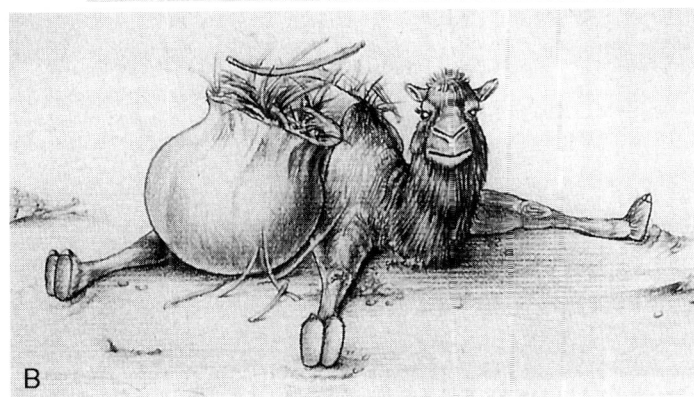

Figure 2. Back pain (the proverbial last straw) relative to total problem of back injury claim. Medical treatment models only attempt to lift the last straw (back pain). (From Bigos, S. J.: Industrial low back pain. Semin. Spine 4:8–9, 1992.)

CONCLUSIONS

Back symptoms are a common and expected part of life. Each year, up to 50% of the work force worldwide admits on surveys to having symptoms or being limited for at least one day by back problems, but only 2% to 5% are expected to file a back injury claim.[43, 68, 74, 75] Obviously, factors other than the presence of symptoms incite the report of a back injury. For example, once a back problem is experienced, the chance of a recurrence and future interference with work probably depends on numerous physical and situational factors. Nonphysical factors such as psychologic distress and negative perceptions of the job have been reported as risk factors for both reports of back pain and work interference.[27, 70] These are not fixed, stable states but dynamic situational factors that can relate to a person's self-perception with respect to his or her environment.

Health care providers must accept that nonphysical stresses in life or work can influence the response to back symptoms. Symbolically, in relation to a back injury claim, back symptoms may be the straw that breaks the back of the already burdened camel (Fig. 2). Concomitantly, not even the most ardent engineer would expect removal of the straw to bounce the camel right back to its feet. Why should concentrating on addressing the back pain alone in an overburdened patient be any more effective? In either case, focusing on only the last straw does not seem to be the answer. Treating back pain alone may not spring the overburdened patient back to his or her feet, to work, or to the previous station in life. Back problems seem many times to be only one aspect of the patient's total predicament.

Adding nonphysical factors to the industrial back problem equation opens the door for a more educated approach to the needs of workers, employers, health care providers, third-party payers, and society. Fortunately, it does so not by identifying unchangeable markers such as age, sex, and specific physical defects, but by identifying situational factors that can be altered to the benefit of everyone by offering insight into the complex health problem of industrial back pain.

REFERENCES

1. Andersson, G. B. J.: Epidemiological aspects of low-back pain in industry. Spine 6:53–60, 1981.
2. Andersson, G., and Svensson, H. O.: Prevalence of low back pain. S.P.R.I. Rapport 22:11–23, 1979.
3. Battié, M. C., Bigos, S. J., Fisher, L. D., et al.: Isometric lifting strength as a predictor of industrial back pain reports. Spine 14:851–856, 1989.
4. Battié, M. C., Bigos, S. J., Fisher, L. D., et al.: A prospective study of the role of cardiovascular risk factors and fitness in industrial back pain complaints. Spine 14:141–147, 1989.
5. Battié, M. C.: The Reliability of Physical Factors as Predictors of the Occurrence of Back Pain Reports: A Prospective Study Within Industry. Thesis. Goteborg, Sweden, Gothenburg University, 1989.
6. Battié, M. C., Bigos, S. J., Fisher, L. D., et al.: The role of spinal flexibility in back pain complaints within industry: A prospective study. Spine 15:768–773, 1990.
7. Battié, M. C., Bigos, S. J., Fisher, L. D., et al.: Anthropometric and clinical measurements as predictors of industrial back pain complaints: A prospective study. J. Spinal Disord. 3:195–204, 1990.
8. Battié, M. C., Hansson, T., Bigos, S. J., et al.: B-scan ultrasonic measurement of the lumbar spine canal as a predictor of industrial back pain complaints and extended work loss. J. Occup. Med. 35:1250–1255, 1993.
9. Battié, M. C., Videman, T., and Sarna, S.: A comparison of risk indicators of osteoarthritis and back-related symptom complaints, hospitalizations, and pension (abstract). International Society for the Study of the Lumbar Spine, Marseilles, France, June 1993.
10. Bergenudd, H., and Nilsson, B.: Back pain in middle age: Occupational workload and psychologic factors: An epidemiologic survey. Spine 13:58–60, 1988.
11. Berkson, M. H., Nachemson, A., and Schultz, A. B.: Mechanical properties of human lumbar spine motion segments. Part II. Responses in compression and shear; influence of gross morphology. J. Biomech. Eng. 101:53–57, 1979.
12. Biering-Sorensen, F.: Physical measurements as indicators for low-back trouble over a one-year period. Spine 9:106–119, 1984.
13. Biering-Sorensen, F., and Thomsen, C.: Medical, social and occupational history as risk indicators for low-back trouble in a general population. Spine 11:720–725, 1986.
14. Bigos, S. J.: Low back pain—potential solution. In Fitzgerald, R. H. (ed.): Orthopaedic Knowledge Update II—Home Study Syllabus Video. Chicago, American Academy of Orthopaedic Surgeons, 1987.
15. Bigos, S. J., and Battié, M. C.: Acute care to prevent back disability. Ten years of progress. Clin. Orthop. 221:121–130, 1987.
16. Bigos, S. J., Battié, M. C., Fisher, L. D., et al.: A prospective study of work perceptions and psychosocial factors affecting the report of back injury. Spine 16:1–6, 1991.
17. Bigos, S. J., Battié, M. C., Fisher, L. D., and Fordyce, W. E.: Pre-morbid risk factors for back pain disability greater than one month (abstract). International Society for the Study of the Lumbar Spine, Chicago, May 1992.
18. Bigos, S. J., Battié, M. C., Fisher, L. D., et al.: A longitudinal, prospective study of industrial back injury reporting. Clin. Orthop. 279:21–34, 1992.
19. Bohart, W. H.: Anatomic variations and anomalies of the spine relative to prognosis and length of disability. JAMA 92:698–701, 1929.
20. Bond, M. B.: Low back injuries in industry. Ind. Med. Surg. 39:28–32, 1970.
21. Cady, L. D., Bischoff, D. P., O'Connell, E. R., et al.: Strength and fitness and subsequent back injuries in firefighters. J. Occup. Med. 21:269–272, 1979.
22. Chaffin, D. B., and Park, K. S.: A longitudinal study of low back pain as associated with occupational weight lifting factors. Am. Ind. Hyg. Assoc. J. 34:513–525, 1973.
23. Cushway, B. C., and Mailer, R. J.: Routine examination of the spine for industrial employees. JAMA 92:701–705, 1929.
24. Dillane, J. B., Fry, J., and Kalton, G.: Acute back syndrome—a study from general practice. Br. Med. J. 2:82–84, 1966.
25. Fitzler, S. L., and Berger, R. A.: Attitudinal change: The Chelsea back program. Occup. Health Saf. 51:24–26, 1982.
26. Fitzler, S. L., and Berger, R. A.: Chelsea back program: One year later. Occup. Health Saf. 52:52–54, 1983.
27. Fordyce, W. E.: Use of the MMPI in the assessment of chronic pain. Clinical notes on the MMPI. In Butcher, M., Gynther, B., and Schofield, W. (eds.): Hoffman-Laroche Monograph Series, Vol. 3. Nutley, NJ, 1979, pp. 1–13.
28. Glover, J. R.: Prevention of back pain. In Jyson, M. (ed.): The Lumbar Spine and Back Pain. Orlando, FL, Grune & Stratton, 1976, pp. 47–54.
29. Green, M., Battié, M. C., and Bigos, S. J.: The role of acute back injuries in lower back pain. J. Spinal Disord. 1989 (submitted).
30. Gyntelberg, F.: One year incidence of low back pain among male residents of Copenhagen aged 40–59. Dan. Med. Bull. 21:30–36, 1974.
31. Haber, L. D.: Disabling effects of chronic disease and impairment. J. Chronic Dis. 24:469–487, 1971.

32. Hellsing, A. L., Nordgren, B., Shcéle, R., et al.: Individual predictability of back trouble in 18-year-old men. Manual Med. 2:72–76, 1986.
33. Hirsch, C., Jonsson, B., and Lewin, T.: Low back symptoms in a Swedish female population. Clin. Orthop. 63:171–176, 1969.
34. Horal, J.: The clinical appearance of low back pain disorders in the city of Gothenburg, Sweden. Acta Orthop. Scand. [Suppl.] 118:1–109, 1969.
35. Huddleson, J. H.: Accidents, Neuroses and Compensation. Baltimore, Williams & Wilkins, 1932.
36. Hult, L.: Cervical, dorsal, and lumbar spinal syndromes. Acta Orthop. Scand. 17(suppl.):1–102, 1954.
37. Hult, L.: The Munksfors investigation. Acta Orthop. Scand. 16(suppl.):1–76, 1954.
38. Johansson, J. A.: Psychosocial Factors at Work and Their Relation to Musculoskeletal Symptoms. Thesis. Goteborg, Sweden, Goteorg University, 1994.
39. Kelsey, J. L.: Epidemiology of radiculopathies. Adv. Neurol. 19:385–395, 1978.
40. Kelsey, J. L., and White, A. A., III: Epidemiology and impact of low back pain. Spine 5:133–142, 1980.
41. Keyserling, W. M., Herrin, G. D., and Chaffin, D. B.: Isometric strength testing as a measure of controlling incidents on strenuous jobs. J. Occup. Med. 22:332–336, 1980.
42. Keyserling, W. M., Herrin, G. D., and Chaffin, D. B.: Establishing an industrial strength testing program. Am. Ind. Hyg. Assoc. J. 41:730–736, 1980.
43. Leavitt, S. S., Johnson, T. L., and Beyer, R. D.: The process of recovery: Patterns in industrial back injury. Part 1. Costs and other quantitative measures of effort. Ind. Med. Surg. 40:7–14, 1971.
44. Leino, P., Aro, S., and Hasan, J.: Trunk muscle function and low back disorders: A ten-year follow-up study. J. Chronic Dis. 40:289–296, 1987.
45. Leino, P., Hasan, J., and Karppi, S.-L.: Occupational class, physical workload, and musculoskeletal morbidity in the engineering industry. Br. J. Ind. Med. 45:672–681, 1988.
46. Leino, P.: Symptoms of stress predict musculoskeletal disorders. J. Epidemiol. Commun. Health 33:293–300, 1989.
47. Leino, P.: Does leisure time physical activity prevent low back disorders? A prospective study of metal industry employees. Spine 18:863–871, 1993.
48. McDonald, E. B., Porter, R., Hibbert, C., and Hart, J.: The relationship between spinal canal diameters and back pain in coal miners. Ultrasonic measurement as a screening test? J. Occup. Med. 26:23–28, 1984.
49. Mostardi, R. A., Noe, D. A., Kovacik, M. E., and Porterfield, J. A.: Isokinetic lifting strength and occupational injury. A prospective study. Spine 17:189–193, 1992.
50. Nachemson, A. L.: The natural history of low back pain. In White, A. A., and Gordon, S. L. (eds.): Symposium on Idiopathic Low Back Pain. St. Louis, C. V. Mosby, 1982, p. 46.
51. Nachemson, A. L.: Spinal disorders. Overall impact on society and the need for orthopedic resources. Acta. Orthop. Scand. Suppl. 241:17–22, 1991.
52. National Safety Council: Accident Facts. Chicago, National Safety Council, 1976.
53. Porter, R., Wicks, M., and Ottewell, D.: Measurement of the spinal canal by diagnostic ultrasound. J. Bone Joint Surg. 60B:481–484, 1978.
54. Porter, R., Hibbert, C., and Wellman, P.: Back-ache and the lumbar spine canal. Spine 5:99–105, 1980.
55. Ready, A. E., Boreskie, S. L., Law, S. A., and Russell, R.: Fitness and lifestyle parameters fail to predict back injuries in nurses. Can. J. Appl. Phys. 18:80–90, 1993.
56. Riihimaki, H., Videman, T., and Tola, S.: Reliability of retrospective questionnaire data on the history of low back trouble (abstract). International Society for the Study of the Lumbar Spine. Kyoto, Japan, 1989.
57. Riihimaki, H., Mattson, T., Zitting, A., et al.: Radiographic changes of the lumbar spine among concrete reinforcement workers and house painters. Spine 15:114–119, 1990.
58. Robertson, L. S., and Keeve, J. P.: Worker injuries: The effects of workers compensation and O.S.H.A. inspections. J. Health Polit. Policy Law 8:581–597, 1983.
59. Roland, M., and Morris, R.: A study of the natural history of low back pain. Part III. Development of guidelines for trials of treatment in primary care. Spine 8:145–150, 1983.
60. Rossignol, M., Lortie, M., and Ledoux, E.: Comparison of spinal health indicators in predicting spinal status in a 1-year longitudinal study. Spine 18:54–60, 1993.
61. Rowe, M. L.: Low back pain in industry. A position paper. J. Occup. Med. 11:161–169, 1969.
62. Rowe, M. L.: Low back disability in industry: Updated position. J. Occup. Med. 13:476–478, 1971.
63. Sachs, B. L., Sohail, S. A., LaCroix M., et al.: Objective assessment for exercise treatment on the B-200 Isostation as part of work tolerance rehabilitation. A random prospective blind evaluation with comparison control population. Spine 19:49–52, 1994.
64. Schussler, T., Kaminer, A. J., Power, V. L., et al.: The preplacement examination. J. Occup. Med. 17:254, 1975.
65. Snook, S. H.: Low back pain in industry. In White, A. A., and Gordon, S. L. (eds.) Symposium on Idiopathic Low Back Pain. St. Louis, C. V. Mosby, 1982, p. 23.
66. Social Security Commission on Evaluation of Pain. Report to Federal Congress (submitted for publication in 1979).
67. Social Security Statistical Supplement, Suppl. Doc. no. HE 3.3/3:979. Washington, DC, U.S. Government Printing Office, 1977–1979.
68. Spengler, D. M., Bigos, S. J., Martin, N. A., et al.: Back injuries in industry: a retrospective study, 1. Overview and cost analysis. Spine 11:241–245, 1986.
69. Svensson, H. O., and Andersson, G. B. J.: Low back pain in forty to forty-seven year old men. I. Frequency of occurrence and impact on medical services. Scand. J. Rehabil. Med. 14:47–53, 1982.
70. Taylor, P. J.: Personal factors associated with sickness absence. A study of 194 men with contrasting sickness absence experience in a refinery population. Br. J. Ind. Med. 15:106–118, 1968.
71. Troup, J. D. G., Martin, J. W., and Lloyd, D. C. E. F.: Back pain in industry: A prospective study. Spine 6:61–69, 1981.
72. Troup, J. D. G., Foreman, T. K., Baxter, C. E., and

Brown, D.: The perception of back pain and the role of psychophysical tests of lifting capacity. Spine 12:645–657, 1987.
73. Valkenburg, H. A., Haanen, H. C. N.: The epidemiology of low back pain. *In* White, A. A., and Gordon, S. L. (eds.): Symposium on Idiopathic Low Back Pain. St. Louis, C. V. Mosby, 1982, p. 9.
74. Vallfors, B.: Acute, subacute and chronic low back pain. Clinical symptoms, absenteeism and working environment. Scand. J. Rehabil. Med. Suppl. 11, 1985.
75. Vicente, P. J.: The Nuprin report: A summary. Part I. Am. Pain Soc. Newsl. 1988.
76. Videman, T., Rauhala, H., and Asp, S.: Patient-handling skill, back injuries, and back pain. An intervention study in nursing. Spine 14:148–156, 1989.
77. Waddell, G.: A new clinical model for the treatment of low back pain. 1987 Volvo Award in Clinical Sciences. Spine 12:632–644, 1987.
78. Weber, H.: Lumbar disc herniation: A controlled, prospective study with ten years of observation. Spine 8:131–140, 1983.
79. Wiesel, S. W., Feffer, H. L., and Rothman, R. H.: Industrial low back—a prospective evaluation of a standardized diagnostic and treatment protocol. Spine 9:199–203, 1984.
80. Wood, D. J.: Design and evaluation of a back injury prevention program within a geriatric hospital. Spine 12:77–82, 1987.

Trunk Performance, Strength, and Endurance: Measurement Techniques and Applications

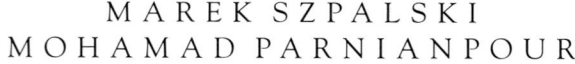

MAREK SZPALSKI
MOHAMAD PARNIANPOUR

Efforts to address the management of patients with low back pain are hampered because of an inability to identify the cause of the symptoms. Indeed, some studies have indicated that a precise cause of nociception cannot be recognized in more than 80% of patients with low back pain.[123, 124] Nachemson suggested that it is likely that the symptom of idiopathic low back pain does not represent a disease process at all, but rather reflects a self-limited physiologic phenomenon. Indeed, idiopathic low back trouble appears to be a functional condition. Furthermore, abnormal radiologic images of the lumbar spine are found in a significant proportion of subjects who have never experienced low back pain.[15] The inability to correlate low back pain with anatomic findings and the difficulties in quantifying pain have directed much effort toward measurement of spinal performance. The problem is made even more complex by the clinician's need to quantify the level of impairment of patients reporting back pain without objective findings.

There are three basic impairment evaluation systems, each having merits and shortcomings: (1) anatomic, based on physical examination findings; (2) diagnostic, based on pathologic changes; and (3) functional, based on performance or work capacity. The earlier systems were anatomic, based on amputation and ankylosis. Although this approach may be applicable to the hand, it is inappropriate for the spine. The diagnosis-based systems are flawed by lack of correspondence between the degree of impairment for a given diagnosis and the resultant disability and even more by the lack of diagnosis. The function-based systems are more desirable. However, the lack of established reliability and reproducibility of performance assessment tools have been substantial obstacles to their development.[92] Lowery and associates[91] showed how the strict application of American Medical Association guidelines, based on range of motion, can lead to unreliable impairment scores.

Clark and Haldeman[x] developed guideline factors for the evaluation of spine disability. They indicated tremendous variations in the disability rating recommended for the 42 case reports that were given to multiple independent medical examiners. It was clear that two or more examiners consulting on the same case often submitted grossly different findings. The average difference between low and high estimates of disability was 43%, and in three cases, the difference was as high as 85%. Their final guideline included 37 factors. There was a poor relationship between the number of factors and the level of disability given by the assessing physician. The measurement of trunk muscles is recommended, but no justification is given for suggesting computerized isokinetic testing as the preferred method. The current lifting capacity measurement is recommended, without an explanation of how it is to be performed.

Assessment of function across various dimensions of performance (e.g., strength, speed, endurance, and coordination) has provided the basis for a rational approach to clinical assessment, rehabilitation strategies, and determination of return-to-work potential for injured employees. To understand the complex problem of trunk performance evaluation of patients with low back pain, the terminology of muscle exertion must first be defined. However, a number of excellent reviews of trunk muscle function and performance have been undertaken.[4, 11, 127, 142] This extensive literature is not reproduced here, as the authors' motivation is to provide a critical analysis that will lead the reader toward an understanding of the future of functional assessment techniques.

MUSCLE ACTION AND QUANTIFICATION OF TRUNK PERFORMANCE

The details of the complex processes of muscle contraction in terms of the bioelectrical, biochemical, and biophysical interactions are under intensive research.[63, 185] Muscle tension is a function of muscle length and its rate of change and can be altered by the level of neural excitation. These relationships are called the length-tension and velocity-tension relationships. The central nervous system (CNS) appropriately excites the muscle, and the generated tension is transferred to the skeletal system by the tendon to cause motion, to stabilize the joint, and/or to resist the effect of external forces on the body. Hence, the functional evaluation of muscles cannot be performed without the characterization of the interfaced mechanical environment (i.e., the nature of the load).

The four fundamental types of muscle exertion or action are isometric, isokinetic, isotonic, and isoinertial. In isometric exertion, the muscle length is kept constant and there is no movement. Although mechanical work is not achieved, physiologic work (i.e., static work) is performed and energy is consumed.[141] When the internal force exerted by the muscle is greater than the external force offered by the resistance, then concentric (i.e., shortening) muscle action occurs; whereas if the muscle is already activated and the external force offered by the resistance exceeds the internal force of the muscle, then eccentric (i.e., lengthening) muscle action occurs.[82, 141] When the muscle moves, either concentrically or eccentrically, dynamic work is performed.[141] If the rate of shortening or lengthening of the muscle is constant, the exertion is called isokinetic.[58, 148] When the muscle acts on a constant inertial mass, the exertion is called isoinertial. Isotonic action occurs when the muscle tension is constant throughout the range of motion.[82, 148]

These definitions are clear for isolated muscles during physiologic investigations. However, terminology employed in the literature of strength evaluation is imprecise and confusing. The terms are intended to refer to the state of muscles, but they actually refer to the state of the mechanical interface (i.e., the dynamometer). Isotonic exertion, as defined, is not as realizable physiologically because muscle tensions change as the efficacy of its lever arm changes despite the constancy of external loads.[148] Isotonic contraction does not occur during any known form of clinical muscle testing or exercise.[152]

Special designs may vary the resistance level to account for changes in mechanical efficiency of the muscles. In addition, the rate of muscle length change may not remain constant, even when the joint angular velocity is regulated by the dynamometer during isokinetic exertions. During isoinertial action, the net external resistance is not only a function of the mass (inertia) but also of the acceleration. The acceleration, however, is a function of the input energy to the mass. Hence, to characterize the net external resistance fully, it is necessary to know the acceleration and the inertial parameters (mass and moment of inertia) of the load and body parts. Currently, scant data are available regarding the inertial properties of the dynamometers, which poses limitations on quantification of muscle activities during nonisometric and nonisokinetic exertions.

For any joint or joint complex, muscle performance can be quantified in terms of the basic dimensions of performance: strength, speed, endurance, steadiness, and coordination. Muscle strength is the capacity to produce torque or work by voluntary activation of the muscles, whereas muscle endurance is the ability to maintain a predetermined level of motor output (e.g., torque, velocity, range of motion, work, and energy) over time. Smidt and colleagues[156] defined muscle strength as the ability of a muscle or muscle group to generate a moment about a body axis, whereas muscle endurance is the ability to generate moments repetitively. Fatigue is considered a process under which the capability of muscles diminishes. However, neuromuscular adjustments take place to meet the task demands (i.e., increase in neural excitation) until there is final performance breakdown-endurance time; this time is specified as the endurance time. Coordination, in this context, is the temporal and spatial organization of movement and the recruitment patterns of the muscle synergies.

Despite the proliferation of various technologies for measurement, basic questions remain unanswered. What has to be measured and how can it best be measured? Strength, one of the most fundamental dimensions of human performance, has been the focus of many investigations. Despite the general consensus about the abstract definition of strength, there is no direct method for measuring muscle tension in vivo. Strength has often been measured at the interface of a joint (or joints) with the mechanical environment. A dynamometer, an external apparatus onto which the body exerts force, is used to measure strength indirectly.

From a physiologic point of view, the measured force, or torque, applied at the interface is a function of

1. The individual's motivation (magnitude of the neural drive for excitation and activation processes)
2. Environmental conditions (muscle length, rate of change of muscle length, nature of the external load, metabolic conditions, pH level, temperature, and so forth)
3. Prior history of activation (fatigue)
4. Instruction and descriptions of the tasks given to the subject
5. The control strategies and motor programs employed to satisfy the demands of the task
6. The biophysical state of the muscles and fitness (fiber composition, physiologic cross-sectional area of the muscle, and cardiovascular capability)

It cannot be overemphasized that these processes are complex and interrelated.[82] Hirsch and associates[57] also listed the following factors that may affect patients' performance: misunderstanding of the degree of effort needed in testing maximum force, test anxiety, depression, nociception, fear of pain and reinjury, and unconscious and conscious symptom magnification. Various modes of strength testing have evolved on the basis of different levels of technologic sophistication. The practical implication of contextual dependencies on the provided mechanical environment of the strength measures is often neglected. To classify the various methods of strength measurement, it is necessary to identify the dependent, independent, controlled, and confounding variables. The independent variables are purposefully manipulated, whereas the dependent variables are quantified to show the effects of such manipulation. Controlled variables are carefully maintained at preestablished conditions to minimize the interference on the relationship of dependent and independent variables. Confounding variables are uncontrolled variables that may interfere with the aforementioned relationship. Kroemer and colleagues[82] provided concrete examples of different types of strength testing and classified variables for prevailing modes of strength testing as well as for some techniques that are not yet used.

The meaning of the objectivity of the performance measurements has also been confused. Strength and endurance performances of the muscles remain psychophysical measures, regardless of the degree of sophistication of the dynamometers used, because the muscles are excited by the CNS under the subject's volition. Hence, all references to maximum capacity should be qualified by maximum voluntary performance. When studying the structural and material properties of specimens, one can quantify their ultimate strength and stress. If such engineering concepts are applied to strength assessment, however, they are not without shortcomings. The best one may hope for is the maximum voluntary performance (assuming that the subject made maximum effort), which has had low correlation with the physical anthropometric findings and the cross-sectional areas of the muscles.[4] In addition, the maximum performance may not be the same as the maximum capability. Hence, assessment results in quantification of performance measures, but not a measure of ultimate strength. The ultimate strength of the structure results in the failure of the structure. It is also teleologically reasonable that subjects would not even approach the ultimate strength of the muscles because microtrauma occurs in the muscle and the surrounding tissues well before the yield strength.

Biomechanical strength models of the trunk are usually based on static maximum strength measurement lasting for long durations.[25, 154] This may be misleading because, in actual work situations, individuals rarely exert lengthy or maximum static effort. In most clinical situations, submaximum protocols are recommended, especially in patients with pain or cardiovascular problems. Also, submaximum testings are less prone to fatigue and injury.[187]

Activities of daily living also involve a great deal of submaximum effort at a self-selected pace. Hence, testing at the preferred rate may be complementary to the maximum effort protocol.[94] The preferred motion was solicited by instructing the subject to perform repetitive movement at a pace and through the range of motion that is subjectively felt to be most comfortable. McIntyre and coworkers[93] showed that patients with low back pain and normal subjects have different characteristics of resisted preferred flexion-extension motion. The maximum effort velocities of 16 normal subjects were predicted on the basis of their preferred motion performance, with R^2 values ranging from .57 to .80.[94]

STATIC AND DYNAMIC STRENGTH MEASUREMENTS OF TRUNK MUSCLES

Weakness of the trunk extensor and abdominal muscles in patients with low back pain was demonstrated with a cable tensiometer.[3, 122] The disadvantage of the cable tensiometer is that it neglects to measure the lever arm distance from the center of trunk motion. Also, cable tensiometers are best used to determine peak isometric torques rather than the stable average torque exerted over a 3-second period, as recommended by some investigators.[21, 28]

Dynamometers used for testing dynamic muscle performances contain either hydraulic or servomotor systems to provide constant velocity (e.g., isokinetic devices) or constant resistance (e.g., isoinertial devices). The isokinetic devices can be further categorized into passive and active types. Robotics-based dynamometers can actively apply force on the body and hence allow eccentric muscle performance assessments, whereas only concentric exertions can be measured by the passive devices. Cybex (Cybex Inc., Lumex, NY) isokinetic dynamometers, which were originally used for the extremities, were adapted by several researchers for measurement of isometric and isokinetic trunk strength.[68, 84, 129, 156] Mayer and associates[109, 110] used the dedicated back isokinetic Cybex dynamometers to measure trunk extension-flexion and torso rotation. Other uniaxial isokinetic dynamometers are Biodex (Biodex Corp., Shirley, NY), Lido (Loredan Biomedical Inc., Davis, CA), and Kin/Com (Chattex Corp., Chattanooga, TN). The only commercial triaxial dynamometer is the Isostation B200 (Isotechnologies Inc., Hillsborough, NC), which simultaneously measures performance in the three cardinal planes. The hydraulic pumps provide independent resistances in each plane, while mechanical locks allow measurement of the isometric exertion at various trunk postures in the sagittal plane. The degree of pelvic stabilization varies with different devices. MedX (Ocala, FL), by the use of specifically designed femur and thigh restraints, stabilizes the pelvis.[45] Gracovetsky and associates[44] emphasized the role of pelvic tilt in reducing compressive stress in the spine, and Gracovetsky[43] strongly objected to testing spinal function with stabilization of the spine. In addition, some technologies allow the testing to be performed in sitting, standing, and semistanding postures, whereas others are limited to the sitting posture.[24]

Studies on healthy male volunteers have shown that trunk motions occur in more than one plane. Buchalter and associates[17] used a three-dimensional, low-frequency magnetic field tracking device to measure the degree of accessory motions present in unrestrained trunk extension. They showed that trunk motion was coupled and that the coupling patterns in the accessory planes were not organized. Both in vivo and in vitro studies have shown the motion of the spine to be highly coupled. Lateral bending accompanies the primary motion of axial rotation. Numerous attempts have been made to measure the segmental range of motion three dimensionally in the lumbar spine, with the purpose of quantifying abnormal coupling and diagnosing instabilities.[33] Weitz[182] found that abnormal axial rotation of a lumbar vertebra, while the patient was bending laterally, had clinical relevance. Most of the existing dynamometers are uniaxial and can measure only in a single plane of exertion at a given time.

Triaxial measurements are important[132] because trunk exertions are highly coupled owing to overlapping anatomic arrangements of the trunk muscles.[34,95] Each unit tension in trunk muscles causes moments in at least two cardinal planes, because they pass eccentrically to the center of rotation of the motion segments. Parnianpour and colleagues[132] using a triaxial dynamometer, showed that trunk torques are coupled in all planes. The torque generation coupling of trunk muscles was more prominent during intended exertions in the coronal and transverse planes.

The concept of kinematic constraints inherent in the design of the dynamometers, and their effects on the performance measurements, has not been adequately explored.[137] Using a triaxial dynamometer, one can test the effect of locking or unlocking the accessory axes during a planar trunk movement. In other words, the effect of using a uniaxial dynamometer for testing a triaxial joint can be explored. Internal loading of the spine depends not only on the external load but also on the recruitment of trunk muscles. Better quantification of spine loading during performance evaluations is vital to an understanding of biomechanical causation and the prevention of spinal disorders. The effect of kinematic constraints (locking the accessory axes) during maximum isometric and isoinertial axial rotation on motor output and the recruitment patterns of the trunk muscles were investigated in 15 normal male subjects using the Isostation B200. During isometric axial trunk maximum voluntary contraction (MVC), the kinematic constraints significantly affected only the activities of abdominal muscles. The net mechanical output in the primary plane of exertion (axial torque) was not affected by whether the accessory axes were locked. The accessory torque generated in the coronal and sagittal planes during isometric exertions was considerable when these axes were locked. The torques generated in the sagittal and coronal planes were 57% and 67% of the maximum torque generated in the transverse planes, respectively (Fig. 1). During dynamic repetitive trunk movements, the motor output (axial torque and velocity) in the primary plane was not affected by the kinematic constraints. However, results indicated that abdominal muscles were significantly affected. The clinical criteria for selection of an appropriate tool for spinal evaluation are far from clear. This study attempted to clarify the effects of kinematic constraints on the recruitment and motor output of trunk muscles. The clinical question can be posed as to whether the accessory axes should be locked or unlocked during functional evaluation of the trunk during axial rotation. The selection could be argued to be only a matter of choice, because kinematic constraint had no significant effect on the primary motor output. However, the large generated coupled torque and significantly different muscle activities point to different loading conditions for the spine. Another variable influencing performances during static or dynamic testing is the trunk position during testing.

Graves and associates[45] used the MedX Lumbar Extension Machine, a computer-monitored dynamometer designed for testing trunk isometric strength in sitting. They

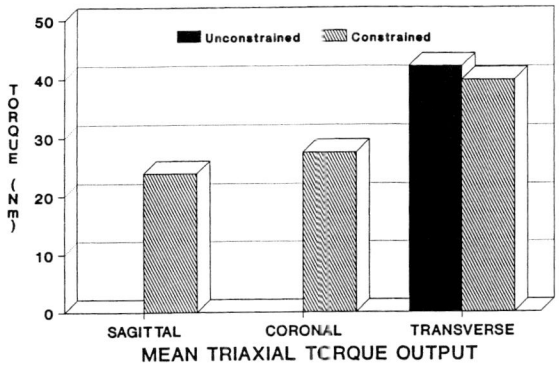

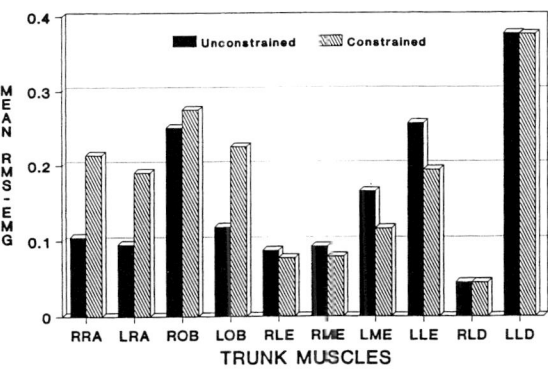

Figure 1. The population (N = 15) mean of RMS-EMG of 10 selected trunk muscles and triaxial torque generated during maximum isometric axial exertion with the accessory axes locked (constrained) or unlocked (unconstrained). The Isostation B200 was used to measure the torques about L5–S1. (LLD, RLD, left and right latissimus dorsi; LLE, RLE, left and right lateral erector spinae; LME, RME, left and right medial erector spinae; LRA, RRA, left and right rectus abdominis; LOB, ROB, left and right oblique; RMS, root mean square. (Adapted from Parnianpour, M., and Hoffer, H.: The effect of kinematic constraints, levels of resistance and directions of exertion during isometric and isoinertial axial trunk rotation on the motor output and muscle activity. Proceedings of 1991 Engineering Systems Design and Analysis Conference, 1992.)

reported that isometric strength increased as the trunk was flexed from 0° to 72°, with an increment of 12°, and that isometric training of the trunk using the device improved isometric trunk strength significantly.

Tan and coworkers[174] tested 31 healthy male subjects for the effects of trunk flexion positions (0, 15, and 35 degrees) in standing on triaxial torques and performed electromyography (EMG) of 10 trunk muscles during isometric trunk extension at 30%, 50%, 70%, and 100% of maximum voluntary exertion (MVE). Trunk muscle strength was significantly increased at a more flexed position.[136] But the accessory torques in the transverse and coronal planes were not affected by trunk postures. The recorded lateral bending and rotation accessory torques were less than 5% and 16% of the primary extension torque, respectively. The rectus abdominis muscles were quiet during all tests. The EMG of the erector spinae muscle varied linearly with higher values of MVE, whereas the latissimus dorsi had a nonlinear behavior. The oblique muscles were coactivated only during 100% of MVE. The neuromuscular efficiency ratio (NMER) was operationally defined as the ratio of the extension torque to the RMS-EMG of the extensor muscles. It was hoped that NMER could be used in clinical settings where generation of the maximum exertion is not indicated. However, the NMER proved to have limited clinical utility because it was significantly affected by the subject's exertion level and posture. The NMER of the extensor muscles increased at a more flexed position.

Marras and Mirka[102] studied the effect of trunk postural asymmetry, flexion angle, and trunk velocity (eccentric, isometric, and concentric) on maximum trunk torque production. It was shown that trunk torque decreased by about 8.5% of the maximum value for every 15 degrees of asymmetric trunk angle. At higher trunk flexion angles, extensor strength increased. Complex significant interaction effects of velocity, asymmetry, and sagittal posture were detected. The studies of range of velocity were more limited (±30 degrees/second) than those customarily used in spinal evaluation.

LIFTING STRENGTH TESTING

In the United States, the National Institute for Occupational Safety and Health[125] recommended static (i.e., isometric) strength measurement as its standard for lifting tasks. This was based on evidence that associated low back pain with inadequate isometric strength.[29, 71, 72] It is assumed that the amount of weight lifted on a job might cause some back injuries.[27] The risk of an individual's sustaining a back injury at work increases threefold when the lifting requirements of a task approach or exceed the individual's strength capacity.[29] However, lifting strength is certainly not a true measure of trunk function, but instead a global measure taking into account arm, shoulder, and leg strength as well as the individual's lifting technique and overall fitness. Indeed, it is a measure of whole-body performance. Chaffin and coworkers[29] and Keyserling[71] showed that strength tests were more valid if they simulated the demands of the job.

Static strength measurements were also reported to underestimate significantly loads on the spine occurring during dynamic lifting.[19, 39, 186] Comparing static and dynamic biomechanical models of the trunk, Leskinen[88] found that, depending on the lifting technique, the predicted spinal loads under static conditions were 33% to 60% less than those under dynamic conditions. The recruitment patterns of trunk muscles, thus internal loading of spine, is significantly different under isometric and dynamic conditions.[101]

Other studies also showed poor correlations between static lifting performances and maximum acceptable weights of lift, as determined by psychophysical tests.[69, 117, 118] In psychophysical lifting tests, one of the task variables (e.g., the weight of the object to be lifted) is under the individual's control. All other variables (e.g., the frequency of lift, the distance and height at which the person must lift, and the size of the object to be lifted) are controlled by the tester. The individual adjusts the amount of weight to be lifted depending on his or her judgment of his or her own strength and endurance level.[162]

The widely conflicting results found in the literature regarding the relationship of an individual's strength to the risk of developing low back pain may be due to inappropriate modes of strength measurements (i.e., lack of job specificity).[9, 134] Furthermore, repetitiveness of lifting effort plays a role, and Mital and coworkers[117, 118] showed that, for jobs requiring lifting more frequently than once per minute, strength does not predict repetitive lifting ability. Despite these controversies, isometric strength testing of the trunk is still widely used, especially in large-scale industrial and epidemiologic studies, because it has been standardized and studied prospectively in industry.[9, 10] Compared with trunk dynamic strength testing protocols, the trunk isometric strength testing protocols are simpler and less expensive.

DYNAMIC TRUNK MOVEMENT AND TRUNK MUSCLE ENDURANCE

A series of these were devoted to quantification of trunk recruitment and motor output under various mechanical conditions and types of movement.[41, 149, 153, 173] Consideration of these results is beyond the scope of this discussion. The CNS recruits muscles with full exploitation of the gravitational field and uses external resistances for both deceleration and stabilization of the spine.[41, 149] Better understanding of normal movement planning and execution may contribute to clinical care and management of patients with low back pain. The phasic patterns of the extensor and flexor muscles are markedly different from the EMG activities during isokinetic exertions.[41] Figure 2 indicates that, during isokinetic trunk extension, the trunk erector spinae and external oblique muscles are activated reciprocally. This is because the subject is relieved of planning for the acceleration and deceleration of the motion. However, during isoresistive exertions, the extensors are activated during deceleration of the flexion phase of movements and continue their activity in the acceleration phase of extension (Fig. 3). Hence, considerable overlap exists when the muscles are coactivated during isoresistive movement. The effect of resistance on the recruitment of trunk muscles during different phases of movement was highly significant. The temporal and spatial organization of the recruitment and movement patterns points to a much richer and more complex medium for the study of low back pain.[41]

Ross[149] investigated the effects of varying resistance levels on patterns of muscle activity and trunk motion during the performance of dynamic trunk extension using Isostation B200. The point-to-point (unidirectional) movement of the trunk from forward flexion to neutral position in standing

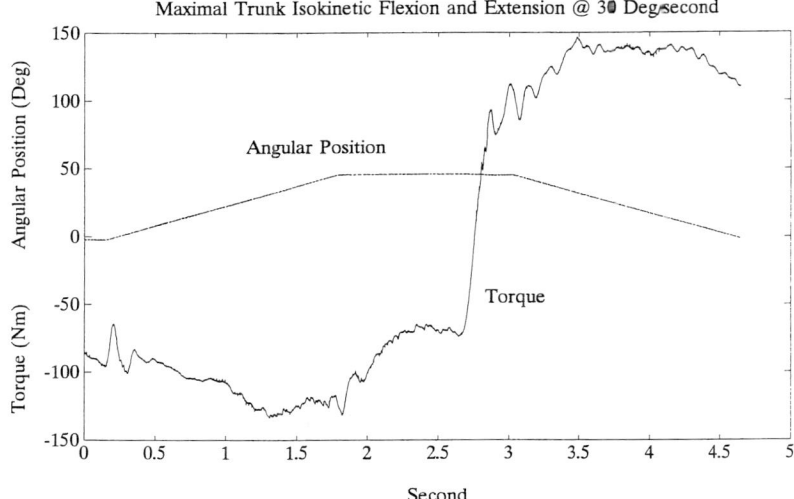

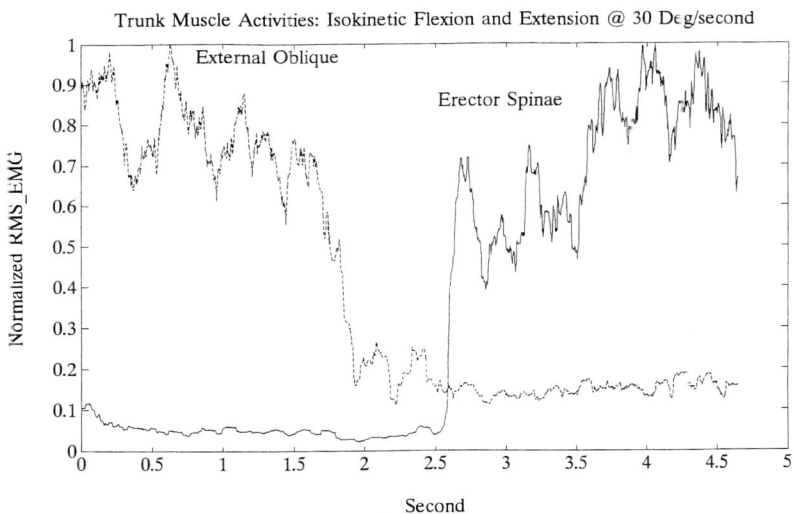

Figure 2. The angular position and maximum sagittal torque about L5–S1 and RMS-EMG activity of erector spinae and external oblique muscles during isokinetic trunk flexion and extension at 30 degrees/second for a normal male subject. The KinCom dynamometer was modified to allow measurement of the isokinetic performances.

was studied. Twenty-five normal female subjects were tested at four resistance levels: nominal resistance and 30%, 50%, and 70% of maximum isometric extension exertion. Peak velocity, acceleration, and deceleration decreased with increased resistance level. The maximum velocity, acceleration, and deceleration were attained at 30% of MVC; no further increases were seen at nominal resistance. This represents the existence of a kinematic soft constraint that limits maximum acceleration despite the availability of the strength and power to perform it. The effect of these constraints on performance warrants further evaluation.

Such a phenomenon would not have been observable under isometric or isokinetic modes of testing. Coactivation of abdominal muscles was present at all resistance levels, although it was greater for the nominal resistance condition than for the other conditions. At nominal resistance, the stabilization gained by coactivation was needed most while the CNS exploited the viscous nature of the higher resistances provided by the dynamometer. The timing of EMG activity of the extensor and abdominal muscles was significantly affected by resistance. With increased resistance level, the EMG activity of the extensor muscles increased in

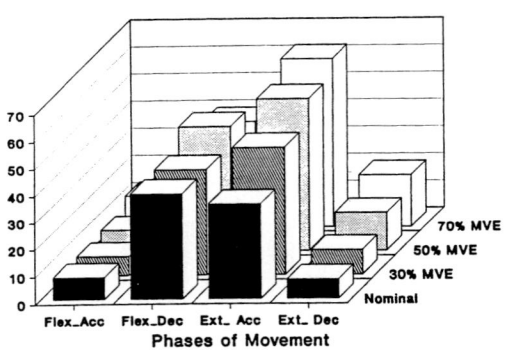

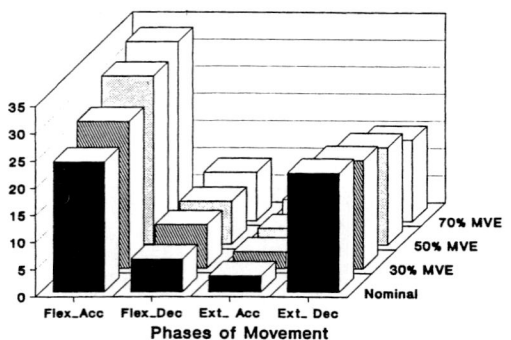

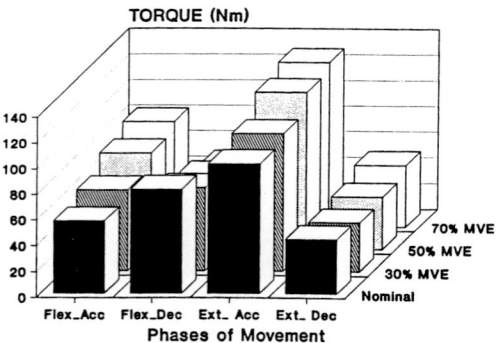

Figure 3. The population (N = 24) mean of the net muscular moment about L5–S1 and RMS-EMG of erector spinae and abdominal oblique muscles during the repetitive sagittal flexion and extension against four resistances during four phases of movement: flexion acceleration and deceleration (Flex-Acc and Flex-Dec) and extension acceleration and deceleration (Ext-Acc and Ext-Dec). Isostation B200 was used to measure the triaxial movement and provided the resistance. (Adapted from Gabriel, R. J.: The Effect of Direction and Resistance Level on Muscle Coordination, Movement Patterns, and Motor Output During Repetitive Isoinertial Trunk Flexion and Extension of Healthy Males. Unpublished Doctoral Thesis. New York, New York University, 1992.)

amplitude, and the peak of the activity occurred later in the movement cycle. Thus, not only the magnitude, but also the time course, of spinal loading varied as resistance was increased. While increased resistance delayed the peak of EMG activity in the extensor muscles, there was a corresponding decrease in the time to peak activity of the abdominal muscles, such that the peak activity of the extensor and abdominal muscles most closely coincided at 50% of MVC, increasing the impulsive loading of the spine.

These results are in contrast to the those of Tan and associates[174] who found no coactivation of the abdominal oblique or rectus abdominis muscles with isometric extension exertions at 30%, 50%, and 70% of MVC. They found coactivation of the abdominal oblique, but not of the rectus abdominis, with 100% of MVC isometric extension. These different patterns of abdominal muscle activity can likely be attributed to the different neuromuscular requirements for controlling dynamic versus isometric activities; again, these findings emphasize the need for study of nonregulated (nonisometric, nonisokinetic) movement to explore the performance of the neuromuscular system of the trunk.

Soft tissues subjected to repetitive loading demonstrate creep and load relaxation because of their viscoelastic properties. The loss of precision, speed, and control of the neuromuscular system reduces their ability to protect the weakened passive structure, which may explain many industrial, clinical, and recreational injury mechanisms. The high percentage of type I fibers of the back muscles, in addition to the better vascularization of these muscle groups, contributes to their superior endurance.[188] Physiologic studies indicate that, at higher utilization ratio (relative load) of muscles, fatigue is detected earlier.[132] These results further indicate the necessity of relating clinical protocol to the job and show how short-duration maximum isometric tests cannot provide the complex functional interaction of strength, endurance, control, and coordination.

Jorgensen and associates[67] also indicated that the isometric endurance of the back muscles is much higher than that of the extremity muscles, because of high numbers of slow-twitch fibers with a considerable number of capillaries in contact with each fiber. The glycogen, as well as the anaerobic and aerobic metabolic key enzymes, are present in paravertebral muscles. The relative slow-twitch cross-sectional area of the longissimus muscle is 71%, compared with 63% in the multifidus muscle and 58% in the iliocostalis muscle. Biomechanically, this may explain the higher activity of longissimus muscle in erect posture, in which the iliocostalis and multifidus muscles are silent. The higher diversity of muscle fibers in the iliocostalis muscle reflects its functional diversity, including rapid correction of spinal movement.

Isometric endurance tests have been used to compute the median frequency of the myoelectrical activities of trunk muscles in both normal subjects and patients with low back pain.[151] The expected decline of the median frequency with fatigue is defined by the intercept (initial median frequency) and the slope of the fall. Klein and associates[76] compared spinal mobility and isometric trunk extensor strength with EMG spectral analysis for discrimination analysis of low back pain. They found that range of motion and isometric strength were less specific and sensitive than spectral variables. Biederman and colleagues[13] discriminated normal subjects from patients with chronic low back pain, classified as avoiders and confronters, by their responses to the Pain Behavior Checklist, using the spectral variables of the selected trunk muscles. The canonic discriminant functions accounted for the 68% variance between the groups and correctly classified normal subjects, confronters, and avoiders at 59.1%, 66.7%, and 88.9%, respectively. These data indicate promising results, but these models must be cross-validated with independent data sets to verify their discriminate functions.

The long-term test-retest reliability of the spectral variables during a constant force contraction was assessed for the multifidus and iliocostalis muscles of sedentary healthy women.[175] It was concluded that initial median frequency of both muscles had high reliability, whereas the left-right difference measures were not stable. The fatigue variables were found to have maximum variations of about 50% between pretests and posttests. It was argued that this variation is within the range of the potentially underlying metabolic processes; however, more research is needed before the clinical utility of this measure is determined.

CORRELATIONS AMONG DIFFERENT ISOMETRIC AND DYNAMIC LIFTING TESTS

General manual materials handling tasks require a coordinated multilink activity that can be simulated using classical psychophysical techniques or the robotics-based lift task simulators. It has been suggested that dynamic lift simulation is close to the actual requirements of lifting tasks encountered in industry.[114, 116, 179] Various lifting tests, including static, dynamic, maximal, and submaximal tests are currently available. Unfortunately, the intercorrelations among these tests are poorly quantified.[11, 40, 130, 138]

Parnianpour and coworkers[130] investigated the intercorrelation among strength measures using various isometric and isokinetic and isoinertial tests for isolated trunk and multilink-coordinated exertions in 43 healthy persons (21 men and 22 women). The testing equipment used was the Lido Active Back System and the Lido Lift Rehabilitation System. The performance variables for isokinetic tests were the peak and the average torque, work, and joint angle at peak torque for flexion, and extension movements at 30, 90, and 120 degrees/second. The variables of the endurance test at 120 degrees/second were total work performed during 1 minute of flexion and extension. The peak power, force, and average work during raising and lowering were selected for isokinetic lift during raising and lowering. The selected variables for isoinertial lift were the maximum load, peak force, velocity, and acceleration during raising and lowering. The magnitude of correlations varied (ranging from nonsignificant correlations to $r = .99$; $p < .0001$), and no single test emerged as the ideal generic test of choice. The results confirmed the theoretic prediction that strength depends on the measurement technique. Because muscle action requires external resistance, the effect of muscle action depends on the nature of the resistance. The implicit assumption is that a generic strength test exists that can be used for preplacement (preemployment) testing of workers and predictions of the risk of injury or future occurrence of low back pain. The results of this study, and others in the literature, point to low correlation among various strength measures.

Mayer and associates[116] found poor correlation among isokinetic lift (at 46 cm/s and 76 cm/s) and isoinertial lifting capacity. The linear correlations ranged from −.09 (not significant) to .62 ($p < .05$). Battié[9] found correlation coefficients to range from .5 to .85 when isometric strength in arm, leg, and torso lift positions was compared. The correlations were significantly higher among women (from .74 to .85) than among men (from .5 to .68). Gagnon and Smyth[42] proposed an approach based on the assessment of total mechanical energy expenditure and its duration throughout body joints as an alternative to biomechanical modeling of the internal loads. They studied lifting and lowering performed at five heights (from 15 to 185 cm) with five loads (from 3.3 to 22 kg). The movement strategies were modified with heavier loads. The heights affected the redistribution of load among different joints. In general, lower extremity participation was minimal.

One outstanding issue during dynamic testing is the unresolved problem of how the wealth of information can be presented in a succinct and informative fashion. One approach has been to compare the statistical features of data with the existing normal data bases. This is crucial because there is not the option of comparing the results with those for a contralateral asymptomatic joint, as with lower or upper extremity joints. Given the large differences between individuals, comparison should be made to job-specific data bases. However, because of the scarcity of such data, comparison of functional capacity with job demand is suggested.

INVERSE AND DIRECT DYNAMICS

A major task of biomechanics has been to estimate the internal loading of musculoskeletal structure and to establish the physiologic loading during various daily activities. The kinematics studies deal with the movement of joints, with no emphasis on the forces involved. However, kinetics studies the effect of forces that generate such movements. Using sophisticated experimental and theoretic stress-strain analyses, hazardous or failure levels of loads have been determined.

The experimental data on the joint trajectories are differentiated to obtain the angular velocity and acceleration. Appropriate inertial properties of the limb segments are used to compute the net external moments about each joint. This mapping from joint kinematics to net moments is called inverse dynamics. Direct dynamics refers to studies that simulate the motion on the basis of the known actuator torques at each joint. The key issue in these investigations is understanding the control strategies underlying the trajectory planning and performance of purposeful motion. A highly multidisciplinary field has emerged to address these unsolved questions. (Berme and Cappozzo[12] present a comprehensive treatment of these issues.)

It is well known that differentiation magnifies the errors inherent in joint angular measurements. Novel techniques have used both vision (motion analysis) systems with accelerometers and digital signal processing to obtain a more accurate estimate of the moments. A typical result from a dynamic analysis of a lifting task during an isokinetic and isoinertial lift using the Lido Lift task simulator is shown in Figures 4 and 5. The maximum simulated isoinertial load for this normal male subject (24 years old, height of 183 cm, weight of 77 kg) was 71 kg. The net muscular power is shown to vary considerably between the two modes of lifting. The contribution of the knee muscles is greatest at the beginning of the isokinetic lift, while the knee contribution for the isoinertial lift peaks much later in the lift cycle. The net torque about L5–S1 and the compressive reaction force are sustained for much longer periods during the isokinetic mode than during the isoinertial mode. Thus, the accumulated load is more severe for the isokinetic lift, although it has slightly lower peak values. These two modes of lifting represent diverse coordination strategies.

Sparto and associates[163] performed a thorough reliability and validity study for Lido Lift in isometric, isokinetic, and isoinertial modes of testing. They also addressed the question of functional equivalence by posing the following questions:

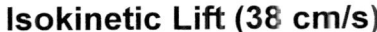
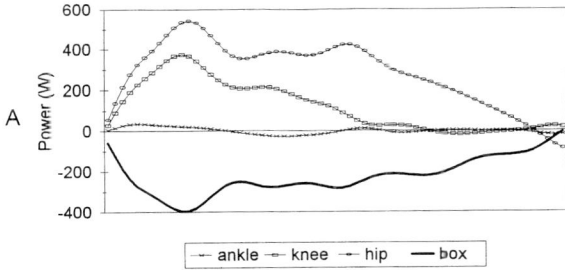
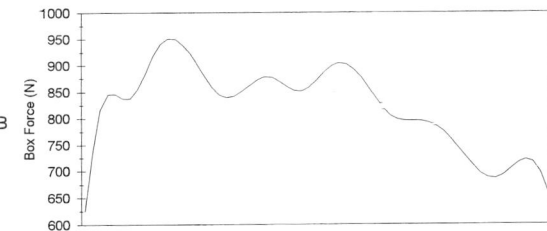
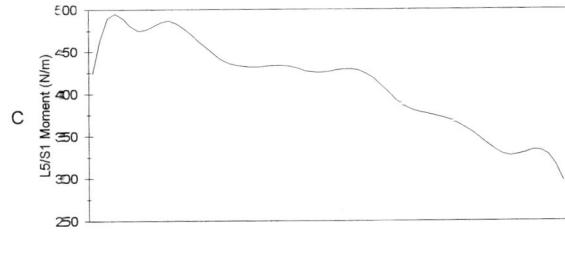
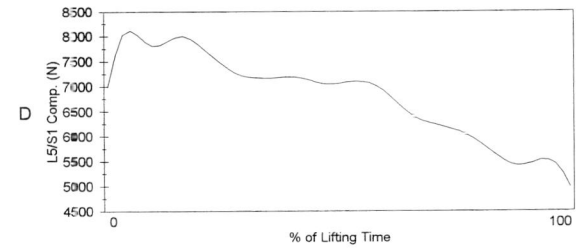

Figure 4. The joint muscular powers (*A*), transmitted force to the box (*B*), net muscular moment at L5–S1 (*C*), and the compressive reaction force at L5–S1 (*D*) during an isokinetic lift (38 cm/s) for a normal male subject. A Lido Lift simulator was used in addition to a six-link biomechanical model to solve the inverse dynamic problem.

1. Which space should be explored for determining normalcy or equivalence?
2. Should one consider the performance of the multilink system in the joint space or end effector (cartesian work space)?

These issues have profound effects on both the development of new technologies and the evaluation of trunk or lifting performance. Careful consideration of these issues and evidence provided in this review do not support the tempting oversimplification of lumping different technologies and modes of testing into a single iso-machine category.[126, 127]

The determination of the external moments about different joints during manual materials handling tasks is based on well-established laws of physics. However, the determination of human performance and the assessment of functional capacity are based on other disciplines (e.g., psychophysics) that are not as exact or well developed. One can describe the job demand, in terms of the required moments about each joint, easily by analyzing the workers performing the tasks. However, one cannot predict the workers' ability to perform arbitrary tasks because of incomplete knowledge of the functional capacities of these workers at

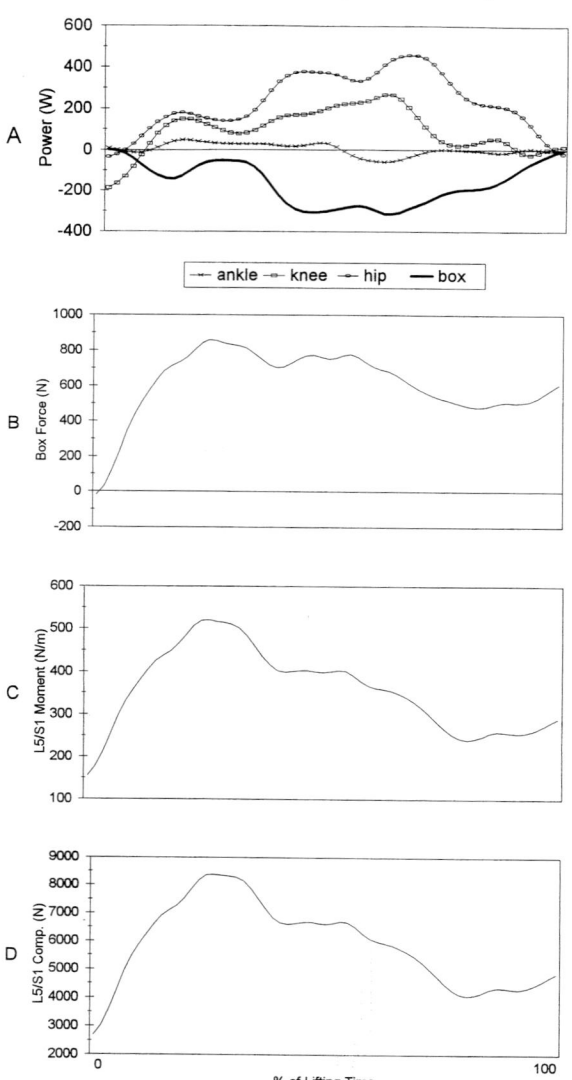

Figure 5. The joint muscular powers (*A*), transmitted force to the box (*B*), net muscular moment at L5–S1 (*C*), and the compressive reaction force at L5–S1 (*D*) during an isoinertial lift (simulated load of 71 kg) for a normal male subject. A Lido Lift simulator was used in addition to a six-link biomechanical model to solve the inverse dynamic problem.

the joint levels. In other words, a task is easily decomposed to its demands at the joint level, but one cannot compose (construct) an arbitrary task on the basis of knowledge of functional capacity. The mapping from high-level task demands on the joint level to functional capacity for a given performance trial is unique. However, the mapping from joint level functional capacity to the high-level task demand is one to many (not unique). The challenge of ergonomics and occupational biomechanics is to establish that missing link. Much of the integration of ergonomics and functional analysis depends on the removal of this obstacle.

The enormous degree of freedom existing in the neuromusculoskeletal system provides the control centers with both the kinematic and actuator redundancies. The redundancies provide optimization possibility. Because a person can lift an object from point A to point B with infinite postural possibilities, certain physical variables may be optimized for the learned movements. The possible candidates for objective function to be optimized are movement time, energy, smoothness, and muscular activities. This approach, although still in its early stage, may be important for spine functional assessment. The given performance can be compared with the optimum performance that is predicted by the model. The flexion and extension of trunk have been modeled, and the predicted position and angular velocity of the trunk have been calculated, for different cost functions. At present, the model is being validated with normal subjects. This approach provides specific goals and gives biofeedback with respect to each individual's performance.[133]

COMPARISON OF TASK DEMANDS AND FUNCTIONAL CAPACITY

Regression analysis was used to model the dynamic torque, velocity, and power output in healthy subjects as a function of resistance level during flexion and extension using the Isostation B200.[134] Results indicated that the measured torque was not a good discriminator of the 10th, 50th, and 90th percentile population. However, velocity and power were shown to discriminate the three populations effectively. On the basis of this data, it was suggested that, during clinical testing, sagittal plane resistance should not be set at higher than 60 foot-pounds to minimize internal loading of the spine while taxing trunk functional capacity. The data in this study were presented in terms of absolute value of resistance rather than normalized with respect to maximum isometric strength, as suggested previously.

This presentation of data may be useful for the physician or the ergonomist in an evaluation of the functional capacity requirements of workplace manual materials handling tasks. For example, a manual materials handling task that requires 60 foot-pounds of trunk extensor strength can be performed by 90% of the population in that data base if the required average velocity of trunk does not exceed 40 degrees/second, whereas only 50% can perform the task if the velocity requirement exceeds 70 degrees/second. A few versions of lumbar motion monitors that can record triaxial motion in the workplace have been used to measure trunk movement requirements.[49, 103, 149]

The more mature debate regarding the strength testing should be about which set of existing modes of testing is needed to assess strength capability with respect to the demands of the workplace. To provide optimum clinical assessment, a set of these tests, as dictated by ergonomic analysis of job demands, may be necessary. However, part of the problem is that no generic job exists. The more diverse the demands of a job are, the more complex the functional assessment is. Unless ergonomists develop tools and techniques that can quantify various dimensions of human performance, the existing confusion could prevail, and clinicians will have to subject themselves to unsystematic trial and error with technologies that have evolved on an ad hoc basis.

RESOURCE ECONOMICS PARADIGM: THE ELEMENTAL RESOURCE MODEL

The resource economics paradigm is reflective of the principal goal of ergonomics: fitting the demands of the task to the functional capability of the worker.[79] The elemental resource model is based on the application of general performance theory, (i.e., a unified theory for measurement, analysis, and modeling of human performance across all different aspects of performance, across all human subsystems, and at any hierarchic level).[79] This approach uses the same bases to describe both the fundamental dimensions of functional capacity and the task demand (available and utilized resources) of each functional unit involved in performance of high-level tasks.

The elegance of the elemental resource model is due to its hierarchic organization, allowing causal models to be generated on the basis of an assessment of the task demands and function capabilities across the same dimensions of performance. The major contributions of Fleishman and Quaintance[36] and others of describing the fundamental abilities from factor analysis and regression-based models have been ineffective owing to population and task (context) dependencies of their results and lack of agreement in definitions of identified abilities among various fields. The covariance of the performance of high-level tasks with the utilization of resources at the level of functional unit must be used toward a more stochastic model of human performance.

At present, Kondraske and Vasta[80] are working on a different approach to address these observed limitations by introducing the nonlinear causal resource analysis. The nonlinear causal resource analysis generates a resource demand profile for a population sample that is subsequently used to predict the high-level task performance, given a new set of performance resource measures for a specific case.

CLINICAL APPLICATIONS OF TRUNK MUSCLE STRENGTH TESTING

Identification of Subjects with Low Back Pain and Predictive Value

The lack of trunk muscle strength has often been described as a contributor to low back pain. Several investigators have published data showing that symptom-free subjects have stronger trunk muscles than do subjects reporting low back pain.* It seems that not only are the muscles weaker but there are also modifications in the extensor/flexor strength ratio. In healthy subjects, trunk extension strength is greater than flexion strength.† In subjects with low back pain, there is a significant loss of both flexor and extensor strength, but the main loss seems to be in extensor muscles.[96, 108-110, 146] These results are reported in isometric as well as isokinetic studies.

Other investigators using isoinertial techniques reported that subjects with low back pain tend to have slower movements than do normal subjects[22, 57, 100, 169] and that velocity in extension shows the main reduction.[22, 169] Those modifications in muscle strength balance results are used to prescribe muscle-strengthening therapies.

Only one study tries to correlate strength measurement with muscle condition. Mayer and colleagues,[115] using an isokinetic device, tested patients 3 months after spinal surgery. They found that strength values were lower than those in a control sample and that there was a greater reduction in extensor than in flexor strength. Single-cut computed tomographic scans showed erector spinae and psoas muscle atrophy through a decrease in muscle density. There was a significant correlation between increased trunk strength performance and higher muscle density on computed tomographic scans.

A few other reports are somewhat contradictory. Addison and Schultz[2] reported that inpatients with severe back disorders had less back strength than did matched symptom-free persons, but outpatients with low back disorders were as strong as normal subjects. Nicolaisen and Jorgensen,[128] studying a group of postal workers, did not demonstrate differences in isometric strength between subjects who experienced back trouble that made work impossible, those who experienced back pain to a lesser degree, and those without any history of back trouble. Balagué and associates,[7] studying 117 schoolchildren, showed no difference in isokinetic strength between those with low back pain and symptom-free children. Newton and associates[126] using an isokinetic device, found that patients with low back pain were weaker than healthy controls, but they found no changes in extension/flexion ratio.

Despite these conflicting results, there seems to be agreement that patients with low back pain have weaker trunk muscles than do symptom-free subjects in a control group. Chronicity may be a supplementary factor. Nachemson and Lindh[122] found that isometric strength is significantly reduced in chronic as compared with acute low back pain. Hultman and associates[62] found a reduction in the isokinetic strength of back muscles in subjects with chronic back pain as compared with those with intermittent pain. But Suzuki and Endo[171] found no differences in isokinetic strength between patients with chronic pain and those without chronic pain.

Most of the published studies report only results of significance statistics (analysis of variance or t-tests) on the basis of mean values. Because of the wide range of values in both normal subjects and patients with low back pain, those ranges tend to overlap, which makes it impossible to discriminate individual subjects and limits the application of this information in clinical practice.

Few studies attempt to assess the real discriminant value of strength measure: sensitivity (the probability of the test being positive when a pathologic condition is present) and specificity (the probability of the test being negative when a pathologic condition is absent). Burdorf and associates,[18] testing

---

*References 2, 3, 14, 55, 62, 96, 109, 122, and 146.
†References 38, 50, 55, 81, 95, 109, and 157.

a limited sample of steel factory workers on an isoinertial device, showed specificity and sensitivity values of about 70%, which means approximately 30% false-positive and false-negative findings. Deutsch,[32] using the same isoinertial device on 104 subjects with low back pain and 124 controls, found a sensitivity of between 76% and 81% (false-negative rate of 19% to 24%) and a specificity of between 75% and 88% (false-positive rate of 12% to 25%).

Masset and associates[105] using the same isoinertial device in steel industry workers, found a specificity and a sensitivity of 82% when the quadratic velocity was computed for the three axes during tests against a resistance of 50% of the corresponding maximum torques. Figure 6 gives the cumulative histograms of the mean quadratic velocity for subjects with and without low back pain. The velocity value that discriminates most effectively is the value for which specificity and sensitivity are the highest. A value of 75 degrees/second could be proposed to discriminate between the two categories of subjects. The sensitivity and specificity of 82% can be compared with those (100% and 70%) provided by the past history of low back pain as discriminant factor.

Newton and colleagues,[126] using an isokinetic device, found a satisfactory average specificity of approximately 85% (false-positive rate of 15%) but an average sensitivity of only 44% to 63%. This means that there was a high false-negative rate (37% to 56%) which is barely permissible in clinical practice. Using a more complete battery of tests, including a lifting task test, they found better discriminant values, but these were only marginally better than clinical evaluation. There were only limited correlations between dynamometric and clinical measures.

These inconsistencies between investigators may be partly due to different methods and types of testing. Nevertheless, there remain a great number of confounding variables, such as the way instructions are delivered to subjects,[107] effort,[51, 146] and training.[54]

The predictive value of strength testing is often discussed, yet few studies have investigated this question. Biering-Sorensen[14] demonstrated that, in a general population without acute back pain, isometric trunk muscle strength was reduced in subjects who experienced recurrence of low back troubles in the follow-up year, as compared with those without recurrence. However, trunk strength in subjects who experienced low back trouble for the first time during the follow-up year did not differ from that of subjects without low back trouble. Mostardi and coworkers[120] studying a group of 174 nurses with an isokinetic device, failed to show any predictive value of strength measures. In this study, they measured lifting strength, which encompasses more factors than trunk strength alone.

Newton and associates[126] tested and followed 66 normal subjects during a 26- to 32-month period. There were no significant differences in isokinetic measures between those subjects in whom low back pain did or did not develop. However, those studies were conducted on small or specific populations, and there is no large-scale prospective study clearly showing that trunk muscle weakness may or may not predispose to back pain, or that it is not the result of painful symptoms.

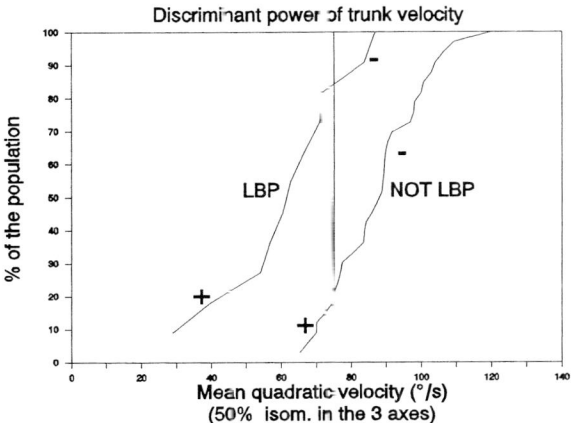

Figure 6. Cumulative histograms of the mean quadratic velocity at 50% of the maximum isometric torques for subjects with and without low back pain (LBP). (Adapted from Masset D., Malchaire, J., and Lemoine, M.: Static and dynamic characteristics of the trunk and history of low back pain. Int. J. Ind. Ergonomics 11:279, 1993.)

Follow-up of Treatment Modalities

Using such information for diagnostic purposes seems to be of limited value. Although lack of strength may be associated with back pain, it reveals little about the underlying diagnosis. The use of this quantitative approach is not easily adaptable to the individual patient. Nevertheless, it may be interesting to assess the efficacy of various treatment modalities for low back pain.

Szpalski and Hayez[169] showed the efficacy of a nonsteroidal antiinflammatory drug compared with placebo in patients with acute low back pain. In this study, velocity of movements and isometric strength in extension showed the greatest improvement. Improvement in trunk function was associated with relief of pain as reported on a visual analog scale.

Klein and Eek[77] demonstrated the lack of effect of low-energy laser when compared with placebo in chronic back pain. Once again, velocity showed the highest level of improvement. Szpalski and Hayez[165] compared two groups of subjects with acute low back pain who were assigned to 3-day or 7-day bed rest. Function testing was performed on day 1 and at the end of bed rest. Having found a similar increase in trunk function and in pain visual analog scale readings in both groups, they concluded that a shorter bed rest period was as efficient as a longer one and therefore preferable.

Holmström and Ulrich[60] investigated the efficacy of lumbar belts in a 2-month study of construction workers with low back pain. They showed an increase in flexor strength, but this was not correlated to any significant degree with modification in pain rating.

Several studies have documented the improvement over time of trunk strength with different regimens of exercise or rehabilitation programs.* This is true for isometric testing,[31, 45, 147, 158, 180] isokinetic testing,[52, 108, 112] and isoinertial testing.[31] Mayer and associates[108, 111, 112] reported that there is an association between isokinetic strength and reduction of pain, reduced disability, and return to work. Risch and associates[147] found that exercises for lumbar extension muscles in patients with chronic low back pain resulted in a significant increase in isometric extension strength and a significant decrease in reported pain and psychosocial dysfunction.

In evaluation of the effectiveness of treatment programs, the homogeneity of patients must be considered. Talo and colleagues[172] classified a heterogeneous group of patients with low back pain into more homogeneous subgroups. Patients were assigned to two rehabilitation programs: functioning activation and a spa program. The functioning activation was more effective in treating patients with personality disorders but good cognitive abilities, whereas the spa resort program more effectively treated the distress of the cognitively and functionally weaker patients. In future, classification of patients may include both behavioral and motion profile information.

This relation between behavior and performance has been further addressed by Cooke and colleagues.[31] They compared subjects with chronic low back pain enrolled in a back school program of therapy with healthy control subjects. The program did not include specific trunk muscle-strengthening exercises. Trunk function was measured at entry in the program and after 2 and 4 weeks using an isoinertial device that assessed isometric strength, range of motion, and velocity. They showed a significant improvement in performances in all measures, above all in dynamic function measured through velocity. However, they found an improvement greater than that expected from the natural history of physical recovery and greater than the strength increase attributable to therapeutic exercises or any training effect. This abnormally high degree of improvement had previously been reported by other researchers.[113, 158]

The improvements measured with dynamometric devices are probably due to an ensemble of physiologic, psychologic, and behavioral factors. Pain certainly plays a major role in the reduction of measured trunk strength, and was also reported by Nachemson and Lindh[122] in early studies and confirmed by later works.[11, 109, 169] Other factors that could hinder maximum strength exertion are fear of reinjury, anxiety, depression, misunderstanding of instructions, and illness behavior or symptom magnification. Spengler and Szpalski[164] showed low performances in patients with nonorganic signs. Hirsch and associates[57] using the same isoinertial devices, investigated the relationship between performance on lumbar dynamometry and several psychologic tests and measures of nonorganic pain behavior in a population with low back pain. They concluded that a poor performance on physical (biomechanical) testing may be a form of abnormal illness behavior that suggests the multifactorial nature of the behavior of low back pa-

---

*References 31, 45, 52, 60, 78, 108, 147, 158, and 180.

tients. The conclusion that the performances cannot be assumed to reflect the true neuromusculoskeletal impairment alone confirms the previous discussion. The population in the study had pain that was relatively chronic, with an average of 131.6 days since injury.

There is some evidence that programs focusing on physical reconditioning through resistive exercises, aerobics, stretching, and postural exercises help some patients with chronic low back pain. This subgroup also show reduction in the behavioral signs, whereas other patients may need psychiatric and behavioral intervention in addition to physical components of the functional restoration to improve.[183] In addition, increase in the physical performance has accompanied inconsistent change in the pain experiences for patients completing the functional restoration program.[145] This reinforces the idea that part of the improvement in the physical measures may be due to cognitive and behavioral factors and that exercise quotas should not be based on the daily experience of pain. Mellin and coworkers[117] showed that intensive physical training and improved physical performance did not play crucial roles in the rehabilitation of patients with chronic low back pain when return to work was used as an outcome measure. The lumbar strengthening exercises increased the trunk extension strength in patients with chronic low back pain more than in the control group.[147] Despite the reduction of pain, psychologic distress was not significantly changed, indicating the need for a behavioral component in rehabilitation programs for patients with chronic low back pain.

In patients with low back pain, dynamometric measures can therefore be considered more as a psychophysiologic test than a measure of true physical capacity. Those measures may not represent a true assessment of muscle strength but rather are an estimate of global trunk function.

Aids to Diagnosis

An interesting and innovative approach would be to conduct a more qualitative study that would examine abnormal movement patterns and profiles. Such research should determine how spinal pathologic changes modify patterns of motion; it can help to identify a spinal signature[133] associated with the pathologic alteration.

The function-based impairment evaluation schemes have traditionally used spinal mobility. Given the poor reliability of range of motion, its large variability among individuals, and the static psychometric nature of range of motion, the use of continuous dynamic profiles of motion with the higher-order derivatives has been suggested.[104] Dynamic performances of 281 consecutive patients from the Impairment Evaluation Center were used. As part of the comprehensive physical and psychologic evaluation, 281 consecutive patients with low back pain underwent isometric and dynamic trunk testing using Isostation B200. Feature extraction and cluster analysis techniques were used to find the main profiles in dynamic performances.[139] The middle three cycles of movements were interpolated and averaged into 128 data points. Thus, the data were normalized with respect to cycle time, and allowed between-individual comparison. Figure 7 presents the main profiles of sagittal trunk angular position. The number of patients in each group is also noted on the graph. Patients in the first (n = 48) and second (n = 55) groups had similar flexion mobility; however, those in the first group had more limited extension mobility. The time to peak sagittal position also varied among the five groups. Forty-seven patients in the fifth group showed extreme impairment in both flexion and extension. The third group, 26 patients, showed differential impairments with respect to direction of motion. A marked improvement over the use of range of motion has been achieved by preserving information in the continuous profiles. The patients with low back pain in this study are heterogeneous with respect to their movement profile. Uniform treatment of these patients is questionable, and rehabilitation programs should consider their specific impairments. Future research should incorporate the clinical profiles with these movement profiles to delineate further the heterogeneity of low back patients.

Marras and associates[104] used similar feature extraction techniques to characterize the movement profiles of 510 subjects belonging to a normal group (n = 339) and 10 patient groups with low back pain (n = 171). Subjects were asked to perform flexion-extension trunk movement at five

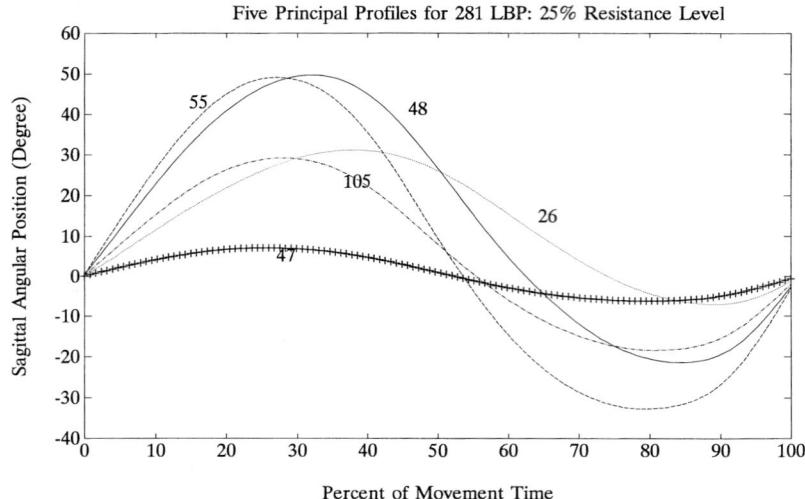

Figure 7. The five principal patterns of sagittal movement during repetitive flexion and extension for 281 patients with low back pain against resistance set equal to 25% of maximum voluntary isometric sagittal exertion using the Isostation B200. (Adapted from Parnianpour, M., Hanson, T., Goldman, S., et al.: Heterogeneity of low back pain patients: Towards consideration of the variability of their dynamic continuous movement profile. North American Spine Society Meeting, Hawaii, April 18–21, 1994.)

levels of asymmetry, while three-dimensional movement of the spine was monitored by the Lumbar Motion Monitor (an exoskeletal goniometer developed at the biodynamics laboratory of Ohio State University). Trunk motions were performed against no resistance, and no pelvic stabilization was required. The quadratic discriminant analysis was able to classify correctly more than 80% of the subjects. Marras and associates[105] have continued their analysis and obtained much better results while requiring only the movement profiles of symmetric sagittal movement. The newer algorithm first classifies the patients and normal subjects and subsequently categorizes the patients in one of the 10 patient groups. The model was capable of identifying more than 94% of patients with low back pain and normal subjects correctly and was also able to classify 70% of the patients into one of the 10 groups in the cross-validation study.

During analysis of motion profiles of normal subjects, they found that the angular velocity, acceleration, and range of motion were correlated. Hence, a pilot study was performed to investigate whether one can reduce the within-group variability of performance measures by controlling the range of motion and the required accuracy of the movement.[74] A much better discrimination capability can be realized by reducing the within-group variance and increasing the between-group differences. The early experiments of Fitts[35] indicated the speed and accuracy tradeoff. The ratio of movement amplitude (A) and the target width (W) defines the index of difficulty [(ID = $\log_2(2A/W)$]. Fitts' law states that the higher the index of difficulty, the longer the movement time is: movement time = intercept + slope * ID. The inverse of the slope signifies the information-processing capability in terms of number of bits per second. Twenty healthy male subjects were asked perform flexion and extension as fast as they could at their preferred range of motion. In addition, they were asked to perform trunk bending as fast and as accurately as possible while they were provided with a visual feedback on the monitor that specified the range of motion and the target width.

By properly selecting the movement amplitude and the target width, 22 additional trials were randomly performed. Figure 8 shows the results of the movement time versus index of difficulty for one of the subjects. Highly significant regression lines were found that specified the intercept and the slope values (R^2 = .77 ± .11). The information processing of the trunk neuromuscular system was found to be 4.23 ± 1.43 bits/

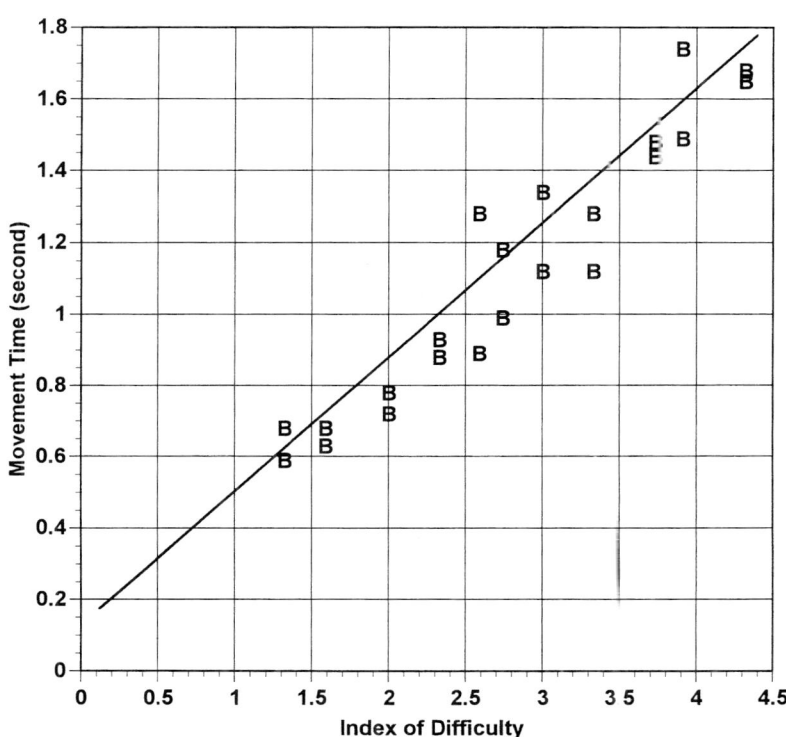

Figure 8. Control capability shown as slope and intercept based on Fitts' law. The movement time plotted against the index of difficulty for one normal male subject for 22 trials of repetitive sagittal trunk flexion and extension. The linear regression determining the intercept and the slope is according to Fitts' law. The target width and movement amplitude were set to get 11 different indices of difficulty. The Lumbar Motion Monitor was used to measure the triaxial trunk movement. (Adapted from Kim, J. Y., Parnianpour, M., and Marras, W. S.: Quantitative measurement of neuromuscular control capability of the trunk during dynamic oscillatory bending movements. In 1993 Advances in Bioengineering, Vol. 26. New York, American Society of Mechanical Engineers, 1993.)

second, which is considerably lower than 23 and 10 bits/second estimated for the wrist and the arm, respectively. Two important results are that neither the slope nor the intercept were correlated with the motion characteristic during maximum performance. Hence, a measure of control and coordination that is independent of the maximum speed and acceleration has been identified. In addition, the coefficient of variation of the trunk flexion and extension velocity were reduced by half, while the accelerations were less affected. The results indicated that, by providing the target and defining the range of motion, it is possible to reduce normal variability in motion measures. Future studies are needed to see if it is possible to generalize this result to the population with low back pain.

Szpalski and coworkers[167, 170] studied three groups of subjects: (1) 13 patients with spinal stenosis, (2) 14 patients with posterior bulging disc associated with facet arthrosis but with a canal diameter remaining within normal limits, and (3) a control population of 30 symptom-free volunteers. An isoinertial trunk testing dynamometric device (Isostation B200) was used. First, the maximum sagittal isometric torque was recorded; then subjects were asked to perform six sagittal flexion-extensions as fast as possible against a resistance set at 50% of the torque measured previously. A phase plane analysis (velocity versus position) was performed for every subject (Fig. 9). An ensemble averaging technique using a Lagrange interpolator[70] was then employed to average the six repetitions of each subject (Fig. 10).

Healthy persons move faster and further than impaired persons; therefore, movement patterns drawn were different in size, making it difficult to compare them. To enable comparison of the different group patterns on the same scale, each individual data set is normalized by assigning a value of 100 to the highest positive value for position as well as velocity. With relative velocity and position values, an average phase plane analysis was then drawn for each group to compare movement shapes. The average

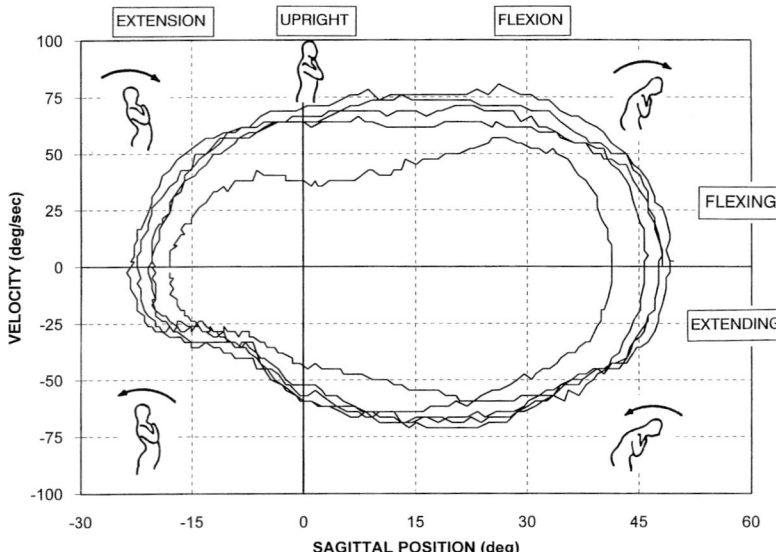

Figure 9. Five consecutive cycles of a velocity-position phase plane graph in test subjects with posterior bulging disc and facet arthrosis. Note the marked decrease of velocity at end of extension. (Reprinted from Clinical Biomechanics, 8, Keller, T. S., Szpalski, M., and Spengler, D. M.: Interpretation and parametrization of dynamic trunk isoinertial movements using an ensemble averaging technique, 220–222, Copyright 1993, with kind permission from Butterworth-Heinemann journals, Elsevier Science Ltd, The Boulevard, Langford Lane, Kidlington OX5 1GB, UK.)

phase plane graph showed three distinct patterns of movement for the three groups (Fig. 11). Velocity was then divided into octiles to quantify and compare its evolution during the different phases of the movement (Fig. 12). Analysis of variance performed on the velocity values confirmed the discriminant nature of the extension phase of the movement. The spinal stenosis group showed lower normalized velocity than did the control subjects during the whole extension phase ($p < .05$), while the bulging disc group demonstrated a significant decrease in normalized velocity on the seventh octile, at the end of extension ($p < .01$).

Liyang and associates[90] demonstrated the reduction of diameter of the normal spinal canal during extension. Penning and Wilmink[140] showed that the marked bulging of a disc appearing in extension may represent a risk of root compression, with possible neurogenic claudication, if associated with facet hypertrophy. Adams and colleagues[1] showed that during extension there is an increase in disc bulging, especially if there are degenerative changes in the apophyseal

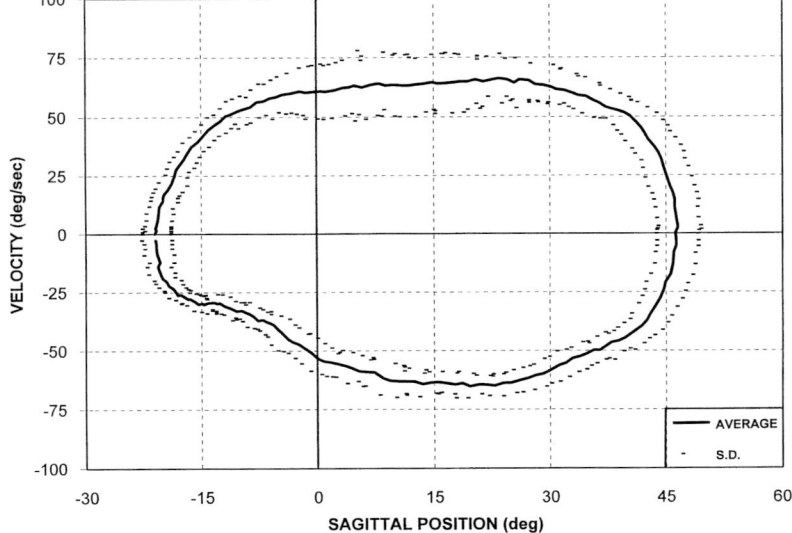

Figure 10. Ensemble average (*solid line*) and standard deviations (*dotted lines*) corresponding to each of the 200 time-normalized points obtained from the data from Figure 9. (Reprinted from Clinical Biomechanics, 8, Keller, T. S., Szpalski, M., and Spengler, D. M.: Interpretation and parametrization of dynamic trunk isoinertial movements using an ensemble averaging technique, 220–222, Copyright 1993, with kind permission from Butterworth-Heinemann journals, Elsevier Science Ltd, The Boulevard, Langford Lane, Kidlington OX5 1GB, UK.)

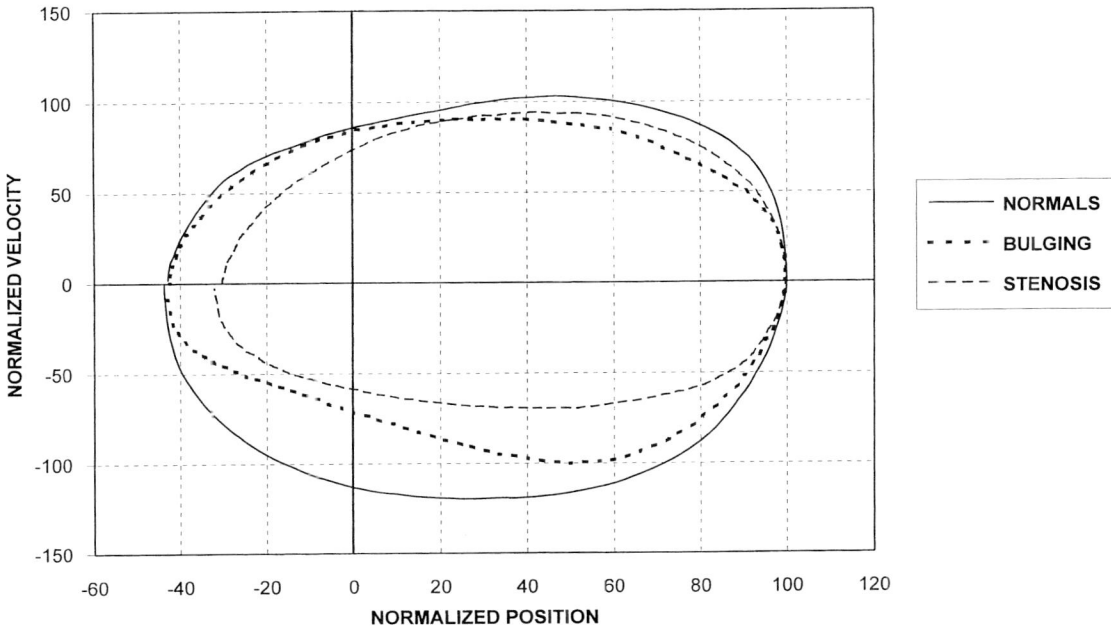

Figure 11. Average movement patterns drawn for the three subject groups. Note the marked differences during the extension phase of the movement (lower half of the graph).

joints. The differences noted in velocity during extension by Szpalski and coworkers[170] can be related to those findings and may represent a form of position-related claudication. This preliminary study shows the relation between some anatomic findings and movement patterns. Such studies are interesting to assess the repercussions of anatomic lesions for function and to determine the responsibility of unclear pathologic findings such as bulging disc and facet syndromes for a patient's symptoms. These

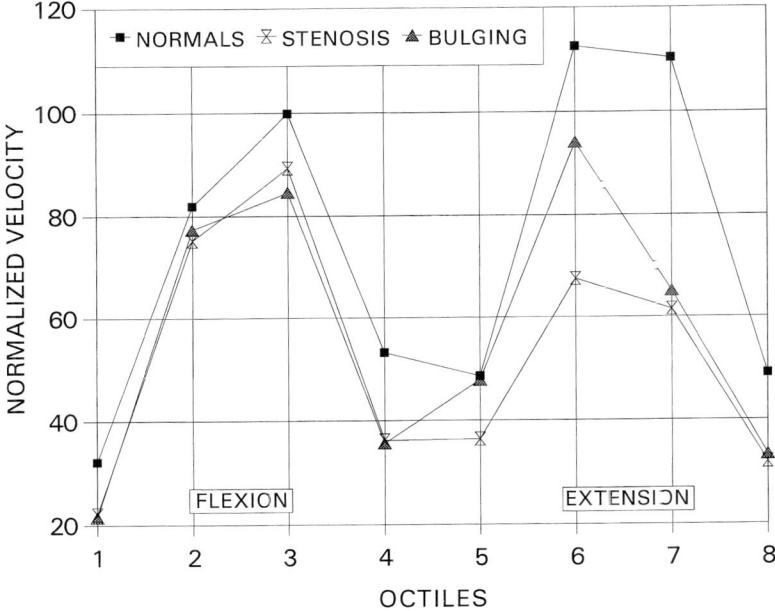

Figure 12. The total motion has been divided in eight segments to quantify the evolution of velocity during the different phases of movement. Note the differences between the groups during the extension phase (octiles 5 through 8).

promising results indicate that diagnosis-specific spinal movement signatures may exist and could bring about the more functional quantitative evaluation tools to aid the diagnosis, prognosis, and effective treatment of low back pain.

OCCUPATIONAL APPLICATIONS OF TRUNK STRENGTH TESTING

Preemployment trunk strength measurement is presented as an important application of quantitative muscle testing. It certainly is an appealing concept. Testing a person before employment appears to be a reasonable way to prevent future back injury. However, most published studies deal with lifting strength, which is not a true measure of trunk function but a global measure that encompasses arm, shoulder, and leg strength and that is based on the individual's lifting technique and overall fitness. Indeed, it is a measure of whole-body performance. The relation between the isometric lifting test and isometric or isokinetic trunk muscle strength is poor.[130]

The factor-limiting performance may reside in any of the involved muscle groups, and not specifically in the trunk muscles. Lifting strength measure is mainly of interest in preemployment testing to determine whether an individual is capable of performing a task involving lifting movements. Isometric lifting strength, which is easy and inexpensive to perform, has been reported as predictive of injury[20, 27, 29, 72] but only if it is job specific.[72] Parnianpour and associates[134] illustrated how isometric tests can miscalculate the risk assessment of demands of a given task with respect to normal population.

Nevertheless, Battié and associates[10] conducted a prospective study to determine the physical risk factors associated with back pain reported among 3020 aircraft manufacturing employees. They found that isometric lifting strength measurements were not predictive of back pain incidence, possibly because the standard isometric lifting tests used were not specific for the job. It seems that the injury predictive capability of isometric strength testing is limited to those jobs requiring the worker to use a high percentage of strength potential.[29, 72]

Isometric lifting strength is a static measure, which poorly reproduces real life tasks. Dynamic lifting tests providing more realistic lifting simulation[118, 119] based on isokinetic[69, 75, 99, 143] or isoinertial[81, 119] principles have been proposed. They allow closer simulation of true job requirements, especially the isoinertial technique. Yet, the only longitudinal dynamic lifting tests study to date, conducted by Mostardi and colleagues[120] on a group of 174 nurses, failed to show any predictive value of isokinetic lifting strength measures.

Another testing method, the submaximum dynamic strength assessment used in psychophysical testing,[6, 86, 150, 161, 179] is a safe way to perform realistic job simulation, but the results may be influenced by psychologic or behavioral factors beyond actual strength. Troup and coworkers[178] showed that psychophysical lifting tests were not good predictors of first-time low back pain incidence during the follow-up year; however, lifting capability was significantly lower in subjects with chronic low back pain. These results tend to invalidate the theory of lack of strength being the cause of low back pain, and then may indicate instead that loss of strength is a process resulting from recurrent low back pain. However, the number of confounding variables associated with psychophysical testing must also be taken in account. Newton and associates[126] in a small sample of 66 symptom-free subjects followed for an average of 30 months, found no difference in initial isometric or psychophysical lifting simulation between subjects in whom back pain did or did not appear. However, testing in this study was not job specific.

Despite certain contradictory results, it seems that lifting strength measurements have a certain predictive value if they are made highly task specific. The use of these tests is further limited to jobs requiring regular lifting movements. Furthermore, few jobs demand that a single lifting task be performed in a single position. No data confirm this limited predictive value regarding long-term evolution.

As for trunk strength testing itself, there are no studies investigating the predictive value of preemployment strength trunk testing. Some studies have investigated the relation between strength measures after injury and return to work. Hazard and associates[52] showed that improvement in isokinetic measures at the end of a functional restoration program did not predict return to work. Mayer and associates[111] found that subjects returning to work after a functional restoration program had improved extensor isokinetic strength compared with that of those who did not resume work. However, they failed to demonstrate that isokinetic measures predicted return to work. At present, the only interest in preemployment trunk strength testing is to provide a baseline of trunk performance at time of hiring. This baseline may then be used to determine a level of return to work after subsequent back injury.

Some other applications of trunk strength testing in occupational settings have been described. Carlier and coworkers[22] showed that pediatric nurses who carry children indifferently in either arm are stronger and have less back pain than those who always carry them on the same side. The same team produced preliminary data suggesting that trunk muscle strength deficit is influenced by working positions.[23]

APPLICATIONS OF TRUNK MUSCLE ENDURANCE TESTING

Fatigue occurs when a contraction can no longer be maintained (isometric fatigue) or when repetitive movements can no longer be sustained at a certain output (dynamic fatigue). Endurance is the period before fatigue occurs. The endurance capacity of the muscles is an expression of their fatigability. It is conceivable that individuals with low trunk muscle endurance are more exposed to postural stress that may lead to incorrect loading of the spine and impaired coordination of the postural muscles resulting in subsequent back trouble. Indeed, it is classically assumed that local muscle fatigue predisposes person to injury.[26] Many reports have been published to indicate that the skill of the worker is affected by fatigue.[5, 8, 59, 65, 83] Chaffin[26] demonstrated that reduction of precise motor control accompanies muscle fatigue.

This tendency to loss of skill and motor control is confirmed by Parnianpour and associates[132] who studied the effect of isoinertial fatiguing of flexion and extension trunk movements on the movement pattern (angular position and velocity profile) and the motor output (torque) of the trunk. They showed that, with fatigue, there is a reduction of the functional capacity in the main sagittal plane. There is also a loss of motor control, enabling a greater range of motion in the transverse and coronal planes while performing the primary sagittal task. The association of sagittal with coronal and transverse movements is considered more likely to induce back injuries[47, 48, 97, 178, 184]; thus the effect of fatigue and reduction of motor control and coordination may be an important risk factor leading to injury-prone working postures. The endurance limit is a more useful predictor of incidence and recurrence of low back disorders than are the absolute strength values.[132]

Potvin[144] examined the effect of fatigue on the mechanisms of injury to the low back during unconstrained repetitive lifting. Eight male subjects performed dynamic sagittal lift of inertial loads at a high intensity (8 lifts/minute; average load of 20 kg) for 20 minutes and at a low intensity (6 lifts/minute; average load of 18 kg) for 2 hours. Fatigue was quantified intermittently in an isometric test contraction apparatus with strength measures and EMG analysis during submaximum exertions, as well as a trunk extensor muscle endurance at the end of each session. The EMG-driven models also assess the kinetics and spine loading. The results indicated different individual adaptations to the quantified fatigue. This documented adapting mechanism has been hypothesized to increase the risk of damaging the posterior ligaments, intervertebral discs, vertebral bodies, or erector spinae muscle. However, no prospective study demonstrates that lack of trunk muscle endurance may predispose to low back trouble. The few existing studies failed to establish this relationship clearly.[14, 66, 128] Biering-Sorensen[14] demonstrated that isometric back endurance was of significance for prediction of first-time occurrence of low back troubles among men in the follow-up year. However, the women showed an insignificant trend in the opposite direction.

Trunk muscle endurance does differ between healthy subjects and those reporting low back pain. During isometric endurance testing,[171] trunk flexors develop fatigue faster than do extensors in symptom-free subjects. The flexor fatigability appeared significantly higher in patients with low back pain as compared with controls, but no difference in extensor endurance was demonstrated.

Chronicity also influences trunk muscle endurance. Hultman and associates[62] showed reduced abdominal isometric endurance in patients with intermittent low back pain as compared with healthy individuals. Patients with chronic low back pain showed reduced abdominal as well as back muscle endurance as compared with the healthy control subjects and lower back muscle endurance as compared with those with the intermittent low back pain. Holmström and colleagues[61] demonstrated a similar loss of extensor endurance in relation to the severity of low back pain. Nicolaisen and Jorgensen[128] found that persons with a history of debilitating low back pain demonstrated less isometric trunk extensor endurance than did either normal persons or patients with history of less severe low back pain.

Magnetic resonance imaging scanning was used to evaluate the recruitment of the trunk muscles in patients with chronic low back pain after the endurance test using the Roman chair extension exercise.[37] Increased signal intensity occurred in the exercised muscles. At rest, the patients with prior surgery (n = 5) had lower intensity than did the normal subjects (n = 5) and the nonsurgical patients (n = 5). The exercise increased the intensity of the multifidus and longissimus or iliocostalis signals. The patients with surgery showed attenuated responses to the exercise. The image intensity of the multifidus muscle was higher than that for the longissimus or iliocostalis muscles after exercise.

Few studies have investigated the evolution of trunk muscle endurance during treatment of low back pain. Holmström and colleagues[60] showed that construction workers with low back pain wearing a weight lifter's belt for 2 months significantly increase their trunk flexor endurance. They also showed an insignificant decrease in extensor endurance. This improved endurance, however, was not related to any significant modifications in pain rating.

A randomized prospective study on patients with nonspecific mechanical low back pain proved that a graded activity program increased the mobility, strength, and endurance of back muscles and returned the workers to work an average of 5.1 weeks earlier than the control group.[89] The number of sick days before return to work in the activity group was negatively correlated with pretreatment measures: the less spinal rotation, less abdominal muscle endurance time, and less lifting capacity observed, the more sick leave was needed before subjects returned to work.

A prospective randomized study among employees in a geriatric hospital showed that exercising during work hours to improve back muscle strength, endurance, and coordination proved cost-effective in preventing back symptoms and absence from work.[46] Every hour spent by the physiotherapist on the exercise group reduced work absence by an average of 1.3 days. In this study, both training and testing equipment were modest.

Dynamic fatigue data were reported by Langrana and Lee[85] and by Smidt and associates[156] using the same protocol. Dynamic endurance was measured as the time needed for the maximum concentric torque to decrease by 25% at an isokinetic speed of 30 degrees/second. They also found a higher fatigability in the abdominal muscles. Women were found to have more endurance than men. Oddly, those studies showed that patients with low back pain had greater endurance than did healthy control subjects. This can be explained by the fact that the critical occluding strength is 60% of MVC for subjects with low strength as opposed to 45% of MVC for high-strength individuals.[56] Low-strength subjects showing less occlusion of blood flow may therefore have more endurance.

Muscle fibers are commonly classified into type I (slow twitch, red, oxidative with high aerobic capacity) and type II (fast twitch, white, glycolytic with high anaerobic capacity) fibers. Type I fibers are considered more fatigue resistant and are predominant in trunk extensor muscles.[64] The dynamic endurance studies using isokinetic devices[84, 156] were performed at slow velocities (30 degrees/second), conditions in which blood flow has enough time to be reestablished between contraction occlusions in the back muscles during the flexion phase of the movement.[130] It also appears that back muscles are able to mobilize a larger blood perfusion at a given relative contraction (percentage of MVC) than other muscles.[16] Furthermore, isokinetic movement is not a natural type of muscle activity. For those reasons, the protocols used in those studies may not be appropriate for true endurance measurement.

Szpalski and associates[168] investigated the endurance of trunk flexor and extensor muscles during isoinertial maximum velocity activity in the sagittal plane. Sixteen male volunteers with no history of low back pain were included in the study. An isoinertial trunk testing dynamometric device (Isostation B200) was used. In the first part of the examination, maximum isometric strength was measured. Then the subjects were asked to perform repeated sagittal flexion-extension movements as fast as possible against a resistance set at 50% of the previously measured maximum isometric torque. The subjects were asked to perform the movements until exhaustion or until a limit of 50 repetitions. The analyzed variables included peak velocity, average velocity, and power in flexion and extension. Individual performances were divided into quartiles on the basis of the number of completed repetitions (Fig. 13). An analysis of variance was realized on the slopes of the regressions lines of performance values versus quartiles. Only five subjects were able to reach the 50-repetition limit. The decrease in performance during the test was 19% in peak flexion velocity, 15.9% in peak extension velocity, 19.6% in average flexion velocity, 21.6% in average extension velocity, 24.3% in flexion power, and 24.2% in extension power. The analysis of variance on the slopes did not show any statistical differences between flexion and extension endurance in any of the measured variables (peak velocity: $p = .86$; average velocity: $p = .57$; and power: $p = .65$). It appears that during a high-velocity isoinertial movement, there is no difference

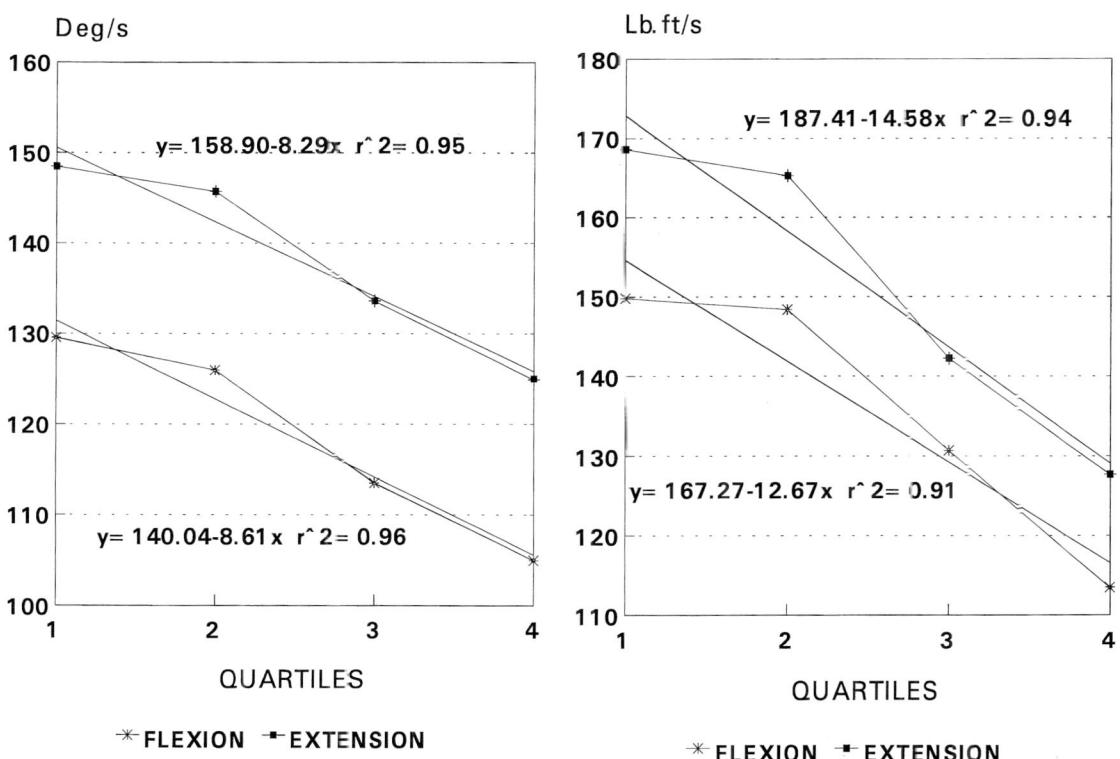

Figure 13. Average decrease (16 subjects) of sagittal flexion and extension peak velocity and power during fatigue test.

in endurance characteristics between trunk flexor and extensor muscles. This contradicts previous studies conducted at low isokinetic velocities during which blood flow could be restored after contraction because of the slow speed of movement. It seems that, when high-velocity movement does not enable this blood flow to be reestablished and an anaerobic condition is created, the predominantly aerobic extensor muscles do not retain their fatigue resistance qualities.

CONCLUSIONS

It appears that by measuring trunk strength one really measures global trunk function, which takes in account many physiologic, psychologic, and behavioral factors that are difficult to control and assess separately. Those measures seem to enable a certain degree of discrimination between normal subjects and populations with low back troubles and to enable measurement of treatment efficacy. There are many conflicting reports on the need for trunk function quantification in the field of occupational applications. The need for strength variable quantification cannot be dismissed before the relationship between the job and the strength variable is critically assessed.

There is an abundance of literature in the field of trunk strength and endurance measurement. Sophisticated techniques of assessment are described, and the evolution of computer technology allows for near-infinite possibilities of analysis and modeling. Those methods should enable more precise modeling of trunk function data, namely patterns of trunk movement, which seem to hold a promising future in determining the influence of back pathologic conditions on the quality of trunk motion.

However, despite the wealth of information and technical possibilities, the major question, which will not be addressed by technical performances, but by prospective clinical epidemiologic studies, remains unanswered: Does poor trunk function, as measured by low muscle strength or endurance, predispose a healthy person to subsequent low back trouble?

Acknowledgement

The authors acknowledge the support from OSURF and NIDRR H133E30009. The authors would like to thank Drs. Elen Ross, Jackson Tan, Robert Gabriel, Robert Crowell, William Marras, Ali Sheikhzadeh, Jung Yong Kim, Sue Ferguson, Patrick Sparto, Heinz Hoffer, Jean-Pierre Hayez, and Jean-Marie Tielemans for invaluable comments and contributions.

REFERENCES

1. Adams, M. A., Dolan, P., and Hutton, W. C.: The lumbar spine in backward bending. Spine 13:1019–1026, 1988.
2. Addison, R., and Schultz, A.: Trunk strength in patients seeking hospitalization for chronic low back disorders. Spine 5:539, 1980.
3. Alston, W., Carlson, K. E., Feldman, D. J., et al.: A quantitative study of muscle factors in chronic low back syndrome. J. Am. Geriatr. Soc. 14:1041, 1966.
4. Andersson, G.: Evaluation of muscle function. In Frymoyer, J. W. (ed.): The Adult Spine. New York, Raven Press, 1991, pp. 271–274.
5. Asmussen, E.: Muscle fatigue. Med. Sci. Sports 11:313, 1979.
6. Ayoub, M. M., Mital, A., Bakken, G. M., et al.: Development of strength and capacity norms for manual materials handling activities. The state of art. J. Hum. Factors 22:271, 1980.
7. Balagué, F., Damidot, P., Nordin, M., et al.: Cross-sectional study of the isokinetic muscle trunk strength among school children. Spine 18:1199, 1993.
8. Bates, B. T., Osternig, L. R., and James, S. L.: Fatigue effects in running. J. Motor Behav. 9:203, 1977.
9. Battié, M.: The Reliability of Physical Factors as Predicted of Occurrence of Back Pain Reports. A prospective study within industry. Unpublished Doctoral Dissertation. Gothenburg, Sweden, Gothenburg University, 1989.
10. Battié, M. C., Bigos, S. J., Fisher, L. D., et al.: Isometric lifting as a predictor of industrial back pain. Spine 14:851, 1989.
11. Beimborn, D. S., and Morrissey, M. C.: A review of the literature related to trunk muscle performance. Spine 13:655, 1987.
12. Berme, N., and Cappozzo, A.: Biomechanics of Human Movement: Applications in Rehabilitation, Sports and Ergonomics. Worthington, OH, Bertec Corporation, 1990.
13. Biedermann, H. J., Shanks, G. L., Forrest, W. J., et al.: Power spectrum analyses of electromyographic activity: Discriminators in the differential assessment of patients with chronic low-back pain. Spine 16:1179, 1991.
14. Biering-Sorensen, F.: Physical measurements as risk indicators for low back trouble over a one-year period. Spine 9:106, 1984.
15. Boden, S. D., Davis, O. D., Dian, T. S., et al.: Abnormal magnetic resonance scans of the lumbar spine in asymptomatic subjects. J. Bone Joint Surg. 72A:403, 1990.
16. Bonde-Petersen, F., Mork, A. L., and Nielsen, E.: Local muscle blood flow and sustained contrac-

tions of human arm and back muscles. Eur. J. Appl. Physiol. 34:43, 1975.
17. Buchalter, D., Parnianpour, M., Viola, K., et al.: Three-dimensional spinal motion measurements. Part 1: A technique for examining posture and functional spinal motion. J. Spinal Disord. 1:279, 1989.
18. Burdorf, A., van Riel, M., and Snijders, C.: Trunk muscle strength measurements and prediction of low-back pain among workers. Clin. Biomech. 7:55, 1992.
19. Buseck, M., Schipplein, O. D., Andersson, G. B. J., et al.: Influence of dynamic factors and external loads on the moment at the lumbar spine in lifting. Spine 13:918, 1988.
20. Cady, L. D., Bischoff, D. P., O'Connell, E. R., et al.: Strength and fitness and subsequent back injuries in firefighters. J. Occup. Med. 21:269, 1979.
21. Caldwell, L. S., Chaffin, D. B., Dukes-Dobos, F. N., et al.: A proposed standard procedure for static muscle strength testing. Am. Ind. Hyg. Assoc. J. 35:201, 1974.
22. Carlier, P., Szpalski, M., Vanderbecken, F., and Hayez, J. P.: Isoinertial functional assessment of low-back disorders in paediatric nurses. Ergonomic and rehabilitation guidelines. J. Occup. Rehabil. 2:131, 1992.
23. Carlier, P., Szpalski, M., Vanderbecken, F., et al.: Differences in isometric torques and velocities in low back pain patients with different professions and working postures. Orthop. Trans. 17:314, 1993.
24. Cartas, O., Nordin, M., Frankel, V. H., et al.: Quantification of trunk muscle performance in standing, semistanding, and sitting postures in healthy men. Spine 18:603, 1993.
25. Chaffin, D. B., and Baker, W. H.: A biomechanical model for analysis of symmetric sagittal plane lifting. AIIE Trans. 2:16, 1970.
26. Chaffin, D. B.: Localized muscle fatigue—definition and measurement. J. Occup. Med. 15:346, 1973.
27. Chaffin, D. B., and Park, K. S.: A longitudinal study of low back pain as associated with occupational weight lifting factors. Am. Ind. Hyg. Assoc. J. 34:513, 1973.
28. Chaffin, D. B.: Ergonomics guide for the assessment of human static strength. Am. Ind. Hyg. Assoc. J. 37:505, 1975.
29. Chaffin, D. B., Herrin, G. D., and Keyserling, W. M. Preemployment strength testing: An updated position. J. Occup. Med. 20:403, 1978.
30. Clark, W., and Haldeman, S.: The development of guideline factors for the evaluation of disability in neck and back injuries. Spine 18:1736, 1993.
31. Cooke, C., Menard, M. R., Beach, G. N., et al.: Serial lumbar dynamometry in low back pain. Spine 17:653, 1992.
32. Deutsch, S. D.: B200 back evaluation system. Version 3.0. Pawtucket, RI, Occupational Orthopaedic Centre, 1989, pp. 127–130.
33. Dvorak, J., Panjabi, M., Chang, G. J., et al.: Functional radiographic diagnosis of the lumbar spine. Flexion/extension and lateral bending. Spine 16:562, 1991.
34. Dumas, G. A., Poulin, M. J., Roy, B., et al.: A three-dimensional digitization method to measure trunk muscle lines of action. Spine 13:532, 1988.
35. Fitts, P. M.: The information capacity of the human motor system in controlling the amplitude of movement. J. Exp. Psychol. 47:381, 1954.
36. Fleishman, E. A., and Quaintance, M. K.: Taxonomies of Human Performance. Orlando, FL, Academic Press, 1984.
37. Flicker, P. L., Fleckenstein, J. L., Ferry, K., et al.: Lumbar muscle usage in chronic low back pain. Spine 18:582, 1993.
38. Flint, M. M.: Effect of increasing back and abdominal strength in low back pain. Res. Q. 29:160–171, 1955.
39. Freivalds, A., Chaffin, D. B., Garg, A., et al.: A dynamic biomechanical evaluation of lifting maximum acceptable loads. J. Biomech. 17:251, 1984.
40. Freivalds, A., and Fotouki, D. M.: Comparison of dynamic strength as measured by the Cybex and Mini-Gym isokinetic dynamometers. Int. J. Ind. Ergonomics 1:189, 1987.
41. Gabriel, R. J.: The Effect of Direction and Resistance Level on Muscle Coordination, Movement Patterns, and Motor Output During Repetitive Isoinertial Trunk Flexion and Extension of Healthy Males. Unpublished Doctoral Thesis. New York, New York University, 1992.
42. Gagnon, M., and Smyth, G.: Muscular mechanical energy expenditure as a process for detecting the risk in manual material handling. J. Biomech. 24:191, 1991.
43. Gracovetsky, S.: The Spinal Engine. Wien, Springer-Verlag, 1988.
44. Gracovetsky, S., Kary, M., Pitchen, L, et al.: The importance of pelvic tilt in reducing compressive stress in the spine during flexion and extension exercises. Spine 14:412, 1989.
45. Graves, J. E., Pollock, M. L., Foster, D. et al.: Effect of training frequency and specificity on isometric lumbar extension strength. Spine 15:504, 1990.
46. Gundewall, B., Liljeqvist, M., and Hansson, T.: Primary prevention of back symptoms and absence from work. Spine 18:587, 1993
47. Gunzburg, R., Hutton, W. C., and Frazer, R. D.: Axial rotation of the lumbar spine and the effect of flexion. An in-vitro and in-vivo biomechanical study. Spine 16:22–28, 1991.
48. Gunzburg, R., Parkinson, R., Moore, R., et al.: A cadaveric study comparing discography, magnetic resonance imaging, histology, and mechanical behavior of the human lumbar disc. Spine 17:417–426, 1992.
49. Haig, A. J., Weismann, G., Haugh, L. D., et al.: Prospective evidence for change in paraspinal muscle activity after herniated nucleus pulposus. Spine 18:926, 1993.
50. Hasue, M., Masatoshi, F., and Kikuchi, S.: A new method of quantitative measurement of abdominal and back muscle strength. Spine 5:143, 1980.
51. Hazard, R. G., Reid, S., Fenwick, J., et al.: Isokinetic trunk strength and lifting strength measurements: Variability as an indicator of effort. Spine 13:54, 1988.
52. Hazard, R. G., Fenwick, J. W., Kalisch, S. M., et al.: Functional restoration with behavioral support: A one-year prospective study of patients with chronic low-back pain. Spine 14:157, 1989.
53. Hazard, R. G., Reeves, V., and Fenwick, J. W.: Lifting capacity. Spine 17:1065, 1992.
54. Hazard, R. G., Reeves, V., Fenwick, J. W., et al.:

Test-retest variation in lifting capacity and indices of subject effort. Clin. Biomech. 8:20, 1993.
55. Herlant, M., Vanvelcenaher, J., Delahaye, H., et al.: Evaluation isocinétique du déficit musculaire chez les lombalgiques. Rev. Med. Ortop. 28:2, 1992.
56. Heyward, V.: Influence of static strength and intramuscular occlusion on submaximal static muscle endurance. Res. Q. 46:393, 1974.
57. Hirsch, G., Beach, G., Cooke, C. et al.: Relationship between performance on lumbar dynamometry and Waddell score in a population with low-back pain. Spine 16:1039, 1991.
58. Hislop, H. J., and Perrine, J. J.: Isokinetic concept in exercise. Phys. Ther. 47:114, 1967.
59. Holding, D. H.: Fatigue. In Hockey, R. (ed.): Stress and Fatigue in Human Performance. New York, Wiley, 1983, pp. 145–165.
60. Holmström, E., and Ulrich, M.: Effects of lumbar belts on trunk muscle strength and endurance: A follow-up of construction workers. J. Spinal Disord. 5:260, 1992.
61. Holmström, E. B., Andersson, M., and Moritz, U.: Trunk muscle strength and back muscle endurance in construction workers with and without low back disorders. Scand. J. Rehabil. Med. 24:3, 1992.
62. Hultman, G., Nordin, M., Saraste, H., et al.: Body composition, endurance, cross-sectional area, and density of MM erector spinae in men with and without low back pain. J. Spinal Disord. 6:114, 1993.
63. Huxley, A. F.: Muscular contraction. J. Physiol. 243:1, 1974.
64. Johnson, M. A., Polgar, J., Weightman, D., et al.: Data on the distribution of fibre type in thirty-six human muscles. An autopsy study. J. Neurol. Sci. 18:111, 1973.
65. Jones, L. A., and Hunter, I. W.: Perceived force in fatiguing isometric contraction. Percept. Psychophysics 33:369, 1983.
66. Jorgensen, K., and Nicolaisen, T.: Trunk extensor endurance: Determination and relation to low-back trouble. Ergonomics 30:259, 1987.
67. Jorgensen, K., Mag, C., Nicholaisen, T., et al.: Muscle fiber distribution, capillary density, and enzymatic activities in the lumbar paravertebral muscles of young men. Spine 18:1439, 1993.
68. Kahanovitz, N., Nordin, M., Verderame, R., et al.: Normal trunk muscle strength and endurance in women and the effect of exercises and electrical stimulation. Part 2: Comparative analysis of electrical stimulation and exercises to increase trunk muscle strength and endurance. Spine 12:112, 1987.
69. Kamon, E., Kiser, D., and Pytel, J. L.: Dynamic and static lifting capacity and muscular strength of steelmill workers. Am. Ind. Hyg. Assoc. J. 43:853, 1982.
70. Keller, T. S., Szpalski, M., and Spengler, D. M.: Interpretation and parametrization of dynamic trunk isoinertial movements using an ensemble averaging technique. Clin. Biomech. 8:220, 1993.
71. Keyserling, W. M.: Isometric Strength Testing in Selecting Workers for Strenuous Jobs. Doctoral Dissertation. Ann Arbor, MI, University of Michigan, University Microfilms International, 1979.
72. Keyserling, W. M., Herrin, G. D., and Chaffin, D. B.: Isometric strength testing as a means of controlling medical incidents on strenuous jobs. Occup. Med. 22:332, 1980.
73. Khalil, T. M., Goldberg, M. L., Asfour, S. S., et al.: Acceptable maximum effort (AME): A psychophysical measure of strength in back pain patients. Spine 12:372, 1987.
74. Kim, J. Y., Parnianpour, M., and Marras, W. S.: Quantitative measurement of neuromuscular control capability of the trunk during dynamic oscillatory bending movements. In 1993 Advances in Bioengineering, Vol 26. New York, American Society of Mechanical Engineers, 1993.
75. Kishino, N. D., Mayer, T. G., Gatchel, R. J., et al.: Quantification of lumbar function. Spine 10:921, 1985.
76. Klein, A. B., Snyder-Mackler, L., Roy, S., et al.: Comparison of spinal mobility and isometric trunk extensor forces with electromyographic spectral analysis in identifying low back pain. Phys. Ther. 71:445, 1991.
77. Klein, R. G., and Eek, B. C.: Low energy laser treatment and exercises for chronic low-back pain: Double blind controlled trial. Arch. Phys. Med. Rehabil. 71:34, 1991.
78. Kohles, S., Barnes, D., Gatchel, R. J., et al.: Improved physical performance outcomes after functional restoration treatment in patients with chronic low back pain: Early versus recent training results. Spine 15: 1321, 1990.
79. Kondraske, G. V.: Quantitative measurement and assessment of performance. In Smith R. V., and Leslie, J. H. (eds.): Rehabilitation Engineering, Boca Raton, FL, CRC, 1990, p. 101.
80. Kondraske, G. V., and Vasta, P. J.: Nonlinear Causal Resource Analysis: Concepts and Design of a Software Tool. Technical Report 91–008R. Arlington, TX, University of Texas, 1991.
81. Kroemer, K. H.: An isoinertial technique to assess individual lifting capability. Hum. Factors 25:493, 1983.
82. Kroemer, K. H. E., Marras, W. S., McGlothlin, J. D., et al.: On the measurement of human strength. Int. J. Ind. Ergonomics 6:199, 1990.
83. Lance, B. M., and Chaffin, D. B.: The effect of prior muscle exertions on simple movements. Hum. Factors 13:355, 1971.
84. Langrana, N., and Stover, C. N.: The correlation of clinical and Cybex isokinetic isometric assessment of back strength and its application to the preemployment physical examination. Proceedings of the 30th Annual Conference on Engineering in Medicine and Biology, 1977, p. 187.
85. Langrana, N. A., Lee, C. K., Alexander, H., et al.: Quantitative assessment of back strength using isokinetic testing. Spine 9:287, 1984.
86. Legg, S. J., and Myles, W. S.: Maximum acceptable repetitive lifting workloads for an 8-hour work day using psychophysical and subjective rating methods. Ergonomics 24:907, 1981.
87. Lehmann, T. R., Spratt, K. F., and Lehmann, K. K.: Predicting long-term disability in low back injured workers presenting to a spine consultant. Spine 18:1103, 1993.
88. Leskinen T. P. J.: Comparison of static and dynamic biomechanical models. Ergonomics 28:289, 1985.
89. Linström, I., Öhlun, C., Eek, C., et al.: Mobility,

strength, and fitness after a graded activity program for patients with subacute low back pain. Spine 17:641, 1992.
90. Liyang, D., Yinkan, X., Wenming, Z., et al.: The effect of flexion-extension motion on the capacity of the spinal canal. Spine 14:523, 1988.
91. Lowery, W. D., Horm, T. J., Boden, S. D., et al.: Impairment evaluation based on spinal range of motion in normal subjects. J. Spinal Disord. 5:398, 1992.
92. Luck, J. V., and Florence, D. W.: A brief history and comparative analysis of disability systems and impairment evaluation guides. Office Pract. 19:839, 1988.
93. McIntyre, D. R., Glover, L. H., Conino, M. C., et al.: A comparison of the characteristics of preferred low-back motion of normal subjects and low-back patients. J. Spinal Disord. 3:90, 1991.
94. McIntyre, D. R., Glover, L. H., and Reynolds, D. C.: Relationship between preferred and maximum effort low back motion. Clin. Biomech. 8:203, 1993.
95. Macintosch, J. E., and Bogduk, N.: The biomechanics of the lumbar multifidus. Clin. Biomech. 1:205, 1986.
96. McNeill, T., Warwick, D., Andersson, G., et al.: Trunk strength in attempted flexion, extension, and lateral bending in healthy subjects and patients with low back disorders. Spine 5:529–538, 1980.
97. Magora, A.: Investigation on the relation between low back pain and occupation: 4. Physical requirements. Bending, rotation, reaching, and sudden maximal effort. Scand. J. Rehabil. Med. 5:186–190, 1973.
98. Mandell, P. J., Weitz, E., Bernstein, J. I., et al.: Isokinetic trunk strength and lifting strength measures: Differences and similarities between low-back injured and noninjured workers. Spine 18:2491, 1993.
99. Marras, W. S., King, A. I., and Joynt, R. L.: Measurement of loads on the lumbar spine under isometric and isokinetic conditions. Spine 9:176, 1984.
100. Marras, W. S., and Wongsam, P. E.: Flexibility and velocity of normal and impaired lumbar spine. Arch. Phys. Med. Rehabil. 67:213, 1986.
101. Marras, W. S., and Reilly, C. H.: Networks of internal trunk-loading activities under controlled trunk motion conditions. Spine 13:661, 1988.
102. Marras, W. S., and Mirka, G. A.: Trunk strength during asymmetric trunk motion. Hum. Factors 31:667, 1989.
103. Marras, W. S., Lavender, S. A., Leurgan, S., et al.: The role of dynamic motion in occupationally-related low back disorders: The effects of workplace factors, trunk position, and trunk motion characteristics on injury. Spine 18:617, 1993.
104. Marras, W. S., Parnianpour, M., Ferguson, S. A., et al.: Quantification and classification of low back disorders based on trunk motion. Eur. J. Med. Rehabil. 3:218, 1993.
105. Marras, W. S., Parnianpour, M., Ferguson, S. A., et al.: The classification of anatomic and symptom based low back disorders using the motion measure model. Spine (in press)
106. Masset, D., Malchaire, J., and Lemoine, M.: Static and dynamic characteristics of the trunk and history of low back pain. Int. J. Ind. Ergonomics 11:279, 1993.
107. Matheson, L., Mooney, V., Caiozzo, V., et al.: Effect of instructions on isokinetic strength testing variability, reliability, absolute value, and predictive value. Spine 17:914, 1992.
108. Mayer, T. G., Gatchel, R. J., Kishino, N., et al.: Objective assessment of spine function following industrial injury. Spine 10:482, 1985.
109. Mayer, T. G., Smith, S. S., Keely, J., et al.: Quantification of lumbar function. Part 2. Sagittal plane trunk strength in chronic low back patients. Spine 10:765, 1985.
110. Mayer, T. G., Smith, S. S., Kondraske, G., et al.: Quantification of lumbar function. Part 3. Preliminary data on isokinetic torso rotation testing. Spine 10:912, 1985.
111. Mayer, T. G., Gatchel, T. J., Kishino, N., et al.: A prospective short-term study of chronic low back pain patients utilising novel objective functional measurement. Pain 25:53, 1986
112. Mayer, T. G., Gatchel, R. J., Mayer, H., et al.: A prospective two-year study of functional restoration in industrial low back injury: An objective assessment procedure. JAMA 258:1763, 1987.
113. Mayer, T. G.: Discussion: Exercise, fitness and back pain. In Bouchard, C. (ed.): Exercise, Fitness and Health: A Consensus of Current Knowledge. Champaign, IL, Human Kinetic Books, 1988, pp. 541–546.
114. Mayer, T., Barnes, D., Kishino, N., et al.: Progressive isoinertial lifting evaluation: I. A standardized protocol and normative database. Spine 13:993, 1988.
115. Mayer, T. G., Vanharanta, H., Gatchel, R. J., et al.: Comparison of CT scan muscle measurements and isokinetic trunk strength in postoperative patients. Spine 14:33, 1989.
116. Mayer, H., Barnes, D., Nichols, G., et al.: Progressive isoinertial lifting evaluation II. A comparison with isokinetic lifting in a disabled chronic low-back pain industrial population. Spine 13:998, 1988.
117. Mellin, G., Harkapaa, K., Vanharanta, H., et al.: Outcome of multimodal treatment including intensive physical training of patients with chronic low back pain. Spine 18:825, 1993.
118. Mital, A., Channaveerajah, C. E., Fard, H. F., et al.: Reliability of repetitive dynamic strengths as a screening tool for manual lifting tasks. Clin. Biomech. 1:125, 1986.
119. Mital, A., Karkowski, W., Mazouz, A. K., et al.: Prediction of maximum acceptable weight of lift in the horizontal and vertical planes using simulated job dynamic strengths. Am. Ind. Hyg. Assoc. J. 47:288, 1986.
120. Mostardi, R. A., Noe, D. A., Kovacik, M. W., et al.: Isokinetic lifting strength and occupational injury. A prospective study. Spine 17:189, 1992.
121. Mundt, D. J., Kelsey, J. L., Golden, A. L., et al.: An epidemiologic study of non-occupational lifting as a risk factor for herniated lumbar intervertebral disc. Spine 18:595, 1993.
122. Nachemson, A., and Lindh, M.: Measurement of abdominal and back muscle strength with and without low back pain. Scand. J. Rehabil. Med. 1:60, 1969.
123. Nachemson, A.: Work for all. Clin. Orthop. 179:77, 1983.

124. Nachemson, A.: Recent advances in the treatment of low back pain. Int. Orthop. 9:1, 1985.
125. National Institute for Occupational Safety and Health (NIOSH): Work Practices Guide for Manual Lifting (DHHS Publication no. 81–122). Washington, DC. U.S. Government Printing Office, 1981.
126. Newton, M., Morag, T., Somerville, D., et al.: Trunk strength testing with iso-machines, Part 2: Experimental evaluation of the Cybex II Back Testing System in normal subjects and patients with chronic low back pain. Spine 18:812, 1993.
127. Newton, M., and Waddell, G.: Trunk strength testing with iso-machines. Part 1: Review of a decade of scientific evidence. Spine 18:801, 1993.
128. Nicolaisen, T., and Jorgensen, K.: Trunk strength, back muscles endurance and low back trouble. Scand. J. Rehabil. Med. 17:121, 1985.
129. Nordin, M., Kahanovitz, N., Verderame, R., et al.: Normal trunk muscle strength and endurance in women and the effect of exercises and electrical stimulation. Part 1: Normal endurance and trunk muscle strength in 101 women. Spine 12:105, 1987.
130. Parnianpour, M., Nordin, N., Moritz, U., and Kahanowitz, N.: Correlation between different tests of trunk strength. In Buckle, P. (ed.): Musculoskeletal Disorders at Work. New York, Taylor & Francis, 1987.
131. Parnianpour, M.: The Effect of Fatiguing Isoinertial Trunk Flexion and Extension Movement on Patterns of Movement and Motor Output. Unpublished Doctoral Dissertation. New York, New York University, 1988.
132. Parnianpour, M., Nordin, M., Kahanovitz, N., and Frankel, V. H.: The triaxial coupling of torque generation of trunk muscles during isometric exertions and the effect of fatiguing isoinertial movements on the motor output and movement patterns. Spine 13:982, 1988.
133. Parnianpour, M., and Laferriere, G.: Minimum jerk and near energy optimal trajectories of sagittal trunk movement. In 1990 Advances in Bioengineering, Vol. 17. New York, American Society of Mechanical Engineers, 1990, p. 159.
134. Parnianpour, M., Nordin, M., and Sheikhzadeh, A.: The relationship of torque, velocity, and power with constant resistive load during sagittal trunk movement. Spine 15:639, 1990.
135. Parnianpour, M., Zkaya, N., Nordin, M., et al.: Phase plane analysis of isoinertial trunk performance: Quantitative measurement of "spinal signature." In 1989 Advances in Bioengineering, Vol. 15. New York, American Society of Mechanical Engineers, 1990, p. 51.
136. Parnianpour, M., Campello, M., and Sheikhzadeh, A.: The effect of posture on triaxial trunk strength in different directions. Int. J. Ind. Ergonomics 8:279, 1991.
137. Parnianpour, M., and Hoffer, H.: The effect of kinematic constraints, levels of resistance and directions of exertions during isometric and isoinertial axial trunk rotation on the motor output and muscle activity. Proceedings of 1991 Engineering Systems Design and Analysis Conference, 1992.
138. Parnianpour, M., Hasselquist, L., Fagan, L., et al.: Correlation among isometric, isokinetic, and isoinertial muscle performance during multi-joint coordinated exertions and isolated single joint trunk exertion. Eur. J. Med. Rehabil. 3:114, 1993.
139. Parnianpour, M., Hanson, T., Goldman, S., et al.: Heterogeneity of low back pain patients: Towards consideration of the variability of their dynamic continuous movement profile. North American Spine Society Meeting, Hawaii, April 18–21, 1994.
140. Penning, L., and Wilmink, J. T.: Posture dependent bilateral compression of L4 or L5 nerve roots in facet hypertrophy. Spine 12:488, 1987.
141. Pitman, M. I., and Peterson, L.: Biomechanics of skeletal muscle. In Nordin, M., and Frankel, V. (eds.): Basic Biomechanics of the Musculoskeletal System, 2nd Ed. Philadelphia, Lea & Febiger, 1989, p. 89.
142. Pope, M. H.: A critical evaluation of functional muscle testing. In Weinstein, J. N. (ed.): Clinical Efficacy and Outcome in the Diagnosis and Treatment of Low Back Pain. New York, Raven Press, 1992, p. 101.
143. Porterfield, J. A., Mostardi, R. A., King, S., et al.: Simulated lift testing using computerized isokinetics. Spine 12:683, 1987.
144. Potvin, J. R.: The Influence of Fatigue on Hypothesized Mechanisms of Injury to Low Back During Repetitive Lifting. Unpublished Doctoral Thesis. Waterloo, Canada, University of Waterloo, 1992.
145. Rainville, J., Ahern, D. K., Phalen, L., et al.: The association of pain with physical activities in chronic low back pain. Spine 17:1060, 1992.
146. Reid, S., Hazard, G. H., and Fenwick, J. W.: Isokinetic trunk strength deficits in people with and without low back pain: A comparative study with consideration of effort. J. Spinal Disord. 4:68, 1991.
147. Risch, S. V., Norvell, N. K., Pollock, M. L., et al.: Lumbar strengthening in chronic low back pain patients: Physiologic and psychological benefits. Spine 18:232, 1993.
148. Rodgers, M. M., and Cavanagh, P. R.: Glossary of biomechanical terms, concepts, and units. Phys. Ther. 64:1886, 1984.
149. Ross, E. C.: The effect of resistance level on muscle coordination patterns and truncal velocity, acceleration and deceleration during isoinertial trunk extension. Unpublished Doctoral Thesis, New York, New York University, 1991.
150. Ross, E. C., Parnianpour, M., and Martin, D.: Timing and amplitude of trunk activity during extension under varying loading conditions. Spine 18:1829, 1993.
151. Roy, S. H., DeLuca, C. J., and Casavant, D. A.: Lumbar muscle fatigue and chronic low back pain. Spine 14:992, 1989.
152. Sapega, A. A.: Muscle performance evaluation in orthopaedic practice. J. Bone Joint Surg. 72A:1562, 1990.
153. Schmitz, T. J.: The Effect of Direction and Resistance Level on Muscle Coordination Patterns and Truncal Velocity, Acceleration and Deceleration During Unidirectional Isoinertial Trunk Flexion and Extension of Healthy Males. Unpublished Doctoral Thesis. New York, New York University, 1992.
154. Schultz, A., and Andersson, G.: Analysis of loads on the lumbar spine. Spine 6:76, 1981.
155. Seeds, R. H., Levene, J. A., and Goldberg, H. M.: Abnormal patient data for the Isostation B100. J. Orthop. Sports Phys. Ther. 9:121, 1988.

156. Smidt, G., Herring, T., Amundsen, L., et al.: Assessment of abdominal and back extensor function: A quantitative approach and results of chronic low back patients. Spine 8:211, 1983.
157. Smidt, G. L., and Blanpied, P. R.: Analysis of strength tests and resistive exercises commonly used for low back disorders Spine 12:1025, 1987.
158. Smidt, G. L., Blanpied, P. R., and White, W. W.: Exploration of mechanical and electromyographic responses of trunk muscles to high-intensity resistive exercise. Spine 14:815, 1989.
159. Snijders, C. J., Van Riel, M. D., and Nordin, M.: Continuous measurements of spine movements in normal working situations over periods of 8 hours or more. Ergonomics 30:639, 1987.
160. Snook, S. H., and Irvine, C. H.: Maximal acceptable weight of lift. Am. Ind. Hyg. Assoc. J. 28:322, 1967.
161. Snook, S. H.: The design of manual handling tasks. Ergonomics 21:963, 1978.
162. Snook, S. H.: Psychophysical acceptability as a constraint in manual working capacity. Ergonomics 28:327, 1985.
163. Sparto, P., Parnianpour, M., and Khalaf, K.: The reliability and validity of a lift simulator and its functional equivalence with free weight lifting task. IEEE Trans. Rehabil. Eng. 3:155, 1995.
164. Spengler, D. M., and Szpalski, M.: Newer assessment approaches for the patient with low back pain. Contemp. Orthop. 21:371, 1990.
165. Szpalski, M., and Hayez, J. P.: How many days of bed-rest for acute low back pain? Objective assessment of trunk function. Eur. Spine J. 1:29, 1992.
166. Szpalski, M., Hayez, J. P. Debaize, J. P., and Spengler, D. M.: Velocity of trunk movements, most sensitive variable of low-back condition. A prospective study. Orthop. Trans. 16:254, 1992.
167. Szpalski, M., Michel, F., and Hayez, J. P.: Sagittal isoinertial movement patterns associated with spinal pathologies. International Society for the Study of the Lumbar Spine, Marseille, June 1993.
168. Szpalski, M., Ray, J., Keller, T. S., et al.: Analysis of trunk flexor and extensor fatigue during isoinertial sagittal movements. Orthop. Trans. 17:332, 1993.
169. Szpalski, M., and Hayez, J. P.: Objective functional assessment of the efficacy of tenoxicam in the treatment of acute low back pain. A double blind placebo controlled study. Br. J. Rheumatol. 33:74, 1994.
170. Szpalski, M., and Hayez, J. P.: L'évaluation fonctionnelle des protrusions discales. In Lucas, P., and Stehman, M. (eds.), Actualités du dommage corporel, Vol. 3. La hernie discale. Brussels, Juridoc, 1994.
171. Suzuki, N., and Endo, S.: A quantitative study of trunk muscle strength and fatigability in the low back pain syndrome. Spine 8:69, 1983.
172. Talo, S., Rytokoski, U., and Puukka, P.: Patient classification, a key to evaluate pain treatment: A psychological study in chronic low back pain patients. Spine 17:998, 1992.
173. Tan, J. C.: The Effect of Sagittal-Standing Trunk Posture on Temporal and Amplitude Recruitment Patterns, and Triaxial Torques of Trunk Muscles During Isometric Trunk Extension. Unpublished Doctoral Dissertation. New York, New York University, 1991.
174. Tan, J. C., Parnianpour, M., Nordin, M., et al.: Isometric maximal and submaximal trunk exertion at different flexed positions in standing: Triaxial torque output and EMG. Spine 18:2480, 1993.
175. Thompson, D. A., and Biedermann, H. J.: Electromyographic power spectrum analysis of the paraspinal muscles: Long-term reliability. Spine 18:2310, 1993.
176. Thorstensson, A., and Nilsson, J.: Trunk muscle strength during constant velocity movements. Scand. J. Rehabil. Med. 14:61, 1982.
177. Toussaint, H. M., van Baar, C. E., van Langen, P. P., et al.: Coordination of the leg muscles in backlift and leglift. J. Biomech 25:1279, 1992.
178. Troup, J. D. G., Martin, J. W., and Lloyd, D. C.: Back pain in industry: A prospective study. Spine 6:61, 1981.
179. Troup, J. D. G., Foreman, T. K. Baxter, C. E., et al.: The perception of back pain and the role of psychophysical tests of lifting capacity. Spine 12:645, 1987.
180. Tucci, J. T., Carpenter, D. M., Pollock, M. L., et al.: Effects of reduced frequency of training and detraining on lumbar extension strength. Spine 17:1497, 1992.
181. Waddell, G., Main, C. J., Morris, E. W., et al.: Normality and reliability in the clinical assessment of backache. Br. Med. J. 284:1519, 1982.
182. Weitz, E. M.: The lateral bending sign. Spine 6:388, 1981.
183. Werneke, M. W., Harris, D. E., and Lichter, R. L.: Clinical effectiveness of behavioral signs for screening chronic low-back pain patients in a work-oriented physical rehabilitation program. Spine 18:2412, 1993.
184. Wilder, D. G., Pope, M. H. Seroussi, R. E., et al.: Sudden unstable rotation responses to an overload in the lumbar spine. Proceedings of the International Society for the Study of the Lumbar Spine, 1987, p. 76.
185. Winters, J. M., and Woos, L. Y.: Multiple Muscle System. New York, Springer-Verlag, 1990.
186. Wood, G. A., and Hayes, K. C.: A kinetic model of intervertebral stress during lifting. Br. J. Sports Med. 8:74, 1974.
187. Yang, J. F., and Winter, D. A.: Electromyography reliability in maximal and submaximal isometric contractions. Arch. Phys. Med. Rehabil. 64:417, 1983.
188. Zhu, X., Parnianpour, M., Nordin M., et al.: Histochemistry and morphology of erector spinae muscle in lumbar disc herniation. Spine 14:391, 1989.

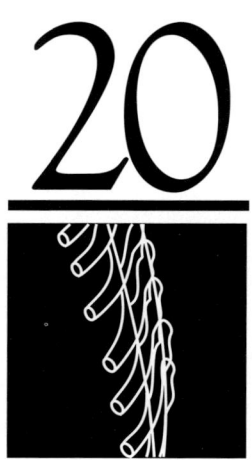

20

Multiply Operated Lumbar Spine: Algorithmic Approach

SAM W. WIESEL
STEPHEN EISENSTEIN
RICHARD DELAMARTER
JOHN DOVE
SCOTT BODEN

Surgery on the lumbar spine is not always successful. The patient who has undergone one or more low back operations with continued discomfort is becoming an ever-increasing problem for the spine physician. It is estimated that 300,000 new laminectomies are performed each year in the United States alone and that 15% of these patients will continue to have significant pain.[19] The inherent complexity of these cases, especially when confounded by the degeneration of the aging spine, necessitates a method of problem solving that is precise and unambiguous.

The best possible strategy for preventing recurrent symptoms after spine surgery is to avoid inappropriate surgery whenever possible. It cannot be overstressed that proper surgical indications must be present before surgery is undertaken. The idea of exploring the low back when the necessary objective criteria are not met is no longer acceptable. In fact, even when there are objective findings, if the patient is psychologically unstable or there are compensation or litigation factors, the outcome of low back surgery is uncertain.[20, 21] Thus, the initial decision to operate is the most important one. Once the situation of recurrent pain after surgery arises, the potential for a solution is limited at best.[9]

In the evaluation of recurrent symptoms after surgery, the first problem confronting the physician is to distinguish mechanical and nonmechanical causes. The common types of mechanical lesions include recurrent herniated disc, spinal instability, and spinal stenosis. These three entities produce symptoms by causing direct pressure on the neural elements and are amenable to surgical intervention. The nonmechanical entities consist of scar tissue (either arachnoiditis or epidural fibrosis), discitis, psychosocial instability, and systemic medical disease. These problems are not helped by any type of additional lumbar spine surgery.

The keystone of successful treatment of the multiply operated spine is to obtain an accurate diagnosis. Although seemingly obvious, this essential step is often not taken. Consequently, rehabilitation of this patient group has been fraught with difficulty. The goals of this chapter are to analyze the significant decision points in the evaluation of the multiply operated lumbar spine patient and to organize this information into a standardized approach for efficiently obtaining an accurate diagnosis. Finally, the technique of revision spine surgery is reviewed.

PATIENT EVALUATION

When a multiply operated back patient first arrives for evaluation, it is important to obtain all the vital information in an organized manner. The use of a standardized approach may lessen the chance of missing significant details. This is important, for these patients are usually difficult to evaluate.

History

The evaluation of the multiply operated low back patient must begin with the history, which can be complicated. Many patients want to relate their entire story to the evaluating physician, and it is best to let them do so. After the patient finishes talking, however, there are three specific historical points that must be elucidated.

The first is the number of previous lumbar spine operations that the patient has undergone. With every subsequent operation, regardless of the diagnosis, the likelihood of good results diminishes. Statistically, the second operation has a 50% chance of success, and beyond two operations, patients are more likely to be made worse than better.[9]

The next important historical point is the length of the pain-free interval after the patient's previous operation. If the patient awoke from surgery with pain still present, it is likely that the nerve root was not properly decompressed or that the wrong level was explored. If the pain-free interval was at least 6 months, the patient's current pain may be caused by recurrent disc herniation at the same or a different level. If the pain-free interval was between 1 and 6 months and recurrent symptoms had a gradual onset, the diagnosis is most often some type of scar tissue, either arachnoiditis or epidural fibrosis.

Finally, the patient's pain pattern must be evaluated. If leg pain predominates, a herniated disc or spinal stenosis is most likely, although scar tissue is also a possibility.[8] If back pain is the main component, instability, tumor, infection, and scar tissue are the major considerations. If both back and leg pain are present, spinal stenosis and/or scar tissue is a likely possibility. Nonmechanical pain, especially in older patients, may be the harbinger of an infectious, neoplastic, or referred process unrelated to the original low back pain.

Physical Examination

Physical examination is the next major step in the evaluation of the multiply operated back patient. The neurologic findings and the existence of a tension sign, such as a positive sitting straight leg raising test, must be noted. It is helpful to have the results of a dependable previous examination so a comparison between the preoperative and postoperative states can be made. If the neurologic picture is unchanged from that before the previous surgery and the tension sign is absent, mechanical compression is unlikely. If, however, a new neurologic deficit has occurred since the previous surgery or the tension sign is positive, pressure on the neural elements is possible. However, one should recognize that epidural or perineural fibrosis can cause a positive tension sign; the tension sign is not pathognomonic of a mechanical lesion in these patients.

Nonorganic physical signs should also be carefully evaluated. In some cases, even if a true mechanical problem exists, the surgical outcome may be less than ideal if nonorganic findings are present. Waddell[21] developed a simple set of nonorganic signs that are easy to assess. If three or more of his signs are present, one should be careful about surgery.

Imaging Modalities

Imaging studies are the last major part of the patient's workup. It is most helpful to have the results of prior studies for comparison of the preoperative and postoperative situations. Often, careful analysis may reveal that the initial operation was not indicated. The following discussion focuses on specific applications of these techniques in evaluating the multiply operated low back patient.

The plain radiograph must be evaluated for the extent and level of previous laminectomies and for any evidence of spinal stenosis. It should not be taken for granted that the correct level was decompressed; the laminectomy level on the plain radiograph must correspond to the level on the preoperative radiographic studies, to the level described in the operative report, and to the neurologic findings demonstrated by the patient. The standing (weight-bearing) lateral flexion-extension radiographs must be assessed for any evidence of abnormal motion (see under Lumbar Instability below).

Water-soluble myelography in the multiply operated back patient with chronic pain can be of some value. Although this test can identify extradural compressions, myelography cannot distinguish between disc material and epidural scar tissue.[2] The major information obtained from myelography is used for confirming arachnoiditis when the diagnosis is otherwise uncertain.[17]

Computed tomographic (CT) scanning after contrast medium injection in the subarachnoid space is also a sensitive test for demonstrating the changes of arachnoiditis. CT scanning is rarely used alone to evaluate the multiply operated back patient. It is usually employed after myelography. The size of the spinal canal, surgical deficits, and hypertrophied bony changes causing stenosis are well visualized.

Magnetic resonance imaging (MRI) scanning is the most useful diagnostic tool to distinguish a recurrent residual disc herniation from epidural scar tissue.[2, 11] Intravenous contrast medium enhancement with gadolinium-labeled pentetic acid (Gd-DTPA) identifies scar tissue because it is vascular. On the other hand, a herniated disc is avascular and does not enhance after the injection of Gd-DTPA. However, for the first 6 months after surgery, a gadolinium-enhanced MRI scan may reveal pathologic changes, including persistent herniated disc material, despite the complete relief of symptoms.[1] There is an orderly progression of imaging changes during the first 6 months after lumbar surgery that limits the interpretation of MRI scanning during this time period. Thus, even in patients who have undergone successful decompression, a residual mass effect on the neural elements may frequently simulate a recurrent or residual disc fragment. MRI scans during the initial 6 months postoperatively, even when enhanced with Gd-DTPA, must be interpreted with extreme caution.

Finally, the MRI scan is also a good screening tool for other types of processes that can cause back pain and that may cause continued symptoms after previous back surgery. These include metabolic abnormalities and other types of infections and tumors of the spine.

DIAGNOSIS

The primary goal in the evaluation of the multiply operated back patient is to identify the specific diagnosis correctly. Although this seems obvious, it is not done in many cases. The most common lesions accounting for failed back surgery syndrome include recurrent or persistent disc herniation (12% to 16%), lateral (58%) or central (7% to 14%) stenosis, arachnoiditis (6% to 16%), epidural fibrosis (6% to 8%), and instability (<5%).[4] The various pathologic entities with their associated signs, symptoms, and radiographic findings are summarized in Table 1. The same data are presented in Figure 1 as an algorithm.

Extraspinal Problems

The first step in the algorithm is to determine whether the patient's symptoms are based on a nonorthopedic cause, such as pancreatitis, diabetes, and an abdominal aneurysm. Thus, a thorough general medical examination should be obtained routinely. If a systemic problem is revealed, it should be treated appropriately. In addition, the patient's psychosocial makeup should also be evaluated, and specific adverse factors, such as alcoholism, drug dependence, and

Table 1

Differential Diagnosis of the Multiply Operated Back

History, Physical Examination, Radiographs	Original Disc Not Removed	Recurrent Disc at Same Level	Recurrent Disc at Different Level	Spinal Instability	Spinal Stenosis	Arachnoiditis	Epidural Scar Tissue	Discitis
Pain-free interval	None	>6 months	>6 months			>1 month but <6 months	>1 month, gradual onset	
Predominant pain: leg vs. back	Leg pain	Leg pain	Leg pain	Back pain	Back and leg pain	Back and leg pain	Back and/or leg pain	Back pain
Tension sign	+ with same pattern	+ with same pattern	+ at different level			May be positive	May be positive	
Neurologic examination	+ with same pattern	+ with same pattern	+ at different level		+ after stress			
Plain films	+ at wrong level				+			±
Lateral motion films				+				
Metrizamide myelogram	+ but unchanged	+ at same level	+ at different level		+	+	+	
CT scan	+	+	+		+	+	+ (IV contrast) + (gadolinium contrast)	+ (IV contrast)
MRI scan	+	+	+		+	+	+	+

From Boden, S. D., Wiesel, S. W., Laws, E. R., Jr., and Rothman, R. H.: The Aging Spine. Philadelphia, W. B. Saunders, 1991.

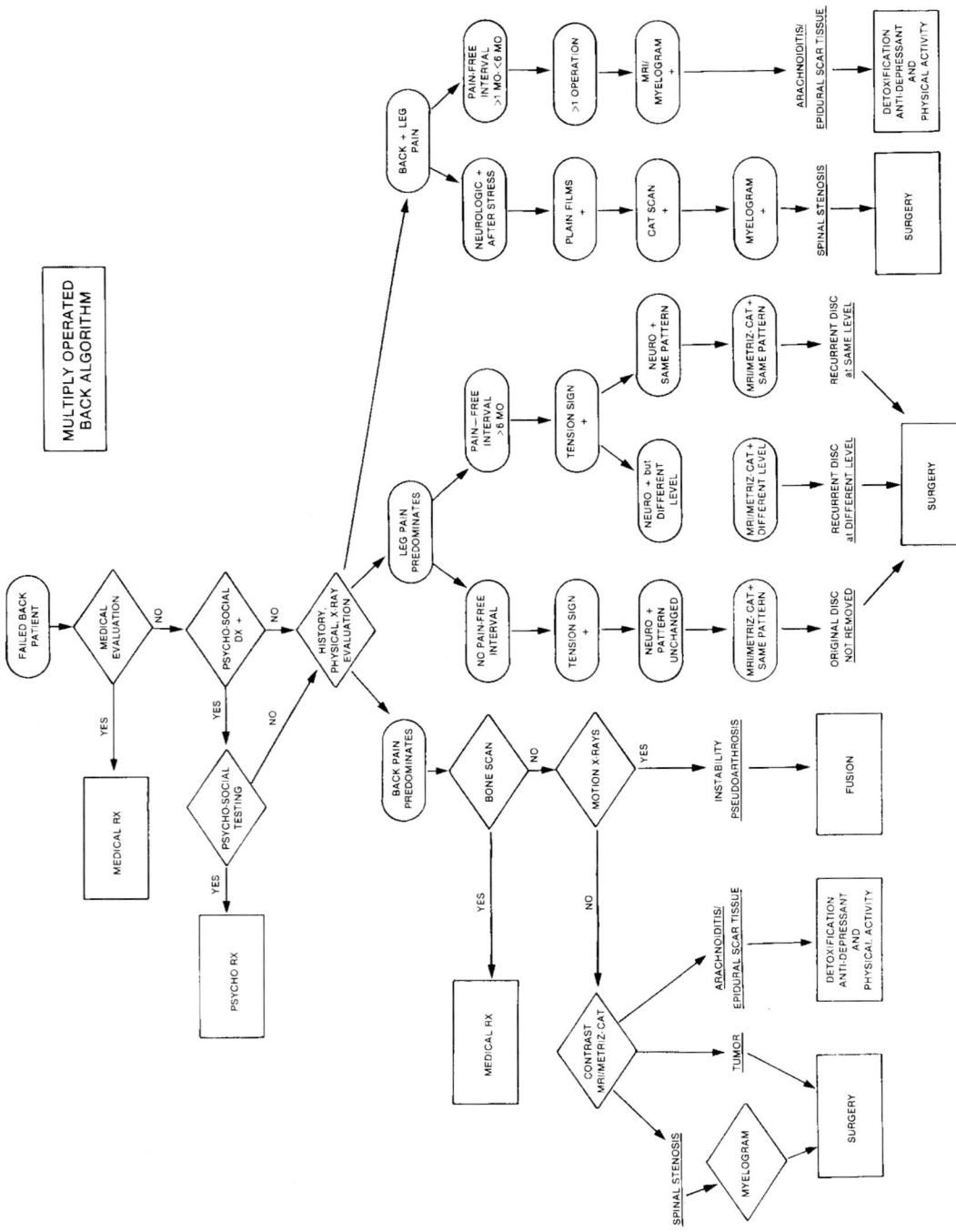

Figure 1. Evaluation of the multiply operated back. (From Boden, S. D., Wiesel, S. W., Laws, E. R., Jr., and Rothman, R. H.: The Aging Spine. Philadelphia, W. B. Saunders, 1991.)

depression, and ongoing compensation or litigation issues should be identified. It has been clearly demonstrated that persons with profound emotional disturbances and those involved in litigation do not derive any significant benefit from additional surgery.[18] Even if a specific anatomic diagnosis is made, psychosocial problems should be addressed first. In many cases, after a patient's underlying psychosocial problem has been treated successfully, the somatic back symptoms and disability significantly lessen or disappear.

After patients with medical and psychosocial problems are identified and eliminated, the physician is left with a group of people who have back pain and/or leg pain. The goal is then to separate patients who have specific mechanical problems from patients whose symptoms are secondary to some form of scar tissue or inflammation. The former may benefit from additional surgery; the latter do not. Surgically correctable problems are rare.

Mechanical Lesions

Herniated Intervertebral Disc

Three possibilities exist if the patient's pain is caused by a herniated disc. First, the disc that caused the original symptoms may not have been satisfactorily removed. This can happen if the wrong level was explored, if the decompression performed was not adequate to free the neural elements, or if a fragment of disc material was left behind. Such patients continue to have pain because of mechanical pressure on and irritation of the same nerve root that caused their initial symptoms. They report predominantly leg pain, and their neurologic findings, tension signs, and radiographic patterns remain unchanged from the preoperative state. The distinguishing feature is that they report no pain-free interval; they awaken from surgery reporting the same pain as experienced preoperatively. Patients in this group are aided by a technically correct laminectomy and discectomy.

A second possibility is that there is a recurrent herniated intervertebral disc at the previously decompressed level. These patients report sciatica and have unchanged neurologic findings, tension signs, and radiographic studies. The distinguishing characteristic is a pain-free interval of longer than 6 months. A repeated operative procedure is indicated in these patients, provided that the MRI scan can demonstrate herniated disc material rather than just scar tissue after 6 months.

Finally, a herniated disc can occur at a completely different level. Such patients generally experience sudden onset of recurrent pain after a pain-free interval of longer than 6 months. Sciatica predominates and tension signs are positive. However, a neurologic deficit, if present, and radiographic signs are seen at a different level than on the original studies. A repeated operation for these patients is beneficial.

Lumbar Instability

Lumbar instability is another mechanical condition causing pain in the multiply operated back patient. Instability is the abnormal or excessive movement of one vertebra on another, causing pain.[12, 22] The origin may be the patient's intrinsic back disease, such a spondylolisthesis, or an excessively wide bilateral laminectomy. Pseudarthrosis resulting from failed spine fusion is included in this category because pain is caused by the instability created by the failed fusion.

Patients with instability usually report predominantly back pain but the physical examination findings may be normal. Sometimes, the key to diagnosis of these patients is weight-bearing, lateral flexion-extension radiography; however, it is often difficult to define precisely the anatomic origin of back pain in the presence of radiographic instability. Relative flexion–sagittal plane translation of greater than 12% of the anteroposterior diameter of the vertebral body and relative flexion–sagittal plane rotation of greater than 11 degrees between segments are the most commonly cited guidelines for instability of the lumbar spine. At the lumbosacral junction, the criteria are slightly different: relative translation of greater than 25% or rotation of greater than 19 degrees indicates instability.[22] These criteria are based on maximum displacements on a single flexion or extension view. However, dynamic measurements of relative translation and rotation from flexion to extension may prove to be a more reliable indication of true instability.

Unfortunately, there is little information explaining why some patients with segmental instability have back pain yet others do not. If there is radiographic evidence of instability in symptomatic patients, spine fusion or repair of the pseudarthrosis may be considered.[5] Additional confirmatory evidence to determine the precise level of origin of the patient's symptoms may be gathered from studies such as facet injections and discography. However, these tests have a substantial rate of false-positive results. Many patients who have known pseudarthrosis are asymptomatic, so one should be extremely careful before assuming that the pseudarthrosis is the origin of the patient's symptoms. This is particularly true if the indications for the original fusion were questionable.

Spinal Stenosis

Spinal stenosis in the multiply operated back patient can mechanically produce back and/or leg pain. The pain may be secondary to progression of inherent degenerative spinal disease, a previous inadequate decompression, or overgrowth of a previous posterior fusion. The physical examination findings are usually inconclusive, although a neurologic deficit may occur after exercise, with reproduction of the patient's symptoms. This phenomenon is termed a positive stress test.[18]

The plain radiographs can be suggestive of and may display facet degeneration, decreased interpedicle distance, decreased sagittal canal diameter, and disc degeneration. A postmyelographic CT scan demonstrates bony encroachment on the neural elements. This is especially helpful in evaluating the lateral recesses and neural foramina. An MRI scan shows compression of the dural sac at the involved levels. Spinal stenosis and scar tissue can coexist.[8] Good results can be expected from surgery in at least 70% of properly selected patients with spinal stenosis, whereas surgery in patients with previous laminectomy and spine fusions is less successful. If definite evidence of bony compression is present, a revision decompression is indicated. However, if substantial scar tissue is present, the degree of pain relief that may be anticipated is uncertain. Selective diagnostic nerve root blocks may be helpful to isolate a level producing particularly severe symptoms. Although this maneuver can help to direct revision surgery to the symptomatic level, it does not distinguish root pain due to mechanical compression from that due to scarring.

Nonmechanical Entities

Scar tissue (arachnoiditis or epidural fibrosis) and discitis are nonmechanical causes of recurrent pain in the multiply operated back patient. Although the causes and specific locations of these lesions differ, they are discussed together because they do not respond to repeated surgical procedure.

Postoperative scar tissue formation can be divided into two main types on the basis of anatomic location. Scar tissue that occurs within the dura is commonly referred to as arachnoiditis. Scar tissue can also form extradurally, either directly on the cauda equina or around the nerve root.

Arachnoiditis

Arachnoiditis is strictly defined as an inflammation of the pia-arachnoid membrane surrounding the spinal cord or the cauda equina.[3, 16] The condition may be present in varying degrees of severity, from mild thickening of the membranes to solid adhesions. The scarring may be severe enough to obliterate the subarachnoid space and block the flow of contrast agents.

The cause of this condition has been attributed to many factors; lumbar spine surgery and previous injections of contrast material seem to be the most frequent precipitating factors.[15] Oil-based dye, formerly used in myelography, is strongly associated with the occurrence of arachnoiditis. Postoperative infection may also play a role in the pathogenesis. The exact mechanism by which arachnoiditis develops from these events is not clear.

There is no uniform clinical presentation for arachnoiditis. The history usually reveals more than one previous operation and a pain-free interval of between 1 and 6 months. Often, these patients report back and leg pain. Physical examination is inconclusive; alterations in neurologic status may be due to a previous operation. As mentioned earlier, CT scanning myelography and MRI scanning can be helpful to confirm the diagnosis.

At present, there is no effective treatment of arachnoiditis. Surgical intervention has not proved effective in eliminating the scar tissue or significantly reducing the pain. Along with much-needed encouragement, various nonoperative measures can be used. The administration of epidural steroids, transcutaneous electrical nerve stimulation, spinal cord stimulation, operant conditioning, bracing, and patient education have all been tried. None of these leads to a cure, but when used judiciously, they provide symptomatic relief for varying periods. Patients should be detoxified from all narcotics, given amitriptyline hydrochloride (Elavil), and encouraged to perform as much physical activity as possible. Treating these patients is a real challenge, and the physician must be willing to devote time and patience to achieve optimum results.

Epidural Scar Tissue

Formation of scar tissue outside the dura on the cauda equina or directly on the nerve roots is relatively common.[15] This epidural scar tissue can act as a constrictive force about the neural elements, and it frequently causes postoperative pain. However, although most patients have some epidural scar tissue, only an unpredictable few become symptomatic.

Patients with epidural scarring may present with symptoms at any time—from several months to a year after surgery. The onset is gradual, and patients generally report back pain and/or leg pain. Commonly, neurologic findings are absent, although a positive tension sign may occur, purely on the basis of scar formation around a nerve root. The diagnosis is best differentiated from a recurrent herniated disc by using contrast-enhanced CT[2] or gadolinium-enhanced MRI scanning.[11]

As with arachnoiditis, there is no definitive treatment of epidural scar tissue. Prevention may be the best answer, and a free-fat graft is sometimes used as an interposition membrane to minimize scar tissue after laminectomy.[15] Once a scar has formed, surgery is not successful because scarring will reform in greater quantity. The treatment program should be similar to that already described for arachnoiditis.

Discitis

Discitis is an uncommon but debilitating complication of lumbar disc surgery. Its pathogenesis is postulated to be direct inoculation of the avascular disc space but is not completely understood.[6] The onset of symptoms is usually 1 month after surgery, and most patients report severe back pain. Physical examination sometimes reveals fever, a positive tension sign, and occasionally a superficial abscess.

If discitis is suspected from the history and physical examination, an erythrocyte sedimentation rate, blood cultures, and a plain radiograph should be obtained. In the acute postoperative period, the C-reactive protein level may be a more specific indicator than the erythrocyte sedimentation rate. Plain radiographs may not demonstrate the changes of disc space narrowing and end-plate erosion in early stages. Contrast-enhanced MRI should confirm the diagnosis.[14]

Effective treatment has been controversial. It is recommended that the patient be restricted to short-term bed rest with immobilization of the lumbar spine, with or without a brace or corset. If the patient experiences progressive pain after adequate immobilization or has constitutional symptoms, a needle aspiration should be performed. If a bacterial organism is identified, administration of antibiotics is indicated. There is no need for open disc space biopsy if the patient responds to conservative therapy. With improvement of symptoms (e.g., pain relief and normal erythrocyte sedimentation rate), the patient may ambulate as tolerated.

SURGICAL TECHNIQUES

Operating on the lumbar spine after it has been operated on previously can be a challenge. The actual technique of a repeated laminectomy is somewhat different from that of the initial operation. The morbidity is certainly greater, with the danger of tearing the dura ever present. The techniques for both a repeated laminectomy and the repair of a dural tear are presented.

Repeated Decompression

The goal of a decompression in the multiply operated back patient is the same as that for the initial procedure: to decompress the neural elements safely but completely without causing excessive hemorrhage. Unfortunately, after the spine has already been operated on, the anatomic features are no longer as distinct, and a great deal of scar tissue can be present. Thus, several technical aspects of performing a repeated laminectomy are different from those for a primary procedure.

The first difference involves the operative approach. The surgeon cannot strip the paraspinal muscles away with impunity because no lamina or ligamentum flavum is present to protect the neural elements at the previously operated sites. This means that one must begin the approach at a new anatomic level, which is normal and protected, to find the correct depth of the cauda equina (neural elements).

The surgeon may also be tempted, after the depth of the neural elements is determined, to remove the extradural scar tissue directly from the dura. Technically, this is difficult, and there is a great deal of hemorrhage and a strong possibility of injury to the dura. Even if the scar tissue is successfully removed, there is no good way to prevent its regrowth. Therefore, it is recommended that, in most cases, the extradural scar tissue should be left intact. Only tissue that is covering the area of pathologic change should be removed. Otherwise, the operative plane should be developed by elevating the scar (and dura) away from the bone at the lateral margin of the old laminectomy.

Finally, the object of the surgical procedure is to visualize the nerve roots laterally and to remove any mechanical pressure on them. This is accomplished by extension of the laminectomy from the new level down the lateral gutters, leaving the central scar tissue as is. As each nerve root is identified, any bony encroachment or herniated disc material at that level can then be easily removed. It is essential not only to visualize the nerve root to the dorsal root ganglion and to enlarge the foramen, but also to ensure that the root is mobile.

A fusion does not necessarily need to be performed routinely in a multiply operated back patient. If there are preoperative signs of instability on the lateral flexion-extension roentgenograms, a fusion is indicated. Also, if the laminectomy is widened during surgery so that, at any level, 50% of the facet joints bilaterally are destroyed or the pars interarticularis is thinned, a potentially unstable situation is created and a fusion should be considered. A bilateral lateral fusion is recommended in these circumstances, and both the patient and the surgeon should be prepared for this possibility.

If a previous fusion has been performed in a patient who is being operated on, the integrity of the bony mass should be checked. This can be extremely difficult to accomplish. Unless there are objective signs on flexion-extension radiographs of instability with horizontal translation, there can be many instances in which a nonunited fusion is missed. After the fusion mass is identified laterally, an osteotome can be used to shave off the outer surface to see whether the bone is contiguous throughout. If a defect is identified, the areas should be decorticated and new bone added. It is difficult, as stated before, to decide whether a patient's symptoms are the result of a nonunion. In many instances, the fusion does not heal, yet the patient is asymptomatic.

Repair of Dural Tears

The risk of causing a dural tear is definitely increased in the multiply operated back patient. Thus, the surgeon should be prepared to deal with this complication. Although each dural tear is different, certain basic principles always should be considered.

A dural tear usually occurs as the surgeon is gaining visualization of the spinal canal. This can result when a small fold of the dura is inadvertently pinched by a bone-biting instrument. Alternatively, the removal of adhesions to the undersurface of bone can also be a cause. When a tear occurs, the wound usually fills quickly with cerebrospinal fluid (CSF), obscuring the extent of the damage. The surgeon's first impulse is to try to see the tear by using suction in the approximate area of the problem. This is a mistake because the individual nerve roots may be sucked up, causing extensive neurologic damage. One should use suction only over a Cottonoid patty so that no further damage is done. After the tear is visualized, the surgeon places a piece of absorbable gelatin sponge (Gelfoam) over the injury site—with a large Cottonoid covering the entire area—and obtains adequate exposure of the tear. The patient's head should be tilted down to decrease the flow of CSF in the wound.

After adequate exposure is obtained, attention can be turned to repair of the dural tear. The goal is to achieve a watertight closure. If this is not accomplished, a CSF fistula can form, raising the risk of meningitis or a subarachnoid cyst that can exert mechanical pressure on the neural elements.

The operative field should be dry, with hemostasis maintained. Magnification loupes and adequate lighting facilitate the repair. The actual technique of closure depends on the size and the location of the dural tear. For simple dural lacerations, 4–0 gauge silk sutures are used on a tapered one-half circle needle. A running locking suture (Fig. 2A) or simple sutures incorporating a free fat graft (Fig. 2B) give a watertight closure. If a large tear is present, a graft from the lumbar fascia is obtained and sutured in place with interrupted dural silk sutures (Fig. 2C). If the defect is in an inaccessible area, a small tissue plug of muscle or fat is introduced

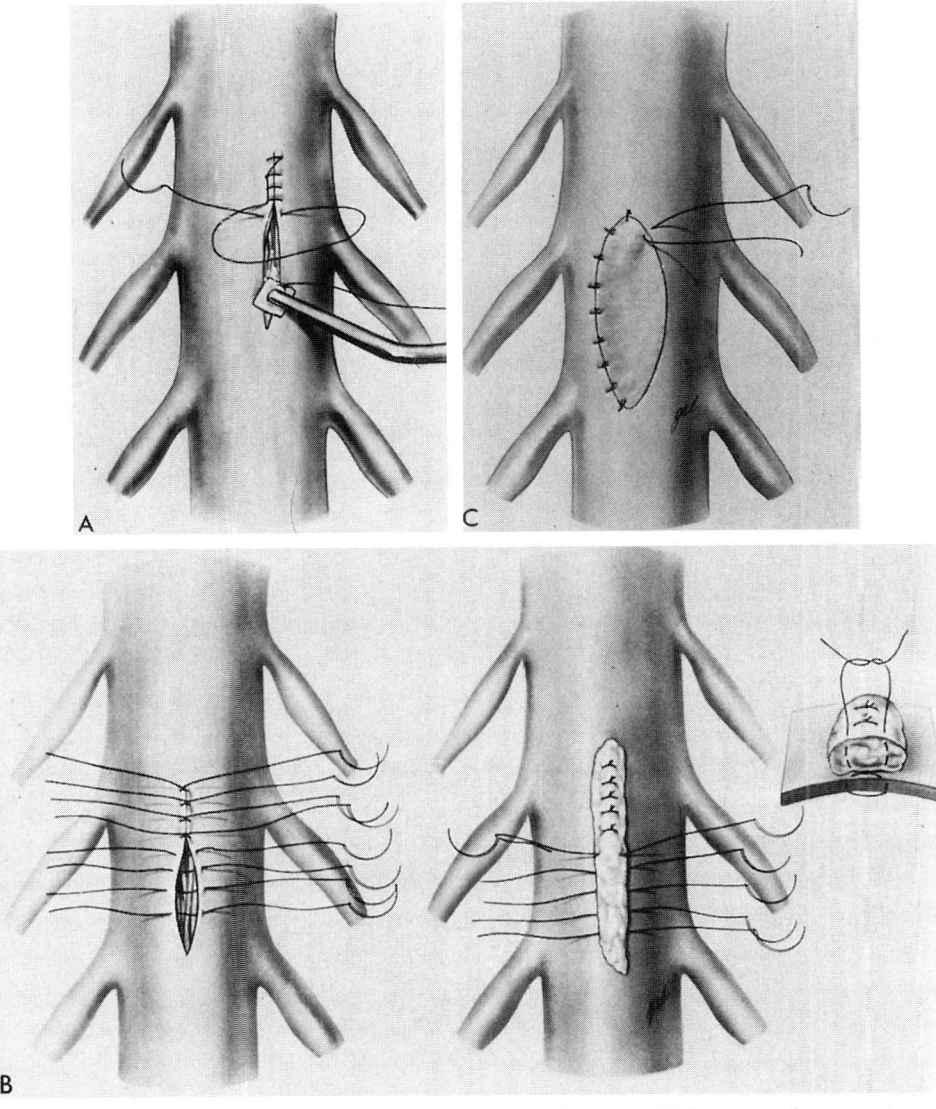

Figure 2. A, Dural repair with a running locking suture. B, Dural repair with interrupted sutures incorporating a free fat graft. C, Large dural tear repaired with a fascial graft. (From Eismont, F. J., Wiesel, S. W., and Rothman, R. H.: Treatment of dural tears associated with spinal surgery. J. Bone Joint Surg. 63A:1132–1137, 1981.)

through a second midline durotomy and pulled against a tear from the inside of the dura.

The repair is tested by placing the patient in the reverse Trendelenburg position and performing the Valsalva maneuver to increase intrathecal pressure. The fascia is closed with a heavy, nonabsorbable suture so that the closure is watertight. Drains should not be used (so a fistula does not form if the dura continues to leak). Postoperatively, the patient should be kept prone for at least 3 days to reduce pressure on the repair while it heals.

The diagnosis of a CSF leak in the postoperative period can be difficult. If relatively clear drainage occurs, the surgeon must consider the possibility of a dural leak. No good noninvasive diagnostic techniques are available at preset. The presence of glucose in the fluid draining from an incision is not a reliable determinant because glucose is normally present in both noninflammatory and inflammatory exudates. The best diagnostic test is a myelogram performed with water-soluble contrast medium; this is recommended if a dural leak is seriously suspected. After the postoperative CSF leak is identified, the patient should be returned quickly to the operating room for dural repair to prevent an infection in the CSF.

A nonoperative alternative treatment of closed subarachnoid drainage may also be used.[13] A subarachnoid shunt can be placed percutaneously into the lumbar canal, which results in the resolution of some CSF leaks. If a shunt is not successful quickly, the patient should be taken to the operating room for an open dural repair.

Prevention of dural tears is best achieved by excellent visualization during exposure. Hemostasis should always be maintained. If there is any question about the presence of dura when a bone-biting instrument is used, a Cottonoid patty can be placed between the dura and the bony structures to prevent dural injury; this is an easy and safe preventive measure.

CONCLUSION

The physician must take an organized approach to the evaluation of the multiply operated back. The origin of the problem in many cases is a faulty decision to perform the original surgical procedure. Further exploratory surgery is not warranted and leads to only further disability. A repeated operative procedure is indicated only when objective findings of a specific diagnosis are present.

The cause of each patient's symptoms must be accurately localized and identified. In addition to the orthopedic evaluation, thorough investigation of the patient's psychosocial and general medical status is needed. When the spine is identified as the source of the patient's symptoms, specific features should be sought in the patient's clinical history, physical examination, and radiographic studies. The number of previous operations, characteristics of the pain-free interval, and predominance of leg pain or back pain are the major historical points. The most important aspects of the physical examination are the neurologic findings and the presence of a tension sign. Plain radiographs, motion films, CT scans, and MRI scans all have specific roles in the workup. When all the information is integrated, the physician can usually separate patients with arachnoiditis, epidural scar tissue, and discitis from those with mechanical problems of the spine.

In the few patients who require an additional operation, the patient should appreciate that it can be complicated and lengthy procedure with certain inherent risks. The surgeon should approach the spine at a previously unoperated level to identify the depth of the neural elements and to visualize the appropriate nerve root or roots laterally, while leaving the midline epidural scar tissue intact. If the dura is injured during the procedure, it should be repaired and the closure should be watertight.

Physicians involved in the treatment of the multiply operated patient must realize that there is little likelihood that these patients will return to a pain-free state. There is usually some form of permanent impairment, depending on the type of previous surgery and the patient's current symptoms. These patients require counseling and must be strongly encouraged to resume as functional a role as possible in society.

REFERENCES

1. Boden, S. D., Davis, D. O., Dina, T. S., et al.: Contrast-enhanced MR imaging performed after suc-

cessful lumbar disc surgery: Prospective study. Radiology 182:59–64, 1992.
2. Braun, I. F., Hoffman, J. C., Davis, P. C., et al.: Contrast enhancement in CT differentiation between recurrent disk herniation and postoperative scar: A prospective study. AJNR 6:607–612, 1985.
3. Burton, C. V.: Lumbosacral arachnoiditis. Spine 3:24–30, 1978.
4. Burton, C. V., Kirkaldy-Willis, W. H., Yong-Hing, K., and Heithoff, K. B.: Causes of failure of surgery on the lumbar spine. Clin. Orthop. 157:191–199, 1981.
5. Byrd, S. E., Cohn, M. L., Biggers, S. L., et al.: The radiographic evaluation of the symptomatic postoperative lumbar spine patient. Spine 10: 652–661, 1985.
6. Dall, B. E., Rowe, D. E., Odette, W. G., and Batts, D. H.: Postoperative discitis: Diagnosis and management. Clin. Orthop. 224:138–148, 1987.
7. Eismont, F. J., Wiesel, S. W., and Rothman, R. H.: Treatment of dural tears associated with spinal surgery. J. Bone Joint Surg. 63A:1132–1137, 1981.
8. Epstein, B. S.: The Spine. Philadelphia, Lea & Febiger, 1962.
9. Finnegan, W. J., Tenlin, J. M., Marvel, J. P., et al.: Results of surgical intervention in the symptomatic multiply-operated back patient. J. Bone Joint Surg. 61A:1077–1082, 1979.
10. Grubb, S. A., Lipscomb, H. J., and Gilford, W. B.: The relative value of lumbar roentgenograms, metrizamide myelography, and discography in the assessment of patients with chronic low-back syndrome. Spine 12:282–286, 1987.
11. Hueftle, M. G., Modic, M. T., Ross, J. S., et al.: Lumbar spine: Postoperative MR imaging with bd-DTPA. Radiology 167:817–824, 1988.
12. Johnson, K. E., Willner, S., and Johnson, K.: Postoperative instability after decompression for lumbar spinal stenosis. Spine 11:107–110, 1986.
13. Kitchel, S. R., Eismont, F. J., and Green, D. A.: Closed subarachnoid drainage for management of cerebral spinal fluid leakage after an operation of the spine. J. Bone Joint Surg. 71A:984–987, 1989.
14. Lahde, S., and Puranen, J.: Disk-space hypodensity in CT: The first radiological signs of postoperative diskitis. Eur. J. Radiol. 5:190–192, 1985.
15. Langenskydd, A., and Kiviluoto O.: Prevention of epidural scar formation after operations on the lumbar spine by means of free fat transplants. Clin. Orthop. 115:92–95, 1976.
16. Quiles, M., Marchisello, P. J., and Tsairis, P.: Lumbar adhesive arachnoiditis: Etiologic and pathologic aspects. Spine 3:45–50, 1978.
17. Ross, J. S., Masaryk, T. J., Modic, M. T., et al.: MR imaging of lumbar arachnoiditis AJNR 8:885–892, 1987.
18. Rothman, R. H., and Simeone, F. A.: The Spine, 3rd Ed. Philadelphia. W. B. Saunders, 1992.
19. Spengler, D. M., and Freeman, D. W.: Patient selection for lumbar discectomy: An objective approach. Spine 4:129–134, 1979.
20. Waddell, G., Kummel, E. G., Lotto, W. N., et al.: Failed lumbar disc surgery and repeat surgery following industrial injuries. J. Bone Joint Surg. 61A:201–207, 1979.
21. Waddell, G.: Failures of disc surgery and repeat surgery. Acta Orthop. Belg. 53:300–302, 1987.
22. White, A. A., Panjabi, M. M., Posner, I., et al.: Spinal stability: Evaluation and treatment. Instr. Course Lect. 30:457, 1981.

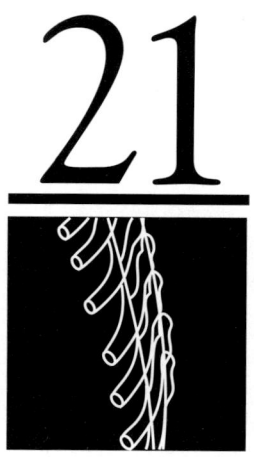

21

Adult Scoliosis

Evaluation and Decision-Making

RICHARD A. BALDERSTON
TODD J. ALBERT

Adult scoliosis can be defined as a spinal deformity with a Cobb angle greater than 10 degrees in the coronal plane in a patient older than 20 years of age. It is convenient to divide patients with adult scoliosis into two groups, (1) patients with onset of deformity before skeletal maturity and with persistence and possibly worsening of the curve after age 20 years and (2) patients with a previously straight spine (Cobb angle < 10 degrees at age 20 years) but with de novo deformity in adult life. Patients in the first category usually have a diagnosis of idiopathic, congenital, or neuromuscular scoliosis made before age 19 years.[28, 30] Patients in the second group usually have scoliosis caused by degenerative disc disease, osteoporosis, osteomalacia, or instability with or without decompressive surgery. This discussion relates primarily to patients with adult scoliosis and with an onset of deformity before skeletal maturity.

EPIDEMIOLOGY AND NATURAL HISTORY

Vanderpool and associates[36] studied a group of adult patients with an average age of 61 years and noted a prevalence of 6% with coronal plane deformity. However, their curve definition was 7 degrees and greater. In patients with osteoporosis, 36% were noted to have a spinal deformity, but more than one third of these patients had evidence that the scoliosis developed de novo. The observation of these investigators was that scoliosis associated with osteoporotic compression fracture was common.

Kostuik and Bentivoglio[19] in 1981 reviewed intravenous pyelograms of 5000 patients and found a prevalence of scoliosis of 3.9%, with curve definition being Cobb angle of 10 degrees or greater. Among cases of deformity in the lumbar spine, 86% were judged to be idiopathic.

The issue of curve progression in the adult patient with an idiopathic curve pattern has been well defined. Several researchers have demonstrated that curves in adult patients frequently progress.[9, 21, 37] In a landmark study by Weinstein and Ponseti,[37] 40-year follow-up data were reviewed for patients with idiopathic curve patterns. Patients with curvatures of between 50 and 75 degrees were at high risk for progression. Thoracic curves with a Cobb angle of 50 to 75 degrees at initiation of the study progressed an average of slightly less than 30 degrees during the 40-year period. Thoracolumbar curves increased an average of 22 degrees during the same period. These figures represent an average for all participants in the study. Although many patients did not have any progression, some progressed 1 to 2 degrees per year during the study. In the lumbar spine, the worst prognosis over long-term follow-up was expected in persons with curves in which the L5 vertebra was seated above the intercristal line and with curves that had lumbar apical rotation greater than 33%. If the lumbar or thoracolumbar curve was not balanced at the beginning of the follow-up period, a higher incidence of progression could be expected.

The issue of back pain and scoliosis with respect to the lumbar spine is as yet poorly defined. Perhaps the best study to date is that by Kostuik and Bentivoglio,[19] who noted a 59% incidence of low back pain in 189 patients with scoliosis recognized with intravenous pyelograms. When these patients were matched for age, sex, and occupation with 100 patients without scoliosis, the incidence of pain was found to be the same in both populations. Of the patients with pain, 44% had mild episodes, 49% had moderate episodes, and 7% had severe pain. The correlation with age was also similar, with the maximum severity appearing between the ages of 40 and 60 years. Kostuik and Bentivoglio[19] noted that, in patients with curves greater than 45 degrees in the lumbar spine, there was a statistically significant increase in incapacitating pain compared with that in patients with curves less than 45 degrees or in the control population.

In patients who have had surgery for idiopathic scoliosis with fusion of their lumbar spine, Cochran and associates[7] defined the risk of low back pain. For patients with fusions ending at the L2 or L3 level, the incidence of low back pain was no different from that found in a control population. For patients with a fusion ending at the level of L4, the occurrence of low back pain increased statistically, and for fusions ending at the L5 level, the incidence approached 100%, although the number of patients in this group was small.

PATIENT EVALUATION

History

For the adult patient with an adolescent curve pattern that arose before skeletal maturity, the history is the most important aspect of the overall evaluation.

The first area of inquiry includes a history of all previous treatment. When was the diagnosis made? What was the Cobb angle, and what were the end vertebrae at the time of the initial assessment? Did the curve progress during adolescence and, if so, to what level? Was observation, bracing, or surgery ever recommended? Most patients who are currently in their 40s or 50s would have been told by their physician that after age 19 years there was little or no chance that the scoliosis would progress, because at that time it was thought that progression did not occur in adults.

A history of curve progression can be ascertained from patients or their close friends and family. Questions for the patient concerning progression should include: Do you feel that you are leaning more to one side? Do you feel you are losing your waistline on one side, or that your hip is becoming more prominent on one side? Do you feel that you have gotten shorter? How tall were you when you graduated from high school compared with your current height? Does it seem that you have gotten fatter without an increase in weight? Do you have to hem your clothes differently or have you had to have them adjusted because you felt that one leg was becoming longer than the other? Often, patients may report increased fatigue because they must expend more energy in their attempts to stand without decompensation. Serial x-ray films should be obtained because they have greater precision than do historical data.

A history of back pain is frequently elicited, and the examiner must ask the patient to be precise in the definition of the location and intensity of the pain. Does the pain originate at the lumbosacral junction, the iliac crests, the sacroiliac joints, or the distal sacrum? Or is the pain associated with a thoracolumbar prominence, a rib hump, or the thoracic or thoracolumbar spine in the midline? How often does the pain occur and how severe is it? What medication is required to achieve some pain relief? Is the patient able to work when the pain occurs? If not, how many days have been missed from work in the past year because of the pain?

Pain occurring in the region of the lumbar spine may also be referred to the posterior buttocks or to the proximal half of the posterior or lateral thigh. True radicular pain may be defined as any pain radiating below the knee or to the anterior thigh. Adult patients with scoliosis frequently have an L3, L4, or L5 radiculopathy related to the concavity of a lumbar curve or to the concavity of the compensatory lumbosacral curve. The examiner must be precise in having the patient define feelings of numbness or sharp pain. How far can the patient walk before the symptoms become severe? Is the pain made better with rest and worse with activity? Does extension of the lumbar spine increase symptoms? A pain questionnaire is a valuable adjunct in patients with back pain and/or radicular pain.

All patients with thoracic or thoracolumbar curves should be evaluated with respect to pulmonary function. All patients should be asked whether they have had increasing shortness of breath during periods of exertion such as climbing stairs and performing aerobic exercise. Certainly, a history of asthma should be ruled out. In patients with congenital or neuromuscular curves, respiratory problems are much more common than in those with idiopathic scoliosis, but pulmonary dysfunction has been documented in patients with thoracic curves greater than 60 degrees.[23] Patients with significant thoracic or thoracolumbar lordosis and an early onset of idiopathic scoliosis are also at high risk for pulmonary compromise. Pulmonary function tests are recommended in any patient with a history of shortness of breath that has been increasing, thoracic curvatures greater than 60 degrees, congenital or paralytic scoliosis, or any concomitant pulmonary disease such as asthma or asbestosis.

One final assessment that should be made for every patient is a psychologic one. Although many patients have learned to live with the deformity, there may be significant life circumstances, such as divorce or a new job, which cause patients to focus on the spine again. Indeed, although there may be no change in the patient's spine, if the patient has a profound alteration in lifestyle the issue of spinal deformity may resurface. Some patients may have depression caused by a multitude of factors. Some assessment must be made with respect to the patient's general feeling of well-being. For many patients, increasing back pain may be a sign of increasing depression and simply treating the depression may improve the back pain.

Physical Examination

Physical examination of the patient with adult scoliosis focuses on several areas. Careful palpation must be performed of the entire spine and pelvis to determine whether there are any tender areas over the rib hump, the thoracolumbar prominence, individual spinous processes of the entire thoracolumbar spine, the iliolumbar ligament, the sacroiliac joint, the sciatic notch, the lateral iliac crests, and the greater trochanters.[38] Often, percussion of the spine is extremely helpful in eliciting a painful segment.

Spinal alignment and deformity are defined in several ways. A plumb line is used to determine the position of the C7 spinous process with respect to the gluteal cleft. In the standing position, the relative heights of the shoulder and the iliac crests are measured. Again, with the patient in the standing position, the degree of rotatory malalignment is noted by measuring any asymmetry of the shoulders in the sagittal plane. The patient is asked to bend forward and the examiner must view the spine from four different directions. The location of a thoracic rib prominence and lumbar asymmetry are noted with respect to level and angulation. With the patient in the standing position, lateral bending of the patient is performed by the examiner to evaluate how supple the curvatures are and to determine whether pain is elicited or reproduced with forced side bending. Any degree of loss of lumbar lordosis, hip flexion, or knee flexion in the standing position should be noted.

A neurologic assessment of the lower extremities should be performed, with an evaluation of each spinal nerve from L3 to S1. In addition, any calf asymmetries, foot deformities, or hyperreflexia should be noted. Some abnormal findings may also be expected with an increased frequency in patients with unusual curve patterns, such as left thoracic idiopathic curves.

Any areas of abnormal skin pigmentation, dimpling, or unusual hair distribution should be noted. Any patient with ocular abnormalities, a high arched palate, and/or hyperlaxity of the joints should be evaluated further for connective tissue disorders.

Radiologic Studies

The roentgenographic assessment of patients with any coronal deformity and a Cobb angle greater than 10 degrees should include posteroanterior and lateral views taken on a 36-inch cassette to evaluate the entire thoracolumbar spine in the standing position. Only with these views can one ascertain completely the degree of deformity with respect to Cobb angle in the standing position and the degree of decompensation in both the coronal and sagittal planes. Spot anteroposterior and lateral films of the lumbar spine with the patient in the supine position should be obtained for any lumbar spinal deformity. In adult patients, supine x-ray films provide more specific assessment of enlarged or subluxated facets, disc narrowing or sclerosis, or subtle congenital anomalies. Spondylolysis or spondylolisthesis should be ruled out in all patients.

Bending films are usually not recommended unless surgery is contemplated. At the authors' center, bending films are usually procured with patients in the supine position. Traction films may be of value to determine whether distraction produces decompensation. In any patient with a kyphotic deformity, the lateral hyperextension view is mandatory. In patients with degenerative disease of the lumbar spine, flexion-extension views in the lateral decubitus position are necessary to rule out subtle degrees of instability that may affect the lower limit of fusion.

For the assessment of low back pain or radiculopathy, magnetic resonance imaging scanning has been extremely helpful in ruling out tumor or infection. Great care must be taken in the diagnosis of herniated disc because of the three-dimensional complexity of the scoliotic curvature. Myelography and postmyelography computed tomographic scanning may be necessary to define the exact position of spinal nerve compression. A bone scan may be helpful in younger patients with a mild painful curve to rule out osteoid osteoma or other tumor. Discography may be used to assess pain levels in patients with scoliosis in whom fusion is being contemplated. Grubb and Lipscomb[15] demonstrated that discs that were painful on discography in patients with adult scoliosis frequently might not be considered for fusion if traditional methods were used to determine the lower limits of fusion. It was Grubb and coworkers'[15, 20] recommendation that patients with painful scoliosis have discography performed so that the fusion levels for scoliosis would extend far enough.

NONOPERATIVE CARE

The primary symptom treated nonoperatively is back pain. There are no reasonable nonoperative interventions for the treatment of curve progression, curve decompensation, respiratory embarrassment, or progressive spinal nerve compromise with motor weakness.

For patients with scoliosis, the chance of having a significant episode of back pain is at best the same risk as in the general population.[19, 32] Ninety percent of these episodes are not directly related to the patient's scoliosis and improve in a manner similar to that for patients with straight spines. For acute exacerbations, a short period of bed rest for 1 or 2 days, the use of analgesics and antiinflammatory medications, and application of heat or cold are appropriate. Thereafter, gradual mobilization with emphasis on antiinflammatory as opposed to analgesic medication is appropriate.

Physical therapy and weight reduction can be successful in controlling back pain in patients with adult spinal deformity, provided that progressive curve worsening or decompensation is not occurring. It is important to emphasize that patients with scoliosis do not have normal motion and thus are not able to perform significant range of motion exercises. This fact may cause extreme frustration for the patient, and the physical therapist should be alerted to this possibility. Paraspinal and abdominal isometric and strengthening exercises are important. Ideally, an aerobic regimen of low-impact aerobics, cycling, or swimming should also be undertaken.

Frequently, in elderly patients, an orthosis may be of value for pain control, especially for pain that originates at the thoracolumbar junction. Often, these patients are kyphotic and may also have compression fractures at the thoracolumbar junction secondary to osteopenia and trauma. However, in elderly patients, great care must be taken that bony prominences are well padded. The purpose of the orthosis is to allow greater mobilization. It may be that the mobilization itself improves the patient's symptoms. The patient must be warned, however, before orthotic management is initiated that the orthosis may not fit well and may have to be abandoned.

INDICATIONS FOR SURGERY

The indications for surgery in adult scoliosis include curve progression, back pain in the area of the spinal curvature unresponsive to nonoperative care, progressive sciatica emanating from the concavity of spinal curvature unresponsive to conservative care, progressive loss of neurologic function, and muscle fatigue due to increasing decompensation in the coronal or sagittal plane.[17, 31, 34]

Progression of lumbar curves, with associated coronal plane decompensation, portends a high risk of future disability and increasing back pain. Patients at the authors' center with 10 degrees of documented progression and a thoracolumbar or lumbar curve greater than 50 degrees are considered for spinal stabilization. Generally, these patients also have increasing fatigue from the muscle imbalance associated with coronal or sagittal plane decompensation.

Patients with significant axial pain in the area of their scoliosis and a curvature of greater than 45 degrees may be helped by spinal stabilization. In these patients, one can expect an 85% to 90% chance of improvement of the pain, but patients must be cautioned that there is a 10% to 15% chance that the back pain will be no better after fusion surgery.[17, 18] Patients with rotatory or lateral listhesis, localized pain, and progressive decompensation may be helped with fusion surgery.

If sciatica surgery is contemplated for a patient with an idiopathic curve pattern, with the decompression planned for an area near the apex of the patient's lumbar curvature, consideration should be given to a fusion of the curvature that stabilizes the spine and prevents future decompensation (Fig. 1).[31] Lumbar decompressive surgery in the apex of a lumbar curvature has a high risk of producing progression if the curve is not stabilized concomitantly.

Lumbosacral symptoms, when present by themselves, are almost never cured by scoliosis fusion.[20] Frequently, these patients have degenerative disc disease of the lumbosacral junction in an area where there is no significant curvature.

DEGENERATIVE ADULT SCOLIOSIS

Coronal plane deformity with Cobb angle measurements greater than 10 degrees may arise de novo in adults.[24, 27] One of the first studies to document progressive scoliosis with a preexisting straight spine was by Vanderpool and associates.[36] They examined a group of patients primarily in the seventh and eighth decades of life who had coronal plane deformities. They identified 14 patients who had documented evidence of no scoliosis (i.e., coronal plane deformity less than 5 degrees) and who, several years later, had spinal curvature. The cause of deformity in this group of patients was primarily compression fractures secondary to osteoporosis or osteomalacia.

Robin and colleagues[27] studied a group of 554 patients, with an average follow-up of 10 years. At final follow-up, 30% of the pa-

---

Figure 1. A 67-year-old woman had progressive low back and left anterior thigh and lateral calf pain. Preoperative posteroanterior *(A)* and lateral *(B)* radiographs. Myelography demonstrated spinal stenosis at the level of the rotatory listhesis at L4–L5. There are six lumbar vertebrae. After decompression surgery from L6 to L3 *(C and D)*, stabilization and bilateral lateral fusion were carried out. Pedicle screw instrumentation was used to maintain foraminal cross-sectional area, especially on the left at L4–L5 and L5–L6. At L3–L4 on the right, complete facetectomy was also performed. At 2-year follow-up, the patient continued to have improved function with diminution of leg and back pain.

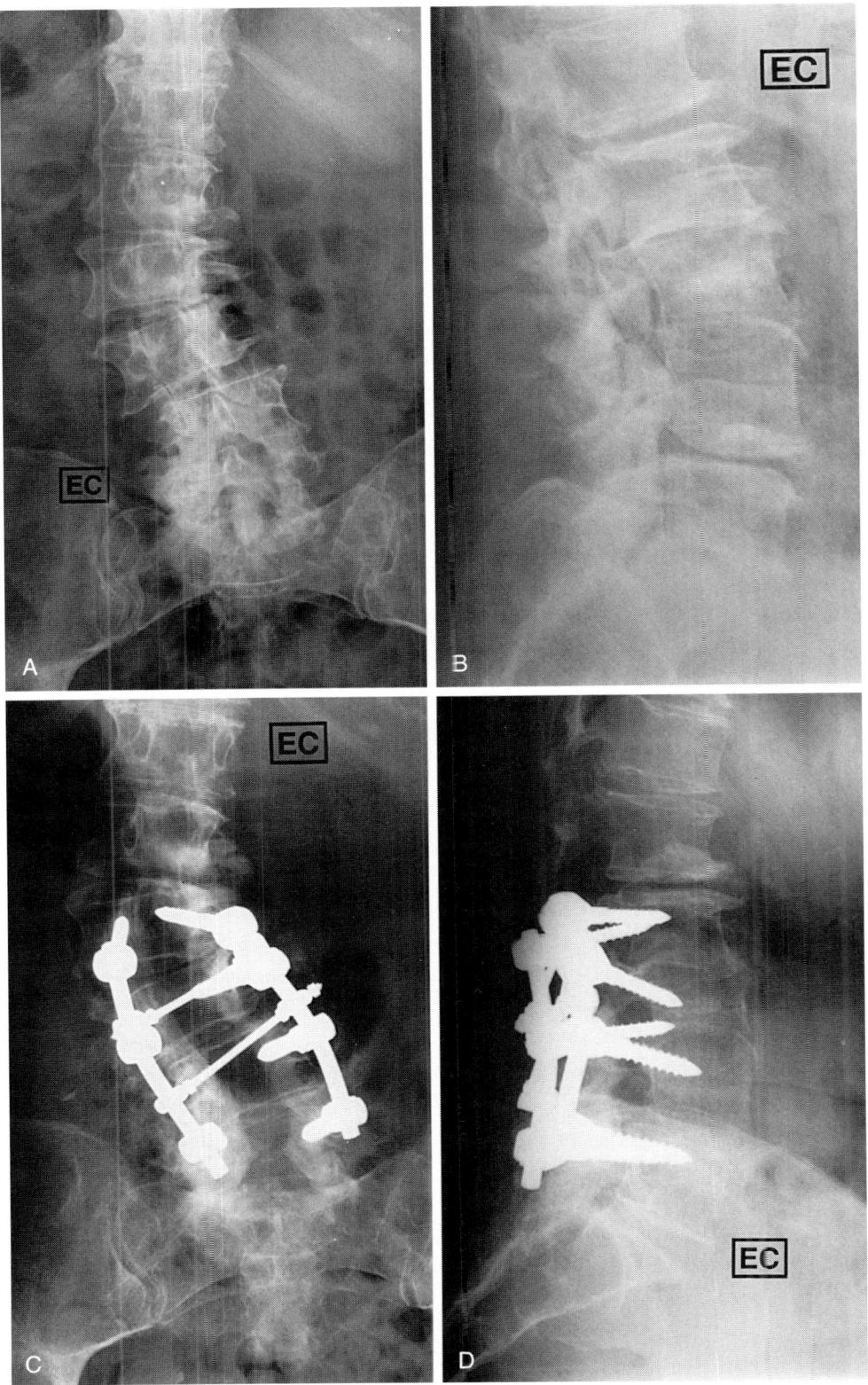

tients had curvature greater than 10 degrees, whereas in 10% of the patients scoliosis had developed de novo. These authors were unable to demonstrate a significant relationship among increased back pain, magnitude of curvature, and progression of deformity.

A more recent study of degenerative lumbar scoliosis was made by Pritchett and Bortel.[24] Their series included 200 patients with degenerative scoliosis. There were 151 women, and the mean age of the cohort was 69 years. Curves were defined as scoliosis if the Cobb angle was greater than 10 degrees. During the study, 41 patients had follow-up x-ray studies at an average of 6½ years, with a range of 5 to 17 years. Degenerative spondylolisthesis was present in 55% of the patients. Lateral listhesis, which averaged 8 mm, was present in 78% of patients. Examination of the sagittal plane revealed that 85% of patients had lordosis that was less than normal levels. For the entire group, the mean lordosis was 18 degrees.

All patients in the series had a history of low back pain, and 72% of patients had symptoms related to the lower extremities. Documented neurologic findings were present in 91 patients, but unfortunately, many of these findings were diminished sensory perception on the lateral aspect of the thigh, a physical finding common to many spinal and extraspinal problems.

Risk factors for curve progression in the 41 patients for whom follow-up was available demonstrated the following: Cobb angle greater than 30 degrees, rotation of grade II or grade III, an intercristal line that passed through L5 as compared with L4, and vertebral translation greater than 6 mm.

The roentgenographic findings in the study by Pritchett and Bortel[24] emphasized the lack of vertebral body asymmetry in adult degenerative scoliosis that characterizes adolescent idiopathic scoliosis. All of the patients studied had significant degenerative disease, with asymmetric disc narrowing and facet hypertrophy. In patients who failed to respond to conservative management, myelography demonstrated significant indentation of the dye column at the level of the apex of the lumbar scoliosis, usually at the L3 level.

The management of back and lower extremity symptoms in patients with degenerative adult lumbar scoliosis includes the usual modalities of rest, the use of antiinflammatory agents and analgesics, and the application of heat during the acute period. Paraspinal strengthening, including abdominal exercises and a general aerobic conditioning program, remains the cornerstone of long-term treatment of these problems. Custom-molded braces may be effective in the patient with significant deformity. However, care must be taken that a physical therapy program is emphasized as well. Especially in female patients, attention should be given to the treatment of osteopenia, and prevention of further mineral loss from the vertebral bodies should be instituted.

The most common indication for surgery in patients with adult lumbar scoliosis is related to the symptoms of neurogenic claudication.[17, 18, 31, 34] Just as in spinal stenosis surgery, the individual L2, L3, L4, and L5 nerves must be examined with the consideration of individual patterns of lateral nerve entrapment. Myelograms and postmyelography computed tomographic scans are the best studies for delineating individual spinal nerve pathologic changes in patients with significant lumbar coronal plane abnormalities. A 6- to 12-week trial of conservative management is definitely indicated before surgery is contemplated.

At the time of surgery, great care must be taken that the individual nerves are entirely decompressed to a point lateral to the lateral aspect of the corresponding pedicles. Although there are no surgical series with control groups of fusion versus no fusion, in the face of decompression with complete facetectomy for lumbar scoliosis, most surgeons recommend at least an in situ fusion at the time of decompression. Currently, the authors use a pedicle screw construct to prevent further Cobb angle progression and subsequent compression of nerves at the apex concavity. Patients have undergone decompression with good results, only to have further symptoms result from apical compression and compression of the spinal nerve between the pedicles. The surgeon should be cautioned that the results of spine fusion for back pain in these patients are not as good as the results of surgery for symptoms related to spinal stenosis.[33]

SPECIAL CONSIDERATIONS IN ADULT SCOLIOSIS SURGERY

The presence of disc degeneration, facet arthritis, and osteopenia are major factors that differentiate adult scoliosis surgery from adolescence scoliosis surgery.[18] For curvatures in which significant correction is achieved, great force is placed on the end vertebra, which may then be subject to fracture or loss of fixation. In adult patients with lumbar spinal deformity, end vertebra fixation may be enhanced by the use of pedicle screw instrumentation.

Patients with adult scoliosis have an increased tendency for progressive kyphosis at the junction of their instrumentation with remaining spinal segments. This situation is particularly evident at the thoracolumbar junction. Preoperative hyperextension lateral x-ray films are recommended for most patients who undergo fusion to correct adult deformity in the lumbar spine.

In patients with significant disc and facet disease, the amount of correction achieved is less than that possible in the corresponding curve in the adolescent. The surgeon should not expect the extent of correction that is usually achieved in a younger patient. Adult patients should be warned of this outcome as well.

Decompensation in the coronal plane is a problem more commonly seen in adults than in adolescents. The discs that are left free in the adolescent often allow the surgeon more room for error by accommodating to the altered structure above. Thus, the patient is able to maintain balance. In the adult patient with significant disc degeneration, coronal plane balance is more likely to result if the configuration of the discs in the lower back is accounted for during preoperative planning.

POSTERIOR INSTRUMENTATION FOR ADULT DEFORMITY OF THORACOLUMBAR AND LUMBAR SPINE

Posterior instrumentation for adult lumbar curvature is used primarily for two types of patients. The first type are patients with significant progression of thoracolumbar curvature and increased decompensation or pain (Fig. 2). In this type of patient, instrumentation is used to correct the deformity within limits and to provide stability in the partially corrected position.[10] The issues of lordosis maintenance, coronal plane balance, and the fate of the remaining, possibly degenerated lumbar open segments are critical. In the second type of patient, surgery is indicated primarily for progressive sciatica. In this situation, because of the removal of posterior elements, the options for fixation are much more limited. Nevertheless, the same considerations are fundamental for this type of patient because issues of loss of balance in the sagittal and coronal planes are always present after decompressive surgery has been performed for degenerative scoliosis.

In the patient with thoracolumbar curvature, the same principles of scoliosis surgery as for the adolescent, should be observed initially. Hook fixation may be used to provide compression on one side of the spine. In general, this compression force allows correction of coronal plane deformity when the force is applied to the convexity of a scoliosis curvature. In addition, a compressive force is used to compensate the spine to the side on which the compression is performed. When hook or pedicle screw fixation is used in the lumbar spine, distraction is almost never applied as an initial force. The reason for this warning is that most patients with loss of lumbar lordosis have a progressive thoracolumbar curve. In many adult patients, distraction of the thoracic spine is a common procedure to correct deformity. However, distraction in the lumbar spine produces only increased lumbar kyphosis. The surgeon must never assume that, because a distraction force is applied in the concavity of a lumbar curve, correction of the coronal curve will occur before sagittal balance is lost.

In adult patients, a minimum of one fixation site is mandatory for each lumbar vertebra attached to a thoracolumbar fusion. For curvatures extended to the L3 or L4 level, where significant postoperative loading is expected, the number of fixation points should be increased.

Patients with degenerative lumbar scoliosis who have sciatica and require decompressive surgery generally do not have significant idiopathic curve patterns. In patients who do not have substantial problems with coronal or sagittal plane balance, fixation and fusion of the lumbar spine may be confined to only the areas where decompressive surgery has been performed. Pedicle screw instrumentation may be used to obtain par-

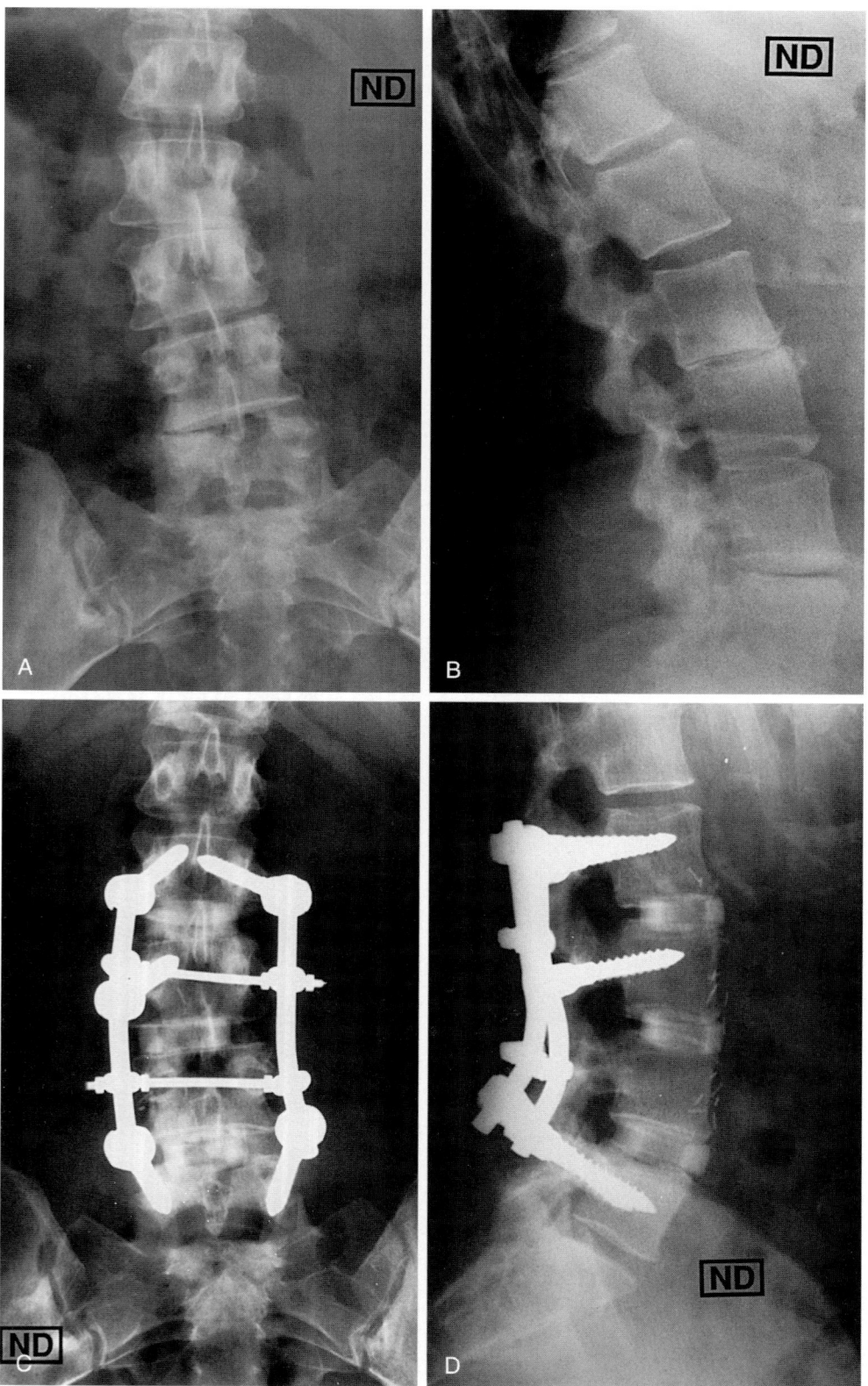

See figure legend on opposite page.

tial correction of coronal Cobb angle deformity, in order to prevent future spinal nerve compression from increasing deformity, which is usually caused by pedicle migration.

MEDICAL COMPLICATIONS OF SCOLIOSIS SURGERY

Respiratory complications of scoliosis surgery in adults can occur from either anterior or posterior surgery.[4, 8, 13, 22, 25, 35] These include atelectasis, pneumonia, pleural effusion, pneumothorax, chylothorax, hemothorax, acute respiratory distress syndrome, respiratory failure, pulmonary thromboembolism, and fat embolism.

Pneumothorax can occur during posterior surgery when dissection is carried out too aggressively in the intertransverse process area of the thoracic spine. Additionally, pointed retractors, when used in the thoracic spine and penetrated too deeply, can injure the pleura and cause a pneumothorax. Treatment is with chest tube insertion and negative pressure suction. Rib resection and thoracoplasty can be associated with the development of a pneumothorax. Familiarity with this complication and surveillance with a chest x-ray film are important. After anterior thoracotomy, all patients have a chest tube placed for anterior drainage to treat the obligatory pneumothorax that occurs with incision of the parietal pleura. Removal of the chest tube occurs when drainage decreases significantly and the residual pneumothorax is resolved. A chest x-ray study is always obtained after the chest tube is removed. Chylothorax and/or chyloperitoneum can occur after anterior approach to the thoracic or lumbar spine.[8, 22, 25] These complications should be recognized at the time of surgery when the stump of the lymphatic duct responsible can be ligated. This complication is difficult to treat postoperatively, and it often requires insertion of drainage catheters and potentially the use of sclerosing agents.

Pulmonary embolism is less common in spinal surgery than in pelvic and extremity surgery.[35] The authors apply thromboembolic stockings and pneumatic compression hose at the time of anesthetia induction for prophylaxis. The diagnosis of pulmonary embolism requires prompt heparinization. In patients with contraindications to anticoagulation, placement of a caval filter may be necessary.

Other postoperative pulmonary problems, such as pneumonia and atelectasis, are more frequent in patients who have anterior thoracotomies or thoracolumbotomies. The frequency of these complications can be decreased by ensuring that the lung is fully inflated after intercostal repair sutures are placed and before final closure of the chest after the anterior procedure. Additionally, aggressive postoperative pulmonary toilet with incentive spirometry and early mobilization when possible also help to prevent these pulmonary complications. Patients at particularly high risk for postoperative pneumonia and/or atelectasis (patients with nonidiopathic scoliosis or with developmental disabilities) should routinely have a preoperative medical consultation.

Postoperative ileus is relatively common after scoliosis surgery, particularly surgery involving violation of the retroperitoneal space. The authors routinely use nasogastric suction intraoperatively and postoperatively in patients requiring anterior lumbar approaches. Nasogastric suction is not discontinued until the patients have active bowel sounds and/or have passed flatus. The slow readministration of oral feedings is undertaken postoperatively, narcotic use is kept to a minimum, and early mobilization and ambulation are encouraged when possible.

Figure 2. *A*, A 51-year-old woman had progressive degenerative scoliosis with decompensation to the left. In addition, she had progressive right anterior thigh pain and left anterior leg pain. *B*, Progressive disc degeneration had caused asymmetric narrowing of the formina on the right at L2–L3 and on the left at L4–L5. In addition, disc height loss had caused mild loss of lordosis. After 6 months of progressive lower extremity pain in spite of nonoperative modalities, this patient underwent anterior and posterior reconstruction. Anterior discectomies were performed from L2 to L5 with insertion of femoral ring allografts cut to the size of the disc space. Posterior surgery consisted of foraminotomies on the left at L4–L5 and on the right at L2–L3 with pedicle screw fixation *(C and D)*. At 1-year follow-up, this patient continued to have significant improvement of her lower extremity symptoms.

All of these interventions help to minimize the risk of prolonged ileus.

Ileus, which can be treated expectantly, should not be confused with true mechanical bowel obstruction. In the patient with scoliosis who has undergone significant correction with instrumentation or casting, superior mesenteric artery syndrome should be thought of when symptoms of nausea and vomiting are present.[1, 3, 5, 16, 29] This can result from an obstruction of the third portion of the duodenum, when the angle between the superior mesenteric artery and the aorta narrows and compresses that portion of the bowel. Barium swallow examination is diagnostic. Superior mesenteric artery syndrome can usually be treated successfully with nasogastric suction, placement in the left lateral decubitus position, and occasionally, modification of the cast if necessary. Surgical intervention is necessary only if prolonged nonoperative treatment fails.

The possibility of acute cholecystitis should be considered when the scoliosis patient presents with acute abdominal pain in the right upper quadrant early in the postoperative period.[12] Diagnosis is made with a cholecystogram or an abdominal ultrasonographic examination, and surgical intervention may be necessary.

Urinary retention and urinary tract infection are the most common medical complications affecting scoliosis patients in the postoperative period. Prolonged use of indwelling catheters or repeated instrumentation of the urinary tract increases the risk of these complications. Prolonged recumbency and the use of narcotics add to this risk. Prompt diagnosis with urinalysis and urine culture are necessary. Appropriate antibiotic treatment should be instituted. Hydronephrosis can be seen remotely, after anterior surgery in the lumbar spine for scoliosis, owing to retroperitoneal fibrosis.[6]

The syndrome of inappropriate antidiuretic hormone secretion has been reported after scoliosis fusion.[2] The patients have hyponatremia, oliguria, and concentrated urine. Treatment involves fluid restriction.

Scoliosis surgery entails large exposures across the spine, with multiple areas of exposed bone. This can lead to excessive blood loss that requires a significant transfusion. The scoliosis surgeon should be aware of the possibility of disseminated intravascular coagulation as a causative factor of excessive bleeding.[26] Additionally, the risks of homologous blood transfusion must be considered before undertaking elective scoliosis surgery. Disseminated intravascular coagulation is diagnosed on the basis of elevated prothrombin and partial thromboplastin times, thrombocytopenia, a low fibrinogen level, and high levels of fibrin split products. Rapid reinfusion of fresh frozen plasma, cryoprecipitate, platelets, and red blood cells is often necessary to treat disseminated intravascular coagulation.

Infection with hepatitis B or C virus, human immunodeficiency virus, or cytomegalovirus is possible with a homologous transfusion of blood or blood products. The authors routinely have patients predonate autologous blood for scoliosis surgery and use Cell Saver autologous blood recovery system intraoperatively. Meticulous surgical technique also helps in preventing excessive intraoperative blood loss.

The risk of retrograde ejaculation exists from an anterior lumbar procedure for scoliosis. This is the result of injury to the sympathetic plexus, usually a plexiform mesh of nerves or a single nerve in the presacral area running anterior to the aorta and coursing down into the pelvis over the bifurcation. The most frequent injury to this plexus occurs during fusions of L5–S1. The sympathetic plexus is responsible for bladder neck closure during ejaculation. Failure of closure of the bladder neck causes the ejaculate to travel in a retrograde fashion into the bladder. Fusion at L5–S1 should be performed with careful predissection bluntly over the discs, the use of Kittner dissectors, and the avoidance of electrocautery at this level. Retrograde ejaculation is rare, and it almost always resolves over time. However, male patients should be warned about this complication preoperatively if they are to undergo anterior lumbar fusions.

REFERENCES

1. Barner, H. B., and Sherman, D. C.: Vascular compression of the duodenum. Surg. Gynecol. Obstet. 117:103, 1963.
2. Bell, G. R., Gurd, A. R., Orlowski, J. P., et al.: The syndrome of inappropriate anti-diuretic hormone secretion following spinal fusion. J. Bone Joint Surg. 68A:720–724, 1986.
3. Bisla, R. S., and Louis, H. J.: Acute vascular compression of the duodenum following cast application. Surg. Gynecol. Obstet. 140:563–566, 1975.
4. Brown, L. P., and Stelling, F. H.: Fat embolism as a

complication of scoliosis fusion. J. Bone Joint Surg. 56A:1764, 1974.
5. Bunch, W., and Delaney, J.: Scoliosis and acute vascular compression of the duodenum. Surgery 67:901, 1970.
6. Cleveland, R. H., Gilsanz, V., Labowitz, R. L., et al.: Hydronephrosis from retroperitoneal fibrosis and anterior spinal fusion. J. Bone Joint Surg. 60A:996, 1978.
7. Cochran, T., Irstram, L., and Nachemson, A.: Long-term anatomic and functional changes in patients with adolescent idiopathic scoliosis treated by Harrington rod fusion. Spine 8:576–584, 1983.
8. Colletta A. J., and Mayer, P. J.: Chylothorax: An unusual complication of anterior thoracic interbodies spinal fusion. Spine 7:46–49, 1982.
9. Collis, D. K., and Ponseti, I. V.: Long-term follow-up of patients with idiopathic scoliosis not treated surgically. J. Bone Joint Surg. 51A:425–445, 1969.
10. Cotrel, Y., Dubousset, J., and Guillaumat, M.: New universal instrumentation in spinal surgery. Clin. Orthop. 227:10–23, 1988.
11. Elster, A. D.: Hyponatremia after spinal fusion caused by inappropriate secretion of anti-diuretic hormone (SIADH). Clin. Orthop. 194:136–141, 1985.
12. Flowman, Y., Micheli, L. J., Barker, W. D., et al.: Acute cholecystitis following the surgical treatment of spinal deformities in the adult. Clin. Orthop. 180:132–134, 1984.
13. Gittman, J. E., Buchaman, T. A., Fisher, B. J., et al.: Fatal fat embolism after spinal fusion for scoliosis. JAMA 249:779–781, 1983
14. Grubb, S. A., Lipscomb, H. J., and Coonrad, R. W.: Degenerative adult onset scoliosis. Spine 13:241–245, 1988.
15. Grubb, S. A., and Lipscomb H. J.: Diagnostic findings in painful adult scoliosis. Spine 17:518–527, 1992.
16. Hughes, J. P., McEntire, J. D., and Setze, T. K.: Cast syndrome. Arch. Surg. 108:230, 1974.
17. Kostuik, J. P., Israel, J., and Hall, J. E.: Scoliosis surgery in adults. Clin Orthop. 93:225–234, 1973.
18. Kostuik, J. P.: Recent advances in the treatment of painful adult scoliosis. Clin Orthop. 147:238–252, 1980.
19. Kostuik, J. P., and Bentivoglio, J.: The incidence of low back pain in adult scoliosis. Spine 6:268–273, 1981.
20. Kostuik, J. P., and Hall, B. B.: Spinal fusions to the sacrum in adults with scoliosis. Spine 8:489–500, 1983.
21. Nachemson, A.: A long-term follow-up study of non-treated scoliosis. Acta Orthop. Scand. 39:466–476, 1968.
22. Nakai, S., and Zielke, K.: Chylothorax—a rare complication after anterior and posterior spinal correction (a report of six cases). Spine 11:830–833, 1986.
23. Nilsonne, U., and Lundgren, K. D.: Long-term prognosis in idiopathic scoliosis. Acta Orthop. Scand. 39:455–465, 1968.
24. Pritchett, J. W., and Bortel, D. T.: Degenerative symptomatic lumbar scoliosis. Spine 18:700–703, 1993.
25. Probst-Proctor, S. L., Riski, L. A., and Bleck, E. E.: The cisterna chyli in orthopaedic surgery. Spine 8:787–792, 1983.
26. Raphael, B. G., Lakner, H., and Ergler, G. L.: Disseminated intravascular coagulation during surgery for scoliosis. Clin. Orthop. 162:41–46, 1982.
27. Robin, G. C., Span, Y., Steinberg, R., et al.: Scoliosis in the elderly. A follow-up study. Spine 7:355–359, 1982.
28. Rogala, E. J., Drummond, D. S., and Gurr, J.: Scoliosis: Incidence and natural history A prospective epidemiological study. J. Bone Joint Surg. 60A:173–176, 1978.
29. Scandalakis, J. E., Akin, J. T., Milsap, J. H., et al.: Vascular compression of the duodenum: Contemp. Surg. 10:33, 1977.
30. Shands, A. R., Jr., and Eisberg, H. B.: The incidence of scoliosis in the state of Delaware. J. Bone Joint Surg. 37A:1243–1249, 1955.
31. Simmons, E. H., and Jackson, R. F.: The management of nerve root entrapment syndromes associated with the collapsing scoliosis of idiopathic lumbar and thoracolumbar curves. Spine 4:533–541, 1979.
32. Simmons, E. H., Jackson, R. F., and Stripinus, D.: Incidence and severity of back pain in adult idiopathic scoliosis. Spine 8:749–756, 1983.
33. Sponseller, P. D., Cohen, M. S., Nachemson, A. L., et al.: Results of surgical treatment of adults with idiopathic scoliosis. J. Bone Joint Surg. 69A:667–675, 1987.
34. Swank, S., Lonstein, J. E., Moe J. H., and Bradford, D. S.: Surgical treatment of adult scoliosis. A review of two hundred and twenty-two cases. J. Bone Joint Surg. 63A:268–287, 1981
35. Uden, A.: Thromboembolic complications following scoliosis surgery in Scandinavia. Acta Orthop. Scand. 50:175–178, 1979.
36. Vanderpool, D. W., James, J. I. P., and Wynne-Davies, R.: Scoliosis in the elderly. J. Bone Joint Surg. 51A:446–455, 1969.
37. Weinstein, S. L., and Ponseti, I. V.: Curve progression in idiopathic scoliosis. J. Bone Joint Surg. 65A:447–455, 1983.
38. Winter, R. B., Lonstein, J. E., and Denis, F.: Pain patterns in adult scoliosis. Orthop. Clin. North Am. 19:339–345, 1988.

Assessment and Treatment

JOHN KOSTUIK

Adult scoliosis has been defined as a presentation of that deformity after skeletal maturity. Some definitions have specified that the patient's age must be 20 years or older when the patient first seeks treatment. Adult scoliosis can further be classified as a curve that starts before skeletal maturity, but for which treatment is sought later, or a deformity that arises de novo after skeletal maturity. The former is usually idiopathic but may have congenital or paralytic causes. The latter is secondary to degeneration, osteoporosis, osteomalacia, or extensive surgical decompression, usually for spinal stenosis. In addition, patients may present as adults who have a later complication of spinal fusion. The most common problems are iatrogenic flat back and accelerated degeneration of mobile adjacent vertebral segments.

Thirty years ago, most experts believed that surgical treatment of these conditions was not warranted, with few exceptions, most commonly a thoracic curve in patients in the third decade of life. Conservative care was advocated by authorities such as Nachemson,[68] who reported the risks of scoliosis surgery in adults. For complicated adult curves, he estimated that the risks were death (5%), neurologic damage (6%), significant loss of correction (20%), deep infection (10%), and medical problems (40%). Numerous clinical investigators showed not only that idiopathic curves could progress in adults, but also that they might become the source of significant clinical symptoms.*

A more aggressive surgical approach to these adult deformities became possible with the advent of Harrington rods[32]; many subsequent improvements in spinal instrumentation followed, such as the devices designed by Dwyer,[16, 22, 23, 32, 75, 109] Luque,† Zielke,[32, 43, 51, 78, 98, 111] and Cotrel and Dubousset.‡ These fixation devices have overcome many of the technical obstacles to successful surgical treatment. At the same time, improvements in preoperative assessment, anesthetic techniques and intraoperative management, and spinal cord monitoring,[11] combined with better understanding of postoperative care, have markedly improved the ability to address the complex problems of adult spinal deformities.[47] Today, this capability is recognized not only by orthopedists but also by family practice physicians and paramedical personnel.

ADULT PRESENTATION OF SCOLIOSIS BEGINNING BEFORE SKELETAL MATURITY

The four basic types are (1) an idiopathic curve, which is by far most common; (2) a congenital curve, usually associated with marked rigidity and kyphosis; (3) a paralytic curve; and (4) myopathic deformities.

Magnitude of the Current Problem

Kostuik and Bentivoglio[48] found that the prevalence of curves involving the adult thoracolumbar and lumbar spine was 3.9% in a review of 5000 intravenous pyelograms. These curves were truly structural and appeared to have commenced in adolescence and progressed in adult life, rather than arising de novo. This figure was similar to that reported by Dewar (unpublished data reported by Shands,[91] who analyzed 10,000 consecutive chest radiographs done for routine hospital admission). The prevalence of true structural curves in that sample was 4%. These figures parallel a classic study by Shands and Eisberg,[91] who studied a representative sample of 194,060 chest radiographs made in the state of Delaware in 1953. This represented 82.2% of the entire population older than age 14 years. They found that 1.9% of the population had a

---
*References 7, 12, 16, 17, 23, 25, 29, 40, 54, 56, 60, 69, 74, 75, 80, 84, 96–101, 103, 110, and 112.
†References 5, 6, 28, 35, 36, 41, 62, and 89.
‡References 10, 11, 14, 15, 18, 19, 43, and 56.

spinal curvature; 1.4% had mild curves (10 to 19 degrees), 0.3% had moderate curves (20 to 29 degrees), and only 0.2% had significant curves (30 degrees or more). The age distribution was fairly consistent. Shands and Eisberg[91] reported that their results were similar to those reported by Niebauer (personal communication cited by Shands and Eisberg[91]), who noted that the prevalence was 2.5 per 100 in the general population, but in the age group 20 to 65 years, this rose to 4.2 per 100.

Perennou and colleagues[82] further defined the frequency and characteristics of lumbar scoliosis in the adult population with low back pain. These were assessed by a clinical and radiologic prospective study. The prevalence was 7.5% and it increased with age: 2% before age 45 years, 15% after 60 years. Eighty-six percent of patients who initially presented with low back pain were subsequently discovered to have a scoliosis on radiologic investigation. The mean Cobb angle was 21 ± 11.4 degrees. A Cobb angle of more than 30 degrees was noted in 16% of the patients with scoliosis. This was 1% of the entire population with low back pain. The proportion of women affected increased with the severity of scoliosis. Right- and left-sided scolioses were equally distributed. A positive correlation was found between Cobb angle and age. The patients with lumbar scoliosis were distinguished by a more advanced age, 62 ± 12.4 years versus 49.6 ± 5.5 years. A great proportion of women, 72% versus 48%, have radicular pain emanating from the L3–L4 levels. Radicular pain was more related to unstable deformities. These investigators also concluded that most cases of degenerative scoliosis seemed to originate from minor childhood scoliosis and evolved because of disc degeneration. This has been the author's experience as well.

Weinstein and Ponseti[109] determined factors that are responsible for continued progression of scoliosis in adult life. Thoracic curves between 50 and 75 degrees at skeletal maturity increased an average of 30 degrees over a lengthy follow-up interval. Thoracolumbar curves of 50 to 75 degrees at skeletal maturity increased an average of 22.3 degrees over the next 40 years. Progression was the greatest when there was a lumbar curve, when the fifth lumbar vertebra was not well seated, and when the apical rotation was greater than 33%. These findings are similar to observations of Kostuik and colleagues.[51] The adolescent patient with the worst prognosis for later difficulty as an adult presents with an imbalanced lumbar or thoracolumbar curve, the fifth lumbar vertebra not parallel to the sacrum, and the curve emanating from the lumbosacral junction (Fig. 1). This curve pattern also presents the greatest technical difficulty for correction in older adults, and it is best treated surgically at an earlier age, if possible.

Other curves with a poor prognosis include those with a pattern in which the apex falls at L2–L3 or L3–L4, a grade III rotation, an unbalanced frontal position, and a secondary compensatory curve that is sharp and angular at L4–L5 and L5–S1. These curves can often be treated in young adults or adolescents by dealing with the compensatory curve at one or two levels rather than with the entire and more proximal curve, which often extends over five to seven levels (see Fig. 1).

Despite increased knowledge about risk factors for progression, the spine surgeon commonly encounters with an adult patient with scoliosis, increasing pain, loss of lumbar lordosis, or truncal imbalance. Accompanying these deformities may be problems associated with osteoporosis and spinal stenosis. These conditions can also be treated (Fig. 2). How often do these problems occur, and in particular, how common is significant axial pain?

In a review of adult patients with idiopathic lumbar and thoracolumbar scoliosis, Kostuik and Bentivoglio[48] found that 60% reported pain. This was similar to the prevalence in 100 age-matched patients without curvature and also to the figures reported in numerous population studies of low back pain. When the curves were greater than 45 degrees, the prevalence and severity of pain symptoms increased significantly. These findings are in contrast to those of Nachemson[68–70] and Nilsonne,[75] who found a similar prevalence of pain but noted that it was rarely a significant clinical problem. All studies seem to agree that thoracic curves are rarely a source of pain, although a hyperlordotic curve may cause significant pulmonary dysfunction.

A variety of factors have been analyzed to determine which may be important in

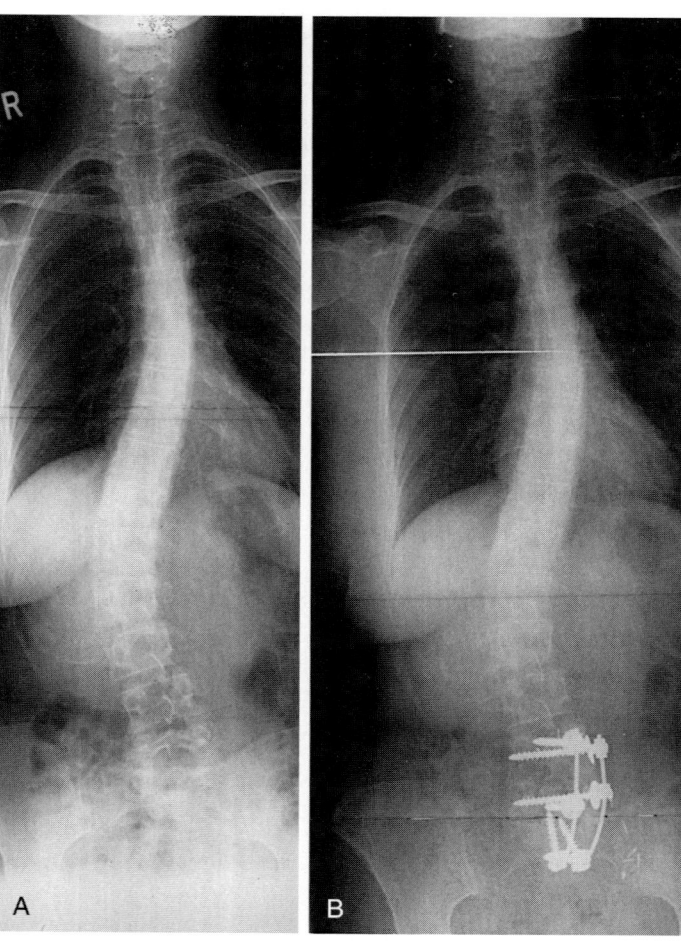

Figure 1. Female patient, age 26 years, with a painful scoliosis. *A*, Note marked imbalance to the left. Pain was reproduced on discography at both L4–L5 and L1–S1 discs. *B*, Rebalance was achieved with relief of pain lateral closing wedges. Note double Zielke rods to control rotational forces.

producing pain. Age is relevant, as in all spinal disorders. Pain appears to reach its maximum between the ages of 40 and 60 years and thereafter, in general, is less of a problem.

The effects of occupation are less well understood, but a patient with a preexisting adolescent curve may select less physically demanding occupations.[48, 88] If a patient has scoliosis and a physically demanding occupation, he or she is more likely to miss time from work or become disabled.[48]

Pain is also associated with curves greater than 45 degrees at skeletal maturity. When the apex of the curve shows radiographically evident degeneration, this is associated with both more pain and greater degeneration at the lumbosacral joint.[48]

Kostuik and Musha[58] analyzed the long-term prognosis after surgery. One hundred ten adult scoliotic patients were independently reviewed as to long-term functional assessment. They had undergone surgery as adults, with follow-up occurring at an average of 12.5 years (minimum, 10-year follow-up). They underwent independent functional assessment with reference to pain, recreation, marriage, childbearing, employment, education, and sexual activity. A lower rate of marriage was noted. There were no unusual childbearing problems. More were employed part-time than in the general population. Education levels were generally higher than normal. Eleven percent of these patients were receiving disability compensation. Seventy percent were involved in recreational activities. Increasing back pain was noted at an average of 5.9 years after surgery but in and of itself was not disabling. Eighty-five percent said that they would have their surgery again, and 64% said surgery fully achieved their goals and expectations. It was believed that the patients' social integration was somewhat

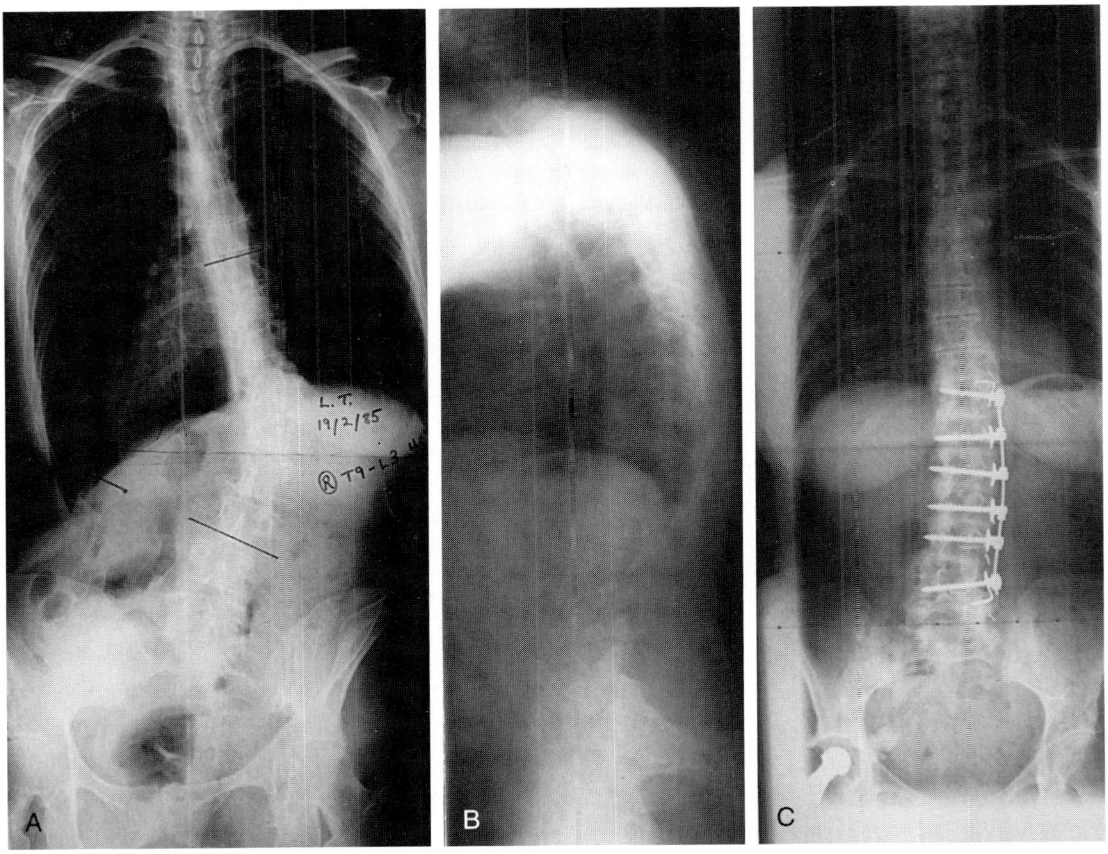

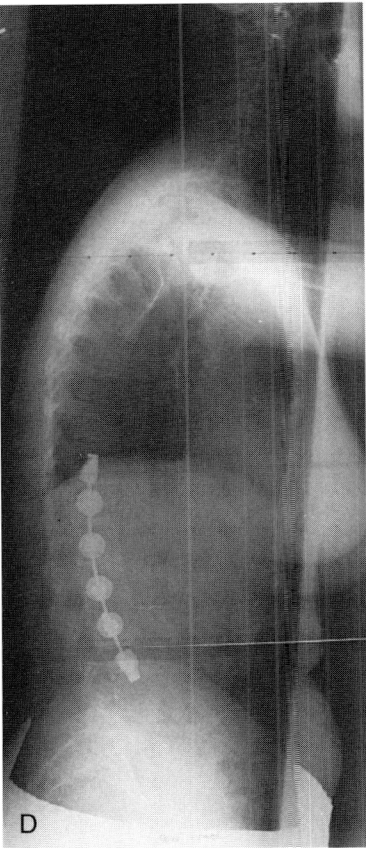

Figure 2. Female patient, age 65 years. *A*, Documented progressive painful curve of 44 degrees. L4–L5 and L5–S1 discs were not painful on discography; L4–S1 and L5–S1 facet blocks did not relieve pain. Note previous total hip replacement. *B*, Preoperative lateral view showing curve of 66 degrees. *C*, Postoperative view of Zielke instrumentation curve corrected to 12 degrees. At 6 years follow-up, there was no pain. *D*, Lordosis has been fully preserved.

significantly impaired, although the vast majority were active and gainfully employed. Working capacity with reference to relevant numbers working full-time or part-time was significantly less than that of the general population. All patients had been treated by Harrington instrumentation. It is anticipated that with advances in all aspects of adult spine surgery, including indications, preoperative evaluation, selection of fusion levels, surgical approach, instrumentation, and rehabilitation, the future long-term results could be significantly improved.

Bartie and associates[3] analyzed 172 patients a minimum of 19 years after spine fusions terminating at L2, L3, L4, or L5. All had been treated by posterior spine fusion and Harrington instrumentation, with a minimum 10-year follow-up. No radiographic measurements or trends could be found statistically to predict a painful outcome. Both patients and control subjects, of whom there were 209, experienced similar back pain. However, control subjects functioned at a higher physical level. In this series, the functional outcome was independent of the lowest level of fusion to L2, L3, or L4. In contrast, Connolly and associates,[13] in a review of adolescent patients who underwent fusion extending into the lumbar spine to L2 or distally, found a higher incidence of low back pain than in a similar control group 10 years after surgery. A higher incidence of degenerative changes was noted with the descending level of fusion for fusions extending into the lower lumbar spine. Alone, degenerative changes were not indicative of a poor result. Sagittal plane imbalance (flat back or junctional kyphosis) was associated with a poor result, which was consistent with previous reports. There was a 29.6% rate of additional surgery. Seventeen percent of patients thought that the goals of initial surgery had not been accomplished. Increased Cobb angels and increased kyphosis were related to the lower spine score.

These signs were more consistent than those of Bartie and associates[3] and were more in keeping with previous studies of Cochran and coworkers[10] and Edgar and Mehta.[23]

Poitras and associates,[83] similarly, did a comparative study of patients treated for adolescent idiopathic scoliosis who were analyzed 10 to 20 years after referral. These investigators noted a higher prevalence of arthritis and heart disease than that in control subjects. Female scoliotic subjects were less likely to become pregnant, with a higher rate of miscarriages and stillbirths. Cesarean section rates were lower in the scoliotic group. Patients with scoliosis had a higher prevalence of respiratory symptoms. Interestingly, scoliotic subjects, particularly women, had a problem with self-image. Overall, the patients with idiopathic scoliosis had more health problems than expected.

A comparison of 1476 patients with idiopathic scoliosis followed into adult life with a slightly larger but similar number of community control subjects was analyzed with reference to back pain.[83] Seventy-three percent of patients with idiopathic scoliosis experienced back pain in the year before analysis, compared with 56% of control subjects. The intensity of pain was greater in the subjects with scoliosis, was more continuous and generalized, and tended to have more of a neurogenic component. Patients with scoliosis were more restricted in usual daily activities compared with control subjects. It was believed that back pain was related to the structural derangement of the spine in patients with idiopathic scoliosis and was responsible for a considerable degree of disability and handicap in later life. These conclusions are similar to those noted by Kostuik and associates reported in 1990.[53]

Patient Evaluation

History

Obviously, it is important to obtain a complete history, as it is for any patient with a spinal disorder. A family history of progressive deformity may give some clue to prognosis. The date of onset of the deformity should be elicited but is usually not, in itself, important. However, the history of curve progression is important. Some measure of progression may be surmised from changes in how clothes fit, an observed increase in rib hump, loss of height, or altered waistline. Ideally, a more precise definition of curve progression can be obtained from serial radiographs; unfortunately, these have often been lost or never taken.

It is also important to discuss and understand how the deformity affects the patient's life. Many adults are reluctant to discuss the aesthetic consequences of their curve unless asked directly. Many have learned to cope with the deformity, but for others it is a source of major concern. This problem was identified in 10% of the patients surveyed.[48]

A careful pain history should also be elicited, which can be aided by the use of pain drawings. Pain at the apex of the curve should be differentiated from pain remote from the apex. Important information is pain duration and its affect on activities of daily living, occupation, social function, recreation, and sexual activities.

Often, a radicular or referred component of the axial pain is present. Sometimes, this is related to the apex of the curve. A thoracic or thoracolumbar curve may present with intercostal neuralgia. Leg symptoms may relate to the primary or the compensatory curve and either can be sclerotomal or have the characteristics of frank sciatica. Any associated bladder or bowel dysfunction is an important diagnostic and prognostic clue. Incontinence, particularly in elderly women, should not be assumed to be secondary to myogenic causes until proven otherwise. Often, spinal stenosis can be causative.

In addition to the history of the deformity and associated pain, the general impact on health should be evaluated. Respiratory malfunction may be a presenting symptom with adult scoliosis,[46, 47, 81] but is far more common in paralytic or severe congenital curves and relatively rare in old idiopathic curves. The author reviewed 200 consecutive adults with idiopathic scoliosis (unpublished data). Functionally important, respiratory dysfunction was not observed, even with curves of 100 degrees or more. However, ventilation was often decreased by up to 25% of normal predicted values. Arterial blood gas values were generally normal. Exceptions to this overall favorable picture are patients with idiopathic scoliosis associated with marked thoracic lordosis.

Nachemson[68, 70] in 1968 reported the risk of death as 5% from pulmonary compromise and 40% from other medically associated problems in adults with spinal deformity secondary to scoliosis. He reported that the loss of ability to breathe properly was first measurable in patients with thoracic curves of about 60 degrees. Death from cor pulmonale usually occurs with curves greater than 100 degrees in patients who are 45 years or older. However, a subsequent prospective report on 200 adult patients with idiopathic scoliosis with thoracic deformities showed no measurable dysfunction in the ability to perform work or daily activities, unless the curve exceeded 100 degrees.[47] In 1988, the same authors reexamined 24 patients who were initially examined or had surgery in 1968.[70] They noted that the decline in spirometric value over the 20 years was of the same magnitude as a predicted decline due to aging. Reduced vital capacity was the strongest predictor of the development of respiratory failure, followed by the scoliotic angle. Respiratory failure occurred only in patients with a vital capacity of less than 45% of that predicted in 1968 and with an angle greater than 110 degrees. Thus, respiratory failure developed in adults with scoliosis who exhibited a large angle and a low vital capacity. Normal aging reduces the ventilatory capacity further. Kesten and associates[44] also noted that the impairment of exercise performance found in adults with moderate scoliosis cannot be attributed to any important ventilatory limitation, abnormality in lung volume, or impaired chemoreceptor sensitivity. They believed that the reduction likely arises from deconditioning and lack of aerobic exercise.

Physical Examination

Again, the elements of the physical examination are comparable to the evaluation of all patients with spinal disorders. Curve assessment includes the following: the three-dimensional characteristics, including kyphosis and lordosis; the rib hump; the degree of decompensation; and flexibility.

The neurologic examination should be complete and should include assessment of subtle neurologic findings. For example, left thoracic idiopathic curves are sometimes associated with syringomyelia. Mild clawing of the toes may indicate a tethered cord.

Imaging Studies

The initial radiographic analysis includes three views: foot, standing posteroanterior, and lateral films. Focal, coned views may be useful in patients with pain to evaluate facets, congenital anomalies, and disc narrowing. Oblique radiographs are taken using Stagnara views, to assess the rotational deformity, particularly when a kyphosis is present.

Lateral bending radiographs indicate the curve's flexibility, but do not predict positively or negatively the degree of surgical correction that might be obtained. For example, the amount of correction obtained by anterior Zielke instrumentation was twice that predicted by the preoperative bending films. Extension views may have greater value in determining whether an associated kyphosis is flexible, whereas flexion views may provide similar information about lordotic deformities. Traction films occasionally may be of value in determining whether distraction will overcome decompensation.

After the routine radiographs are obtained, a variety of ancillary imaging studies may be considered. Bone scans are rarely indicated, except in young adults with pain and minor curvature. In this instance, the bone scan may reveal an alternative cause, particularly osteoid osteoma.

If there are neurologic findings or surgical correction is contemplated, myelography is the imaging modality of choice. Its particular importance is to determine any areas of actual or potential compression, which become important when corrective forces are applied. Computed tomographic scans have little use, except when combined with myelographic enhancement. The role of magnetic resonance imaging appears promising, but its usefulness remains uncertain for the evaluation of spinal deformities because of its inability to obtain views parallel or 90 degrees to the dural sac.

Other Ancillary Tests, Discography, and Facet Blocks

One of the major issues in the adult with scoliosis and pain is to determine the source of symptoms. When surgery is contemplated, one needs to assess accurately which spinal levels to include in the fusion. In the author's early experience with adult deformities, 30% to 35% of patients had persisting pain after a solid fusion was attained. Since that time, the results appear to have improved, which is attributed in part to the use of discography.[46, 47] Specifically, the L3–L4, L4–L5, and L5–S1 levels are evaluated, but rarely is the test performed at the apex of the curve. Although the ideal approach is posterolateral, the rotational deformity may necessitate a transdural approach (Fig. 3).

Facet blocks are also employed, usually at the same lower lumbar levels. If discography produces pain and facet blocks relieve it, the author's opinion is that the fusion should incorporate that level. This is believed to be particularly important when the lumbosacral level fulfills these criteria. Conversely, if discograms do not reproduce the patient's pain and facet blocks do not relieve it, this level is not incorporated.

Magnetic resonance imaging scans may be used to assess the water content of an L5–S1 disc in T2-weighted images, but they do not correlate with pain. Therefore, discography continues to be performed in the area of the lumbosacral junction.

Nonoperative Care

The basic approach to nonoperative care is similar to that for the treatment of all chronic, painful spinal disorders. This includes exercise and the use of nonsteroidal, antiinflammatory drugs. Physiotherapeutic modalities and exercises do not prevent curve progression, but may maintain flexibility. Activities such as low-thrust aerobics, cycling, and swimming are useful adjuncts and are particularly important in preventing osteoporosis. It is also important to use the other preventive measures for postmenopausal osteoporosis, including estrogen and calcium administration.

The role of orthotics is unknown, and there is no evidence to suggest that they prevent curve progression in adults. Orthotics seem to be useful in elderly patients, but the equipment should be rigid and fitted

Figure 3. Female patient, age 58 years. A, Progressive painful thoracolumbar curve. The pain was diffuse and clinically appeared to originate from the apex of the deformity and the lumbosacral curve. B, Discography at L5–S1 reproduced the lumbosacral pain. C, Fusion to the sacrum was performed with an excellent result. D, The Jackson intrasacral technique of sacral fixation was used. The sacral screws are angled across the proximal S1 end plate, enhancing fixation. The rods are intrasacral and are buttressed by the iliac wings.

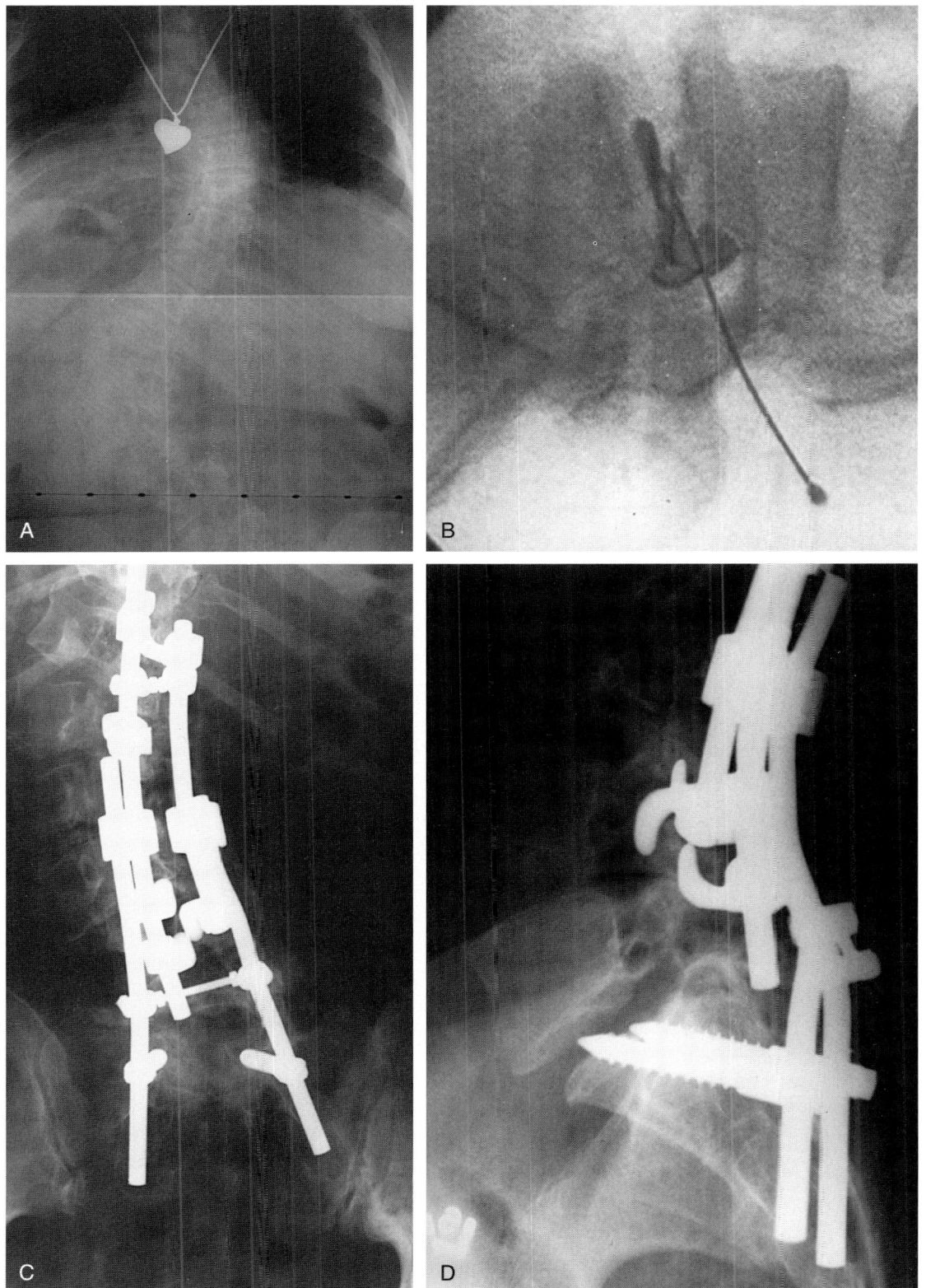

See figure legend on opposite page.

carefully to the patient's deformity. However, these devices are frequently poorly tolerated.

Surgery

Surgical Indications

The indications for surgery in an adult with an idiopathic curve are

1. To obtain pain relief
2. To prevent further progression of deformity
3. To manage current significant neurologic dysfunction or later dysfunction in a patient at risk
4. To improve cosmetic appearance

PAIN

Pain is the most common indication, occurring in about 85% of surgical cases. Determining the sources of pain and predicting its surgical relief are a great challenge. The prevalence of pain and the use of a variety of testing techniques, such as discography, have been discussed. As for any spinal disorder, the more certain one is of the cause of pain, the more likely one is to have a successful outcome.

PROGRESSING DEFORMITY

An even greater question than who should undergo fusion for pain relief is who should undergo fusion to prevent further progression of deformity. It is the author's opinion that two groups of patients are candidates. First, fusion is performed for adults younger than 35 years with an obviously increasing deformity, in particular those with lumbar or thoracolumbar curves that measure 45 degrees or greater. Inevitably, these curves progress and become painful. In women, especially those with secondary degenerative changes, scoliosis with retention of lumbar lordosis may convert to a kyphoscoliosis. If this deformity becomes rigid, it requires a two-stage surgical correction. In comparison, younger adults can be treated by a one-stage anterior or posterior correction and fusion with Zielke or Texas Scottish Rite Hospital instrumentation or other forms of posterior segmental instrumentation with minimum morbidity (see Fig. 3).

Second, fusion is performed for younger patients with truncal imbalance of 4 cm or more. This group of patients is characterized by a major curve of 40 degrees or more that extends to L3 or L4, accompanied by a compensatory curve at L4, L5, or the sacrum. The primary curve in this instance may be reduced significantly by rebalancing of only the lower compensatory curve. This approach should be employed if the lower curve is painful. The patient should be aware that extension of the fusion may be required at a later date. To date, the author has used this technique in 16 patients. The average degree of correction of the major curve has been more than 40% (see Fig. 1). This technique is discussed in more detail under Lateral Lumbar Circumferential Osteotomy with Imbalanced Adult Scoliosis below.

NEUROLOGIC DEFICIT

Neurologic deficits are occasionally an indication for surgical intervention in a patient with preexistent curvature who presents as an adult. In a review written in 1979, only 5 of 227 patients treated surgically required decompression.[47] However, with an increasingly aged population, it is possible that a greater number of patients will be seen who have associated spinal stenosis (Fig. 4). Of 101 adults treated by Cotrel-Dubousset instrumentation between 1986 and 1989, 22 required decompression. Most were older than 50 years.

Jackson and Simmons[40] described a subset of patients with radicular symptoms arising from a compensatory rather than a primary curve. They noted significant improvement of these symptoms after anterior stabilization of the major curve. This approach has been less successful in the author's experience.

COSMESIS

Cosmesis is generally thought to be an uncommon indication in the adult with scoliosis, with the exception of the young adult who has an imbalanced curve. However, this may be an underestimation. Johnson and Holt[41] followed 100 patients for more than 10 years after spine fusion. Retrospectively, patients reported that body image and cosmesis had played a greater role in their deci-

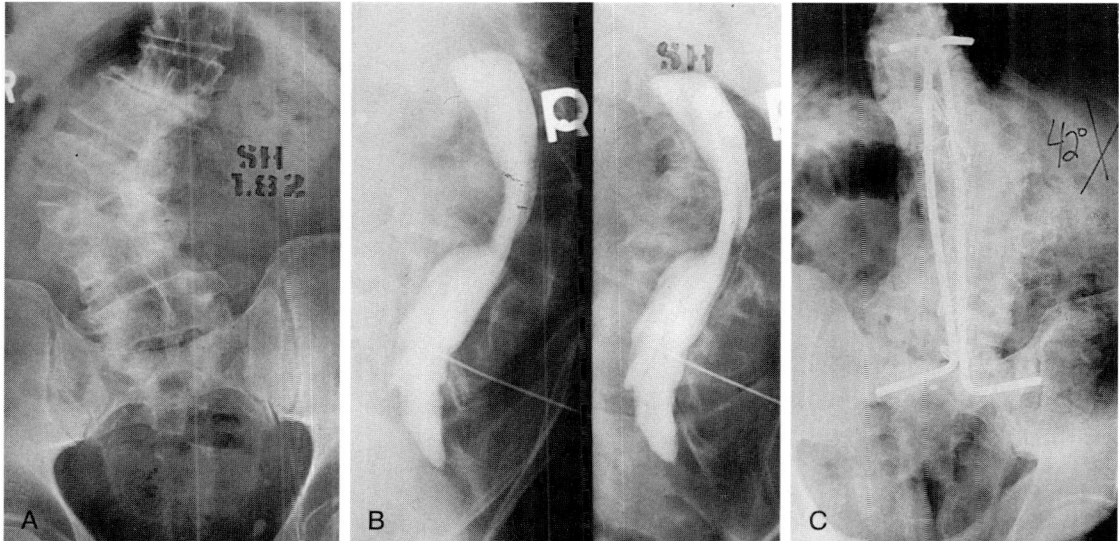

Figure 4. Male patient, age 56 years. *A*, Curve of 68 degrees. The patient had marked symptoms and mild signs of spinal stenosis. *B*, Preoperative myelogram indicates severe compromise of the canal of the apex of the curve. *C*, Postoperative anteroposterior (AP) view showing curve of 42 degrees. Five years later, the patient is pain free and working.

sion to have surgery than was evident at the time of the operation.

If a patient's goal is predominantly cosmetic, surgical intervention may be warranted after repeated discussions with the patient and his or her close relatives. Posterior segmental instrumentation is particularly helpful, especially if the patient is hypokyphotic, and excellent cosmetic correction can be obtained. The use of thoracoplasty (partial rib excision over four to six levels) may be an additional means to improve that outcome. Thoracoplasty has gained popularity. The morbidity is minimum. Rib excision should extend to the posterior axillary line. Pulmonary function is not compromised by thoracoplasty.

Surgical Techniques

Harrington posterior instrumentation is rarely indicated in the treatment of adult scoliosis. Loss of lumbar lordosis inevitably occurs with this distracting device, even with the use of sacroalar hooks, contouring, or square-ended rods. Three basic strategies are available: anterior fusion using internal fixation,[32, 47, 77] posterior fusion using posterior segmental instrumentation,[15] and Cotrel-Dubousset instrumentation with combined anterior-posterior approaches.[8, 39, 41, 105] The author prefers the latter.

Lumbar and thoracolumbar curves with good lumbar lordosis may be treated with anterior instrumentation using the Zielke, Texas Scottish Rite Hospital, or Universal system technique.[111] However, this method is not useful if there is an associated true kyphosis or a small degree of lumbar lordosis as measured from L1 to S1. The kyphosis increases with this approach. This possibility is best evaluated by oblique Stagnara views.

In patients with kyphosis or loss of lordosis, pain relief and restoration of balance should be accompanied by restoration of lumbar lordosis. At present, this objective is best achieved in rigid curves by a two-stage procedure. An anterior approach is used, followed by multiple-level discectomies and fusion with instrumentation. A posterior fusion is performed using Cotrel-Dubousset instrumentation (Figs. 5 and 6) either at the same time or at a later stage.

On the other hand, if the kyphoscoliosis is mobile, correction can be achieved by a single-stage procedure using the Cotrel-Dubousset technique or other newly developed posterior segmental systems. The advantage of this instrumentation is its ability to derotate the spine, especially in the lumbar area,

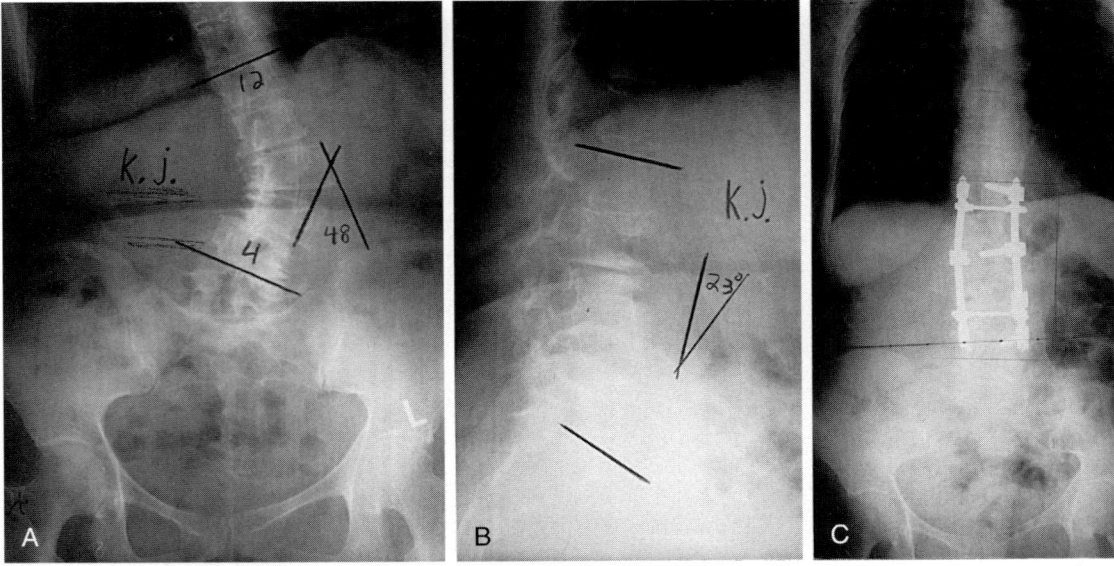
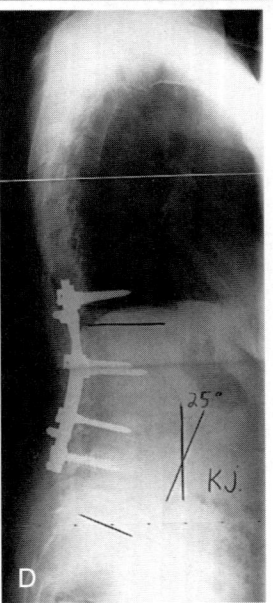

Figure 5. Female patient, age 62 years. *A*, Progressive painful curve. *B*, Preoperative lateral view. Note significant loss of lordosis (−23 degrees measured from L1 to S1). *C*, Postoperative AP view. *D*, Postoperative lateral view. Two-stage surgery was performed. Stage 1: Multiple anterior discotomies with morcellized bone graft. Stage 2: Cotrel-Dubousset instrumentation and fusion. Note significant return of lumbar lordosis owing to derotation and anterior release (increase of 48 degrees).

and to restore lordosis when there is curve mobility. An alternative is the use of contoured Luque rods combined with the Galveston technique.* Although this technique initially showed great promise, pain related to the sacroiliac joint has been reported in the presence of solid lumbar fusion. There is also a risk of neurologic damage associated with passage of the sublaminar wires. For these reasons, the author has abandoned this technique.

ANTERIOR INSTRUMENTATION

In scoliosis surgery, the indications for anterior instrumentation are curve corrections and lumbosacral fusion.

The first indication for this approach is a thoracolumbar or lumbar curve that does not require lumbosacral fusion, is mobile on

---

*References 1, 11, 22, 27, 28, 30, 31, 34, 36, 42–45, 49, 52, 59, 61, 62, 73, 88, and 102.

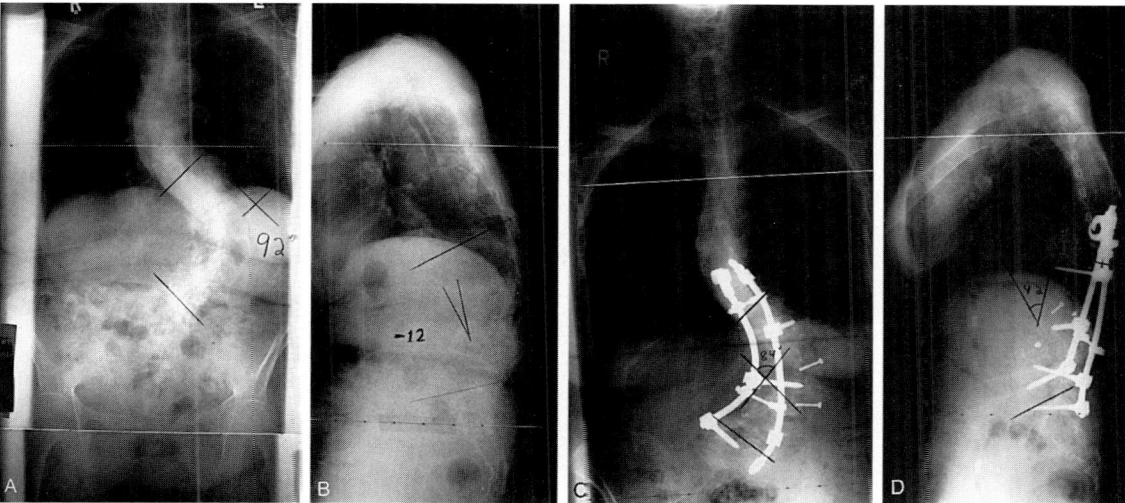

Figure 6. Female patient, age 57 years. *A,* Progressive kyphoscoliosis, curve of 92 degrees. *B,* Preoperative lateral view showing −12 degrees of lordosis. *C,* Postoperative AP view. There is minimal correction. *D,* Postoperative lateral view. Two-stage surgery was performed. Stage 1: Multiple anterior discotomies with morcellization of L2–L3. Stage 2: Cotrel-Dubousset instrumentation and fusion. There is marked restoration of lordosis to 42 degrees (gain of 54 degrees).

bending films, and preserves lordosis.* The entire curve should be spanned in adults. In comparison, the adolescent spine may require a fusion of lesser extent. The systems most commonly used include the Zielke system and the Texas Scottish Rite Hospital system.

After the levels to be fused have been exposed, the disc spaces are cleared, including the end plates, back to the posterior longitudinal ligaments. This exposure is essential so that an accurate angle of insertion can be obtained for the screws. If at all possible, the screws should be angled toward the contralateral junction of the pedicle with the vertebral body. To ensure that the opposite cortex is penetrated, a depth gauge is placed on the exposed disc space to determine the pathway and length of the screw. Arbitrarily, the author adds 2 mm of additional length, which is particularly important when there is lipping of the vertebral margins secondary to degeneration. If there is significant osteoporosis, methyl methacrylate is used. In these instances, the screw hole is enlarged with a curet to retain the cement and to enhance screw fixation (Fig. 7). The use of low-viscosity or cooled cement increases the working time. This technique is particularly

*References 32, 36, 39, 43, 47, 51, 52, 57, 66, 77, 78, and 98.

useful in the most proximal screw. Rather than adding an extra level across an unfused level, the author now routinely uses cement at the upper level (Fig. 8). The use of a derotator is now almost routine, because it has the capability to reproduce lordosis in the lumbar spine or to reduce kyphosis in the thoracolumbar spine.

Autogenous bone graft is used, usually consisting of excised ribs cut up into small fragments. To increase the lordosis, block or minced grafts are selectively placed anteriorly in the disc space. The average blood loss with this technique has been 1750 ml.

Limitations of Technique. The technique is possible from L5 to T9 or T10. Further extension above that level is rarely of value, because the disc spaces are so narrow that little correction can be obtained in an adult, although its efficacy has been shown in the thoracic spine of adolescents. Although fusion can be extended across the lumbosacral junction, this is usually combined with a posterior fusion.

Postoperative Care. Prolonged recumbency is not required; patients usually become ambulatory by the third or fourth postoperative day. Patients with thoracolumbar curves are fitted to a total contact orthosis, a modular Boston overlap-type brace, or a

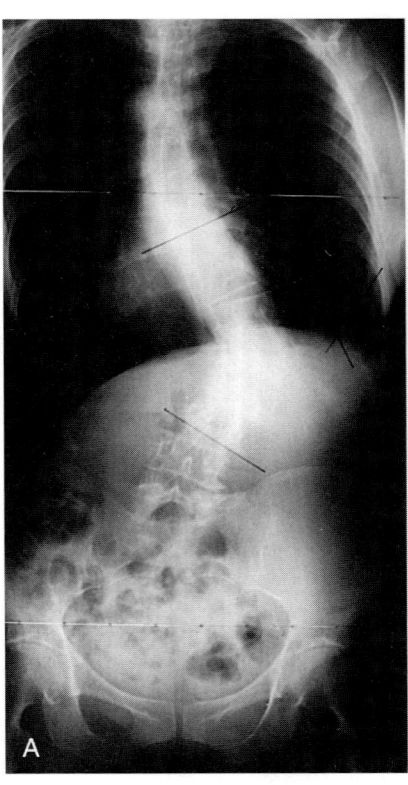 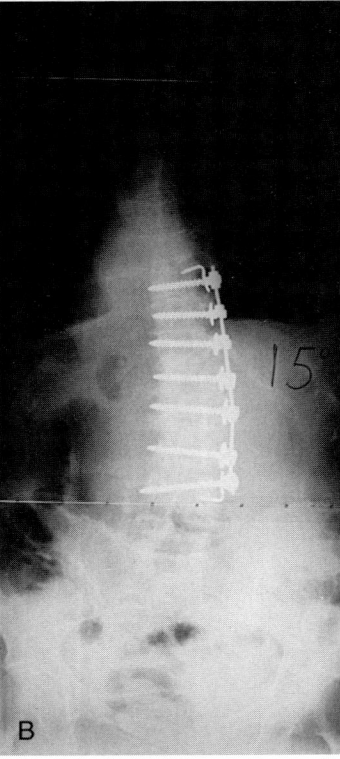

Figure 7. Female patient, age 72 years. *A*, Severe incapacitating painful curve of 75 degrees. *B*, Postoperative curve of 15 degrees. Methyl methacrylate is used to hold the screws. The patient has been pain free for 7 years postoperatively.

molded plastic corset. Thoracic curves require no exterior support.

Results. The results obtained with Zielke instrumentation have markedly improved on the results obtained with Dwyer and other posterior instrumentation techniques. Kostiuk and colleagues[51, 52] reviewed the results in the first 57 patients and found that the average correction was 70%, compared with 45% obtained with Dwyer instrumentation. Moreover, there were no pseudarthroses. In double idiopathic curves, the average correction was 62% initially. Twenty-four months postoperatively, the mean loss of initial correction was 3.4 degrees (4%). Noninstrumented proximal thoracic curves improved 28%, and there was no deterioration during the 2-year follow-up. Correction in the frontal plane for patients younger than 50 years of age was 72% and correction for patients older than age 50 years was 60%.

The use of derotation devices has further improved curve correction in the sagittal and anteroposterior planes. Rotational deformity improved by one grade with the use of the Nash-Moe method.[72]

Complications. No major complications or deaths were encountered in the 57 patients studied. General complications were limited to 10 cases of atelectasis and pleural effusion, which resolved without major treatment. Short-term local complications included three lateral femoral cutaneous nerve entrapments, one of which required later surgical decompression, and two postthoracotomy syndromes. Later complications were the following: one case of instrument failure occurred, which required later posterior surgery; there was one case of proximal staple pullout at two levels, and five additional patients had partial staple disengagement, none of which required treatment; the nuts backed out of the screw head in 10 cases without loss of correction or rod displacement; and rod disengagement from the screw head was present in six cases without loss of correction.

The Texas Scottish Rite Hospital system has been used for indications similar to those for anterior Zielke instrumentation. The advantages are that the Texas Scottish Rite Hospital system is more rigid.

Trammell and associates,[104] in an analysis

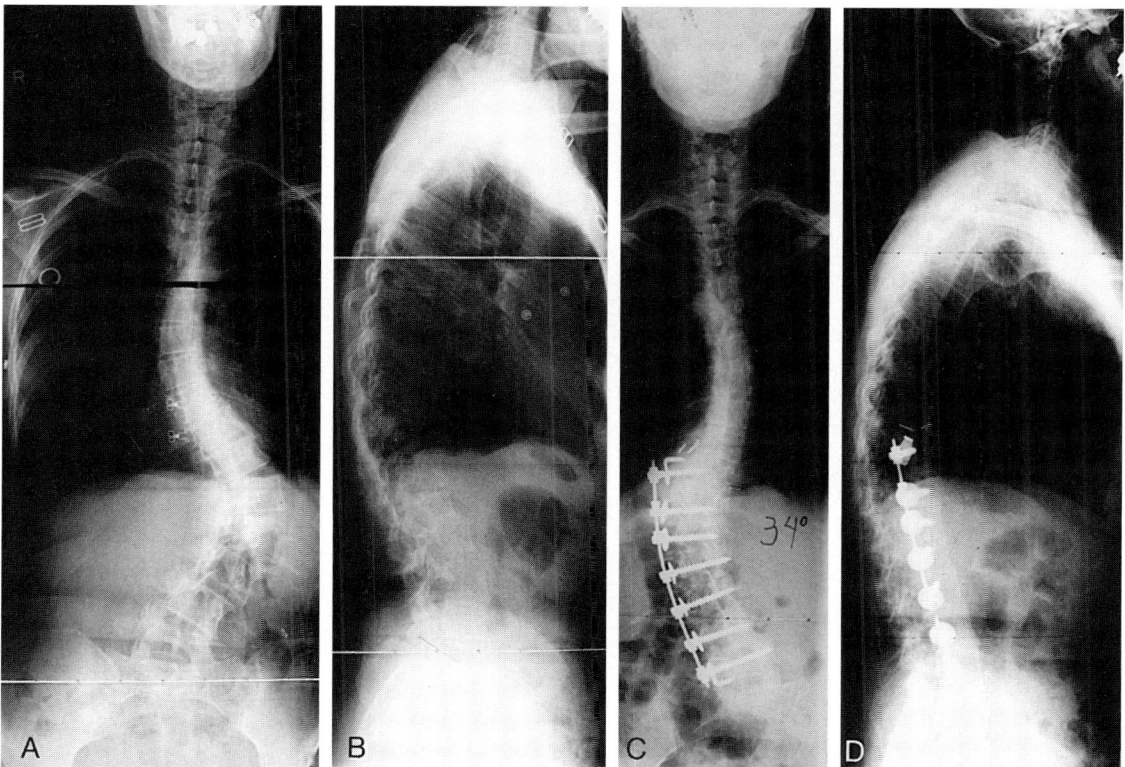

Figure 8. Female patient, age 52 years. *A,* Curve of 68 degrees that was painful, progressive, and rigid. *B,* Preoperative lordosis of 50 degrees measured from L1 to S1. *C,* Postoperative curve of 34 degrees. Note the proximal hook pullout. *D,* Postoperative lateral view showing lordosis of 38 degrees, good long-term result.

of surgery in 26 adults with an average age 41 years who underwent correction by Zielke instrumentation, noted an average correction of 63%. These researchers believed that high-risk groups were patients with a curve greater than 60 degrees or those older than age 50 years with rigid deformity. There were eight cases of instrumentation failure.

Krismer and colleagues,[59] in an analysis of results in 97 patients, noted an average of 79% correction with 11% loss of correction in the first year and 2% subsequently. These investigators believed that Zielke instrumentation was the apparatus of choice for thoracolumbar and lumbar scoliosis, but noted a mild tendency to increase kyphosis. Krismer and colleagues'[59] results appear to be somewhat better than those reported by Trammell and coworkers,[104] Kostuik and colleagues,[51] and others.[43, 67, 78, 95]

POSTERIOR SEGMENTAL INSTRUMENTION

Although popularized by Luque,[62, 63] posterior segmental instrumentation using sublaminar wires (Fig. 9) has been replaced by the use of multilevel hooks and/or pedicle screws. Cotrel-Dubousset instrumentation is the other major option for patients with scoliosis or mobile kyphoscoliosis. Other similar devices are now available. This device combines the rigidity of segmental fixation with derotation, which is particularly effective in the lumbar spine.

The surgical technique for this instrumentation has been described in detail elsewhere.[14, 15] Adjuncts to this basic approach are anterior releases in rigid curves, posterior releases when there has been prior posterior surgery, and rib excision to improve cosmetic outcome when there is significant curve rigidity and a rib hump (Fig. 10).

An independent analysis was performed studying 123 adults who underwent correction of their idiopathic scoliosis with Cotrel-Dubousset instrumentation between 1985 and 1991, with a minimum 2-year follow-up.[55] The average age was 41 years, ranging from 20 to 75 years, with 43 patients older

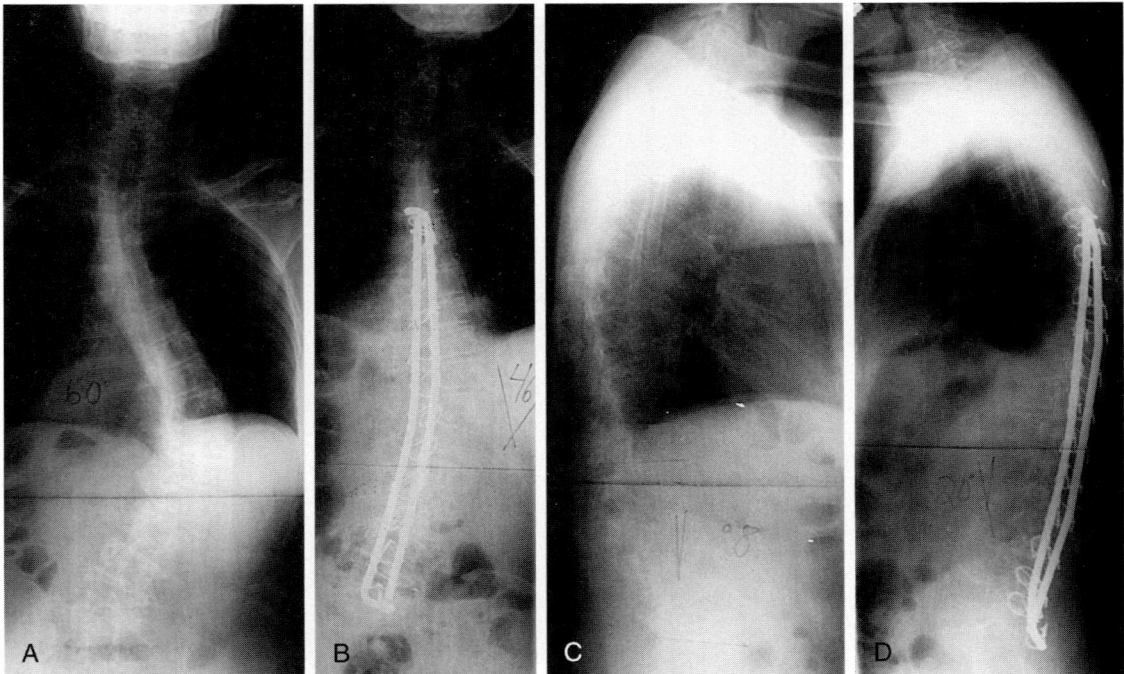

Figure 9. Luque segmental sublaminar wiring. *A*, A painful progressive thoracolumbar curve of 60 degrees. *B*, Reduction of the curve to 46 degrees with pain alleviation. Fusion was to L5. *C*, Lordosis was measured from L1 to S1 (8 degrees). *D*, Lordosis was increased to 20 degrees.

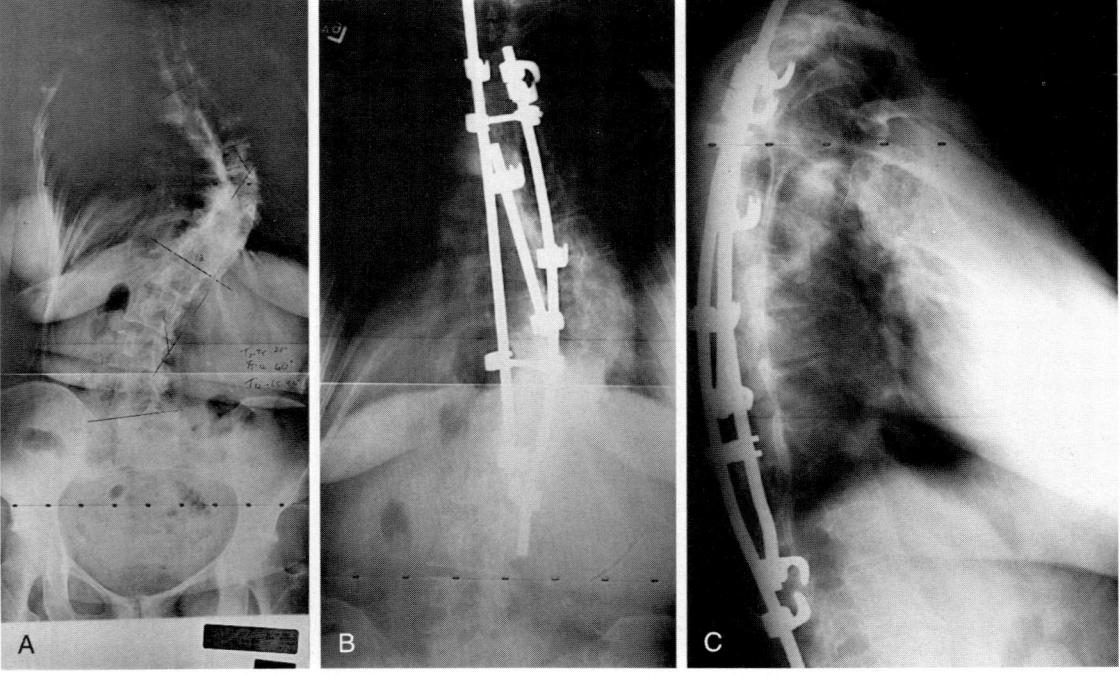

Figure 10. Female patient, age 48 years, with progressive deformity. *A*, The deformity measured 60 degrees and was rigid. *B*, Postoperative AP view. *C*, Postoperative lateral view. The deformity has been reduced to 38 degrees. A thoracoplasty was performed as well as osteotomies of the posterior fusion mass.

than 50 years. Curve types included 39 primary thoracic curves, 37 primary lumbar curves, 35 double major curves, and 12 thoracolumbar curves. Twenty-eight patients had undergone previous surgical procedures consisting of short-segment fusions and/or decompressive surgery. The indications for current surgery included disabling back pain or disabling back pain with neurologic symptoms in 114 patients. In the nine remaining patients, the indication for surgery was progression of the deformity. Preoperatively, thoracic curves measured an average 55 degrees; lumbar curves, 56 degrees; thoracolumbar curves, 64 degrees; thoracic double curves, 65 degrees; and lumbar double curves, 78 degrees.

Pain was considered disabling when it was constant and unrelieved by posture or recumbency, muscle strengthening and other exercises, local application of heat, transcutaneous electrical stimulation, or the use of analgesics with a minimum of 30 mg of codeine more than three times daily.

In general, for thoracic curves, the selection of fusion levels was described by King. Patients with severe rigid thoracic curves greater than 90 degrees underwent anterior and/or posterior releases before instrumentation. Preoperative measurement of thoracic curves was 53 degrees and was 35 degrees at final follow-up (Fig. 11).

The treatment of thoracolumbar and lumbar curves depended on where the pain was located and whether the lumbosacral area was a source of pain on discography, as well as the degree of flexibility and the presence or absence of associated lumbar kyphosis secondary to degenerative changes.

If the L5–S1 disc was part of the pain complex, fusion to the sacrum was necessary and required both anterior and posterior surgery. If the curve was flexible and L5–S1 was not a source of pain, a single-stage procedure was performed using posterior Cotrel-Dubousset instrumentation and fusion. If kyphosis was present, an anterior release was performed to allow the rigid curve to become more flexible. This was followed by a second-stage posterior Cotrel-Dubousset instrumentation procedure to derotate the spine and to restore lordosis. On the basis of discography, flexibility, and kyphosis, thoracolumbar and lumbar curves were divided into four groups.

- Group A had a flexible curve with good lordosis. These patients were treated by simple posterior Cotrel-Dubousset seg-

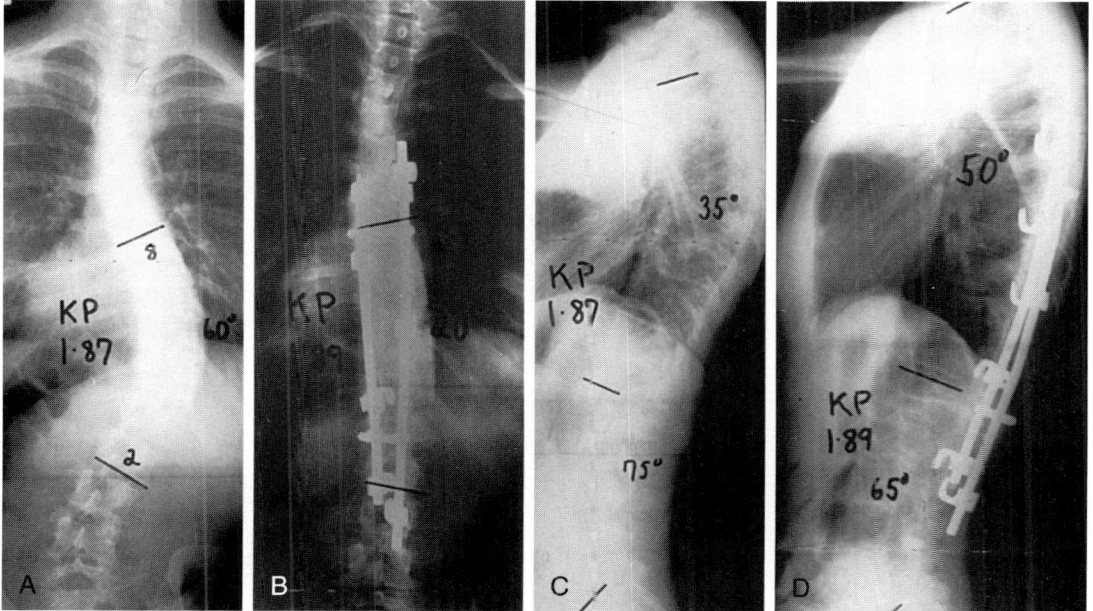

Figure 11. Female patient, age 32 years. *A*, Progressive 60-degree flexible curve. *B*, The deformity has been reduced to 20 degrees with good sagittal alignment. *C*, Preoperative lateral view. *D*, Postoperative lateral view.

mental instrumentation and fusion with autogenous grafting (Fig. 12).

- Group B patients had rigid kyphoscoliosis but a painless L5–S1 disc on discography. Treatment consisted of an anterior release through multiple disc spaces with the application of morcellized graft, usually from the rib, taken at the time of the thoracoabdominal approach. Either on the same day or at a later stage, posterior Cotrel-Dubousset instrumentation and fusion were carried out again using autogenous graft (Fig. 13).
- Group C consisted of patients with lumbar or thoracolumbar scoliosis that was flexible but that involved a painful L5–S1 disc on discography. These patients underwent anterior fusion at the L4–L5 and L5–S1 disc spaces using block autogenous graft from the iliac crest and anterior instrumentation consisting of the use of long 6.5-mm AO screws, short threaded, which were passed from the superior surface of the L5 vertebral body across the L5–S1 space into the sacrum to emerge just through the anterior cortex of the sacrum. Block grafts were also used at the L4–L5 space together with anterior instrumentation, usually consisting of a Yuan I-beam plate (Fig. 14). A second-stage procedure was performed 7 or 8 days later or on the same day and consisted of posterior Cotrel-Dubousset instrumentation and grafting. This instrumentation was used to derotate the spine and to restore lordosis.
- Group D consisted of patients with rigid lumbar kyphoscoliosis and a painful L5–S1 disc. In the first stage, these patients underwent an anterior release at multiple levels through a thoracoabdominal approach. Morcellized grafts were implanted at levels proximal to L4 and block iliac crest grafts and anterior instrumentation, as described above, were used from L4 to the sacrum. A later second-stage posterior Cotrel-Dubousset instrumentation and fusion was carried out to derotate the spine and to restore lordosis (Fig. 15).

More recently, at the L4–L5 and L5–S1 levels, to decrease iliac crest morbidity, femoral ring allografts packed with autogenous cancellous iliac crest bone taken from the inner aspect of the ilium have been used as block grafts (Fig. 16).

A total of 36 patients required both anterior and posterior staged surgery. Eighteen patients had fusions extending to the sacrum.

The preoperative scoliosis averaged 64 de-

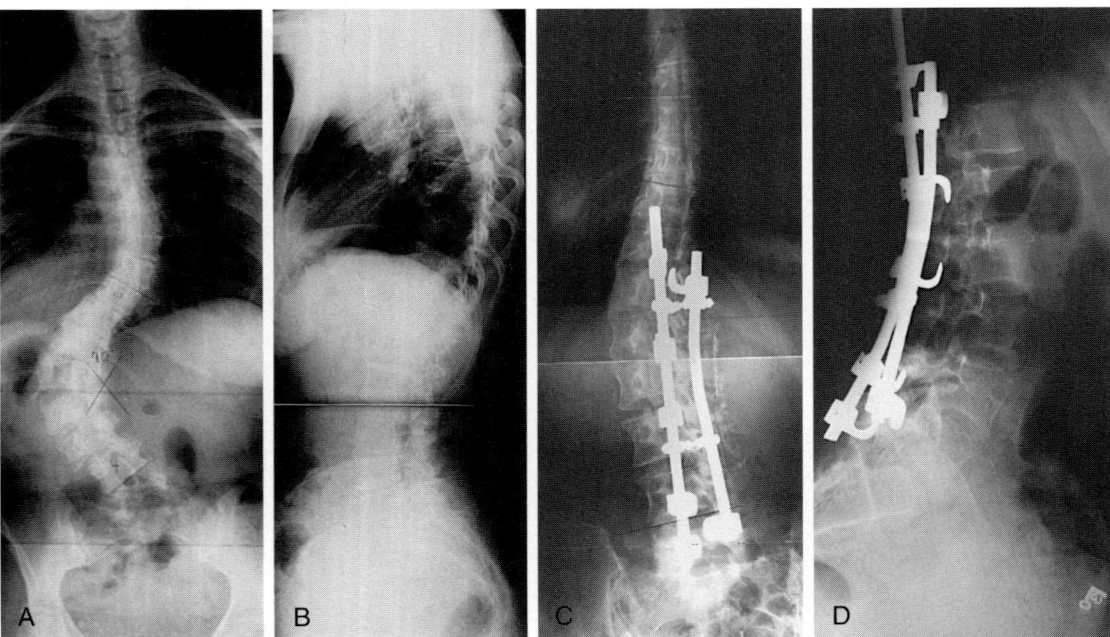

Figure 12. *A, B,* A painful thoracolumbar curve in a 34-year-old female patient. *C, D,* The deformity has been partially corrected, with resultant pain relief.

Assessment and Treatment 1147

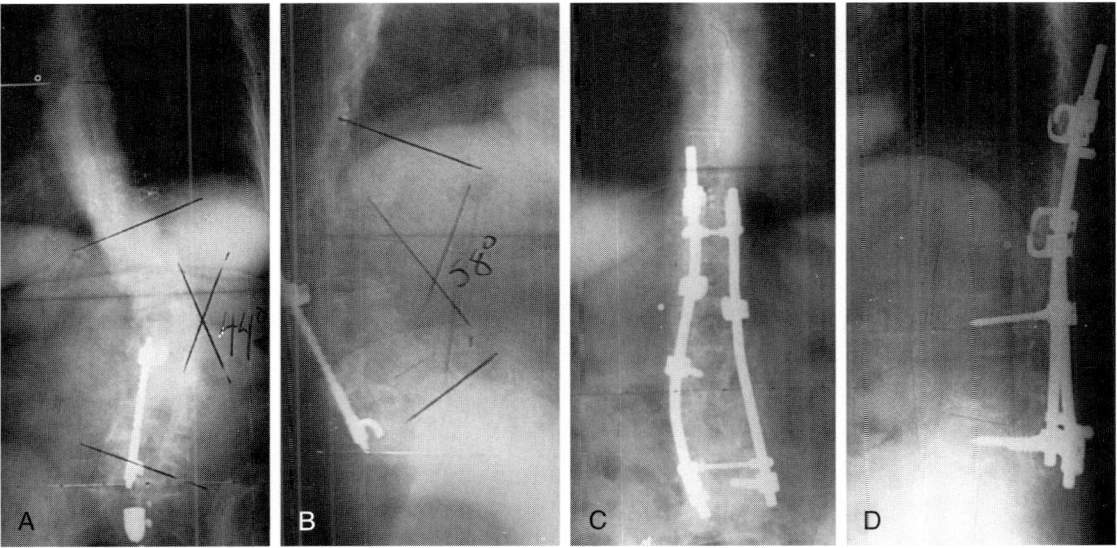

Figure 13. Patient, age 54 years. The curve is rigid. *A,* The lumbosacral disc was painless and normal on discography. A previous attempt at pain relief was employed, elsewhere, by fusing from L2 to L5. *B,* The kyphosis was not addressed and the patient remained painful with a significant kyphoscoliosis. *C,* The old fusion was osteotomized and the scoliosis was almost completely corrected. *D,* The kyphosis from L1 to S1 was reduced from 58 degrees to 20 degrees of lordosis with pain relief.

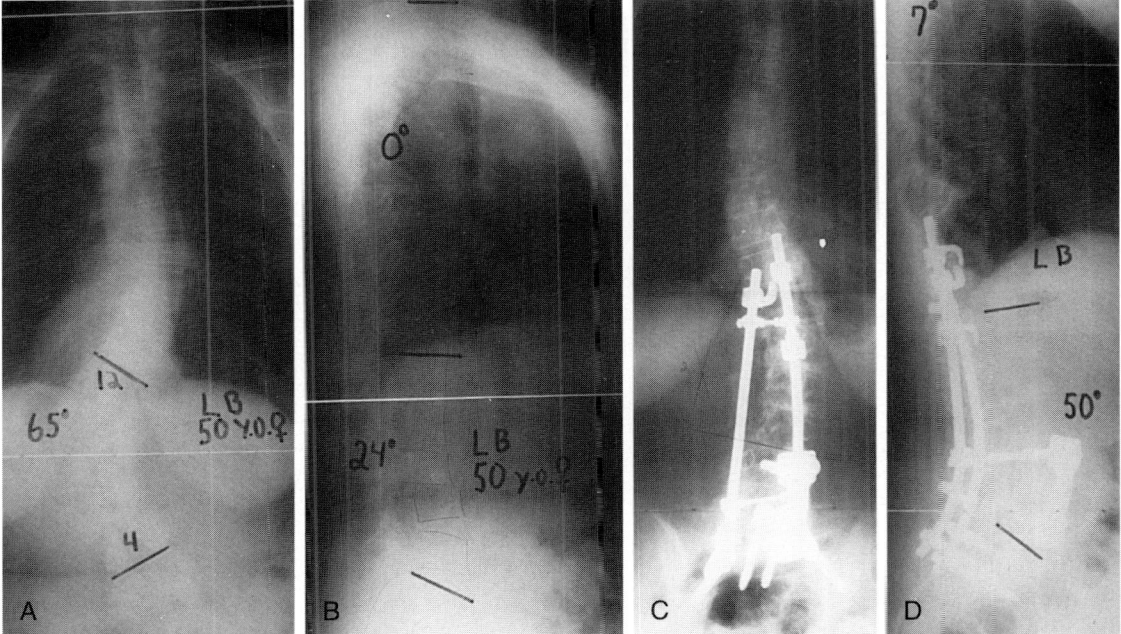

Figure 14. Female patient, age 50 years. *A, B,* Painful, progressive deformity measuring 65 degrees with 24 degrees of lordosis from L1 to S1. The L5–S1 disc was painful on discography. *C, D,* The deformity was corrected and lordosis increased to 50 degrees from L1 to S1. Both anterior and posterior procedures were performed the same day.

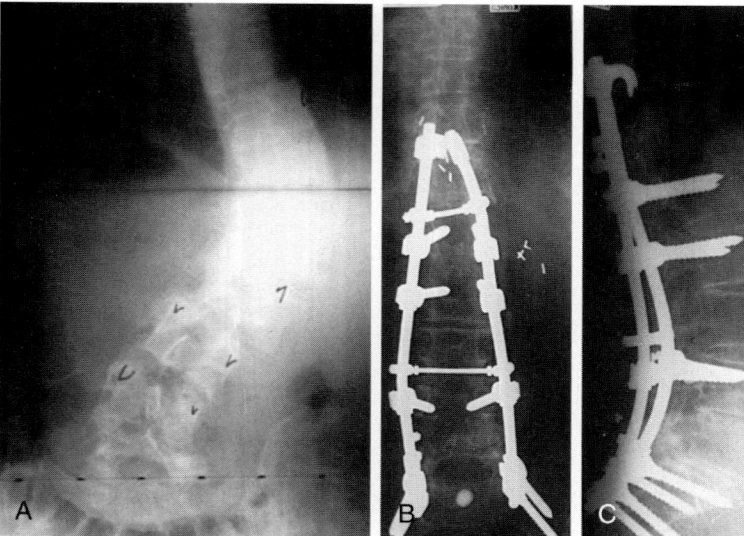

Figure 15. *A*, A painful rigid deformity in a 56-year-old female patient. The L5–S1 disc was part of the pain complex as proved by discography. *B, C*, A two-stage procedure was performed consisting of an anterior thoracolumbar release and anterior fusion to the sacrum. A second stage segmental instrumentation was done, to reduce the deformity and to restore lordosis.

grees, and postoperatively it averaged 38 degrees, for a 42% correction. Thoracic curves measured an average 53 degrees preoperatively and 35 degrees postoperatively; lumbar curves measured 56 degrees preoperatively and 29 degrees postoperatively on average; and thoracolumbar curves measured on average 64 degrees preoperatively and 56 degrees postoperatively.

Sagittal curve correction was most dramatic in the hypokyphotic thoracic and hypolordotic lumbar spine. The average amount of correction for the thoracic hypokyphotic curve was 173%, and for the kyphotic or hypolordotic lumbar spine, it was 133%. For the hypokyphotic thoracic spine, which measured less than 20 degrees preoperatively, the average amount of correction was approximately 100%. Little change occurred for curves measuring between 20 and 60 degrees preoperatively in the sagittal plane. In excessively kyphotic spines (mea-

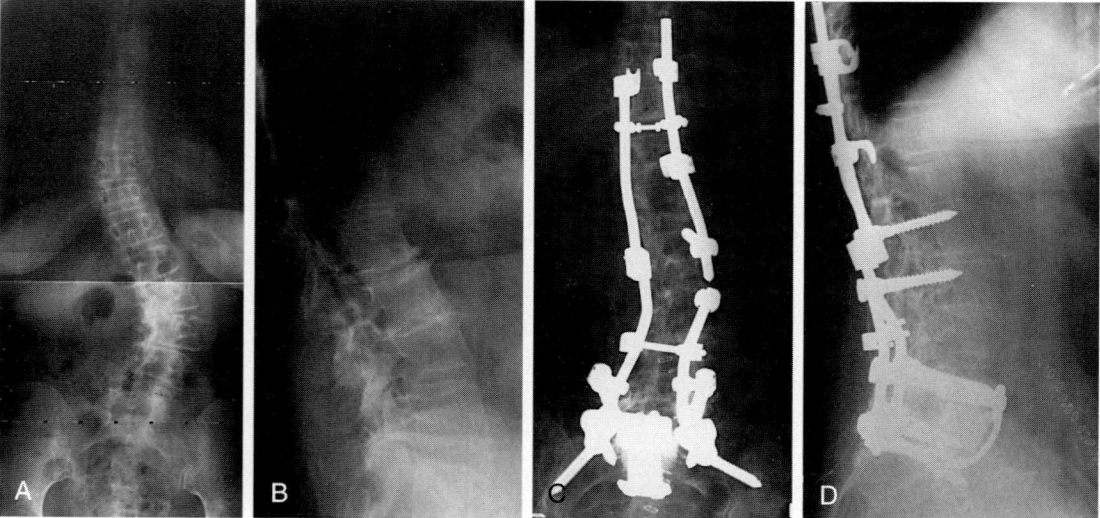

Figure 16. *A*, A painful thoracolumbar curve in a 60-year-old female patient. The L5–S1 disc was painful on discography. *B*, Kyphosis was developing secondary to degenerative disc changes and narrowing. *C, D*, Fusion was performed to the sacrum. Anterior fixation at L5–S1 was used together with a femoral ring allograft, filled with autogenous iliac crest cancellous bone. Lordosis has been restored and pain abbreviated.

suring an average of 73 degrees), the thoracic kyphosis was decreased an average of 16 degrees. Similarly, in relatively kyphotic lumbar spines with less that 20 degrees of lordosis from L1 to S1, there was an average improvement of 107%. In lumbar spines measuring preoperatively between 20 degrees and 50 degrees lordosis, improvement averaged only 14%, and in relatively hyperlordotic lumbar spines measuring greater than 50 degrees, lumbar lordosis was decreased an average of 11%.

There was significant loss of correction in the frontal plane of greater than 5 degrees in 16 patients. This ranged from 6 to 28 degrees.

Apical vertical rotation, as measured by the method of Nash and Moe,[71] improved an average of one half of one grade. Preoperatively, 65 patients had imbalance and, in the follow-up, only 10 patients remained imbalanced. Shoulder imbalance commonly encountered in adolescents does not appear to be a problem postoperatively in adults.

Total blood loss for the whole series averaged 1600 ml. For patients older than 50 years, the blood loss was 1900 ml (1300 ml for patients younger than 50 years). Patients began ambulation on the second or third day after surgery. A thoracolumbar sacral orthosis was used in only elderly osteoporotic patients in whom fixation of the instrumentation was thought to be at risk.

Eighty-six percent of the 92 patients with disabling pain before surgery had pain relief; 62 of these patients experienced complete relief and required no form of analgesia. Decreased pain occurred in 17 additional patients. Pain was the same or worse in 13 patients, including all patients with a pseudarthrosis. The pseudarthrosis rate was 5%. Complications tended to be somewhat more frequent in patients older than 50 years (Figs. 17 to 20). Twenty-two complications occurred in 43 patients older than age 50 years. Loss of fixation due to lumbar laminar fracture and hook pullout occurred in eight patients, six of whom were older than 50 years. Fixation was salvaged in these cases by the reapplication of pedicle screws. It is recommended that, in patients older than 50 years or in any patient with osteopenia, pedicle screws rather than hooks be used in the lumbar spine. There were no major neurologic complications in the total group of patients, but two nerve root neuropraxias occurred and were attributed to instrumentation. These resolved with the passage of time. The only more common complication in the patients younger than 50 years was soft tissue irritation from instrumentation. Other complications included two pneumothoraces, one case of pancreatitis, and five urinary tract infections. One dural tear occurred intraoperatively and was closed primarily without sequelae. One superficial wound infection occurred and responded to local care. One hemothorax occurred, requiring a complete thoracotomy. Two patients developed postthoracotomy pain syndrome, which responded to blocks.

One patient required extension of the fusion to the sacrum 18 months after the original surgery. She had undergone Harrington instrumentation at age 16 years but later developed pain attributable to multiple pseudarthrosis in the lumbar region. Continued pain after Cotrel-Dubousset instrumentation and re-fusion led to reevaluation by discography. The original surgery was carried down to L5. Discography revealed a painful L5–S1 disc and this resolved following extension of the fusion to the sacrum. Although the complications are numerous, they are less than those reported in previous series of adult surgery. There was a 40% incidence of complications overall. This is less than the 62% incidence reported by Swank and colleagues[102] and Hall.[97]

This experience, which is ongoing, suggests that Cotrel-Dubousset instrumentation is a versatile device that provides a means to deal with complex adult structural deformities. However, there is a steep learning curve, a real "fiddle" factor, and the rate of complications is significant. These disadvantages, which can be overcome with experience, are outweighed by the ability it provides to deal with the complex three-dimensional anatomy of scoliosis in adults.

Special Problems in Adults with Scoliosis

Some special problems may be encountered in the adults with scoliosis and influence both the approach and the results. Special considerations are called for in cases of severe rigidity, paralysis, and age over 50 years.

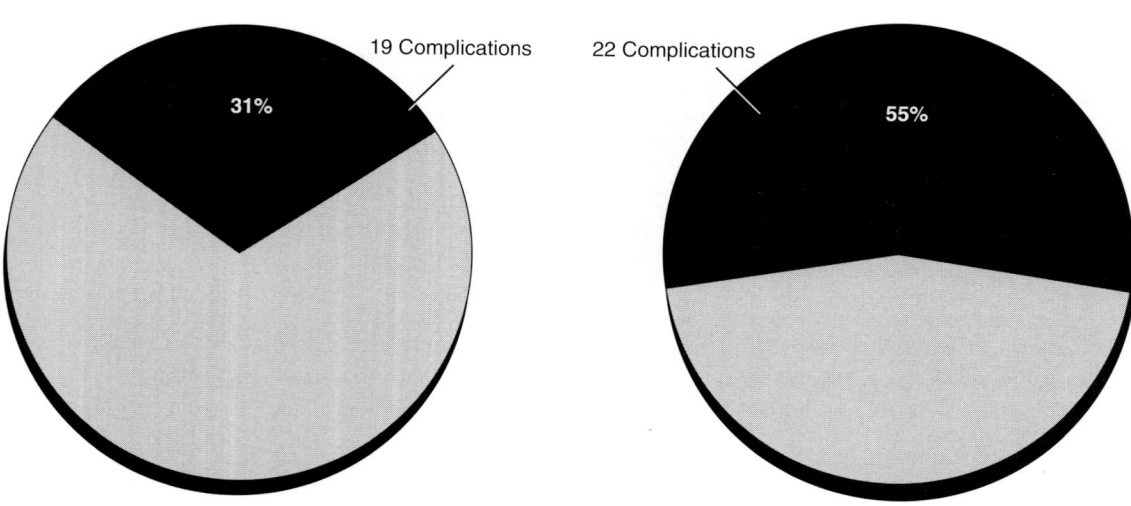

Figure 17. Complications of Cotrel-Dubousset instrumentation and fusion.

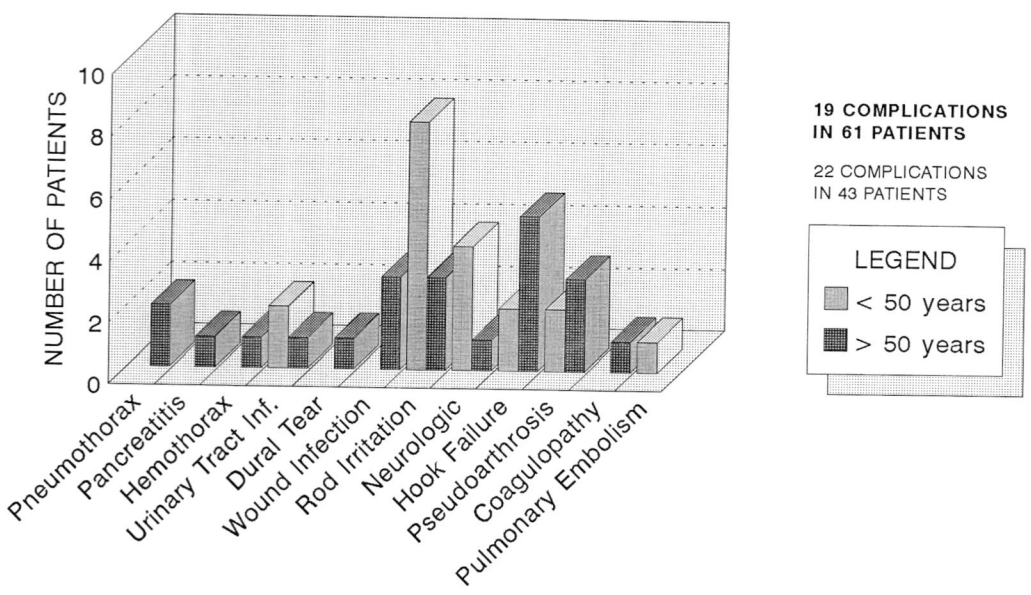

Figure 18. Adult scoliosis complications of Cotrel-Dubousset instrumentation and fusion.

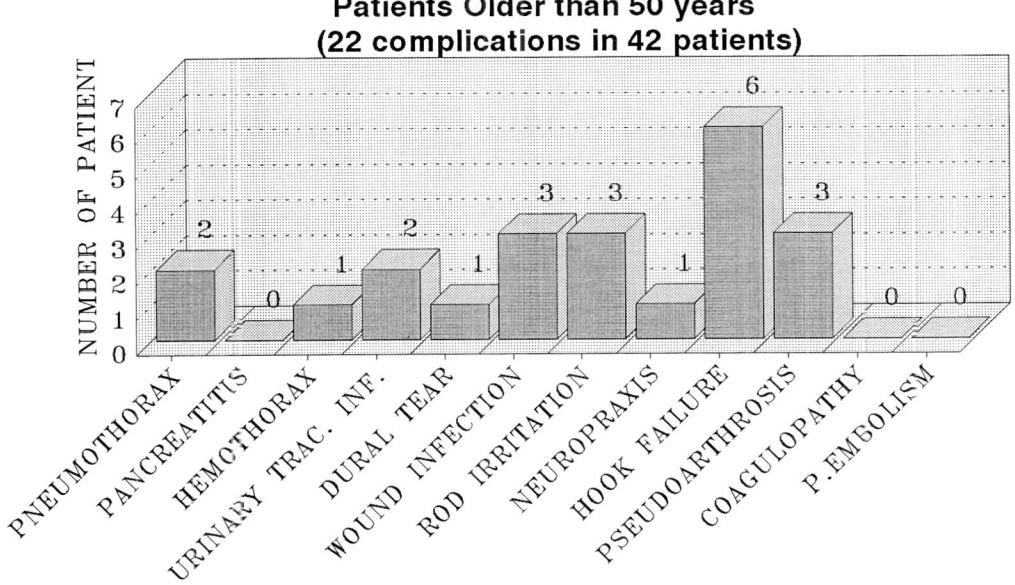

Figure 19. Treatment of adult idiopathic scoliosis. Complications of Cotrel-Dubousset instrumentation and fusion in patients older than 50 years (22 complications in 43 patients).

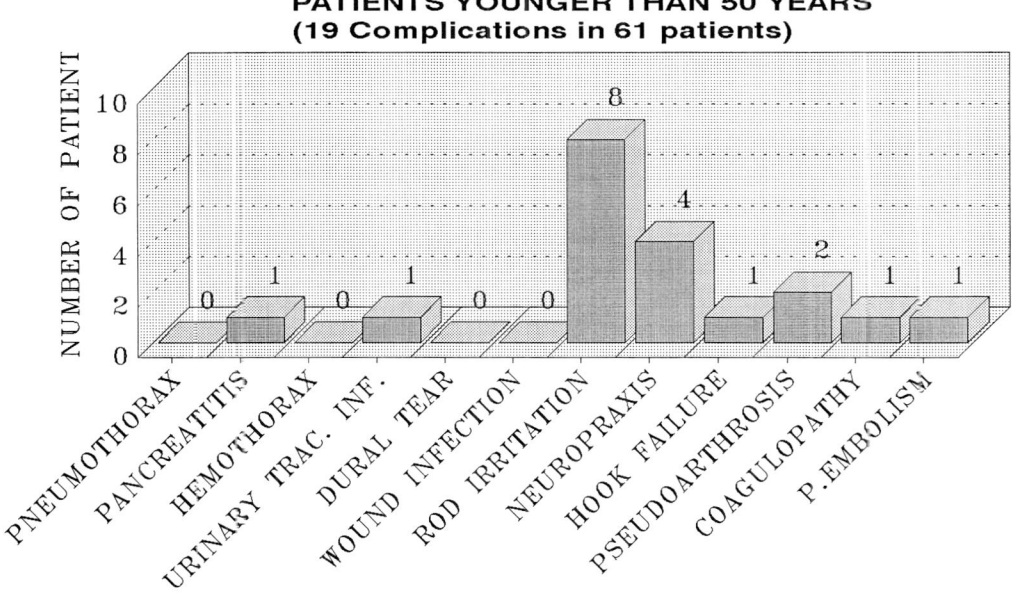

Figure 20. Treatment of adult idiopathic scoliosis. Complications of Cotrel-Dubousset instrumentation and fusion in patients younger than 50 years (19 complications in 61 patients).

Severe Rigid Scoliotic Deformities

Patients with severe rigid structural deformities may present as a consequence of an idiopathic or, much less commonly, a congenital curve, usually associated with significant or severe kyphosis. The author's initial experience with 85 patients with these challenging deformities was reported in 1979.[47] The age range was from 20 to 55 years. The curves ranged from 75 to 180 degrees, and all were rigid, as determined by bending radiographic criteria. Of these 85 patients, 15 had primarily kyphosis, 42 had idiopathic curves, and 28 had congenital curves. In addition to the 28 patients with congenital curves due to failures of segmentation, four patients had spontaneous fusions. An additional 20 patients had undergone previous arthrodeses, and thus 52 had rigidity from a congenital or previous surgical fusion.

The approach in all patients was a posterior release including, if necessary, osteotomies of surgical or congenital fusion. The usual number of osteotomies required was four, often associated with rib releases over three to four levels on the curve concavity, transverse process osteotomies, and rib resections on the convexity, usually involving five or six ribs. Forty patients required anterior osteotomies as well.

After the preliminary releases were accomplished, traction was applied. In the first 32 patients, halo-femoral traction was used. Later, halo-pelvic distraction became the method of choice. Most recently, the author has tended to use halo-dependent traction in either the CircOlectric bed positioned for 30 degrees of dependency or the wheelchair device.

The second-stage procedure, done 2 weeks later, used Harrington instrumentation, superceded first by sublaminar wiring techniques and, most recently, by Cotrel-Dubousset instrumentation.

Results. The initial degree of correction obtained after anterior and/or posterior releases and traction was 40% with halo-pelvic traction and 32% with halo-femoral traction. In patients treated by Harrington instrumentation, a further 8% correction occurred. The overall correction obtained was 40%. As expected, the improvement was less for congenital curves, which averaged a total of 33% correction, as compared with idiopathic curves, which were corrected an average of 48%. Similar results with a lesser degree of pseudarthrosis and earlier ambulation have been achieved with the use of Cotrel-Dubousset instrumentation.

Paralytic Curves

Patients with a paralytic curve may find sitting at a desk or in a wheelchair difficult because of marked pelvic obliquity, accompanied by either kyphosis or hyperlordosis (Fig. 21). Hyperlordosis is encountered, particularly in patients who have had peritoneal shunts. In addition, collapsing curves are often associated with respiratory dysfunction, which can be improved by correction and stabilization. The mechanism by which pulmonary function is improved is lifting of the diaphragm out of the abdomen, which results in enhanced diaphragmatic breathing. A preoperative trial of dependent traction helps one to estimate the degree of improvement in pulmonary function that might be anticipated.

The author has advocated a combined anterior and posterior approach to eliminate the need for postoperative immobilization and to facilitate a return to wheelchair function. At present, there is insufficient information to recommend a posterior approach alone, even with the availability of Cotrel-Dubousset instrumentation.

Spinal Deformities in Patients Older Than Fifty Years

Adults older than 50 years present special challenges. Their deformities are often rigid and may be associated with significant imbalance and loss of normal lumbar lordosis; the bone is more apt to be osteopenic, and spinal stenosis is more often present. Because of these problems, and the greater risk of neurologic or even vascular injury, these deformities in earlier days were usually stabilized posteriorly, without any effort at correction. The approach the author uses is basically the same as that for younger patients with curve rigidity. When there is good preservation of lordosis, the anterior Zielke approach is used (see Fig. 7). In the presence of rigid kyphoscoliosis, a two-stage procedure is preferable, as described previously. Methyl methacrylate is used to enhance screw fixation for the anterior devices, but is

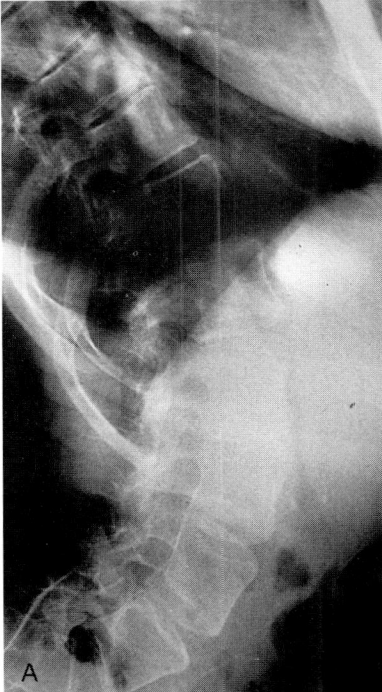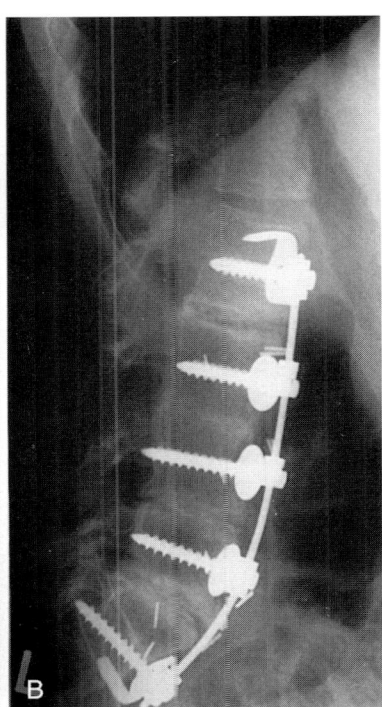

Figure 21. *A,* Marked paralytic hyperlordosis. *B,* Lordosis has been reduced to 60 degrees from L1 to S1 by anterior Zielke instrumentation. Note the anteroposterior orientation of the screws.

avoided in the pedicle with posterior screw fixation because of the risk of cement extrusion and potential neurologic injury. Age is no contraindication when the main indication for surgical intervention is pain and the patient's health is otherwise satisfactory (Fig. 22). The oldest patient treated surgically to date was 82 years of age.

Results. The author has reviewed a subset of 80 patients undergoing surgery for spinal deformity after age 50 years.[47] Fifty had idiopathic curves and the remainder had congenital curve, paralytic curve, or pure kyphotic deformity. Of the 50 idiopathic curves, 12 were thoracic, nine were thoracolumbar, 17 were lumbar, and 12 were double primary curves.

The major indication for all 80 patients was pain; all patients had significant back pain and 16 had associated nerve root pain. Additional factors were progressive pulmonary dysfunction, usually related to increasing kyphosis (eight patients) or evidence of progression of greater than 10 degrees in the preceding 3 years (46 patients).

The 80 patients underwent 100 procedures. Twenty (25%) had staged anterior and posterior surgery for enhanced stabilization, and 12 had simultaneous anterior and posterior operations. This latter group was largely patients who had a flat back deformity (discussed below).

The overall results obtained were 12.5% excellent, 56.5% good, 6% fair, and 25% poor. Complete pain relief occurred in 27 (34%) of the 80 patients, but root pain was relieved in all patients. The curve correction obtained was analyzed with respect to type of instrumentation used. The results were Harrington instrumentation, 22%; sublaminar wired Harrington rods, 22%; Harrington rods combined with L rods, 21%; double L rods, 33%; Cotrel-Dubousset, 50%; Dwyer, 42%; and Zielke, 67%. Although the numbers in each category are small and the indications for the various devices somewhat different, the Zielke correction appears to be the greatest. Moreover, the results obtained with the Zielke devices in the patients older than 50 years were similar to the results obtained in all adults older than 20 years.[36, 39]

The general complications included pulmonary problems in 24%, such as pneumonia, atelectasis, and adult respiratory distress syndrome. Infection occurred in 1%. One patient became paraparetic with partial but incomplete recovery.

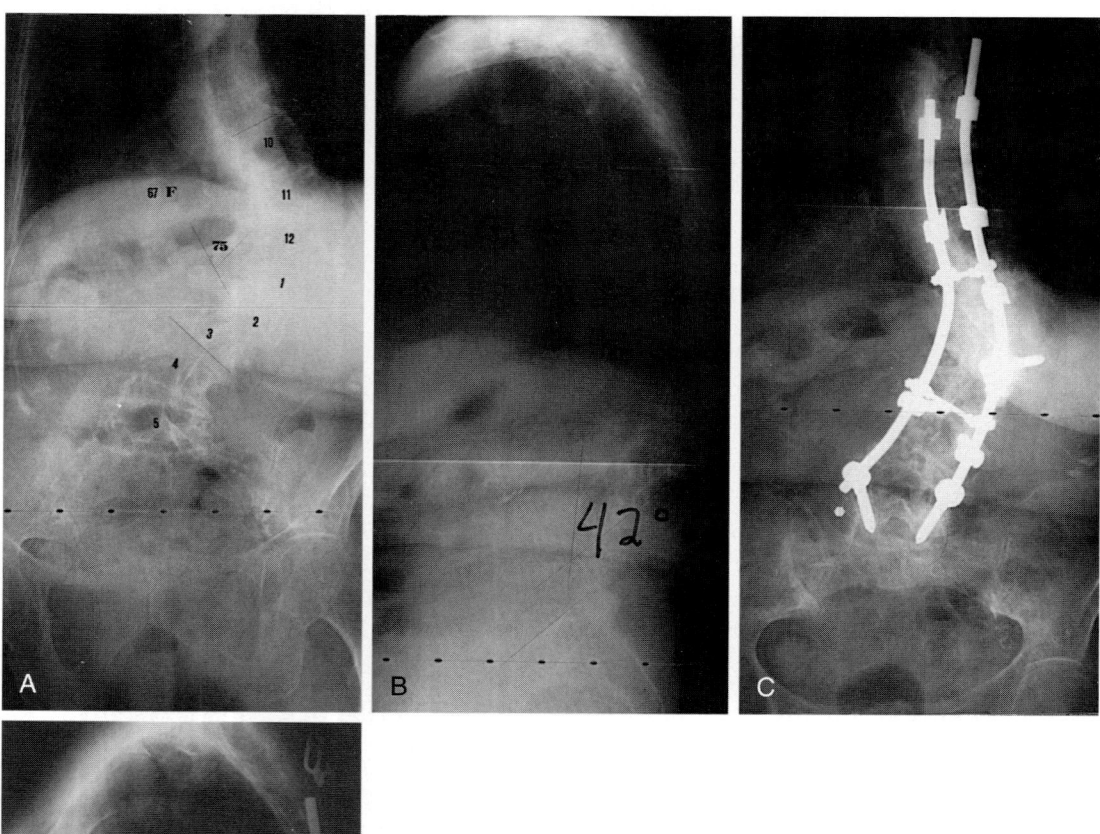

Figure 22. Female patient, age 67 years. *A,* Painful progressive deformity. *B,* A thoracolumbar kyphosis has developed. *C,* The deformity has been partially corrected and stabilized, achieving pain relief. *D,* A marked improvement in the kyphosis has been achieved and the lordosis improved from 42 degrees to 65 degrees. Note the thoracic pedicle screws, which aid in preventing proximal pullout and subsequent loss of correction. Occasionally, four screws or a screw-hook combination is necessary.

The local complications observed were significant and to some degree dependent on the approach and the device. Thirteen of the patients treated with Harrington instrumentation alone developed flat back deformity. Four have undergone later single-stage anterior and posterior osteotomy. Intraoperative fracture of either lamina or vertebral bodies occurred in an additional seven cases and was overcome by the use of methyl methacrylate.

Later instrument failures occurred in 11 of the 80 patients and included six Harrington rod fractures and one rod displacement, two L rod migrations, one anterior screw breakage, and one other rod failure. An additional nine patients later had increased kyphosis above the fusion secondary to osteoporotic compression fractures.

The pseudarthrosis rate was 21%, most of which occurred in the Harrington rod constructs. By vertebral level, fusions carried to L5 had a 25% failure, and those carried to the sacrum had a 24% failure rate. All of these pseudarthroses occurred prior to the two-stage approach now used when fusion is carried to the sacrum. To date, Zielke[51] and Cotrel-Dubousset[55] devices have been associated with pseudarthrosis. A more recent analysis of 43 patients older than age 50 years treated with Cotrel-Dubousset instrumentation and followed for longer than 2 years revealed a rate of 0% for Zielke instrumentation and 7% for Cotrel-Dubousset instrumentation. There was an increased complication rate compared with that in 61 patients younger than 50 years. The overall complication rate was 40% for 104 patients treated by Cotrel-Dubousset instrumentation (see Fig. 17). The incidence in patients older than age 50 years was 55%, and the incidence for patients younger than 50 years of age was 31% (see Fig. 17). Except rod irritation, complications were generally more frequent in all groups older than age 50 years. Presumably this is because of the greater level of activity postoperatively in younger patients (see Figs. 17 to 20).

It appears that a successful outcome can be obtained in patients older than 50 years, but great care must be taken to improve or preserve lumbar lordosis, osteopenia must be managed, and the operative approach must be specifically tailored, often with the use of combined approaches. Moreover, there is a high rate of potential complications, both generally and locally, although major neurologic problems and death fortunately have not been a significant issue to date.

Problems Related to Adjacent Motion Segments Following Previous Fusion for Scoliosis Beginning Before Maturity

Patients who have had previous fusions for scoliosis are at risk for degeneration in adjacent motion segments. The risk increases proportionally to the extent of the prior fusion into the lumbar spine.[10, 17, 23, 26, 34] These patients may require extension of fusions if nonoperative means fail to control the symptoms. It is also common for the problem to be progressive and associated with some degree of spinal stenosis (see Fig. 12).

Paonessa and Engler[80] analyzed 103 patients fused with Harrington instrumentation to L3 or more distally compared with a control group of 92 patients fused to L2 or proximally. Those fused more distally exhibited a higher rate of secondary surgical complications or late degenerative changes. They experienced a higher back pain score and more difficulty with normal daily activities, required more regular pain medication administration, and had more episodes of back pain. This was particularly true of patients 30 years or older at the time of initial surgery. The degree of remaining lumbar lordosis correlated significantly with the difficulty of normal daily activities.

Connolly and associates[13] performed a linear regression analysis of factors influencing pain 10 years after Harrington instrumentation into the lumbar spine in idiopathic adolescent scoliosis. A higher incidence of low back pain was noted for fusion done to L2 or more distally, similar to the findings of Cochran and colleagues,[10] and was greater than that in a control group.

A higher incidence of degenerative changes was noted with the descending level of fusion for fusions into the lower lumbar spine. Sagittal plane imbalance was associated with a poor result (flat back or functional kyphosis). There was a 29.6% rate of additional surgery. Seventeen percent of patients thought that the goals of initial surgery had not been accomplished. Increased Cobb angles related to a lower spine score. Increased kyphosis related to a lower spine score.

Evaluation. After history and physical examination, investigative studies may include myelography, computed tomographic scanning, and magnetic resonance imaging, as well as discography and facet blocks. The plain radiographic and bending films frequently show abnormal translational motion, which varies according to the fusion extent. The presence of retrospondylolisthesis correlates with pain, but little relationship has been reported to the degree of lordosis or disc space height.[34] The choice of test depends on the pattern of referred pain, neurologic involvement, and extent of back pain.

Operative Approach. The approach is dictated by whether the lumbosacral joint must be included in the fusion. When the lumbosacral joint is not involved, anterior or posterior fusion with instrumentation suffices. However, extension of the fusion to the sacrum, requires a combined approach.[5] Today, this is done with anterior instrumentation and posterior pedicle fixation. To improve lordosis, some of the posterior laminae at L3–L4, L4–L5, or L5–S1 may be removed, together with pars resection and compression applied to increase lordosis. The important principle in the anterior approach is to use interbody grafts applied at the front of the disc space to increase lordosis further. Anterior instrumentation appears to improve the rate of fusion.

Results. The author has surgically treated and reviewed 81 scoliotic patients who required extension of a fusion, previously terminating at L3, L4, or L5 and who required extension of their fusion to the sacrum. Fifty-six patients have had a follow-up of longer than 2 years. The average age of the patients was 48 years, with a range from 20 to 70 years. Fifty-one patients were women, 46 patients had idiopathic scoliosis, six had paralytic curves, and three had congenital curves. These patients were treated between 1975 and 1990. Presenting symptoms included pain in 91 and sciatica in 62. The average number of previous procedures was two. Time interval from previous surgery in adolescence was 137 months, with a range of 7 to 540 months. The termination of the previous fusion was L3 in 16%, L4 in 41%, L5 in 31%, and the sacrum in 12%. All patients previously fused to the sacrum had pseudarthroses.

Because of neurologic problems, decompression with fusion was done in 32% of patients. Decompression alone should never be done. Initially, most patients were treated in two single stages, but more recently, all patients have been treated on the same day.

There was an evolution of treatment ranging from posterior fusions only to anterior and posterior fusions as well as an evolution in instrumentation.

Between 1975 and 1978, six patients underwent posterior Harrington instrumentation with extension of the fusion to the sacrum. Initially, 5 of the 6 patients developed pseudarthroses, of which two were salvaged by further surgery. For this reason, posterior fusion and instrumentation, even with prolonged postoperative recumbency, was not a satisfactory solution to the problem. Accordingly, between 1978 and 1982, an additional 18 patients were treated with a variety of anterior and posterior instrumentation (Fig. 23). The rate of pseudarthrosis in this group was only 11%. In patients who required increased lordosis, a posterior osteotomy through the pars interarticularis, usually at the L4–L5 level was carried out. With the development of more rigid pedicle fixation and better anterior fixation after 1986, further improvement was obtained in 32 patients. The pseudarthrosis rate in these 32 patients was 6% (two patients). Anterior instrumentation included the use of L5–S1 AO 6.5-mm screws, short threaded, which were passed from the superior part of body of L5 across the disc space of L5–S1 into the anterior sacrum. Block iliac crest grafts were used at the L5–S1 space. Further instrumentation at either L4–L5 or L3–L5 consisted of the use of Yuan I-beam plates (Fig. 24). Posterior instrumentation usually consisted of AO plates or, more recently, Cotrel-Dubousset instrumentation with pedicle screws and the use of a Chopin sacral block or a sacral Harrington bar (Fig. 25). Procedures have been performed in an additional 35 cases since 1990, with similar satisfactory results. Overall pain relief, including that in initial patients treated with Harrington instrumentation, was good in 82%, fair in 18%, and poor in 10%, based on both subjective and objective analyses. Poor re-

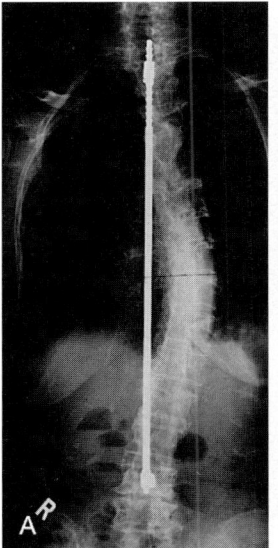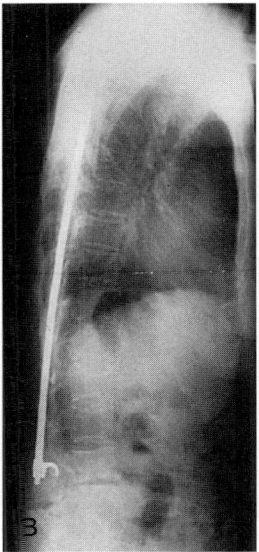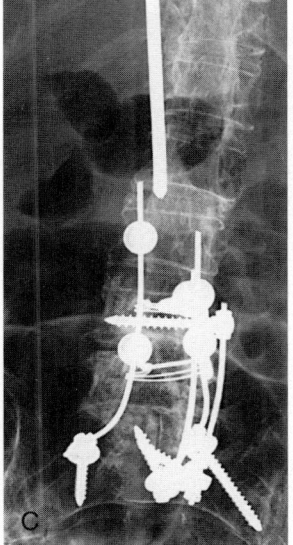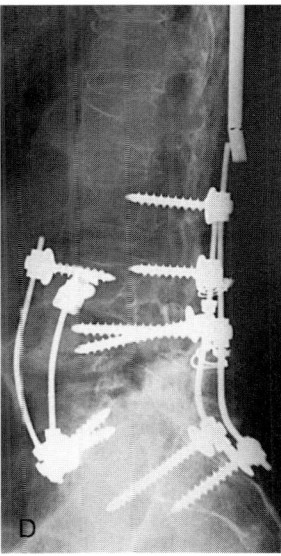

Figure 23. Female patient, age 56 years. Previous fusion had been performed 25 years ago. *A,* AP view demonstrates marked degenerative changes at L4–L5 and L5–S1 with a flat back. *B,* Lateral view. *C,* Postoperative AP view. *D,* Postoperative lateral view. Extension of fusion to S1. Note the restoration of lordosis. Preoperative discography had reproduced pain at L4–L5 and L5–S1. Relief was obtained with facet blocks.

sults were generally related to persistence of pseudarthroses. Complications included intravascular operative tears that were usually venous. Minor neurapraxia developed in seven patients and resolved postoperatively. One patient experienced a major neurologic problem, which only partially resolved, as a result of a tear in the dura over a significant area in the posterior aspect. One patient had bleeding greater than 5000 ml. There was one posterior infection that cleared with the use of dressings. One patient had thrombophlebitis. In six patients, respiratory difficulties developed postoperatively, requiring intubation for longer than 1 day. One patient had pancreatitis, and two patients had urinary obstruction due to retroperitoneal fibrosis. This has not been encountered in other cases of anterior surgery. In two patients, sacral iliac joint pain of a temporary nature developed, which resolved with the use of antiinflammatory drugs.

Iatrogenic Flat Back Deformities

Fusions to the sacrum using Harrington instrumentation result in a 50% loss of lumbar lordosis. Many of these patients require later restorative surgery.* This may not be apparent in the early years after fusion in an adolescent, but it becomes a significant problem when the patient reaches the third, fourth, or fifth decade of life. Onset of symptoms is heralded by reports of low back fatigue, followed by symptoms of increasing pain despite a solid fusion. The increasing loss of lordosis causes the patient to walk with a hip and knee flexion contracture.[33] The deformity that results may be striking and disabling (Fig. 26).

The etiologic factors, in descending order of frequency, are distraction instrumentation of the lumbar spine that ends caudally at the L5 or S1 level; a thoracolumbar junction kyphosis of greater than 15 degrees, especially if it is associated with a hypokyphotic thoracic spine; and degenerative changes above and/or below the previous fusion. If pseudarthrosis is a component of the deformity, repair without correction of lordosis does not relieve the symptoms.

There are two approaches to this problem, one preventive and the other restorative.

Prevention

Throughout this discussion, the importance of maintaining lumbar lordosis when

---

*References 6, 9, 19, 20, 26, 34, 37, 42, 45, and 59.

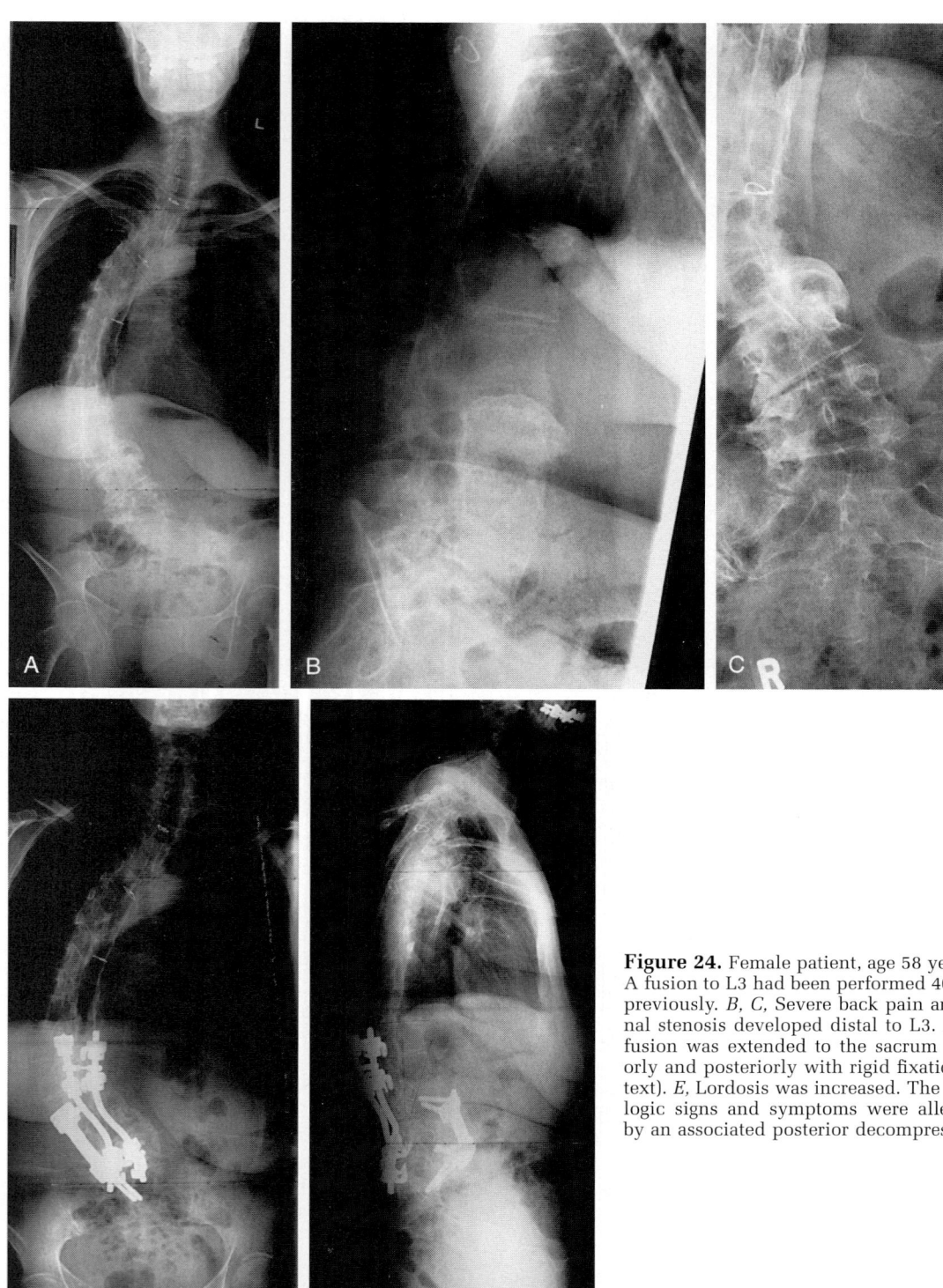

Figure 24. Female patient, age 58 years. *A*, A fusion to L3 had been performed 40 years previously. *B, C*, Severe back pain and spinal stenosis developed distal to L3. *D*, The fusion was extended to the sacrum anteriorly and posteriorly with rigid fixation (see text). *E*, Lordosis was increased. The neurologic signs and symptoms were alleviated by an associated posterior decompression.

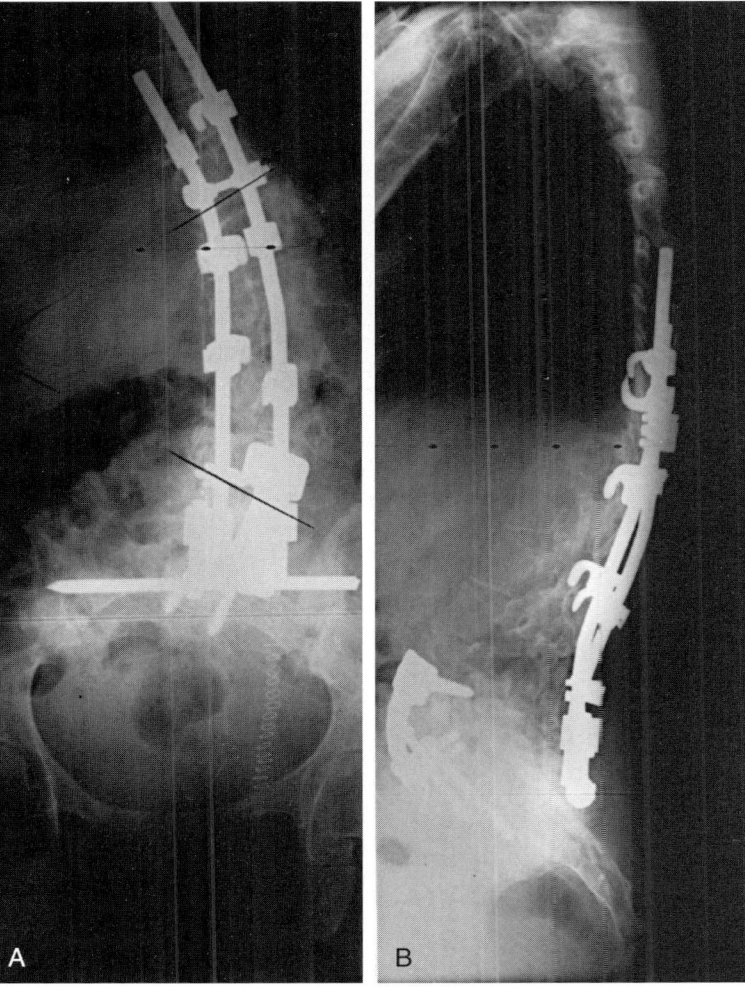

Figure 25. *A, B,* An alternative technique of sacral fixation. A Harrington sacral bar is passed between the iliae over which Cotrel-Dubousset rod connectors have been fitted, to which proximal Cotrel-Dubousset rods are attached by dominoes.

dealing with adult scoliosis has been emphasized. A review in 1978 revealed that 4% of all fusions in adolescents for scoliosis resulted in significant loss of lumbar lordosis when posterior instrumentation was used.[47] When the fusions extended into the lumbosacral joint, this figure rose to 50%, and one half required later surgery.[2] Historically, attempts to overcome this risk included contouring of the Harrington rod,[9] together with use of square-ended Moe rods and sacral-alar hooks. However, the rate of pseudarthrosis remained at 40%. The Luque rod appeared to offer an improvement and reduced the rate of pseudarthrosis to 20% and the rate of flat back deformities to 15%.[49, 50] The Cotrel-Dubousset instrumentation appears to have further improved these results. However the author prefers a two-stage procedure that varies according to curve mobility.

An independent assessment was made of 21 adults with fusion extending to the sacrum using a combination of anterior and posterior surgery together with posterior Cotrel-Dubousset instrumentation. These patients were treated between 1985 and 1990. All patients had a minimum of 2 years of follow-up. The average age of patients was 46 years, with a range from 21 to 63 years, and all were female. Nineteen had idiopathic scoliosis. Indications for surgery were pain and progression of deformity in 20 patients and pain alone in one patient. Eight patients had associated radicular pain. In all cases, pain was further defined at the L5–S1 disc by discography. Nine patients had proven spinal stenosis on myelography.

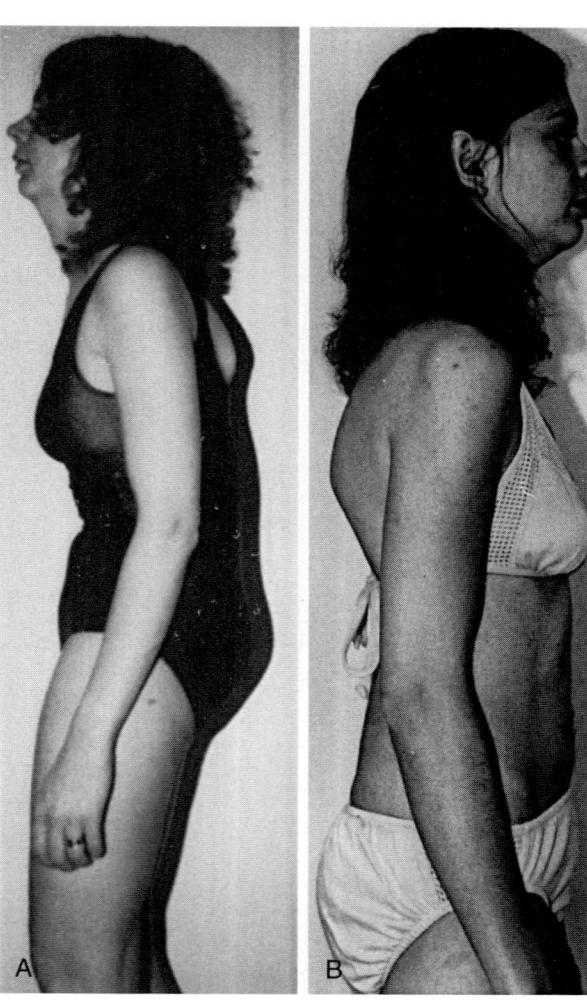

Figure 26. Female patient, age 24 years. *A*, Previous lumbar fusion. Note marked kyphosis (flat back) secondary to distraction. *B*, Postoperative view. Note restoration of lordosis.

Eight patients underwent decompressive surgery at the time of fusion. Anterior and posterior surgery was performed on the same day in 19 patients, and 1 week apart in two patients. The number of anterior levels fused averaged five, with a range of two to eight; posterior approaches averaged eight levels, with a range from three to 14. Autogenous graft was used in 14 patients and a mixture of autogenous graft and allograft was used in seven patients. Blood loss in single-stage surgery averaged 1750 ml and blood loss in patients undergoing two-stage surgery averaged 3600 ml.

There were two treatment groups. First, 19 patients with rigid curves and loss of lordosis underwent anterior release. Morcellized autogenous graft was used at all levels to L4. Block iliac crest grafts were used at L4–L5 and L5–S1 with anterior instrumentation, as described previously. Posterior Cotrel-Dubousset instrumentation was used to derotate the spine and to increase lordosis. Sacral fixation was usually accomplished using four sacral screws initially. More recently, in good-quality bone, Chopin sacral block has been used. In more osteoporotic bone, either the Jackson intrasacral technique of fixation has been used or hooks around a Harrington sacral bar have been used (Figs. 25 to 28).

The second group consisted of two patients with flexible curves. The first-stage Cotrel-Dubousset instrumentation was used with similar sacral fixation to derotate the spine and to increase lordosis, followed by an anterior L4–L5 and L5–S1 interbody fusion with the anterior fixation as previously described.

Curves measured in the frontal plane pre-

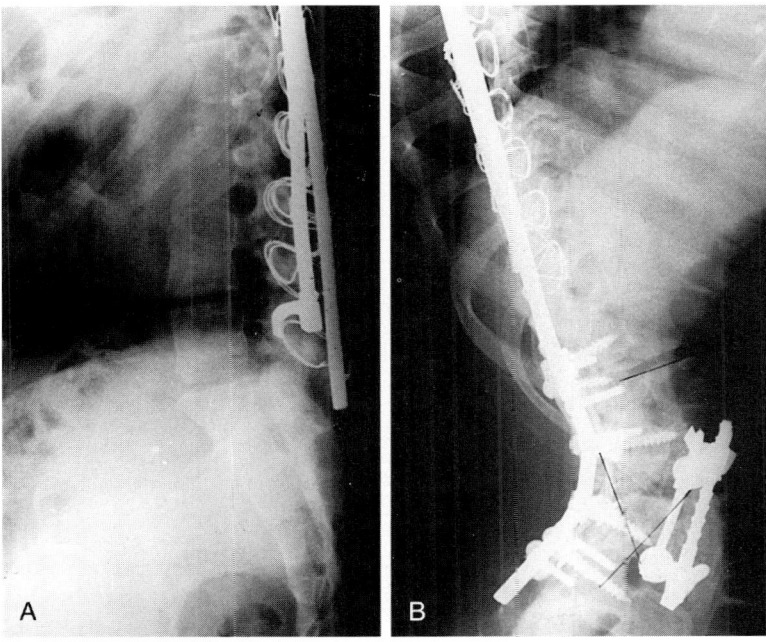

Figure 27. A patient previously underwent fusion to L5. *A,* Lordosis was lost, pain and fatigue persisted. Preoperative discography revealed a normal, painless L5–S1 disc. *B,* A combined single-stage osteotomy, anterior and posterior, was done to restore lordosis with good alleviation of symptoms. If the L5–S1 had been painful, fusion would also have extended to the sacrum (as in Fig. 28).

operatively averaged 55 degrees, with a range from 37 to 92 degrees. Curves measured postoperatively measured an average of 31 degrees with a range from 23 to 55 degrees and an average correction of 33%. Lordosis from L1 to measured the top of S1 measured 37 degrees preoperatively and 48 degrees postoperatively, for an overall average of 30% improvement. Imbalance in the frontal plane was present in 21 patients. Postoperatively, one patient was slightly worse, 12 were fully rebalanced, and eight remained the same.

Excellent to good pain relief occurred in 85% of patients. None required analgesics. Those who were working preoperatively returned to work. Those who were homemakers returned to their preoperative duties. Fair to poor relief occurred in 15%, mainly among patients with pseudarthroses. The pseudarthrosis rate was 8%. One patient had a flat back as a result of a pseudarthrosis. Complications included blood loss greater than 5,000 ml in one patient, a minor neurapraxia that partially resolved in one patient, and atelectasis in five patients. Hook pullout occurred in one patient, reflecting the importance of the use of pedicle screws rather than hooks in the lumbar spine, particularly in the elderly. One deep infection occurred that resolved with débridement and a flap rotation. One patient had pancreatitis. One patient had cardiac difficulties postoperatively, which resolved with appropriate treatment. Since 1990, a further 36 patients have been treated similarly with comparable results.

Devlin and associates[19] reported on 27 adults with fusion of the sacrum using Cotrel-Dubousset instrumentation. Most of their patients were treated with posterior instrumentation only. Problems with instrumentation were encountered in 70% of patients, and the pseudarthrosis rate was 26%, with flat back occurring in 19%. Patients who require fusions to the sacrum, because of the long lever-arm, require rigid fixation posteriorly in the sacrum (see above) as well as anterior surgery to minimize the risk of pseudarthrosis.

Using these approaches, the rate of pseudarthrosis has been reduced to 7% in the author's experience with the most recent 30 cases. Saer and colleagues,[89] in an analysis of long fusions to the sacrum using the Luque-Galveston technique, noted no significant loss of lumbar lordosis and a 12% incidence of pseudarthrosis. They noted that the best results occurred in patients with two-stage procedures consisting of an anterior lumbar fusion to the sacrum with instrumentation followed by posterior segmental instrumentation using the Galveston technique of fixation to the pelvis.

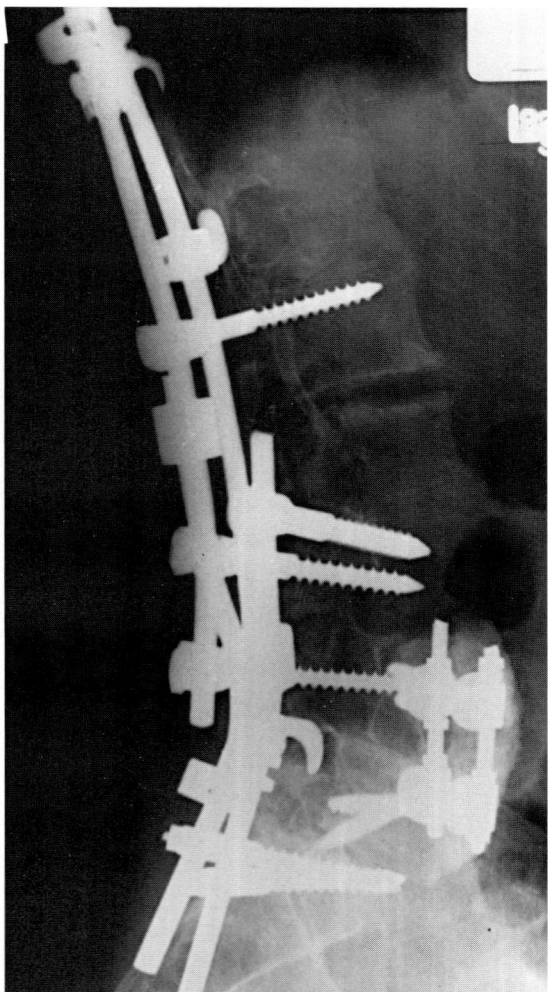

Figure 28. The Jackson technique of intrasacral fusion has been employed because the patient required extension of the fusion to the sacrum as well as an osteotomy at L4–S1 anterior and posterior, to restore lordosis. Cotrel-Dubousset instrumentation has been used posteriorly instead of Dwyer cables and plates.

Boachie-Adjei and coworkers[5] also reported their experience using combined anterior-posterior arthrodesis with the Luque-Galveston technique of posterior instrumentation in 25 patients. They noted reduction of pain in 63% of cases. The pseudarthrosis rate was 41%, and the complication rate was 82%.

Shufflebarger and Clark[93] addressed the problem of loss of lumbar lordosis following correction of thoracolumbar and lumbar curves in patients with sagittal plane imbalance. They corrected the deformity in the area of the thoracolumbar junction with the use of posterior osteotomies alone. Frequently, more than one osteotomy was necessary. All deformities were fixed intraoperatively with Cotrel-Dubousset instrumentation. However, lumbar lordosis increased only 9 degrees. Thoracic kyphosis improved from 87 degrees to 41 degrees.

The author believes that this is a satisfactory procedure for major deformities showing a kyphosis at the thoracolumbar junction. It is not, however, without significant risk in the area of the cord. In a true flat back deformity in the lumbar spine, a single-stage anterior-posterior osteotomy with internal fixation (described above) is preferred.

Boachie-Adjei and associates[6] described the use of Cotrel-Dubousset iliosacral fixation for long fusions in adult spinal deformity requiring extension of fusion to the sacrum. In two of 11 patients studied, pseudarthroses developed. Six patients continued to experience mild to moderate pain in the area of the sacroiliac joint complex. In at least three of these, the problem was due to internal fixation devices and subsequent removal of the iliosacral screws resulted in improved pain. There was one L5–S1 neurologic deficit and no infections. In the sagittal plane, lumbar lordosis averaged 33 degrees preoperatively and 44 degrees postoperatively. These investigators concluded that the use of iliosacral fixation was better than conventional sacral alar screw fixation.

Restoration of Lordosis in Patients with Iatrogenic Flat Back

A combined approach with anterior and posterior osteotomies is preferable, as opposed to a posterior osteotomy alone[26, 40, 42, 50, 59] (see Fig. 27). This is because greater correction can be obtained and it is unnecessary to immobilize patients postoperatively. Moreover, in cases treated by posterior osteotomy alone, recurrence of deformity has occurred.

Surgical Indications. The indications for surgery are pain and loss of lordosis, particularly when the symptoms and deformity are increasing. As previously indicated, a pseudarthrosis, if present, cannot be assumed to be the cause of the symptoms.

Surgical Approach. The approaches used vary according to the type of deformity identified. If there is imbalance in the anteroposterior plane, a quadrilateral wedge osteotomy is done anteriorly and posteriorly to correct that deformity (Fig. 29). The technique used is similar to that described by Smith-Peterson for the treatment of ankylosing spondylitis. When the fusion is solid, this is usually performed at the L3–L4 level. If a pseudarthrosis is present, the osteotomy is simply enlarged. The nerve roots at the level of osteotomy must be clearly identified. A variety of posterior fixation devices have been used.

Initially, Dwyer screws are inserted into the lateral fusion mass, combined with cables to close the osteotomy. Four screws are placed proximal and four screws are placed distal to the osteotomy. However, the cables are not tightened at this time. Following the posterior approach, an anterior approach is immediately carried out corresponding in level to the posterior osteotomy. An opening wedge osteotomy is performed through the disc or through a previous anterior fusion mass, if present. Simultaneous with the anterior opening of the osteotomy, the posterior cables are tightened anteriorly and a bicortical or tricortical graft is then impacted. A posterior, midline, contoured AO plate may be added to control rotation, with at least two screws placed proximal and distal to the osteotomy if there has been no previous laminectomy. If there has been a previous laminectomy, Cotrel-Dubousset instrumentation is preferred (Fig. 30).

Surgical Results. In 1988, Kostuik and coworkers[50] reported on 54 patients treated with this technique. Pain was relieved in 48 (90%). Nonunion occurred in three patients owing to anterior graft collapse, and one of these patients requested reoperation. Neurologic complications occurred in two patients, one of whom had permanent dorsiflexion and plantar flexion weakness and inconsistent bladder control.

The minimum follow-up interval was 4 years. The average preoperative lordosis was 21.5 degrees, which was restored to 49 degrees. The average correction was 29 degrees, with a range from 24 to 64 degrees. A further 21 patients have undergone similar treatment with equally good results.

Hu and Bradford[38] described an L5 opening wedge osteotomy in the treatment of lumbar scoliosis. They proposed this treatment for patients with adult scoliosis with fixed oblique takeoff but without significant degenerative changes in the lumbosacral area. This was thought to be an option that would avoid fusion across the lumbosacral junction and prevent neutralization of L4. These researchers described their technique in 10 patients (average age of 45 years) with an average fractional curve of 29 degrees. An L4–L5 osteophyte, if present, was removed anteriorly. An L5 subchondral osteotomy was then performed to achieve mobility. Postoperatively, the average fractional curve was decreased to 8 degrees. One patient required revision for instrumentation failure; one patient had mild low back pain 10 years postoperatively; and radicular pain and a proximal junctional kyphosis developed in one patient. All others had relief of their symptoms and improvement of their deformity with spinal balance.

Horton and associates[37] described a tricolumnar osteotomy for patients with fixed sagittal and/or coronal imbalance of the lumbar spine. This was performed using a one-stage posterior three-column osteotomy in 14 patients with fixed spinal imbalance. There were no pseudarthroses in the follow-up period. Lordosis increased an average of 32 degrees. Coronal imbalance was also improved in all but one patient. Complica-

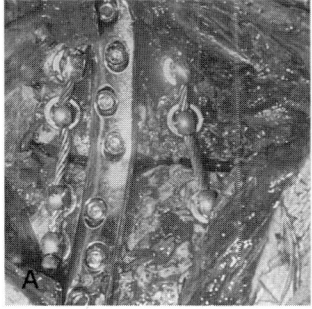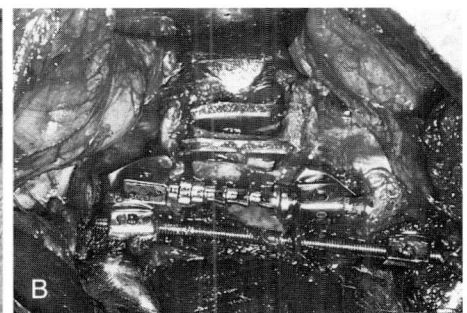

Figure 29. *A*, Posterior osteotomy has been closed by the application of Dwyer screws in the lateral fusion mass and an AO plate has been added in the midline to help to control rotation. *B*, Simultaneous to posterior closure, the anterior osteotomy site is opened with Kostuik-Harrington instrumentation. Iliac crest grafts are added and a second Kostuik-Harrington compression rod is added to enhance stability.

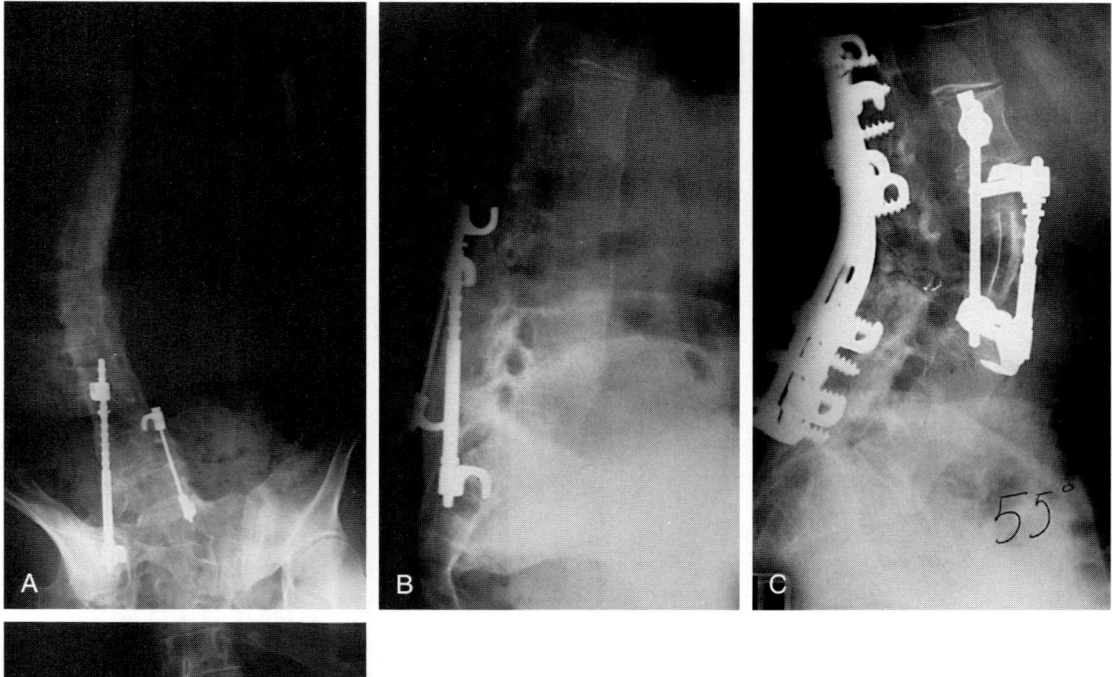
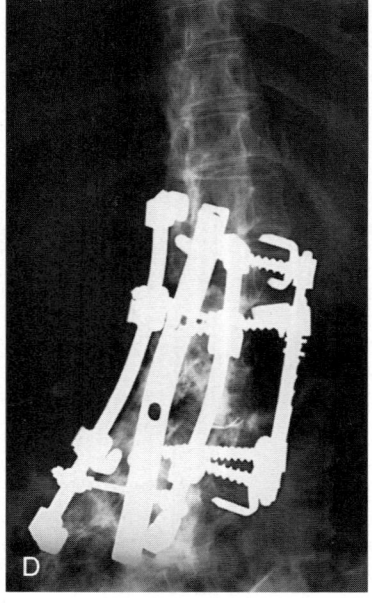

Figure 30. *A,* This 52-year-old patient had had a previous fusion to L3 as an adolescent. The fusion was extended to the sacrum at another institution. *B,* Lordosis was decreased, and although the fusion was solid, pain persisted, owing to the loss of lordosis. *C,* Lordosis was increased to 55 degrees from L1 to S1 using a single-stage anterior-posterior osteotomy. *D,* Cotrel-Dubousset instrumentation was used posteriorly to close the osteotomy. Kostuik-Harrington instrumentation was used anteriorly to open the osteotomy anteriorly.

tions, however, occurred in 10 of 14 patients.

Lateral Lumbar Circumferential Wedge Osteotomy for Imbalanced Adult Scoliosis

Patients have significant imbalance secondary to either a compensatory lumbosacral deformity or a previously fused thoracolumbar and lumbar deformity. There may be pain only in the compensatory lumbosacral curve or pain in both the primary and the compensatory curve. Kostuik and Masha[57] described a technique of lateral lumbar circumferential wedge osteotomy using a combined anterior and posterior approach to achieve rebalance in the following patients:

1. Patients previously untreated, who

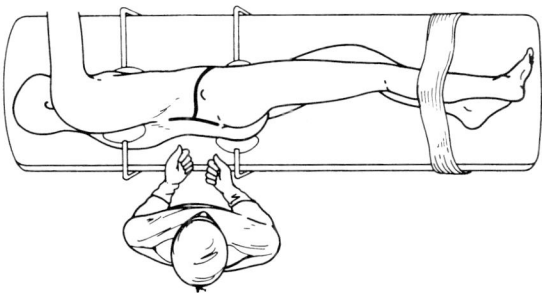

Figure 31. The incision for a lateral wedge circumferential osteotomy. This allows simultaneous access to both the anterior and the posterior spine.

have pain in the compensatory lumbosacral curve and who have imbalance greater than 4 cm

2. Patients who present with pain in both the compensatory curve and the primary curve, who require rebalancing as well as treatment of the primary deformity
3. Patients who remain imbalanced as a result of previous surgery

This is usually performed at the L3–L4, or L4–L5 level, with closing wedge osteotomy fixed anteriorly by Kostuik-Harrington compression and instrumentation and fixed posteriorly by Cotrel-Dubousset instrumentation. A T-incision (Fig 31) is performed. The psoas muscle is mobilized together with the lumbar roots.

This procedure has been performed a total of 24 times. The first group consisted of six patients who were treated for painful compensatory lumbosacral curves. After rebalancing, the proximal curve was reduced approximately 40% (Fig 32). Long-term follow-up revealed that in 5 of 6 patients, balance was maintained. One patient subsequently has had the primary curve corrected. In this group of patients, pain was proved to emanate from the lumbosacral compensatory curve on the basis of discography. In the third group, 10 patients who had previous surgery but remained imbalanced underwent similar osteotomies for rebalancing (Fig. 33).

The second group of patients, eight in number, have had the compensatory curve corrected at a first stage to achieve rebalance. Because they had problems relating to their proximal deformity and pain, they underwent a second-stage correction of the primary deformity usually 1 to 2 weeks later (Fig. 34).

The degree of imbalance ranged from 4 to 13.5 cm. The average correction was 8.5 cm. One patient remained uncorrected for technical reasons. Two patients had partial recurrence of the deformity. The remaining patients maintained the correction, with the exception of the one patient in the first group in whom the proximal thoracolumbar curve became worse.

Complications included two minor neurapraxias that resolved in two patients. One patient experienced significant blood loss of greater than 5000 ml. Adult respiratory distress syndrome developed in one patient.

The technique is recommended only

Figure 32. Female patient, age 28 years. *A*, A painful deformity was noted. Discography reproduced pain at L4–5 and L5–S1 but not at L3–4. *B*, An anterior closing wedge L4–5 wedge osteotomy was done with extension of the fusion to S1, using Zielke instrumentation. The proximal deformity has been reduced and remains so 8 years later. The patient had been advised of possible proximal disc degeneration and/or increased proximal deformity in later life but still has a relatively flexible lumbar spine.

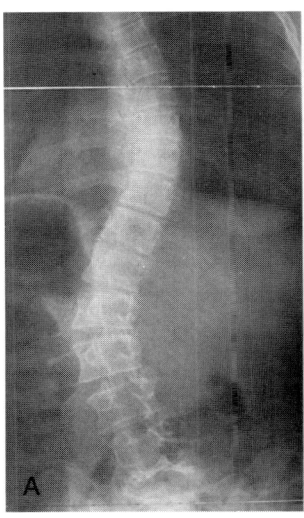
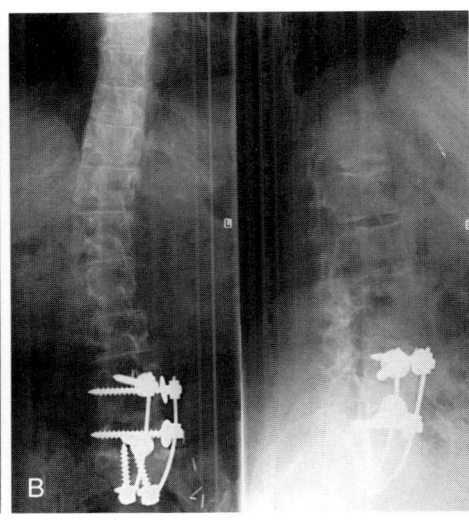

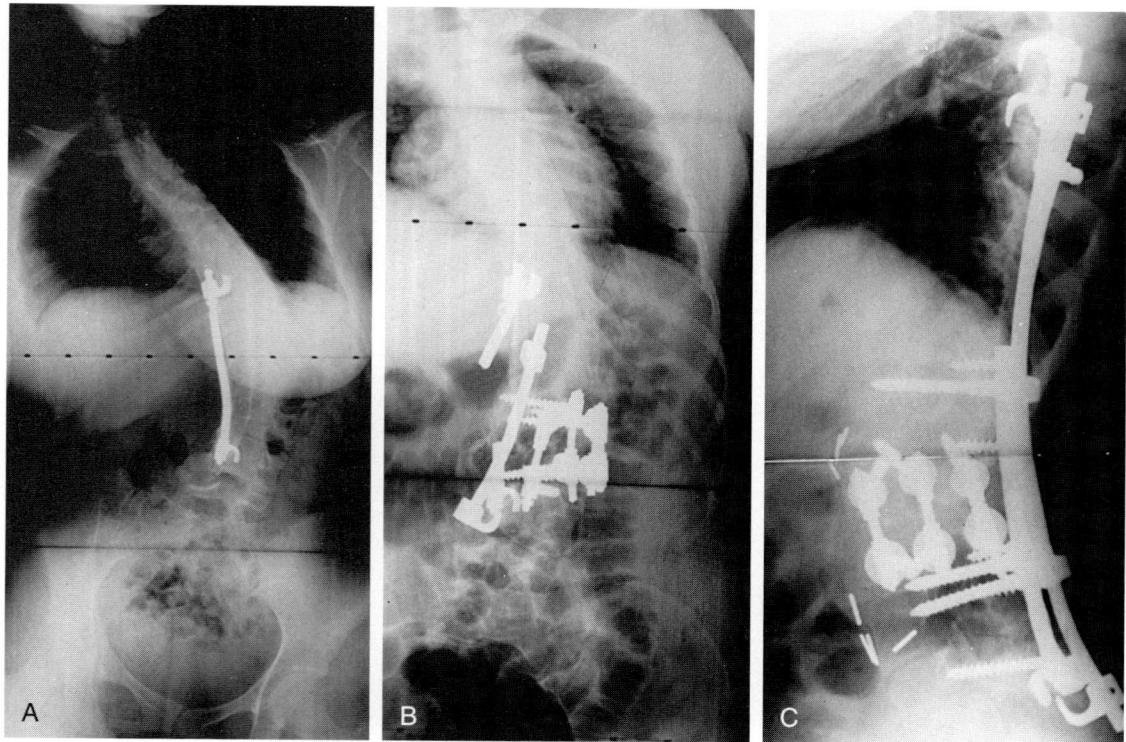

Figure 33. *A*, The patient, age 26 years, had undergone a previous thoracolumbar operation, elsewhere, but remained markedly imbalanced. *B*, A combined circumferential lateral wedge using anterior and posterior instrumentation (posterior Cotrel-Dubousset instrumentation and anterior Kostuik-Harrington compression rods) corrected the imbalance. *C*, The lateral view demonstrates the anterior fixation. Lordosis has been restored as well.

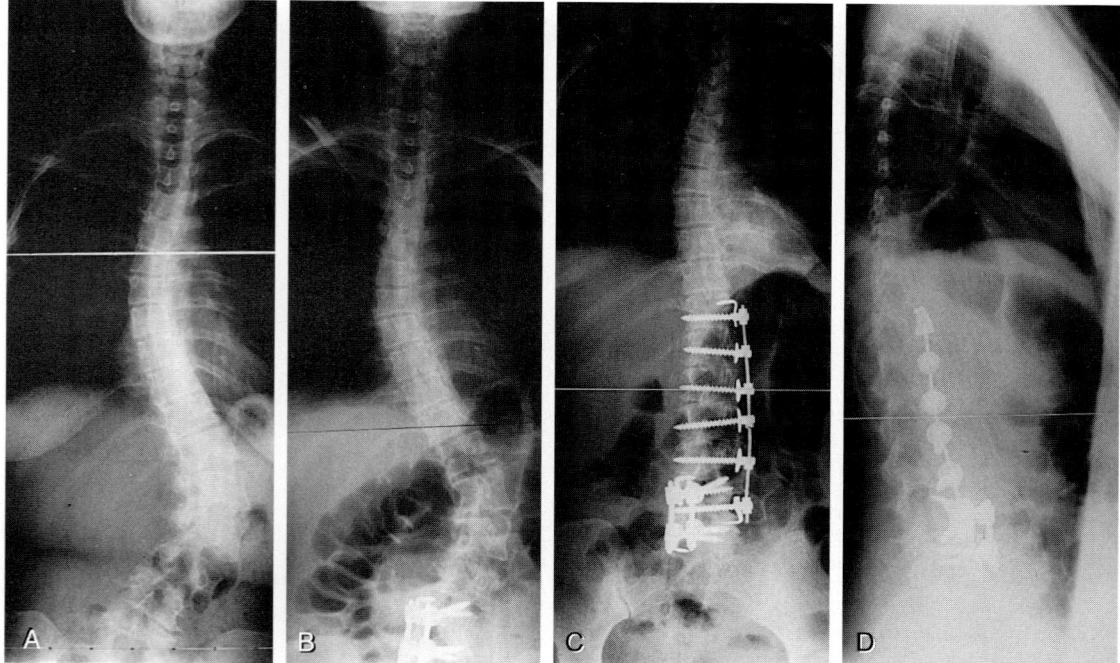

Figure 34. *A*, A patient, age 34 years, presented with a markedly imbalanced, painful lumbar scoliosis. *B*, The patient was rebalanced at the first stage by an anterior-posterior, lateral closing wedge circumferential osteotomy at L4–S1. *C*, Because the deformity was so severe and pain was also located at the apex of the deformity, an anterior Zielke procedure was done 1 week later. L5–S1 was normal on discography. *D*, Postoperative lateral view.

when the patient has imbalance greater than 4 cm, when the lumbosacral compensatory curve is rigid and painful, or when patients have undergone fusion previously and remain imbalanced, if the fusion has extended into the lumbosacral area.

DEGENERATIVE (DE NOVO) ADULT SCOLIOSIS

Prevalence

The other major category of adult scoliosis is deformity presenting de novo in an adult. This has been referred to as collapsing scoliosis[95] or senescent lumbar scoliosis.[24] Exactly how often this occurs is unknown. The only certain proof that a patient has a new curve rather than a progression of a previously unrecognized curve, is a normal spinal radiograph taken sometime in the past. For this reason, it is impossible to determine precisely the prevalence of de novo scoliosis. Vanderpool and associates[107] were the first to study this problem carefully. In the control group (average age of 61.4 years), the prevalence of scoliosis was 6%, but most curves were mild (7 to 15 degrees). A similar finding was observed in adult relatives of patients with scoliosis. In an osteoporotic group, 36% had curvature. The average age was 71 years. These investigators were able to identify 14 of 36 patients who had unequivocal evidence that they were free from scoliosis at an earlier age. The average age at onset was 40 years. An episode of back pain was usually the identified point at which scoliosis began and was usually secondary to an osteoporotic compression fracture. The curves were, in general, mild and ranged from 7 to 53 degrees. The distribution in the spine involved all levels equally. A similar finding was present in 24 patients with osteomalacia; 38% had a curvature, but it was generally mild and involved little or no rotation. On the basis of this analysis, the investigators concluded that adult-onset curves were secondary to osteomalacia and osteoporosis.

A different perspective was advanced by Robin and associates.[87] They followed a group of 554 subjects for intervals of 8 to 13 years. Some degree of scoliosis was found in 70% of subjects, and 30% had curves of greater than 10 degrees. In 10% of their patients, scoliosis developed during follow-up. However, they concluded that there was little relationship of progression to osteoporosis, or degenerative changes in the spine. Their conclusion is intriguing: "Since scoliosis in the elderly seldom becomes a clinical problem of significance, there would appear to be no valid reason for more extensive study of this condition at this time."[87]

This conclusion is striking in its contrast to the experience of Epstein and colleagues,[24] Benner and Ehni,[4] Grubb and coworkers,[28, 29] and Perennou and associates.[82] Their findings were that scoliosis can arise de novo in the adult, is probably degenerative in etiology, and can be the source of severe symptoms.

Idiopathic Versus Degenerative Scoliosis

Grubb and coworkers[27, 29] attempted to differentiate the adults with preexistent but progressive scoliosis from those with a new curve. Significant differences and similarities are present:[75]

Demographics. All of the group with idiopathic scoliosis were female, with a mean age of 42 years, whereas the sex distribution was equal in the group with degenerative disease and the mean age was 60 years.

Pain. Low back pain was equivalent in both groups, radiating into the buttock and upper thighs. However, 90% of the patients with degenerative scoliosis had symptoms indicative of spinal stenosis, compared with 31% of the idiopathic group. The major attribute of the stenotic pain was aggravation by spinal extension. Unlike the case with typical degenerative stenosis, patients often were not able to relieve pain by sitting down. Rather they had to support body weight with their arms.

Magnitude of Curve. The curve was greater in the idiopathic group and averaged 52 degrees, with a range from 34 to 78 degrees. The degenerative group curve average was 28 degrees, with a range from 15 to 53 degrees. However, the average 9-degree deformity per vertebral level was the same in both groups. An additional finding in the degenerative group was lateral translation, a finding emphasized by Epstein and associates.[24]

Myelographic Defects. Myelographic defects were most commonly seen within the compensatory lumbosacral curve in the idiopathic group. In comparison, the degenerative group showed most myelographic defects within the primary curve.

Discography. The adult-onset group had grossly degenerative changes within the curve, but pain frequently was not produced by discography. In comparison, reproduction of pain by discography was common in the idiopathic group, an observation made earlier.[47] It is speculated that, when degeneration is so advanced, injection does not distend the disc and pain does not result.

Conservative Management

The management is similar to that described for patients who have idiopathic curves presenting in adulthood. It consists of the administration of nonsteroidal antiinflammatory medications, exercise (usually with avoidance of extension), and general aerobic conditioning. Braces and corsets may offer temporary relief, but no studies prove their efficacy over time. Treatment of existent osteoporosis and prevention of further bone loss are encouraged, particularly in female patients.

Surgery

Operative Indications

The most common indication for surgery in adult-onset scoliosis is nerve root symptoms and spinal stenosis. Back pain is currently a less common indication. The debate about who can be treated by decompression alone and who requires decompression with fusion is unresolved. The author believes that decompression without fusion can be done when it is limited to one nerve root and the facets can be preserved. If greater decompression is necessary or facets are sacrificed, the operation should include a fusion in situ or correction of the deformity plus fusion but only if lordosis has been preserved, which is unusual. If kyphotic, lordosis must be restored; as noted earlier, a patient fused in kyphosis is not satisfied. Otherwise, progression and increasing pain are major future problems (Fig. 35). This perspective is not shared by others. For example, Epstein and coworkers[24] thought that patients with significant osteophytes might be treated by decompression alone, a perspective advocated by Nachemson.[69]

Preoperative Evaluation

All of the preoperative tests recommended for the idiopathic group may be necessary for patients with degenerative scoliosis. However, pulmonary dysfunction is rarely an issue unless the patient has some other coexistent disease.

If fusion is to be done, there is a question about how many vertebrae to include in the fusion. Nash and associates[72] analyzed whether the criteria for fusion extent in adolescents are applicable to adults. The criteria selected were the stable zone, the central sacral line, neutrally rotated vertebra, degenerative arthritis, displaced wedging, rotatory subluxation, and hemisacralization. They concluded that multiple factors should be considered in selecting the extent of fusion and that no single measurement had particular predictive value. The stable zone and the central sacral line were of little use in comparison with the situation in an adolescent patient with scoliosis. However, it was relevant when the fusion included L2, L3, and L4.

The most important factors were the magnitude of degeneration and its extent into the lower lumbar levels. Incorporation of vertebral levels with rotatory subluxation, disc space narrowing, and wedging seemed to be important. All of these findings were common and were seen in at least 50% of patients. An oblique L5 takeoff and hemisacralization were seen in 25% of patients and were relevant to the decision to include the lumbosacral joint. When all criteria were applied, Nash and associates[72] reported significant pain reduction in 89% of patients. It is the author's opinion that the important factor is to incorporate all painful areas into the fusion, which is best determined by preoperative discography and facet blocks.

Simmons and Jackson[94] reported on spinal stenosis associated with scoliosis. In a review of 40 patients, all treated by posterior decompression and pedicle screw fixation, with an average age of 61.5 years, marked reduction of pain was noted in 93%. The

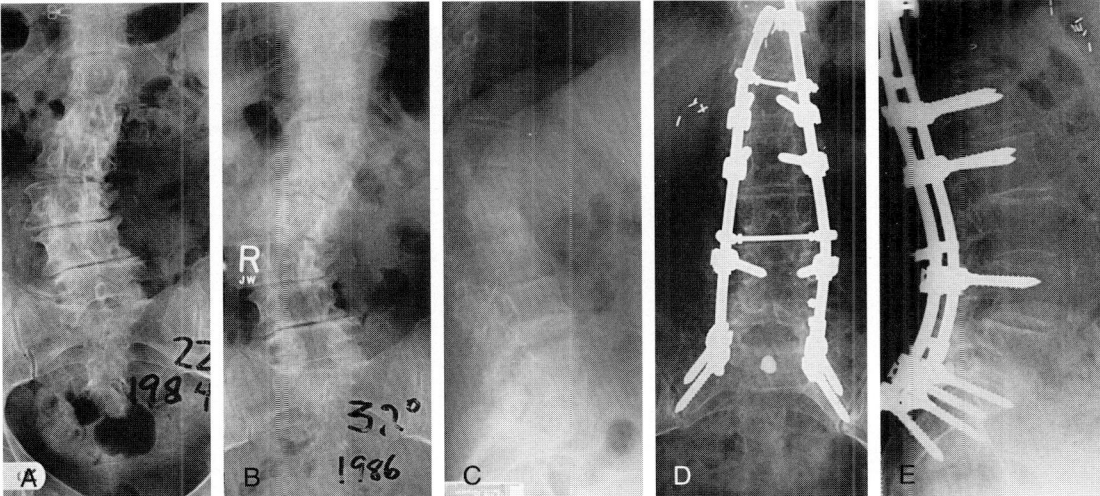

Figure 35. Female patient, age 65 years. *A*, Prelaminectomy scoliosis remained at 22 degrees. *B*, After decompression, the deformity increased to 32 degrees, together with totally disabling back pain, and subsequently to 50 degrees. *C*, Note loss of lordosis post decompression. *D, E,* Two-stage surgery restored lordosis and relieved pain. The first stage consisted of multiple anterior discectomies and bone graft. The second-stage Cotrel-Dubousset instrumentation and fusion corrected the deformity and restored lordosis.

average degree of deformity preoperatively was 37 degrees, postoperatively it was 19 degrees. There were no associated deaths, instrumentation failures, or pseudarthroses. Marchesi and Aebi[64] also reported on the use of pedicle fixation in the treatment of degenerative adult lumbar scoliosis. The average correction was just over 50%. Satisfactory results were obtained in 86%. Pseudarthrosis occurred in 4%. The mean age was 60 years.

This author agrees that, in patients with degenerative scoliosis, age is not a contraindication to surgery. Restoration of lumbar lordosis is paramount, and the use of pedicle fixation on osteoporotic bone makes this possible.

Grubb and associates,[29] in a series of 53 adults with scoliosis, including idiopathic and degenerative cases, noted an 80% reduction in pain among those with idiopathic scoliosis and a 70% reduction in patients with degenerative scoliosis. The rate of pseudarthrosis was 4% in idiopathic disease and 33% in degenerative disease. All pseudarthroses were in patients fused to the sacrum with posterior procedures alone. Preoperative assessment included the use of discography.

Surgical Approaches

The first important decision is whether decompression is necessary, as assessed by the preoperative findings and imaging studies. Unfortunately, no one criterion establishes that adequate decompression has been accomplished, unless the patient has specific nerve root findings localized to one or two levels. The criteria that are considered are the levels of involvement seen by myelography and the myelographically enhanced computed tomographic scan, the restoration of pulsatile dura, and the patency of the foramina. Intraoperative evoked somatosensory potentials have also been reported to be useful. Some surgeons often take a radical approach, including removal of the facets, pars, and portions of the pedicles to ensure adequate decompression.[92, 94, 95]

If fusion is selected, many of the same basic strategies apply as described above. Fusion in situ may be done, although it seems likely, but is not yet proved, that a lower rate of pseudarthrosis will result with instrumentation (Fig. 36). In general, pedicle systems that incorporate rigid linkages, particularly plates, are less suitable because they are less adaptable to the three-dimensional curve characteristics. This difficulty can be overcome with Cotrel-Dubousset instrumentation or posterior Zielke apparatus, as described by Simmons and Capicotto.[95] Using that technique, a 100% fusion rate was obtained in a patient cohort with a mean age of 62 years, who had a variety of

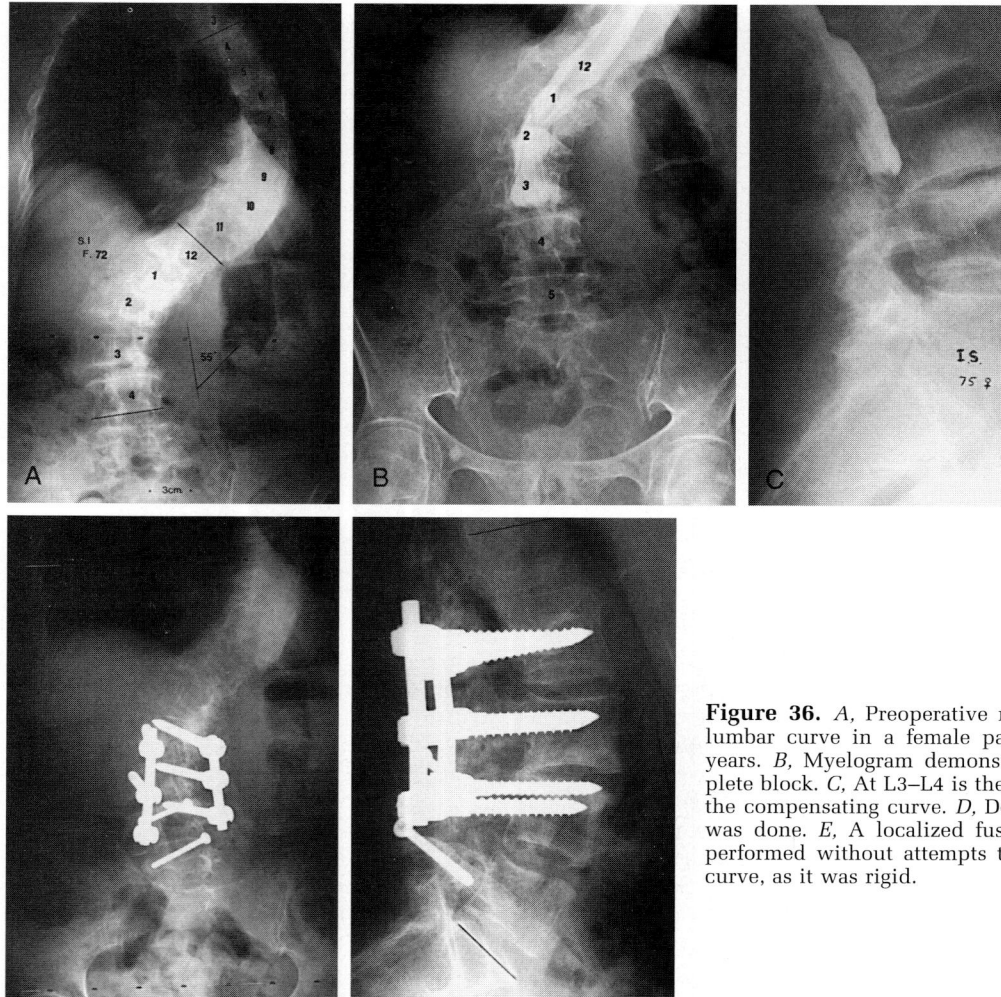

Figure 36. *A,* Preoperative rigid thoracolumbar curve in a female patient, age 72 years. *B,* Myelogram demonstrates a complete block. *C,* At L3–L4 is the beginning of the compensating curve. *D,* Decompression was done. *E,* A localized fusion was also performed without attempts to correct the curve, as it was rigid.

conditions, including degenerative scoliosis. The author remains convinced that it is still important to combine anterior and posterior approaches, particularly at unstable levels and particularly at the lumbosacral junction, and to restore lumbar lordosis.

Degenerative Scoliosis Following Decompression for Spinal Stenosis

There is no question that an increased curve can follow decompression in a patient with previous degenerative scoliosis. The question is how common scoliosis is after decompression of spinal stenosis if there were normal spinal curves preoperatively. At present, there is no information to provide a precise answer to this question (see Fig. 35).

COMPLICATIONS IN ADULT SCOLIOSIS (Table 1)

Complications in surgical treatment of adult scoliosis are based on numerous factors. These include the approach, the level of the deformity, and the age of the patient. McDonnell and associates,[65] in analysis of preoperative complications of all forms of anterior spine surgery, noted a 26% incidence of complications for patients between the ages of 3 and 20 years (9% major and

Table 1
Complications of Adult Scoliosis Surgery

Category / Complication	Rate
Hematologic	
Excessive blood loss	
Coagulopathy	
Disseminated intravascular coagulopathy	
Vascular	
Thrombophlebitis	0.25%
Pulmonary embolism	5%
Vascular injury (great vessels) (minor)	~50%
Negative effects of sympathectomy	<<1%
Cerebrovascular accident	0%
Respiratory	
Pneumonia	1–2%
Atelectasis	3–7%
Pneumothorax	1%
Adult respiratory distress syndrome	1–2%
Postthoracotomy syndrome	5%
Urologic	
Retrograde ejaculation (anterior)	<1%
Ureteric injury (repeated surgery—anterior)	~1%
Urinary tract infection	5–10%
Retroperitoneal fibrosis → hydronephroses	<<<1%
Neurologic	
Nerve root injury	
Minor	3%
Major	<1%
Nerve root dysesthesia	~5%
Spinal cord injury	~0.25% or less
Cauda equina injury	<<0.25%
Cluneal nerve problem	~5%
Lateral femoral cutaneous nerve	~5%
Osseous	
Pseudarthrosis: posterior	
Thoracic	~1%
Thoracolumbar	~3%
Lumbar	~5%
Lumbosacral	7%
Pseudarthrosis: anterior	3%
Hook pullout	
Thoracic	5%
Lumbar	5–10%
Pedicle screw pullout	
Thoracic	~5%
Lumbar	<1%
Sacral	3%
Laminar fracture	
Thoracic	5%
Lumbar	5–10%
Iliac crest fracture (anterior)	~3–5%
Donor site pain, persistent (usually mild)	10%
Sacroiliac instability	<0.5%
Postthoracotomy shoulder stiffness	5–10%
Gastrointestinal	
Ileus > 3 days	~5%
Duodenal obstruction	<<<1%
Ulcer	~0%
Pancreatitis	<<<1%
Lymphocele	0–<<<1%
Cholecystitis	<<<1%
Abdominal wall weakness (anterior—elderly)	5%
Infection	
Superficial	7–10%
Deep (primary wound)	
Acute	1%
Persistent sinus	<<<1%
Donor site	1%
Wound dehiscence	<1%
Psychologic	
Pseudoparalysis (conversion reaction)	0.5%
Depression	10%
Psychosis	<1%
Dermatologic	
Skin breakdown	
Minor	2–3%
Major	<1%

<<, much less than; <<<, very much less than.

20% minor), a 27% incidence for ages 21 to 40 years (6% major and 21% minor), a 41% incidence of complications for ages 41 to 60 years (14% major and 27% minor), and a 64% incidence for patients aged 61 to 85 (32% major and 40% minor). However, complication rates were lower in idiopathic scoliosis (16%, including 3% major and 4% minor) in contrast to those for fracture (25%), adult scoliosis (44%, with 11% major and 33% minor), neuromuscular scoliosis (49%), revision procedures (38%), general scoliosis (36%), tumor (33%), infection (63%), and kyphosis (23%). The incidence of complications in the thoracic spine was 5%, and in the thoracolumbar area the incidence was 24%. An analysis of patients undergoing vertebrectomy and fusion in contrast to those undergoing discectomy and fusion showed that blood loss was twice as great in the former, but the complication rate for vertebrectomy fusion was 31% and for discectomy fusion, 32%. Major and minor complications were not differentiated in this study.

Minchew and associates[56] analyzed the risk of hyponatremia and syndrome of inappropriate antidiuretic hormone secretion after adult spine surgery. They believed that spine patients are at risk for syndrome of inappropriate antidiuretic hormone secretion and hyponatremia, with an incidence of 6.9%. Patients undergoing revision surgery were at approximately 2 to 4 times greater risk than those having primary surgery. Also, there is an additional increased risk of inappropriate antidiuretic hormone secretion with greater percentage of blood loss. A normal antidiuretic hormone level did not preclude the diagnosis of the syndrome of inappropriate antidiuretic hormone secretion. Blood loss replacement with colloid solutions was not protective against the development of the syndrome.

Reports of morbidity committees generally note the occurrence of lie infections in scoliosis surgery at between 1% and 2%. The incidence of infection is somewhat higher in adult scoliosis patients (approximately 3%). Dubousset and coworkers[21] also noted a 1% incidence of late infection after segmental instrumentation with Cotrel-Dubousset instrumentation. It was thought to be due to micromotion between various forms of instrumentation. This resulted in threading corrosion and the development of inflammatory response. In their analysis, 18 of 18 patients had swelling, pain, and often spontaneous drainage. Presurgical cultures were generally negative, as were intraoperative cultures. A few positive cultures consisted of *Staphylococcus epidermidis*. They believed that the majority of these were simply inflammatory.

In a general review of complications of adult reconstructive spine surgery for spinal deformity, Nelson and Trammell[73] noted that 80% of patients had at least one complication. Sixty-seven percent were considered minor and 33% major. There was a mortality rate of 3%. Increasing age, decreased pulmonary function, increasing degree of deformity, and surgical approach correlated with increased complication rates. With reference to outcome, the author noted an average score of patient satisfaction of 81.5 of 100 and 88% of patients who had surgery previously with similar circumstances. This correlated with similar larger numbers reported by Kostuik and colleagues[53] in 1990. In Nelson and Trammell's[73] study, the estimated blood loss was 5 ml/minute of surgical time and averaged 2060 ml per case. The average hospital stay was 20.5 days, which is 7 days longer than that reported by Kostuik and colleagues.[53]

Lauerman and associates[61] reported on the analysis of pseudarthrosis after arthrodesis of the spine in idiopathic scoliosis. Sixty-three repairs were performed in 51 patients with an average age of 30 years. Indications were surgical pain and progression of deformity combined with radiographic changes. Failure of instrumentation was noted in only 27 of 63 procedures. Pseudarthrosis was diagnosed an average of 2.8 years after arthrodesis. Sixty-eight percent of defects were noted on plain x-ray films, and 32% were identified at the time of surgery. Curvature had increased an average of 7 degrees in the anteroposterior view and kyphosis had increased by mean of 10 degrees from the time of original arthrodesis to time of pseudarthrosis repair. The most frequently used instrumentation was Harrington distraction instrumentation, and it was most commonly used for repair together with autogenous graft.

Staging of Surgery

Controversy exists as to the staging of surgery for patients requiring anterior and posterior procedures. A review by Jeffrey and associates[39] compared 11 patients who underwent staged surgery and 13 who underwent a combined single-stage procedure. Morbidity from infection was less frequent, and costs were 30% less in those undergoing single-stage combined procedures. The amount of blood transfusion and operating times were similar for both groups. Shufflebarger and associates[92] interviewed 35 patients and reached similar conclusions. Protein and calorie malnutrition in both these groups increased the risk of postoperative morbidity for staged procedures.

The author concurs with the conclusions reached by these investigators, except for patients older than the age of 50 years. In this age group undergoing single-stage surgery, morbidity was significantly increased because of extensive blood loss after long operating time and coagulopathy. If the patient is not morbidly obese and is younger than 50 years, a single-stage procedure may be considered if it does not include a thoracotomy. Otherwise, in patients older than 50 years in whom thoracotomy is required as well as an extensive posterior procedure, staged surgery with an interval of 7 to 10 days during which the patient receives parenteral nutrition may be of value.

SUMMARY

Adult scoliosis comprises a diverse group of conditions, whose commonality is their presentation in adulthood. Regardless of etiology, the important issues are back pain and neurologic symptoms, which are more common in those with degenerative curves. These two symptoms are the most common indications for surgery, although curve progression and occasionally cosmesis may be important factors. If surgery is necessary, a critical issue is the restoration or maintenance of lumbar lordosis. The surgical management of an iatrogenic flat back is a major undertaking. Fusion often may have to extend into the lumbosacral joint. The author believes that it is important to assess that need not only from plain radiographs and other imaging studies, but also by discography. In general, a combined anterior-posterior approach is advocated when the lumbosacral joint is included in the fusion. The addition of internal fixation devices adds to the predictability of fusion, and properly selected devices allow the maintenance of lumbar lordosis. Using these techniques and principles, a high rate of symptomatic relief and fusion can be achieved. However, the complication rate is significant. With continued refinements in technique, the rate of success and the reduction of complications can be predicted.

REFERENCES

1. Allen, B. L., Jr., and Ferguson, R. L.: The Galveston technique for L-rod instrumentation of the scoliotic spine. Spine 7:276–254, 1982.
2. Balderston, R. A., Winter, R. B., Moe, J. H., et al.: Fusion to the sacrum for nonparalytic scoliosis in the adult. Spine 11:824–829, 1986.
3. Bartie, B. J., Lonstein, J. E., Winter, R. B., et al.: Long-term follow-up of idiopathic scoliosis patients after spinal fusion An outcome analysis. Presented at the 28th Annual Meeting of the Scoliosis Research Society, Dublin, September 18–23, 1993.
4. Benner, B., and Ehni, G.: Degenerative lumbar scoliosis. Spine 4:548–552, 1979.
5. Boachie-Adjei, O., Dendrinos, G. K., Ogilvie, J. W., and Bradford, D. S.: Management of adult spinal deformity with combined anterior-posterior arthrodesis and Luque-Galveston instrumentation. J. Spinal Disord. 4:131–141, 1991.
6. Boachie-Adjei, O., Gupta, M., and Marrero, G.: C-D sacro-pelvic fixation for adult spinal deformity. Results of primary and salvage reconstruction. Presented at the 28th Annual Meeting of the Scoliosis Research Society, Dublin, September 18–23, 1993.
7. Bradford, D. S.: Adult scoliosis: Current concepts of treatment. Clin. Orthop. 229:70–87, 1988.
8. Byrd, J. A., III, Scoles, P. V., Winter, R. B., et al.: Adult idiopathic scoliosis treated by anterior and posterior spinal fusion. J. Bone Joint Surg. 69:843–850, 1987.
9. Casey, M. P., Asher, M. A. Jacobs, R. R., and Orrick, J. M.: The effect of Harrington rod contouring on lumbar lordosis. Spine 12:750–753, 1987.
10. Cochran, T., Irstam, L., and Nachemson, A.: Long-term anatomic and functional changes in patients with adolescent scoliosis treated by Harrington rod fusion. Spine 8:576–584, 1983.
11. Coe, J. D., Becker, P. S. McAfee, P. C., and Gurr, K. R.: Neuropathology with spinal instrumentation. J. Orthop. Res. 7:359–370, 1989.
12. Collis, D. K., and Ponsetti, I. V.: Long term follow-up of patients with idiopathic scoliosis not treated surgically. J. Bone Joint Surg. 51A:425–445, 1969.
13. Connolly, P. J., von Schroeder, H. P., Johnston, G. E., and Kostuik, J. P.: Idiopathic adolescent scoliosis: A long-term (minimum 10 years) follow-up following Harrington instrumentation into the lumbar spine. Presented at the 28th Annual Meeting of the Scoliosis Research Society, Dublin, September 18–23, 1993. (To be published in J. Bone Joint Surg. (A), Autumn 1995.)
14. Cotrel, Y.: Instrumentation for Surgery of the Spine. Paris, Freud Publishing House, 1986.
15. Cotrel, Y., Dubousset, J., and Guillaumat, M.: New universal instrumentation in spinal surgery. Clin. Orthop. 227:10–22, 1988.
16. Cummine, J. L., Lonstein, J. E., Moe, J. H., et al.: Reconstructive surgery in the adult for failed scoliosis fusion. J. Bone Joint Surg. 61A:1151–1161, 1979.
17. Dawson, E. G., Caron, A., and Moe, J. H.: Surgical management of scoliosis in the adult. J. Bone Joint Surg. 55A:437, 1973.
18. Denis, F.: Cotrel-Dubousset instrumentation in the treatment of idiopathic scoliosis. Orthop. Clin North Am. 19:291–311, 1988.
19. Devlin, V. J., Boachie-Adjei, O., Bradford, D. S., et al.: Treatment of adult spinal deformity with fusion to the sacrum using CD instrumentation. J. Spinal Disord. 4:1–14, 1991.
20. Doherty, J. H.: Complications of fusion in lumbar scoliosis. J. Bone Joint Surg. 55A:438, 1973.
21. Dubousset, J., Schufflebarger, H. L and Wenger, D.: Late "infection" with CD instrumentation. Presented at the 28th Annual Meeting of the Scoliosis Research Society, Dublin, September 18–23, 1993.
22. Dwyer, A. F.: Experience of anterior correction of scoliosis. Clin. Orthop. 93:191–214, 1973.
23. Edgar, M. A., and Mehta, M. H.: A longterm review of adults with fused and unfused idiopathic scoliosis. Orthop. Trans. 6:462–463, 1982.
24. Epstein, J. A., Epstein, B. S., and Jones, M. D.: Symptomatic lumbar scoliosis with degenerative changes in the elderly. Spine 4:542–547, 1979.
25. Goldstein, J. M., Nash, C. L., and Wilham, M. R.: Selection of lumbar fusion levels in adult idio-

pathic scoliosis patients. Spine 16:1150–1154, 1991.
26. Grobler, L. J., Moe, J. H., Winter, R. B., et al.: Loss of lumbar lordosis following surgical correction of thoracolumbar deformities. Orthop. Trans. 2:239, 1978.
27. Grubb, S. A., Lipscomb, H. J., Coonrad, R. W.: Degenerative adult onset scoliosis. Spine 13:241–245, 1988.
28. Grubb, S. A., Lipscomb, H. J., and Coonrad, R. W.: Diagnostic findings in painful adult scoliosis. Presented at a meeting of the Scoliosis Research Society, Amsterdam, 1989.
29. Grubb, S. A., Lipscomb, H. J., and Suh, P. B.: Results of surgical treatment of painful adult scoliosis. Presented at the 28th Annual Meeting of the Scoliosis Research Society, Dublin, September 18–23, 1993.
30. Haher, J. E., Devlin, V., Freeman, B., and Rondon, B.: Long-term effects of sublaminar wires on the neural canal. Orthop. Trans. 11:106, 1987.
31. Hall, J. E.: Dwyer instrumentation in anterior fusion of the spine. J. Bone Joint Surg. 63A:1188–1190, 1981.
32. Harrington, P. R., and Dickson, J. H.: An eleven-year clinical investigation of Harrington instrumentation. A preliminary report on 578 cases. Clin. Orthop. 93:113–130, 1973.
33. Hasday, C. A., Passoff, T. L., and Perry, J.: Gait abnormalities arising from iatrogenic loss of lumbar lordosis secondary to Harrington instrumentation in lumbar fractures. Spine 8:501–511, 1983.
34. Hayes, M. A., Tompkin, S. F., Herndon, W. A., et al.: Clinical and radiological evaluation of lumbosacral motion below fusion levels in idiopathic scoliosis. Spine 13:1161–1167, 1988.
35. Herndon, W. A., Sullivan, J. A., Yngve, D. A., et al.: Segmental spinal instrumentation with sublaminar wires. J. Bone Joint Surg. 69A:851–859, 1987.
36. Herring, J. A., and Wenger, D. R.: Segmental spinal instrumentation. A preliminary report of 40 consecutive cases. Spine 7:285–298, 1982.
37. Horton, W. G., Heller, J. G., Whitesides, T., et al.: Tricolumnar osteotomy for fixed sagittal and/or coronal imbalance of the lumbar spine. Presented at the 28th Annual Meeting of the Scoliosis Research Society, Dublin, September 18–23, 1993.
38. Hu, S. S., and Bradford, D.: L5 opening wedge osteotomy in the treatment of lumbar scoliosis: A new technique to restore coronal balance and avoid arthrodesis to the sacrum. Presented at the 28th Annual Meeting of the Scoliosis Research Society, Dublin, September 18–23, 1993.
39. Jeffrey, D., Boachie-Adjei, O., and Wilson, M.: One stage versus two stage anterior and posterior spinal reconstruction in adults: Comparison of outcomes including nutritional status, complication rates, hospital costs and other factors. Spine 17:S310–S316, 1992.
40. Jackson, R. P., Simmons, E. H., and Stripinis, D.: Incidence and severity of back pain in adult idiopathic scoliosis. Spine 8:749–756, 1983.
41. Johnson, J. R., and Holt, R. T.: Combined use of anterior and posterior surgery for adult scoliosis. Orthop. Clin. North Am. 19:361–370, 1988.
42. Johnston, C. E., II, Happel, L. T., Jr., Norris, R., et al.: Delayed paraplegia complicating sublaminar segmental spinal instrumentation. J. Bone Joint Surg. 68A:556–563, 1986.
43. Kaneda, K., Fujiya, N., and Satoh, S.: Results with Zielke instrumentation for idiopathic thoracolumbar and lumbar scoliosis. Clin. Orthop. 205:195–203, 1986.
44. Kesten, S., Garfinkel, S. K., Wright, T., and Rebuck, A. S.: Impaired exercise capacity in adults with moderate scoliosis. Chest 99:663–666, 1991.
45. Kostuik, J. P., and Hall, B. B.: Spinal fusions to the sacrum in adults with scoliosis. Spine 8:489–500, 1973.
46. Kostuik, J. P., Israel, J., and Hall, J. E.: Scoliosis surgery in adults. Clin. Orthop. 93:225–234, 1973.
47. Kostuik, J. P.: Decision making in adult scoliosis. Spine 4:521–525, 1979.
48. Kostuik, J. P., and Bentivoglio, J.: The incidence of low back pain in adult scoliosis. Spine 6:268–273, 1981.
49. Kostuik, J. P.: Treatment of scoliosis in the adult thoracolumbar spine with special reference of fusion to the sacrum. Orthop. Clin. North Am. 19:371–381, 1988.
50. Kostuik, J. P., Maurais, G. E., Richardson, W. J., and Okajimay, Y.: Combined single stage anterior and posterior osteotomy for correction of iatrogenic lumbar kyphosis. Spine 13:257–266, 1988.
51. Kostuik, J. P., Carl, A., and Ferron, S.: Anterior Zielke instrumentation for spinal deformity in adults. J. Bone Joint Surg. 72A:898–912, 1989.
52. Kostuik, J. P., Maurais, G. E., and Richardson, W. J.: Primary fusion to the sacrum using Luque instrumentation for adult scoliotic patients. Orthop. Trans. 13:30, 1989.
53. Kostuik, J. P., Worden, H. R., and Salo, P.: Long term functional outcome following surgery for adult scoliosis. Presented at a meeting of the American Orthopaedic Association, Boston, 1990.
54. Kostuik, J. P.: Adult scoliosis. In Frymoyer, J. (ed.): The Adult Spine. New York, Raven Press, 1991.
55. Kostuik, J. P., Connolly, P. J., and Munting, E.: Lumbar circumferential lateral wedge osteotomy: Descriptions of technique and review of surgical experience. Presented at the 28th Annual Meeting of the Scoliosis Research Society, Dublin, September 18–23, 1993.
56. Kostuik, J. P., Mhaidli, H., Finkenberg, J., et al.: The surgical results of the first 100 adult idiopathic scoliosis patients treated with Cotrel-Dubousset instrumentation. Presented at a meeting of the Scoliosis Research Society, Kansas City, MD, 1993. Submitted for publication.
57. Kostuik, J. P., and Musha, Y.: Extension of previous fusion to the sacrum in adult scoliosis. Presented at the Annual Meeting of the Scoliosis Research Society, Portland, OR, September 1994.
58. Kostuik, J. P., and Musha, Y.: Fusion to the sacrum in adult idiopathic scoliosis using Cotrel-Dubousset instrumentation (1986–1990). Presented at the Annual Meeting of the Scoliosis Research Society Portland, OR, September 1994.
59. Krismer, M., Bauer, R., and Sterzinger, W.: Scoliosis correction by Cotrel-Dubousset instrumentation. Spine 17:263–269, 1992.
60. Lagrone, M. O., Bradford, D. S., Moe, J. H., et al.: Treatment of symptomatic flatback after spinal fusion. J. Bone Joint Surg. 70A:569–580, 1988.
61. Lauerman, W. C., Bradford, D. S., Ogilvie, J. W.,

and Transfeldt, E. E.: Results of lumbar pseudarthrosis repair. J. Spinal Disord. 5:149–157, 1992.
62. Luque, E. R.: The anatomic basis and development of segmental spinal instrumentation. Spine 7:256–259, 1982.
63. Luque, E. R.: Segmental spinal instrumentation for correction of scoliosis. Clin. Orthop. 163:192–198, 1982.
64. Marchesi, D. G., and Aebi, M.: Pedicle fixation devices in the treatment of adult lumbar scoliosis. Spine 17:S304–S309, 1992.
65. McDonnell, M. F., Glassman, S. D., Dimar, J. R., et al.: Perioperative complications of anterior spine surgery. Presented at the 28th Annual Meeting of the Scoliosis Research Society, Dublin, September 18–23, 1993.
66. Minchew, J. T., Callewart, C. C., Kanim, L. E., et al.: Hyponatremia/syndrome of inappropriate antidiuretic hormone secretion in adult spinal surgery. Presented at the 28th Annual Meeting of the Scoliosis Research Society, Dublin, September 18–23, 1993.
67. Moe, J. H., Purcell, G. A., and Bradford, D. S.: Zielke instrumentation (VDS) for the correction of spinal curvature. Analysis of results in 66 patients. Clin. Orthop. 180:133–153, 1983.
68. Nachemson, A.: A longterm follow-up study of non-treated scoliosis. Acta Orthop. Scand. 39:466–476, 1968.
69. Nachemson, A.: A longterm follow-up study of non-treated scoliosis. J. Bone Joint Surg. 50:203–204, 1969.
70. Nachemson, A.: Adult scoliosis and back pain. Spine 4:513–517, 1988.
71. Nash, C. L. Jr., and Moe J. H.: A study of vertebral rotation. J. Bone Joint Surg. 51A:223–229, 1969.
72. Nash, C. L., Goldstein, J. M., and Wilham, M. R.: Selection of lumbar fusion levels in adult idiopathic scoliosis patients. Presented at a meeting of the Scoliosis Research Society, Amsterdam, 1989.
73. Nelson, L. M., and Trammell, T. R.: Complications and outcome of adult reconstructive spinal surgery. Presented at the 28th Annual Meeting of the Scoliosis Research Society, Dublin, September 18–23, 1993.
74. Nicastro, J. F., Hartjen, C. A., Traina, J., and Lancaster, J. M.: Intraspinal pathways taken by sublaminar wires during removal. An experimental study. J. Bone Joint Surg. 68A:1206–1209, 1986.
75. Nilsonne, U., and Lundgren, K. D.: Longterm prognosis in idiopathic scoliosis. Acta Orthop. Scand. 39:455–465, 1968.
76. Nuber, G. W., and Schafer, M. F.: Surgical management of adult scoliosis. Clin. Orthop. 208:228–237, 1986.
77. O'Brien, M., Bridwell, K., Lenke, L., et al.: Adult onset de novo 'degenerative scoliosis.'' Guidelines for evaluation and treatment. Presented at the 28th Annual Meeting of the Scoliosis Research Society, Dublin, September 18–23, 1993.
78. Ogiela, D. M., and Chan, D. P. K.: Ventral derotation spondylodesis. A review of 22 cases. Spine 11:18–22, 1986.
79. Opitz, G., and Zielke, K.: 10 year results following surgery of idiopathic scoliosis using the Harrington technique (work by the Conference of German-language Spinal Surgeons). Z. Orthop. 128:482–489, 1990.
80. Paonessa, K., and Engler, G.: Back pain and disability after Harrington rod fusion to the lumbar spine for scoliosis. Spine 17:S249–S253, 1992.
81. Pehrsson, K., Bake, B., Larsson, S., and Nachemson, A.: Lung function in adult idiopathic scoliosis: a 20 year follow up. Thorax 46:474–478, 1991.
82. Perennou, D., Marcelli, C., Herisson, C., and Simon, L.: Adult lumbar scoliosis: Epidemiologic aspects in a low-back pain population. Spine 19:123–128, 1994.
83. Poitras, B., Mayo, N., Goldberg, M., et al.: The Ste-Justine adolescent idiopathic scoliosis (AIS) cohort study III. Surgical correction and back pain. Presented at the 28th Annual Meeting of the Scoliosis Research Society, Dublin, September 18–23, 1993.
84. Ponder, R. C., Dickson, J. H., Harrington, P. R., and Erwin, W. D.: Results of Harrington instrumentation and fusion in the adult idiopathic scoliosis patient. J. Bone Joint Surg. 57A:797–801, 1975.
85. Ponsetti, I. V.: The pathogenesis of adult scoliosis. In Zorab, P. A., Cansation, E., and Livingston, S. (eds.): Proceedings of the Second Symposium on Scoliosis. Edinburgh, Churchill Livingstone, 1968.
86. Reckling, C., Ogilvie, J., and Cohen, M.: Lumbar fusions in the elderly. Presented at the 28th Annual Meeting of the Scoliosis Research Society, Dublin, September 18–23, 1993.
87. Robin, G. C., Span, Y., Steinberg, R., et al.: Scoliosis in the elderly. A follow-up study. Spine 7:355–359, 1982.
88. Rogala, E. J., Drummond, D. S., and Gurr, J.: Scoliosis: Incidence and natural history. A prospective epidemiological study. J. Bone Joint Surg. 60A:172–176, 1978.
89. Saer, E., Winter, R., and Lonstein, J.: Long scoliosis fusion to the sacrum in adults with nonparalytic scoliosis: an improved method. Spine 15:650–653, 1990.
90. Schrader, W. C., Bethem, D., and Scerbin, V.: The chronic local effects of sublaminar wires—an animal model. Orthop. Trans. 11:106, 1987.
91. Shands, A. R., Jr., and Eisberg, H. V.: The incidence of scoliosis in the state of Delaware. J. Bone Joint Surg. 37A:1243–1249, 1955.
92. Shufflebarger, H. L., Grimm, J. O. Bui, V., and Thomson, J. D.: Anterior and posterior spinal fusion: Staged versus same-day surgery. Spine 16:930–933, 1991.
93. Shufflebarger, H. L., and Clark, C. E. Thoracolumbar osteotomy for postsurgical sagittal imbalance. Spine 17:S287–S290, 1992.
94. Simmons, E. H., and Jackson, R. P.: The management of nerve root entrapment syndromes associated with the collapsing scoliosis of idiopathic lumbar and thoracolumbar curves. Spine 4:533–541, 1979.
95. Simmons, E. H., and Capicotto, W. N.: Posterior transpedicular Zielke instrumentation of the lumbar spine. Clin. Orthop. 236:180–191, 1989.
96. Simmons, E. D., Jr., and Simmons, E. H.: Spinal stenosis with scoliosis. Spine 17:S117–S120, 1992.
97. Sponseller, P. D., Cohen, M. S., Nachemson, A. L., et al.: Results of surgical treatment of adults with idiopathic scoliosis. J. Bone Joint Surg. 69A:667–675, 1987.

98. Stagnara, P.: Scoliosis in adults. Surgical treatment of severe forms. Paris, Excerpta Medica Foundation International Congress Series no. 192, 1969.
99. Stagnara, P., Jouvinoux, P., Peloux, J., et al.: Cyphoscoliosis essentielles de l'adulte. Formes severe de plus de 100. Redressment partial et arthrodese. Presented at the XISICOT Congress, Mexico City, 1969.
100. Stagnara, P.: Utilization of Harrington's device in the treatment of adult kyphoscoliosis above 100 degrees. In Fourth International Symposium. Stuttgart, George Thieme Verlag, 1971.
101. Stagnara, P., Fleury, D., Fauchet, R., et al.: Major scoliosis over 100 degrees, in adults. 183 surgically treated cases. Rev. Chir. Orthop. 61:101–122, 1975.
102. Swank, S., Lonstein, J. E., Moe, J. H., and Bradford, D. S.: Surgical treatment of adult scoliosis. A review of 222 cases. J. Bone Joint Surg. 63A:268–287, 1981.
103. Thompson, G. H., Wilber, R. G., Shaffer, J. W., et al.: Segmental spinal instrumentation in idiopathic scoliosis. A preliminary report. Spine 10:623–630, 1985.
104. Trammell, T. R., Benedict, F., and Reid, D.: Anterior spine fusion using Zielke instrumentation for adult thoracolumbar and lumbar scoliosis. Spine 16:307–316, 1991.
105. van Dam, B. E., Bradford, D. S., Lonstein, J. E., et al.: Adult idiopathic scoliosis treated by posterior spinal fusion and Harrington instrumentation. Spine 12:32–36, 1987.
106. van Dam, B. E.: Nonoperative treatment of adult scoliosis. Orthop. Clin. North Am. 19:347–351, 1988.
107. Vanderpool, D. W., James, J. I. P., and Wynne-Davies, R.: Scoliosis in the elderly. J. Bone Joint Surg. 51A:446–455, 1969.
108. Vaughan, J. J., Holt, R. T., and Dopf, C. A.: Degenerative lumbar scoliosis treated by combined anterior and posterior spinal fusion. Presented at the 28th Annual Meeting of the Scoliosis Research Society, Dublin, September 18–23, 1993.
109. Weinstein, S. L., and Ponsetti, I. V.: Curve progression in idiopathic scoliosis. J. Bone Joint Surg. 65A:447–455, 1983.
110. Wilber, R. G., Thompson, G. H., Shaffer, J. W., et al.: Postoperative neurological deficits in segmental spinal instrumentation. A study using spinal cord monitoring. J. Bone Joint Surg. 66A:1178–1187, 1984.
111. Winter, R. B.: Combined Dwyer and Harrington instrumentation and fusion in the treatment of selected patients with painful adult idiopathic scoliosis. Spine 3:135–141, 1978.
112. Winter, R. B., Lonstein, J. E., and Denis, F.: Pain patterns in adult scoliosis. Orthop. Clin. North Am. 19:339–345, 1988.
113. Zielke, K., Stunkat, R., and Beujean, F.: Ventrale derotations-spondylodese. Arch. Orthop. Unfallchir. 85:257–277, 1976.

22

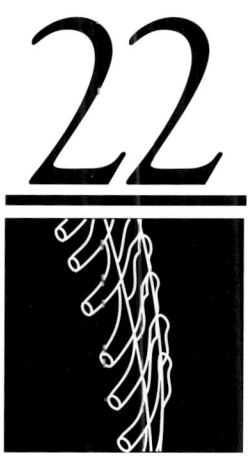

Spinal Instrumentation

Biomechanics of Transpedicle Spine Fixation

■

MARTIN KRAG

Extensive interest has developed in spinal instrumentation that uses transpedicle screws as the method of vertebral attachment. This interest has been stimulated by certain major advantages that this approach provides, although much remains to be learned concerning its limitations and the best methods for avoiding potential complications. Many of these issues are related to biomechanics. This discussion presents a history of the development of these devices as well as a review of transpedicle fixation, which is organized by biomechanical issues and which includes the current understanding as well as certain remaining questions.

DEVELOPMENT OF TRANSPEDICLE IMPLANTS

Attachment sites other than the pedicles were used for a number of decades for spinal implants. The spinous processes were the attachment sites for the upper and lower ends of pairs of tin-plated steel rods implanted by Lange[106, 107] in 1910 for treating "spondylitis." The plates first used by Wilson and Straub[191] in 1943, and by Williams[190] in 1956, were bolted together on each side of four or five spinous processes for stabilization after injury or lumbosacral degeneration. A similar approach was used by Reimers[146] and Sicard and Menegaux.[163] A wire loop passed around adjacent spinous processes for thoracolumbar fracture-dislocations was described by Stanger.[166]

At about this same time, the facet joints were used as attachment sites for metal screws placed across the joints for partial immobilization of the lower lumbar and lumbosacral spine. In the early 1940s, apparently independently, both Toumey[176] and King[81, 82] described the same method almost simultaneously, which was then also used by others.[14, 139, 175] A fairly high pseudarthrosis rate with this method led Boucher[21] to redirect the screws more medially so that they still went across the facet joint but continued into the pedicle, rather than exiting the lateral cortex of the superior articular process. Other researchers[4, 139] reported their experience with this method. Yet another method, described by Magerl[123, 124] and also used by Jacobs and colleagues,[75] was to increase the angulation of the screw in the opposite direction so that it was oriented more laterally: the screw enters at the base of the spinous process on the contralateral side, passes through the ipsilateral lamina, crosses the facet joint, and exits the lateral cortex of the superior articular process. This probably gave a stronger grip on the inferior articular process, which appears to be the weak link in the other facet screw methods. Casey and Jacobs[28] showed that this method provides stiffness in the lumbosacral region comparable with that provided by Luque rods (see below).

A different line of development was based on attachment of implants to the laminae. Harrington distraction rods were described in 1962.[65] The choice of hook attachment site was based upon strength testing of various possible attachment sites. This implant was designed for realignment of scoliosis but was also used for spondylolisthesis[67, 68] and for trauma[6] and other causes of instability.[66] The history of this device has been described elsewhere.[68, 69]

As experience with Harrington rods grew, problems with their use were identified.[60] The range of their usefulness was explored, and clinical problems that posed greater biomechanical demands were treated. A number of refinements and modifications resulted:

1. The hook shape was modified.[45, 56]
2. Two or more upper hooks on each rod were used.[20, 133]
3. An enclosed two-part hook was developed.[75, 76]
4. The ratchets on the rod were replaced by threads[75, 76, 177, 192] or eliminated altogether.[179]
5. The lower rod end was made square to prevent rotation of the rod after it was bent into lordosis.[34, 130]
6. A plastic spacer between the lamina and the central portion of the rod was used to allow increased lordosis without bending the rod.[44, 50]
7. Wires passed through the bases of the spinous processes spanned by the rods were used to increase the number of attachment sites of the implant.[42, 43, 170]
8. The length of the rods was increased to the third vertebra above and third vertebra below with either no graft[47] or a short graft,[27, 74, 76] which caused some concern regarding the spanned but ungrafted facet joints.[78, 79]

In conjunction with the Harrington distraction rods, compression rods were also developed.[65] These, too, have been subsequently modified[80] and mechanically tested (e.g., by Laborde and colleagues[105]). These rods were initially intended to be used in combination with distraction rods for realignment of scoliotic spines, but have also been used in combination for stabilization of traumatized spines.[159]

Other devices have been attached to the laminae by means of hooks. Beginning in 1961, Knodt and Larrick[87] used a threaded rod to produce distraction between a pair of hooks. Attenborough and Reynolds[13] stretched a spring between a pair of hooks to achieve compression and extension. Weiss,[186] apparently independently of Attenborough and Reynolds and extending the work of Gruca,[62] devised a similar system.

Another method of attachment to the laminae was described by Luque.[118, 119] Wires were passed around the laminae and tied to a longitudinal smooth L-shaped rod dorsal to the laminae. The major features of this method were that (1) it allowed multiple vertebrae to be attached to the implant (previously described by Resina and Alves,[147] based on their experience with a similar system used since 1963), and (2) it allowed long segment deformities such as scoliosis and kyphosis to be corrected gradually by transverse rather than longitudinal forces.

One variation of this method is to join the two L rods into a solid rectangle.[22, 40] Another variation is to replace the wires with synthetic fabric (Mersilene) tapes, which are much more flexible and thus safer to pass around the laminae.[61] Yet another approach has been to use the circumlaminar wires with Harrington distraction rods instead of L rods.[3, 24, 41, 57, 150] Various techniques for wire closure have been described and mechanically tested.[183] Comparisons between wires placed around the lamina and those placed through the spinous processes have also been performed.[184, 187] The risk that wire passage around or removal from the lamina may cause neural damage is significant,[41] particularly when the wires are used with Harrington distraction rods[41] or compression rods,[150] although other investigators have not emphasized this.[3, 24] Mersilene tapes may be significantly safer in this regard.[61]

Use of the pedicle specifically as an attachment site for spinal implants to the vertebra has a history of more than 25 years. In 1969, Harrington and Tullos[67] described two patients with L5 spondylolisthesis, operated on in 1967, in whom lag screws were placed through each of the pedicles and into the body of L5 and then wired to Harrington distraction rods to produce and maintain a partial reduction (Fig. 1A, B). Because these investigators believed that this method was not particularly helpful for this problem,[69] they stopped using it. Since 1970, however, Roy-Camille and coworkers,[151, 152] under the initial guidance of Judet (according to Louis[117]), reported an extensive positive experience using transpedicle screws (which apparently they began using in 1963) to attach specially designed posterior plates for spine stabilization in various conditions. Other researchers have described their experience with this implant system as well.[19, 32, 71, 83] The extensive and pioneering work by Roy-Camille appears to have been directly or indirectly the origin for most of the current transpedicle fixation systems.

Plates and screws were thus the first really successful transpedicle screw–based spinal implants, and a family of such implants has developed. Louis, drawing on his experience with the Roy-Camille system, modified the design.[115–117] Since at least 1979, use of tibial dynamic compression plates (AO-DCP) has been described[132, 173] for posterior spinal fixation; the use of a somewhat different AO plate (notched plate) has also been described.[19, 35] Steffee also made modifications of "standard AO neutralization plates,"[167–169] so that the screw could be adjusted along the plate and could be clamped perpendicularly to it by means of

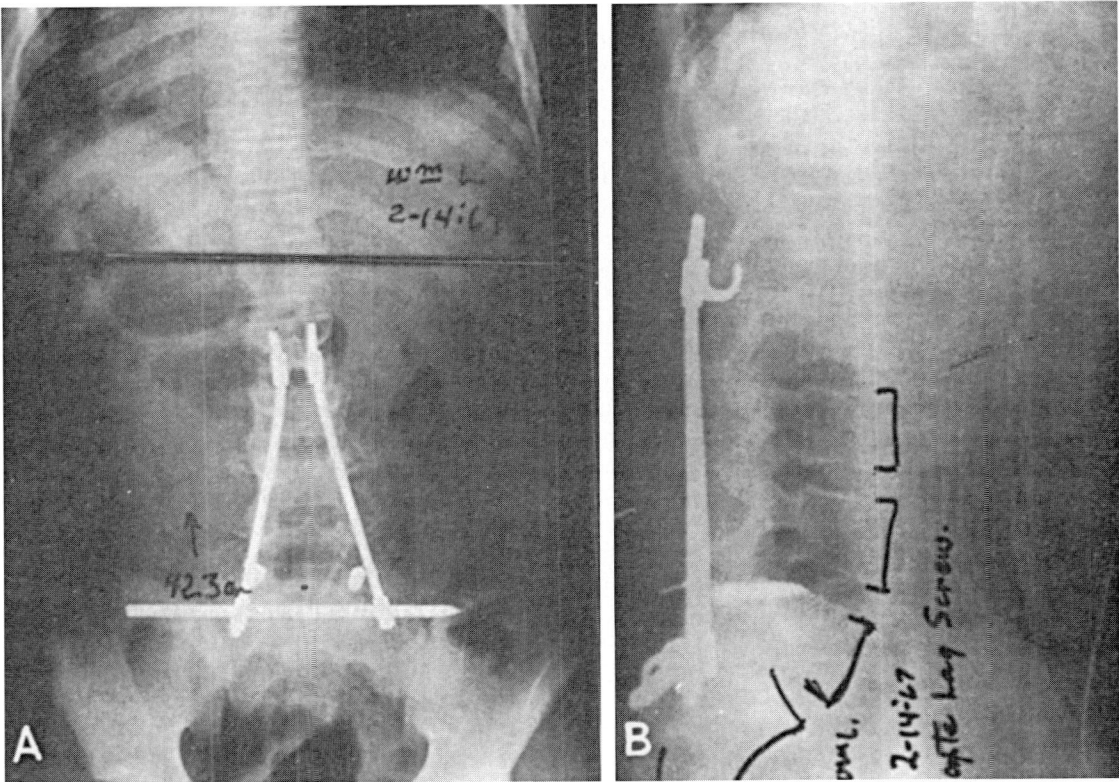

Figure 1. The earliest report (1969) of the use of transpedicle screws for attachment to a vertebra by Harrington and Tullos.[67] A, An (AP) x-ray film shows transpedicle screws in L5 medial to the rods. B, A lateral x-ray film shows screws into the L5 vertebra, attached by wires to Harrington distraction rods from L1 above to a sacral bar below. (From Harrington, P. R., and Tullos, H. S.: Reduction of severe spondylolisthesis in children. Reprinted by permission from Southern Medical Journal 62:1–7, 1969, Figure 5).

nuts both anterior and posterior to the plate. Other workers have reported their experience with this method.[72, 73, 145, 188] The longitudinal adjustability of the screw along the plate introduced by Steffee has been further increased by Luque and Rapp.[121]

In another large family of transpedicle screw–based implants, rods are used as the longitudinal element. It may be useful to consider these in two subgroups: (1) those in which the screws provide supplemental fixation sites for rods that are also attached by either hooks or circumlaminar wires and (2) those in which the screws alone are used for rod attachment. In the first subgroup, a number of systems were devised specifically for obtaining and maintaining reduction of spondylolisthesis. Harrington and Tullos,[67] Sijbrandij,[164] Vercauteren and DeGroote,[179] and Zielke and Strempel[196] attached the transpedicle screw to a Harrington distraction rod between the upper and lower hooks. In contrast, placement of the screw above two attachment points to the sacrum was the approach used by Schöllner,[160] Edwards,[48] and Matthias and Heine.[126] Vidal and associates[180] described yet a different use for transpedicle screws: as an attachment point for the lower hook of a Harrington distraction rod to the sacrum. Other devices in this subgroup were not specifically designed for management of spondylolisthesis. Kostuik[89, 90] used a screw that attaches to a Harrington distraction rod in the same way as standard Harrington hooks. Although he used this for anterior stabilization, apparently it was originally intended for posterior stabilization in the presence of myelomeningocele, in which no lamina was available for hook attachment. Luque[120] described screws that were wired to Luque L-shaped rods, which was somewhat analogous to the early work of Harrington and Tullos.[67] Similarly, Mehdian and coworkers[127] wired Dwyer screws to a Luque rectangular frame. Edwards and Weigel[51] used compression rods to join a proximal hook to a sacral screw bilaterally for low lumbar nonunions. In 1988, Cotrel and coworkers[31] described a system in which various screws or hooks are attached along a knurled rod. Others, such as Birch and associates,[18] also reported their experience with this system.

In the second of the two subgroups of implants, screws alone are used for rod attachment. Because these systems are typically used with at least three screws on each side, in general either the rods must be bent to contact the screws[64, 138, 143, 144, 161, 165] or care must be taken to align the posterior ends of the screws collinearly.[161] On the basis of publication date and length of patient follow-up, two such systems, both of which use threaded rods, have apparently been used since the early 1980s: the Zielke system[144, 165] and the Balgrist system,[161] the latter inspired by experience with Roy-Camille and Louis plates. Since 1985, the Wilste system has been used and a fairly extensive experience has been acquired.[64, 138, 174] In 1987, Puno and colleagues[143] presented mechanical testing of a newer system.

A third family of transpedicle screw–based implants is the fixators, the two major characteristics of which are (1) three-dimensional positional adjustability between the screw and the longitudinal linking component without bending of either one, and (2) three-dimensional positional control of each screw (and thus of each vertebra). Two subgroups of this family have developed: external fixators and internal fixators. For the former, Magerl[123, 124] certainly was the pioneer. He apparently combined the idea of transpedicle screw attachment popularized by Roy-Camille and the idea of external fixation for limb fractures, the use of which had been evolving for decades. Substantial experience with this spinal external fixator was acquired in Western Europe.[32, 86, 123, 124] Arnold,[7, 8] in Leipzig, developed one modification of this device, and Ölerud and coworkers,[135] in Uppsala, adapted a Hoffman fixation frame for temporary lumbosacral fixation as a diagnostic test for degenerative instability. A special mattress was used to accommodate the posteriorly protruding device. Also, pin track infections can develop as with any external fixator, and accidental penetration of the pins through the anterior vertebral cortex is possible. These disadvantages have inhibited widespread use of these devices.

Development of internal spinal fixators began almost simultaneously along two independent lines, both directly influenced by the work of Magerl. According to Dick,[35, 37] Magerl suggested such an internal fixator. Dick and coworkers subsequently designed the system in late 1982 and first used it in December 1983. The first report of its use appeared in Gorman in 1984,[35] and it first was reported in the English-language literature in 1985.[36] More extensive clinical experience has since been reported by Dick[37, 112] as well as by others.[1, 2, 32, 54, 172] Experience with this device was the basis for its modification by Kluger and Gerner[86] from West Germany in 1985, whose design has also been used by others.[19] Similarly, Olerud and colleagues from Uppsala described their modification, apparently in use since late 1985.[136]

The other separate line of internal fixator development was stimulated not only by Magerl but also by Roy-Camille. In 1981, the author met with Roy-Camille concerning his internal plate and screw system, and with Magerl and Schläpfer regarding their work on the external fixator. These visits helped to solidify ideas concerning how best to internalize an external fixator. Only after publications from the author's laboratory on this topic in 1985[91] was it learned through published reports, of the efforts of others (see above) who pursued the same basic goal. Because in 1981 even the basic morphometric issues needed further research, a program of implant design development, extensive biomechanical testing,[91, 92, 94, 95, 97, 99, 100] and anatomic studies[98] was begun that eventually led to the initial clinical implantation[96, 99, 101, 103, 104] of the Vermont spinal fixator in July of 1986.

It seems clear that further testing and design development in the area of transpedicle screw–based spinal implants will continue. Improved understanding of the various benefits, complications, and risks associated with such devices is needed, which in turn will help guide future design improvements. Because biomechanical issues play a central role in this development, some of these topics are reviewed below.

MORPHOMETRY

The limiting factor to the diameter of a transpedicule screw is the mediolateral width of the pedicle. Saillant[155] reported important cadaver data; however, these findings have certain limitations. First, only average values were given and not the ranges or standard deviations. Second, the reported length of the screw that could be implanted was for a purely sagittal placement; other screw placement angles may be preferable,* and their

use would usually have an influence on this length. Third, only the pedicle diameter perpendicular to the pedicle axis was reported; screws not oriented along the pedicle axis may encounter an effectively smaller diameter. Finally, no clinically usable radiographic confirmation of the caliper measurements from the cadaver specimens was provided.

For these reasons, a study was undertaken to provide the desired data,[92, 98] some of which is shown in Figure 2 and Table 1. Additional morphometric data subsequently have confirmed or extended this work. Zindrick and coworkers[199] measured pedicle widths not only T9 to L5, but also from T1 to T8, and included sagittal height and angulation of the pedicles. Berry and associates[17] studied T2, T7, T12, and L1 to L5. They included a number of other measurements relative to the vertebral body, spinous process, and spinal canal. Banta and colleagues[15] compared pedicle dimensions of cadaveric vertebrae obtained from AP and lateral x-ray films, as well as direct measurement with calipers. Although they concluded that lateral x-ray films are not helpful (pedicle height/width ratios are not constant), they unfortunately did not report the correlation between width measurements from AP x-ray films and those from calipers. Misenheimer and colleagues[129] confirmed the accuracy of CT scanning, showed that sequential insertion of probes of increasing diameter into the pedicle did not give an accurate assessment of pedicle endosteal diameter, and showed that pedicle cortical disruption did not occur if screw diameter was less than endosteal diameter or less than 80% of cortical diameter. Various aspects of sacral morphometry have been investigated. Screw path lengths of various sacral sites were described by Asher and Strippgen[11] and Dohring and Krag.[39] The relative locations of major neurovascular structures were reported by Dohring and Krag,[39] Esses and coworkers,[53] and Mirkovic and associates.[128] The anteromedial (promontory) path length is longer and thus presumably stronger than is the anterolateral (alar). Only small regions across which no major neurovascular structures pass ("safe zones") exist along the arcuate line.

TRANSPEDICLE SCREW DESIGN

Even though there is a fairly extensive literature characterizing the strength of vari-

---

*References 85, 86, 91, 92, 95–97, 99–101, 123, and 124.

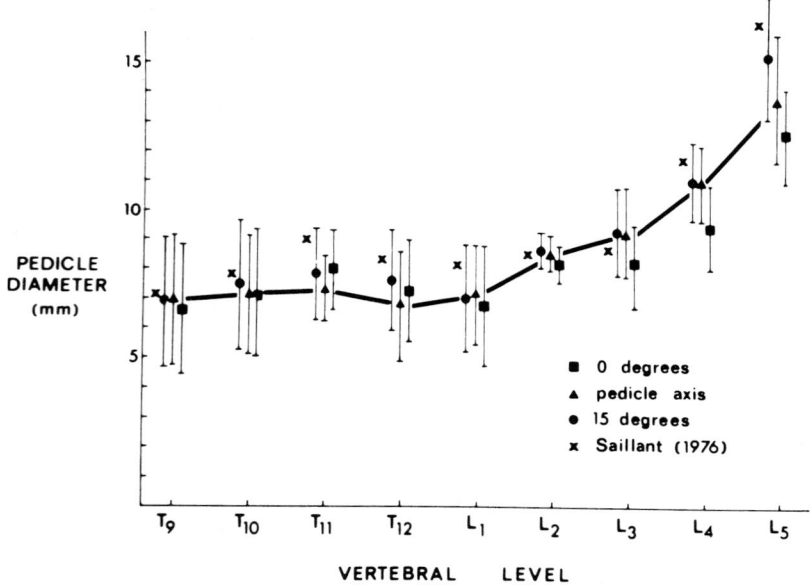

Figure 2. Mean pedicle diameters ± 1 SD for each vertebral level, measured from transverse plane computed tomographic (CT) images. Effective diameter was measured parallel to the frontal plane (0 degrees), perpendicular to the pedicle axis (pedicle axis), or in a plane 15 degrees anterolateral from the frontal plane (15 degree). The data means given by Saillant[155] are provided for comparison. (From Krag, M. H., Beynnon, B. D., Pope, M. H., et al.: An internal fixator for posterior application to short segments of the thoracic, lumbar, or lumbosacral spine: Design and testing. Clin. Orthop. 203:75–98, 1986.)

ous screws implanted into limb bones, only one study has been done that independently varied the different screw design features of tooth profile, pitch, and minor diameter.[33] Bechtol[16] compared pullout strength of screws from dog limb bones with screws in which eight different tooth profiles were done in a way that did not allow the effect of this variable to be isolated. Koranyi and colleagues,[88] in a study using dog or cattle femora, reported equal pullout strengths for both V-toothed Sherman screws and buttress-toothed AO screws. However, neither the major nor the minor diameters were specified, although tooth heights were the same. Diehl and coworkers[38] concluded that the pullout strengths of AO cortical and cancellous screws were approximately the same when these were inserted into epiphyseal or metaphyseal sites (i.e., those that were predominantly cancellous bone). Lyon and colleagues,[122] Nunamaker and Perren,[134] and Schatzker and coworkers[156] each studied various groups of different commercially

Table 1

Pedicle Diameter and Distribution by Size

Level	Mean	SD	Number	3–3.9 mm (%)	4–4.9 mm (%)	5–5.9 mm (%)	6–6.9 mm (%)	7–7.9 mm (%)	8–19.4 mm (%)
T9	6.88	2.23	14	14	7	14	21	7	35
T10	7.47	2.24	18	11		11	39		39
T11	7.83	1.56	22			14	18	14	55
T12	7.63	1.79	24			21	21	12	46
L1	7.01	1.84	22	9		18	18	14	41
L2	8.67	0.64	14					7	92
L3	9.30	1.51	24				8	12	79
L4	11.03	1.36	24						100
L5	15.15	1.97	20						100

available screws, but their study designs did not allow the individual effects of pitch, major diameter, and minor diameter to be segregated.

Martin and associates[125] focused attention on a feature of screw design other than just axial or pullout loads, namely flexural rigidity (i.e., bending stiffness). In the case of screws used to hold plates against tubular long bones, sufficient friction must be present to shield screws from such flexural loads. However, when loosening (e.g., screw backout and resorption of bone under the plate) occurs, such shielding may break down, leading to the failure of the screws, which were not designed to tolerate such loads.[30, 137, 140, 194] Shielding of screws from flexural loads may be especially difficult to maintain under plates applied to the spine posteriorly, because the surface is fairly irregular, even if the facet joints are partially removed. Herrman[71] emphasized the relationship between facet trimming and plate contact area. Failure to design screws to tolerate flexural loads may be the explanation behind the high rates of screw breakage or bending encountered with the use of various implant systems.[72, 151-153, 168, 188]

Studies specifically directed at transpedicle screws are few. Only one such study[92, 95] has systematically varied pitch, minor diameter, and tooth profile. In screw pullout strength tests, this showed that (1) the V-tooth and buttress-tooth profile were the same; (2) 2-mm-pitch screws were only somewhat (21%) stronger than 3-mm-pitch screws in only one of three subgroups tested; and (3) smaller minor diameter screws (3.8 mm) were only somewhat stronger (19%–26% depending on subgroup) than larger minor diameter screws (5 mm), but that this was offset by a reduction to less than half $[(3.8/5)^3 = 44\%]$ of the flexural rigidity of the 5-mm minor diameter screws.

Other issues concerning transpedicle screw design have also been studied. Liu and colleagues[113] showed experimentally that the above-described and predictable sensitivity of flexural rigidity to minor diameter was in fact present increasing the minor diameter of Steffee screws from 3 mm to 3.8 mm doubled the static and fatigue strength $[(93.8/3.0)^3 = 2.04]$. The author determined[94] the fatigue response of Vermont Spinal Fixator screws and showed that the limiting factor for fatigue life was not the clamps that joined the screw to the rod, but rather the first thread root Liu and coworkers[114] showed that implantation of nitrogen ions into the metal of 7-mm Steffee screws could improve fatigue life by 98% (significant, $p < .05$) at lower bending loads (3.96 N·m or 35 inch-pounds), although it only improved 20% (insignificant, $p < .01$) at higher bending loads (5.09 N·m or 45 inch-pounds). Geiger and coworkers[58] measured four-point bending fatigue strengths of a number of screw types subjected to various cyclic loads (haversine pattern, 2.9 – 10.8 N·m, lever arm of 28 mm, frequency of 4 Hz). The screws studied were Cotrel-Dubousset 5 mm, Ölerud 5 mm, Steffee 5.5 mm, AO modified 6.5 mm, Luque 6.5 mm, and Steffee 7 mm without and with integral nuts. Geiger and coworkers noted the importance of avoiding stress risers in screw design and the lack of correlation between major diameter and fatigue life. Unfortunately, the minor diameters of the screws tested were not specified: this measure may correlate fairly well with fatigue life. It has also been emphasized[72] that bending the screws may significantly decrease screw fatigue life and thus should clearly be avoided during either reduction maneuvers or during attachment between the screw and the longitudinal linking device (plate or rod). It seems clear that further work in the area of transpedicle screw design remains to be done.

TRANSPEDICLE SCREW PLACEMENT

The basic principles involved in optimum screw placement include (1) the strength of the resulting bone-metal interface, (2) the avoidance of damage to neurologic structures by screw penetration through pedicle cortex or vertebral body cortex, (3) the avoidance of damage to the adjacent facet joint, and (4) the ease and convenience of implantation. Various aspects of screw implantation are considered with these four principles in mind.

Entry Site and Orientation

Because the desired orientation affects the entry site, these are considered together. Two different approaches have been advocated. Roy-Camille and coworkers[151, 152] adopted the motto of "straight ahead," based on their recommendation (followed by others[111, 117, 136, 167, 168]) that transpedicle screws be placed parallel to the sagittal plane as well as to the vertebral end plates. The resulting entry point (Fig. 3A) is at the intersection between a transverse line bisecting the transverse process and a longitudinal line bisecting the facet joint. In contrast, Magerl[123, 124] and later other clinicians* used an "inward," or anteromedial, approach. For this, the longitudinal guideline for the entry site (Fig. 3B) is along the lateral aspect of the superior articular process rather than through the facet joint. Through this entry site the screw is oriented along the pedicle axis, obliquely to the sagittal plane, but parallel to the end plate.

An even further departure from the straight-ahead approach that the author has found useful may be described as "up and in" (Fig. 3C). The entry site is as far lateral as in the Magerl approach, but is also somewhat lower, along a transverse line between the upper two thirds and lower one third of the transverse process. The orientation is still medially angulated along the pedicle axis, but it is also inclined somewhat cephalad, although not so far as to intersect the superior end plate. This up and in approach allows the dorsally protruding screw head to remain down and out, relative to the superjacent facet joint (also mentioned by Levine and Edwards[111]). This in turn has at least three implications. First, there is less interference with the superjacent facet joint,[96] which may be a more important factor than implant stiffness in causing the accelerated degeneration of the superjacent motion segment that has been reported.[73] Second, a screw placed along the oblique path can be

---

*References 1, 2, 35–37, 92, 97, 104, and 185.

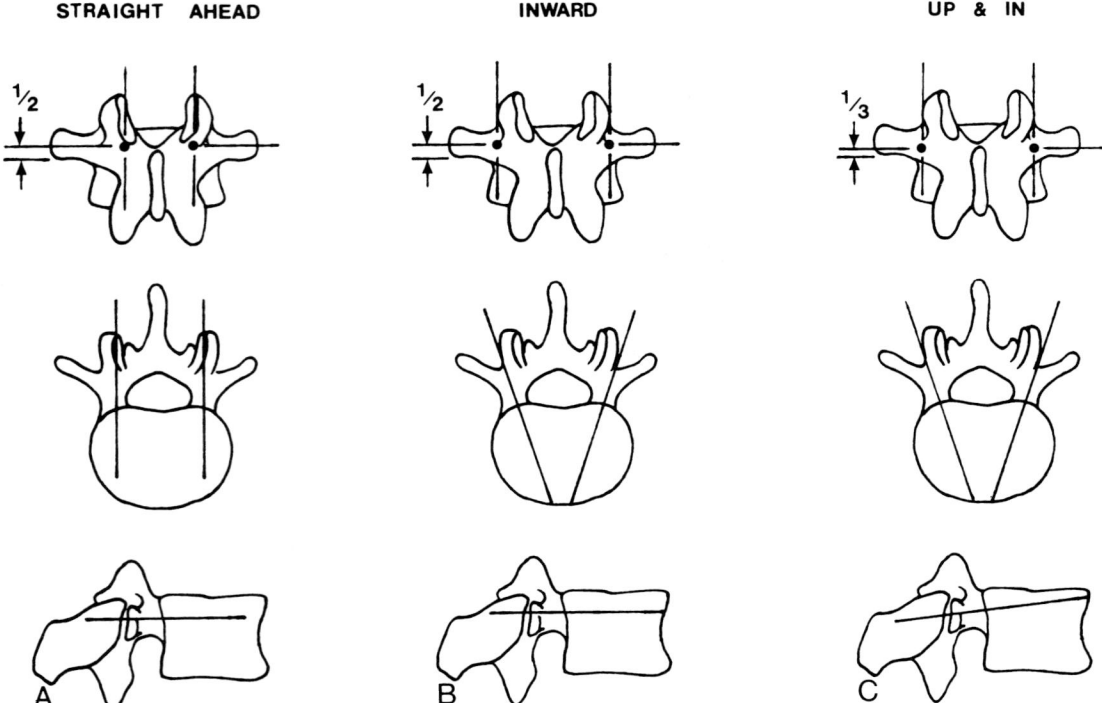

Figure 3. Entry point and orientation alternatives for transpedicle screws. *A*, Straight ahead. The entry point is the intersection of a line that bisects the transverse process and a line that bisects the facet joint. Orientation is parallel to the sagittal plane and parallel to the end plates. *B*, Inward. The entry point is more lateral and the orientation is anteromedial along the pedicle axis. The longitudinal line is along the lateral aspect of the facet joint (superior articular process). *C*, Up and in. The entry point is more lateral (as in *B*) and is also lower (caudad). The transverse line divides the upper two thirds and lower one third of the transverse process. The orientation is still anteromedial, but also anterocephalad (up and in), although not enough to intersect the superior end plate.

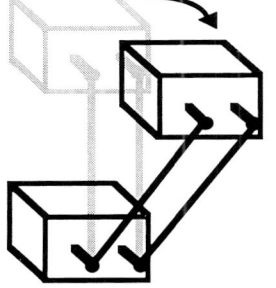
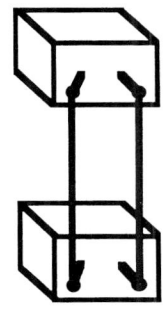

Figure 4. Orienting the screws straight ahead causes the screws to be parallel, and thus lateral shifting meets with little resistance (friction between screw and bone). Orientating the screws up and in causes an interlocking, or toenailing, effect that resists this lateral shifting.

longer than one placed along the straight-ahead path,[98, 199] without anterior cortex penetration, thereby increasing the bone-metal interface strength.[97, 109] Third, the extent to which the vertebral body can function as a cross-bridge is substantially increased (the exact extent is presently under investigation), both to resist anteroposterior forces[102] and lateral "pushover" (Fig. 4).

Placement of screws into the sacrum poses a particular problem because of the unique anatomy in this region and the somewhat greater difficulty of intraoperative visualization of structures, even radiographically. Perhaps for these reasons, a variety of recommendations has been given for screw entry site and orientation (Table 2).

Data to help select among these recommendations are limited. Asher and Strippgen[11] measured the path lengths of various screw placements in the sacrum. The length anteromedially to the sacral promontory was 47 and 50 mm in women and men, respectively, whereas the length anterolaterally into the S1 ala was 37 and 39 mm, respectively. Using these lengths as a basis, these investigators conjectured that the stronger screw would be the one directed anteromedially into the promontory. However, no measurements of strength were made to confirm this. Zindrick and colleagues[198] performed strength measurements

Table 2

Methods for Sacral Screw Placement

Author	Level	Entry Site	Transverse Plane Angle*	Sagittal Plane Angle†	Depth
Cotrel et al.[31]	S1	Midpoint between L5–S1 facet and S1 foramen	30 degrees lat	?	?
Edwards et al.[46]	S1	Base of L5–S1	From inferodorsal corner of L5 spinous process to entry site		Through anterior cortex
Guyer et al.[64]	S1	Caudal and just lateral to S1 superior articular process	25 degrees med	?	To anterior cortex
Krag[96]	S1	Center of S1 pedicle seen by x-ray film oriented along S1 pedicular axis	Toward midline (from preoperative CT)	Toward promontory	To anterior cortex
Louis[117]	S1	Lateral to L5–S1 facet and S1 foramen	35–45 degrees lat	35–45 degrees caud	?
Magerl[123]	S1	Intersection of lines along lateral and inferior edges of S1 superior articular process	15–20 degrees med	Toward promontory	To anterior cortex
Roy-Camille et al[152]	S1	?	30 degrees lat	?	?
Steffee et al.[167]	S1	Just below S1 superior articular process	0 degree	0 degree	To anterior cortex
Guyer et al.[64]	S2	Midway between 1st and 2nd dorsal foramina	40–50 degrees lat	10–15 degrees ceph	?
Steffee et al.[167]	S2	?	45 degrees lat	?	?

*Lat, anterolateral; med, anteromedial.
†Ceph, anterocephalad; caud, anterocaudal.

using 6.5-mm screws placed into various sites in the sacrum. Unfortunately, they noted a high interspecimen variation and yet did not do right-left comparisons of different screw sites within the same specimen. Thus, it is not clear whether the mean differences observed between screw sites were significantly different or not. Also, the type of load used was pullout of the screw along its own axis, yet this does not appear to be an important failure mode clinically. Dohring and Krag[39] (also reported elsewhere[102]) compared the strength of an anteromedially directed screw in one S1 pedicle with the strength of an anterolaterally directed screw in the opposite S1 pedicle of the same specimen. A flexion load was used rather than pullout along the screw axis, because the former is believed to be more clinically relevant. Torque for 0.1-degree deflection was the same for both orientations, but for 1.0-degree deflection, the anteromedial orientation was significantly stiffer (15 N·m versus 6 N·m; $p < .01$).

A final issue concerning screw entry and orientation is that of monitoring this process to ensure safe and accurate placement of screws through the pedicles. The most direct approach is to remove the posterior elements completely, down to the pedicles, so that the process of screw placement into the pedicle is continuously visible.[72, 120, 168] A smaller amount of resection still allows direct palpation of the borders of the pedicle with a curved probe, which enables semidirect visualization; various guides for assisting this process have been described.[72] Yet another approach, without bone resection, is to use posterior anatomic landmarks to guide an initial insertion of a drill bit, an awl, or a guide wire, and then to obtain an x-ray film to identify proper (or improper) placement. Even in experienced hands, however, this method has been reported to yield miss rates (screw out of pedicle) that are disturbingly high. Saillant[155] in 1976 reported a 10% miss rate and Roy-Camille[153] in 1987 reported a 13.5% rate, although elsewhere Roy-Camille and colleagues[152] described the rate in their experience with trauma as "near to nil." Robbins and Gertzbein[148] described the use of image intensification to guide screw replacement (but did not describe which x-ray views were used), and they reported a miss rate of 28.8%. Even though a miss may not cause neurologic deficit, it probably does affect the screw-vertebra interface strength.

An alternative to using surface landmarks alone is to use x-ray films to locate and orient the drill bit (or guidewire) accurately even before insertion is accomplished. For this, however, the choice of x-ray technique may be important. Using AP and lateral views alone, Weinstein and colleagues[185] showed a miss rate of approximately 21% for screws implanted into cadaveric spine specimens. However, other x-ray views are also possible.[96] If the central x-ray beam is positioned obliquely to pass along the axis of the pedicle (the orientation of which is readily available either accurately from preoperative CT scans or approximately from morphometric data[17, 92, 98, 155, 199]), the pedicle cortex can be clearly seen as an oval. The drill bit tip can then be positioned in the middle of this oval. Next, the drill bit shaft (with no driver attached) is rotated up to an orientation parallel to the x-ray central beam: the drill bit then appears as a spot in the center of the pedicle (bull's-eye, or pedicle coaxial, x-ray view) as shown in Figure 5. The image intensifier can then be rotated aside and the driver (power or manual)

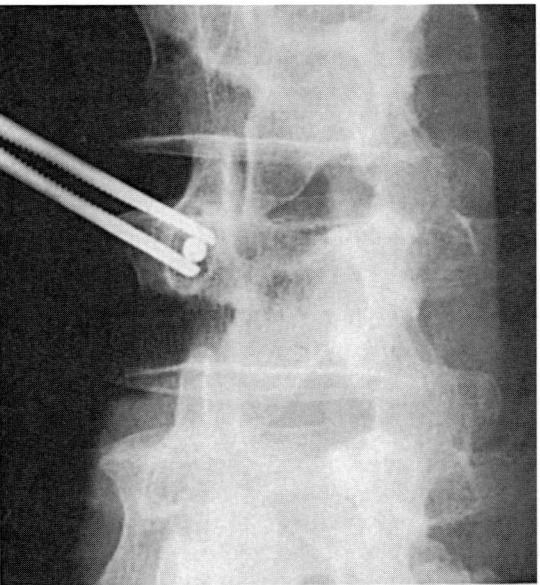

Figure 5. Coaxial, or bull's-eye, x-ray view. Oblique view of L3 vertebra with central beam along left pedicle axis. The drill bit is seen end on as a spot, centered within the oval cortex of the pedicle, adjacent to the left L2–L3 facet joint. The drill bit is held by the jaws of a Kocher clamp.

attached to the drill bit, which is then advanced to the desired depth. The author has used this method since 1986 and routinely probes all four quandrants of the drill hole before screw placement to establish cortical intactness. In 53 patients (212 screws), there have been two pedicles with cortical disruption (one of which was deliberate: a 6-mm screw in a 6-mm-diameter pedicle). Although these results have obviously not been confirmed by transecting the pedicles (as in a cadaver study), postoperative CT scans have been obtained on many of these patients. The probe and CT scan results have established that the miss rate can be low when this specific x-ray view is used instead of the more traditional AP and lateral views.

Depth of Penetration

The optimum depth of screw penetration through the pedicle and into the vertebral body is not yet well established. A variety of clinically based opinions have been reported. Roy-Camille,[152] for example, described it as "dangerous and pointless" to insert the screw so deeply that it contacts the anterior cortex of the vertebral body. In contrast, Magerl[123, 124] and Dick[37] recommended placement of the screw tip close to the anterior cortex.

Although the relationship between strength and screw penetration depth has been well established for tubular bones,[5, 16, 88, 178] few studies have been done for transpedicle screws. Lavaste[108, 109] measured pullout strength of various commercially available screws and concluded that depth of penetration was not an important determinant of strength. However, his analysis failed to take advantage of the right-to-left comparisons that were possible with his data, and thus his conclusions were heavily influenced by interspecimen variability, which he emphasized was large. A reanalysis of his data,[97] based upon his 10 specimens that allowed right-to-left comparison, led to a conclusion the opposite of that which he drew: that an increase in depth of only 5 mm produced a significant ($p < .05$) increase in pullout strength.

Zindrick and coworkers[198] conducted both pullout and cyclic transverse displacement testing. In pullout tests, the "through anterior cortex" group had a mean strength of 220% for the 4.5-mm cortical screw, and 130% for the 6.5-mm cancellous screw, compared with that in the "to anterior cortex" group. In contrast, there was no significant difference between the mean strengths of the to anterior cortex group and the 50% depth group. Whether younger specimens (the mean age was 74.5 years in that study) or a different analysis (e.g., matched-pairs t-test) would have altered the results is not clear. For the cyclic transverse displacements, both the through cortex versus to cortex and the to cortex versus 50% depth comparisons showed the deeper screws to be significantly stronger. The clinical significance of this test mode, however, is not clear, as is discussed in more detail elsewhere.[97]

The author compared the peak strength of screws at 50% versus 80% depth of penetration and 80% versus 100% depth of penetration, using a right-left comparison within each vertebral specimen.[97] Each pair of screws was exposed to a load mimicking vertebral flexion or axial rotation. Matched-pairs t-testing was used and showed that strength varied approximately linearly with penetration depth (Fig. 6) for both load types. The strength of screws at 50% depth was 75% to 77% (depending on load type) that of screws at 80% depth. Strength for screws at 100% (to cortex) depth was 124% to 154% that of screws at 80% depth.

Thus, on the basis of at least the reanalysis[97] of Lavaste's data[108] and the author's work, it can be concluded that deeper screw insertion provides increased screw-vertebra interface strength. Of course this also increases the risk of anterior vertebral cortex penetration. The optimum balancing between these two features must take into account the skill and experience of the surgeon, the availability of an adequate x-ray visualization source, the anticipated postoperative loading, and other factors as well.

Particularly with the deeper screw penetration, monitoring of the depth by one or more methods is desirable to avoid breaking through the anterior cortex. One method is based on the increased resistance to further drill bit or screw advancement that can sometimes be felt when the cortex is reached. Another method[100] is to insert the drill bit or probe almost to the anterior cortex and then to tap lightly on it with a mallet; a distinct change in sound (rise in pitch)

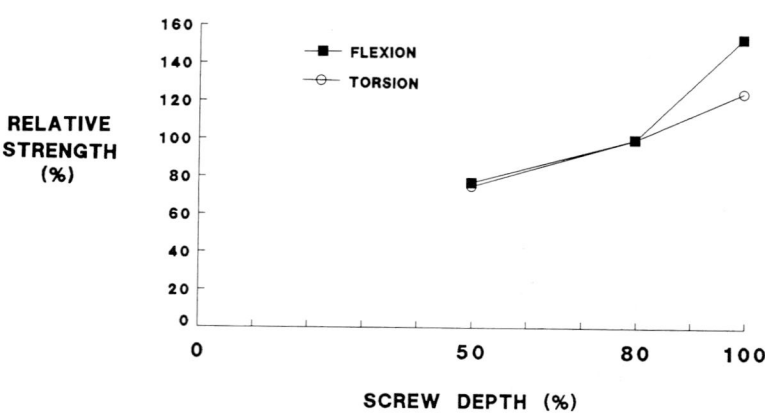

Figure 6. Mean strength of screws at 100% and 50% depth of penetration relative to the mean strength of screws at 80% depth. A screw was implanted in each vertebra either at 80% and 50% depth, or at 80% and 100% depth. Relative strength is plotted against percentage of depth of penetration, both for flexion and for torsion loads. (From Krag, M. H., Beynnon, B. D., DeCoster, T. A., and Pope, M. H.: Depth of insertion of transpedicular vertebral screws into human vertebrae: Effect upon screw-vertebra interface strength. J. Spinal Disord. 1:287–294, 1988.)

and increased vibration in the instrument shaft may be detected when the tip of the instrument contacts the anterior cortex. In osteopenic bone, however, caution must be used; neither method may be dependable.

A third method is to use x-ray films to provide a direct assessment of the distance between screw tip and anterior cortex. However, the choice of x-ray view is important in avoiding a misleading appearance. This same problem can occur during internal fixation of the hip[23, 110, 149, 162, 181, 182] and knee[52] and has been described in more detail elsewhere[100] for transpedicle screw placement. The lateral view may be inaccurate, as has been suggested by some investigators[111, 123, 136] and shown clearly by Whitecloud and colleagues.[189] The latter noted that, of those screws that appeared on lateral x-ray films to have an apparent depth of penetration of 80%, in fact 30% of those at L4 and 10% at L5 had actually perforated the anterior vertebral body cortex. As shown in Figure 7, if the screw tip is contacting the anterior cortex at a location away from the midline, the lateral view gives a false reading: the apparent distance from screw tip to cortex is greater than the actual distance, because the screw tip is over the horizon. When the beam is tangential to that point on the anterior cortex at which the screw would penetrate, the distance from screw tip to cortex is at a minimum (near-approach view).

Hole Preparation Method

There are four phases of hole preparation. The first phase is to break through the posterior cortex overlying the pedicle. Tools for accomplishing this vary from drill bit to rongeur to air-driven dental bur. The second phase is to deepen the hole past the narrow waist, or middle portion, of the pedicle. This can be done by drill bit,[96, 97, 123, 124, 151, 152] curet,[49, 109] curved probe,[64, 167] or straight probe or guidewire.[136] The third phase is to complete the hole to the maximum desired depth. Here, the options are drill, curved probe, or straight probe. The fourth phase is to use a tap for cutting threads in bone, if desired.

Various methods for accomplishing these four phases of hole preparation have been recommended and are summarized in Table 3. Although each method should be assessed for safety, ease or speed of insertion, and the effect on screw-vertebra interface strength, few of these variables have actually been studied. Concerning the issue of tapping, no data from vertebral testing appear to be available. Although Zindrick and colleagues[197] mentioned that they studied this matter, little difference overall was seen; there was no benefit in osteopenic bone, and a decrease in strength was noted in some specimens. For sites other than the spine, Nunamaker and Perren[134] showed that, in bovine cancellous limb bone, tapping added no strength, and Koranyi and coworkers[88] and Vangsness and associates[178] showed similar results for screws placed across the femoral diaphysis. Thus, there appear to be no data in support of tapping to increase screw strength and some data against it. On the subject of probe versus drill bit, on a small number of specimens the use of a drill bit versus a straight 2-mm cylindric probe (with blunt conical tip) produced no sig-

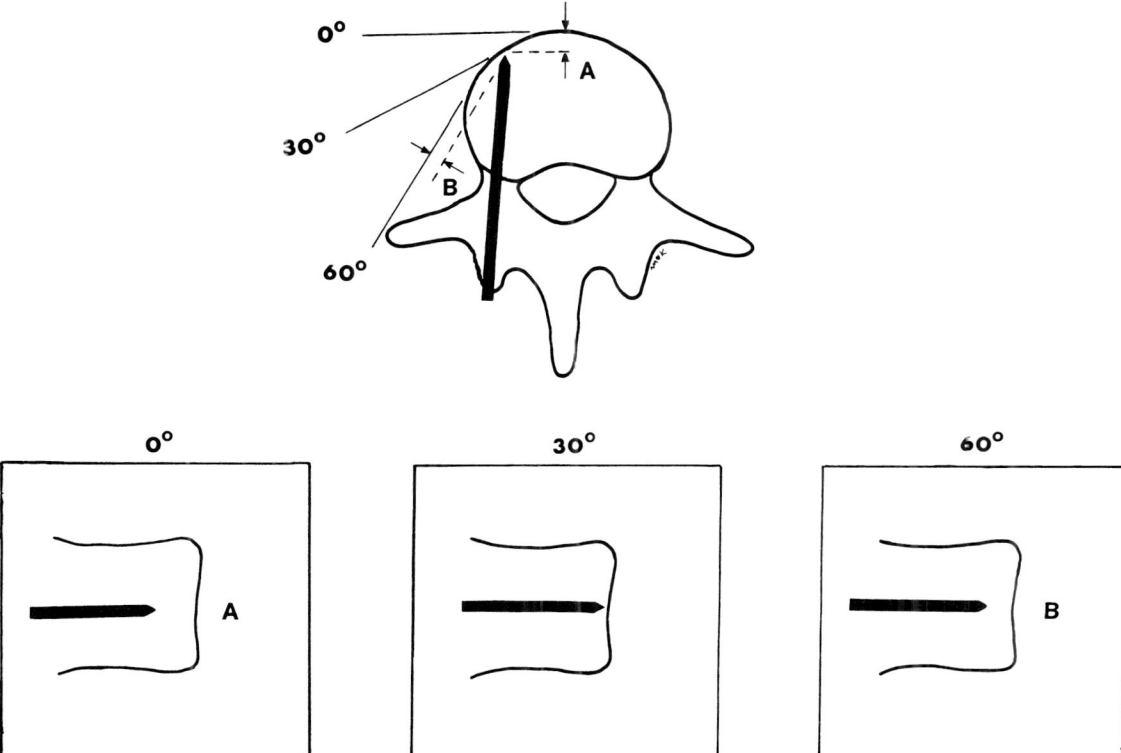

Figure 7. Near-approach x-ray view to decrease likelihood of anterior penetration. When the drill (or screw or probe) tip is actually at the anterior cortex, the lateral view (0 degree) misleadingly shows the tip to still be some distance away from the cortex (A). At too oblique an angle of view (60 degrees), the tip again misleadingly appears to be some distance away from the cortex (B). Only when the view is tangential to the point of penetration (30 degrees in this case) does the tip appear most nearly to approach actual breakthrough.

nificant difference for transpedicle screw pullout.[59] In choosing between these two methods, not only these laboratory results, but also the important issues of safety, dependability of the method, and speed should be considered. Regarding pilot hole depth, no specific data are available for vertebrae, but the work of Lyon and coworkers[122] (with limited data) suggested that this may be an important issue for screw strength in human femora. For pilot hole diameter as well, there has been no specific testing on vertebrae. Banta and colleagues[15] raised the concern that use of a hole that is too small may lead to pedicle blowout during screw insertion. This may bear on the choice between probe and drill to form the pilot hole: the former compacts bone, whereas the latter removes it. Whether this significantly affects the blowout tendency remains to be established.

Insertion of the screw after hole preparation is complete requires proper orientation of the screw with the central axis of the hole. Because the cortical bone is thin, because the cancellous bone does not provide substantial resistance to screw malalignment, and because the deep end of the hole is not visible for use as a guide, the screw does not necessarily follow the hole. A useful technique is to insert a short Kirschner wire into an adjacent bony prominence (e.g., spinous process and posterior ilium), approximately parallel to the drill bit or probe. This provides a visual guide for correct screw orientation, even after the drill bit or probe is removed.

Polymethyl Methacrylate Augmentation

Questions remain about whether the screw-vertebra interface should be prophylactically strengthened by the insertion of polymethyl methacrylate (PMMA) into the

Table 3

Pilot Hole Preparation Techniques for Transpedicle Screws

Author	Method
Dick[37]	1. 2-mm Kirschner wire into body (approximately 3-cm deep) 2. 3.5-mm drill 5–10 mm deep 3. Screw under x-ray study control
Edwards[49]	1. Develop hole with 3–0 curet 2. Replace with guidewire; x-ray study control 3. Screw
Guyer et al.[64]	1. Awl 2. Pedicle probe through pedicle 3. Blunt Kirschner wire driven in under x-ray study control 4. Kirschner wire removed; tap threads to 2 cm 5. Screw
Krag[96]	1. Bur to enter cortex, centered on pedicle by x-ray film coaxial view 2. Drill along pedicle axis to anterior cortex; monitor by x-ray film near-approach view 3. Screw; orient with nearby guidewire; depth by x-ray film near-approach view
Louis[117]	1. 2.8-mm drill (depth?) 2. Screw
Luque and Rapp[121]	1. Enter pedicle (use drill?) 2. Curet through pedicle 3. Drill in blunt Kirschner wire to anterior cortex 4. Cannulated tap over Kirschner wire 5. Cannulated screw over Kirschner wire
Magerl[124]	1. 3.5-mm drill approximately 4-cm deep 2. Replace with Kirschner wire; x-ray control 3. Screw to anterior cortex; monitor with x-ray studies
Ölerud et al.[136]	1. Kirschner wire and x-ray film to define entry site 2. Drill through cortex 3. Screw to anterior cortex; monitor with lateral view
Roy-Camille et al[152]	1. Awl to locate entry 2. 3.2-mm drill 3. Screw
Steffee et al.[167]	1. Awl or probe through pedicle 2. Tap through pedicle 3. Screw

pilot hole before screw insertion into osteopenic bone and whether, if a screw becomes loose intraoperatively, PMMA should be inserted or the screw should be redirected or moved to another site. Few data relevant to these questions have been reported. Kleeman and coworkers[84] tested human calcanei and tibiae into which screws were inserted in the usual fashion, pulled out using an Instron materials testing machine, reinserted after the holes had been manually filled with PMMA, and then again pulled out after the PMMA had set. The pullout force for reinforced screws was 226% of the initial pullout force. Zindrick and colleagues[198] performed similar testing on human cadaveric vertebrae with transpedicle screws and also tested the effect of PMMA pressurization before screw reinsertion. They showed that PMMA placement without pressurization provided a screw strength approximately equal to normal values (with the contralateral pedicle used as a control), whereas PMMA placed under pressure provided a strength approximately twice normal values. The authors cautioned, however, against the possibility of nerve root or cord damage from PMMA extrusion through any cortical defects that may be present, especially when pressurization is used. Pfeifer and colleagues[141] showed after deliberate screw pullout that pullout strength could be reconstituted (relative to initial stripout of the pedicle) to 149% of original strength with PMMA.

The difficulty of PMMA removal (e.g., for débridement of infection) is a sobering counterbalance to the fairly large gain in strength achieved in this fashion. Perhaps placement of the screws all the way to, or even slightly through, the anterior cortex would be a better option. The above study by Pfeifer and colleagues[141] showed reconstitution using morcellized bone graft to produce a strength that was 70% of the initial value. How best to deal with screw stripout remains to be established. Avoidance of stripout by measurement of screw insertion torque has been investigated by a number of researchers,[25, 29, 142, 193, 195] as discussed in Complications of Transpedicle Spine Fixation by Hsu and colleagues.

LONGITUDINAL LINKAGE BETWEEN SCREWS

Transpedicle screw–based fixation devices are still under active development and will likely undergo further changes. Other than the screw itself, the linkage between the screw and the longitudinal component (rod or plate) is the most varied design feature in current devices and it will probably continue to be a focus of future improvement. Thus, certain general aspects of this linkage may be worth considering.

Positional Adjustability

The choice of screw entry sites and orientations in the pedicle is fairly limited, and screw bending causes a significant loss of fatigue life.[131] Thus, alignment of the screw to the plate or rod requires either bending of the plate or rod or some sort of adjustable linkage. A wide variety of methods have been used. For plates with individual, separate, circular holes,* any mediolateral and cephalocaudad angulation of the screw is allowed, but longitudinal translation is stepwise adjustable in fairly coarse intervals, for example, 13-mm increments with Roy-Camille plates.[152] Mediolateral translation is adjustable only by bending of the plate in the coronal plane if there are two other screws already fixing the plate in position. Finer stepwise adjustability of longitudinal translation (a few millimeters) is provided by the Steffee[167] and Luque[121] plates, and Edwards rods.[45] These plates use longitudinal slots instead of circular holes, and have scalloped edges (or "screw nests") to provide some mechanical interlocking between the screw head and the plate. The Edwards rods are ratcheted for stepwise adjustment. In the case of the Steffee system, the continuous adjustability of angulation between the screw and the plate is restricted by the use of a nut on each side of the plate to lock these two components together. If the screw is not positioned in the vertebra to be perpendicular to the adjacent segment of the plate, tightening of the lock nut tends to bend the screw shaft (thereby weakening it) or loosen the screw in the vertebra.[72] A 5-degree wedge-shaped washer provides an alternative angular position for the screw.

The Balgrist,[161] Cotrel-Dubousset,[31] Edwards,[45] Puno,[143] Wiltse,[64] and Zielke[144] systems all require a perpendicular orientation between the screw and the longitudinal linking component. However, because these systems use a rod instead of a plate, two adjustability restrictions are lessened: (1) bending of the rod is significantly easier than bending of the plate within the coronal plane (mediolateral direction) and (2) a wider range of difference in mediolateral angulation between adjacent screws is allowed, because the range of this angulation for the screw about the rod is greater than that for the screw within the plate hole (mediolateral toggle).

Full three-dimensional adjustability between the screw and the rod is allowed by the internal fixators (Dick,[37] Kluger,[86] Ölerud,[136] and Vermont[92, 99, 101, 103, 104]). These devices combine the cephalocaudad angular adjustment of some of the plate systems, with the continuous adjustability of longitudinal translation in the previously described rod systems, and yet maintain the mediolateral angular adjustability. Cephalocaudad angulation is adjustable in 6-degree increments (maximum mismatch is ±3 degrees) for all of these internal fixators, except for the Ölerud, which allows continuous adjustability. Mediolateral angulation is continuously adjustable in all of these fixators except for the Dick device, which is adjustable in 6-degree increments.

Positional Control

Control between the vertebra and the screw is determined by the screw design

---

*References 19, 115–117, 132, 151, 152, and 173.

and bone strength, as discussed above. Positional control between the screw and the longitudinal component has a range across devices that is as great as that for positional adjustability.

For most of the plate and screw systems,* the screw is free to toggle within the plate and is only prevented from doing so by the ligamentous interconnections between adjacent vertebrae, the friction between the plate and subjacent bone, and friction between the plate and the screw head. The first of these control elements is subject to soft tissue elongation or stretching, which is one of the problems associated with Harrington distraction rods. The second control element, plate-bone friction, is subject to bone resorption, especially if the bone surface is irregular. Bone graft placed underneath the plate may also add to this problem. The final control element, friction between the screw head and the plate, has a minor effect. Because of the above, toggling of the screw in the plate may be a fairly likely occurrence. This allows the screws to be subjected to bending loads, which in turn can cause screw breakage, especially if the screws have not been specifically designed to tolerate such loads. In addition, such motion may contribute to nonunion of the bone graft. It probably is relevant that 25% (21 of 84) of patients with trauma had distal screws break with Roy-Camille instrumentation;[152] that 24% (5 of 21) of patients with trauma had a loss of reduction measuring 10% to 12% at follow-up with this same implant system;[83] and that a 53% rate of solid union in primary operations, an 11% (5 of 46 patients) rate of screw loosening, and a 6.5% (3 of 46 patients) rate of screw breakage and nonunion were seen with DCP plates.[173] Blauth and colleagues[19] referred to screw toggle as "a major disadvantage."

Substantial but incomplete positional control of the screw or the rod is provided by the Edwards[45] and the Puno[143] implants. Edwards[47] conjectured that the partial motion allowed between the screw and the rod may protect the system from peak loads. Puno and colleagues[143] described micromotion between the screw and the rod and speculated that this may lessen the degree of stress shielding of the bone graft by the implant. Whether such motion actually occurs in vivo and, if so, whether it produces either of these effects remains to be established.

Complete positional control between the screw and the longitudinal linking component is provided by the Balgrist,[161] Cotrel-Dubousset,[31] Dick,[37] Kluger,[86] Ölerud,[136] Steffee,[167] Vermont,[92] and Wiltse[64] devices. These devices allow only motion that occurs by elastic deflection or (if the loads are high enough) plastic deformation of bone, screw, or longitudinal linking component. Carlson and associates[25] demonstrated the improved strength that results when a sacral screw is securely attached to the longitudinal element rather than being allowed to toggle. Secure attachment provides a more uniform load distribution along the screw in response to compressive loads along the rod; toggling allows stress to concentrate along the posterior cortex and thus the screw has a lower failure strength. Future research will have to determine the amount of positional control that provides the optimum balance between all of the biologic and mechanical factors affected by it.

Stiffness

The stiffnesses of the assembled implants vary considerably. On the basis of dimensions, the Steffee device is probably the stiffest, and the Wiltse single-rod construct is the least stiff, although full data have not been published. Geiger and colleagues[58] tested some of the longitudinal components in four-point bending: the Steffee plate is 11.6 kN/mm, and the Cotrel-Dubousset rod is 7 kN/mm, or 60% that of the Steffee. The stiffness level that is optimum remains to be established in terms of preventing dangerous intervertebral deflections before healing, facilitating development of bony union during healing, and preventing excessive stress shielding after healing. Whether implant stiffness also affects the rate of degeneration at adjacent motion segments (as conjectured by Hsu and associates[72, 73] and discussed in Complications of Transpedicle Spine Fixation) remains to be established. Bony fusion alone produces a segmental stiffness that is so much greater than that of a normal disc that the incremental stiffness from the addition of hardware may be relatively small.[102]

---

*References 19, 115–117, 121, 132, 151, 152, and 173.

Fatigue Strength

Typically, the fatigue strength of a structure is determined by repeatedly applying a specific load to it until either it fails or a sufficiently high number of load cycles is reached. This is then repeated on other test specimens using a number of different load amounts to characterize the fatigue strength of that structure. The results of such testing have not been published for plates and rods intended for connection between transpedicle screws. However, limited testing at a single load amount (24.1 N·m at a frequency of 4 Hz) has been performed by Geiger and colleagues,[58] who showed a wide range of cycles to failure for different devices. Differences between the Cotrel-Dubousset rod (65,000 cycles), the Ölerud rod (80,000 cycles), and the Luque plate (100,000 cycles) were not significant. The Steffee plate (210,000 cycles) and Harrington ¼-inch rod (220,000 cycles) were also not significantly different from each other, but were both stronger than the former group.

Performance of Reduction

If a fusion in situ is to be performed, no alteration in the relative position of one vertebra with respect to another (reduction or realignment) is produced. If realignment is performed, it must be accomplished either before or after the transpedicle screws are inserted into the vertebra and attached to the longitudinal link (rod or plate). For systems in which the longitudinal link must be positioned before screw insertion,[117, 121, 152] reduction must be accomplished either by traction on or positioning of the patient (described in further detail elsewhere[117, 152]) or by means of a temporarily implanted device, such as Harrington distraction rods (although this may require additional dissection). If the longitudinal link can be applied after screw insertion, it then becomes possible to use the screw as a handle for controlling vertebral position and performing the reduction. In some cases, this may allow a successful reduction to be performed that otherwise might be attempted only through a separate anterior approach.[117]

Various instruments that attach to individual screws have been mentioned,[72, 86, 121] and the dorsally protruding shaft of a Schanz pin can be used in this fashion before it is cut off.[37, 124] Positioning of such screw extensions to produce realignment can be accomplished either manually or by means of an instrument. Whatever method is used, caution must be exercised that excessive force is not placed on any one screw, because screw-vertebra loosening or screw bending can occur. To decrease the chance of this complication, the author's approach has been to develop a reduction frame that rigidly links together the right and left screws at each vertebral level thereby producing balanced load sharing between the screws. The biomechanical relevance of this is indicated by the results of cadaveric testing performed by Kling and colleagues,[85] which showed that such cross-linked screws are more than twice as strong as a single screw alone ($p < .05$).

The use of this reduction frame (1) provides an accurate control of position; (2) allows slower, more gradual reductions with less chance of excessive transient loads than might be feasible during manually driven reductions in difficult cases; (3) may be used to provide bridging between right and left screws for load equalization; (4) frees up surgical hands for other tasks; and (5) allows the implanted device to remain simple: the tool used for the reduction is not implanted in the patient.

One special consideration exists for reduction of spondylolisthesis, because this is a situation in which an unusually large amount of anteroposterior force may be needed. An obliquely placed screw probably can resist a posteriorly directed pull better than a screw placed along the AP axis. Still, as it begins to pull out, the obliquity and the associated resistance tend to be lost. If right and left obliquely placed screws are securely cross-linked, this loss of strength does not occur.

Other Characteristics

The design used for connection between screws and longitudinal links is one of the major determinants of the bulk of the implant, the simplicity of the device, and the ease of assembly. Although these aspects are not as readily quantified as mechanical characteristics (such as positional adjustability, stiffness, and fatigue strength), they nonetheless may be important. Bulky devices may encroach on adjacent facet joints, displace muscle tissue away from its normal position, produce increased dead space (possible increase in the rate of infection), cause tenderness from adjacent tissue irritation, and occupy space otherwise available to the bone graft. Devices that are not simple and easy to assemble may be associated with longer operative times, increased risk of holes in sterile gloves, greater chance for incorrect implantation, and an overall greater "fiddle" factor.

TRANSVERSE CONNECTION BETWEEN RIGHT AND LEFT IMPLANTS

Transverse connectors were initially used to improve deformity correction for scoliosis. The history for this has been reviewed by Asher and colleagues.[10] Attention has been focused on using such connectors to improve the overall stiffness of implants, although testing apparently has not yet been done on transpedicle screw–based implants. Asher and coworkers[10] measured the improved stiffness from cross-bridging between Harrington distraction rods without and with circumlaminar wires; Ashman and associates[12] studied Luque and Cotrel-Dubousset rods attached by such wires. The effect of the cross-bridging was to increase stiffness in response to certain load types but not to others. The relationship of these results to transpedicle screw–based devices is not clear: the interface between a screw and the vertebral pedicle or body is different from that between a hook and the lamina.

For transverse connectors attached to transpedicle screw–based devices, Gurr and coworkers[63] described biomechanical testing of whole implants attached to fresh calf lumbar spines that had the laminae excised and that were exposed to torsional and flexural loads. Carson and colleagues[26] studied the effect of screw obliquity angle on the strains on the screws themselves. Cotrel-Dubousset implants spanning three or five vertebrae were tested without and with transverse connectors. No significant stiffening effect was produced by these connectors. Ruland and coworkers[154] showed that the strength of cross-bridged right and left pedicle screws was stronger than that of a single screw, but it is unclear why the strength was less than that of two individual screws added together, as would have been expected. Thus, statements based on clinical experience that such connectors are important[31] do not yet have an experimentally validated basis.

Another type of connector involves the use of diagonal wires in an X pattern attached to the dorsal ends of the screws. This has been described by Dick[37] and Ölerud and colleagues[136] and is intended to increase implant resistance to lateral shifting of the upper vertebra relative to the lower. The same kind of resistance provided by the wires may instead be accomplished by orienting the screws up and in (see Fig. 4), which allows the vertebral body to function substantially as a cross-bridge and also provides other benefits (see under Entry Site and Orientation above). If the screws are angulated parallel to one another (e.g., narrow, parasagittally oriented pedicles), only friction between screw and bone resists the lateral shifting, which reduces the vertebral cross-bridging effect to a negligible amount. In this circumstance, especially in the case of a highly unstable fracture, the diagonal wiring may be helpful. The combination of these two methods may provide even more stiffening than either one alone, because the force distribution between screw and bone produced by a laterally directed load is different for each method.

BIOMECHANICAL TESTING OF WHOLE IMPLANTS

The testing of individual components such as screws, rods, and plates does not yield information concerning either the connecting device between the screw and the longitudinal component or the interface between the screw and the vertebra. Such information can be obtained by testing the entire assembled device implanted into some appropriate model. Human cadaveric spines can be used, but interspecimen variation can be a problem. Animal spines can be obtained that are more consistent in their properties, but their relevance to the human situation may be an issue. Nonbiologic specimens, such as plastic blocks, are highly consistent but differ even more from the human specimens. Not only does each model have its own special drawback, but all have in common the absence of muscle and ligament forces, which may be the major feature of these models that makes their application to the in vivo situation difficult.

As an example of how such forces may be important, an axial compressive load along the central axis of the vertebral bodies tends to produce substantial bending loads in the implanted screws, even if the middle column or posterior portion of the vertebral bodies and discs was intact to function as a fulcrum. When posterior muscle forces are present, however, the bending loads are converted into shear loads, to which the screws are much more resistant. The knowledge about such loads in humans is limited,[93] as is the understanding of the relationship between human and nonhuman spinal loads; thus, simulating such loads is difficult. Even less is known of the load distribution in various injury states[157] or the relationship between experimental models of such injuries and the reality in vivo. These model limitations should not preclude such testing but should be kept clearly in mind during the interpretation of results and the application of conclusions.

Table 4 summarizes certain major features of reports on in vitro static testing of various transpedicle screw–based implants. In most cases other devices were also tested (not shown in Table 4) to provide a comparison. Some work using fatigue testing has also been done. Tencer and colleagues,[171] in addition to the static loads indicated in Table 4, also exposed each construct to 4320 cycles at 0.5 Hz (over 6 hours) of a combined compression, flexion, and lateral bending load. Although full details are not provided in the abstract, the transpedicle screw–based devices appear to have fared substantially better than the hook and wire–based devices. Fatigue testing was performed on assembled implants attached to plastic blocks (simulating vertebrae) used to model a highly unstable injury (no interconnections).[94] Up to 1 million cycles of various magnitudes of a combined flexion-compression load were applied. In no case did clamp

Table 4

Static Tests of Whole Implants In Vitro

Author	Device	Specimen	Injury Model	Loads Type	Loads Amount	Outcome Measures
Asazuma et al.[9]	Steffee VSF Zielke	Pig (L5, L6, L7, S1)	Intact	Flexion Extension Lateral bend Torsion	<11.2 N·m <11.2 N·m <11.2 N·m <11.2 N·m	3 rotations and 3 translations for each
Ashman et al.[12] Herring and Ashman[70]	Steffee	Calf (L5, L6, S1, S2)	Spondylolisthesis (cut pars and disc)	Compression Flexion Torsion	? ? ?	Major motion for each
Falahee et al.[55]	Dick	Human (T10–L3)	Trauma (L1 burst, cut multiple ligaments)	Flexion Extension Lateral bend Torsion	10 N·m 10 N·m 10 N·m 10 N·m	3 rotations and 3 translations for each
Gurr et al.[63]	Cotrel-Dubousset Steffee	Calf (L1, S1)	Laminectomy (L4 and L5, partial L4–L5 and L5–S1 facetectomy, L4–L5 discectomy)	Compression Flexion Torsion	100, 200 N (5 cm) 5 N·m	Major motion for each
Jacobs et al.[76]	Roy-Camille	Human (T9–L3)	Trauma (flex to failure)	Flexion	25 N·m	Flexion
Puno et al.[143]	Steffee Screw-rod fixator	Human (L4–S2)	Intact	Compression Flexion Extension Lateral bend Torsion	450 N 31.2 N·m 31.2 N·m 31.2 N·m 11.2 N·m	Energy absorption to failure for each
Schläpfer et al.[158]	Magerl	Human (T11–L5)	Trauma (wedge osteotomy and cut posterior ligaments; also cut anterior ligaments)	Flexion	≤40 N·m	Flexion
Tencer et al.[171]	Roy-Camille VSF	Human (T10–L2)	Trauma (remove anterior two thirds body and cut posterior ligaments; remove rest of body)	Flexion Extension Lateral bend Torsion	<310 N <310 N <310 N <18 N·m	Rotation; AP and lateral translation each

loosening occur, although at high loads screw failure was eventually seen at the root of the first thread.

As can be seen, these reports of both static and fatigue tests involve a wide variety of devices, applications (spine specimen and injury model), and methods (loads and outcome measures). From this diversity, certain conclusions may be drawn:

1. Transpedicle screw–based devices definitely convey better overall positional control than do other devices.

2. One component of this improved positional control is the improved security of the screw–pedicle or body interface compared with the hook-lamina or the wire-lamina interface.

3. Devices that provide secure three-dimensional positional control between the screw and the longitudinal element can return normal stiffness to an injury model even if only applied to one vertebra above and one vertebra below the injury site (rather than two or three above and below as with other devices). They also provide greater resistance to longitudinal loads because of better load distribution along the screw.

4. When a failure of the screw-vertebra interface occurs, it tends not to threaten neural elements (i.e., the spinal canal and foramina remain intact).

5. The significance of different mechanical characteristics must be kept in mind in the clinical situation. Ultimate strength is an important measure because it may describe screw-bone failure, but stiffness is also important, because the amount of deflection may affect bone or disc fragment motion.

6. The overall response of an implant to a variety of load types should be assessed, because device response may be load type dependent, and in vivo loads likely are varied.

7. Much remains to be learned concerning in vivo load reality and the applicability of various experimental injury models to clinical situation.

POSTOPERATIVE MANAGEMENT

The major issues that are generally considered important in postoperative management are length of bed rest; the type and duration of external support, if any; and restrictions on activities. Reports that address these topics are summarized in Table 5. The extent to which mechanical loads are affected by such intervention is by no means clear. Available clinical studies are sufficiently varied that generalizations concerning these particular issues cannot yet be made. The spectrum of bracing recommended (from none to total contact trunk orthosis with a thigh cuff for 3 months) is

Table 5

Postoperative Management

Orthosis						
Type	Weeks	Restrictions	Device	Diagnosis	Site*	Report
None	—	?	Ölerud	Trauma	T/L	Ölerud et al.[136]
None		?	Steffee	Various	L, L/S	Steffee et al.[167]
Corset	12	Walking ≤1 mile Minimal sitting	Steffee	Degeneration	L, L/S	Hsu et al.[72]
Chairback	≤12	Cautious exercise	AO plates	Degeneration	L, L/S	Thalgott et al.[173]
Jewett	8	?	Kluger	Trauma	T, L	Blauth et al.[19]
Jewett	8	?	Dick	Various	T, L	Dick et al.[37]
Lumbar brace	8	?	Dick	Trauma	T, L	Aebi et al.[1]
Lumbar brace	≤12	?	Roy-Camille	Trauma	T, L	Kinnard et al.[83]
Lumbar brace	25	Progressive over 3 months	Vermont	Various	L/S	Krag et al.[96]
Lumbar brace	25	No sitting (? no. of weeks)	Louis	Various	L/S	Louis[117]
Lumbar brace	≤16	?	Roy-Camille	Various	T/L, L	Roy-Camille et al.[152]
Brace and thigh Thigh out	12 12	?	Edwards	Trauma	Low L	Levine and Edwards[111]
Bed rest, then brace	12 12	?	Roy-Camille	Spondylolisthesis	L/S	Roy-Camille et al.[152]

*T, thoracic; T/L, thoracolumbar; L, lumbar; L/S, lumbosacral.

sufficiently wide that some conclusions should be forthcoming. Little information has been given in available reports concerning activity restrictions. Although patient compliance with recommended restrictions may be difficult to assess, some description concerning this in future clinical reports would probably be useful.

IMPLANT REMOVAL

Consensus has by no means been reached regarding the risks and benefits of hardware removal. Many clinical reports do not mention this topic, although concern has been raised about a number of issues that retained implants present, such as (1) impairment of fusion solidity assessment,[19, 117] (2) impairment of visualization by diagnostic radiographic techniques, (3) accelerated degeneration or altered function at adjacent motion segments,[72, 73] (4) prolonged stress shielding of the fusion mass, (5) irritation to overlying tissue, (6) hematogenous spread of infection in the site, (7) altered local damage in the event of future regional trauma, and (8) long-term metal toxicity. Ölerud[136] does not remove devices before at least 1 year. Dick[37] and Kinnard and colleagues[83] recommend routine removal if discs are spanned that have not also been grafted. Only the long-term results will establish which approach provides the best balance between the risks and costs of an additional surgical procedure for device removal and the benefits to function thereby achieved.

CONCLUSION

A high level of interest has developed over the past few years in transpedicle screw fixation. Clearly such fixation can be used in a way that is effective and safe, as demonstrated by a growing number of patients who have had extremely satisfactory outcomes and yet who have not been condemned to a lifetime of dealing with an unnecessarily long segment of fused spine. Equally clearly, such fixation brings with it certain demands and risks. The challenge is to find ways to meet the demands and simultaneously to reduce the risks.

To accomplish this will require further research not only in the area of biomechanics (e.g., implant design, materials, fabrication techniques, testing methods, and in vivo measurements), but also in the area of clinical practice (surgical indications, implantation techniques, patient function, and satisfaction outcome studies). As in any relatively new field, there are far more good questions than there are good answers, but at least a substantial start has been made, and part of that start is the biomechanical research already completed.

REFERENCES

1. Aebi, M., Etter, C., Kehl, T., and Thalgott, J.: Stabilization of the lower thoracic and lumbar spine with the internal spinal skeletal fixation system: Indications, techniques, and first results of treatment. Spine 12:544–551, 1987.
2. Aebi, M., Etter, C., Kehl, T., and Thalgott, J.: The internal skeletal fixation system: A new treatment of thoracolumbar fractures and other spinal disorders. Clin. Orthop. 227:30–43, 1988.
3. Akbarnia, B. A., Fogarty, J. P., and Tayob, A. A.: Contoured Harrington instrumentation in the treatment of unstable spinal fractures: The effect of supplementary sublaminar wires. Clin. Orthop. 189:186–194, 1984.
4. Andrew, T. A., Brooks, S., and Piggott, H.: Long-term followup evaluation of screw-and-graft fusion of the lumbar spine. Clin. Orthop. 203:113–119, 1986.
5. Ansell, R. H., and Scales, J. T.: A study of some factors which affect the strength of screws and their holding power in bone. J. Biomech. 1:279–302, 1968.
6. Armstrong, G. W. D.: Harrington instrumentation for spinal fractures. In Proceedings of the Scoliosis Research Society Annual Meeting, Toronto, 1976. Orthop. Trans. 1:133, 1977.
7. Arnold, W.: Early surgical treatment using an external fixation device in traumatic paraplegia. Beitr. Orthop. Traumatol. 32 6–14, 1985.
8. Arnold, W.: Early surgical treatment of traumatic paraplegia with an external fixation device and diagonal vertebroplasty. Unfallchirurg 88:293–298, 1985.
9. Asazuma, T., Stokes, I. A. F., Moreland, M. S., and Suzuki, N.: An intersegmental spinal flexibility with lumbo-sacral instrumentation: In vitro biomechanical investigation. Spine 15:1153–1158, 1990.
10. Asher, M., Carson, W., and Heinig, C.: A modular spinal rod linkage system to provide rotational stability. Spine 13:272–277, 1988.
11. Asher, M. A., and Strippgen, W. E.: Anthropometric studies of the human sacrum relating to dorsal transsacral implant designs. Clin. Orthop. 203:58–62, 1986.
12. Ashman, R. B., Birch, J. G., Bone, L. B., et al.: Mechanical testing of spinal instrumentation. Clin. Orthop. 227:113–125, 1988.
13. Attenborough, C. G., and Reynolds, M. T.: Lumbosacral fusion with spring fixation. J. Bone Joint Surg. 57B:283–288, 1975.

14. Baker, L. D., and Hoyt, W. A.: The use of interfacet vitalium screws in the Hibbs fusion. South. Med. J. 41:419–426, 1948.
15. Banta, C. J., King, A. G., Dabezies, E. J., and D'Ambrosia, R.: Direct measurement of effective pedicle diameter. In Proceedings of the North American Spine Society Annual Meeting, Banff, Canada, 1987.
16. Bechtol, C. O.: Internal fixation with plates and screws. In Bechtol, C. O., Ferguson, A. B., Jr., and Laing, P. B. (eds.): Metals and Engineering in Bone and Joint Surgery. Baltimore, Williams & Wilkins, 1959, pp. 152–171.
17. Berry, J. L., Moran, J. M., Berg, W. S., and Steffee, A. D.: A morphometric study of human lumbar and selected thoracic vertebrae. Spine 12:362–367, 1987.
18. Birch, J. G., Herring, J. A., Roach, J. W., and Johnston, C. E.: Cotrel-Dubousset instrumentation in idiopathic scoliosis. Clin. Orthop. 227:24–29, 1988.
19. Blauth, M., Tscherne, H., and Haas, N.: Therapeutic concept and results of operative treatment in acute trauma of the thoracic and lumbar spine: The Hannover experience. J. Orthop. Trauma 1:240–252, 1987.
20. Bobechko, W. P.: The instant Harrington. In Proceedings of the Scoliosis Research Society Annual Meeting, Montreal, 1981. Orthop. Trans. 6:25, 1982.
21. Boucher, H. H.: A method of spinal fusion. J. Bone Joint Surg. 41B:248–259, 1959.
22. Bridwell, K. H.: The treatment of flexion/distraction spinal fractures with SSI and Luque rectangles. In Proceedings of the Scoliosis Research Society Annual Meeting, Orlando, FL, 1984.
23. Brodsky, J. W., Barnes, D. A., and Tullos, H. S.: Unrecognized pin penetration of the hip joint. Contemp. Orthop. 9:13–20, 1984.
24. Bryant, C. E., and Sullivan J. A.: Management of thoracic and lumbar spine fractures with Harrington distraction rods supplemented with segmental wiring. Spine 8:532–537, 1983.
25. Carlson, D. G., Abitbol, J. J., Anderson, D. R., et al.: Screw fixation in the human sacrum: An in vitro study of the biomechanics of fixation. Spine 17:S196–S203, 1992.
26. Carson, W., Duffield, R. C., Arendt, M., et al.: Internal forces and moments in transpedicular spine instrumentation. Spine 15:893–901, 1989.
27. Casey, M., Jacobs, R. R., and Asher, M.: The rod long-fuse short technique in the treatment of thoraco-lumbar and lumbar spine fractures. In Proceedings of the Scoliosis Research Society Annual Meeting, Orlando, FL, 1984. Orthop. Trans. 9:121, 1985.
28. Casey, M. P., and Jacobs, R. R.: Internal fixation of the lumbosacral spine: A biomechanical evaluation. In Proceedings of the International Society for Study of the Lumbar Spine Meeting, Montreal, 1984.
29. Coe, J. D., Warden, K. E., Herzig, M. A., et al.: Influence of bone mineral density on the fixation of thoracolumbar implants: A comparative study of transpedicular screws, laminar hooks and process wires. Spine 15:902–907, 1990.
30. Cordey, J., and Perren, S. M.: Limits of plate on bone friction in internal fixation of fractures. In Proceedings of the Orthopaedic Research Society Annual Meeting, Las Vegas, NV, 1985, p. 186.
31. Cotrel, Y., Dubousset, J., and Guillaumat, M.: New universal instrumentation in spinal surgery. Clin. Orthop. 227:10–23, 1988.
32. Daniaux, H.: Transpedikuläre Reposition and Spongiosaplastik bei Wirbelkörperbrüchen den unteren Brust- und Lendenwirbelsäule. Unfallchirurg 89:197–213, 1986.
33. DeCoster, T., Jones, W., and Heetderks, D.: Bone screw pullout strength as a function of thread design. In Proceedings of the Orthopaedic Trauma Association Annual Meeting, Dallas, TX, 1988, p. 89.
34. Denis, F., Ruiz, H., and Searls, K.: Comparison between square-ended distraction rods and standard round-ended distraction rods in the treatment of thoracolumbar spinal injuries: A statistical analysis. Clin. Orthop. 189:162–167, 1984.
35. Dick, W.: Innere Fixation von Brust- und Lendenwirbelfrakturen. Bern, Hans Huber, 1984.
36. Dick, W., Kluger, P., Magerl, F., et al.: A new device for internal fixation of thoracolumbar and lumbar spine fractures: The "fixateur interne." Paraplegia 23:225–232, 1985.
37. Dick, W.: The "fixateur interne" as a versatile implant for spine surgery. Spine 12:882–900, 1987.
38. Diehl, K., Hanser, U., Hort, W., and Mittelmeier, H.: Biomechanische Untersuchungen uber die maximalen Vorspannkräfte der Knochenschrauben in verschiedenen Knochenabschnitten. Acta Orthop. Unfallchirurg. 80:89, 1974.
39. Dohring, E. J., and Krag, M. H.: Sacral screw fixation: a morphologic, anatomic and mechanical study (8208.23). In Proceedings of the American Academy of Orthopaedic Surgeons 58th Annual Meeting, Anaheim, CA, March 8, 1991, p. 114.
40. Dove, J.: Internal fixation of the lumbar spine: The Hartshill rectangle. Clin. Orthop. 203:135–140, 1986.
41. Dove, J.: Segmental wiring for spinal deformity. A morbidity report. Spine 14:229–231, 1989.
42. Drummond, D., Narechania, R., Wenger, D., et al.: Wisconsin segmental spinal instrumentation. In Proceedings of the Scoliosis Research Society Annual Meeting, Montreal, 1981. Orthop. Trans 6:22–23, 1982.
43. Drummond, D. W., Guadagni, J., Keene, J. S., et al.: Interspinous process segmental spinal instrumentation. J. Pediatr. Orthop. 4:397–404, 1984.
44. Edwards, C. C., Griffith, P., Levine, A. M., and DeSilva J. B.: Early clinical results using the spinal rod sleeve method for treating thoracic and lumbar injuries. In Proceedings of the American Academy of Orthopaedic Surgeons Annual Meeting, New Orleans, 1982. Orthop. Trans. 6:345–346, 1982.
45. Edwards, C. C.: Sacral fixation device: Design and preliminary results. In Proceedings of the Scoliosis Research Society 19th Annual Meeting, 1984.
46. Edwards, C. C., Levine, A. M., York, J. J., and Holt, E. S.: A new spinal hook: Rationale and clinical trials. In Proceedings of the Scoliosis Research Society Annual Meeting, 1984.
47. Edwards, C. C.: New method for direct sacral fixation: Rationale and clinical results. In Proceedings of the International Society for Study of the Lumbar Spine Meeting, Dallas, 1986. Orthop. Trans 10:541–542, 1986.

48. Edwards, C. C.: Reduction of spondylolisthesis: Biomechanics and fixation. *In* Proceedings of the International Society for Study of the Lumbar Spine Meeting, Dallas, 1986. Orthop. Trans. 10:543–544, 1986.
49. Edwards, C. C.: Spinal screw fixation of the lumbar and sacral spine: Early results treating the first 50 cases. *In* Proceedings of the Scoliosis Research Society 21st Annual Meeting, Hamilton, Bermuda, 1986. Orthop. Trans. 11:99, 1987.
50. Edwards, C. C., and Levine, A. M.: Early rod-sleeve stabilization of the injured thoracic and lumbar spine. Orthop. Clin. North Am. 17:121–145, 1986.
51. Edwards, C. C., and Weigel, M. C.: A prospective study of 51 low lumbar nonunions. *In* Proceedings of the International Society for Study of the Lumbar Spine Meeting, 1988.
52. El-Khoury, G. Y., and McWilliams, F. E.: A simple radiological aid in the diagnosis of small avulsion fractures of the knee. J. Trauma 18:275–277, 1978.
53. Esses, S. I., Botsford, D. J., Huler, R. J., and Rauschning, W.: Surgical anatomy of the sacrum: A guide for rational screw fixation. Spine 16:S283–S288, 1991.
54. Esses, S. I.: The AO spinal internal fixator. *In* Proceedings of the North American Spine Society 3rd Annual Meeting, Colorado Springs, CO, 1988.
55. Falahee, M., Mann, K., Yuan, H., et al.: Biomechanical evaluation of augmented anterior and posterior short segment internal fixation for thoracolumbar burst fractures. *In* Proceedings of the International Society for Study of the Lumbar Spine Meeting, 1988, pp. 65–66.
56. Freedman, L. S., Houghton, G. R., and Evans, M.: Cadaveric study comparing the stability of upper distraction hooks used in Harrington instrumentation. Spine 11:579–582, 1986.
57. Gaines, R. W., Breedlove, R. F., and Munson, G.: Stabilization of thoracic and thoracolumbar fracture-dislocations with Harrington rods and sublaminar wires. Clin. Orthop. 189:195–203, 1984.
58. Geiger, J. M., Udovic, N. A., and Berry, J. L.: Bending and fatigue of spine plates and rods and fatigue of pedicle screws *In* Proceedings of the American Academy of Orthopaedic Surgeons Annual Meeting, 1989.
59. George, D. C., Krag, M. H., Johnson, C. C., Van Hal, M. E., et al.: Hole preparation techniques (drill versus probe) for transpedicular screws: Effect upon pullout strength from human cadaveric vertebrae. Spine 16:181–184, 1991.
60. Gertzbein, S. D., MacMichael, D., and Tile, M.: Harrington instrumentation as a method of fixation in fractures of the spine: A cortical analysis of deficiencies. J. Bone Joint Surg. 64B:526–529, 1982.
61. Grobler, L. J., Kempff, P. G., and Gaines, R. W., Jr.: Comparing Mersilene tape (M. T.) and stainless steel wire (S.S.W.) during segmental spinal instrumentation—evaluation of the macroscopical and microscopical tissue response in the baboon (*Papio urinus*). *In* Proceedings of the Scoliosis Research Society Annual Meeting, Vancouver, BC, 1987.
62. Gruca, A.: Pathogenesis and treatment of idiopathic scoliosis: A preliminary report. J. Bone Joint Surg. 40A:570–584, 1958.
63. Gurr, K. R., McAfee, P. C., and Shih, C. M.: Biomechanical analysis of posterior instrumentation systems following decompressive laminectomy: An unstable calf model. J. Bone Joint Surg. 70A:680–691, 1988.
64. Guyer, D. W., Wiltse, L. L., and Peek, R. D.: The Wiltse pedicle screw fixation system. Orthopaedics 11:1455–1460, 1988.
65. Harrington, P. R.: Treatment of scoliosis. Correction and internal fixation by spine instrumentation. J. Bone Joint Surg. 44A:591–610, 1962.
66. Harrington, P. R.: Instrumentation in spine instability other than scoliosis. South Afr. J. Surg. 5:7–12, 1967.
67. Harrington, P. R., and Tullos, H. S.: Reduction of severe spondylolisthesis in children. South. Med. J. 62:1–7, 1969.
68. Harrington, P. R.: The history and development of Harrington instrumentation. Clin. Orthop. 93:110–112, 1973.
69. Harrington, P. R., and Dickson, J. H.: Spinal instrumentation in the treatment of severe progressive spondylolisthesis. Clin. Orthop. 117:157–163, 1976.
70. Herring, J. A., and Ashman, R. B.: Biomechanical testing of instruments for the fixation of spondylolisthesis. *In* Proceedings of the Scoliosis Research Society 21st Annual Meeting, Hamilton, Bermuda, 1986. Orthop. Trans. 11:98–99, 1987.
71. Herrman, H. D.: Transarticular (transpedicular) metal plate fixation for stabilization of the lumbar and thoracic spine. Acta Neurochir. (Wien) 48:101–110, 1979.
72. Hsu, K., Zucherman, J. F., White, A. H., and Wynne, G.: Internal fixation with pedicle screws. *In* White, A. H., Rothman, R. H., and Ray, R. C. (Eds.): Lumbar Spine Surgery: Techniques and Complications. St. Louis, C. V. Mosby, 1987.
73. Hsu, K. Y., Zucherman, J., White A., et al.: Deterioration of motion segments adjacent to lumbar spine fusions. *In* Proceedings of the North American Spine Society Annual Meeting, Colorado Springs, CO, 1988.
74. Jacobs, R. R., Nordwall, A., and Nachemson, A.: Stability and strength provided by internal fixation systems for dorso-lumbar spinal injuries. Clin. Orthop. 171:300–308, 1982.
75. Jacobs, R. R., Dahners, L. E., Gerzbein, S. D., et al.: A locking hook–spinal rod: Current status of development. Paraplegia 21:197–200, 1983.
76. Jacobs, R. R., Schlaepfer, F., Mathys, R., Jr., et al.: A locking hook spinal rod system for stabilization of fracture-dislocations and correction of deformities of the dorsolumbar spine: A biomechanic evaluation. Clin. Orthop. 189:168–177, 1984.
77. Jacobs, R. R., Montesano, R. X., and Jackson, R. P.: Enhancement of lumbar spine fusion by use of translaminar facet joint screws. Spine 14:12–15, 1989.
78. Kahanovitz, N., Arnoczky, S. P., Levine, D. B., and Otis, J. P.: The effects of internal fixation on the articular cartilage of unfused canine facet joint cartilage. Spine 9:268–272, 1984.
79. Kahanovitz, N., Bullough, P., and Jacobs, R. R.: The effect of internal fixation without arthrodesis on human facet joint cartilage. Clin. Orthop. 189:204–208, 1984.
80. Keene, J. S., Drummond, D. S., and Narechania,

R. G.: Mechanical performance of the Wisconsin compression system. *In* Proceedings of the Orthopaedic Research Society 26th Annual Meeting, Atlanta, GA, 1980.
81. King, D.: Internal fixation for lumbosacral fusion. Am. J. Surg. 66:357–361, 1944.
82. King, D.: Internal fixation for lumbosacral spine fusions. J. Bone Joint Surg. 30A:560–565, 1948.
83. Kinnard P., Ghibely, A., Gordon, D., et al.: Roy-Camille plates in unstable spinal conditions: A preliminary report. Spine 11:131–135, 1986.
84. Kleeman, B. C., Gerhart, T. N., and Hayes, W. C.: Augmenting screw fixation in osteopenic trabecular bone. *In* Proceedings of the Society of Biomaterials Annual Meeting, New York, 1987.
85. Kling, T. F., Jr., Vanderby, R., Jr., Belloli, D. M., and Thomsen, E. L.: Cross-linked pedicle screw fixation in the same vertebral body: A biomechanical study. *In* Proceedings of the Scoliosis Research Society Annual Meeting, Hamilton, Bermuda, 1986. Orthop. Trans. 11:98, 1987.
86. Kluger, P., and Gerner, H. J.: Das Mechanische Prinzip des Fixateur Externe zur Dorsalen Stabilisierung der Brust- und Lendenwirbelsäule. Unfallchirurg 12:68–79, 1986.
87. Knodt, H., and Larrick, R. B.: Distraction fusion of the spine. Ohio State Med. J. 60:1140–1142, 1964.
88. Koranyi, E., Bowman, C. E., Knecht, C. D., and Janssen, M.: Holding power of orthopaedic screws in bone. Clin. Orthop. 72:283–786, 1970.
89. Kostuik, J. P.: Anterior fixation for fractures of the thoracic and lumbar spine with or without neurologic involvement. Clin. Orthop. 189:103–115, 1984.
90. Kostuik, J. P.: Anterior Kostuik-Harrington distraction systems. Orthopaedics 11:1379–1391, 1988.
91. Krag, M. H., Beynnon, B. D., Pope, M. H., and Frymoyer, J. W.: Vermont spinal fixator for posterior thoracic, lumbar, or lumbosacral spinal stabilization: Initial mechanical testing and implantation. *In* Proceedings of the International Society for Study of the Lumbar Spine Meeting, Sydney, Australia, 1985.
92. Krag, M. H., Beynnon, B. D., Pope, M. H., et al.: An internal fixator for posterior application to short segments of the thoracic, lumbar, or lumbosacral spine. Clin. Orthop. 203:75–98, 1986.
93. Krag, M. H., Pope, M. H., and Wilder, D. G.: Mechanisms of spine trauma and features of spinal fixation methods. Part I: Mechanisms of injury. *In* Ghista, D. (ed.): Spinal Cord Medical Engineering. Springfield, IL, Charles C Thomas, 1986, pp. 133–157.
94. Krag, M. H., Beynnon, B. D., Frymoyer, J. W., and Haugh, L. D.: Fatigue testing of an internal fixator for posterior spinal stabilization. *In* Proceedings of the American Academy of Orthopaedic Surgeons 54th Annual Meeting, San Francisco, CA, 1987.
95. Krag, M. H., Frymoyer, J. W., Beynnon, B. D., and Pope, M. H.: An internal fixator for posterior application to short segments of the thoracic, lumbar, or lumbosacral spine: Design and testing. *In* White, A. H., Rothman, R. H., and Ray C. D. (eds.): Lumbar Spine Surgery: Techniques and Complications. St. Louis, C. V. Mosby, 1987, pp. 339–367.
96. Krag, M. H.: Lumbosacral fixation with the Vermont spinal fixator. *In* Lin, P. M., and Gill, K. (eds.): Lumbar Interbody Fusion: Principles and Techniques of Spine Surgery. Rockville, MD, Aspen, 1988.
97. Krag, M. H., Beynnon, B. D., DeCoster, T. A., and Pope, M. H.: Depth of insertion of transpedicular vertebral screws into human vertebrae: Effect upon screw-vertebra interface strength. J. Spinal Disord. 1:287–294, 1988.
98. Krag, M. H., Weaver, D. L., Beynnon, B. D., and Haugh, L. D.: Morphometry of the thoracic and lumbar spine related to transpedicular screw placement for surgical spinal fixation. Spine 13:27–32, 1988.
99. Krag, M. H.: Internal fixation of the lumbosacral spine, experience with the Vermont spinal fixator. *In* Lin, P. M., and Gill, K. (eds.): Lumbar Interbody Fusion. Principles and Techniques of Spine Surgery. Rockville, MD, Aspen, 1989, pp. 251–260.
100. Krag, M. H., Van Hal, M. E., and Beynnon, B. D.: Placement of transpedicular vertebral screws close to anterior vertebral cortex: Description of methods. Spine 14:879–883, 1989.
101. Krag, M. H.: Spinal fusion: Overview of options and posterior internal fixation devices. *In* Frymoyer, J. W. (ed.): The Adult Spine. New York, Raven Press, 1991, pp. 1919–1946.
102. Krag, M. H.: Biomechanics of thoracolumbar spinal fixation. Spine 16(3S):S84–S99, 1991.
103. Krag, M. H.: The Vermont Spinal Fixator. *In* Lonstein, J., and Arnold, D. (eds.): Internal Pedicular Fixation of the Lumbar Spine. Spine: State of the Art Review. Philadelphia, Hanley & Belfus, 1992.
104. Krag, M. H.: The Vermont spinal fixator. *In* An, H. S., and Cotler, J. M. (eds.): Spinal Instrumentation. Baltimore, Williams & Wilkins, 1992, pp. 237–255.
105. Laborde, J. M., Bahniuk, E., Bohlman, H. H., and Samson, B.: Comparison of fixation of spinal fractures. Clin. Orthop. 152:303–310, 1980.
106. Lange, F.: Support for the spondylitic spine by means of buried steel bars attached to the vertebrae. Am. J. Orthop. Surg. 8:344–361, 1910.
107. Lange, F.: Support for the spondylitic spine by means of buried steel bars attached to the vertebrae. (Reprinted from the original.) Clin. Orthop. 203:3–6, 1986.
108. Lavaste, F.: Etude des Implants Rachidiens. Mémoire de Biomécanique. Thèse Ingénieur, Ecole Nationale Supérieure des Arts et Métiers à Paris, 1977.
109. Lavaste, F.: Bioméchanique du Rachis Dorso-Lombaire. Deuxième Journées d'Orthopédie de la Pitie 19–23, 1980.
110. Lehman, W. B., Grant, A., Rose, D., et al.: A method of evaluating possible pin penetration in slipped capital femoral epiphysis using a cannulated internal fixation device. Clin. Orthop. 186:65–70, 1984.
111. Levine, A. M., and Edwards, C. C.: Low lumbar burst fractures. Orthopaedics 11:1427–1432, 1988.
112. Lindsey, R. W., and Dick, W.: The fixateur interne in the reduction and stabilization of thoracolumbar spine fractures in patients with neurologic deficit. Spine 16:S140–S145, 1991.
113. Liu, Y. K., Njus, G. O., and Singerman, R.: Improvement in the mechanical properties of pedi-

cle screws used in spinal internal fixation. *In* Proceedings of the International Society for Study of the Lumbar Spine Meeting, Dallas, TX, 1986.
114. Liu, Y. K., Njus, G. O., Bahr, P. A., and Geng, P.: Fatigue life improvement of nitrogen-ion implanted pedicle screws. *In* Proceedings of the International Society for Study of the Lumbar Spine Meeting, Miami, FL, 1988.
115. Louis, R., and Maresca, C.: Les arthrodèses stables de la charnière lombo-sacrée (70 cas). Rev. Chir. Orthop. 62(suppl. II):70–79, 1976.
116. Louis, R., and Maresca, C.: Stabilisation Chirurgical avec Réduction des Spondylolyses et des Spondylolisthésis. Int. Orthop. 1:215–25, 1977.
117. Louis, R.: Fusion of the lumbar and sacral spine by internal fixation with screw plates. Clin. Orthop. 203:18–33, 1986.
118. Luque, E. R.: Anatomic basis and development of segmental spinal instrumentation. Spine 7:256–259, 1982.
119. Luque, E. R., Cassis, N., and Ramirez-Wiella, G.: Segmental spinal instrumentation in the treatment of fractures of thoracolumbar spine. Spine 7:312–317, 1982.
120. Luque, E. R.: Interpeduncular segmental fixation. Clin. Orthop. 203:54–57, 1986.
121. Luque, E. R., and Rapp, G. F.: A new semirigid method for interpedicular fixation of the spine. Orthopaedics 11:1445–1450, 1988.
122. Lyon, W. F., Cochran, J. R., and Smith, L.: Actual holding power of various screws in bone. Ann. Surg. 114:376–384, 1941.
123. Magerl, F.: External spinal skeletal fixation. *In* Weber, B. G., and Magerl, F. (eds.): The External Fixator. New York, Springer-Verlag, 1985.
124. Magerl, F. P.: Stabilization of the lower thoracic and lumbar spine with external skeletal fixation. Clin. Orthop. 189:125–141, 1984.
125. Martin, D., Cordey, J., Rahn, B. A., and Perren, S. M.: Bone screw displacement under lateral loading. *In* Proceedings of the 2nd Meeting of the European Society of Biomechanics, Strasbourg, France, 1979.
126. Matthiass, H. H., and Heine, J.: Surgical reduction of spondylolisthesis. Clin. Orthop. 203:34–44, 1986.
127. Mehdian, H., Jaffray, D., and Eisenstein, S. M.: Dwyer/Hartshill transpedicular segmental fixation. *In* Proceedings of the International Society for Study of the Lumbar Spine Meeting, Miami, FL, 1988.
128. Mirkovic, S., Abitbol, J., Steinman, J., et al: Anatomic considerations for sacral screw placement. Spine 16:S289–S294, 1991
129. Misenhimer, G. R., Peek, R. D., Wiltse, L. L., et al.: Anatomic analysis of pedicle cortical and cancellous diameter as related to screw size. *In* Proceedings of the International Society for Study of the Lumbar Spine Meeting, Dallas, TX, 1988.
130. Moe, J. H., and Denis, F.: The iatrogenic loss of lumbar lordosis. *In* Proceedings of the Scoliosis Research Society Annual Meeting, Toronto, 1976. Orthop. Trans. 1:131, 1977.
131. Moran, J. M., Berg, W. S., Berry, J. L., et al.: Transpedicular screw fixation. J. Orthop. Res. 7:107–114, 1989.
132. Müller, M. E., Allgöwer, M., Schneider, R., and Willenegger, H.: Fractures of the spine. *In* Müller, M. E., et al. (eds): Manual of Internal Fixation; Techniques Recommended by the AO Groups, 2nd Ed. Berlin, Springer-Verlag, 1979, pp. 304–305.
133. Nasca, R. J., and Johnson, L. P.: Harrington-Bobechko instrumentation in the treatment of scoliosis: A preliminary report. Spine 13:246–249, 1988.
134. Nunamaker, D. M., and Perren, S. M.: Force measurements in screw fixation. J. Biomech. 9:669–675, 1976.
135. Ölerud, S., Sjöström, L., Karlström, G., and Hamberg, M.: Spontaneous effect of increased stability of the lower lumbar spine in cases of severe chronic back pain: The answer of an external transpeduncular fixation test. Clin. Orthop. 203:67–74, 1986.
136. Ölerud, S., Karlström, G., and Sjöström, L.: Transpedicular fixation of thoracolumbar vertebral fractures. Clin. Orthop. 227:44–51, 1988.
137. Pawluk, R. J., Musso, E., Tzitzikalakis, G. I., and Dick, H. M.: Effects of internal fixation techniques on altering plate screw strain distribution. *In* Proceedings of the Orthopaedic Research Society Annual Meeting, Las Vegas, NV, 1985, p. 185.
138. Peek, R. D., Thomas, J. C., Weinstein, J., et al.: Lumbar spine fusion with pedicle screw and rods. *In* Proceedings of the International Society for Study of the Lumbar Spine Meeting, Dallas, TX, 1988.
139. Pennal, G. F., McDonald, G. A., and Dale, G. G.: Method of spinal fusion using internal fixation. Clin. Orthop. 35:86–94, 1964.
140. Perren, S. M., Cordey, J., Enzler, M., et al.: Mechanics of bone screw with internal fixation plates. Unfallheilkunde 81:211–218 1978.
141. Pfeifer, B., Krag, M., and Johnson, C.: Repair of failed transpedicle screw fixation: A biomechanical study comparing polymethylmethacrylate, morcellized bone, and matchstick bone reconstruction. *In* Proceedings of the International Society for the Study of the Lumbar Spine Meeting, Heidelberg, Germany, 1991.
142. Pfeifer, B. A., Krag, M. H., Johnson, C. C.: A biomechanical study comparing insertion torque with pullout strength in pedicle screws. *In* Proceedings of the North American Spine Society 7th Annual Meeting, Boston, July 9–11, 1992, pp. 108–109.
143. Puno, R. M., Bechtol, J. E., Byrd, J. E., et al.: Biomechanical analysis of five techniques of fixation for the lumbosacral junction. *In* Proceedings of the Orthopaedic Research Society Annual Meeting, San Francisco, CA, 1987, p. 366.
144. Puschel, J., and Zielke, K.: Transpedicular vertebral instrumentation using VDS instruments in ankylosing spondylitis. *In* Proceedings of the Scoliosis Research Society 19th Annual Meeting, Orlando, FL, 1984. Orthop. Trans. 9:139, 1985.
145. Reed, S., and Wagner, T.: Preliminary report on lumbo-sacral fusion with pedicle screws and Steffee plates. *In* Proceedings of the Scoliosis Research Society 21st Annual Meeting, Hamilton, Bermuda, 1986. Orthop. Trans. 11:99–100, 1987.
146. Reimers, C.: Die Dorsale Spannverstrebung von Wirbelsäulenabschnitten mittels innerer Schienung. Chirurgie 17:10, 1956.
147. Resina, J., and Alves, A. F.: Technique of correction and internal fixation for scoliosis. J. Bone Joint Surg. 59B:159–165, 1977.

148. Robbins, S., and Gertzbein, S.: Accuracy of pedicle screw placement in vivo. In Proceedings of the Orthopaedic Trauma Association Annual Meeting, Dallas, TX, 1988, pp. 27–28.
149. Rooks, M. D., Schmitt, E. W., and Drvaric, D. M.: Unrecognized pin penetration in slipped capital femoral epiphysis. Clin. Orthop. 234:82–89, 1988.
150. Rossier, A. B., and Cochran, T. P.: The treatment of spinal fractures with Harrington compression rods and segmental sublaminar wiring: A dangerous combination. Spine 9:796–799, 1984.
151. Roy-Camille, R., and Demeulenaere, C.: Ostéosynthèse du rachis dorsal, lombaire et lombosacrée par plaque métalliques vissées dans les pédicules vertébraux et les apophyses articulaires. Presse Med. 78:1447–1448, 1970.
152. Roy-Camille, R., Saillant, G., and Mazel, C.: Internal fixation of the lumbar spine with pedicle screw plating. Clin. Orthop. 203:7–17, 1986.
153. Roy-Camille, R.: Experience with Roy-Camille fixation for the thorocolumbar and lumbar spine. Acute spinal injuries: Current management techniques. University of Massachusetts Continuing Medical Education Course, Sturbridge, MA, October 1987.
154. Ruland, C. M., McAfee, P. C., Warden, K. E., Cunningham, B. W.: Triangulation of pedicular instrumentation: A biomechanical analysis. Spine 16:S270–S276, 1991.
155. Saillant, G.: Étude Anatomique des Pédicules Vertébraux: Application Chirurgicale. Rev. Chir. Orthop. 62:151–160, 1976.
156. Schatzker, J., Sanderson, R., and Murnaghan, P. J.: The holding power of orthopaedic screws in vivo. Clin. Orthop. 108:115–126, 1975.
157. Schläpfer, F., Magerl, F., Jacobs, R., et al.: In vivo measurements of loads on an external fixation device for human lumbar spine fractures. Institute of Mechanical Engineers C131/80:59–64, 1980.
158. Schläpfer, F., Wörsdörfer, O., Magerl, F., and Perren, S. M.: Stabilization of the lower thoracic and lumbar spine: Comparative in vitro investigation of an external skeletal and various internal fixation devices. In Uhthoff, H. K., and Stahl, E. (eds.): Current Concepts of External Fixation of Fractures. New York, Springer-Verlag, 1982.
159. Schlicke, L., and Schulak, J.: The simultaneous use of Harrington compression and distraction rods in a thoracolumbar fracture-dislocation. J. Trauma 20:177–179, 1980.
160. Schöllner, O.: Ein neues Verfahren zur Reposition und Fixation bei Spondylolisthesis. Orthop. Praxis 4:270, 1975.
161. Schreiber, A., Suezawa, Y., and Jacob, H. A. C.: Preliminary report of 40 patients. Dorsal spinal fusion with a transpedicular distraction and compression system. Orthop. Rev. 15:93–96, 1986.
162. Shaw, J. A.: Preventing unrecognized pin penetration into hip joint. Orthop. Rev. 13:142–152, 1984.
163. Sicard, A., and Menegaux, J.: L'Abord Anterieur de l'Articulation Sacroiliaque. J. Chir., 77:29, 1959.
164. Sijbrandij, S.: A new technique for the reduction and stabilisation of severe spondylolisthesis. J. Bone Joint Surg. 63B:266–271, 1981.
165. Simmons, E. H., and Capicotto, W. N.: Posterior Zielke instrumentation of the lumbar spine with transpedicular fixation. In Proceedings of the Scoliosis Research Society Annual Meeting, Hamilton, Bermuda, 1986. Orthop. Trans. 11:100, 1987.
166. Stanger, J. K.: Fracture-dislocation of the thoracolumbar spine. With special reference to reduction by open and closed operations. J. Bone Joint Surg. 29:107–118, 1947.
167. Steffee, A. D., Biscup, R. S., and Sitkowski, D. J.: Segmental spine plates with pedicle screw fixation: A new internal fixation device for disorders of lumbar and thoracolumbar spine. Clin. Orthop. 203:45–53, 1986.
168. Steffee, A. D., and Sitkowski, D. J.: Posterior lumbar interbody fusion and plates. Clin. Orthop. 227:99–102, 1988.
169. Steffee, A. D., and Sitkowski, D. J.: Reduction and stabilization of grade IV spondylolisthesis. Clin. Orthop. 227:82–89, 1988.
170. Tello, C. A.: Early results with a variation of spinal instrumentation. In Proceedings of the Scoliosis Research Society Annual Meeting, Orlando, FL, 1984.
171. Tencer, A. F., Ferguson, R. L., Woodard, P. L., and Allen, B. L., Jr.: Biomechanical evaluation of posterior fixation of spine fractures. In Proceedings of the Orthopaedic Research Society 33rd Annual Meeting, San Francisco, CA, 1987.
172. Thalgott, J. S., Aebi, M., and LaRocca, H.: Internal spinal skeletal fixation system. Orthopaedics 11:1465–1468, 1988.
173. Thalgott, J. S., LaRocca, H., Aebi, M., et al.: Reconstruction of the lumbar spine using AO DCP plate internal fixation. Spine 14:91–95, 1989.
174. Thomas, J. C., Jr., Haye, W., Wiltse, L. L., et al.: Review of deep wound infection complicating pedicle screw fixation of the lumbar spine. In Proceedings of the International Society for Study of the Lumbar Spine Meeting, Miami, FL, 1988.
175. Thompson, W. A. L., and Ralston, E. L.: Pseudarthrosis following spine fusion. J. Bone Joint Surg. 31A:400–405, 1949.
176. Toumey, J. W.: Internal fixation in fusion of the lumbo-sacral joints. Lahey Clin. Bull. 3:188–191, 1943.
177. Trias, A., Bourassa, P., and Massoud, M.: Dynamic loads experienced in correction of idiopathic scoliosis using two types of Harrington rods. Spine 4:228–235, 1979.
178. Vangsness, C. T., Carter, D. R., and Frankel, V. H.: In vitro evaluation of the loosening characteristics of self-tapped and non–self-tapped cortical bone screws. Clin. Orthop. 157:279–286, 1981.
179. Vercauteren, M., and DeGroote, W.: Reduction of spondylolisthesis with severe slipping. Acta Orthop. Belg. 47:502–511, 1981.
180. Vidal, J., Fassio, B., Buscayret, C., and Allieu, Y.: Surgical reduction of spondylolisthesis using a posterior approach. Clin. Orthop. 154:156–165, 1981.
181. Volz, R. G., and Martin, M. D.: Illusory biplane radiographic images. Radiology 122:695–697, 1977.
182. Walters, R., and Simon, S. R.: Joint destruction: A sequel of unrecognized pin penetration in patients with slipped capital femoral epiphysis. In Proceedings of the Eighth Open Scientific Meeting of the Hip Society. St. Louis, C. V. Mosby, 1980.
183. Wang, G. J., Reger, S. I., Jennings, R. L., et al.: Variable strengths of wire fixation. Orthopaedics 5:435–436, 1981.
184. Ward, J. J., Nasca, R. J., and Lemons, J. E.: Biomechanical evaluation of the neural arch. In Proceed-

ings of the Scoliosis Research Society Annual Meeting, Orlando, FL, 1984.
185. Weinstein, J. N., Spratt, K. F., Spengler, D., and Brick, C.: Spinal pedicle fixation: reliability and validity of roentgenogram-based assessment and surgical factors on successful screw placement. Spine 13:1012–1018, 1988.
186. Weiss, M.: Dynamic spine alloplasty (spring-loading corrective devices) after fracture and spinal cord injury. Clin. Orthop. 112:150–158, 1975.
187. Wenger, D., Miller, S., and Wilkerson, J.: Evaluation of fixation sites for segmental instrumentation of the human vertebra. In Proceedings of the Scoliosis Research Society Annual Meeting, Montreal, 1981. Orthop. Trans. 6:23–24, 1982.
188. Whitecloud, T. S., Butler, J. C., Cohen, J. L., and Candelora, P. D.: Complications with the variable spinal plating system. Spine 12:472–476, 1989.
189. Whitecloud, T. S., III, Skalley, T., Cook, S. D., and Morgan, E. L.: Roentgenographic measurement of pedicle screw penetration. Clin. Orthop. 245:57–68, 1989.
190. Williams, E. W. M.: Traumatic paraplegia. In Matthews, D. N. (ed.): Recent Advances in Surgery of Trauma. London, Churchill, 1963, pp. 171–186.
191. Wilson, P. D., and Straub, L. R.: Lumbosacral fusion with metallic-plate fixation. Instr. Course Lect. 9:53–57, 1952.
192. Yamagata, M.: Biomechanical study of posterior spinal instrumentation for scoliosis. J. Japan. Orthop. Assoc. 58:523–534, 1984.
193. Yamagata, M., Kitahara, H., Minami, S., et al.: Mechanical stability of pedicle screw fixation systems for the lumbar spine. Spine 17S:51–54, 1992.
194. Zand, M. S., Goldstein, S. A., and Matthews, L. S.: Fatigue failure of cortical bone screws. J. Biomech. 16:305–312, 1983.
195. Zdeblick, T. A., Kunz, D. N., Cocke, M. E., et al: Pedicle screw pullout strength: Correlations with insertional torque. Spine 18:1673–1676, 1993.
196. Zielke, K., and Strempel, A. V.: Posterior lateral distraction spondylodesis using the twofold sacral bar. Clin. Orthop. 203:151–158, 1986.
197. Zindrick, M. R., Wiltse, L. L., Holland, W. R., et al.: Biomechanical study of intrapeduncular screw fixation in the lumbosacral spine. In Proceedings of the International Society for Study of the Lumbar Spine Meeting, Sydney, Australia, 1985.
198. Zindrick, M. R., Wiltse, L. L., Widell, E. H., et al.: Biomechanical study of interpeduncular screw fixation in the lumbosacral spine. Clin. Orthop. 203:99–111, 1986.
199. Zindrick M. R., Wiltse, L. L., Doornik, A., et al.: Analysis of the morphometric characteristics of the thoracic and lumbar pedicles Spine 12:160–166, 1987.

Complications of Transpedicle Spine Fixation

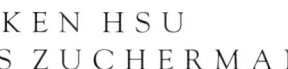

KEN HSU
JAMES ZUCHERMAN
MARTIN KRAG

INTRAOPERATIVE COMPLICATIONS

Neurologic

Neural injury is of particular concern when pedicle screws are used because neurologic structures are close to the pedicle and inserting the pedicle screw instrumentation is often technically demanding. Neural injuries can occur intraoperatively during hole preparation and screw insertion from burring, drilling, probing, curetting, misdirecting the screw out of the pedicle, or using a screw with a diameter that is too large. Intraoperative injuries such as screw stripout, pedicle fracture, and bone graft displacement by a longitudinal plate, can also result during hardware assembly. These are less likely to occur with articulated screw-and-rod systems with three-dimensional adjustability, such as the Olerud,[31] the fixateur interne,[6, 7] and the Vermont spinal fixator.[17, 23, 28] Finally, postoperative injuries can occur from late screw cutout or pedicle erosion. These injuries include dural tears, nerve root irritation or mechanical damage, and lumbar or lumbosacral plexus injuries.

Dural tears can be caused by misdirected screws or other instruments inserted medial to the pedicle. Cerebrospinal fluid pressure may keep the tear open and lead to pseudomeningocele or fistula formation. This increases the risk of infection or neurologic compromise. The misdirected screw probably should be removed as soon as possible, although the exact level of urgency is not clear. Surgical closure of dural tears is recommended whenever feasible and especially when nerve rootlets are extravasated. The extravasated rootlets should be returned to within the dural sac. If leakage of cerebrospinal fluid persists, a subarachnoid catheter inserted percutaneously to relieve cerebrospinal fluid pressure should allow dural healing in many cases. Rarely, a patient may have to be returned to the operating room for surgical closure.

The nerve roots are the structures that are most at risk for damage by screws placed out of the pedicle. Each nerve root passes along the medial and caudal cortices of the pedicle, then courses out through the superior third of the intervertebral foramen to become the spinal nerve, which runs lateral to the subjacent pedicle. Thus nerve root damage can occur by screw penetration at any of these sites (although screw penetration by no means necessarily causes nerve damage).

How best to reduce the risk of intraoperative pedicle cortex penetration is not clear. The use of anteroposterior and lateral radiographs is not helpful. In a cadaver study by Weinstein and colleagues,[46] anteroposterior and lateral view C-arm monitoring during screw placement resulted in a 21% incidence of pedicle penetrations, and 60% of these were not detected on these x-ray views. Roy-Camille and coworkers,[34] using anteroposterior and lateral x-ray films after screw placement, reported a 10% rate of screws out of the pedicle. Davne and Myers[5] reported lateral cortical breakthrough to be their most common technical problem. However, in contrast to this, using a coaxial oblique x-ray view along the pedicle (described in Biomechanics of Transpedicle Spine Fixation) Krag and associates[21] had an out of pedicle rate of only 0.5% (1 of 212 screws).

Another alternative is sufficient laminectomy to allow palpation and direct visualization of the medial pedicle wall and nerve root, although this still does not allow visualization of lateral cortical penetration. The pedicle may fracture with insertion of a screw with a diameter too close to that of the pedicle. Tapping may help prevent this, although the use of a smaller screw is preferable. Morphometric studies have shown considerable variations in diameter, length, shape, and angulation of human pedicles.[19, 22] Appropriate preoperative radiographs and computed tomographic scans are helpful in recognizing these pedicle features, especially in a spine that is abnormal or was previously operated on, in which bony surface landmarks may be difficult or impossible to identify reliably.

Late screw cutout from pedicle erosion or fracture can also injure the nerve roots. The involved screw should be removed if symptoms are significant. In one clinical study, eight of 30 patients developed leg pain 1 to 2 months after variable screw-plate placement.[56, 58] This was presumably a result of nerve root irritation and was relieved by selective root blocks, epidural blocks, or application of a brace. This problem occurred early in the series when vertebrae with instrumentation were locked in distraction, which probably led to pedicle erosion or fracture.

Parts of the lumbosacral plexus are located anterior to the sacral ala. The lumbar plexus is found anterior to the L5–S1 disc and sacral promontory. Therefore, anterior perforation of the sacral cortex may injure either of these structures. Such injuries are prevented by limiting the depth of penetration beyond the sacral cortex or by avoiding it altogether. Mirkovic and associates[28] believed that the potential for lumbosacral trunk impingement or injury is as high as 55% with an S1 screw insertion through the cortex at a lateral angle of 45 degrees. They proposed that a more medial 30-degree S1 insertion is safer because of a wider safe zone. Dohring and Krag[8] found that the safe zones for both anterolaterally oriented alar screws or anteromedially oriented promontory screws were unusably small and pointed out that the neurovascular structures near the midline were less important than those in front of the ala. In addition, they showed that anteromedial screws have a bone-screw interface stiffness that is twice as great as that of anterolateral screws.

The question of whether the risk of neurovascular damage from anterior cortical penetration is large enough to offset the presumed benefit of the greater strength that is probably achieved has not yet been answered. However, risk reduction can be achieved by certain intraoperative steps. Steffee[41] recommended inserting a Steinmann pin slowly and carefully to and then through the anterior sacral cortex using a mallet. At each strike of the mallet, the sound pitch, the vibration detected by the fingertips holding the pin, and the amount of pin advancement are monitored; at pin contact with the anterior cortex, the pitch rises, the vibration increases, and the advancement slows.[20] At cortical breakthrough, the pitch and vibration are reduced. At this point, the Steinmann pin is advanced no further. The intent is to engage the anterior sacral cortex without perforating the periosteum (although Weinstein and colleagues[47] recommended inserting the screw tip 1 to 2 mm anterior to the cortex). This technique may be less reliable in osteoporotic bone. In more than 500 cases of bicortical sacral screw fixation, the authors have had no complications related to screw insertion using this method.

Using a drill in the sacrum should be avoided. Using a tap when the anterior cortex is crossed should also be avoided. Mirkovic and coworkers[28] recommended the use of self-tapping screws with recessed flutes. They also advised palpating the medial side of the hole with the foot of the depth gauge until it emerges on the anterior cortex. The screws inserted past the sacral alar anterior cortex should not be sharp, but rather blunt tipped, and should have tapered distal threads.

During spine surgery in which pedicle screws are used, neurologic complications can be caused by events other than pedicle screw insertion. They may occur when a spinal deformity such as scoliosis or spondylolisthesis is corrected. The potential for such a complication is greater with pedicle screw systems because of the improved mechanical control that they provide of vertebral realignment. In the case of scoliosis or spondylolisthesis, distraction may result in excessive stretching of neural elements. In the case of spondylolisthesis, the risk of nerve root compression from osteophytes, fibrous tissue, and disc material is increased, especially with long-standing higher-grade spondylolisthesis and secondary changes such as severe foraminal stenosis. Meticulous examination, canal exploration, and adequate decompression must be performed before and after reduction and instrumentation. If reduction is planned, it should be carried out gradually and carefully.

It is important to remember that neural injuries are known complications of spine surgery even when no implants are used. During fracture reduction and stabilization, the spinal cord, the conus, and the cauda equina as well as the nerve roots may be injured further, especially when they are already inflamed and swollen from the initial injury. All neural elements are sensitive to manipulation and retraction. Increased epidural bleeding may also compound the problem. Spinal cord or conus retraction should be avoided. Instead, a pedicle may be removed or an alternative surgical approach used. Other injuries can occur in the course of spinal canal exploration, decompression, and fracture reduction. Nerve root compressions from bone graft and even paraplegia from postoperative epidural hematoma have been reported.[32, 42]

Vascular

Pedicle screw strength has been shown by Krag and colleagues[18, 20, 22] to increase gradually with depth of vertebral penetration up to the anterior cortex. The strength of screw placement through the cortex was not tested. The authors conjectured that a closer approach by the tip of the screw (or drill or tap) to the anterior cortex presented a greater risk of unintentional penetration through it. To reduce this risk, they described an intraoperative radiographic method ("near-approach" view).[20] Anterior cortex penetration carries the risk of injury to vascular, visceral, neural, and ureteral structures. The depth or distance of anterior perforation, the mobility of the adjacent structures, the size of the screw, and the sharpness of the screw thread or screw tip all have an influence on this risk.

The incidence of anterior perforation by pedicle screws is not known. It is probably higher than usually appreciated. Whitecloud and associates[51] and Krag and coworkers[20] showed that a true lateral roentgenogram is not accurate for detecting pedicle screw penetration of the vertebral anterior cortex. Whitecloud and associates[51] showed that the greatest discrepancy between roentgenographic appearance and actual penetration was for screw insertions at the L4 and L5 levels. At 50% apparent depth of penetration on lateral roentgenograms, the screw may be safely assumed not to have perforated the anterior cortex. At 80% apparent depth, there is a 30% probability of cortical perforation at L4 and a 10% probability at L5. At 100% apparent depth, there is almost a 100% probability of perforation.

Inadvertent puncture of a major blood vessel often causes bleeding, which may result in death. Formation of a hematoma, a false aneurysm, or a fistula may also occur. Thrombus formation and embolism[1] may result from vascular irritation by the part of the screw inside the blood vessel.

Perforation of an artery may result in rapid hemorrhage, which can be fatal if an emergency laparotomy is not performed to repair the vessel. Injuries to the aorta occur at or above the L4 level. Injuries to the common iliac arteries can occur at L5 or S1 from perforations of the anterolateral cortex.[1] Much smaller arteries are present at the midline than at the alar portion of the sacrum.[8]

In the case of venous perforation, the intravascular pressure may affect the outcome. Intravenous pressure is influenced by different patient positions. Wayne[45] showed that the lowest pressure is found with the patient in the tuck position or knee-elbow prone position. Lower intravenous pressure results in less bleeding. Anda and colleagues[1] showed that the inferior vena cava and common pelvic veins have large transverse diameters and lie closer to the vertebral cortex than do the arteries. These major venous structures form a broad band. Their walls are much thinner than the walls of arteries and thus they are probably injured more frequently in spine surgery. Injury to both a vein and artery may result in arteriovenous fistula. Anda and coworkers[1] demonstrated six typical configurations of the vascular anatomy to explain the types of vascular complications seen at the L3–L4 and L4–L5 levels. They also showed the transverse prevertebral vascular anatomy at the L5–S1 level. Usually at the L3 level the vena cava and the aorta have not divided, so at this level a right pedicle screw perforation tends to injure the vena cava and a left pedicle screw the aorta. Arterial or venous injuries can occur at the L4 or the L5 level, although the venous injuries are probably more likely.

Visceral

In addition to vascular and neural structures, visceral and ureteral structures can also be damaged by anterior cortical penetration by pedicle screws. The sigmoid colon is located anterior to the L5, S1, and S2 levels. The colon with its mesentery enters the pelvis from the left and remains mobile at the level of S1 and S2. At about the S3 level, the mesentery is no longer found and the rectosigmoid colon is located directly over the sacral surface anteriorly.[28] Bowel perforations can occur with deeply inserted sharp probes, drill bits, depth gauges, taps, and screws and may cause peritonitis. Gas-filled intestine was found by Anda and colleagues[1] to be located closer to the spine when the patient was in the prone position than in other positions. Presumably, sharp instruments and pedicle screws may perforate an air-filled gut more readily than a deflated gut not only because the former is located more posteriorly, but also because it has a larger diameter and its wall is under more tension. In spine surgery, most gut injuries occur at the L5–S1 level.[15, 37–39]

TECHNICAL COMPLICATIONS

In addition to screw penetration through the cortex of the pedicle or the anterior part of the vertebral body, other technical problems encountered in the use of pedicle screw instrumentation include screw breakage, bending, loosening, or cutout; nut loosening; coupling failure; rod breakage; and insufficient screw length, size, or thread type.

The design, material, and manufacturing methods for screws may each contribute to early failure of the implant. In the case of the Steffee system, screw failure was common with the early-generation devices. Steffee and colleagues reported eight implant problems out of 128 cases.[42] These included screw breakage, loosening, and migration. Zucherman and coworkers reported broken screws in 23% of 77 cases in an early series.[56] Screw breakage seems to occur more commonly with greater intervertebral motion, a greater disc height, or less anterior

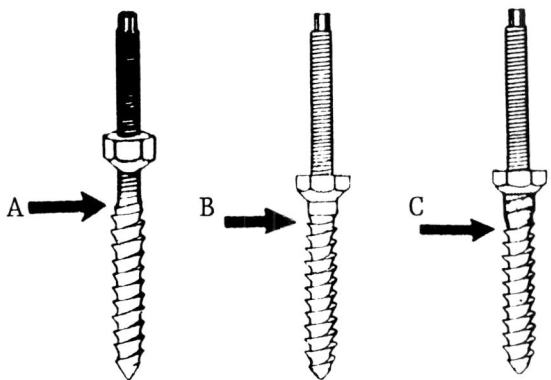

Figure 1. *A*, With the first-generation screw, which did not contain an integrated nut, failure occurred at the junction of the bone and the machine threads. *B*, With the second-generation screw, which contained the integrated nut, failure occurred at the junction of the bone thread and the integrated nut. *C*, With the third-generation screw, which has a tapered root diameter in the bone thread area adjacent to the nut, failure occurs at the end of the taper.

column load sharing. These circumstances probably contribute to greater stresses on both the screws and the screw-plate junction. In another study of the Steffee system, Davne and Myers[5] reported screw breakage after 4.3% of their 533 surgical procedures (1.1% of the 2642 screws placed). Screw design improvements explain the higher rate of breakage early in the series and the reduced rate later in the series.[44] The first-generation screw (Fig. 1A), which did not have an integral ventral nut, typically failed at the junction of the bone and the machine threads. The second-generation screw (Fig. 1B), which did have an integral nut, typically failed at the junction of the bone thread and the nut. The third-generation screw (Fig. 1C) has a root diameter that gradually tapers down from the nut to a point partway along the screw shaft and then does not decrease further. For this screw, breakage typically occurred at the end of the taper. Anterior or posterior interbody bone grafts probably reduce stress on the implant. Yashiro and colleagues[53] showed a 14% screw breakage rate with posterolateral grafts and no breakage with posterior interbody grafts. Tradeoffs between the increased morbidity from the additional surgery and the biomechanical benefits remain to be established. Also, improvement of implant design to reduce screw breakage without additional grafting is another avenue that remains open.

It is commonly assumed that a secure connection between the screw and the plate or rod leads to a greater risk of fatigue failure, although this has not yet been established. Certainly, systems with less secure connections are also subject to this problem. In a series of 84 patients treated with the Roy-Camille system of plates and unlocked screws, Roy-Camille and colleagues[34] reported 25% of the distal screws broke 5 to 24 months after stabilization of lumbar fractures and that sacral screws failed most frequently. In his series of 101 cases treated with a similar system, Louis[25] reported that eight screws broke and six screws loosened in the first 36 months after surgery. It is unknown whether implant failure causes nonunion, whether nonunion causes implant failure, or whether no cause-and-effect relationship exists.

It is important not to weaken the screw by bending it.[29] For implant systems in which the screw is locked to the plate, this can happen if the screw is not locally perpendicular to the plate (Fig. 2). Even if plastic deformation of the screw does not occur, the greater the deviation from the perpendicular, the greater is the cantilever bending load applied to the screw when the locking nut is tightened (Fig. 3). In actual clinical practice, perpendicular alignment is rarely achieved. Matsuzaki and coworkers[26] demonstrated that the application of a 32-kg force at a distance of 27 mm from the plate resulted in a 5-degree deviation of the screw away

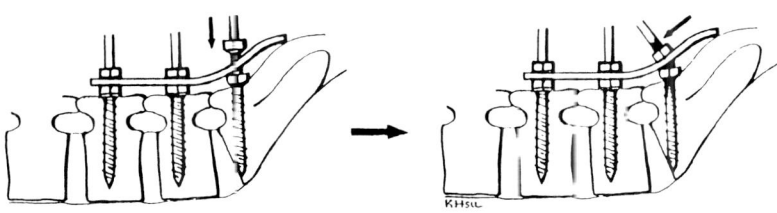

Figure 2. Variance of plate screw angle from 90 degrees can result in screw weakening and bending.

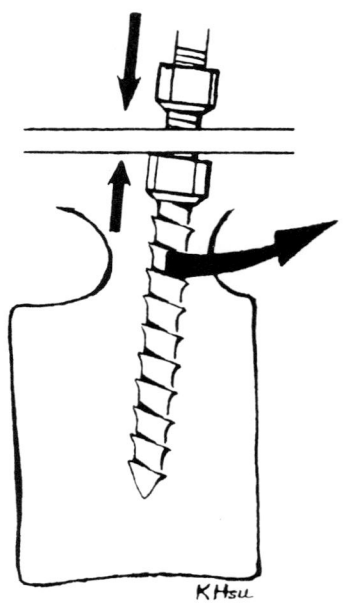 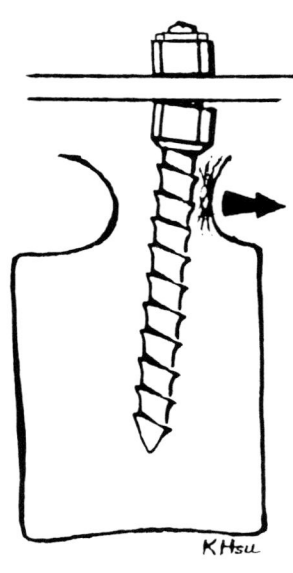

Figure 3. Tightening of the nuts when the screw is set in position varying from 90 degrees in relationship to the plate results in a unidirectional torque that may cause screw weakening and delayed pedicle erosion or fracture.

from perpendicular. Thus, if the screw-plate malalignment is 5 degrees, after the lock nut is tightened the screw tip is exposed to a load of 32 kg. To reduce this problem, they recommended a number of practical improvements.[26] One of these was to increase the width of the slot by 1 mm to accommodate screws that are less than perfectly aligned. Another recommendation was to develop a spherical "nest" in the plate or to recess both the upper and lower surfaces of the plate to allow more choice in alignment of a screw, the integral nut of which would have an upper surface that is spherical (Fig. 4).

Rather than cause screw bending, tightening of the locking nut on a nonperpendicular screw may instead change the intervertebral alignment, which may result in foraminal stenosis (Fig. 5). It is important that the nerve root foramen be examined and gently probed after completion of the instrumentation to be sure that no stenosis is produced and also that bone graft has not been squeezed into the lateral neural canal by the plate. If questions remain, the nerve root should be inspected carefully and adequate decompression performed, if necessary. The nerve root is followed out past its foramen to ensure adequate decompression. Steffee recommended nerve root decompression until a 6-mm probe can be passed through the neural foramen.[42, 44]

The plate should be contoured appropriately to maintain normal lumbar lordosis and to prevent undesirable hardware prominences, especially over the sacrum. Wedged washers (Fig. 6) are helpful in obtaining good plate alignment and fit. Washers of appropriate height can also prevent plate impingement on the adjacent normal facet joints (Fig. 7).

In the authors' early experience, the vertebrae with instrumentation were locked in distraction.[56] It was suspected that distraction placed a constant unidirectional torque on the screw against one wall of the pedicle, possibly resulting in erosion, migration of the screw, or pedicle fracture (Fig. 8). Pedicle fracture occurred intraoperatively in some osteopenic patients. Distraction at one segment may cause compression of adjacent segments that are included in the construct (Fig. 9), resulting in disc narrowing and foraminal stenosis to the instrumented level above or below.

The use of rod systems, even those without three-dimensional adjustability between the screw and the rod (e.g., Isola), may be less likely to result in screw bending, because the rod can be more easily contoured than a plate. Rod systems with three-dimensional adjustability (e.g., Vermont spinal fixator) virtually eliminate the screw bending problem, because any screw-rod align-

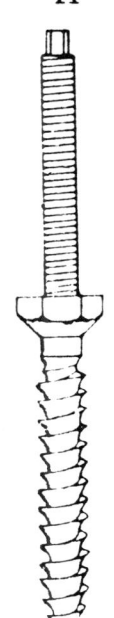 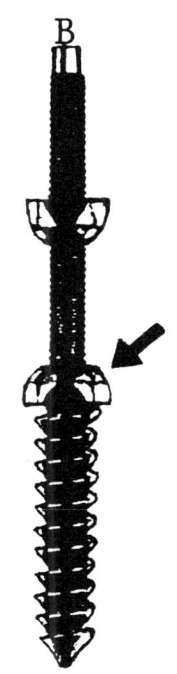

Figure 4. *A*, Standard VSP screw. *B*, Modified pedicle screw with nuts containing spherical upper surfaces to fill the nest on the lower surface of the plate. These may be tightened in different directions, not even perpendicular to the plate.

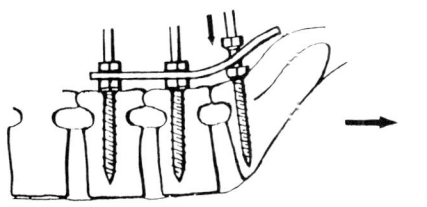 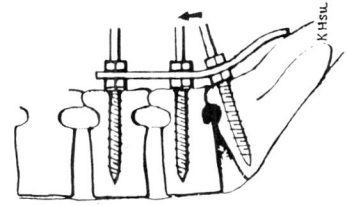

Figure 5. Nuts do not lock until the screw finds a stable position over a sharply curved plate. Foraminal stenosis may be produced by this mechanism.

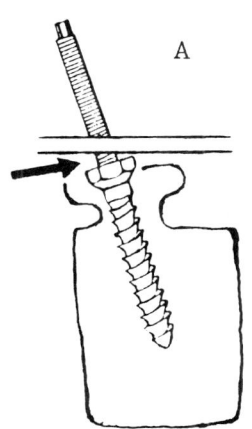 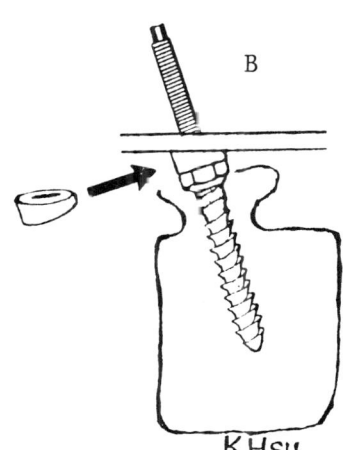

Figure 6. *A*, When the screw is not perpendicular to the plate, eccentric torque stress is generated against the pedicle. Significant bending stress is also generated against the screw when the posterior nut is tightened to the plate. *B*, A wedge-shaped washer improves the fit of the screw nut to the plate and reduces such stresses.

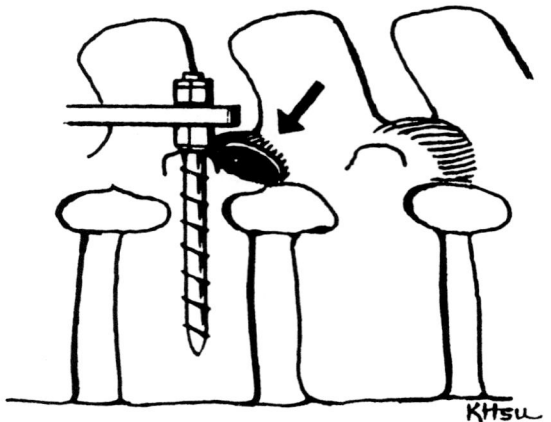

Figure 7. When a screw is inserted into the pedicle, the adjacent facet is often violated.

ment is accommodated even without any component bending.

Screw-plate loosening was reported by Davne and Myers[5] to occur in 5.6% of screws in their series. This problem may be simply a result of inadequate tightening of the nuts or other connectors to the rods or plates. As mentioned previously, secure screw-plate fixation with the Steffee system can be achieved by use of an appropriate washer (angled or straight). Perhaps pedicle fracturing or erosion contributes to screw-plate loosening (by causing increased loading of the screw-plate interface), although it is also possible that fracturing or erosion tends to happen with screws that are malaligned to the plate and not securely attached to the plate initially. For systems in

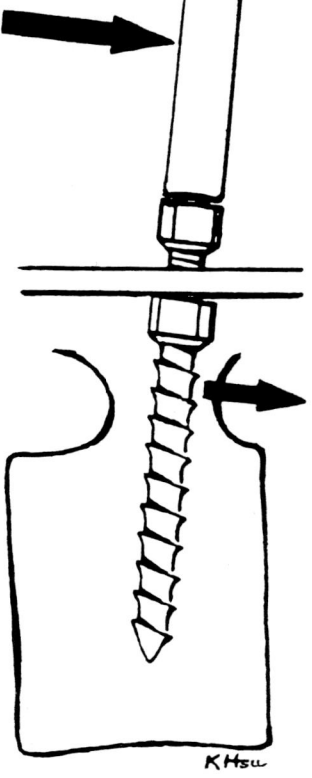

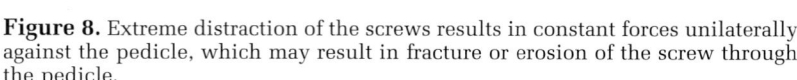

Figure 8. Extreme distraction of the screws results in constant forces unilaterally against the pedicle, which may result in fracture or erosion of the screw through the pedicle.

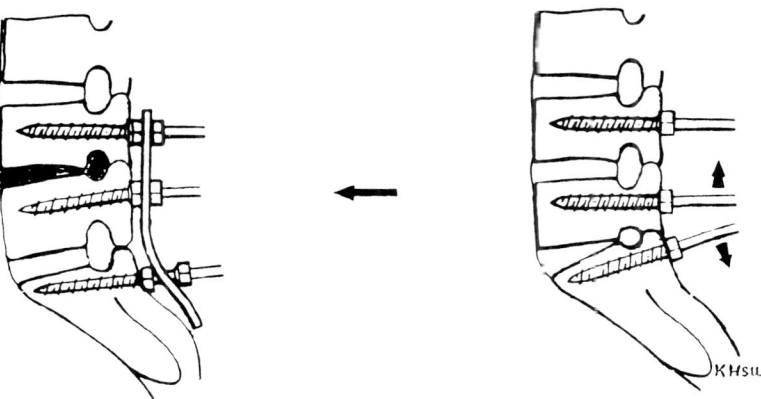

Figure 9. Distraction of one vertebral segment may result in stenosis of adjacent segments.

which three-dimensional adjustability exists between the screw and the rod, malalignment is generally a much smaller problem, because the rod can meet the screw at any angle. If only two screws per side are used, no rod bending is required. With the Steffee system, the nut sometimes cannot be adequately tightened to the plate or the rod because the screw tends to rotate or loosen in the bone. The cannulated wrench (Fig. 10) is useful in controlling this problem by holding the screw stationary while the nut is tightened to the proper torque.

Screw-bone interface loosening is another technical problem that can occur, usually in the absence of screw-rod or screw-plate loosening. A contributing factor in the Steffee system may be the application of high cantilever bending loads when the nut is tightened on a screw that is not perpendicular to the plate (see Fig. 3). Another factor is screw placement through the pedicle cortex: even though no neurologic damage may result, the screw-bone interface is weakened. Yet other factors may be screw length and diameter, which provide insufficient screw-bone interface strength successfully to resist the loads imposed on the vertebra. The importance of each of these factors remains to be clearly established. Yet another factor is bone quality (discussed below).

POSTOPERATIVE COMPLICATIONS

Infection

Infection rates have tended to be high, about 4% to 8%, especially in the initial clinical series on transpedicle fixation systems.[11, 42, 50, 56] More recent series show improvements of 0.5% to 2%.[2, 5, 10, 48, 49] Esses and associates, in a 1992 polling of American Back Society surgeons, found an incidence of 4.2% in more than 600 cases.[10]

The probable reasons for increased infections are many in this population and include the large surface area of the implants, the long operative time, the use of image intensifiers, multiple previous operations with poorly vascularized tissue, occult pre-existing indolent infections, a vast array of instrumentation on the back table used for the procedures, the large wounds necessary for adequate exposure, tissue necrosis from retractors, and postoperative hematoma.[50, 56]

Efforts at preventing infection should be performed as carefully as those for total joint arthroplasty. Measures that may be helpful include using laminar flow rooms, presoaking implants in antibiotic solution, keeping implants covered before use, and débriding devitalized tissue adjacent to retractors before closure. Careful hemostasis should help to reduce hematoma size. Careful closure to reduce dead space is also probably important. Suction drains are widely used, although their benefit here or in total joint replacement surgery has not been clearly established in the literature. Preoperative and postoperative administration of antibiotics is indicated. If the C-arm image intensifier is used, it should be sterilely draped and contamination carefully avoided. Operating room traffic should be minimized.

An important cause of failed back surgery in patients who undergo multiple procedures is an indolent infection that does not

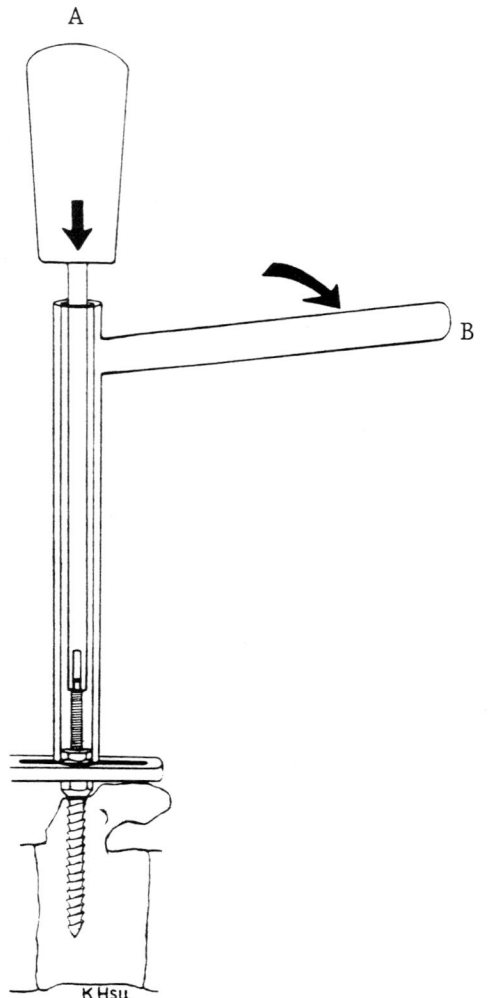

Figure 10. To prevent the screw from stripping and rotating in the bone, the double-wrench technique is effective. The pedicle screw is held stationary by wrench A, which is inside a larger wrench B, which tightens the posterior tapered nut.

produce the usual clinical symptoms or signs. Such infections are usually caused by anaerobic bacteria. An indolent infection may be manifested only by edematous fibrotic tissue in the previous surgery site. A high level of suspicion should be maintained and specimens for cultures should be routinely taken in this situation. Direct consultation with microbiology personnel prevents organisms such as diphtheroids, which are frequently presumed to be contaminants, from not being reported in the culture results, even though they may be present.[35, 57] Aggressive, specific antibiotic treatment may well result in good relief of back pain.

Pseudarthrosis

Although a pseudarthrosis is not necessarily painful, the chances for pain relief are greater when a solid fusion is achieved. However, fusion solidity is frequently difficult to evaluate and is even more difficult to assess when metallic pedicle implants are in place. The posterolateral gutters are obscured by overlying instrumentation, and bending x-ray films are often not helpful because the amount of motion lag by the implants is too minimal to be appreciated. This minimum motion, however, is frequently not clinically tolerated.[12, 59] Imaging studies are obscured by the metallic implants. Anteroposterior radiographs may show confluent fusion masses, yet the anterior elements are not immobilized if they are not really joined to the fusion masses. Even direct open posterior exploration of the fusion masses may be deceptive for the same reason. All of these factors suggest that the rate of bony solid fusions may not be as high as reported.[59]

In patients with persistent postoperative problems, symptoms related to maintaining a static posture or a clicking sound at the surgical site may indicate pseudarthrosis, even though it may not be demonstrated by radiographic studies.[5] Other indicators of pseudarthrosis are delayed periscrew lucency ("windshield wiper" effect) and implant fracture.

Steffee suggested the use of interbody bone grafting along with pedicle fixation. This results in anterior load sharing and much less load transfer to the implant. Using this technique, Hsu and Zucherman[13] reported solid fusion in 49 of 50 failed back surgery cases with multiple procedures, as judged by interbody graft confluence. This compares favorably with other series of mixed patient populations in which the pseudarthrosis rates were greater than 11%[56]; 32%[11]; 11%[2]; and 16%.[48] Interbody grafting should be considered in addition to pedicle fixation when the anterior column is destabilized by fracture, tumor, or extensive discectomy.

Juxtafusion Deterioration

The long-term effect of spinal fusion on adjacent motion segments is an increasing concern, especially with the use of rigid metal fixation. Symptoms may eventually develop at the proximal or the distal end of a fusion. They may be caused by disc degeneration, herniation, facet arthropathy, degenerative stenosis, segmental instability, spondylolisthesis or retrospondylolisthesis at the adjacent unfused segment.[14] The biomechanical processes that promote this accelerated juxtafusion deterioration have been studied in vitro as well as in vivo.[22]

Hsu and Zucherman[14] observed more early juxtafusion breakdown in patients with rigid metal fixation compared with those with no fixation. Whether this quicker onset of breakdown is a result of implant rigidity or instead is caused by surgically induced or implant-induced facet degeneration remains to be established. Bony fusion alone may produce a segmental stiffness so much greater than that of a normal disc that the incremental stiffness from addition of metal fixation is relatively small.[22]

Compression fractures at the adjacent unfused vertebrae have occurred in three of the authors' patients after multilevel fusions with pedicle screw fixation. Juxtafusion stress concentration is greater in multilevel fusions. Loss of normal lumbar lordosis greatly accelerates juxtafusion breakdown, probably because of compensatory hyperextension of the adjacent unfused segment with resultant facet overload and degeneration. Sacroiliac irritation, degeneration, or instability may also develop when a lumbar fusion is extended distally into the sacrum.

The normal facet joint proximal to the instrumented fusion must be protected. The facet joint may be violated during pedicle screw insertion because of the close proximity of the facet joint to the pedicle. The inferior aspect of the facet joint is located directly over the pedicle. Avoidance of this facet joint may be aided by using an entry point as inferolateral as possible (without breaking out through the pedicle cortex) and an orientation that is cephalad and medial ("up and in") as described in Biomechanics of Transpedicle Spine Fixation. Facet impingement (see Fig. 7) may also be aggravated by a larger screw or plate. The application of spacing washers below the plate prevents plate impingement on the normal facet joints.

If the anterolateral orientation for sacral screws is used, care should be exercised to avoid placing the screws too far lateral into the sacroiliac joint. Louis[25] reported four sacroiliac penetrations in his series. Violation of the sacroiliac joint may result in postoperative pain or eventual degenerative arthritis.

OTHER FACTORS

Osteoporosis

Screw loosening, pedicle fracture, loss of alignment, and pseudarthrosis all appear to be more likely after pedicle screw fixation into osteopenic bone than into normal bone. Bone mineral density has been shown to correlate with screw pullout strength.[3, 4, 33, 40, 52, 54] Pullout strength and cycles to failure were linearly related to insertional torque, which may provide a useful intraoperative method for assessing screw-holding capacity.[3, 4, 40, 52, 54] Zdeblick and colleagues[54] did not use pedicle fixation if screw insertion torque was less than 4 inch-pounds. They also showed the importance of pedicle diameter: small pedicles provide greater strength by thread purchase in the endosteal cortex; large pedicles probably provide the highest risk for implant loosening.[54] Coe and associates[4] found lamina hooks resisted posteriorly directed forces better than did pedicle screws in osteoporotic patients. Okayama and coworkers[30] and McBroom and colleagues[27] found quantitative computed tomographic scanning to be more accurate than dual-energy absorptiometry. Vertebrae with an average bone mineral density of 95 mg/ml present a high risk for transpedicle screw loosening, and those with a density of 130 mg/ml present a moderate risk.[30] Pfeifer and coworkers[33] found that midinsertion torque provided a good assessment of the strength produced by reconstruction of a stripped-out thread using cancellous morcellized bone graft.

These studies suggest that preoperative evaluation of pedicle size and bone mineral density may be helpful in the treatment of osteoporotic patients. Polymethyl methacrylate can be used to strengthen the screw insertion site; however, there is risk of thermal or mechanical injury to neural elements and other problems discussed previously.[16, 47, 55] Screw placement techniques are especially important in osteoporotic patients, and careful visualization (directly or radiographically) of the caudal, medial, and cephalic aspects of the pedicle is important in optimum screw placement.

Sacral screw fixation strength has been shown to be increased by anterior cortex engagement, and Weinstein and coworkers[47] believe that it is appropriate in osteoporotic patients.[47] Some surgeons routinely engage the anterior cortex by an anteromedial approach in situations in which there is possibly inadequate sacral fixation. The risk of vascular and neural damage should be kept in mind during screw placement through the anterior sacral cortex.

A suggestive relationship between osteoporosis and pseudarthrosis has been shown by Schofferman and coworkers.[36] If this turns out to be significant and if an underlying cause of osteoporosis can be identified and corrected preoperatively, the pseudarthrosis risk should be lowered.

Implant Intolerance

Although most of the pedicle screw systems are relatively bulky, in general implants are well tolerated by patients. Occasionally, the instrumentation must be removed because of significant prominence, painful bursa formation, metal sensitivity, or impingement on the adjacent unfused level.

Some spinal implants may be excessively prominent in thin individuals and may cause pressure problems. Skin irritation or a pressure sore may be aggravated by external immobilization. Screw and rod ends as well as plates curved over the sacrum sometimes create such problems. Further lowering of the hardware profile is desirable. Careful attention should be paid to implant prominence during surgery before the wound is closed. Where relevant, the bolt ends should be cut as short as possible using appropriate end or side bolt cutters. Special pedicle screw cutters (AcroMed, Synthes) are now available. Screw ends can also be filed or burred with a diamond tip, although the debris in the wound is undesirable. Implant prominence may be increased by pelvic or spinal deformity. Postoperative braces should be carefully adjusted accordingly.

A prominent implant may lead to significant aching and tenderness, often with formation of a bursa. Injection of local anesthetic into the bursa often reproduces the pain initially, followed by relief.

Persistent discomfort may be the result of metal sensitivity or an allergic reaction. Unusual dermatitis may also develop, although this is rare. Tissue reaction to metal ions may cause problems in perhaps 1% of cases, possibly because of the nickel in the stainless steel, according to Edwards and coworkers.[9] Implant removal should provide relief. Titanium-based alloys may produce an even lower incidence of tissue reaction. They are more resistant to mechanical fatigue and to corrosion in a chloride environment. The protective surface of titanium is highly inert and re-forms rapidly after damage. The modulus of elasticity of titanium is lower than that of stainless steel. The effect of titanium on postoperative magnetic resonance imaging scans is less problematic than that of stainless steel. There is ongoing research in the improved use of different alloys in spinal instrumentation.

Removal of the implant may be useful when it impinges on adjacent unfused segments. However, implant removal should be delayed, if feasible, until the fusion is solid. Edwards and coworkers[9] believe that surgical removal should be deferred beyond the time when newly formed bone remains plastic, usually more than 12 months postoperatively.

REFERENCES

1. Anda, S., Aakhus, S., Skaanes, K., et al.: Anterior perforations in lumbar discectomies. A report of four cases of vascular complications and a CT study of the prevertebral lumbar anatomy. Spine 16:54–60, 1991.
2. Blumenthal, S.: Complications of the Wiltse pedicle screw fixation system. Spine 18:1867–1871, 1993.
3. Carlson, G. D., Abitbol, J. J., Anderson, D. R., et al.: Screw fixation in the human sacrum. Spine 17:S196–S203, 1992.
4. Coe, J. D., Warden, K. E., Herzig, M. A., et al.: Influence of bone mineral density on the fixation of thoracolumbar implants. Spine 15:902–907, 1990.
5. Davne, S., and Myers, D.: Complication of lumbar spine fusion with transpedicular instrumentation. Spine 17:S184–S189, 1992.
6. Dick, W.: The "fixateur interne" as a versatile implant for spine surgery. Spine 12:882–900, 1985.

7. Dick, W., Kluger, P., Magerl, F., et al.: A new device for internal fixation of thoracolumbar and lumbar spine fractures: The "fixateur interne." Paraplegia 23:225–232, 1985.
8. Dohring, E. J., and Krag, M. H.: Sacral screw fixation: A morphologic, anatomic, and mechanical study. In Proceedings of the American Academy of Orthopaedic Surgeons 58th Annual Meeting, Anaheim, CA, March 8, 1991, p. 144.
9. Edwards, C., Boston, C. Levine, A., et al.: Complications associated with posterior instrumentation for thoracolumbar injuries and their prevention. Semin. Spine Surg. 5:108–122, 1993.
10. Esses, S. I., Sachs, B. L., and Dreyzin, V.: Complications associated with the technique of pedicle screw fixation. Spine 18:2231–2239, 1993.
11. Horowitch, A., Peek, R. D., Thomas, J. C., Jr., et al.: The Wiltse pedicle screw fixation system: Early clinical results. Spine 14:461–467, 1989.
12. Hsu, K. Y., and Zucherman, J. F.: Pseudarthrosis of lumbar spine fusions—origin of pain and treatment (abstract). In Proceedings of the International Society for Study of the Lumbar Spine, Toronto, May 1989.
13. Hsu, K. Y., and Zucherman, J. F.: Combined anterior interbody and posterior lateral lumbar spine fusion with plate fixation for severe instability and resistant pseudarthrosis. Presented at the Fifth International Conference on Lumbar Fusion and Stabilization, Osaka, Japan, November 8, 1991.
14. Hsu, K. Y., and Zucherman, J. F.: The long-term effect of lumbar spine fusion: Deterioration of adjacent motion segments. In Yonenobu, K., Ono, K., and Takemitsu, Y. (eds.): Lumbar Spinal Fusion and Stabilization. Berlin, Springer-Verlag, 1993, pp. 54–64.
15. Kollbrunner, F.: Dickdarmstenose nach Laminektomie. Gastroenterologia 92:239–251, 1959.
16. Kostuik, J. P., Errico, T. J., and Gleason, T. F.: Techniques of internal fixation for degenerative conditions of the lumbar spine. Clin. Orthop. 203:219–231, 1986.
17. Krag, M. H., Beynnon, B. D., Pope, M. H., et al.: An internal fixator for posterior application to short segments of the thoracic, lumbar, or lumbosacral spine: Design and testing. Clin. Orthop. 203:75–98, 1986.
18. Krag, M. H., Beynnon, B. D., and Pope, M. H.: Depth of insertion of transpedicular vertebral screws into human vertebrae: Effect upon screw-vertebrae interface strength. J. Spinal Disord. 1:287–294, 1988.
19. Krag, M. H., Weaver, D. L., Beynnon, B. D., and Haugh, L. D.: Morphometry of the thoracic and lumbar spine related to transpedicular screw placement for surgical spinal fixation. Spine 13:27–32, 1988.
20. Krag, M. H., Van Hal, M. E., and Beynnon, B. D.: Placement of transpedicular vertebral screws close to anterior vertebral cortex: Description of methods. Spine 14:879–883, 1989.
21. Krag, M. H., Van Hal, M. E., and Beynnon, B. D.: Clinical experience with Vermont spinal fixator (VSF): Initial 46 cases. In Proceedings of the North American Spine Society 4th Annual Meeting, Quebec City, Quebec, 1989, pp. 126–127.
22. Krag, M. H.: Biomechanics of transpedicle spinal fixation. In Weinstein, J. N., and Wiesel, S. (eds.): The Lumbar Spine. Philadelphia, W. B. Saunders, 1990, pp. 916–940.
23. Krag, M. H.: The Vermont spinal fixator. In An, H. S., and Cotler, J. M. (eds.): Spinal Instrumentation. Baltimore, Williams & Wilkins, 1992, pp. 237–255.
24. Krag, M. H.: The Vermont spinal fixator. In Lonstein, J., and Arnold, D. (eds.): Internal Pedicular Fixation of the Lumbar Spine. Spine: State of the Art Review. Philadelphia, Hanley & Belfus, 1992.
25. Louis, R.: Fusion of the lumbar and sacral spine by internal fixation with screw plates. Clin. Orthop. 203:18–33, 1986.
26. Matsuzaki, H., Tokuhashi, Y., Matsumoto, F., et al.: Problems and solutions of pedicle screw plate fixation of lumbar spine. Spine 15:1159–1165, 1990.
27. McBroom, R. J., Hayes, W. C. Edwards, W. T., et al.: Prediction of vertebral body compressive fracture using quantitative computed tomography. J. Bone Joint Surg. 67A:1206–1214, 1985.
28. Mirkovic, S., Abitbol, J., Steinman, J., et al.: Anatomic consideration for sacral screw placement. Spine 16(suppl. 6):S289–S294, 1991.
29. Moran, J. M., Berg, W. S., Berry, J. L., et al.: Transpedicular screw fixation. J. Orthop. Res. 7:107–114, 1989.
30. Okayama, K., Suto, K., Abe, E., et al.: Stability of transpedicle screwing for the osteoporotic spine. Spine 18:S242–S245, 1993.
31. Ölerud, S., Karlström, G., and Sjöström, L.: Transpedicular fixation of thoracolumbar vertebral fractures. Clin. Orthop. 227:44–51, 1988.
32. Peek, R. D., Thomas, J. C., Weinstein, J., et al.: Lumbar spine fusion with pedicle screw and rods. Presented at the International Society for the Study of the Lumbar Spine Meeting, Bal Harbour, FL, April 1988.
33. Pfeifer, B. A., Krag, M. H., and Johnson, C. C.: A biomechanical study comparing insertion torque with pullout strength in pedicle screws. In Proceedings of the North American Spine Society 7th Annual Meeting, Boston, July 9–11, 1992, pp. 108–109.
34. Roy-Camille, R., Saillant, G., and Mazel, C.: Internal fixation of the lumbar spine with pedicle screw plating. Clin. Orthop. 203:7–17, 1986.
35. Schofferman, L., Schofferman, J., Zucherman, J. F., et al.: Occult infection causing persistent low-back pain. Spine 14:417–419, 1989
36. Schofferman, J., Zucherman, J. F., Schofferman, L., et al.: Metabolic bone disease in lumbar pseudarthrosis. Spine 15:687–689, 1990.
37. Schwartz, A. M., and Brodskey, J. S.: Bowel perforation following microsurgical lumbar discectomy. Spine 14:104–105, 1989.
38. Shaw, E. D., Scarborough, J. T., and Beals, R. K.: Bowel injury as a complication of lumbar discectomy. J. Bone Joint Surg. 63A:478–480, 1981.
39. Smith, R. A., and Estridge, M. N.: Bowel perforation following lumbar disc surgery. J. Bone Joint Surg. 46A:826–828, 1964.
40. Soshi, S., Shiba, R., Kondo, H. and Murota, K.: An experimental study on transpedicular screw fixation in relation to osteoporosis of the lumbar spine. Spine 16:1335–1341, 1991.
41. Steffee, A. D.: Personal communication, 1984.
42. Steffee, A. D., Biscup, R. S., and Sitkowski, D. J.: Segmental spine plates with pedicle screw fixation:

A new internal fixation device for disorders of the lumbar spine and thoracolumbar spine. Clin. Orthop. 203:45–53, 1986.
43. Steffee, A. D., and Sitkowski, D. J.: Posterior lumbar interbody fusion and plates. Clin. Orthop. 227:99–102, 1988.
44. Steffee, A. D., and Brantigan, J. W.: The variable screw placement spinal fixation system. Spine 18:1160–1172, 1993.
45. Wayne, S. J.: The tuck position for lumbar disc surgery. J. Bone Joint Surg. 49A:1195–1198, 1967.
46. Weinstein, J. N., Spratt, K. F., Spengler, D., et al.: Spinal pedicle fixation: Reliability and validity of roentgenogram-based assessment and surgical factors on successful screw placement. Spine 13:1012–1018, 1988.
47. Weinstein, J. N., Rydevik, B. L., and Rauschning, W.: Anatomic and technical considerations of pedicle screw fixation. Clin. Orthop. 284:34–46, 1992.
48. West, J. L., III, Bradford, D. S., and Ogilvie, J. W.: Results of spinal arthrodesis with pedicle screwplate fixation. J. Bone Joint Surg. 73A:1179–1184, 1991.
49. West, J. L., III, Ogilvie, J. W., and Bradford, D. S.: Complications of the variable screw plate pedicle screw fixation. Spine 16:576–579, 1991.
50. Whitecloud, T. S., III, Butler, J. C., Cohen, J. L., et al.: Complications with the variable spinal plating system. Spine 14:472–476, 1989.
51. Whitecloud, T. S., III, Skalley, T., Morgan, E., et al.: Roentgenographic measurement of pedicle screw penetration (abstract). International Society for Study of the Lumbar Spine, Kyoto, Japan, May 1989.
52. Yamagata, M., Kitahara, H., Minami, S., et al.: Mechanical stability of the pedicle screw fixation systems for the lumbar spine. Spine 17:S51, 1992.
53. Yashiro, K., Homma, T., Hokari, Y., et al.: Steffee variable screw placement system using different methods of bone grafting. Spine 16:1329–1334, 1991.
54. Zdeblick, T. A., Kunz, D. N., Cooke, M. E., et al.: Pedicle screw pullout strength, correlation with insertional torque. Spine 18:1673–1676, 1993.
55. Zindrick, M. R., Patwardhan, A., and Lorenz, M.: The effect of methylmethacrylate augmentation upon pedicle screw fixation in the spine. Presented at the International Society for Study of the Lumbar Spine, Dallas, TX, 1986.
56. Zucherman, J. F., Hsu, K., White, A., et al.: Early results of spinal fusion using variable spine plating system. Spine 13:570–579, 1988.
57. Zucherman, J. F., Schofferman, L., Gunthorpe, H., et al.: Diphtheroid and associated infections as a cause of failed lumbar instrumentation procedures (abstract). In Proceedings of the International Society for the Study of the Lumbar Spine, April 1988.
58. Zucherman, J. F., Hsu, K., Picetti, G., III, et al.: Clinical efficacy of spinal instrumentation in lumbar degenerative disc disease. Spine 17:834–837, 1992.
59. Zucherman, J. F., Brack, S., Hsu, K. Y., et al.: Myth of the solid posterior lateral fusion. In Yonenobu, K., Ono, K., and Takemitsu, Y. (eds.): Lumbar Spinal Fusion and Stabilization. Berlin, Springer-Verlag, 1993, pp. 10–15.

Internal Fixation: Indications, Technique, and Results

BRUCE FREDRICKSON
HANSEN YUAN

Instrumentation of the lumbar spine and lumbosacral junction has become more commonly accepted over the past 15 years. Instrumentation systems are available that can be implanted either anteriorly or posteriorly or in various combinations. These systems can be classified in several ways on the basis of location, rigidity (load sharing), or segmental characteristics. Anterior systems generally are implanted from an anterior approach and posterior systems from a posterior approach. There are systems, such as the BAK cage, that can be implanted from either the front or the back. Selection of an anterior or posterior device generally depends on the diagnosis and the surgical approach. Rigid implants do not rely on the ligaments or articulations of the spine for their support. Rigid implants decrease the load on the vertebrae and may lead to a relative osteoporosis. Semirigid implants derive some of their stability from the normal articulations and ligamentous attachments of the individual motion segments. Their design characteristics require some degree of load sharing. Systems that are segmental allow attachment of the device to each individual vertebra. The method of attachment may be rigid (pedicle screws) or semirigid (hooks or wires).

The implant may provide either or both of the following functions. First, the implant may be used strictly to maintain the position of the vertebrae relative to each other to enhance fusion. Second, the implant may be used to change the spatial relationships of vertebrae (i.e., to reduce a fracture). An implant that allows a change of spatial relationships is usually of greater complexity.

The indications for use of specific implants vary by diagnosis. In degenerative diseases of the lumbar spine, devices have been used to increase the fusion rate and to improve alignment. Their use in cases of spondylolisthesis has been to enhance the rate of fusion and at times to reduce the deformity. In scoliosis devices have commonly been used for correction of the deformity and maintenance of position while a fusion is consolidating. In the case of trauma to the lumbar spine, devices have been used to afford reduction of the injury and to stabilize it while a fusion is taking place. Specific problems such as osteomyelitis, Pott's disease, and metastatic disease of the spine have required various combinations of anterior and posterior devices to provide stability while the basic pathologic process is being treated. Internal fixation is rarely used by itself. A solid fusion is required in all cases of instrumentation or the device will eventually fail.

HISTORY

The first use of internal fixation in the spine was by Hadra in 1891.[18] He used a wire to fix a cervical fracture-dislocation posteriorly. The history of internal fixation of the spine is then intimately associated with the history of spine fusion itself from the time of Hibbs and Albe in the early 1900s. Attempts at fixation of the spine were carried out by various surgeons in the early 1900s. Lange[38] was the first to implant a metal rod in an attempt to increase spine stability. Jenkins[28] of New Zealand in 1936 used a peg of tibia to fix L5 to S1 anteriorly in a case of spondylolisthesis. Mercer[46] in 1936 and Speed[55] in 1938 described similar procedures involving the use of a bone peg as a form of internal fixation at the L5–S1 junction for spondylolisthesis.

The first extensive use of posterior internal fixation was by King in 1948.[33] He used screws placed across the facet joints to increase the fusion rate in lumbosacral fusions. Boucher[4] in 1959 and Andrew[1a] in 1986 described a similar procedure. Wilson and colleagues[60] in 1952 described the use of a metal plate held to the spinous processes by a series of bolts. They listed four specific objectives in their use of internal fixation: (1) to provide absolute immobilization of the operative area while fusion was occurring, (2) to shorten the period of postoperative recovery, (3) to reduce postoperative discomfort and (4) to reduce the number of failed fusions.

Anterior fixation techniques through the 1950s continued to rely on the use of rigid implants of bone rather than metallic implants. The work of Wiltberger[61] and Harmon[20] illustrates the two approaches taken. Harmon advocated an anterior approach to the intervertebral disc space, whereas Wiltberger recommended the posterior interbody technique. Both techniques relied on fixation by graft itself.

The report of Harrington[21] in 1962 marked the beginning of the application of the current techniques of internal fixation of the lumbar spine. His device was used posteriorly and relied on hooks placed around the lamina for purchase on the spine. Fixation was not segmental, and the construct was classified as semirigid.

Modifications of the Harrington device have been made by several investigators. A distraction rod was specifically developed for the lumbar spine by Knodt and reported on by Beattie.[2] It was designed for use over one or two segments and formed a semirigid construct. Jacobs and colleagues[26] reported on a stronger threaded device with a proximal locking hook in an attempt to decrease the incidence of hook dislodgment and rod breakage.

White and colleagues,[59] Selby,[53] and Lee and deBari[39] reported on their results using the Knodt device. Kaneda and coworkers[30, 31] reported on a similar device supplemented with compression hooks to help further with stability. Edwards[11] increased the torsional stability of the basic Harrington rods by the addition of rod sleeves.

Segmental posterior systems were introduced to North American orthopedists by Luque.[41] Fixation was by sublaminar wires twisted to solid contoured rods. The technique is segmental but only semirigid.

Segmental techniques involving purchase by transpedicle screws were initially developed in Europe by Roy-Camille and associates[52] and later popularized by Louis.[40] An external pedicle fixation system was introduced by Magerl,[41a] modified by Dick,[8] and reported by Aebi.[1] The pedicle systems are all segmental and provide rigid immobilization, with the exception of the Edwards, which is semirigid. The initial systems using the transpedicle technique in North America include those developed by Steffee and colleagues,[56] Edwards,[12] Wiltse,[17] and Krag and coworkers.[37] Numerous systems are now available that rely on pedicle screw fixation.

The development of anterior fixation devices generally has lagged behind that of posterior instrumentation. Dwyer and colleagues[10] developed the first commonly used device for anterior fixation. This was a flexible device and was used for correction of spinal deformity only. Hall[19] reviewed its status in spine surgery in 1981. Zielke and coworkers[64] modified the Dwyer technique to include a rod rather than a flexible cable. Their design is semirigid and has greater applicability to severe spinal deformities and injuries. Kaneda and associates[32] have reported on its use.

Anterior devices have been developed by other surgeons for specific problems. Humphreys and coworkers[25] reported on the use of an anterior plate for either one-level or two-level anterior spine fusions. Werlinich[58] reported on the use of an anterior staple for single-level fusions. Kostuik[34, 35] reported on the development of an anterior device using Harrington distraction rods and modified Dwyer screws. He cautioned that the device did not provide good control of rotation and lateral bending and recommended the use of a supplementary external orthosis. Dunn[9] described the evolution of an anterior fixation system from a semirigid to rigid classification. This device subsequently was removed from the market because of several reported instances of aortic erosion with its use. Kaneda and colleagues[29] described an anterior device similar to that of Dunn with two solid threaded rods placed laterally over the vertebrae. This device was further modified to include a cross-link to provide enhanced torsional stability. To date, there have been no reported instances of aortic erosion with this device.

There are many systems for both anterior and posterior use being developed and tried on a clinical basis. They generally rely on segmental fixation and are either rigid or semirigid.

GOALS AND DEFINITIONS

The goals of any fixation device used in the spine are the same: (1) the device should allow correction of deformity if present and prevent deformity during the postoperative period; (2) the fusion rate should be at least equal to that without the device in place and preferably better; and (3) early mobilization of the patient should be possible with the use of less external immobilization.

To meet the above goals, certain characteristics must be present in the implant. No single implant can be used for every problem; however, the overall characteristics of the implants should be the same:

1. The implant itself should be compatible with the body. Currently used materials include stainless steel and titanium. Titanium has the advantage of not interfering with postoperative computed tomographic and magnetic resonance imaging scanning. Materials that allow ingrowth of bone have been used on an experimental basis. Porous ingrowth devices are advantageous if the device is not to be removed. A significant defect in the spinal column will result if bone ingrowth has occurred, and the device must be removed.

2. The device must allow segmental fixation.

3. The device should be at least semirigid, and preferably rigid, so that it can be used either with or without intact ligamentous and bony structures. Further development in the area of disc replacement would change this, making a flexible implant advantageous for some applications.

4. Space must be left for the application of an adequate bone graft for solid fusion if

needed. Only in specific instances such as metastatic disease can the device be expected to remain stable during a patient's anticipated life span.

5. Implantation of the device must be safe and easy. Instrumentation systems that require a great deal of specialized instrumentation and manual dexterity tend not to be implanted appropriately and greatly prolong the surgical time.

6. The device must be adaptable to various situations and allow correction of deformity if present.

7. The degree of load sharing must be appropriate to prevent segmental osteoporosis.

BIOMECHANICS

The actual loads that a spinal implant is expected to support in the spine are not known. Attempts to assess these loads have been carried out by various techniques. These include the work of Nachemson[47-49] and others,[38] who have measured the in vitro hydrostatic properties of the nucleus pulposus in various positions of the body. Other investigators have used Harrington rods with strain gauges and implanted them in patients and animal models. Numerous researchers using various mathematic models have computed loads on the lumbar spine.[16]

A different approach to this problem was taken by Krag and coworkers.[37] They suggested that the answer to the question of how strong an implant and the implant-bone junction need to be could be answered by looking at the available implants and their relative strengths. They reasoned that an implant in current use and with both a low breakage rate and a high fusion rate must be meeting the biologic demands of the spine.

The work of Nachemson[47-49] and Hirsch and Waugh[24] showed that a posteriorly applied spinal implant must be able to support forces up to 245 N in compressive loading if there are intact bony ligamentous structures. The work of Krag and coworkers[37] suggests that 4.5-mm screws applied through the pedicles are large enough to resist the physiologic forces in an intact spine. Care should be taken in interpreting all of these in vivo data because they were gathered with basically intact spines and not with a major disruption of either the osseous or ligamentous structures. Research such as that of Peek and colleagues[51] and McGowan and associates[42] provided some data on instrumentation loads in destabilized spinal segments.

Testing techniques in the laboratory to assess the actual strength of implants and the implant-bone complex have varied among investigators. The earliest techniques were simple tests to failure. Techniques used since have included the relative stiffness of implanted devices,[44] stress measurements of implanted devices loaded to physiologic forces with secondary mathematic modeling of failure modes,[16] and cyclic testing of implanted devices loaded to physiologic stresses.[50]

INDICATIONS

Each device that can be used for fixation of the lumbar spine, be it anterior or posterior, has advantages and disadvantages. Some devices have had significant complications related to either their implantation or late failure. In the first category are the Knodt and standard Harrington rods. Both of these produce unacceptable kyphosis of the lumbar spine and are contraindicated. Modifications of the standard Harrington system such as Moe square-ended rods and Jacobs[26] ratcheted rods allow control of the lumbar lordosis and therefore have some use in the lumbar spine. An example of the second complication category is the type-3 Dunn device and its association with late vascular erosion.

Surgeons today believe that certain guidelines should be followed when using instrumentation in the lumbar spine. The fewest possible segments in the lumbar spine should be instrumented for any particular problem. Instrumentation extending below the thoracolumbar junction should stop at L3 if at all possible to reduce the incidence of late degenerative changes in the lumbar spine. Fusions of the lumbosacral junction should include as few segments as possible and lordosis must be maintained. Devices currently available that allow segmental instrumentation include sublaminar wires, pedicle screws, and hook-rod constructs that use the claw technique.

Most anterior fixation systems are segmental. The difference among systems is the degree of deformity that can be corrected and the stiffness of the total construct.

The selection of a specific internal fixation device to be used in the lumbar spine depends on the goals of a particular surgical procedure, the approach, the experience of the surgeon, and the limitations of the device. Current indications for use of a particular device are also changing as the capabilities of a device along with its limitations become better known.

Degenerative Disease

Degenerative disease of the lumbosacral junction is the most common diagnostic category currently being treated. Diagnoses include primary discogenic pain, segmental instability, and degenerative deformities.

Primary discogenic pain as defined by Crock[5a] must be proved by discography before fusion.[36] An alternative method of diagnosis is the use of a rigid external fixator as proposed by Ölerud.[50a] Internal fixation devices are always indicated. A fusion that includes both the anterior disc and posterior elements (360 degrees) gives optimum results.[64] Disc excision should be followed by a fusion incorporating either solid bone grafts or some form of implant to prevent collapse of the disc space. The most commonly accepted anterior alternatives include allograft (fibular or iliac crest) and devices such as the BAK system (Fig. 1). The posterior fusion must include an autogenous bone graft but need not be augmented with internal fixation if solid fixation is obtained anteriorly. If any question of stability is present, a pedicle screw system should be placed.

Segmental instability can be treated adequately with a posterior procedure. The preferred method of fixation would be either a pedicle screw system or facet screws (Fig. 2).

Fusion for discogenic pain or segmental instability requires careful analysis of the levels above and below the pathologic segment. In most cases, failure to include a degenerative level in the fusion leads to recurrent symptoms (Fig. 3). The authors currently recommend surgery for only one-level and two-level disease. The results of fusion of three or more segments are uncertain, and such fusions are reserved for isolated cases.

Degenerative listhesis and scoliosis are definite indications for instrumentation. Systems that provide pedicle screw fixation are required because in most cases some form of laminectomy has been or must be carried out at the same time. In cases of fixed deformity, an anterior release and grafting may be required.

Trauma

Fractures of the lumbar spine are treated surgically if one or more of the following criteria are present: (1) neurologic deficits are present and compression of the neural elements is seen; (2) the kyphosis is more than 20 degrees; or (3) the degree of bony or soft tissue canal compromise is greater than

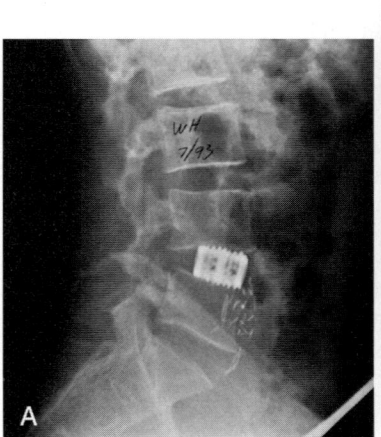
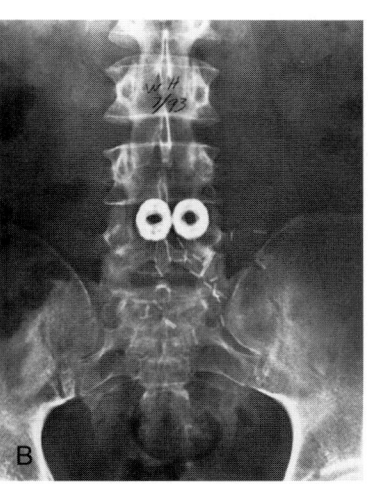

Figure 1. *A, B,* Fusion for discogenic pain should include some form of anterior disc excision and fusion combined with a posterior fusion. The BAK system provides good immediate fixation and prevents some of the anterior collapse seen with the use of either allograft or autograft.

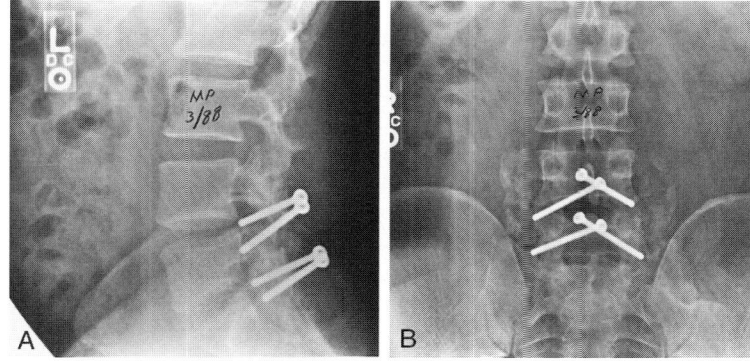

Figure 2. A, B, Facet screws are a useful technique to improve the fusion rate in cases of segmental instability. Their low profile allows better contact between bone graft and muscle to aid with fusion. They are not satisfactory fixation devices if significant anterior support is not present.

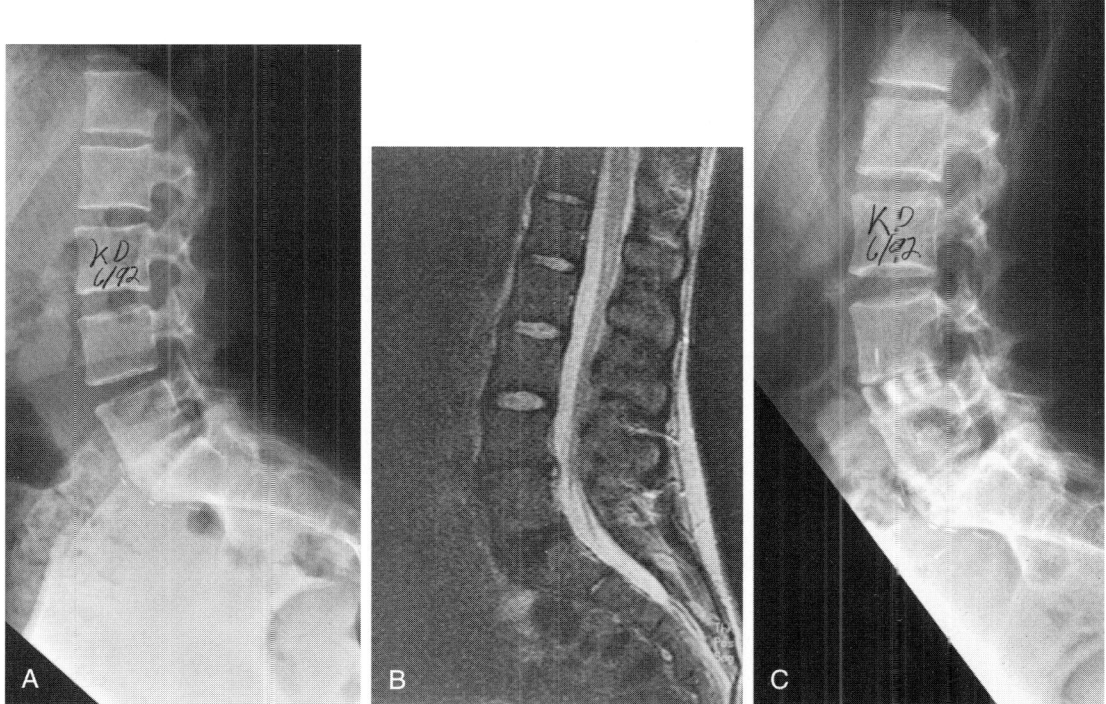

Figure 3. A, This patient had her initial fusion at L5–S1 with excellent relief of discogenic pain. Preoperative discography was abnormal at L4–L5 and L5–S1, with pain produced only at the L5–S1 level. One year after fusion, she redeveloped pain in her low back with radiation to the proximal thighs. B, A T2-weighted MRI scan illustrating the bright spot in the posterior annulus at L4–L5 as described by Aprill.[1b] Discography 1 year after fusion confirmed L4–L5 to be painful. C, Immediately after her second surgery, the patient had excellent resolution of her pain pattern. Fusions for discogenic pain should always include all degenerative levels. Leaving a degenerative level adjacent to a fused segment in most cases leads to the development of pain in the future.

50%[54] (Fig. 4). A posterior approach can be carried out in cases treated within the first 24 to 48 hours with the use of the AO internal fixator or a similar device[7, 8, 13] (Fig. 5). In a small percentage of cases, this does not afford reduction of the intracanal fragment and an anterior approach has to be carried out.[11, 12, 42] A primary anterior approach is used in cases in which more than 72 hours have passed since injury or those involving greater than 75% canal compromise[29, 34, 62] (Fig. 6). Posterolateral fusions are always carried out in conjunction with the instrumentation. Transpedicle grafting of the vertebral body should be considered to prevent late collapse in conjunction with the posterior approach.[8]

Metastasis

Metastatic disease requires an individualized approach to each problem. In cases in which there is an impending pathologic fracture or actual fracture, some form of internal fixation is definitely indicated.[35, 63] The patient's projected life span is an important consideration in determining the type of fixation and whether it is combined with bone grafting or supplemental use of methyl methacrylate. A projected life span of 3 months or longer justifies surgical intervention. The anterior approach is preferred for isolated cases of metastasis[63] (Fig. 7). Fixation is obtained with a lateral plate in conjunction with either a bone graft or methyl methacrylate as indicated above. In cases involving multiple level disease, posterior fixation is generally preferable. Some form of segmental posterior fixation should be obtained with appropriate use of pedicle screws and laminar hooks. External support is required in most cases to prevent failure of the fixation device or the bone-metal junction.

Spondylolisthesis

Spondylolisthesis of L5 in children or adults is generally treated with an isolated in situ posterolateral fusion. Postural reduction, as reported by Bradford,[4a] is used in some cases with a high slip angle. Adolescents and young adults with a high-grade slip (3 or higher) or with an unacceptable slip angle (≥40 degrees) are considered candidates for reduction. The technique is that advocated by Edwards utilizing a pedicle screw system that allows for distraction and posterior translation[12, 43] (Fig. 8). Neurologic deficits including L5 root dysfunction and cauda equina syndrome have been reported with reduction. This technique should be used with caution in patients older than 20 years. Resection of the sacral dome may be required. In extreme cases, L5 corpectomy through an anterior approach may be indicated before reduction as advocated by Gaines and associates.[15]

Scoliosis

Internal fixation devices are definitely indicated in the treatment of lumbar scoliosis whether it is primary or caused by degenerative changes. Treatment of an adolescent with a primary lumbar curve is best carried out with an anterior device such as the ven-

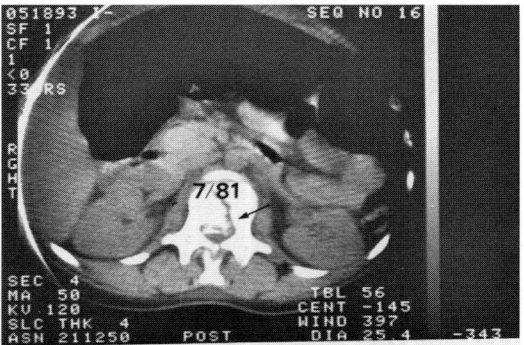

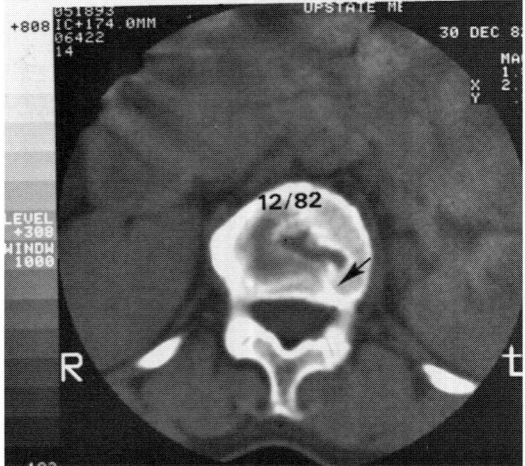

Figure 4. This case illustrates the potential for remodeling of the spinal canal with conservative care. Top, This patient had none of the criteria that would require surgical intervention. Bottom, She was treated with 3 months of extension and bracing. Arrows indicate fracture line.

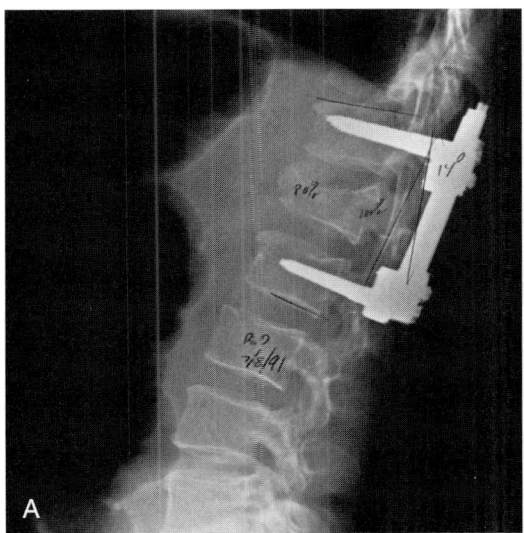
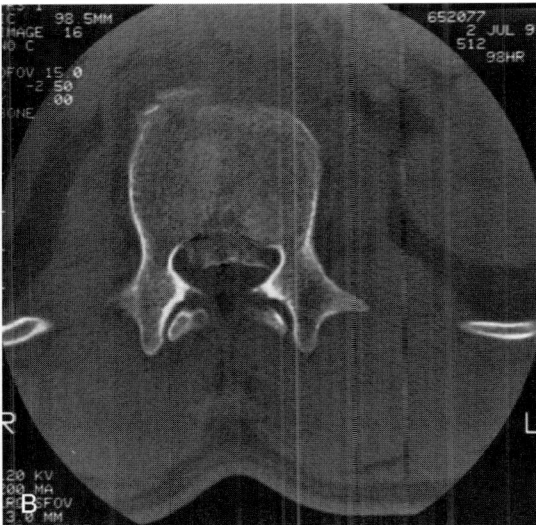
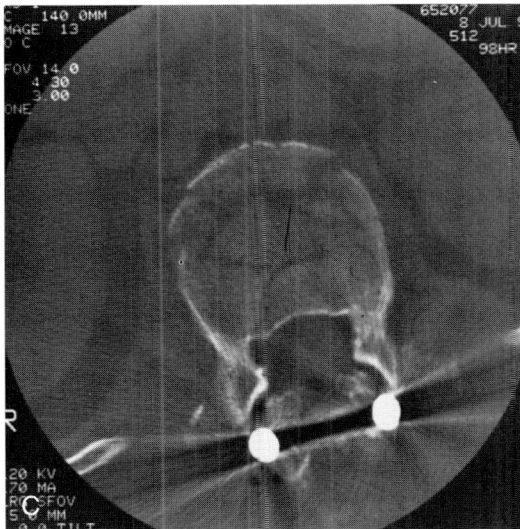

Figure 5. This patient had an incomplete neurologic deficit, 50% canal compromise, and a kyphosis of 30 degrees. *A*, The immediate postoperative reduction. *B*, Preoperative CT scan *C*, CT scan showing the degree of canal reduction obtained by the indirect method.

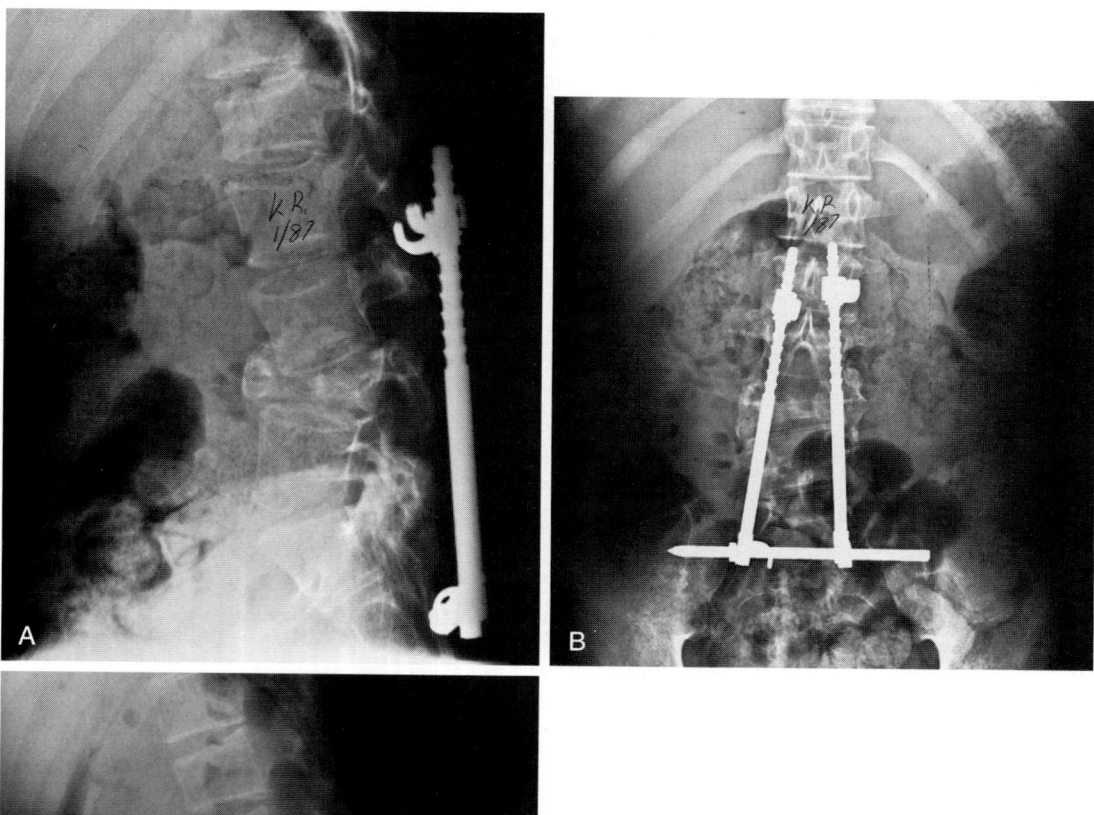
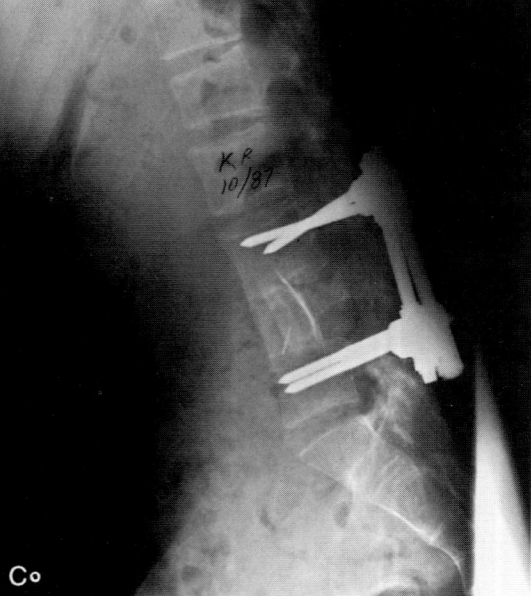

Figure 6. *A, B,* An attempted posterior reduction for a burst fracture of L4. Harrington rods are contraindicated for this fracture because they produce kyphosis of the normal lordotic lumbar spine. *C,* The postoperative picture after removal of the Harrington instrumentation, anterior corpectomy, and posterior internal fixation. Posterior indirect reduction could not be carried out in this case because it was now more than 2 weeks after the original injury.

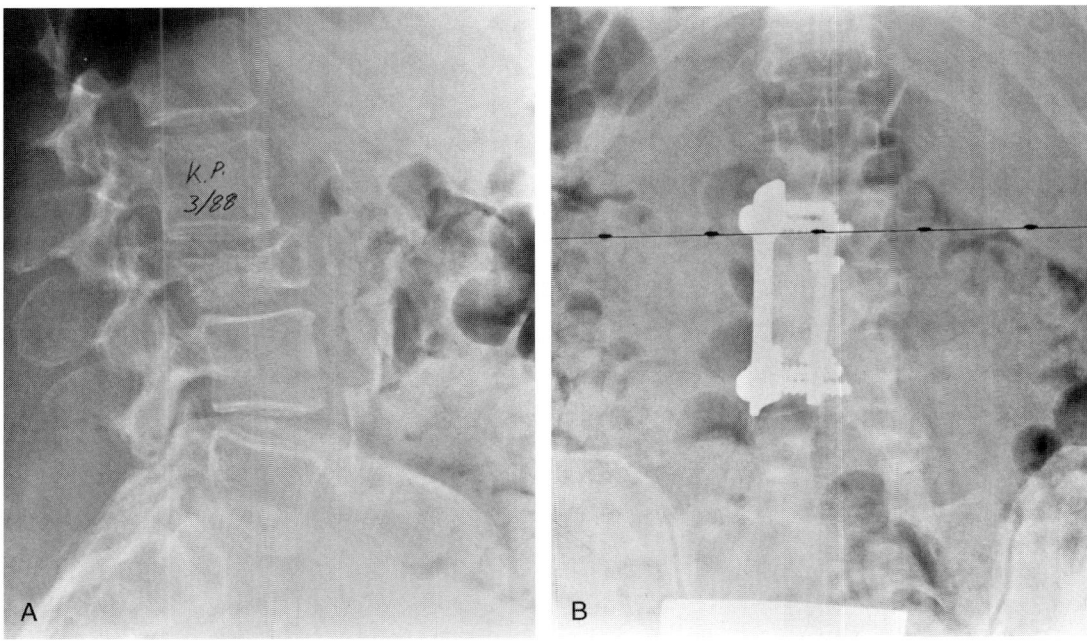
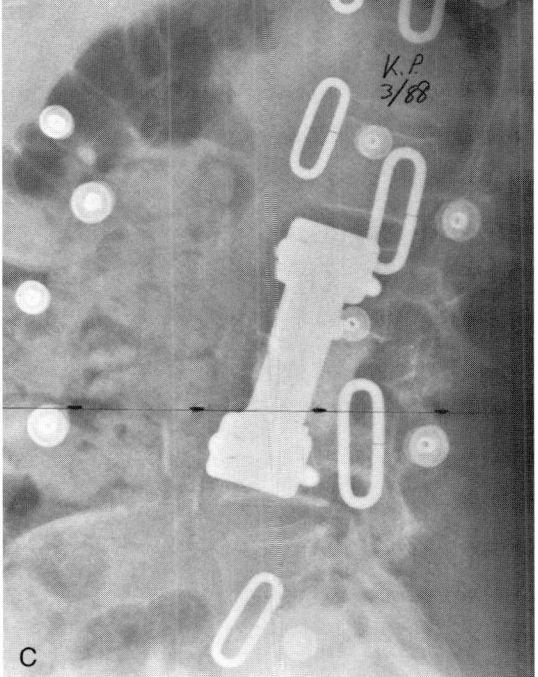

Figure 7. Isolated spinal metastasis can be treated with resection of the vertebral body and internal fixation. *A*, The lesion is at the ideal level for treatment. *B, C*, The lesion was treated with an anterior approach consisting of resection of the tumor and replacement with methyl methacrylate and a plate.

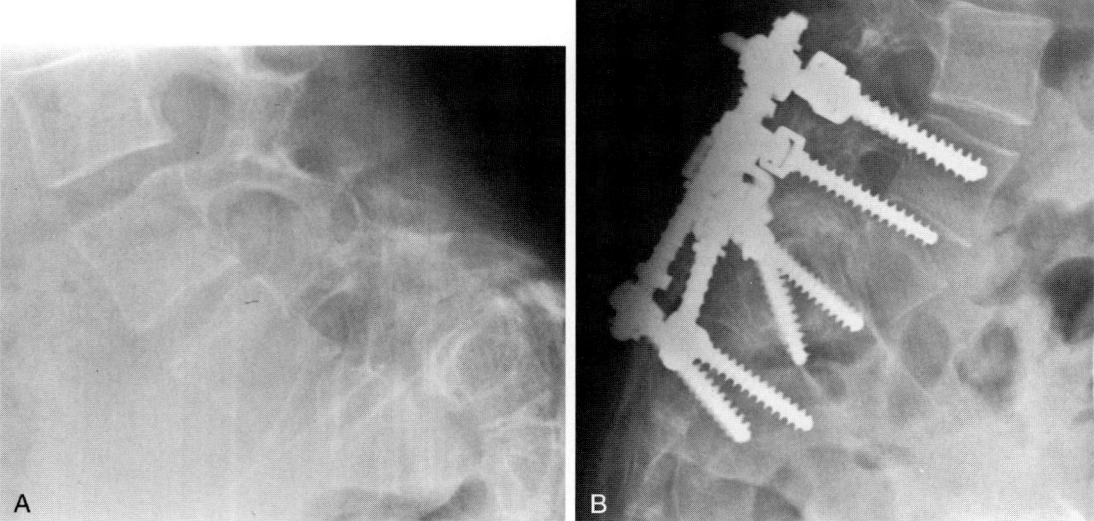

Figure 8. *A, B,* Reduction of a high-grade spondylolisthesis is possible with the pedicle screw devices. The L5 nerve root must be totally decompressed and distraction should be avoided.

tral derotation system (VDS).[32] This limits the length of the fusion and can save an important one or two levels that would have to be fused with more conventional techniques. The development of the Cotrel-Duboussett[5, 14] system and later the Texas Scottish Rite Hospital (TSRH), Isola, and Modulock systems allowed segmental posterior instrumentation. They also help to maintain or produce lumbar lordosis. An adult with either primary lumbar scoliosis or degenerative lumbar scoliosis is best managed with a two-stage procedure. The authors currently perform an anterior discectomy combined with a second-stage implantation of a posterior pedicle screw system. The posterior system used is one of the segmental rigid systems. This allows a circumferential fusion and better correction of the overall deformity rather than attempting to treat the problem through an isolated anterior or posterior approach. Maintenance of or creation of a lumbar lordosis is extremely important in the treatment of this problem (Fig. 9).

TREATMENT RESULTS

The use of posterior segmental instrumentation has resulted in higher rates of fusion when compared with spines in which no device is used. The incidence of pseudarthrosis in uninstrumented fusions has varied from 5% to 25% or more.[6] A rate of 5% to 10% for single-level fusions and 10% to 20% for two-level fusions is accepted by most surgeons. Researchers have reported consistent nonunion rates of 5% for single-level fusions and 10% for two-level fusions with segmental fixators.[3, 23, 27]

Specific problems are encountered when attachment to the sacrum is required. Luque rods should not be attached to the lamina of S1. The lamina does not support the forces applied and the S1 root is vulnerable to damage. The Galveston technique is a useful alternative in cases of neuromuscular deformity.[57] The newer sacral fixation technique of Jackson[25a] needs more evaluation but may provide a more secure method of attachment to the sacrum with fewer complications.

The ability of surgeons to correct deformities in either the sagittal or the coronal plane has been greatly improved with pedicle screw fixation. The complication rate in cases of osteoporotic deformities and high-grade spondylolistheses requires further development of devices and techniques.

All anterior devices currently in use are rigid. They attach to the vertebrae with screws that are either unilateral or bilateral. They differ in their ability to correct deformity. Excellent rates of bone fusion have been reported with all designs.

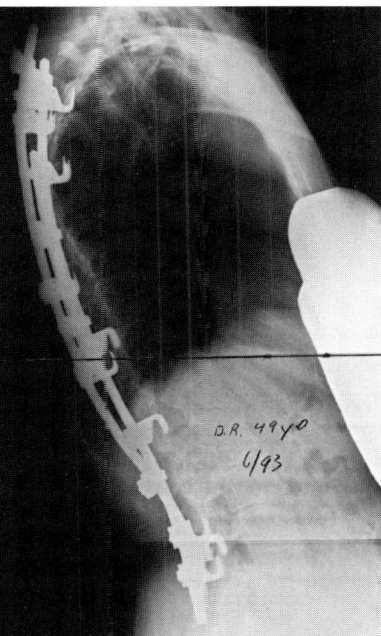

Figure 9. Attention must be paid not only to the coronal plane but also to the sagittal plane when instrumenting the spine. This is demonstrated in a plain film of an adult with idiopathic scoliosis that required instrumentation down to the lower lumbar segments. Careful attention to the sagittal plane contour of the rod allowed maintenance of the patient's normal lordosis.

The results of treatment with the current segmental devices, be they anterior or posterior, show an improved rate of fusion. Other advantages include decreased use of external immobilization, a faster rate of mobilization, and better correction of deformity if present at the time of surgery. These results justify the continued use of these devices.

REFERENCES

1. Aebi, M., Etter, C., Kehl, T., and Thalgott, J.: Stabilization of the lower thoracic and lumbar spine with the internal spinal skeletal fixation system. Spine 12:544–551, 1987.
1a. Andrew, T. A., Brooks, S., Piggott, H., et al.: Long-term follow-up evaluation of screw-and-graft fusion of the lumbar spine. Clin. Orthop. 203:113–119, 1986.
1b. Aprill, C., and Bogduk, N.: High-intensity zone: A diagnostic sign of painful lumbar disc on magnetic resonance imaging. Br. J. Radiol. 65(773):361–369, 1992.
2. Beattie, F. C.: Distraction rod fusion. Clin. Orthop. 62:218–222, 1969.
3. Bernhardt, M., Swartz, D. E., Clothiaux, P. L., et al.: Posterolateral lumbar and lumbosacral fusion with and without pedicle screw internal fixation. Clin. Orthop. 284:109–115, 1992.
4. Boucher, H. H.: A method of spinal fusion. J. Bone Joint Surg. 41B:248–259, 1959.
4a. Bradford, D. S.: Closed reduction of spondylolisthesis. An experience in 22 patients. Spine 13(5):580–587, 1988.
5. Cotrel, Y., and Dubousset, J.: Nouvelle technique d'osteosynthese rachidienne segmentarie par voie posterieure. Rev. Chir. Orthop. 70:489–494, 1984.
5a. Crock, H. V.: Internal disc disruption. In Practice of Spinal Surgery. New York, Springer-Verlag, 1983, pp. 35–92.
6. DePalma, A. F., and Rothman, R. H.: The nature of pseudarthrosis. Clin. Orthop. 59:113–118, 1968.
7. Dick, W.: Spinal system: the "Fixateur interne" (F.I.). AO/ASIF Dialogue 1(3), 1987.
8. Dick, W.: Acute management of spinal injuries. The thoracic and lumbar spine, surgical therapy. Langenbecks Arch. Chir. (Suppl.) 2:261–265, 1988.
9. Dunn, H. K.: Anterior stabilization of thoracolumbar injuries. Clin. Orthop. 189:116–124, 1984.
10. Dwyer, A. F., Newton, N. C., and Sherwood, A. A.: An anterior approach to scoliosis. Clin. Orthop. 62:192–202, 1969.
11. Edwards, C. C., and Levine, A. M.: Early rod-sleeve stabilization of the injured thoracic and lumbar spine. Orthop. Clin. North Am. 17:121–145, 1986.
12. Edwards, C. C.: Low lumbar burst fractures. Reduction and stabilization using the modular spine fixation system. Presented at the Scoliosis Research Society Meeting, Vancouver Canada, September 1987.
13. Esses, S. I.: The AO spinal internal fixator. Spine 14:373–378, 1989.
14. Farcy, J. P., Weidenbaum, M., Michelson, C., et al.: A comparative biomechanical study of spinal fixation using Cotrel-Dubousset instrumentation. Spine 12:877–881, 1987.
15. Gaines, R. W., Jr., et al.: Treatment of spondyloptosis by staged resection and fusion (Gaines procedure). Presented at the North American Spine Society Meeting, Boston, July 9–11, 1993.
16. Goel, V. K., Lin, T. H., et al.: Effects of rigidity of an internal fixation device. A comprehensive biomechanical investigation Spine 16(Suppl. 3):S155–161, 1991.
17. Guyer, D. W., et al.: The Wiltse pedicle screw fixation system. Orthopedics 11:1455–1460, 1988.
18. Hadra, B. E.: Wiring of the vertebrae as a means of immobilization in fracture and Pott's disease. Med. Times Reg. 22:423, 1901.
19. Hall, J. E.: Current concepts review Dwyer instrumentation in anterior fusion of the spine. J. Bone Joint Surg. 63A:1188–1190, 1981.
20. Harmon, P. H.: Anterior excision and vertebra body fusion operation for intervertebral disk syndromes of the lower lumbar spine: Three to five year results in 244 cases. Clin. Orthop. 26:107–127, 1963.
21. Harrington, P. R.: Treatment of scoliosis. J. Bone Joint Surg. 44A:591–634, 1962
22. Harrington, P. R., and Dickson, J. H. Spinal instrumentation in the treatment of severe progressive spondylolisthesis. Clin. Orthop. 117:157–163, 1976.
23. Heggeness, M. H., and Esses, S. I. Translaminar facet joint screw fixation for lumbar and lumbosacral fusion. A clinical and biomechanical study. Spine 16(suppl. 6):266–269, 1991.
24. Hirsch, C., and Waugh, T.: The introduction of

force measurements guiding instrumental correction of scoliosis. Acta Orthop. Scand. 39:136–144, 1968.
25. Humphries, A. W., Hawk, W. A., and Berndt, A. L.: Anterior interbody fusion of lumbar vertebrae: A surgical technique. Surg. Clin. North Am. 41:1685–1700, 1971.
25a. Jackson, R. P., and McManus, A. C.: The iliac buttress. A computed tomographic study of sacral anatomy. Spine 18:1318–1328, 1993.
26. Jacobs, R. R., Schlaepfer, F., Mathys, R., Jr., et al.: A locking hook spinal rod system for stabilization of fracture-dislocations and correction of deformities of the dorsolumbar spine. Clin. Orthop. 189:168–177, 1985.
27. Jacobs, R. R.: Enhancement of lumbar spine fusion by use of translaminar facet joint screws. Spine 14:12–15, 1989.
28. Jenkins, J. A.: Spondylolisthesis. Br. J. Surg. 24:80–85, 1936.
29. Kaneda, K., Abumi, K., and Fujiya, M.: Burst fractures with neurologic deficits of the thoracolumbar-lumbar spine. Results of anterior decompression and stabilization with anterior instrumentation. Spine 9:788–793, 1984.
30. Kaneda, K., Satoh, S., Nohara, Y., and Oguma, T.: Distraction rod instrumentation with posterolateral fusion in isthmic spondylolisthesis, 53 cases followed for 18–89 months. Spine 10:383–389, 1985.
31. Kaneda, K., Kazama, H., Satoh, S., and Fujiya, N.: Follow-up study of medial facetectomies and posterolateral fusion with instrumentation in unstable degenerative spondylolisthesis. Clin. Orthop. 203:159–167, 1986.
32. Kaneda, K., Fujiya, N., and Satoh, S.: Results with Zielke instrumentation for idiopathic thoracolumbar and lumbar scoliosis. Clin. Orthop. 205:195–203, 1986.
33. King, D.: Internal fixation for lumbosacral fusion. J. Bone Joint Surg. 39A:560–565, 1948.
34. Kostuik, J. P.: Anterior fixation for fractures of the thoracic and lumbar spine with or without neurologic involvement. Clin. Orthop. 189:103–115, 1984.
35. Kostuik, J. P.: Anterior spinal cord decompression for lesions of the thoracic and lumbar spine; techniques, new methods of internal fixation, results. Spine 8:512–531, 1985.
36. Kostuik, J. P., Errico, T. J., and Gleason, T. F.: Techniques of internal fixation for degenerative conditions of the lumbar spine. Clin. Orthop. 203:219–231, 1986.
37. Krag, M. H., Beynnon, B. D., Pope, M. H., et al.: An internal fixator for posterior application to short segments of the thoracic, lumbar, or lumbosacral spine. Clin. Orthop. 203:75–98, 1986.
38. Lange, F.: The classic support for the spondylitic spine by means of buried steel bars, attached to the vertebrae. Clin. Orthop. 203:3–6, 1986.
39. Lee, C. K., and deBari, A.: Lumbosacral spinal fusion with Knodt distraction rods. Spine 11:373–375, 1986.
40. Louis, R.: Fusion of the lumbar and sacral spine by internal fixation with screw plates. Clin. Orthop. 203:18–33, 1986.
41. Luque, E. R.: Segmental spinal instrumentation: A method of rigid internal fixation of the spine to induce arthrodesis. Orthop. Trans. 4:391, 1980.
41a. Magerl, F. P.: Stabilization of the lower thoracic and lumbar spine with external skeletal fixation. Clin. Orthop. 189:125–141, 1984.
42. McGowan, D. P., Mann, K. A., Yuan, H. A., et al.: A biomechanical study of anterior spinal fixation for thoracolumbar burst fractures with varying degrees of posterior disruption. Presented at the International Society for the Study of the Lumbar Spine, Rome, 1987.
43. McGuire, R. A., and Amundson, G. M.: The use of primary internal fixation in spondylolisthesis. Spine 18:1662–1672, 1993.
44. Mann, K. A., Found, E. M., Yuan, H. A., et al.: Biomechanical evaluation of the effectiveness of anterior spinal fixation systems. Presented at the 33rd Annual Meeting of the Orthopaedic Research Society, San Francisco, January 19–22, 1987.
46. Mercer, W.: Spondylolisthesis: With a description of a new method of operative treatment and notes of ten cases. Edinburgh Med. J. 43:545–572, 1936.
47. Nachemson, A.: The load on lumbar discs in different positions of the body. Clin. Orthop. 45:107–122, 1965.
48. Nachemson, A. L., Schultz, A. B., and Berkson, M. H.: Mechanical properties of human lumbar spine motion segments. Influences of age, sex, disc level, and degeneration. Spine 4:1–8, 1979.
49. Nachemson, A. L.: Disc pressure measurements. Spine 6:93–97, 1981.
50. Nasca, R. J., Hollis, M., Lemons, J. G., and Cool, T. A.: Cyclic axial loading of spinal implants. Spine 10:792–798, 1985.
50a. Ölerud, S., Sjöström, L., Karlström, G., and Hamberg, M.: Spontaneous effect of increased stability of the lower lumbar spine in cases of severe chronic back pain: The answer of an external transpedicular fixation test. Clin. Orthop. 203:67–74, 1986.
51. Peek, R. D., Wiltse, L. L., Widell, E. H., et al.: Biomechanical effects of decompressive laminectomy on internal fixation of the lumbosacral spine. Presented at The North American Spine Society Meeting, Banff, Alberta, Canada, June 1987.
52. Roy-Camille, R., Saillant, G., and Mazel, C.: Internal fixation of the lumbar spine with pedicle screw plating. Clin. Orthop. 203:7–17, 1986.
53. Selby, D.: Internal fixation with Knodt's rods. Clin. Orthop. 203:179–184, 1986.
54. Selby, D.: The role of anterior lumbar fusion for internal disc disruption. Presented at the International Society for the Study of the Lumbar Spine, Dallas, TX, 1986.
55. Speed, K.: Spondylolisthesis: Treatment by anterior bone graft. Arch. Surg. 37:175–189, 1938.
56. Steffee, A. D., Biscup, R. S., and Sitkowski, D. J.: Segmental spine plates with pedicle screw fixation: A new internal fixation device for disorders of the lumbar and thoracolumbar spine. Clin. Orthop. 203:45–53, 1986.
57. Swank, S. M., Cohen, D. S., and Brown, J. C.: Spine fusion in cerebral palsy with L-rod segmental spinal instrumentation. A comparison of single and two-stage combined approach with Zielke instrumentation. Spine 14:750–759, 1989.
58. Werlinich, M.: Anterior interbody fusion and stabilization with metal fixation. Int. Surg. 59:269–273, 1974.
59. White, A., Wynne, G., and Taylor, L. W.: Knodt rod distraction lumbar fusion. Spine 8:434–437, 1983.
60. Wilson, P. D., Straub, L., and Ramsay, M. D.: Lum-

bosacral fusion with metallic-plate fixation. Instr. Course Lect. 9:53–65, 1952.
61. Wiltberger, B. R.: Intervertebral body fusion by the use of posterior bone dowel. J. Bone Joint Surg. 39A:284, 1957.
62. Yuan, H. A., Mann, K. A., Fredrickson, B. E., and Lubicky, J. P.: Anterior decompression of burst fractures with spinal I-plate fixation: A clinical and experimental study. Presented at the American Spinal Injury Association Meeting, San Francisco, 1986.
63. Yuan, H. A., Mann, K. A., Found, E. M., et al.: Early clinical experience with the Syracuse I-plate: An anterior spinal fixation device. Spine 12:278–285, 1988.
64. Zielke, K., and Stunkat, R.: Derotation and fusion: Anterior spinal instrumentation (abstract). Orthop. Trans. 2:270, 1978.

23

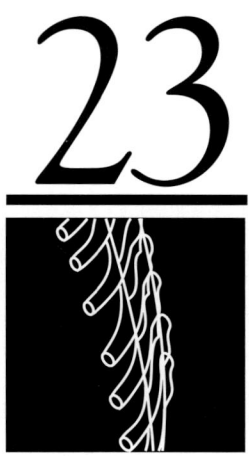

Surgical Approaches

Laminectomies

C. J. M. GETTY
THOMAS S. WHITECLOUD, III

The term laminectomy is often used to describe any spine procedure involving decompression of the spinal cord or nerve roots from the posterior aspect of the spine. In modern parlance, the term is to some extent a misnomer. In degenerative disorders of the lumbar spine, the symptom most effectively relieved by surgical intervention is leg pain of radicular origin. In the preoperative assessment, every attempt is made to establish that the leg pain is of root origin and to identify the specific root responsible for the pain. The aim of this assessment is to allow the operative procedure to be planned carefully and surgical trauma to be kept to a minimum. In turn, the preoperative assessment leads to the development of more limited surgical procedures, the aim being to decompress the affected neural tissue adequately with a minimum of trauma. In cases of spinal cord compression, identifying the specific level responsible for symptoms is also often possible, and accordingly, the surgeon can decompress that level alone instead of performing a classic extensive decompression.

The concept of a carefully planned spine procedure is partly derived from the introduction of advanced technology, such as magnetic resonance imaging (MRI) and computed tomography (CT); more important, it results from an increased appreciation of certain clinical and causal factors that play a part in degenerative disorders of the lumbar spine, in which neurologic function is compromised. A true laminectomy is now much less commonly employed than formerly. As more attention is directed toward the root and as the importance of identifying a specific organic lesion before offering surgical intervention is increasingly appreciated, the term laminectomy should possibly be discarded because it is misleading.

Patient selection for surgical intervention has thus become much more stringent in light of these developments.

DEFINITION

Many terms are used by lumbar spine surgeons to describe various operative procedures. It is useful to consider what some of these terms actually mean. Laminectomy is the most commonly used term for the approach to the disc in which the entire lamina on both sides and the spinous process are removed. It may be performed at more than one level for such conditions as tumors and herniated discs. Hemilaminectomy refers to the excision of only the left or the right lamina.

A laminotomy is the formation of a hole in the lamina to approach the intervertebral disc without destruction of the continuity of the entire lamina.

The term fenestration indicates the removal of the ligamentum flavum in an interlaminar space, whereas laminotomy fenestration implies removal of ligamentum and a small amount of lamina in a cephalic direction and/or a caudal direction. This is the commonest approach for the removal of a herniated disc.

The term discectomy is also a misnomer in that one does not remove the entire disc. Spengler[57] indicated that limited disc excision in selected patients is as effective as the classic radical clearance. Numerous other techniques of discectomy have been developed; all are considered minimally invasive surgical interventions. They include chemical discectomy, automated percutaneous discectomy, percutaneous laser discectomy, and endoscopic manual discectomy. Endoscopic techniques can be combined with other procedures, such as laser discectomy.

The use of enzymes, such as chymopapain and collagenase, was popular in the United States in the early 1980s. However, several problems existed with this technique, including the frequent occurrence of increased pain and muscle spasm after chemonucleolysis and the occasional occurrence of an anaphylactic reaction to the enzyme. Although the use of chymopapain remains relatively popular in Canada and Europe, it is used less frequently in the United States.

The techniques of endoscopically assisted disc excision are gaining in popularity but generally require the insertion of two working portals. This process requires the insertion of much larger instruments into the disc than is necessary for a chemical or laser discectomy.

Automated percutaneous discectomy inserts a motorized probe into the disc space under fluoroscopic control. This technique has been criticized, because occasionally, relatively little disc material is actually removed.

As with the injection of an enzyme, laser discectomy can be performed through a small-bore needle. Various lasers have been evaluated for clinical use. All produce a defect in the center of the nucleus pulposus and obviously do not expose the patient to the risk of anaphylactic reaction. In the United States, two laser wavelengths have been approved by the Food and Drug Administration for this application—the 2.1-mm holmium:yttrium-aluminum-garnet laser and the 532-mm KPT laser.[55]

All of these procedures have their proponents and opponents. When compared with open discectomy, these procedures have clinical results that are usually similar if patients are properly selected. Minimally invasive procedures should be used for patients with sciatica who fail to respond to a trial of nonoperative therapy. The patient should have a prolapsed or a protruded disc. A sequestered fragment is a contraindication to this procedure. Because the natural history of this pathologic process is resolution of symptoms within 2 to 3 months, intervention, even minimal, is unnecessary early in the disease process.

The dominance of the concept of the disc as the prime source of nerve root irritation in the lumbar spine has been usurped by the realization that bony entrapment, usually resulting from osteoarthrosis of the facet joint complex, is the commonest cause of sciatica in older patients. This has resulted in the development of alternative operative procedures designed to decompress the nerve roots in such circumstances. Complete facetectomies have been used, but they are virtually unnecessary because of the development of the technique of partial undercutting facetectomy, which preserves stability and the depth of the spinal canal.[16]

Although it is not discussed in detail here, simultaneous spinal arthrodesis is undertaken at the time of spine decompression by some surgeons. Occasionally, this procedure is performed as an alternative to spine decompression as a means of treating acute disc prolapses.

In summary, the tendency in the treatment of degenerative disorders of the lumbar spine has been to move from the more extensive to the more limited surgical procedures and to concentrate on a specific lesion as identified by the preoperative assessment.

DIAGNOSTIC CRITERIA AND TECHNIQUES

Clinical Assessment

Current philosophy regarding treatment demands careful delineation of the site and type of lesions before surgery. Before an operation is undertaken, stringent diagnostic criteria must be met. The usual indication for operative intervention is evidence of the need to decompress a compromised nerve root.

Irrespective of whether the underlying cause of the degeneration is a herniated disc, facet joint arthritis, or spinal stenosis, the surgeon must determine whether the pain results from neural compromise. The distinction between referred and radicular pain must be established. The attempted distinction between these two types of pain constitutes the basis of clinical assessment of patients with suspected lumbar nerve root entrapment, yet it is often poorly understood, and its importance is rarely fully appreciated.

As a result of electrical stimulation of lumbar nerve roots, McCulloch and Waddell[36] showed that referred pain rarely radiated beyond the upper calf, tended to be dull and poorly localized, and had rarely been described as paresthesia. Radicular pain resulting from L5 and S1 irritation, conversely, nearly always radiates to the ankle or below it, and it is sharp, well localized, and often associated with paresthesia (Table 1). The presence of paresthesia and the extent of the radiation of leg pain are valuable in clinically distinguishing radicular from referred pain.

The actual distribution is less reliable. McCulloch and Waddell[36] showed that pain patterns of L5 and S1 are often difficult to identify. Below the ankle, they tend to follow the recognized dermatomal distribution, whereas above the ankle, the patterns overlap. Kortelainen and coworkers,[32] who analyzed the symptoms and signs of sciatica in relation to the level of lumbar disc protrusion, noted that pain projection into the L5 dermatome was important in establishing L5 root irritation; however, pain projection into the S1 dermatome was less reliable, particularly if two roots were involved. In patients with two roots compromised, pain projection into the L5 dermatome was usually referred to an L4–L5 disc. To establish a clinical diagnosis of S1 root involvement, multiple signs were necessary for a diagnosis of the correct level of a lumbosacral prolapse.

A further important feature of clinical assessment is the recognition of spinal or neurogenic claudication, which may be present in patients with spinal stenosis, bony entrapment, or cauda equina compression and occasionally in those with lateral disc herniation. It is a condition that is often overdiagnosed.[48] The distinction between neurogenic and vascular claudication is important. In some patients, the two conditions coexist, in which case, Doppler testing may be of value.[26]

Patient examination also affords useful diagnostic information. When allied to patients' symptoms, this information provides a basis from which a diagnosis can often be determined without the need for extensive sophisticated investigations.

Nerve root tension is a sign that is often misdiagnosed. It is essential to note the important features of the two commonly used diagnostic tests, the femoral stretch and the straight leg raising tests, as described by Macnab and McCulloch,[38] before a diagnosis of root tension is reached. The femoral stretch test is carried out with the patient prone and is helpful only if pain is reproduced down the front of the thigh. The straight leg raising test involves five components (Fig. 1). In the authors' opinion, all five components of the straight leg raising test should be carried out. Macnab and McCulloch[38] indicated that reproduction of back or leg pain is irrefutable evidence of root compression when the bowstring test is applied.

A careful neurologic examination is essential to the assessment of any patient with a suspected lumbar spinal disorder. However,

Table 1

Clinical Features Useful in Differentiating Radicular from Referred Pain

Radicular pain
  Commonly radiates beyond upper calf
  Often associated with paresthesias
Referred pain
  Seldom radiates beyond upper calf
  Rarely described as paresthesias

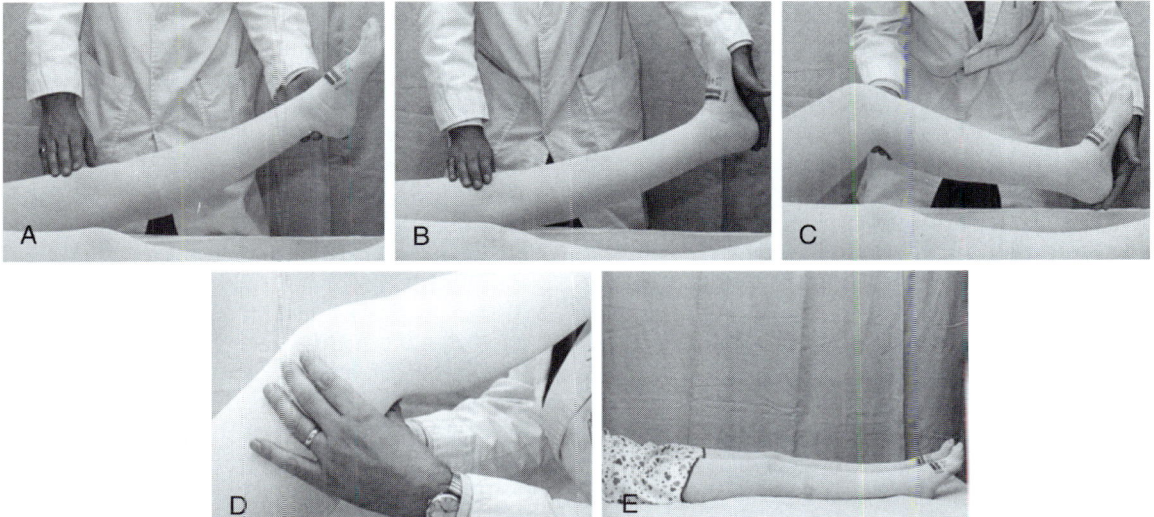

Figure 1. Straight leg raising test—five components: *A*, Straight leg raise, *B*, Dorsiflexion of foot. *C*, Flexion of knee until relief occurs. *D*, Bowstring test. *E*, Verification of straight leg raising limitation obtained by asking the patient to sit up with the legs straight.

the absence of neurologic signs does not exclude a diagnosis of nerve root pain.

The three components of neurologic assessment are motor function, sensory function, and reflex activity. Identification of the compromised nerve root depends on the segmental innervation of the lower limb muscles, which is still controversial. In a detailed study of perioperative lumbar nerve root stimulation, Young and coworkers[71] confirmed that the accepted patterns are essentially reliable. It was also shown that a dual innervation is present for most muscles, with one root being dominant, as is shown in Table 2.

An important feature of this study was the demonstration that in the presence of bony segmentation anomalies, variations in innervation patterns may be present, especially if sacralization of the fifth lumbar vertebra has occurred. Thus, the interpretation of neurologic signs must be allied to analysis of plain lumbar spine x-ray studies and, in particular, to the determination of the number of mobile lumbar vertebrae. A spine surgeon should be aware that Young and coworkers[71] recommended that, in the presence of segmental anomalies, the L5 and S1 roots should be explored at operation. An L5 sensory deficit is strong evidence of an L4–L5 prolapse, whereas S1 sensory changes should be analyzed with care.[32]

Whether the use of diagnostic nerve root blocks and the newer imaging techniques may allow even more preoperative diagnostic accuracy to be achieved remains to be seen.

An analysis of the reflex pattern of the lower limbs should be interpreted with care. The absence of ankle jerks is not unusual in the elderly or in individuals in whom a previous episode of S1 embarrassment has occurred that may have been subclinical.

Table 2

Segmental Innervation of Seven Muscles in the Lower Limb*

Muscle	Root	
Tibialis anterior	L5	
Extensor hallucis longus	L5	
Extensor digitorum brevis	L5	(80%)
	S1	(20%)
Gastrocnemius		
Caput laterale	L5	(75%)
	S1	(25%)
Soleus	S1	
Gastrocnemius		
Caput mediale	S1	
Abductor hallucis (mainly)	S1	

*The roots given are the dominant supply.
From Young, A., Getty, J., Kirwan E., et al.: Variations in the pattern of muscle innervation by the L5 and S1 nerve roots. Spine 8:616–624, 1983.

The ankle jerk is of multiple-root origin, and the absence of an ankle jerk alone is of limited diagnostic value. Kortelainen and colleagues[32] demonstrated that alteration in the status of the knee reflex is of no value in diagnosing the level of low lumbar lesions, nor is its alteration typical for high prolapses.

Clinical Syndromes of Nerve Root Compromise

The three commonest causes of lumbar nerve root compromise are disc prolapse, bony entrapment, and spinal stenosis.

The clinical presentation of prolapsed disc is well established. It is now appreciated in older patients that the commonest cause of sciatica, which is leg pain of root origin, is a degenerative change in the posterior joint complexes. The clinical presentation is different from that of a disc prolapse and has been described by Macnab and McCulloch[38] and by Getty and colleagues.[16]

Patients with bony entrapment tend to be at least 40 years of age, and they often have a long history of backache and subsequently have root pain in the leg. Spinal claudication may be present. Examination in most patients reveals no limitation of straight leg raising, and spinal movements are relatively free.

The clinical features of spinal stenosis have previously been well documented.[15, 64] This condition is better thought of as a clinical spectrum rather than a syndrome. The presentation may be variable.

A useful summary of the symptoms and signs of root entrapment resulting from these three different causes is presented in Table 3. In all three conditions, the commonest presenting symptom is low back and/or leg pain. Rydevik and colleagues[52] indicated that differences in the clinical picture of this disorder may result from the different types of neural deformations produced in the various conditions.

The most important recent advance in patient assessment is the appreciation of the importance of the functional contribution to disability. The commonest cause of a failed laminectomy is an incorrect diagnosis, leading to an inappropriate operation. One cannot assess patients on the basis of physical signs alone, or through sophisticated technologic investigations, without noting the functional contribution to their disability. The identification of the so-called nonorganic physical signs (Table 4) in low back pain, as described by Waddell and coworkers,[65] allows the clinician to recognize the presence of a possible functional contribution. In turn, this information helps to identify patients who require further psychosocial assessment.

The identification of such a functional contribution to the patient's disability enables the surgeon to avoid unnecessary investigation and therapy and accordingly to plan an appropriate management program, which may involve a multidisciplinary ap-

Table 3

Clinical Presentation of Disc Prolapse, Bony Entrapment, and Spinal Stenosis

Characteristic	Disc Prolapse	Bony Entrapment	Spinal Stenosis
Age at presentation			
Range	16–58 years	23–75 years	18–75 years
Mean	77% < 40 years	44.8 years	52 years
Mean duration of symptoms	77% < 5 years	10.6 years	5.8 years
Paresthesias	70%	58%	26%
Claudication	?	17%	39%
Reduction in spinal mobility	100%	71%	39%
Decreased straight leg raising ability	99%	29%	23%
Motor deficit	96%	49%	52%
Sensory deficit	80.6%	38%	58%
Reflex deficit	78%	42%	71%

Data from Getty, C. J. M.: Lumbar spinal stenosis. J. Bone Joint Surg. 62B:481–485, 1980; Getty, C. J. M., Johnson, J. R., Kirwan, E. O., and Sullivan, M. F.: Partial undercutting facetectomy for bony entrapment of the lumbar nerve root. J. Bone Joint Surg. 63B:330–335, 1981; O'Connell, J. E. A.: Protrusions of lumbar invertebral disc. J. Bone Joint Surg. 33b:8–30, 1951.

Table 4

Nonorganic Physical Signs in Low Back Pain*

Detection of tenderness
   Superficial or nonanatomic
Stimulation testing causing low back pain
   Axial loading on the skull
   Rotation of shoulders or pelvis as one unit
Inappropriate straight leg raising
Regional weakness and/or sensory deficit
Overreaction

*For clinical significance, three or more of the five signs should be present.

proach. The value of the nonorganic physical signs is to alert the surgeon that the possible functional contribution to the patient's overall disability should be further carefully assessed by appropriate experts. The presence of these signs does not necessarily always imply that operative intervention is inappropriate.

If a significant organic lesion is established, further investigation may be indicated to confirm the diagnosis and to establish which therapy should be offered. Each patient must receive treatment that is based on the characteristics of his or her individual disorder.

Investigations

Most patients with low back pain undergo plain radiography of the lumbar spine. Nachemson[42] indicated that clinically unsuspected abnormal findings are unusual in patients between the ages of 20 and 50 years. In the context of assessing patients for surgical treatment, the most important value of a plain x-ray study is the determination of the number of mobile lumbar vertebrae. The possibility of anomalous root innervation in the presence of bony segmental anomalies has already been mentioned.[71] Plain x-ray studies in patients who have had previous operative therapy often provide information as to the level in the spine of the previous procedure and give some indication as to its nature.

The introduction of CT and MRI revolutionized the investigation of the lumbar spine. However, as with myelography, these techniques should probably be used in only patients who are under serious consideration for operative intervention on the basis of their clinical assessment. Additionally, it is also well established that interpreting images involves observer bias. Despite popular claims, no single imaging technique has exclusive superiority over the others. One should understand that the information provided is often complementary rather than alternative.

Formerly, myelography was the imaging technique of choice in the investigation of the lumbar spine. This technique involves the introduction of a contrast medium into the subarachnoid space, the aim being to identify and confirm the level of neural compromise and to exclude the presence of neoplasm. Although the role of this investigation in the diagnosis of disc prolapse is well established, its place in identifying root canal stenosis remains less clear.[35]

Euinton and coworkers[13] found that in only one half of patients with bony entrapment did the myelographic and operative findings correlate exactly. They suggested that the reason for this failure was that the contrast-filled root sheaths did not extend far enough distally to allow the contrast medium to outline the site of entrapment (Fig. 2).

In patients for whom revision laminectomy is being considered, myelography has a limited role, largely because of the common existence of postoperative extradural fibrosis.[23] Myelography may also identify root anomalies, knowledge of the existence of which is important for the planning of surgical decompression.[29]

CT scanning is a noninvasive method of visualizing the vertebral canal and its contents. Care is required in the interpretation of CT scans. The incidence of false-positive results of CT scans is less well appreciated than that of false-positive myelographic results. In a comparison of CT and myelography in the diagnosis of bony entrapment, Stockley and coworkers[60] noted that, although myelography correctly identified root entrapment in 54% of patients undergoing primary or revision laminectomy, the accuracy of CT was higher, at 75%. Although they considered CT the method of choice in degenerative disease of the lumbar spine, they stressed that CT and myelography were complementary, not alternative, investigations.

For patients who have had previous sur-

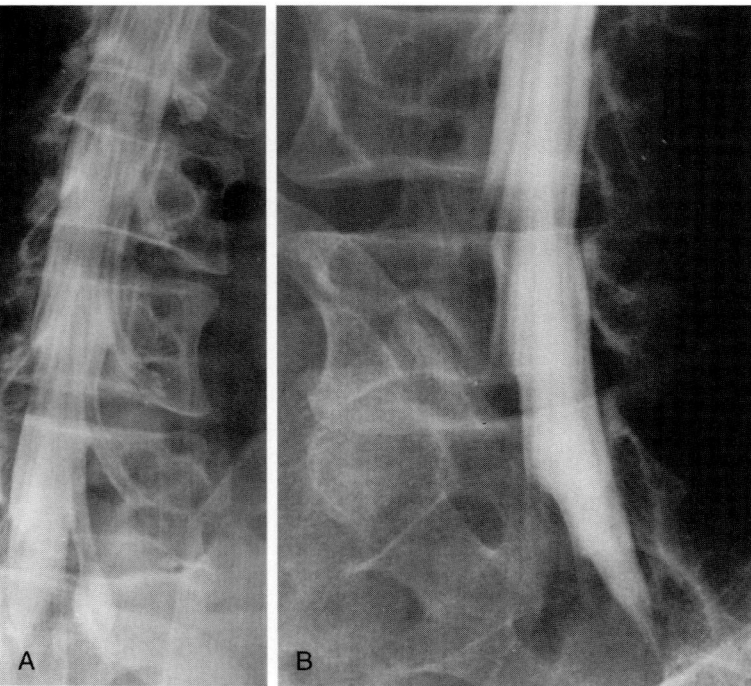

Figure 2. *A*, Root sleeves in this patient are long; thus, bony entrapment is likely to be demonstrated. *B*, Short root sleeves are present; thus, bony entrapment is unlikely to be demonstrated.

gery, CT also provides valuable information, outlining the extent of previous surgery and allowing the surgeon to plan the subsequent surgical intervention. The differentiation of scar tissue from disc material can be difficult. Contrast-enhanced CT was developed to aid in this situation.[61]

MRI as an imaging modality for the assessment of disorders of the lumbar spine is now much more readily available than formerly. It is likely to become the second imaging modality of choice, after routine radiography, for the evaluation of spinal dysfunction. It is a rapidly evolving technique and has the obvious advantage of not using ionizing radiation. The disadvantages are the long acquisition time and the variations of different MRI units in the quality of the images produced. An additional important problem can be the inability to use this modality in patients who are susceptible to claustrophobia.

Burton[4] indicated that the information provided by MRI relates more to the quality and nature of a tissue than to its structural delineation. Regarding the role of MRI in the identification of the level of nerve root involvement, Boumphrey and colleagues[3] found MRI to be more accurate in the diagnosis of disc degeneration, whereas they found CT to be more accurate in the diagnosis of root canal compression. MRI also seems to have a further role in assessing spinal canal dimensions and, in turn, in diagnosing spinal stenosis. A more detailed discussion of MRI in the lumbar spine is included in Magnetic Resonance Imaging of the Lumbar Spine in Chapter 6.

Bischoff and associates[2] reported on the sensitivity, specificity, and accuracy of CT-myelography, MRI, and myelography in the diagnosis of herniated nucleus pulposus and spinal stenosis. This retrospective study evaluated 59 surgical procedures performed on 57 patients who underwent all three tests before surgery. Overall, CT-myelography was the most accurate and the most sensitive test for the diagnosis of herniated nucleus pulposus, whereas myelography was the most specific. In making the diagnosis of spinal stenosis, CT-myelography and MRI were equally accurate and sensitive, whereas myelography was the most specific. In patients who had undergone previous surgery, the accuracy, sensitivity, and specificity in the diagnosis of spinal stenosis or herniated nucleus pulposus were highest with MRI.

This series indicated that CT-myelography was the most sensitive and accurate test for diagnosing both herniated nucleus pulposus and spinal stenosis, whereas myelography was the most specific. However, MRI compared favorably with CT-myelography in most instances, particularly in evaluating patients who had undergone previous spinal surgery, and it may become the diagnostic procedure of choice because of its noninvasiveness and lack of side effects.

Numerous other diagnostic techniques are also available in the preoperative assessment of patients. Nerve root injection studies have had a limited application, despite Macnab and McCulloch's[38] contention that the abolition of leg pain after root sheath infiltration is powerful evidence of the level of lesion. The technique has the advantage of identifying the level involved but does not identify (1) the underlying cause or (2) the reversibility of that cause. The technique is time consuming, and personal experience has indicated that its effectiveness depends on its regular use by the investigator. The advantage of nerve root injection seems to be that, in most patients with spondylosis, as Kikuchi and coworkers[31] demonstrated, abolition of root pain and intermittent claudication can be achieved by a single root infiltration. This result is obviously a great advantage in establishing the level of operative intervention and in minimizing the surgical trauma to the patient.

The experience in the Sheffield Problem Back Unit tends to confirm the last finding.[59] In addition, nerve root injection studies are valuable for determining whether the leg pain is referred or radicular. With the help of these studies, Stanley and coworkers[59] identified 56% of their patients with leg pain that was not predominantly of root origin. In patients undergoing operative treatment, the findings of nerve root injection studies and surgical evaluation correlated closely in 72%, bony entrapment being the main cause in the group studied. The investigators had one false-positive result. Although this test is time consuming and can be uncomfortable for the patient, one author (C. J. M. G.) has used it increasingly in older patients with spondylosis and suspected root involvement for which the level is uncertain.

Ongoing analysis of over 400 nerve root injection studies in the Sheffield Problem Back Unit continues to support this concept and its use, particularly as defined below under The Authors' Approach.

The results of controlled electromyography (EMG) studies, particularly in patients with bony entrapment, have not supported earlier claims for the success at the levels reported for this technique.[33] Jarrett and coworkers,[25] in a preliminary report and subsequently on further analysis, indicated that EMG can determine the presence of root compression, but it has limited value in identifying the level involved. EMG is also useful in patients with diabetes who present with a lumbar radiculopathy because it helps to distinguish the radiculopathy from diabetic neuropathy. The potential importance of this distinction is highlighted in the poor results reported by Simpson and colleagues[56] of lumbar spine surgery in patients with diabetes in whom EMG was not routinely used.

In the experience of one of the authors (T. S. W.), EMG is also beneficial for assessing patients who have undergone previous surgery. EMG abnormalities above the area of surgical intervention may indicate arachnoiditis if no other space-occupying lesions have developed. EMG is also of value in the evaluation of patients with failed back surgery syndrome who have developed arachnoiditis.

Dermatomal sensory evoked potentials have also been found useful in patients with disc prolapses, and they have approximately an 86% accuracy in determining the level.[10] Their role in bony entrapment has yet to be defined.

Liquid crystal tomography has been recommended by several investigators for diagnosing spinal root syndromes[47] Although attractive as a noninvasive technique, it is of no significant value in the diagnosis of these syndromes.[40]

In conclusion, although the aim of diagnostic criteria and techniques is to establish the presence and level of nerve root involvement or level of symptomatic stenosis, undoubtedly the overriding component is the clinical assessment of the patient. Plain x-ray studies and routine blood tests are commonly employed for most patients under investigation. Currently, MRI is probably the imaging investigation of choice. EMG provides a useful method of screening for the presence of radicular pain, particularly in older patients. Nerve root injection studies can provide valuable information, not only in determining the presence or absence of root pain but also in identifying the level involved.

TREATMENT VERSUS SPONTANEOUS RESOLUTION

The success of the treatment of disorders of the lumbar spine is difficult to evaluate because most patients improve spontaneously. The natural history of nerve root compromise, therefore, becomes extremely important. Three main conditions are associated with nerve root compromise in degenerative disorders of the lumbar spine: (1) herniated nucleus pulposus, (2) bony entrapment of nerve roots, and (3) stenosis of the lumbar spine. The diagnostic features of these conditions are considered above.

O'Connell[46] and Weber[67] wrote classic papers on the subject of the herniated nucleus pulposus. O'Connell thought that a history of a definite and remembered injury was important in determining the cause of a lumbar disc herniation.[46] In his opinion, the greatest problem was not establishing the diagnosis but rather deciding on the correct treatment regimen, because of the tendency to spontaneous recovery. He advised rest during the acute phase, followed later by exercise for the lumbar muscles and joints. Surgery was considered only when such a regimen failed. His personal series of 500 discs that were operated on represented only a small proportion of patients seen in his outpatient department in whom the clinical diagnosis of lumbar disc herniation had been made. He believed that determining exactly what proportion of patients with disc protrusions required surgery was difficult, but his estimate was that only one fifth of the patients referred to the outpatient clinic (a preselected population) underwent surgical intervention.

Weber[67] carried out a controlled prospective study of lumbar disc herniation over a 10-year period. For most patients, conservative therapy is preferred initially; surgical intervention is considered only if recovery is delayed. However, because the indications for operative intervention vary among physicians, Weber thought it important to compare the results of operative and nonoperative treatment in two randomized groups with disc herniation. Other investigators reported no significant difference in final outcome between surgery and conservative therapy after follow-ups ranging from 7 to 20 years.[20, 44] Weber studied 126 patients, aged between 25 and 55 years, who after 14 days of rest still had radicular pain and indications of increased dural tension. The choice of further treatment in these patients was debatable, and Weber thought it reasonable to assign them randomly to two groups, one for operative treatment and one for conservative treatment.

Subsequent analysis of the results indicated several important factors that have a major influence on the decision of whether to undertake surgery. No profession showed a striking tendency regarding the onset of low back pain and the onset of sciatica. Psychosocial problems were noted in nearly a third of the individuals, which is the same as the proportion found in the general Scandinavian population.[67]

Weber[67] assessed his patients on the basis of their ability to work, presence or absence of neurologic deficit, pain, and mobility of the spine. The overall assessment at follow-up examination indicated that, after 1 year, the results were significantly better in the surgically treated group. Comparison after 4 years did not show a statistically significant difference, although the surgically treated group still tended to have a more favorable outcome. At 10 years, hardly any difference existed in the results between the two treatment groups. The mean duration of recurrences in the two groups was the same. The rehabilitation period after leaving the hospital was shorter in the conservatively treated group. Restoration of muscle strength was found to be unrelated to the treatment modality and continued over several years. Sensory function followed a similar pattern. No difference was noted in either group with reference to pain or spinal mobility.

After 10 years of observation, only age was found to correlate with unsatisfactory results; older patients had poor results compared with those in younger patients. All other variables were noted to be without prognostic importance.

This carefully controlled study is important because it demonstrates the natural history of the disorder and the influence of conservative treatment and surgical intervention. In summary, in a group of patients who have disc herniation and debatable operative indications, the results of surgical treatment compared with conservative treatment are significantly better after 1 year, but during the course of the following 9 years, the difference becomes less pronounced. Moreover, as Weber also noted, the natural course of radiculopathies in disc disease is more encouraging than one might anticipate.

The relevance of these observations to newer techniques of operative management (e.g., percutaneous nuclectomy and laser discectomy) of disc prolapse remains to be defined.

Natural History of Bony Entrapment

The importance of bony entrapment of lumbosacral nerve roots has become increasingly apparent. Porter and colleagues[49] described the natural history of root entrapment syndrome. They noted that the clinical findings of this syndrome are distinct from those of an acute disc lesion. Root entrapment syndrome was diagnosed in approximately one tenth of patients attending Porter's Back Pain Clinic, which was an incidence higher than that of patients with a disc lesion. Although root symptoms were severe, signs were less common. Spinal movement was freer than in patients with an acute disc prolapse.

No specific therapy was offered in nearly 80% of the patients because they were either improving or were prepared to wait, having had the diagnosis explained. Approximately 10% were treated operatively. Assessment of the operated patients 1 year after surgery indicated that the pain was completely relieved in three patients, less severe in 15, but no better in six.

The progress of the patients who were not operated on and had been seen 1 to 4 years previously was assessed by a postal questionnaire. Most had root pain, but the vast majority of the conservatively treated patients were sufficiently satisfied, in spite of discomfort, not to have sought treatment elsewhere.

Thus, bony encroachment on a lumbar nerve root does not usually seem to require specific intervention. Porter believed that, after root symptoms were sufficiently severe to require hospital assessment, the condition was likely to become chronic, and only one in four patients would be asymptomatic 12 months later. However, most of the remainder found their pain to be manageable. This is certainly the author's (C. J. M. G.) impression. Interestingly Getty and colleagues[16] reported a mean time of 10.5 years from the onset of symptoms to operation in this group of patients; the corresponding time for disc prolapse is much shorter.

The cause of nerve root compromise in different age groups is shown in Table 5.

Natural History of Spinal Stenosis

The natural history of spinal stenosis is less clear. The commonest cause is degenerative spinal stenosis (Fig. 3). Wiltse and coworkers[70] believed that some degree of spinal stenosis was common in humans. Symptoms do not usually develop until the seventh decade of life,[58] and an insidious onset of slowly progressive symptoms is characteristic. Once severe symptoms are established in this condition, the patient is unlikely to improve with time, as, for example, does the younger patient with a disc herniation. Surgical intervention is often the only effective therapy. Undoubtedly for many patients, spinal stenosis goes undetected, and they are diagnosed as having mechanical back pain sometimes with referral to the legs.

The natural history of spinal stenosis was studied by Wardlaw and Macnab,[66] particularly in patients with spinal claudication treated conservatively. The conservative treatment regimen consisted of rest, administration of a nonsteroidal agent, an epidural injection, and application of a rigid lumbar brace. Patients who responded to this treatment had backache of less than 5 years' duration and leg pain of less than 6 months' duration, whereas those with backache lasting longer than 1 year and a tendency for

Table 5
■

Cause of Root Compromise in Different Age Groups

Age	Cause
0–40 years	Herniated nucleus pulposus
40–50 years	Herniated nucleus pulposus and bony entrapment
≥50 years	Bone

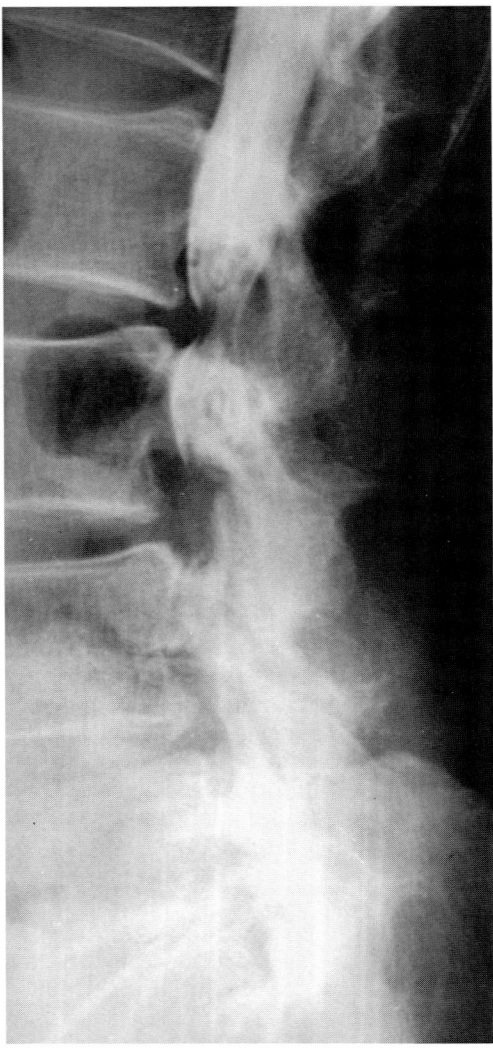

Figure 3. Myleogram of degenerative lumbar spinal stenosis.

bilateral symptoms remained the same or deteriorated. All the patients in this study had radicular leg pain. On the basis of this assessment, the investigators therefore believed that conservative treatment had a reasonable rate of success in patients with spinal stenosis and a history of backache of less than 5 years' duration and of leg pain of less than 6 months' duration. However, once symptoms and signs are established in this condition, operative intervention is often indicated.

Another study by Johnsson and coworkers[27] confirmed the natural history of this disease process. Thirty-two patients with a mean age of 60 years who had spinal stenosis were followed-up for 4 years. Initially, 57% of the patients had spinal claudication. At the end of 4 years, the same number of patients had some claudication, but the symptoms were milder. The authors believed that the symptoms in 70% of the cases were unchanged, 15% showed improvement, and 15% worsened. No proof existed of severe deterioration at the time of the 4-year follow-up.

Conservative Treatment of Sciatica

The evaluation of conservative treatment of sciatica is fraught with difficulty, owing to the spontaneous recovery of most patients. This is apparent from the foregoing analysis of the natural history of the main causes. For most patients, once a diagnosis of sciatica has been established, conservative therapy is offered initially.

Not all the methods available to treat sciatica are described here. The regimen advocated by Bell and Rothman[41] uses the two methods that seem to provide the most effective means of relieving root pain. This regimen consists of a period of bed rest, which may be 2 weeks, although many investigators recommend 3 weeks. The patient is provided with an antiinflammatory agent. Bed rest is followed by 7 to 10 days of mobilization, at which stage a program of back care and exercise is encouraged. In the absence of a definite indication for surgical intervention, up to 3 months of conservative treatment is thought to be reasonable before operative intervention is considered.

In patients without deteriorating neurologic or sphincter function, the authors advise 10 days of rest. Patients are allowed to get up to use the bathroom if they wish. Most patients can be treated at home, and many patients find this more relaxing than being confined to a hospital environment. Sphincter function must be checked at the initial assessment, the patient must be fully advised about disturbance of urinary and bowel control, and the general practitioner must be agreeable to visiting the patient during the period of conservative therapy.

A nonsteroidal antiinflammatory agent is used together with a muscle relaxant, if necessary, over the 10-day period. The nonsteroidal agent can be provided parenterally in the first 24 to 48 hours, and the agent can continue to be given thereafter in oral form. Administration of the drug is continued during the initial mobilization period. Additionally, a laxative is provided until the patient is mobile.

In patients with neurogenic claudication, the regimen of Wardlaw and Macnab[66] is used. The administration of calcitonin has proved unreliable in this situation and is no longer used by the author (C. J. M. G.).[48]

In patients with chronic sciatica, it is essential to define the exact disability, including an assessment of the patient's psychologic profile, if so indicated. If the disability is significant, a period of ambulant treatment and administration of a nonsteroidal agent, often with attention to spinal hygiene, exercise, and possibly a course of physiotherapy, may provide relief to the extent that the patient does not require additional treatment. If the treatment fails, further investigation may be indicated.

Surgical Treatment of Sciatica

It is important to define the indications for ceasing conservative therapy and undertaking a different treatment modality (Table 6). Although up to 3 months of conservative treatment have been advocated, the duration of treatment depends on the prevailing circumstances. In degenerative disorders of the lumbar spine, operative intervention undoubtedly produces the best results when undertaken for proven root entrapment syndromes.

An analysis of the outcome of any therapy for disorders of the lumbar spine is affected by the surgeon's selection criteria and by the therapeutic methods used in the surgeon's practice. In the International Society for the Study of the Lumbar Spine, a constant goal is to achieve an objective assessment of the patient's sciatica and thereby to provide a rationale for the treatment offered. However, every surgeon has his or her proven method for excising a disc, for decompressing a nerve root in cases of bony entrapment, and for decompressing a spinal stenosis.

The decision to operate on a patient is based on an overall assessment. Surgeons tend to rely too heavily on investigations and not to appreciate that the main factor in deciding whether to operate is the clinical assessment of the patient. Morris and coworkers,[41] in a prospective study of 185 patients undergoing primary lumbar spine surgery, compared the accuracy of clinical criteria and myelographic results in predicting the operative findings. They stated that, although surgeons agree in principle that diagnosis and decisions to operate should be based on an overall assessment of the patient and that investigations should be used to complement and not to replace clinical judgment, to their knowledge this study was the first that actually showed that clinical diagnosis supplemented by radiology was still better than radiology alone.

The advent of new technologic advances in imaging may incorrectly lead to decisions to operate, as undoubtedly occurred in the early days of the use of CT. It is essential for the surgeon to appreciate this possibility when he or she interprets the results of therapy.

Treatment of Disc Prolapse

As a compromise between conservative treatment and surgical intervention, other techniques mentioned earlier have gained great popularity. These techniques include chemonucleolysis, percutaneous nuclectomy, and laser discectomy and endoscopic manual discectomy. They are considered in detail in other sections of this book. The two longest established treatments are chemonucleolysis and percutaneous nuclectomy.

In chemonucleolysis, many different agents have been used, the most popular of which is chymopapain. McCulloch and Macnab[37] described in detail the pathophysiology and the arguments for and against the use of this agent. It is useful to assess the results reported by McCulloch and Macnab,[37] who indicated that the procedure was effective in relieving sciatic pain in 70% of properly selected patients. The results,

Table 6
■

Indications for Surgical Decompression of Lumbosacral Nerve Roots

Progressive neurologic deficit
Root pain interfering with function—failure to respond to conservative treatment
Impending cauda equina syndrome

however, were blighted by the occurrence of neurologic complications well documented in the literature to the extent that many lumbar spine surgeons have abandoned the use of this technique. In most cases, it is probably true that needle misplacement was responsible, but in many cases, the complications remain inexplicable.

Postacchini and colleagues[51] conducted a prospective study comparing the results of chemonucleolysis and surgery in 156 patients with lumbar disc herniation that was considered suitable for chemonucleolysis. They found the success of chymopapain injection in patients with large herniations to be significantly less than that of surgery. Chemonucleolysis was apparently the treatment of choice in most patients with small disc herniations. Thus, chymopapain was recommended as an effective alternative to surgery in most patients with medium-sized herniations when the preoperative clinical pattern indicated slight or moderate root compression. However, surgery was preferable in patients with large, small, or medium-sized herniations who had severe nerve root impingement.

Percutaneous nuclectomy offers an alternative method of decompressing the disc prolapse. This method has been recommended for the treatment of uncomplicated, "contained" herniated discs.[9] No significant complications have been reported to date, although obvious risks include nerve root damage, dural tears, and possible damage to retroperitoneal structures. The long-term results of percutaneous nucleotomy remain to be defined.

If these techniques and similar methods prove effective, the advantage is that the spinal canal is not broached. Some investigators claim that subsequent surgical intervention in the case of nuclectomy, if indicated, is no different from a primary procedure, and the results are as effective. This has certainly been the experience of the author (C. J. M. G.).

The least invasive of the classic surgical techniques is microlumbar discectomy, which was developed specifically for patients with surgically undisturbed lumbar anatomy who had a soft disc herniation without any lumbar spinal stenosis.[69] The aim was to decompress only that part of the disc that produced nerve root pressure in a minimum amount of time with minimum blood loss and tissue morbidity. In Williams'[69] hands, the operating time averaged approximately half an hour and the postoperative stay was 3 days. Fourteen percent of the patients in his series required reoperation, usually because of a true recurrent disc. In only 0.3% of patients was the cause a missed disc, whereas 17 (2%) of the 903 patients in his series had recurrent sciatica resulting from adhesions. Williams claimed a 99.1% surgical cure in his series at 12 years. He noted that most of the disc reherniations occurred within 9 months of the initial procedure. Further investigations led him to conclude that rigorous restrictions should be placed on the "lumbar" activities for 1 year after surgery in patients who underwent microlumbar discectomy in an attempt to prevent new lumbar injury.

The aim of decompressing a nerve root is to decompress with a minimum of trauma. Surgeons using microdiscectomy techniques emphasize that the benefits are a better operating field, a shorter procedure, the smaller incision used, and the more rapid rehabilitation. However, the limited access may produce difficulties in identifying the level involved unless radiologic techniques are used. In addition, the risk of leaving herniated disc material outside the operative field is increased, and a risk of failing to decompress stenotic canals adequately exists.[22] Radiologic techniques such as MRI and CT may allow more accurate patient selection. In a comparison of chemonucleolysis and microsurgical discectomy, the results for the group treated with chemonucleolysis were less successful than those for the group treated with microsurgical lumbar discectomy.[72] The rate of treatment success was lower, and the rate of patient morbidity was higher in the chemonucleolysis group.

Considerable variation exists among surgeons in the extent to which they excise disc material from within the disc space. Some favor an extensive exploration with thorough curettage; other surgeons remove only the disc prolapse. Spengler[57] reported the results of a study of 54 patients who underwent a limited discectomy. If the disc was sequestered, the free fragment was removed, and the annulus was not entered. In extruded disc herniations, the extruded fragment was excised, and loose fragments near the annular defect were removed with a small rongeur. In the case of a protruded disc, the annulus was incised, and all loose disc material was removed. The neural foramen was treated, as appropriate, in each case after disc excision. The results indicate that the technique was reliable, safe, and effective in selected patients with disc herniation. The prior concern that the incidence of recurrent disc herniation would increase with limited disc excision was not borne out.

The classic technique of lumbar disc excision was described by O'Connell.[46] In his series, 92% of the patients were completely symptom free or were significantly improved after surgery. O'Connell reported that postoperative recurrent symptoms requiring reoperation occurred in 2% of cases.

The role of simultaneous fusion is controversial. In a prospective study, White and colleagues[68] compared two groups receiving bilateral lumbar laminectomy and disc excision; one group had an intratransverse fusion with internal fixation. Both groups were studied approximately 3 years after the operation, at which time the investigators found that, although the general success rate in both groups was 87%, the best results were in the nonfusion group. Thus, simultaneous fusion appears to be unnecessary in patients with a simple herniated lumbar disc, but with the advent of internal fixation devices, the long-term results of simultaneous fusion in this situation have not been clearly determined.

Although this discussion concerns the posterior approach, disc prolapses may be excised anteriorly with interbody fusion.

Occasionally, the herniated nucleus pulposus is located in the foramen or is extraforaminal. In the past, some surgeons have considered it reasonable to excise the facets to gain access, thereby creating potentially symptomatic instability. However, Jackson and Glah[24] clearly showed that this measure is not necessary. Adequate exposure is invariably gained by a partial facetectomy and foraminotomy. If it is not, a lateral exposure through the intratransverse ligament should be considered, while keeping the facetal complex intact.

Posterior lumbar interbody fusion is used by some surgeons in the treatment of disc herniation. Cloward[5] quoted a success rate ("long-term cures") of 85%. The exact long-term success rate in other surgeons' hands remains to be clearly elucidated. Cloward[6] recommended posterior lumbar interbody fusion for patients with low back pain, with or without sciatica, due to lumbar disc disease as the ultimate answer to the treatment of disease of the lumbar spine. He stated that simple discectomy, decompression, laminectomy, and chemonucleolysis should be eliminated. This is a controversial view and remains to be proved.

The current treatment of choice in patients with simple lumbar disc protrusion, after appropriate investigation and a trial of conservative treatment, appears to be surgical decompression by microdiscectomy, limited lumbar discectomy, or a classic lumbar discectomy with curettage of the disc space through a laminotomy fenestration. Chemonucleolysis has fallen into some disrepute but may, with better understanding of the biochemistry and pathophysiology, be restored to an appropriate place in the treatment of this disorder. The long-term results of alternative techniques already mentioned, such as percutaneous nuclectomy, laser discectomy, and arthroscopically assisted discectomy, remain to be established. Overall, simultaneous fusion does not appear to have a significant role in the treatment of patients with simple lumbar disc protrusion.

The authors do not subscribe to the concept of a routine bilateral procedure, which is based on the idea that the patient may develop problems on the opposite side in the future. The operative therapy should be directed specifically toward the demonstrated site of pathologic change in most cases. This method is in keeping with the concept of minimum surgical trauma to achieve relief of the compromised root. Less radical decompressions are associated with a reduced likelihood of instability and thus fewer immediate or long-term potential problems on the opposite side.

A bilateral exploration of the lumbar spine may be indicated in the case of a central disc prolapse. Imaging techniques such as MRI, however, allow more careful preoperative planning, thereby helping to reduce the extent of surgical exposure. The final decision is, of course, always dictated by the surgeon's judgment at operation.

Treatment of Bony Entrapment

The findings at operation in patients with bony entrapment are often more subtle than those in patients with a true disc prolapse.

As previously mentioned, although in the older patient facetal arthritis is the commonest cause of root compromise, in patients 40 to 50 years of age, root compromise is frequently produced by a mixture of disc prolapse and bone. Defining the causal lesion may be impossible until the time of surgery, particularly in this older group. The decision to carry out a partial undercutting facetectomy, with or without disc excision, is often made at surgery. Likewise, in this group, the appearance of the nerve root is extremely variable; often, it is invisible until the partial undercutting facetectomy has been carried out. Microsurgery does not appear to yield acceptable results in patients with lateral recess stenosis.[14]

The results of operation in patients with bony entrapment were reported previously.[16] The mean age at operation in this group of 78 patients was 45 years, and leg pain was the predominant symptom. In half of the patients, evidence of motor involvement was present. The decompression is carried out by means of a partial undercutting facetectomy, which essentially preserves stability and helps maintain the tent of the spinal canal (Fig. 4). Eighty-five percent of the patients in this group were satisfied with the outcome of the surgery.

In this series, the cause of nerve root compromise was a degenerative change in the posterior joint complex. Although in one third of the patients the disc was removed simultaneously with the decompression, subsequent experience has been associated with a much lower incidence of disc excision. Because degenerative change occurs in the spine, patients with bony entrapment are advised that the aim of the procedure is to ease leg pain. Interestingly, however, in the initial period, a substantial proportion of patients gained relief from the back pain. Surgery should always be directed toward the symptomatic root. Prophylactic bilateral decompression is not indicated: little evidence exists to support its routine use, especially if a partial facetectomy is used.

A long-term analysis for spinal decompression for lumbar lateral recess stenosis was carried out independently at the Sheffield Unit.[53] Sixty-six consecutive patients who had a partial undercutting facetectomy for degenerative lateral recess stenosis between 1982 and 1988 were reviewed. Fifty-seven (86%) were available for examination 5 to 11 years after surgery, with a mean of 8.4 years. The fall-out in this study is important in that three patients had died of unrelated causes, and six were not traceable or were unable to attend.

Ninety-one percent of patients presented with sciatica and 5% with neurogenic claudication. The primary indication for surgery was leg pain, although all patients had back pain.

Interestingly, 18 patients had an associated disc prolapse. The commonest site of lateral recess stenosis was at L4–L5; this occurred in 35 patients (61%). No fusions were performed, and discs were removed in only the 18 patients with a prolapse.

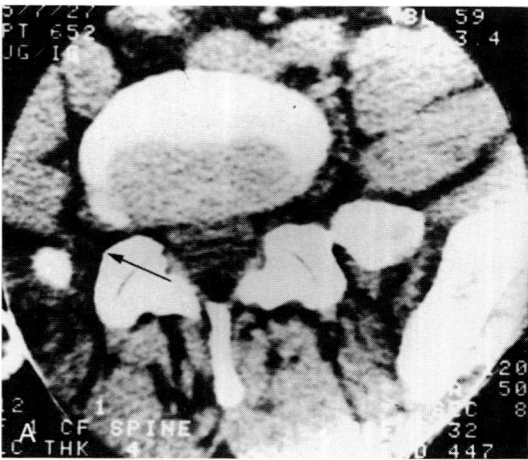 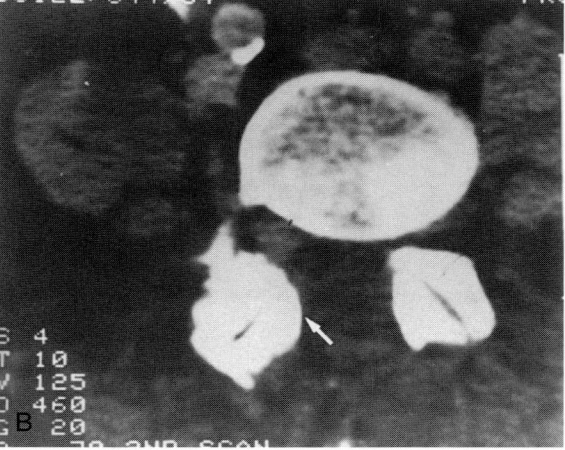

Figure 4. *A*, The arrow indicates the direction of the osteotomy cut in a partial undercutting facetectomy. *B*, CT appearance after a partial undercutting facetectomy.

In the long-term assessment performed a mean of 8.4 years after surgery, approximately 75% had an excellent result, with complete relief of leg pain or occasional mild pain. Nine (16%) had a fair result, and seven (12%) had a poor result.

Back pain was not included in the outcome measure, because it was not the indication for surgery; nevertheless, when the presence of back pain was assessed independently, mild or no back pain was present in approximately two thirds of the patients. In addition, no cases of increased olisthesis were reported after surgery, and no evidence of bone regrowth existed.

Treatment of Spinal Stenosis

The third condition causing sciatica is spinal stenosis, the clinical spectrum of which has already been considered. It may be congenital, developmental, or acquired. Here, treatment of acquired stenosis is discussed. Conservative therapy for this disorder has already been outlined. Once symptoms are firmly established and cause disability, operative treatment is usually indicated. In the past, unnecessarily wide and extensive decompressions have been performed, often with a poor outcome. Such procedures are now seldom indicated because it is understood that one level alone is often responsible for symptoms, despite the presence of extensive stenosis. Additionally, the introduction of newer surgical techniques, such as partial facetectomy, has eliminated the need of most patients for wide, destructive laminectomies, which are often associated with postoperative symptomatic instability. This concept also applies in patients with degenerative spondylolisthesis. Similarly, no statistically significant evidence exists to indicate that prophylactic decompression of the opposite side in patients with unilateral symptoms is routinely warranted, especially when these newer operative techniques are used. Further perioperative refinements, such as monitoring with sensory evoked potentials, remain controversial as a means of determining the required extent of operative therapy.

Spengler[58] reported that after posterior decompression, he did not have to carry out a stabilization procedure in any patient with acquired degenerative spinal stenosis. This author's (C. J. M. G.) experience is similar. Although postoperative slipping in degenerative spondylolisthesis may occur, it does not appear to influence the outcome of surgery.

The results of surgical treatment of idiopathic developmental lumbar spinal stenosis were reported in a classic paper by Verbiest.[64]

Getty[15] reported on a series of 31 patients treated for spinal stenosis. In 28 (90%) of the patients, degenerative change was the principal cause. After therapy, the condition of over 50% of the patients was classified as good, and that of 84% was satisfactory. Partial undercutting facetectomies were used for the lateral decompression, and spinal fusion was not carried out either simultaneously or subsequently in the patients studied in the series. A relatively long decompression was commonly performed in this group over several levels.

Sanderson and Wood,[54] in their study of surgery for lumbar spinal stenosis in elderly patients in a mixed series of 31 patients aged 65 years or older, concluded that the long-term outcome of decompressive surgery in the elderly was good and did not differ from that reported for younger patients.

Nasca[43] reported on a heterogeneous group of patients who had spinal stenosis: 71% of the patients obtained good results from their surgical treatment. The role of fusion was not clearly defined in the various groups. Natelson[45] noted that, in patients who had osteoporosis and a small compression fracture with spinal stenosis, decompression intensified the stenosis, and the compression fractures increased. He considered simultaneous bilateral fixation and fusion to be beneficial to this group.

There has been growing concern among some spinal surgeons about the long-term results of therapy for spinal stenosis. In a report by Katz and associates,[30] the initial good or excellent results found at 1-year follow-up in a series of 88 patients who underwent laminectomy for degenerative lumbar stenosis had begun to deteriorate. Ten of the original group of patients had an unsatisfactory result at 1 year. At 4 years after surgical intervention, 17% of the original 88 patients had to undergo a repeat operation, and 21% of patients who could be evaluated by questionnaire reported severe pain. Katz and associates noted that factors associated with a poor long-term outcome included the presence of a coexisting illness, failure to follow up, and initial laminectomy being performed at only one interspace. In one of the author's (T. S. W.) own series, similar findings were noted. In a series of 27 patients who underwent decompressive laminectomy for spinal stenosis, the initial good or excellent result at 2-year follow-up was 81%, but at 5-year follow-up, only 63% of patients felt they had a good result, and 22% of the original group had undergone another operation in an attempt to relieve the symptoms.

In 1985 and 1991, Herno and coworkers[21] carried out assessments of 108 patients who had undergone surgery for lumbar spinal stenosis. They found that at a mean of 6.8 years the results, when compared with those in 1991 (which was a mean of 12.8 years post surgery), of the patients improved during the course of the longitudinal follow-up time of 7 and 13 years. They felt the chances of a patient's undergoing reoperation after surgery for lumbar spinal stenosis were low. These patients were originally operated on between 1974 and 1981. Interestingly, surgical technique consisted of bilateral laminectomy extended laterally, decompressing the nerve roots. In most cases, lateral decompression was achieved by partial facetectomy, but the whole facet was removed if necessary.[21]

Postacchini and colleagues,[50] in an assessment of the surgical treatment of central lumbar stenosis, concluded that multiple laminotomy was recommended for all patients with developmental stenosis and for those with mild to moderate degenerative stenosis or degenerative spondylolisthesis. They concluded that total laminectomy is preferred for patients with degenerative stenosis or marked degenerative spondylolisthesis.

Tile,[62] in a discussion of how wide and how long a spinal decompression should be, indicated that the nerve should be fully decompressed. In most patients, this process did not necessitate a complete facetectomy. He also believed that long laminectomies were no longer indicated, because the symptoms of spinal stenosis were segmental. Although a limited approach was favored in this context, he believed that surgical judgment was required for the final decision.

However, the use of nerve root infiltration allows the surgeon to be more precise. Macnab and associates[39] reported that most patients with spinal stenosis present with clinical evidence of a single unilateral root compression, which can be confirmed by nerve root injection. In their series, more than 90% of patients had a satisfactory outcome after decompression of the offending root, and the results were maintained over time. He found that the existence of stenosis at other levels did not influence the results of a single root decompression and rarely caused subsequent symptoms.

Thus, conflict exists regarding the treatment of spinal stenosis. Identification of the symptomatic segmental level must be carried out, together with an adequate decompression, which usually involves a laminectomy with adequate decompression of the root canal. The latter can be achieved by using a partial undercutting facetectomy without simultaneously destroying spinal stability.

In cases of spinal stenosis in which so-called instability is evident, simultaneous fusion is indicated. The results of multilevel decompression are generally poor because of excessive fibrosis. Of course, in the assessment of the results of degenerative lumbar spinal disease with particular reference to spinal stenosis, it is important to realize that the degeneration in the spine is an ongoing process at several levels, and one may therefore reasonably expect that further decompression may be required at additional levels at a later stage. In patients with degenerative scoliosis in addition to their stenosis, stabilization in the affected area is usually indicated if a significant lateral listhesis of the apical vertebra is present.

In summary, several techniques of therapy have changed. An attempt has been made to limit the extent of surgical exposure by identifying the symptomatic levels preoperatively in an attempt to minimize scarring and the problems subsequently created in the spine. It is not so much the introduction of advanced technology that has led to these changes but rather the appreciation of certain clinical and causal factors. As previously stated, the decision to operate is ultimately based on clinical assessment.

REVISION SURGERY

In terms of revision surgery and success rates, the prospective consecutive 2-year evaluation of repeated decompression of lumbar nerve roots carried out by Jonsson and Stromqvist[28] provides interesting information. In their study, 93 patients who had had previous lumbar spine surgery were assessed, having undergone repeated decompression for persistent or recurrent back and leg pain.

Jonsson and Stromqvist[28] noted that the results were significantly related to the diagnosis; specifically, in the case of recurrent disc herniation or bony compression, nerve root compression responded well to repeated surgical procedure. In patients with a single root compression, results were similar to those claimed in primary surgery. However, these investigators confirmed a well-known observation that sciatica due to nerve root scarring was seldom improved by the repeated procedure.

Undoubtedly, the advent of MRI with gadolinium enhancement has greatly facilitated the identification of patients in whom the cause of recurrent leg pain of radicular origin is scarring. Both authors subscribe to the foregoing concepts and believe that the critical element in the assessment of patients for revision lumbar spine surgery is a careful clinical assessment. The clinical findings must be closely correlated with the radiologic findings. As with all aspects of lumbar spine surgery, careful counseling of the patient before revision surgery, in particular discussing expectations, is critical.

THE AUTHORS' APPROACH

When a surgeon is asked to describe his or her approach to the treatment of a specific problem, naturally the account is likely to be somewhat eclectic. Understandably, surgeons believe their philosophy to be correct in order to justify their practices.[7]

To understand a surgeon's approach to a specific disorder, one has to understand his or her conception of the problem. Surgeons are concerned with relieving nerve root compromise, whether by conservative therapy, minimally invasive therapy, or surgical intervention. The symptom that they are best equipped to treat is radicular leg pain. (Fusion is not discussed at length here, because this topic is outside this context.)

Table 7 outlines the factors contributing to the authors' philosophy in the treatment

Table 7

The Authors' Philosophy in the Treatment of Lumbosacral Nerve Root Dysfunction

Patients have back symptoms, not problem backs.
"Think root."
Clinical assessment dominates decision-making.
Leg pain is the symptom most effectively treated.
Extensive investigations are unwarranted unless the presence of root dysfunction is established and further treatment is indicated.
In most imaging techniques, the radiologist should be blinded to the suspected lesion until after reporting the results to obviate subjective interpretation.
Treat the symptomatic lesions.
Prophylactic decompressions are seldom indicated.

of lumbosacral nerve root dysfunction. Diagnostic criteria, techniques, current treatment options and their results, and the natural history of the conditions encountered are referred to above. The clinical assessment mentioned earlier is closely followed by the authors. A treatment protocol for lumbar spine decompressive surgery is outlined in Figure 5.

The value of plain x-ray studies has already been mentioned with regard to the segmental pattern of the lumbar spine, but they are also useful in the identification of the presence of an unsuspected spondylolisthesis or a degree of degenerative change not previously anticipated. Rarely does one find a lesion more sinister than already anticipated.

In bony segmental anomalies, sometimes one finds during clinical assessment an apparent overlap of the clinical symptoms and signs, suggesting multiple root involvement. Simple plain x-ray films may solve what initially seems to be a rather confusing pattern. In this context, the furcal nerve also requires consideration.[31]

Irrespective of the cause, the conservative treatment of root entrapment is as already outlined; a period of bed rest, the use of a nonsteroidal antiinflammatory agent, and then a period of mobilization. For most patients, this regimen is adequate, but further investigation is undertaken if symptoms fail to settle and the disability is sufficient to warrant it.

The investigation of choice for the lumbar spine is either MRI or CT, but one should consider these investigations complementary rather than alternative to each other.

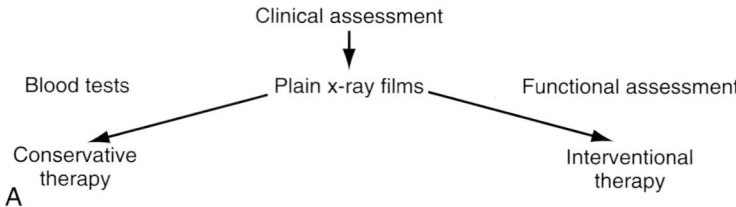

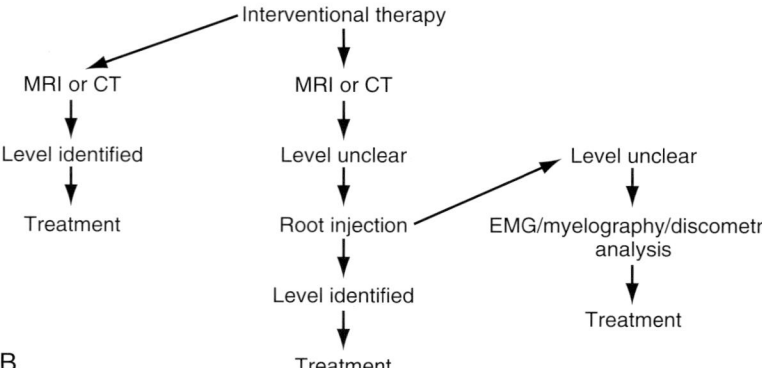

Figure 5. Diagnosis (*A*) and treatment (*B*) protocol for lumbar spine decompressive surgery.

Myelography still has a role to play, as demonstrated in Figure 5, particularly in cases in which the level of disease is unclear after root injection. Usually, the information gained from MRI or CT—and in some cases, root injection as well—is sufficient to complement the clinical assessment and to allow the surgeon to plan for the operation, if one is indicated on clinical grounds.

The value of nerve root injections has already been mentioned in terms of patients with apparent multilevel disease. This investigative tool is used in an attempt to identify the specific level or levels involved.

In the opinion of both authors, as a result of their experience in these groups, nerve root infiltration should be considered as a front-line investigative tool.

Other investigations, such as EMG, may be used in cases in which the level of root entrapment is unclear. EMG evaluation is particularly useful in the assessment of patients with diabetes who have lumbar spine problems.

In the case of an acute disc or bony entrapment, the preparations for surgery, if indicated, are similar after the patient's lesion has been formally identified. A general medical assessment is carried out. The orthopedic surgeon determines whether the patient is fit for the knee-chest position or some variation of the same (Fig. 6). Contraindications for this position include significant cervical spondylosis, obesity, and peripheral vascular disease. The authors use this position routinely, if it is considered safe for the patient. This position permits the best interlaminar exposure. It ensures free respiration and a low intraabdominal pressure, and it prevents venous congestion in the extradural space.[11] Serious complications with the position are rare and largely avoidable.

Positioning the patient is important and requires an adequate number of experienced staff members. The patient is anesthetised on the bed, rolled to the prone position on the operating table, and then lifted to the

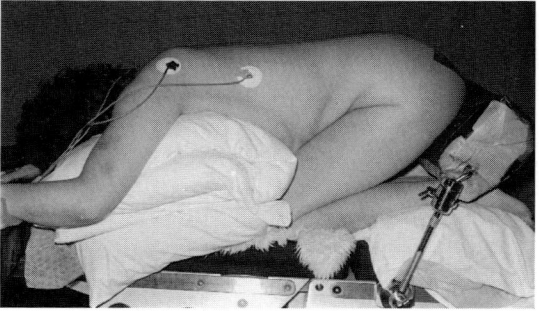

Figure 6. Patient in knee-elbow position.

knee-chest position. The abdomen must lie free. The position of the head is controlled at all times by the anesthetist, and the neck must not be twisted, because of the potential risk of vertebral artery thrombosis.

Preoperative Planning

In preoperative planning, the surgeon must be aware of the number of mobile vertebral bodies, the level of the lesion, and the symptomatic side. It is the author's (C. J. M. G.) practice to mark the symptomatic leg from behind because it is easy to forget that sides change when the patient is turned to the prone position. This is a small but costly cause of failed back surgery.

Surgical Decompression

With induction of anesthesia, a broad-spectrum antibiotic is given, usually cephalosporin, which is routinely administered 8 and 16 hours after operation. The authors do not routinely infiltrate the skin with lidocaine and epinephrine.

Diathermy is used to divide the muscle from the spinous processes, staying close to these processes and thereby ensuring a bloodless plane. Muscle is swept out to expose the appropriate operative field. The level is identified by direct visualization, and the sacrum identified. If any doubts exist regarding the disc level, a radiograph should be obtained. Identification of the pars interarticularis facilitates the extent of the dissection. The spinal canal is then entered. Routinely, a head lamp and loupes are used to facilitate the surgery.

Discectomy

For discectomy, a laminotomy fenestration is usually adequate. The principle of nerve root decompression is to mobilize the neural tissue and to retract it but disturb it as little as possible, while at the same time achieving an adequate decompression. Once exposure is adequate, the nerve is identified and mobilized, and the disc is excised. It is the authors' practice to excise the disc on the basis of a limited discectomy.[57] Vigorous curettage of the disc space is usually unrewarding and potentially dangerous. The production of an intervertebral hematoma caused by scraping of the bone ends can create a potential site of bacterial infection. After the nerve root is adequately decompressed, the surgeon must search carefully in all directions for free fragments.

At the end of decompression, positive-pressure ventilation by the anesthetist is undertaken to detect dural leaks. If any are present, they should be repaired and sealed with a fascial graft if necessary. A fat graft is then placed over the laminotomy fenestration site and sutured to prevent it from dropping into the canal.

Fat grafting appears to be the most effective means of minimizing scar formation,[63] but meticulous hemostasis is essential throughout the procedure. Hypotensive anesthesia is also essential.

If anomalous roots, which are often detectable by the preoperative imaging, are present, they must not be damaged. In the authors' experience iatrogenic trauma to such roots can be avoided when mobilizing and removing the disc or, in the presence of bony entrapment, decompressing the root. It may be necessary to extend the laminotomy fenestration to a wider exposure to allow access to the disc prolapse. In this context, adequate exposure is vital.

Closure of the muscles is performed in layers. Draining the laminectomy wound is not usual.

Postoperative mobilization is largely determined by the patient's progress, straight leg raising is encouraged at once, and the patient is allowed to stand as soon as pain control is adequate, usually within the first 12 to 24 hours. Sitting is allowed after several days, after the patient has control of his or her back and feels comfortable. Instructions in back hygiene are supplied. Excessive physical activity is to be avoided for at least 3 months to facilitate healing.

Intermittent catheterization is undertaken, if necessary, and an appropriate antibiotic is given until 24 hours after voiding of urine is established.

Treatment of Bony Entrapment

The technique of partial undercutting facetectomy may be used in patients with isolated bony entrapment.[16] Osteotomes ranging from 1 to 10 mm in width are used. The direction of the cut is always in the longitudinal axis of the nerve. It is important that no instruments, such as punches, are forced beneath the facets because the nerve may become crushed and damaged. After the partial facetectomy has begun, however, one can use fine punches to complete the decompression.[12] At the conclusion of decompression, the nerve must lie free throughout the root canal, from its origin at the dural sac to its passage through the intervertebral foramen. Occasionally, the pedicle must be shaved with an osteotome to achieve this goal. In true bony entrapment, the disc need not usually be violated. However, in cases of mixed bone and disc disorders, the disc is removed; the ultimate decision for this step is made perioperatively.

The same principles of closure and mobilization are used as for discectomy. A nonsteroidal antiinflammatory agent is used during the postoperative period for 2 to 3 weeks.

To date, bony regrowth has not proved to be a problem.[53] Undoubtedly, preoperative identification of the level involved will serve to minimize surgical trauma and, one hopes, to improve the results.[31, 59]

Treatment of Spinal Stenosis

The identification of the symptomatic root or segmental level has revolutionized the surgical treatment of spinal stenosis. Multisegmental laminectomy is seldom performed unless, obviously, it is indicated from the preoperative investigations. An adequate central decompression must be carried out. A lateral decompression may be accomplished by a partial undercutting facetectomy. Fat grafts are used, and the postoperative regimen is essentially the same as for bony entrapment.

In patients with degenerative spondylolisthesis, a similar technique is used. It has not been the authors' practice to perform simultaneous fusion in such patients routinely, although this topic is still a matter of debate.[8, 34]

THE FUTURE

Much progress has been made in recent years, with the increasing emphasis on the root and the development of newer investigative modalities to delineate the site and cause of nerve root compromise. Refinements in surgical techniques and the introduction of minimally invasive procedures will undoubtedly continue.

Future research continues in the pathophysiology of nerve root compromise. An attractive long-term proposition is the possibility of medication to counteract this compromise.

The role of fusion in treating the entire range of patients with degenerative lumbar spinal disease is still a matter of debate, largely because of ignorance about the pathophysiology and recognition of symptomatic lumbar instability. The situation may be summarized simply: patient selection, not implant selection, is important. Undoubtedly, research in this area will continue.

A major area of concern remains the assessment of the adequacy of nerve root decompression perioperatively. This assessment is largely subjective, and a reliable objective method remains to be developed.

In patients presenting with lumbar spinal disorders, a precise anatomic diagnosis is seldom achieved. As a result, the term problem back has evolved, which is unfortunate because patients should be treated on the basis of their specific disorders. Some of the confusion surrounding this group of patients could be readily dismissed. Ideally, one should not talk of a problem back but of a patient with a back symptoms.[17]

REFERENCES

1. Bell, G. R., and Rothman, R.: The conservative treatment of sciatica. Spine 9:54–56, 1984.
2. Bischoff, R., Rodriguez, R., and Gupta, K., et al.: A comparison of computed tomography–myelography, magnetic resonance imaging, and myelography in the diagnosis of herniated nucleus pulposus and spinal stenosis. J. Spinal Disord. 6:289–295, 1993.
3. Boumphrey, F. R. S., Modic, M., and Bell, G.: Nuclear magnetic resonance of the lumbar spine. Presented at the International Society for the Study of the Lumbar Spine Meeting, Montreal, 1984.
4. Burton, C. V.: High-resolution CT scanning: Present and future. Orthop. Clin. North Am. 14:539–551, 1983.
5. Cloward, R. B.: Posterior lumbar interbody fusion. Treatment of ruptured lumbar intervertebral disc by vertebral body fusion. Indications, operative technique, aftercare. Clin. Orthop. 193:5–15, 1985.
6. Cloward, R. B.: Posterior lumbar interbody fusion, updated. Clin. Orthop. 193:16–19, 1985.

7. Colton, C. L.: Slipped upper femoral epiphysis. In Catterall, A. (ed.): Recent Advances in Orthopaedics. Edinburgh, Churchill Livingstone, 1987, pp. 61–77.
8. Dall, B. E., and Wroe, D. E.: Degenerative spondylolisthesis, its surgical management. Spine 10:668–672, 1985.
9. Davis, G. W.: Personal communication, 1988.
10. Dvonch, V., Scarff, T., Bunch, W. H., et al.: Dermatomal somatosensory evoked potentials: Their use in lumbar radiculopathy. Spine 9:291–293, 1984.
11. Eie, N., Solgaard, T., and Kleppe, H.: The knee/elbow position in lumbar disc surgery. A review of complications. Spine 8:897–900, 1983.
12. Epstein, J.: Personal communication, 1981.
13. Euinton, H. A., Locke, T. J., Barrington, N. A., et al.: Is water soluble radiculography accurate in predicting the level of bony entrapment of lumbosacral nerve roots? J. Bone Joint Surg. 67B:499, 1985.
14. Feldman, R. J., and McCulloch, J. A.: Microsurgical experience in the treatment of degenerative lumbar spine disorders. Presented at the International Society for the Study of the Lumbar Spine Meeting, Rome, 1987.
15. Getty, C. J. M.: Lumbar spinal stenosis. J. Bone Joint Surg. 62B:481–485, 1980.
16. Getty, C. J. M., Johnson, J. R., Kirwan, E. O., and Sullivan, M. F.: Partial undercutting facetectomy for bony entrapment of the lumbar nerve root. J. Bone Joint Surg. 63B:330–335, 1981.
17. Getty, C. J. M.: Management of the problem back. In Catterall, A.: Recent Advances in Orthopaedics. Edinburgh, Churchill Livingstone, 1987, pp. 79–100.
18. Gibson, M. J., Szypryt, E. P., Buckley, J. H., et al.: Magnetic resonance imaging of adolescent disc herniation. J. Bone Joint Surg. 69B:699–703, 1987.
19. Gill, G. G., Scheck, M., Kelley, E. T., and Rodrigo, J. J.: Pedicle fat grafts for the prevention of scar in low back surgery. Spine 10:662–667, 1985.
20. Hakelius, A.: Prognosis in sciatica. A clinical follow-up of surgical and non-surgical treatment. Acta Orthop. Scand. [Suppl.] 129:1, 1970.
21. Herno, A., Airaksinen, O., and Saari, T.: Long term results of surgical treatment of lumbar spinal stenosis. Spine 18:1471–1474, 1993.
22. Hudgins, W. R.: The role of microdiscectomy. Orthop. Clin. North Am. 14:589–603, 1983.
23. Irstam, L.: Differential diagnosis of recurrent lumbar disc herniation and post operative deformation by myelography. Spine 9:759–763, 1984.
24. Jackson, R. P., and Glah, J. J.: Foraminal and extra foraminal disc herniation: Diagnosis and treatment. Spine 12:577–585, 1982.
25. Jarratt, J. A., Getty, C. J. M., Stockley, I., et al.: Electromyography and bony sciatica. J. Bone Joint Surg. 67B:499, 1985.
26. Johansson, J. E., Barrington, T. W., and Ameli, M.: Combined vascular and neurogenic claudication. Spine 7:150–158, 1982.
27. Johnsson, K., Rosen, I., and Uden, A.: The natural course of lumbar spinal stenosis. Clin. Orthop. 279:82–100, 1992.
28. Jonsson, B., and Stromqvist, B.: Repeat decompression of lumbar nerve roots. J. Bone Joint Surg. 75B:894–897, 1993.
29. Kadish, L. J., and Simmons, E. H.: Anomalies of the lumbar sacral nerve roots. J. Bone Joint Surg. 66B:411–416, 1984.
30. Katz, J., Lipson, S., Larson, M., et al.: The outcome of decompressive laminectomy for degenerative lumbar stenosis. J. Bone Joint Surg. 73A:809–816, 1991.
31. Kikuchi, S., Hasue, M., Nishiyama, K., and Tsukasa, I.: Anatomic and clinical studies of radicular symptoms. Spine 9:23–30, 1984.
32. Kortelainen, P., Puranen, J., Kolvisto, E., and Lahde, S.: Symptoms and signs of sciatica and their relation to the localisation of the lumbar disc herniation. Spine 10:88–92, 1985.
33. Leyshon, A., Kirwan, E. O. G., and Wynn Parry, C. B.: Electrical studies in the diagnosis of compression of the lumbar root. J. Bone Joint Surg. 63B:71–75, 1981.
34. Lombardi, J. S., Wiltse, L. L., Reynolds, J., et al.: Treatment of degenerative spondylolisthesis. Spine 10:821–827, 1985.
35. Love, B. R., Davies, A. A., Kirwan, E. O., and Sullivan, M. F.: The normal radiculogram. The relation between operative findings and clinical and electrical investigations. J. Bone Joint Surg. 64B:135, 1982.
36. McCulloch, J. A., and Waddell, G.: Variations of the lumbo-sacral myotomes with bony segmental anomalies. J. Bone Joint Surg. 62B:475–480, 1980.
37. McCulloch, J. A., and Macnab, I.: Sciatica and Chymopapain. Baltimore, Williams & Wilkins, 1983.
38. Macnab, I., and McCulloch, J. A.: Backache. Baltimore, Williams & Wilkins, 1989.
39. Macnab, I., McBroom, R. J., Wardlaw, D., and Parrott, T.: Unilateral root decompression in lumbar spinal stenosis. Presented at the International Society for the Study of the Lumbar Spine, Rome, 1987.
40. Mills, G. H., Davies, G. K., Getty, C. J. M., and Conway, J.: The evaluation of liquid crystal thermography in the investigation of nerve root compression due to lumbo-sacral lateral spinal stenosis. Spine 11:427–432, 1986.
41. Morris, E. W., Di Paola, M., Vallance, R., and Waddell, G.: Diagnosis and decision making in lumbar disc prolapse and nerve entrapment. Spine 11:436–439, 1986.
42. Nachemson, A. L.: The lumbar spine. An orthopaedic challenge. Spine 1:59–61, 1976.
43. Nasca, R. J.: Surgical management of lumbar spinal stenosis. Spine 12:809–316, 1987.
44. Nashold, B. S., and Hrubec, Z.: Lumbar Disc Disease: A 20-Year Clinical Follow-up Study. St. Louis, C. V. Mosby, 1971.
45. Natelson, S. E.: The injudicious laminectomy. Spine 11:966–969, 1986.
46. O'Connell, J. E. A.: Protrusions of lumbar intervertebral disc. J. Bone Joint Surg. 33B:8–30, 1951.
47. Pochaczevsky, R., Wexler, C. E., and Meyers, E. N., et al.: Liquid crystal thermography of the spine and extremity: Its value in the diagnosis of spinal root syndromes. J. Neurosurg. 56:386–395, 1982.
48. Porter, R. W., and Hibbert, C.: Calcitonin treatment for neurogenic claudication. Spine 8:585–592, 1983.
49. Porter, R. W., Hibbert, C., and Evans, C.: Natural history of root entrapment syndrome. Spine 9:418–421, 1984.
50. Postacchini, F., Cinotti, G., Perugia, D., and Gumina, S.: Surgical treatment of central lumbar stenosis. J. Bone Joint Surg. 75B:386–392, 1993.
51. Postacchini, F., Lami, R., and Massobrio, M.: Che-

monucleolysis versus surgery in lumbar disc herniation. Correlation of the results to pre-operative clinical pattern and size of the herniation. Spine 12:87–96, 1987.
52. Rydevik, B., Brown, M. D., and Lundborg, G.: Pathoanatomy and pathophysiology of nerve root compression. Spine 9:7–15, 1984.
53. Sanderson, P. L., and Getty, C. J. M.: The long term results of partial undercutting facetectomy for a lumbar lateral recess stenosis. J. Bone Joint Surg. 76B(Orthopaedic Proceedings, Suppl. 1 and 2): 133, 1994.
54. Sanderson, P. L., and Wood, P. L. R.: Surgery for lumbar spinal stenosis in old people. J. Bone Joint Surg. 75B:393–397, 1993.
55. Sherk, H. (ed.): Laser discectomy. Spine 7:xii, 1993.
56. Simpson, J. M., Silveri, C. D., Balderson, R. A., et al.: The results of operations on the lumbar spine in patients who have diabetes mellitus. J. Bone Joint Surg. 75A:1823–1829, 1993.
57. Spengler, D. M.: Lumbar discectomy, results with limited disc excision and selective foraminotomy. Spine 7:604–607, 1982.
58. Spengler, D. M.: Degenerative stenosis of the lumbar spine. J. Bone Joint Surg. 69A:305–308, 1987.
59. Stanley, D., McLaren, M. I., Euinton, H. A., and Getty, C. J. M.: A prospective study of nerve root infiltration in the diagnosis of sciatica: A comparison of radiculography, computer tomography and operative findings. Spine 15:540–543, 1990.
60. Stockley, I., Getty, C. J. M., Dixon, A. K., et al.: Lumbar lateral canal entrapment: Clinical, radiculographic and computed tomographic findings. Clin. Radiol. 39:144–149, 1988.
61. Teplick, J. G., and Haskin, M. E.: Intravenous contrast-enhanced CT of the post operative lumbar spine. AJR 143:845–855, 1984.
62. Tile, M.: The role of surgery in nerve root compression. Spine 9:57–64, 1984.
63. Van Akkerveekan, P. F., Van De Kraan, W., and Muller, J. W. T. H.: The fate of the free fat graft. Spine 11:501–504, 1986.
64. Verbiest, H.: Results of surgical treatment of idiopathic developmental stenosis of the lumbar vertebral canal. J. Bone Joint Surg. 59B:181–188, 1977.
65. Waddell, G., McCulloch, J. A., Kummel, E., and Venner, R. M.: Non-organic physical signs in low back pain. Spine 5:117–125, 1980.
66. Wardlaw, D., and Macnab, I.: The natural history of spinal stenosis. Presented at the International Society for the Study of the Lumbar Spine, Cambridge, 1983.
67. Weber, H.: Lumbar disc herniation. A controlled prospective study with ten years of observation. Spine 8:131–140, 1983.
68. White, A. H., Von Rogov, P., Zucherman, J., and Heiden, D.: Lumbar laminectomy for herniated disc. A prospective controlled comparison with internal fixation fusion. Spine 12:305–307, 1987.
69. Williams, R. W.: Micro lumbar discectomy: A twelve year statistical review. Spine 11:851–852, 1986.
70. Wiltse, L. L., Kirkaldy-Willis, W. H., and McIvor, G. W. D.: The treatment of spinal stenosis. Clin. Orthop. 115:83–91, 1976.
71. Young, A., Getty, J., Kirwan, E. O. G., et al.: Variations in the pattern of muscle innervation by the L5 and S1 nerve roots. Spine 8:616–624, 1983.
72. Zeiger, H. E.: Comparison of chemonucleolysis and microsurgery discectomy for the treatment of herniated lumbar discs. Spine 12:796–799, 1987.

Anterior Surgical Approach to the Thoracolumbar, Lumbar, and Lumbosacral Spine

■

ROBERT G. WATKINS

After deciding that an anterior approach is needed, the surgeon must choose exactly what type of anterior approach is best. The position of the patient and the location of the skin incision are the first considerations. The flank approach with the patient in the lateral decubitus position is commonly used for thoracolumbar junction pathologic changes. The approach that allows the greatest area of exposure is the 10th rib thoracoabdominal approach. The 10th rib thoracolumbar approach is the universal approach to the thoracolumbar junction; it is transpleural, transdiaphragmatic, and retroperitoneal. The best exposure for the L1–L2 area is via the 12th rib approach. When poor visualization is anticipated on an approach to the upper lumbar spine or ease of approach is sought, the lateral position is used, the kidney rest is raised, the table is cracked in the middle, the 12th rib is removed, and the 12th rib bed is opened extrapleurally and retroperitoneally.

For L1–L2 access, the lateral position is used with a 12th rib excision. The incision begins over the 12th rib, is extended to the 12th rib tip, and is then curved down along the rectus sheath as far distally as needed. To expose the L2–L3 disc space, the supine position is used for the patient, the incision begins in the midlateral line over the 12th rib, and a curvilinear incision is extended to just above the umbilicus. To expose L3–L4 and below, the incision begins equidistant between the 12th rib and the iliac crest. The curvilinear incision ends at the umbilicus for L3–L4, at the junction of the upper and middle third of the distance between the umbilicus and the pubis for exposure of L4–L5, and at the junction of the middle and lower third of that distance for exposure of L5–S1.

The lateral position for obese patients allows the pannus to fall away from the spine, even over the edge of the table, leaving a minimum of tissue between the skin and the spine. If the skin incision begins in the midlateral line, the flank approach allows easy recognition of the peritoneum for the retroperitoneal approach. Gravity assists with retraction of the peritoneal sac when a flank approach is used.

In the supine approach, the patient is positioned on his or her back over the kidney rest. The medialmost extent of the skin incision is to the midline at the same point as explained for the flank approach. It is usually extended 10 to 14 cm toward the midlateral line above the iliac crest.

Cosmetically, the transverse, low, short incision is best, but the curvilinear incision, especially in the upper lumbar spine, gives the area greater exposure, thereby permitting the surgeon better access.

The chief advantage of using the supine position rather than the lateral position is the ability to extend the table, thereby opening the disc space and giving a greater distraction and visibility of the disc space. Extending the table with the patient in the lateral decubitus position also opens the disc space and allows grafts to be held under tension. Also, the space may open unevenly with the patient in the lateral position, more on the left than on the right. Disc space distraction and graft fixation are facilitated by having the patient in the supine position. For reduction of a major deformity, the flank approach may offer advantages. In scoliosis, the convexity is positioned up and excellent exposure of the apex is obtained. In reduction of a spondylolisthesis, the position is determined by the method of reduction to be used. This author usually uses the supine approach, but other surgeons use the flank approach.

Visualization of the posterior disc space and the spinal canal is important in certain operations. In the flank approach, the patient is rotated up to 45 degrees out of the true lateral decubitus position to allow better direct visualization of the spine. With the patient in the supine position, the spine exposure is more directly anteroposterior but is limited by the extent to which the rib cage may be retracted cephalad in the upper lumbar spine or whether the peritoneal sac can be retracted far enough to the right to get a true anteroposterior view in the supine position. Cutting the rectus sheath and rectus muscle and extending the skin incision across the midline can enhance exposure in the midline, if needed. Knowing how to use the retractors is critical to direct anteroposterior visualization with either approach. Exposure of the dural sac from the anterior approach can be accomplished in either of two ways. One is by approaching the canal laterally, exposing a pedicle and the lateral annulus and separating the annulus from the dura laterally. This method is commonly used in the thoracic spine by following the rib to the rib head, to the disc space, and to the canal.

The second method is to make the incision directly down the middle, exposing the back of the vertebral body end plate and dissecting the annulus off the dura as the disc is excised anterior to posterior—much like an anterior cervical fusion with canal exploration. The flank approach may be more suitable when using the first method, and the supine approach more appropriate to the second. The author prefers using the supine approach with maximum table extension and direct annular excision in cases in which the canal is to be exposed in the lumbar spine, and the lateral approach when operating on the thoracic or thoracolumbar spine.

As for the retroperitoneal versus a transperitoneal approach, the retroperitoneal approach has fewer complications and is easier to use. The transperitoneal exposure is used for some difficult cases. In extreme lumbar lordosis, the disc space is angled caudally, making full visualization of the space difficult. A midline transperitoneal approach allows exposure as distally as possible and gives the best direct anteroposterior view. Extreme retroperitoneal scarring may necessitate a transperitoneal approach. Although the retroperitoneal approach is preferred because it is fast and effective, permits retraction of the ureters with the sac, and allows easy exposure to the vessels, the transperitoneal approach allows good visualization in difficult cases.

For approaches to the thoracolumbar junction (T10–L1), Hodgson and Yau[4] recommend a ninth rib resection. Dwyer and colleagues[3] advocated a 10th rib resection with the standard thoracolumbar approach. For T12–L1 exposure, Perry[7] recommended a 10th rib resection. The rules for the best rib to resect for exposure are much the same in this area as in the rest of the thoracic spine. Ideally, choosing the rib in the midaxillary line opposite the lesion or the apex of a curve allows adequate proximal exposure for working down, or caudad, on the lesion.

For maximum exposure of T10–T11, transthoracic resection of the ninth rib is usually best; at T11–L1, a 10th rib thoracoabdominal approach is preferred. These approaches involve detaching the diaphragm at its circumference. In patients in whom the diaphragm must not be taken down, or in whom less exposure is needed (such as in those requiring resection of one disc with grafting), the 12th rib extrapleural retroperitoneal approach is preferred.

Three additional approaches have use in special situations. The 11th rib approach is the highest practical extrapleural retroperitoneal anterior approach for exposure of T10–L2. It is a more demanding approach than any of the others, presenting less expansive exposure, but it avoids opening of the pleural cavity and cutting of the diaphragm in cases with high risk of morbidity.

The posterior costotransversectomy is a viable alternative for limited extrapleural exposure with low morbidity. If the 12th subcostal nerve is followed to T12–L1, the vertebral body and spinal canal can be exposed. The visualization needed for total discectomy, vertebrectomy, and strut grafting is inferior in this approach when compared with that afforded by the anterior approach, unless at least two levels are included in costotransversectomy.

The 10th rib thoracolumbar approach is used for long exposures of the thoracic and lumbar spine. This approach allows proximal and distal extension for multilevel operations and optimum exposure for bony work.

For thoracolumbar approaches, the anatomy of the diaphragm is most important. The diaphragm itself is markedly dome shaped, arching cephalad to approximately the T7 level. It is attached distally to the sternal part of the xiphoid process, the costal part to the inner surface of the costal cartilages, and ribs six through 12. It is also attached to the lumbocostal arches, the crus of the diaphragm, and the lumbar vertebra. Medial and lateral lumbocostal arches are present. The medial lumbocostal arch extends from the crus of the diaphragm and the vertebral body, arches over the cephalad portion of the psoas major muscle, and inserts on the anterior surface of the transverse process of L1. The lateral lumbocostal arch extends from this transverse process of L1, arching over the quadratus lumborum muscle to the tip of the 12th rib. The crura of the diaphragm consists of a large right crus extending down the right side of the L1, L2, and L3 vertebral bodies and a smaller left crus attaching to L1 and L2. These crura extend cephalad and anterior to approximately the T11–T12 area medially in the midline to form the aortic hiatus. The esophageal hiatus and vena cava foramen lie in the anterior wall of the diaphragm. The aortic hiatus itself also gives passage to the azygos vein and the thoracic duct as well as the aorta. The esophageal hiatus at the approximate level of the 10th thoracic vertebra transmits the vagus nerves and hemiazygos vein. The sympathetic trunk usually enters under the medial lumbocostal arch.

The innervation of the diaphragm is of a central origin, and resection should be circumferential, approximately 1 inch from the outer perimeter, leaving enough diaphragm to reattach. This should avoid interfering with innervation of the diaphragm or its function.

The fascial lining of the undersurface of the diaphragm is the transversalis fascia. Its counterpart inside the thorax is the endothoracic fascia, which is the internal investing fascia of the entire inner thoracic cavity. Just as the transversalis fascia covers all muscles (i.e., the psoas muscle and the quadratus lumborum), as well as all vascular and bony structures in the abdomen, the endothoracic fascia covers the internal surfaces of the ribs, the superior surface of the cephalad rib, and the interthoracic portion of the diaphragm. The endothoracic fascia also includes the paravertebral fascia covering the vertebrae and discs. In a cephalad direction, the endothoracic fascia is continuous with the transversalis fascia, or endoabdominal fascia, as it is sometimes called. The insertion of the diaphragm into the ribs interdigitates with the insertion of the transverse abdominal muscle. These interdigitating slips can be used to reapproximate the original positioning of the slips of the diaphragm with their anchoring attachments, especially at the tips of the 11th and 12th ribs. Division of the diaphragm should proceed to the crus of the diaphragm. Elevating the crus of the diaphragm off the involved vertebral bodies to be worked on usually allows a cephalad retraction of the diaphragm to enable work on vertebral bodies through L2. By placement of small stay sutures, the location of reattachment areas can be marked as they are taken down. Any costal cartilage that is divided off the tip of the rib on combined thoracoabdominal approaches can, of course, be reapproximated.

The pleural cavity extends over most of the 11th rib and the midportion of the 12th rib.

TENTH RIB APPROACH

The patient is placed in the lateral decubitus position (Fig. 1). The surgeon approaches from the convexity of the scoliosis or from the left side, when possible. A left-sided approach is preferred because the aorta is more easily mobilized than is the vena cava. In addition, splenic retraction is easier than hepatic. The skin and subcutaneous tissue are incised from the lateral border of the paraspinous musculature over the 10th rib to the junction of the 10th rib and

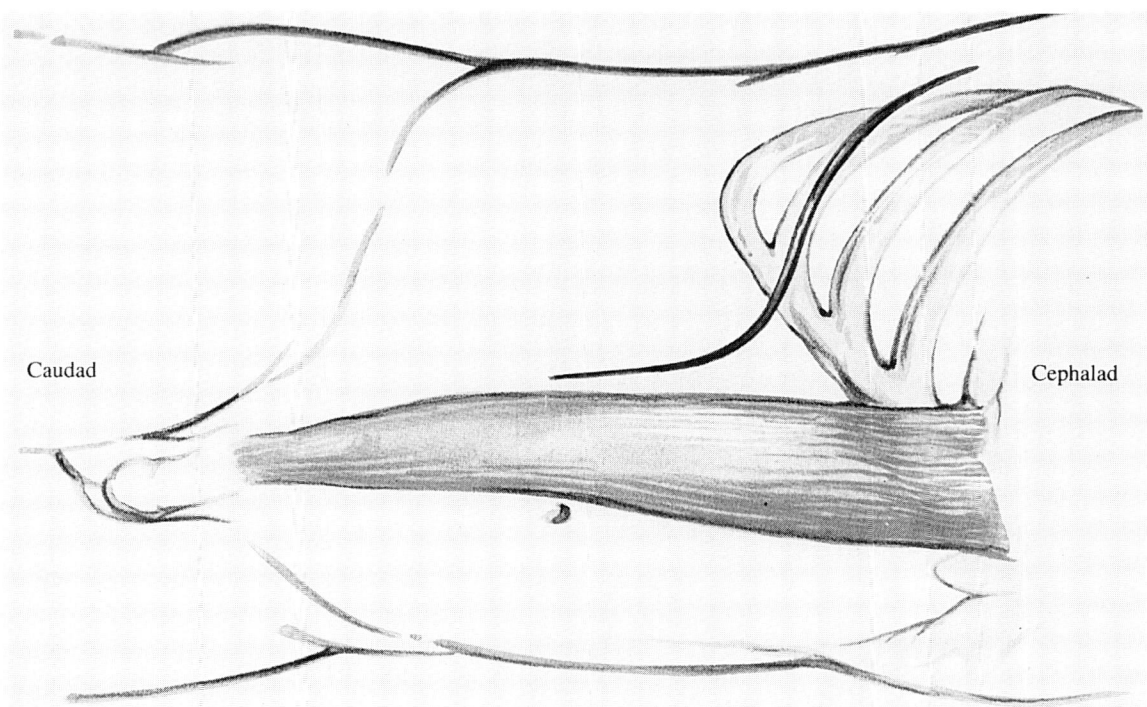

Figure 1. Place the patient in a lateral decubitus position. Approach from the convexity of the scoliosis or from the left side as indicated. A left-sided approach is preferred because the aorta is more easily mobilized than is the vena cava.

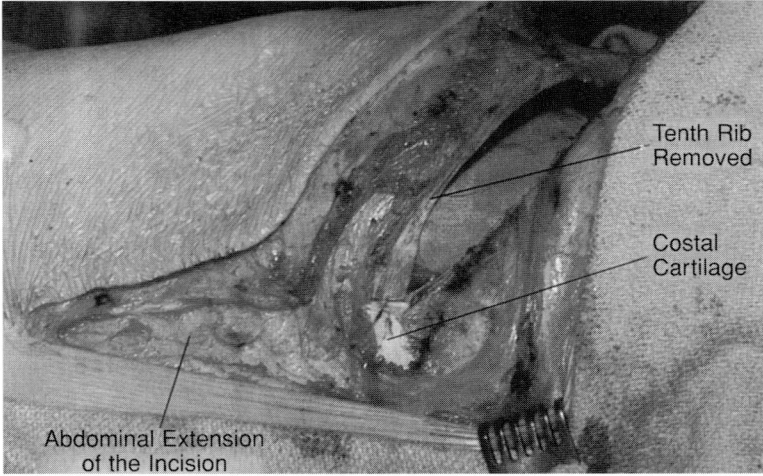

Figure 2. With the rib removed, carefully delineate the costal cartilage. At this point, the intrapleural cavity is opened; the retroperitoneal cavity is still closed.

the costal cartilage. The incision is curved anteriorly from the tip of the 10th rib to the lateral rectus sheath and distally down the edge of the sheath as far as necessary for exposure. The wound is extended slowly through each muscle layer with electrocautery. The assistant aggressively picks up bleeders with two Adson forceps.

The superficial periosteum of the 10th rib is opened to the costal cartilage (Fig. 2). A sharp, curved periosteal elevator is used to remove the superficial and deep periosteum off the rib. Care is taken to avoid the neurovascular bundle on the inferior surface of the rib. A cut is made posteriorly at the angle of the rib and at the junction of rib and costal cartilage. The rib is removed. On opening of the pleural space, the lung is retracted, and the rib bed opened fully with scissors.

The costal cartilage is split with a knife along its length (Fig. 3). The undersurface of the costal cartilage is opened, and the two tags of cartilage are retracted[2, 3, 8] (Fig. 4).

Blunt dissection is performed under the retracted split tips of costal cartilage to identify the retroperitoneal space. The light areolar tissue of the retroperitoneal fat is the guide to the retroperitoneal space.

The peritoneum is bluntly dissected off the inferior surface of the diaphragm (Fig. 5). A sponge is used to sweep away the peritoneum from the undersurface of, first, the diaphragm and then the transversalis fascia and abdominal wall.

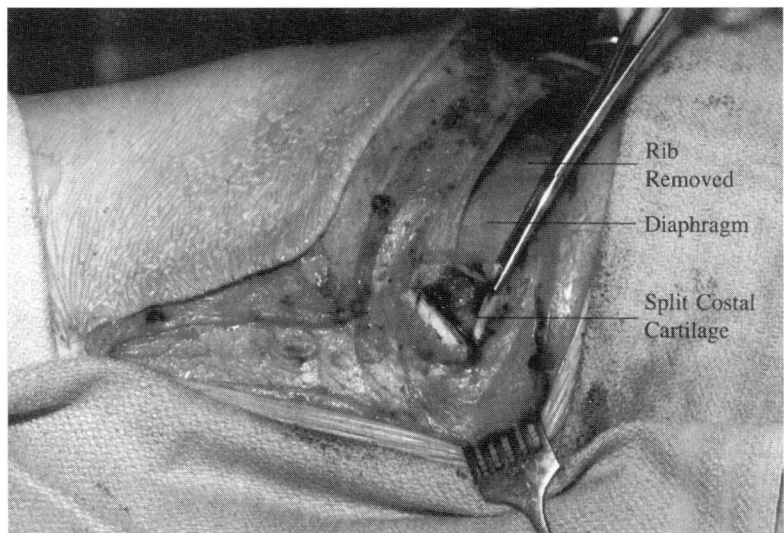

Figure 3. Split the costal cartilage. Open only the most superficial layer of soft tissue under the costal cartilage enough to allow retraction of the cartilage tips.

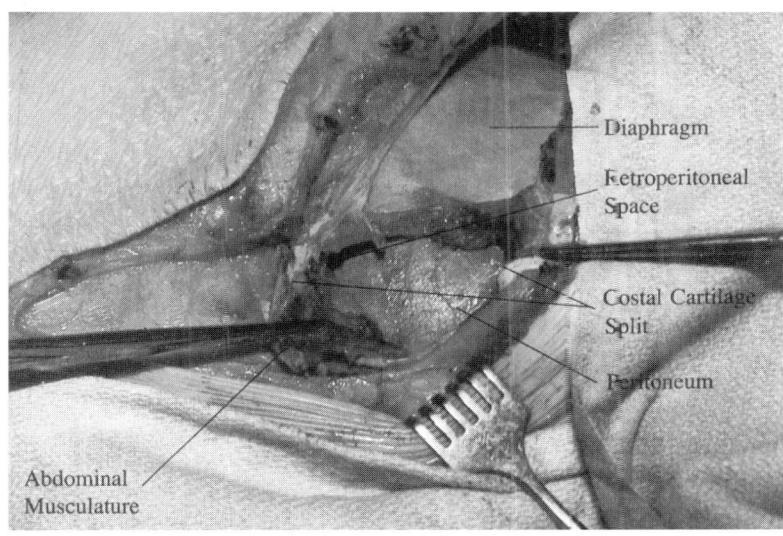

Figure 4. Retract the split tips of costal cartilage. Identify the insertion of the diaphragm into the cephalad cartilage tip and the insertion of the abdominal musculature into the caudad cartilage tip. Bluntly dissect under the retracted tags of cartilage and attached musculature to locate the peritoneum and the retroperitoneal space. The light areolar texture of the retroperitoneal fat is the guide to the retroperitoneal space.

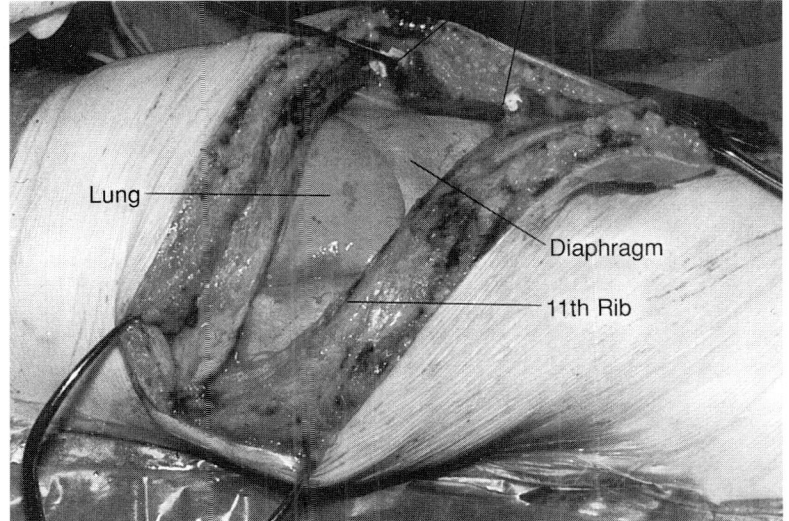

Figure 5. The peritoneum and lung are protected to allow division of the diaphragm.

With the periosteum thus retracted, the abdominal musculature (the external oblique, the internal oblique, and the transversus abdominis muscles) is opened carefully, one layer at a time, with complete hemostasis. At this point, the chest and retroperitoneal space are open, and the diaphragm is the intervening structure in the wound.

The diaphragm is incised from inside the chest with clear visualization under the diaphragm in the retroperitoneal space. The incision is extended in the diaphragm circumferentially 1 inch from its peripheral attachment to the chest wall.[9]

Marker clips are used throughout the takedown of the diaphragm to allow accurate reapproximation.

For work on T12–L1, the diaphragm is resected to the spine. The crus of the diaphragm is cut and elevated off the spinal column. Protected Deaver retractors are used to retract the peritoneal sac anteriorly. A large rib retractor, such as a Feochetti, is used to open the 10th rib incision in the chest. The spine is visualized from approximately T6 as far distally in the lumber spine as is necessary. In the lumbar spine, the attachments of the psoas and the crus of the diaphragm are removed from the spine for proper visualization. In the thoracic spine, the parietal pleura is opened as in the standard thoracotomy approach. Each intercostal artery and vein is tied and ligated to allow mobilization of the major vascular trunks. When necessary, the thoracic duct, which usually crosses right to left around T4–T5, is tied off and the sympathetic plexus is avoided. After the intercostal vessels are removed, a cut is made directly to the spine (Fig. 6). The spine is dissected to remove the soft tissue laterally.

Closure

The key to closure is the reapproximation of the costal cartilage. After the diaphragm is resutured with multiple interrupted sutures and the split cartilage is reapproximated, the chest tube is inserted in the eighth intercostal space, and it is passed posterosuperiorly. Attached to the cephalad half of the costal cartilage is the insertion of the diaphragm and the interthoracic fascia. Inserting into the distal split of costal cartilage is the abdominal transversalis fascia and attachment for the abdominal musculature. With reapproximation of the costal cartilage, the layers of the abdominal musculature are much better defined. Each layer of the abdominal wall is closed separately when possible, and the chest is closed as in a standard thoracotomy.

ELEVENTH RIB APPROACH

A standard skin incision is made over the entire length of the left 11th rib. The incision is extended from the rib tip inferiomedially to the edge of the rectus sheath (Fig. 7). The incision can be expanded by curving

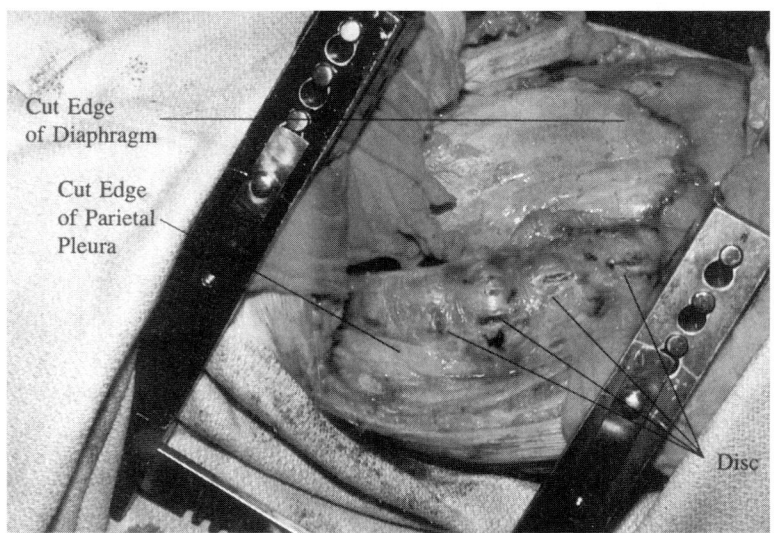

Figure 6. After the diaphragm is detached and retracted, expose the spine. Identify the disc space and clear tissue from it, isolating the intercostal arteries and severing and ligating each over the vertebral bodies.

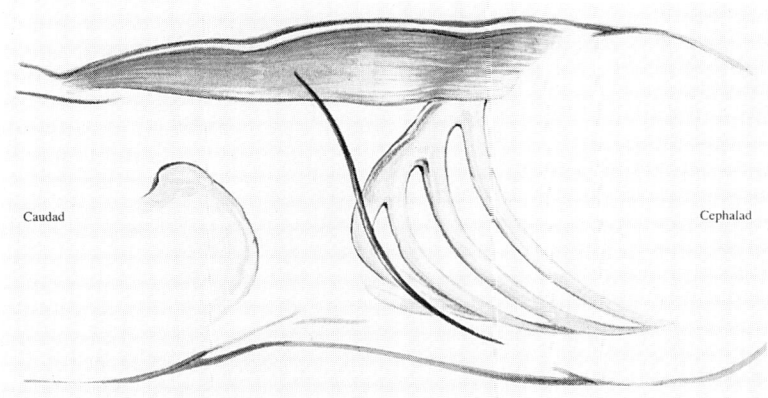

Figure 7. Make a standard incision over the left 11th rib, extending from the tip of the 11th rib to the edge of the rectus sheath. Remove the 11th rib and split the costal cartilage. Separate the split cartilaginous tips, and bluntly dissect with utmost care the separating leaves of tissue. Dissect the parietal pleura from the undersurface of the rib bed, starting at the split cartilage.

the posterior arm cephalad to allow removal of additional rib and by extending the anterior arm down the abdominal wall vertically to expose more of the lumbar spine retroperitoneally.

The 11th rib is resected from the angle of the rib to the junction of the rib and costal cartilage, leaving the rib bed intact.

The most crucial step of the operation is to remain in the extrapleural and retroperitoneal plane at this point.

The costal cartilage is split. The insertion of the diaphragm is into the cephalad edge of the costal cartilage and adjacent rib bed; likewise, the insertion of the transversus abdominis musculature and transversalis fascia is into the caudad portion. The pleura and the pleural cavity are under the rib bed.

The key is to open the split cartilage and dissect carefully under the costal cartilage several inches toward the rib bed to protect the parietal pleura. The pleura must not be damaged while the retroperitoneal space is being opened.

The upper cartilage tag is bluntly dissected cephalad, and the lower tag, caudad. At this point, the retroperitoneal space and the peritoneum are identified. The incision is extended 3 inches from the level of the costal cartilage medially. Each muscle layer (external oblique, internal oblique, transversus abdominis) is divided from the tip of the 11th rib. The muscle layers thin out dramatically medially, and entering the peritoneum is not difficult. If this happens, it is repaired immediately with purse-string sutures. After the peritoneum is reached, it is bluntly dissected from the undersurface of the transverse fascia, the fascia is opened, and the peritoneum is retracted

After the peritoneum is exposed, the parietal pleura must be identified and dissected free, intact (Fig. 8). Occasionally, the pleura extends to the tip of the 11th rib, but it

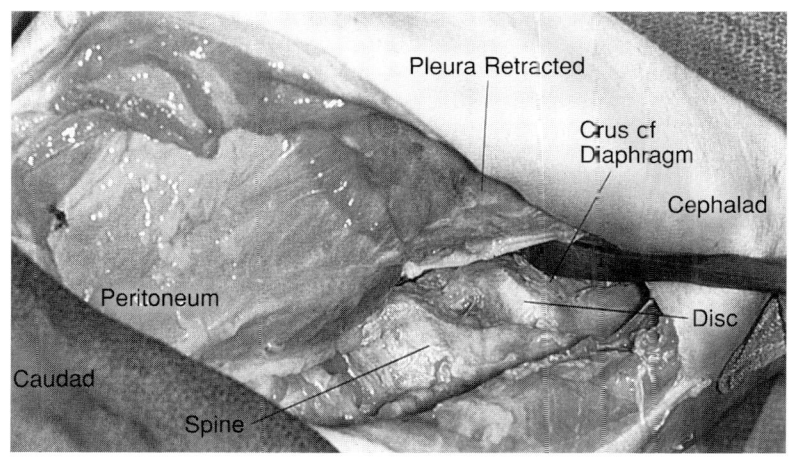

Figure 8. Exposure of the spine consists of identification of disc spaces, blunt dissection on the disc space, isolation of the intercostal arteries and veins, and removal of the insertion of the crus of the diaphragm. Be aware of the 12th intercostal artery and vein under the crus of the diaphragm.

usually passes slightly more proximal to the tip of the 11th rib and across the midportion of the 12th rib. The rib bed has three layers: periosteum, endothoracic fascia, and parietal pleura. Only the periosteum and muscle of the rib bed are opened. The parietal pleura is identified. The crucial dissection of pleura is begun from the endothoracic fascia of the rib bed. Cotton gloves or gauze wrapped around the dissecting finger is used to dissect bluntly toward the spine under the rib bed. While the soft tissue is pushed off, the undersurface of the rib bed is dissected carefully. If the pleura is damaged, it should be sutured. After the pleura is dissected, the rib bed is opened with scissors. The strong fascia of the rib bed prevents exposure. After the rib bed is opened, the Feochetti retractor is inserted. If the Feochetti retractor is ineffective because the lower rib is too small to retract against, a Deaver retractor is used. The diaphragm is attached to the tip of the 12th rib. Often, this is a direct tether to adequate expansion of the wound. With the pleura having been reflected off the undersurface of the diaphragm in this area, the insertion of the diaphragm is cut off the tip of the 12th rib.

The surgeon must remember that this approach is under the diaphragm, which has been retracted cephalad. The peritoneum is bluntly dissected from the undersurface of the diaphragm. The peritoneum and its contents are retracted anteriorly. The retroperitoneal space is entered and the psoas muscle is identified over the transverse processes.

The origin of the psoas muscle is identified over the transverse processes and bodies of T12 and L1. The transverse process of L1, which is the uppermost insertion of the psoas muscle and is the junction of the medial and lateral lumbocostal arches, is also identified. The crus of the diaphragm over L1 is identified.

The attachment of the lumbocostal arches is cut from the transverse process of L1.

The left crus of the diaphragm is cut and elevated from the vertebral bodies of L1 and L2 (Fig. 9). Segmental vessels are identified and ligated at each vertebral body level. The surgeon should not neglect the segmental vessels over L1. Blunt dissection can be carried proximally on the spine to the level of T11. The pleura often extends into the costophrenic sulcus medially at the 12th vertebral body. A danger of entering the pleura with the proximal blunt dissection is present, even after the pleura has been identified under the 11th rib bed.

Often, the psoas muscle bulges medially and obscures the spine and the crus of the diaphragm. Finger palpation is used to differentiate the texture of the intervertebral disc from the vertebral bodies. The psoas is taken down from its insertion onto the body of T12–L1. The bleeding is controlled in the attachments of the psoas by electrocautery on a low setting. The T11–L1 vertebral bodies are exposed in the wound extrapleurally and retroperitoneally. The surgeon must remember to protect the psoas muscle. Retraction should be avoided. The lumbar nerve roots and the lumbar plexus are under the psoas.

Closure

The lung is expanded before closure so that the surgeon can observe any air leaks. The lumbocostal arch is then attached to the transverse process of L1, the crus of the diaphragm to the vertebral body, and the insertion of the diaphragm into the tip of the 11th and 12th ribs.

Again, the key to closure is reapproximation of the costal cartilage on the tip of the 11th rib. The rib bed is closed with interrupted suture, and then each layer is closed with running absorbable suture.

The surgeon should be aware of the muscle-covered intercostal vessels crossing the midbody of T12 and should not damage the pleura over the vertebral body when dissecting proximally toward T11–T12. The crus of the diaphragm forms a sling anteriorly, at which is the aortic hiatus. The thoracic duct enters through the aortic hiatus anterior to the aorta. The renal artery and the kidney have been reflected anteriorly and to the right from this left lateral approach.

The sympathetic chain is in its paraspinous location entering the diaphragm. Although the chain is often sectioned in the approach, it sometimes can be identified and preserved. No permanent sequelae should result from unilateral transection of the sympathetic chain.

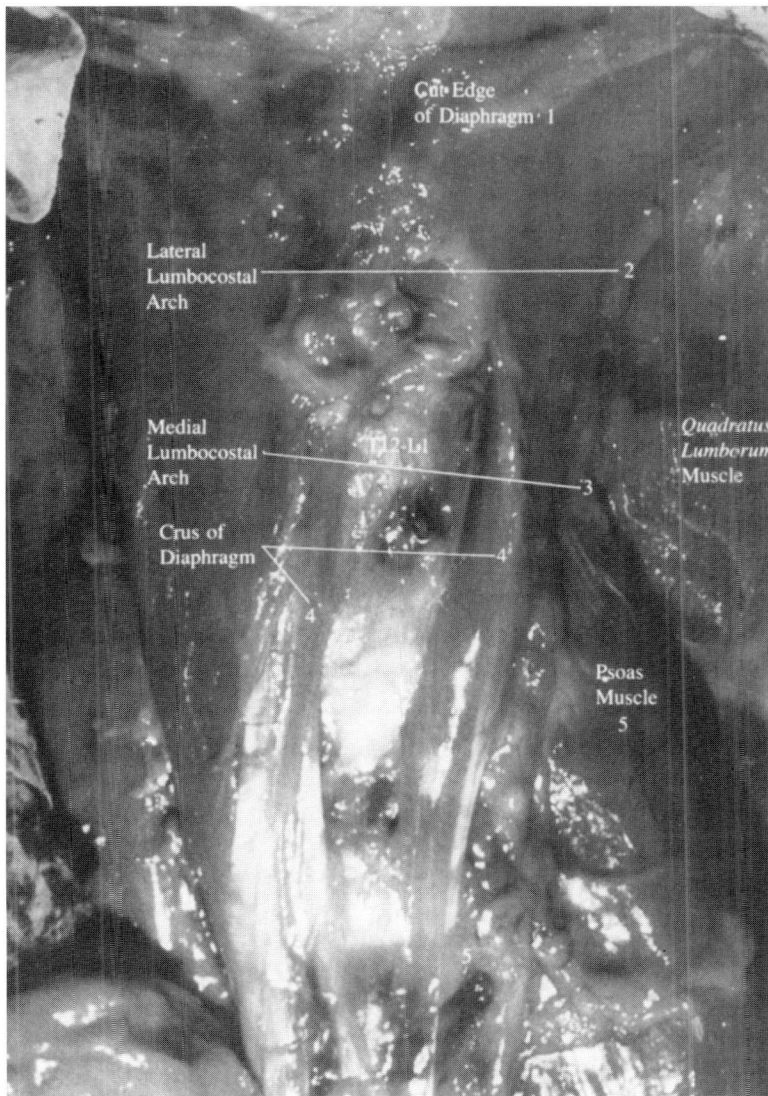

Figure 9. Remove the crus of the diaphragm (4) from the vertebral body. The right crus of the diaphragm is large and extends down the right side of the L1, L2, and L3 vertebral bodies. The left crus extends anteriorly into the substance of the diaphragm, forming the aortic hiatus. The insertion of the diaphragm (1) into the transverse process of L1 is in the form of a medial and lateral lumbocostal arches. The medial lumbocostal 3) arch extends from the crus of the diaphragm and vertebral body, arches over the cephalad portion of the psoas major muscle (5), and inserts into the anterior surface of the transverse process of L1. The lateral lumbocostal arch (2) expands from this transverse process of L1, arching over the quadratus lumborum muscle to the tip of the 12th rib. Be aware of the intercostal vessels over T12–L1 and L1–L2 when removing the diaphragmatic crura.

TWELFTH RIB APPROACH

The 12th rib resection with flank incision was developed to allow better exposure of the kidney.[4,5] The 12th rib and its periosteal bed are joined at the rib's tip by the insertion of the diaphragm and of the transversus abdominis muscle and the transversalis fascia. They form an anchoring point to resist cephalad retraction. By removing the 12th rib, opening the 12th rib bed, and freeing the muscle insertions of the tip of the 12th rib, the surgeon has greater exposure for cephalad retraction when exposing the kidney, retroperitoneal space, or spine. Resection of the rib and the periosteum of the rib bed allows release of the posterior lumbocostal ligament, which is a strong tether against cephalad retraction and frees the fibers of the internal and external oblique muscles. With the added exposure, the L1 vertebral body and distal segments can be adequately visualized.

One of the major complications of the thoracolumbar approach is damage to the pleura in the region of the 12th rib. The relationship of the pleura to the 12th rib, as presented by Hughes,[5] begins with classification of the 12th rib into a long type of 11 to 14 cm and a short type of 1.5 to 6 cm. In the commoner long rib, the pleura is usually on the undersurface of the posterior 6 cm of the rib. The pleura may extend over the T11–T12 interspace anteriorly as far as 10 to 11 cm from the midline. With short 12th ribs, the entire length of the rib should be considered to be covered with pleura. With this location of the pleura in mind, the surgeon may follow the four steps outlined by Digby[1] for avoiding the pleura:

1. Study the maximum-inspiration chest x-ray film taken before the operation and showing the lower extent of the pleura.
2. Expose the periosteum on the outer side of the rib before incising it, avoiding deep plunges that can section the pleura off the rib surface.
3. Avoid leaving sharp projecting fragments on the stump of the last rib, and cover the stump with a tethered gauze roll.
4. Make the longitudinal incision in the periosteum and inner aspects of the last rib sufficiently far out to be below and beyond the pleura reflection.

The patient is placed in the right decubitus position over the break in the table, which increases the distance between the iliac crest and the costal margin and aids in the exposure (Fig. 10).

The skin and subcutaneous tissue are incised from the costotransverse junction to 6 inches anterior to the tip of the 12th rib. The muscle layers are divided with the electrocautery to the surface of the 12th rib. Care is taken to cut the latissimus dorsi and serratus posterior musculature directly in line with the incision to the rib. The surgeon should not slide off the rib inferiorly and damage the subcostal nerve and vessels.

The periosteum of the rib is opened, and the superficial and deep surfaces of the periosteum are elevated off the rib.

The rib is cut at the costotransverse junction, and the cut rib is elevated with a bone clamp from the rib bed, leaving it attached anteriorly. Attached to the tip of the 12th rib is the diaphragm superiorly and the transverse abdominal musculature and fascia inferiorly. The pleura is safely protected under the rib bed. The safest area to enter the rib bed of the 12th rib is at the tip. If it is a short rib, the pleura is at the tip of the 12th rib.

While the rib is elevated, the tissue is split on the tip of the 12th rib, and the rib is removed. The diaphragmatic insertion is retracted slightly cephalad, and the abdominal musculature, caudad.

The foamy fat of the retroperitoneal space is identified. This area is opened carefully and the peritoneum is identified. The peritoneum is bluntly dissected from the undersurface of the abdominal wall for further opening of muscle layers.

The incision is extended through the external oblique and internal oblique musculature with electrocautery (Fig. 11). The transversus abdominis musculature is identified and the muscle is carefully spread to expose the transverse fascia.

The peritoneum is retracted anteriorly, and the retroperitoneal space is exposed.

The endothoracic fascia lines the undersurface of the rib bed. The pleura is dissected bluntly from the endothoracic fascia. The pleura is swept off from the tip proximally. With the pleura removed from the undersurface, the rib bed is opened.

The 12th intercostal nerve runs under and through the internal oblique muscle. In

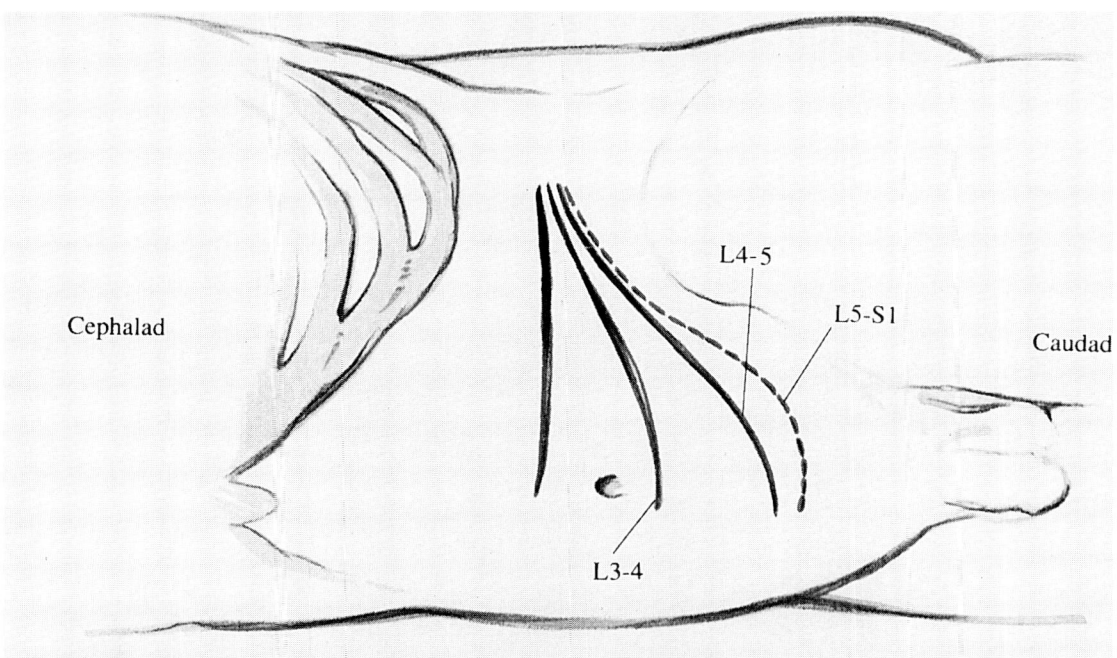

Figure 10. The patient is placed in the left lateral decubitus position. Using the radiopaque beanbag for positioning allows adequate intraoperative radiographic visualization. Slightly flex the patient's knees, place the axillary pad, and support the head sufficiently. Too much hip flexion at this point limits the exposure anteriorly. Ensure that the left hip is only slightly flexed. Begin the incision equidistant between the lowest rib and superior iliac crest in the midaxillary line (it may be closer to the crest for lower levels), and extend it proximally to the edge of the rectus sheath. The level of incision varies according to the level of the spine approached. L5–S1 is in the lower half of the distance between the umbilicus and the symphysis pubis, and L4–L5 lies in the upper half of this distance. L3–L4 is at the umbilicus, and L2–L3 is above the umbilicus. Incise through the skin and subcutaneous tissue, retracting with self-retaining retractors.

opening the abdominal musculature, the 12th intercostal nerve is identified and protected. Then, the retroperitoneal space, the opened rib bed, the cephalad-retracted diaphragm and pleura, each layer of the abdominal musculature, the peritoneum, and the psoas are identified (Fig. 12).

Locating the psoas muscle is the critical step at this point (Fig. 13). Deaver retractors are used to hold the peritoneal sac and its contents anteriorly. Care is taken not to enter the retropsoas space, which is a blind pouch.

With the kidney retracted forward, the ureter is identified on the undersurface of the peritoneum. It need not be dissected free and is retracted with the peritoneum. The spine is palpated to find the soft prominent disc spaces. The retroperitoneal soft tissue is bluntly spread on the first identifiable disc. The surgeon should work solely on the surface of the disc, staying clear of the vertebral body, where the intercostal vessels are. After one disc is cleared a needle is inserted for radiographic confirmation of the level. The psoas frequently bulges over the midline and obscures the spine as it inserts on the 12th and first bodies and on the lumbocostal arches. The psoas muscle is removed initially from the disc area, then from the vertebral bodies.

Vascular structures are cauterized or tied in the midportion of the vertebral body, and bleeding is controlled from the origin of the psoas. The crus of the diaphragm is cut from the spine and elevated in a cephalad direction with the periosteal elevator. With the crus of the diaphragm elevated cephalad and the psoas muscle retracted laterally and inferiorly, the T12–S1 discs should be well visualized. The insertion of the lumbocostal arch on the transverse process of L1 is removed for additional visualization cephalad. Theoretically, this area can be expanded to the 10th thoracic vertebra, but the exposure is confining in any level above T12.

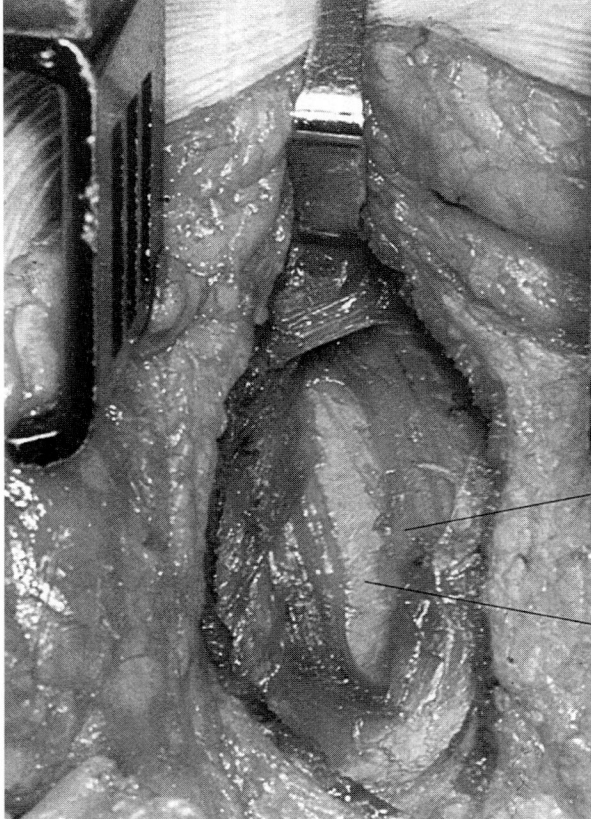

Figure 11. The transversus abdominis muscle layer, often the thinnest of the three muscle layers of the abdominal wall, must be opened carefully. The transversalis fascia underneath the transversus abdominis muscle should also be opened carefully because the peritoneum is the next most immediate layer under the transversalis fascia. Spread through the transversalis muscle, identify the transversalis fascia, penetrate the transversalis fascia in the more lateral aspect of the wound, and identify the peritoneum.

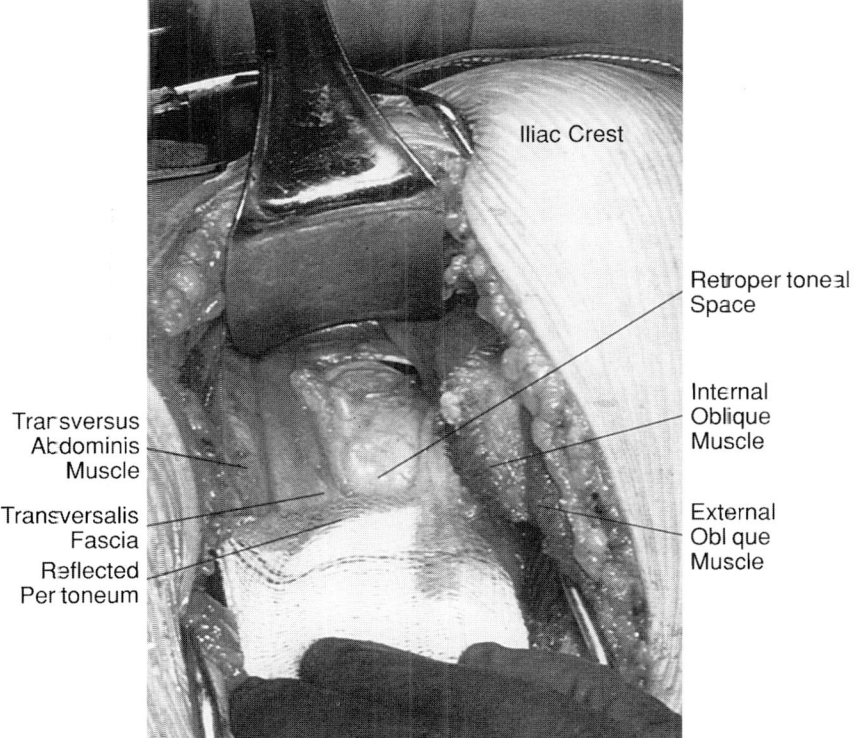

Figure 12. Identify the fatty layer of the retroperitoneal space as the peritoneal sac and cavity is brought medially. Bluntly penetrate the retroperitoneal space with the hand. In addition, remove the peritoneum from the remaining transversalis fascia medially by having the surgeon in the anterior position lift the abdominal wall and the assistant in the posterior position peel the peritoneum off the undersurface of the fascia with a 4 × 4 sponge and extend the incision medially after the peritoneum has been safely removed from under the remaining musculofascial layers of the abdominal wall.

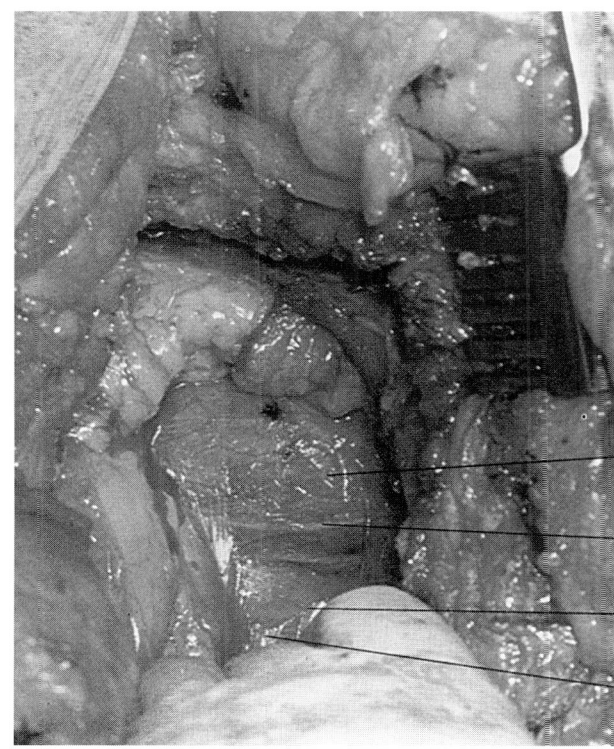

Figure 13. Identification of the psoas muscle is the key to working in the retroperitoneal space. Pass indirectly through the retroperitoneal space to the psoas muscle. Avoid opening the retropsoas space, which is a blind pouch. The dissection must proceed medial to the psoas muscle, not lateral. The genitofemoral nerve can be identified coursing on the psoas muscle. The spine is just medial to the psoas and can be partially hidden by it. Palpate the spine medial to the psoas, and locate the raised intervertebral disc surface with the finger by slowly moving from left to right across the disc surface.

The pleura in the sulcus is immediately over the spine and the rib heads. Blunt dissection of the pleura is continued toward the spine until the pleura is sufficiently elevated.[6]

Closure

The rib bed is closed, the cartilaginous tip of the rib is approximated, and each abdominal muscle layer is closed.

For the standard anterior retroperitoneal flank approach to an L4–L5 exposure of the lumbar spine, the patient is positioned supine on the table with the top of the iliac crest positioned at the flexion point and the kidney rest of the table. The heels and lower extremities are carefully padded. Thromboembolic disease hose are applied before the patient enters the operating room.

The surgeon stands on the patient's left, the assistant, on the patient's right. The level of the incision varies according to the level of the spine approached. L5–S1 exposure starts at the midline at the junction of the lower third and middle third of the distance between the umbilicus and the pubis. L4–L5 in the midline is at the junction of the upper and middle third of that distance, L3–L4 just below the umbilicus, and L2–L3 just above. The length of the incision varies from 8 to 14 cm. The incision is extended laterally on a line equidistant between the lowest rib and the superior iliac crest. The skin incision is made to the midline. With self-retaining retractors, the skin is spread and the subcutaneous tissue opened. The electrocautery is used to cut down to the outer fascial layers of the abdominal wall.

The subcutaneous tissues are incised to the fascia extending beyond the ends of the skin incision, especially laterally to expose the external oblique aponeurosis.

The rectus sheath is incised obliquely from medial to lateral and at the lateral edge is incised vertically for 1 to 2 cm to allow adequate mobilization of the rectus muscle. This incision is then carried laterally to incise the external oblique fascia, which fuses with the rectus sheath near its lateral border and should stop as the aponeurosis becomes muscular. The rectus muscle is then mobilized without being transected and with care being taken not to injure inferior epigastric vessels. The muscle is then retracted toward the midline, and the posterior rectus sheath is carefully incised. This layer is at times tenuous, and care must be exercised to prevent laceration of the peritoneum. This incision should be as close to the lateral edge of the rectus sheath as possible without cutting into the internal oblique muscle. With careful blunt dissection, the peritoneum is then separated from the posterior rectus sheath toward the midline first and then laterally under the internal oblique muscle. At this point, the dissection turns posteriorly, and the peritoneum is mobilized medially until the psoas muscle is identified. The dissection then continues along that plane toward the midline until the left iliac artery is identified. The ureter is usually identified at this point and is carried upward with the peritoneum as the peritoneum is swept off the retroperitoneal structures.

In most cases, both L4–L5 and L5–S1 may be approached from the left of the left iliac vessels. When this tactic is not possible, L4–L5 may be exposed from the left, and L5–S1, from within the bifurcation.

For isolated exposure of L5–S1, the dissection is usually continued anterior to the left iliac artery within the bifurcation. At this point, the L5–S1 disc is palpated, and dissection is carried toward it with a sharp and blunt dissection between the iliac vessels. The left iliac vein is identified below and medial to the artery and is swept away from the anterior surface of the spine using careful dissection to expose the left side of the disc. Care is taken here to preserve any sympathetic fibers that may be encountered just anterior to the disc. Dissection is then carried to the right side of the disc to expose it fully. A needle is then inserted into the disc, and an x-ray study is performed to verify the level.

For exposure to L4–L5, the prevertebral structure is approached medially from the psoas. The dissection is taken deep and lateral to the iliac artery to expose the iliac vein. Further deep dissection is carried out to expose the iliolumbar vein or veins, which can then be doubly ligated and transected (Fig. 14). This process allows medial mobilization of both iliac vessels, exposing the left side of the disc. The dissection is then carried anterior to the disc toward the right side to expose the area properly. Again, a needle is inserted into the disc, and an x-ray study is performed to verify the level (Fig. 15). Si-

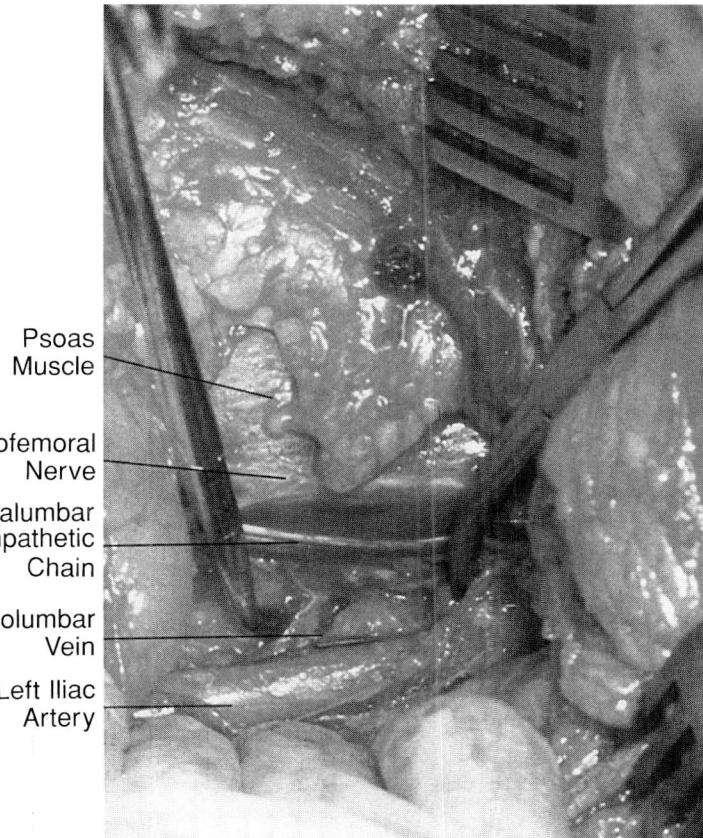

Figure 14. For the lumbar approach to L4–L5 and above, the aorta and vena cava are swept left to right off the spine. The iliolumbar vein is an important direct tether to this left-to-right dissection. This lumbar vein crosses from the vena cava to approximately the level of the L5 body. Any dissection that exposes L4–L5 to the left of the left common iliac and vena cava requires identification, ligation, and division of the iliolumbar vein. Find the L4–L5 disc, and dissect distally to the L5 body to identify the iliolumbar vein.

multaneous exposure of L4–L5 and L5–S1 can usually be obtained with this approach because, once the iliolumbar veins are transected, the vessels can be mobilized far enough to the right to allow such exposure.

Exposure for L3–L4 is similar to that for L4–L5 except that, occasionally, the iliolumbar veins may not have to be transected for adequate exposure.

In addition to knowing the disc level, the surgeon must discern the location of the bifurcation of the aorta. With a high bifurcation of the aorta, approaching the L4–L5 disc within the bifurcation is sometimes necessary, but in most instances, the bifurcation is at L5 or lower, and the approaches to L4–L5 and L3–L4 are to the left of the aorta and vena cava.

Dissection on the anterior surface of the spine consists of gentle stretching and pulling of structures, usually blunt dissection rather than sharp, cutting dissection. Because electrocautery should be used to the minimum extent possible, direct pressure over small bleeders typically produces hemostasis. Branches are present between the preaortic and paraspinous sympathetic chains. Often, these branches must be divided but should be preserved if possible. With identification of the disc space, the vessels and retroperitoneal tissue are swept from left to right and held to the right side of the spine. The author's standard method of retraction is to use a malleable retractor of appropriate width and have the tip turned up in the opposite direction. This turned-up tip is fitted to the opposite side of the spine from the approach, usually the right side with the left approach, and allows adequate retraction and full, clear visibility of the spine. If the abdominal contents obscure direct work on the disc space, then enlarging the skin incision may be necessary. By placing this malleable retractor and several others around the spine, it is possible to isolate the disc space and to allow adequate visibility for the work that needs to be performed. These retractors can be relaxed when work

1268 Surgical Approaches

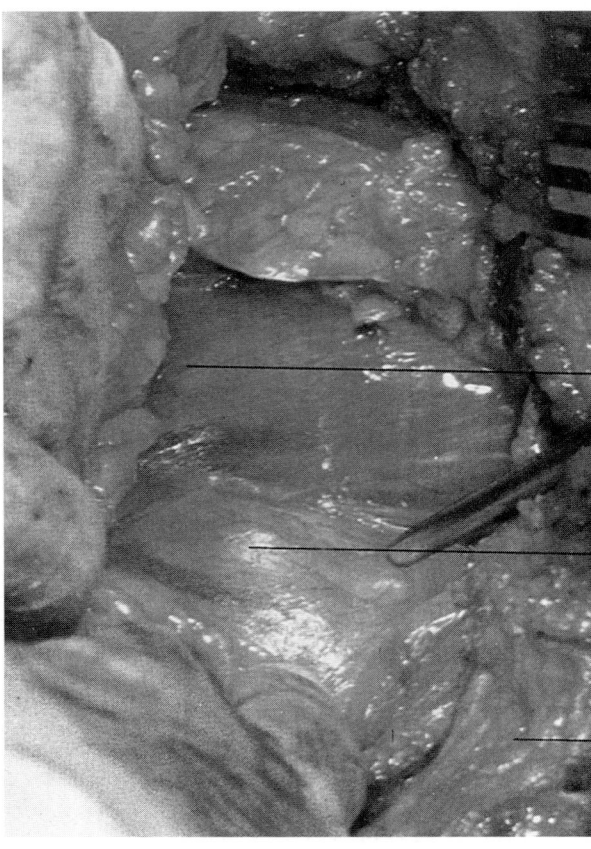

Figure 15. Dissection sweeps the prevertebral tissue off the disc space first because this area is more avascular. Use a sponge-covered finger or blunt instrument. Always obtain radiographic confirmation of the level.

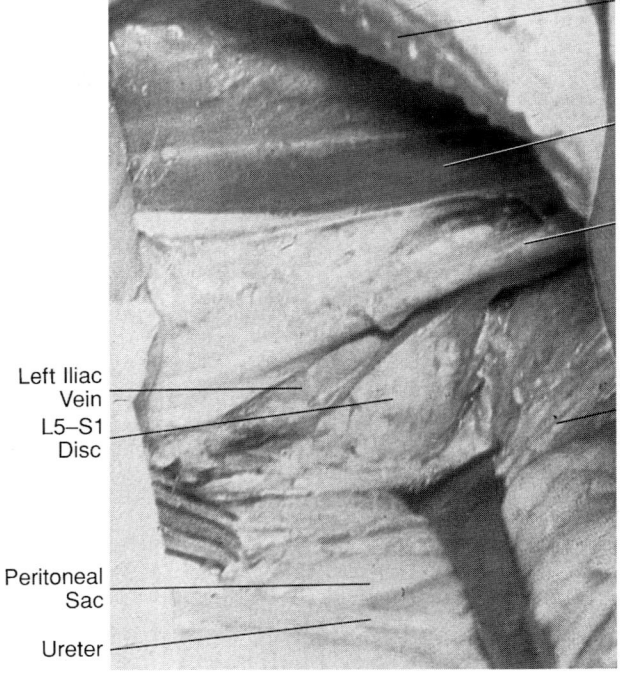

Figure 16. Sweep the prevertebral tissue bluntly off of the front of the L5–S1 disc. The superior hypogastric plexus may be a diffuse plexiform nerve formation that is retracted with the other tissue, or it can be a discrete, well-defined presacral nerve.

is not being directly carried out in the disc space. They also provide protection from instruments that could slip out of the disc space and injure the retracted vessel.

An alternative method of retraction fixes retractors to the spine. Free body Steinmann pin retractors have rubber sleeves and are mounted on a Steinmann pin holder. Four of these pin retractors can be placed into the vertebral bodies adjacent to the disc space—two retractors left and two right. The pin should be stabilized on the tip of the finger and laid directly on the vertebral body under direct vision so the wall of the vena cava or left iliac vein cannot be punctured at the time of insertion of the Steinmann pin tip. With the surgeon holding the pin, the assistant hammers it into the vertebral body The surgeon should remember that the angle of the pin should not be directed toward the disc space or the pin will project into the disc space and obscure the work on the disc space. At the same time, it should be far enough away from the disc space to allow adequate retraction of the soft tissue. Excellent combination pin and blade retractors are available that have the advantage of stationary, broad blade, protective retraction.

The order of placement is usually superior right, then inferior right, then superior left, and then inferior left, if needed. Some of the left pins are not always needed for the exposure, and the right pins carry the great burden of retracting the major vessels. Often, it is advisable to pad the pins and to use malleable retractors between the Steinmann pins to add additional protection to the vascular structures. The most frequent use of the point blade retractor is on the left side of L5 for an L5–S1 approach with the bifurcation.

ANTERIOR RETROPERITONEAL TRANSVERSE APPROACH TO L5–S1

The approach is similar to that of the L4–L5 disc except the skin incision begins at the junction of the middle and distal third of the distance between the symphysis and the umbilicus and extends laterally for approximately 12 cm toward the iliac crest. The anterior retroperitoneal transverse approach can be summarized as follows:

1. Divide the abdominal musculature.
2. Identify and reflect the peritoneum.
3. Identify the psoas muscle.

After identification of the psoas muscle, it is usually best to proceed directly medially to identify the spine As the peritoneal sac is bluntly dissected off the retroperitoneal structures, the spine and blood vessels are identified. The ureter comes with the peritoneal sac and is found on the back of the retracted sac. First, a higher disc is palpated to the left of the vessels in the area of L4–L5 to allow the surgeon to find the spine and get oriented. The pulsations of the aorta and left iliac artery are felt gently. The surgeon must now determine the approximate level of bifurcation of the aorta. Most of the time, the bifurcation is over the L4–L5 disc or the L5 vertebral body. The surgeon identifies the aorta and left iliac artery and proceeds to the bifurcation of the aorta. This area is evaluated visually and with palpation. The disc bifurcation is felt, even if it is through the left iliac vein. After the left common iliac artery is palpated, it is passed over immediately to the L5–S1 disc, and the disc is again identified by its raised white, softer feel. The plane is developed just to the right of the left common iliac artery by blunt dissection. Blunt and occasionally sharp dissection is used to develop the plane down to the intervertebral disc surface (Fig. 16).

The surgeon must be aware of the structures that lie within the bifurcation of the aorta. The first structure, the superior hypogastric plexus, is a continuation of the preaortic, sympathetic chain extending down from the thoracic area, anterior to the aorta and spine in the retroperitoneal space (Fig. 17). The inferior hypogastric plexus is approximately at L3, and the superior hypogastric plexus extends from L4 down over the promontory of the sacrum. The size and consistency of the superior hypogastric plexus vary considerably. A plexiform of multiple strands of nerve tissue or a single large nerve trunk may be present. When one nerve trunk is prominent, it is referred to as the presacral nerve. This plexus extends over the sacral promontory into the pelvis. The superior hypogastric plexus contains sympathetic nerve fibers that course to the urogenital mechanism in the perineal area.

Ejaculation is a combined sympathetic and parasympathetic function, whereas erection is a parasympathetic function through

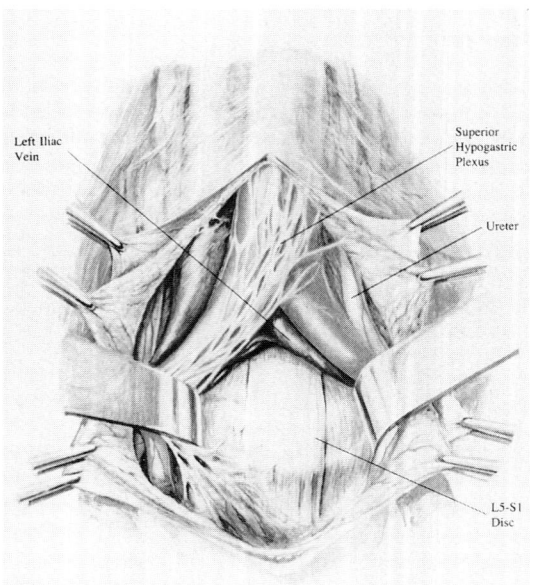

Figure 17. The superior hypograstric plexus within the bifurcation of the aorta. Methods to avoid damaging the hypogastric plexus follow. (1) Use blunt dissection, retraction, and spreading to remove the prevertebral tissue from the sacral promitory. (2) For transperitoneal midline approach, carefully open the posterior peritoneum, and bluntly dissect the prevertebral tissue from right to left. (3) With spreading and blunt dissection, attempt to retract the middle sacral vein and artery without electrocautery. Avoid electrocautery on the anterior surface of L5-S1. When this vessel is of considerable size, use vascular clips or ligation. (4) Opening the posterior peritoneum higher over the bifurcation and extending the opening down over the sacral promontory may allow the surgeon to better visualize and retract these tissues.

control of the seminal muscle and vasculature. Disruption of the sympathetic plexus may result in retrograde ejaculation. These sympathetic fibers have some effect on the motility of the vas deferens, which is important in the transportation of spermatozoa from the epididymis to the seminal vesicle, but the main effect of interruption of the superior hypogastric plexus is a lack of closure of the bladder neck with ejaculation. This aperture allows the semen to be ejected into the bladder rather than out the penis. Technically, if the retrograde ejaculation persists, sterility is the consequence, but any ejaculation problem occurs rarely. The prognosis for recovery from retrograde ejaculation, when it does occur, is excellent.

Impotence or failure of erection is not produced by damage to the superior hypogastric plexus. The parasympathetic fibers responsible for erection for the urogenital system are supplied by the L1-L4 nerve roots and arrive to that area through the pelvic splanchnic nerves. Somatic function from the S1, S2, S3, and S4 levels is carried through the pudendal nerve.

Methods to avoid damage to the superior hypogastric plexus are as follows:

1. Always use blunt dissection: open the prevertebral tissue in the bifurcation of the aorta longitudinally first, just to the left of the left iliac artery, then dissect bluntly from left to right across the L5-S1 disc, longitudinally spreading and retracting, dissecting left to right until the prevertebral tissue is removed intact from the front of the disc space.

2. Use no electrocautery in the aortic bifurcation or on the L5-S1 disc.

Electrocautery produces symptoms much more frequently in this sympathetic tissue. Transverse scalpel cuts should not be made on the front of the L5-S1 disc until the annular tissue is clearly identified.

The second structure is the left iliac vein, which courses in the bifurcation of the aorta, from right to left, cephalad to caudad. It can be easily damaged and must be carefully identified. It is often compressed by the left iliac artery and may be prominent in the wound. Anomalous formation of this vein can produce a huge three-vessel structure that demands careful handling for approach to the L5-S1 disc. Usually, the left iliac vein must be retracted cephalad and is usually tightly draped around the retractor. Care must be taken to protect the left iliac vein as much as possible.

The third structure is the middle sacral artery and vein. These structures are small and are rarely the cause of significant bleeding. These vessels can be bluntly dissected with the superior gastric plexus swept to the side and retracted without risk of major bleeding. If this is a prominent structure, it should be clipped with vascular clamps and ligated, not cauterized. The last of the soft tissue is dissected off the spine with the fingertips or a blunt dissector. To use the Steinmann pin or the pin-blade retractors, the surgeon puts the tip of the pin between the fingers and holds it against the vertebral body. First, the pins are inserted into L5, right then left. This process safely retracts the left iliac vein. Often, only the left pin is needed. The tip of the pin is inserted carefully so that it does not injure the vein. After the L5 pins are placed, a malleable retractor is softly placed over S1. These retractors can be positioned to isolate the veins from the disc space.

Special precautions in exposure should be taken for discs that have a large, reactive anterior lipping. The vena cava is often adherent to the anterior surface of the disc because of prior or current inflammation. The vena cava can be easily torn unless special precautions are taken in anticipation of adhesions between the vena cava and the surface of the inflammatory disc. Large osteophytic spurs and anterior lipping are associated with technical difficulties in the exposure. In cases with calcification in the aortic bifurcation, great care must be taken to avoid clotting of arterial structures during retraction. A special structure of concern is the left iliac artery because this vessel is often tightly retracted during the procedure. Under these circumstances, a malleable retractor should be used, and the compression on the aorta should be frequently released. Especially when pin-stay retractors are necessary, the surgeon must be certain to evaluate the pulse in the artery at the time the retractors are removed.

REFERENCES

1. Digby, K. H.: 12th rib incision as an approach to the kidney. Surg. Gynecol. Obstet. 73:84–85, 1941.
2. Dwyer, A. F.: Experience of anterior correction of scoliosis. Clin. Orthop. 93:192–201, 1973.
3. Dwyer, A. F., Newton, N. C., and Sherwood, A. A.: Anterior approach to scoliosis. Clin. Orthop. 62:192–202, 1969.
4. Hodgson, A. R., and Yau, A. C. M. C.: Anterior surgical approaches to the spinal column. In Apley, A. G. (ed.): Recent Advances in Orthopedics. Baltimore, Williams & Wilkins, 1964, pp. 289–323.
5. Hughes, J.: Urology 61:159–162, 1949.
6. Johnson, R. M., and Southwick, W. O.: Surgical approaches to the spine. In Rothman, R. H., and Simeone, F. A.: The Spine. Philadelphia, W. B. Saunders, 1975, pp. 124–125.
7. Perry, J.: Surgical approaches to the spine. In Pierce, N., and Nichol, V. (eds.): The Total Care of Spinal Cord Injuries. Boston, Little, Brown, 1977, pp. 53–79.
8. Riceborough, E. J.: The anterior approach to the spine for correction of the axial skeleton. Clin. Orthop. 93:207–214, 1973.
9. Scott, R.: Innervation of the diaphragm and its practical aspects in surgery. Thorax 20:357–361, 1965.

Anterior Extraperitoneal Lumbar Discectomy Without Fusion

■

TOHRU NAKANO
KAORU NAKANO
NOBORU NAKANO

For the surgical treatment of lumbar disc lesions, the posterior approach has been customarily used. Some surgeons try to restrict the exposure; problems with hemostasis and nerve root relations in patients with facet arthrosis make surgical exposure difficult. Wide exposure for laminectomy invites irritation of the dura, and arachnoid adhesions produce instability of the lumbar spine. Achieving good results is not always easy. Microsurgery and percutaneous nucleotomy have been recommended to improve the results; however, microsurgery equipment is expensive, and with percutaneous nucleotomy, sometimes the L5–S1 disc is difficult to reach. Once a correct diagnosis is made by myelography or other methods, it is more logical to remove the disc by approaching it from the front, without disturbing the spinal canal. Anterior extraperitoneal lumbar discectomy and fusion have been performed using this approach.

Excellent results were obtained by simply removing the disc without fusion in one young patient (anterior lumbar interbody fusion could not be performed because of severe adhesion of the iliac vessels). This procedure was then tried in other young patients and was then used with even older patients.

The authors performed anterior discectomy without fusion in 450 patients with low back pain and/or sciatica. There were no complications after anterior surgical exposure. Follow-up studies were performed on 352 patients at least 3 years after the surgery, with a mean follow-up of 8.7 years.

Narrowing of the intervertebral disc space was found to occur but could not be equated with poor clinical results, because satisfactory results were obtained in most patients (excellent grade) (see Table 2) without any residual pain or numbness in 90.6%. Retrograde ejaculation with or without poor erection was not seen in this series. Usually, with correct clinical diagnosis refined by myelography, computed tomography, and magnetic resonance imaging, surgeons can confidently remove the disc from the front. With this method, the large posterior muscles are not disturbed, and the spinal canal is not entered. The surgical technique and long-term follow-up procedures are presented here.

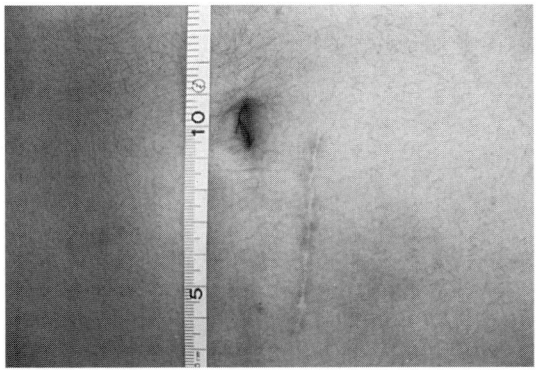

Figure 2. A 5- to 7-cm slightly oblique left abdominal incision is good for L4–L5 and L5–S1.

SURGICAL TECHNIQUE

The instruments needed for this procedure are deep retractors, placenta forceps with sponge, and Kelly forceps with peanut sponge. Special instruments are not necessary (Fig. 1). The patient is in the supine position under general anesthesia after muscle relaxants have been used to secure abdominal muscle relaxation. A left paramedian extraperitoneal approach is used. A 5- to 7-cm slightly oblique left abdominal incision is made (Fig. 2). The anterior layer of the sheath of the rectus abdominis muscle is incised, and the rectus abdominis is retracted laterally (Fig. 3). Then, the posterior sheath of the rectus abdominis muscle is incised after it is separated from the anterior surface of the peritoneum with a small stick sponge (Fig. 4). The peritoneum and its contents are pulled to the right side. As the peritoneum is mobilized, it is easily lifted from the anterior surface of the psoas muscle (Fig. 5). The exposure of the L4 disc is made from the left anterolateral aspect.

The sympathetic chain and the fourth lumbar ganglion lie in the lateral gutter and are not disturbed, but the branches communicating with the hypogastric plexus are pushed out of the way. Ligating the lumbar vessels is usually unnecessary because wide exposure does not require removing the disc. The peripheral disc ligament annulus is opened, and a small hole of 5 to 7 mm

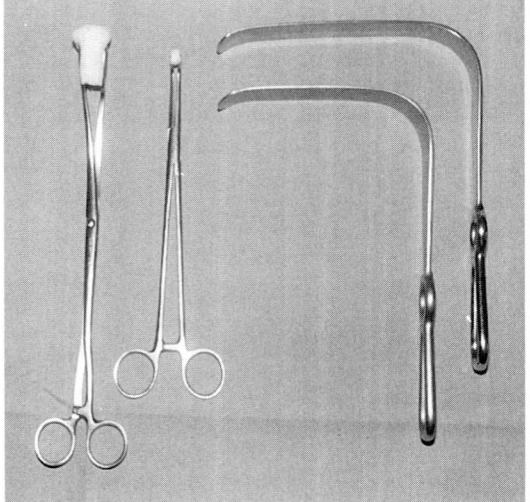

Figure 1. The instruments needed for anterior extraperitoneal lumbar discectomy are deep retractors, placenta forceps, and Kelly forceps.

Anterior Extraperitoneal Lumbar Discectomy Without Fusion

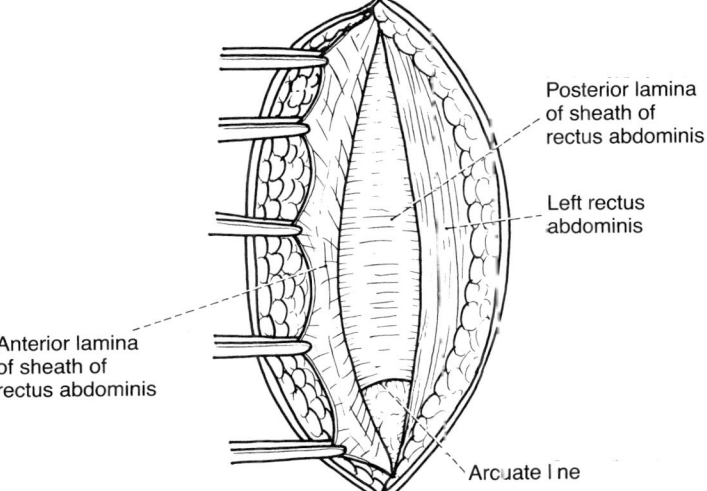

Figure 3. The anterior layer of the sheath of the rectus abdominis muscle is incised, and the rectus abdominis is retracted laterally.

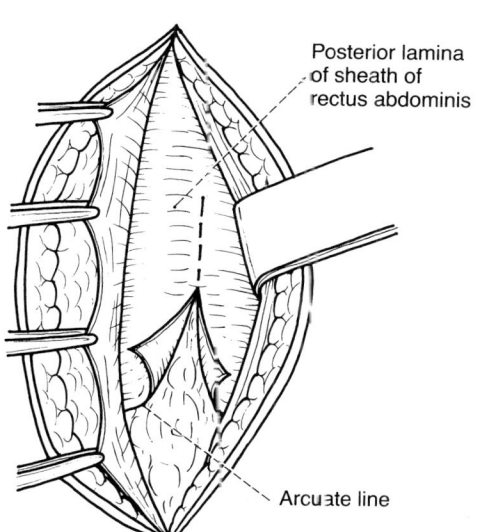

Figure 4. The posterior sheath of the rectus abdominis muscle is incised as laterally as possible.

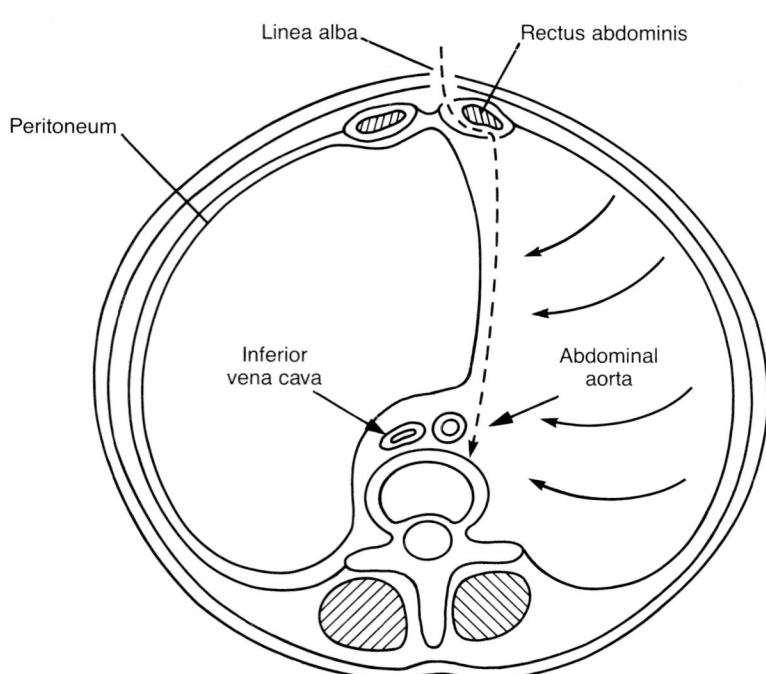

Figure 5. The peritoneum and its contents are pulled to the right side.

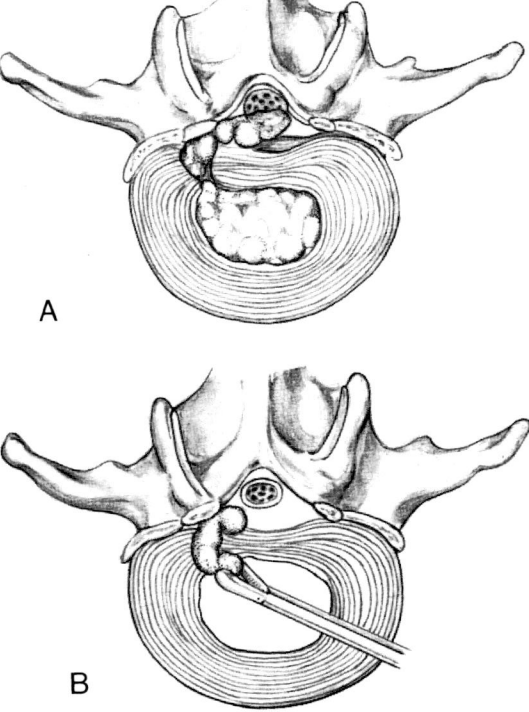

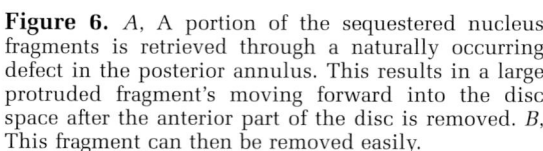

Figure 6. *A*, A portion of the sequestered nucleus fragments is retrieved through a naturally occurring defect in the posterior annulus. This results in a large protruded fragment's moving forward into the disc space after the anterior part of the disc is removed. *B*, This fragment can then be removed easily.

Anterior Extraperitoneal Lumbar Discectomy Without Fusion   1275

Table 1

Age and Sex of Patients Who Underwent Anterior Extraperitoneal Lumbar Discectomy Without Fusion

Age Range (years)	Number of Males (%)	Number of Females (%)	Total Number (%)
9–19	23 (7.1)	17 (13.6)	40 (8.9)
20–29	100 (30.8)	17 (13.6)	117 (26.0)
30–39	85 (26.2)	17 (13.6)	102 (22.7)
40–49	69 (21.2)	32 (25.6)	101 (22.4)
50–59	31 (9.5)	32 (25.6)	63 (14.0)
60–80	17 (5.2)	10 (8.0)	27 (6.0)
TOTAL	325 (72.2)	125 (27.8)	450 (100)

in diameter is created. Residual annulus is removed with care, especially from the posterior area of the disc (Fig. 6). In the case of the L5 disc, sometimes the large vein is in the way, but it is easy to push it upward after the small terminal sacral vessels are ligated. The hypogastric sympathetic plexus is carefully displaced.

SUBJECTS

This operation has been performed on 450 patients, 325 males and 125 females, at Nakano Orthopaedic Hospital between February 1967 and June 1993. The age distribution was from 9 to 80 years, averaging 36.7 years (Table 1).

C A S E ■ 1

A 46-year-old man had been treated by pelvic traction elsewhere, but he became unable to walk because of severe low back pain and sciatica with 20-degree straight leg raising (Fig. 7). Metrizamide myelography revealed a complete defect at the level of the L4 disc (Fig. 8). Extraperitoneal anterior lumbar discectomy was performed, and one large disc fragment with a degenerative disc, weighing 5.6 g, was removed from a posterior protruded pocket on the right side (Figs. 9 through 11). Straight leg raising was improved to up to 85 degrees on both sides 1 week after the operation (Fig. 12).

Myelography was performed 2 months after the operation and showed some improvement, but a filling defect was still recognized. Clinical symptoms, however, disappeared completely (Fig. 13). The patient has since worked without difficulty on a fishing boat for 13.7 years.

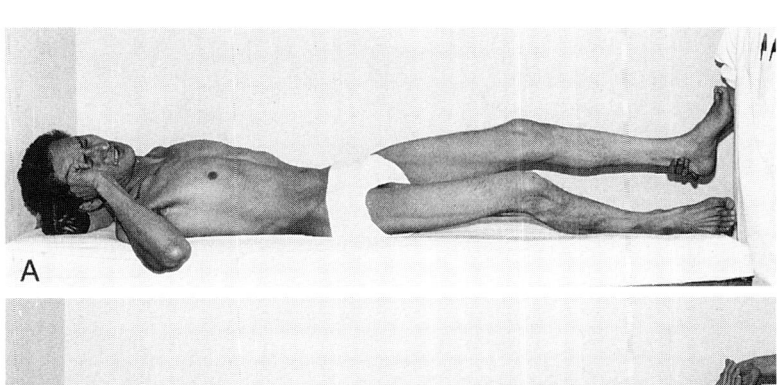

Figure 7. *A, B,* A 46-year-old man who had severe low back pain and sciatica had straight leg raising of only 20 degrees bilaterally.

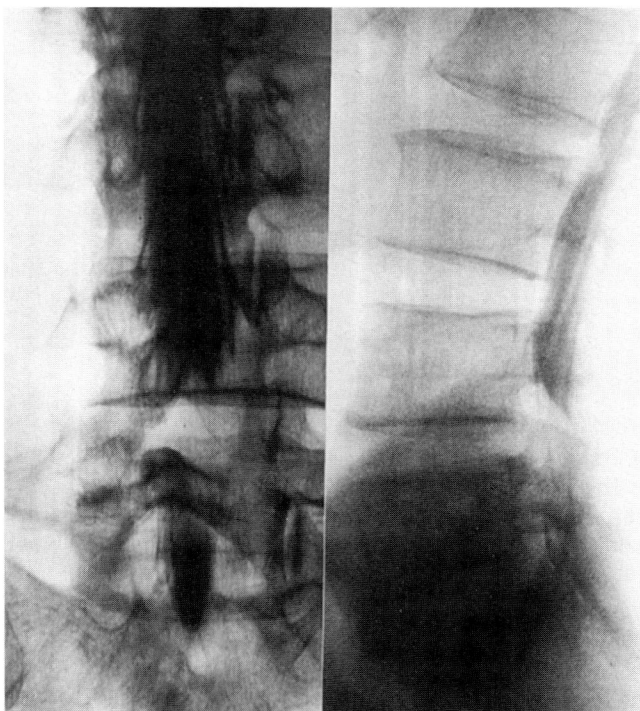

Figure 8. Metrizamide myelograms revealed a complete defect at the level of the L4 disc.

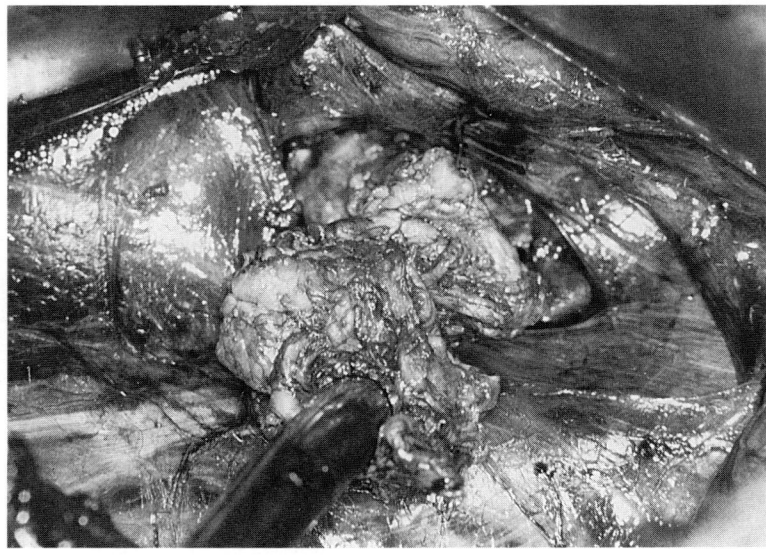

Figure 9. The peripheral disc ligament-annulus is opened, creating a small hole, 5 to 7 mm in diameter. Fragments of degenerated annulus are removed easily.

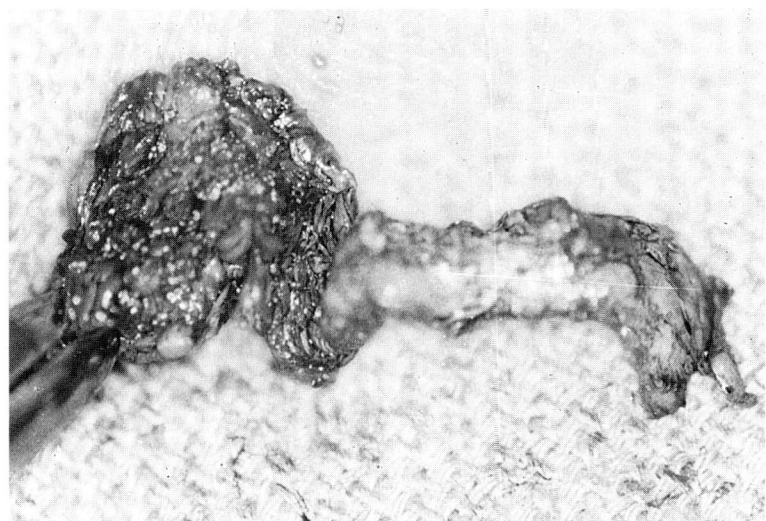

Figure 10. This large disc fragment was removed last.

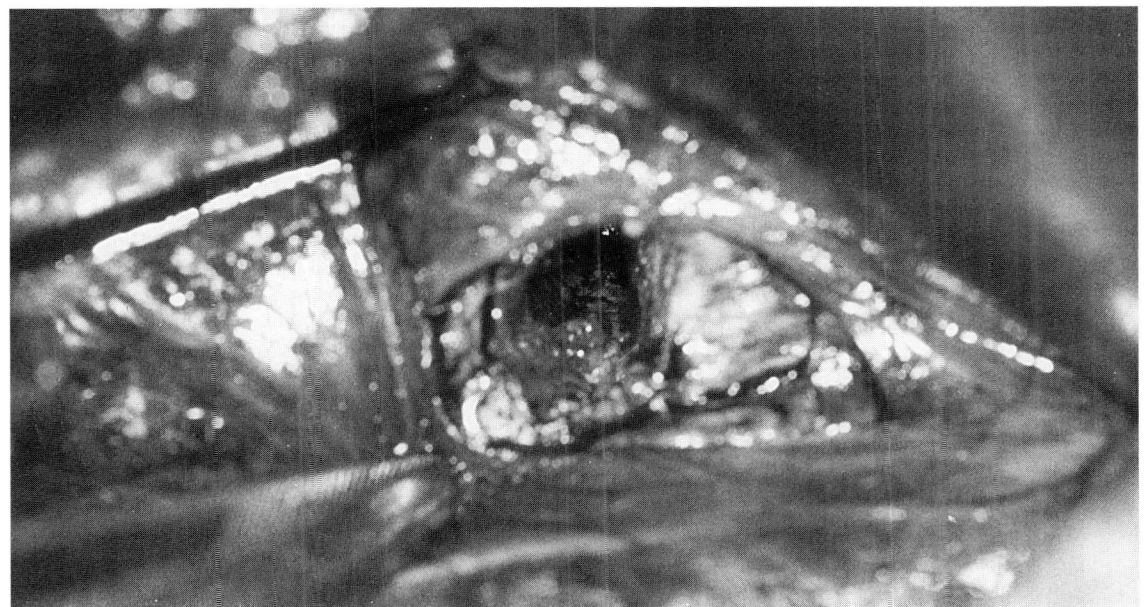

Figure 11. The normal part of the disc was not removed.

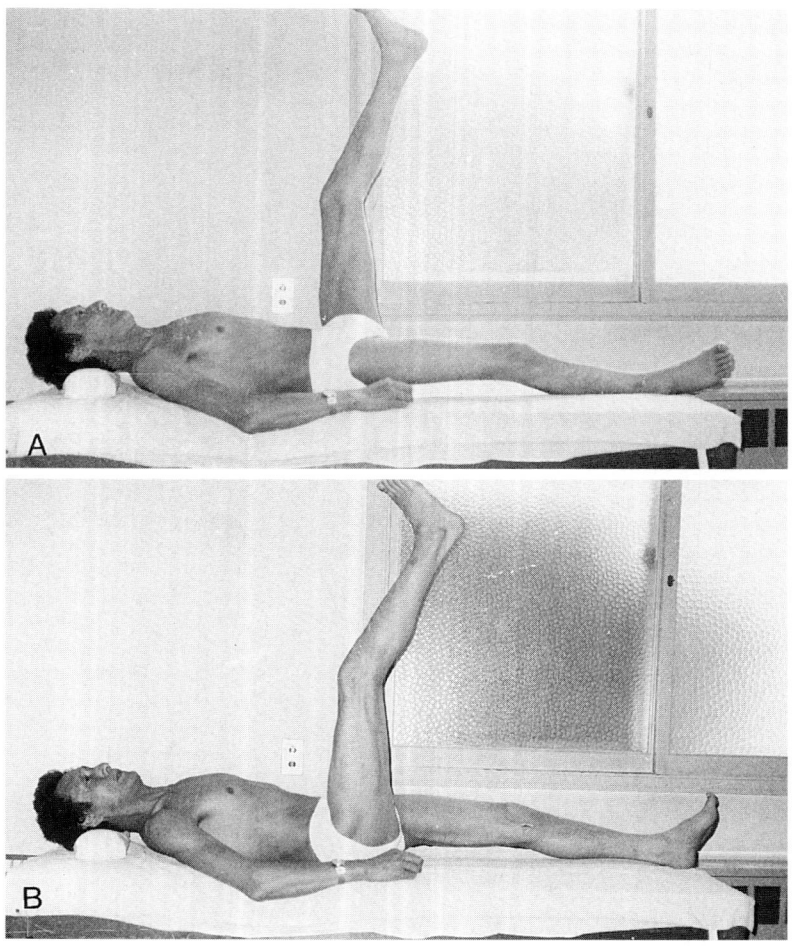

Figure 12. *A, B,* Straight leg raising was improved up to 85 degrees on both sides 1 week after the operation.

RESULTS

Operating time ranged from 30 to 305 minutes, averaging 69.6 minutes. Blood loss ranged from 7 to 337 ml, averaging 61.8 ml. The weight of the removed nucleus and degenerated annulus ranged from 0.5 to 10 g (mean, 2.8 g) at L4–L5. The weight ranged from 0.4 to 5 g (mean, 2 g) at L5–S1. No relation existed between age of the patient and weight of the removed disc.

Narrowing of the disc had progressed as far as it was going to in most patients by 6 months after operation. This narrowing averaged 33% at the L4–L5 disc space and 32.2% at the L5–S1 disc space after 12 years (Fig. 14).

After anterior discectomy was performed, slight instability was seen in seven patients (2%), but no further operation has been required in any patient. Figure 15 is a postoperative radiograph of a patient who was operated on at the L3–L4 and L4–L5 disc spaces. Figure 16 is a 17 years' postoperative flexion-extension x-ray film, which shows no instability; the patient has been working as a carpenter without any difficulty.

Complications

Two superficial infections and one deep one were recognized. In the case of the deep infection, repeated anterior discectomy was performed, and infection might have occurred during the first operation, which was performed at another hospital. Retrograde ejaculation was not seen in any patient in this series.

Eleven patients underwent reoperation posteriorly, seven of whom were operated on at the same level. Two patients were op-

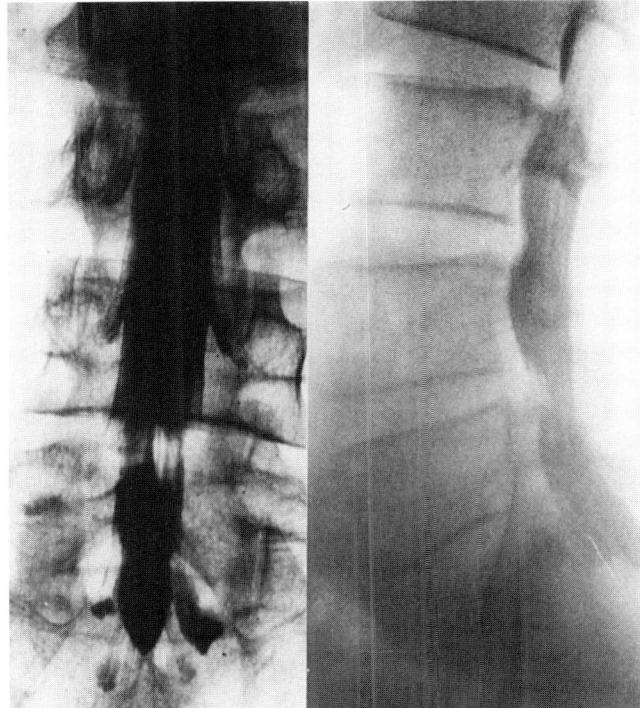

Figure 13. Postoperative myelography was performed 2 months after the operation, but a filling defect was still recognized. Clinical symptoms, however, had disappeared completely.

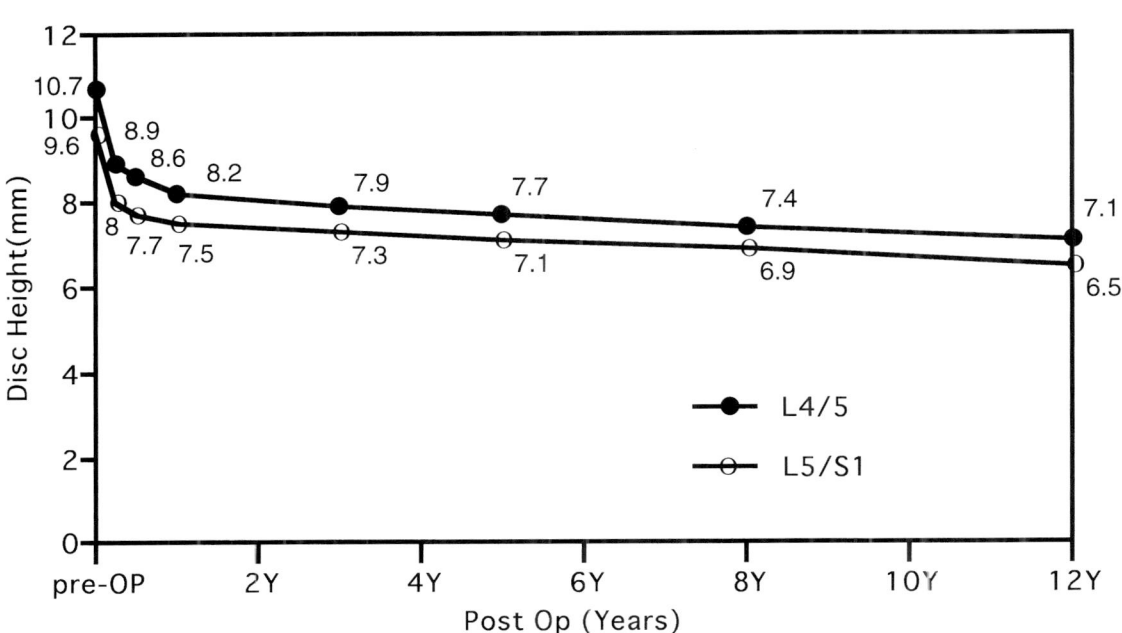

Figure 14. Narrowing of the disc postoperatively in 450 patients who underwent anterior extraperitoneal lumbar discectomy without fusion.

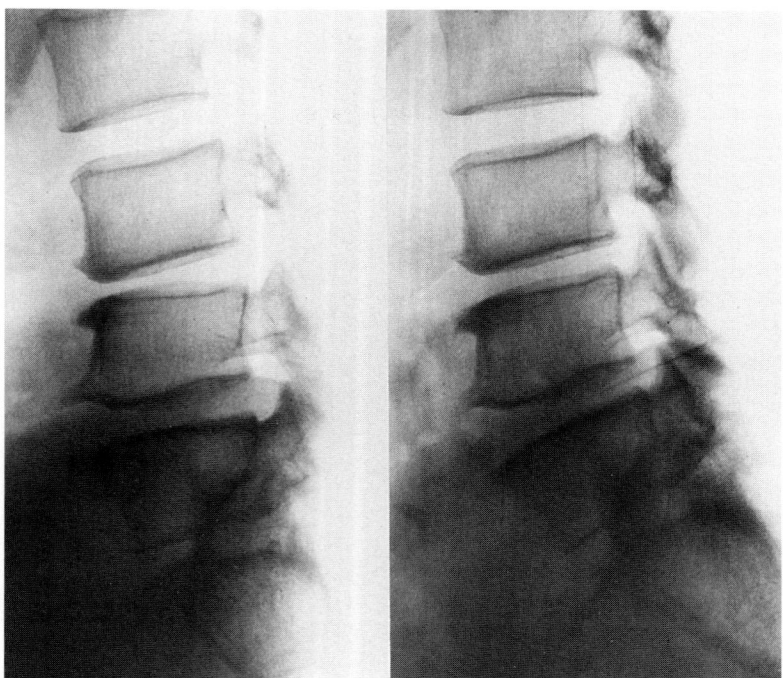

Figure 15. Slight instability was seen by flexion at L4–L5 15 years after surgery, but the patient has worked as a heavy laborer without symptoms.

Figure 16. A 17-year-old male was scheduled to undergo anterior interbody fusion at L5–S1, but because adhesion of big vessels was severe, only anterior discectomy was performed. This is a 17 years' postoperative flexion-extension x-ray film, which shows no instability.

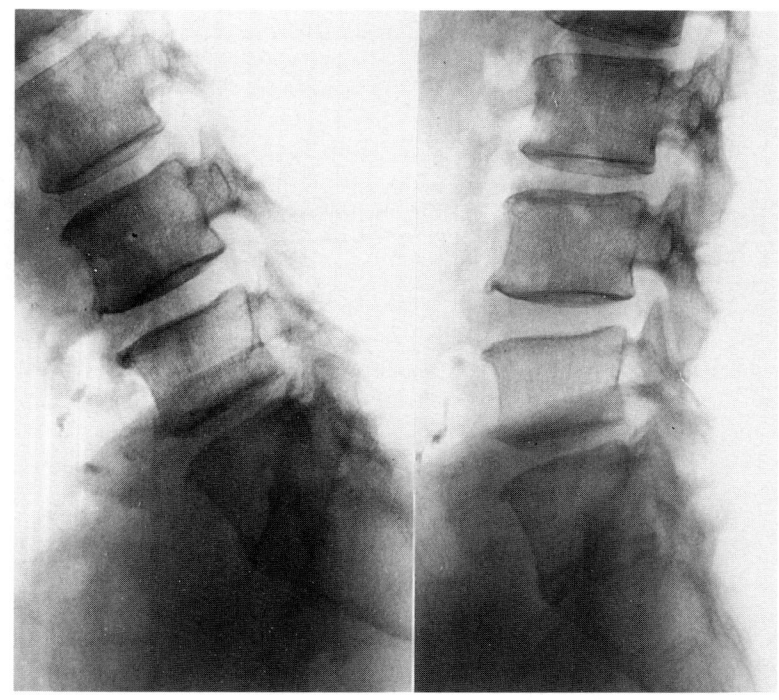

Table 2

Criteria for Clinical Results of Low Back Pain

Results	Criteria
Excellent	All symptoms disappear, and patients can work without difficulty.
Good	Occasional low back pain exists, not sufficient to disturb daily life.
Fair	Symptoms are the same as they were before surgery or have slightly improved.
Poor	Symptoms have worsened.

erated on after 10 years, four after 5 years, and one within 1 year. Recurrence in four patients was at a different level. One patient was unsatisfied, owing to misdiagnosis.

Clinical Evaluation

The criteria used for the postoperative clinical evaluation are shown in Table 2, and the results of the series are presented in Figure 17.

The relationship between the results and patient age is shown in Figures 18 and 19. Women in their 40s received "excellent" ratings in 82% of cases. All but three patients went back to their original occupations, including heavy labor.

Discussion

Hult[3] reported on anterior discectomy with lumbar sympathetic ganglionectomy performed on 30 patients who had chronic low back pain with sciatica and negative myelographic results (degenerated disc without protrusion or extrusion). He thought that the addition of sympathectomy produced better results. Unfortunately, much disagreement exists about the combining of an anterior operation and this surgery; no reports have been published on this method.

Excellent results were obtained by simply removing the disc in a young patient for whom anterior lumbar interbody fusion had been planned but was not performed because adhesion of the iliac vessels was severe. As a result, this procedure was tried in patients with sciatica and low back pain and has produced satisfactory results.

The anterior extraperitoneal lumbar discectomy has been performed after failure of conservative treatments on patients with positive myelography and more than two of the following symptoms: low back pain, pain or numbness in the lower extremity, positive results on the straight leg raising test, muscle weakness of the lower extremity, and disturbance of urinary bladder function. These are, similarly, indications for posterior discectomy without fusion.

Some surgeons pointed out that extruded fragments might be impossible to remove anteriorly. Occasionally, portions of the sequestered nucleus fragments are retrieved through a naturally occurring defect in the posterior annulus. This sometimes results in a large protruded fragment's moving forward into the disc space because of reduced

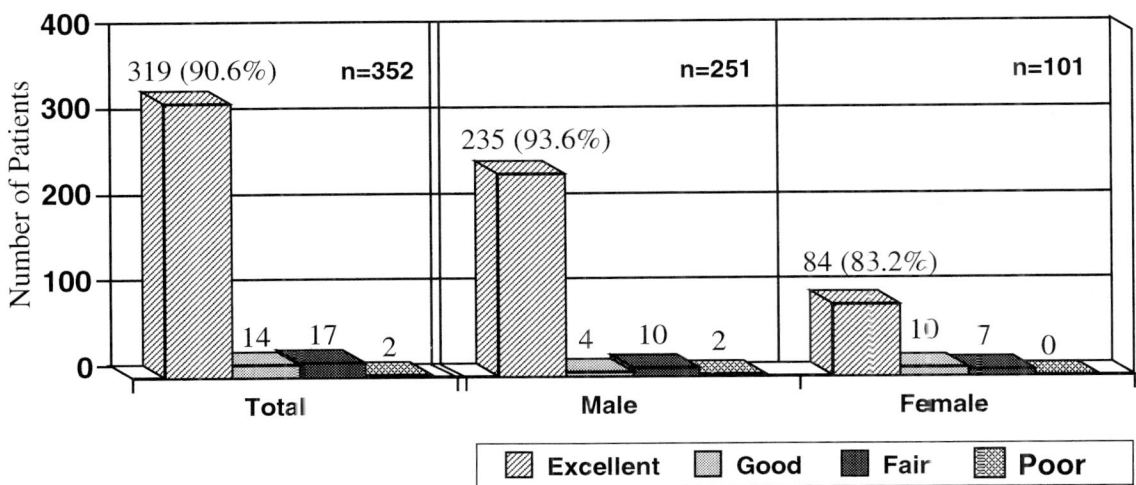

Figure 17. Results of anterior extraperitoneal lumbar discectomy without fusion performed in 352 patients.

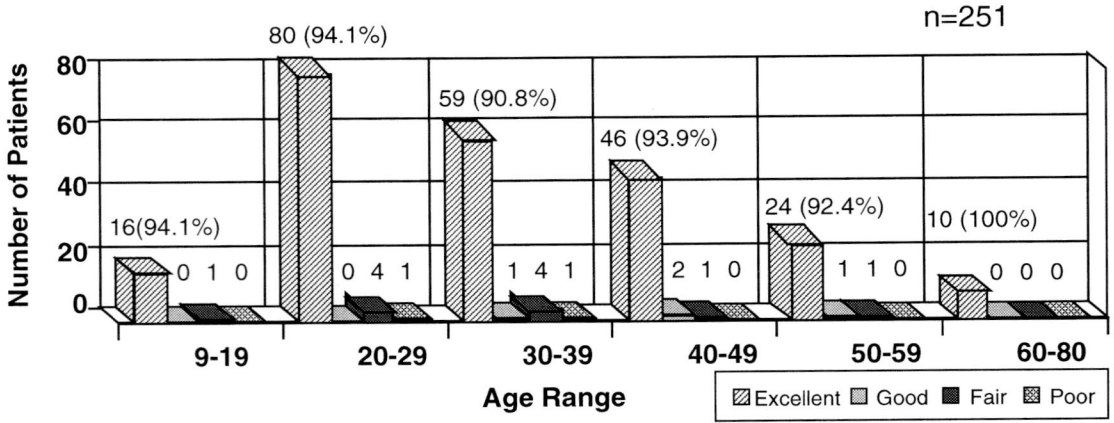

Figure 18. Results according to age of patient of anterior extraperitoneal lumbar discectomy without fusion performed in 251 males.

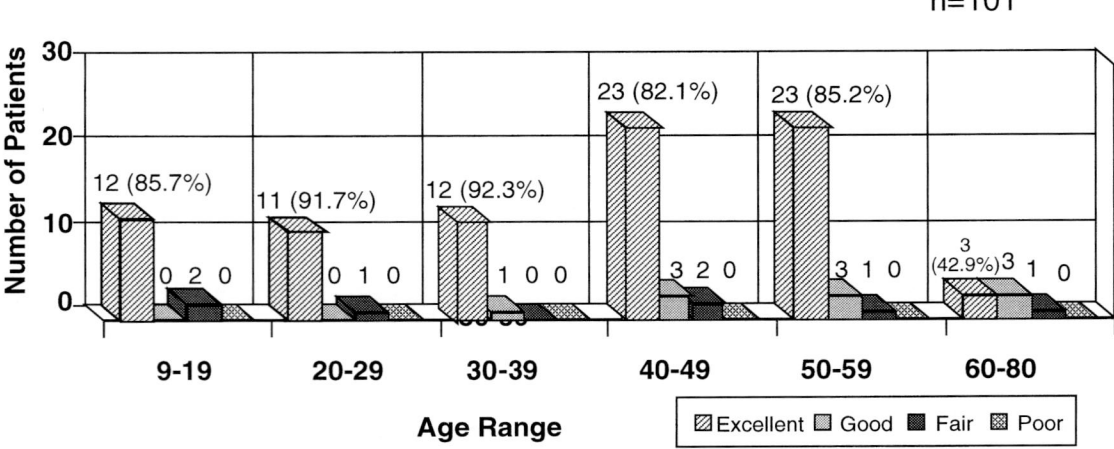

Figure 19. Results according to age of patient of anterior extraperitoneal lumbar discectomy without fusion performed in 101 females.

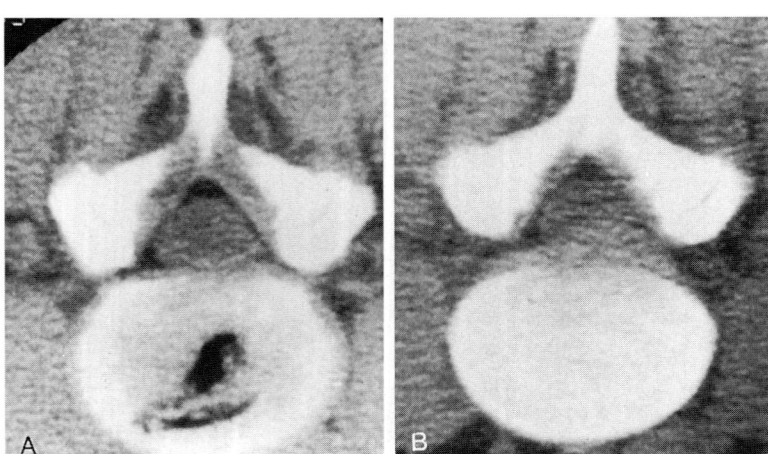

Figure 20. Computed tomographic scans taken after (*A*) and before (*B*) anterior discectomy. It can be seen that the disc was removed anteriorly.

pressure in the disc space after the anterior area of the disc has been removed. This fragment can then be removed easily. Therefore, removal of disc materials from the spinal canal should not be attempted[5-10] (Fig. 20). Extensive laminectomy and rough handling of the dura produced some poor results.[4] Anterior discectomy with interbody fusion became an accepted operation,[2] but some cases of male sterility were reported after this procedure. Flynn and Hogue[1] put this complication into proper focus, finding that surgeons who have performed a large number of anterior discectomies and fusion operations do not experience this complication. It is now believed that most poor results and complications from an anterior operation are due to unfamiliarity with retroperitoneal anatomy and to poor exposure.

The anterior approach is more appropriate than the posterior one because portions of a disc can be removed, without disturbing the spinal canal, for decompression of the posterior disc area. Low back pain and sciatica are caused by a combination of posterior disc protrusion or high intradiscal pressure, produced by degeneration, nucleus absorption, or a segmented disc annulus pressing against the posterior longitudinal ligament.

No statistical correlation exists between narrowing of the space and clinical results, because the decompression of the posterior longitudinal ligament relieves the symptoms. After anterior discectomy, flexion-extension x-ray films were taken of every patient to reveal any instability. Slight instability was recognized in seven patients, but no further operation was required.

An excellent result among women in their 50s occurred more frequently than for other groups (see Figs. 18 and 19). This result may be related to menopause and an incorrect indication for surgery.

This method does not disturb the muscle at all. Therefore, it is a good procedure for athletes with low back pain and sciatica. Postoperative regimens, however, are important for these patients, as they are in all lumbar spine surgery. These regimens include light postural exercise, muscle strengthening of both anterior and posterior muscle groups, and care in lifting, stooping, and twisting. A limitation should be placed on riding in motor vehicles, and the patient should undergo a rest period of a minimum of 4 weeks before resuming normal activities.

REFERENCES

1. Flynn, J. C., and Hogue, M. A.: Anterior fusion of lumbar spine: End result study with long-term follow-up. J. Bone Joint Surg. 61A:1143–1150, 1979.
2. Harmon, P. H.: Anterior extraperitoneal lumbar disc excision and vertebral body fusion: A study of long-term results. Clin. Orthop. 18:169–185, 1961.
3. Hult, L.: Retroperitoneal disc fenestration in low back pain sciatica. A preliminary report. Acta Orthop. Scand. 20:342–348, 1950.
4. Nakano, N.: Multiple back operations. J. West. Pacific Orthop. Assoc. 14:67–74, 1977.
5. Nakano, N.: Anterior extraperitoneal discectomy in lumbar disc herniation. J. Jpn Orthop. Assoc. 52:1530–1531, 1978.
6. Nakano, N., and Tomita, T.: Results of surgical treatment of low back pain: A comparative study of the anterior and posterior approach. Int. Orthop. 4:101–106, 1980.
7. Nakano, N.: Lower lumbar anterior discectomy without fusion: A several year follow-up indicating usefulness of this procedure in surgery of the lower lumbar spine—a report of 110 cases. J. Jpn Orthop. Assoc. 57:321–328, 1983.
8. Nakano, N., and Nakano, T.: Surgical technique of anterior extraperitoneal lumbar discectomy to the lumbar disc herniation. Operation 41:1–6, 1987.
9. Nakano, N., Nakano, T., and Nakano, K.: Long term results of anterior extraperitoneal lumbar discectomy. Acta Orthop. Belg. 53:291–292, 1987.
10. Nakano, N., Nakano, T., and Nakano, K.: Anterior extraperitoneal lumbar discectomy and the results. J. Spine Spinal Cord 7:49–54, 1994.

24

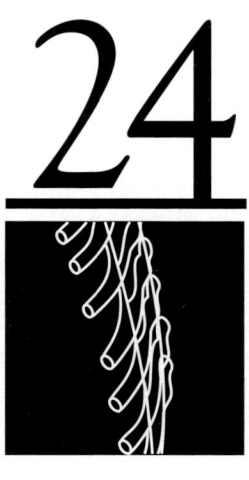

Fusion

Biology of Lumbar Spine Fusion and Bone Graft Materials

SCOTT D. BODEN
JEFFREY H. SCHIMANDLE

Spine fusion may be defined as the elimination of movement across an intervertebral motion segment by bony union. It is one of the most commonly performed, yet incompletely understood, procedures in spine surgery. The concept of spine fusion surgery was first reported on in 1911 by Albee,[1] who sought to inhibit tuberculous spread in Pott disease by providing mechanical support and stability to involved vertebrae, and by Hibbs,[74] who used fusion surgery to halt the progression of scoliotic deformity. The rate of nonunion has since been reported to range from 5% to 35%,[42, 175] and many factors are thought to affect this rate, including local biomechanical factors (e.g., instability and loading), local and systemic biologic factors (e.g., blood supply, hormones, drugs, and smoking), and bone graft factors (e.g., source, type, and quantity of graft, and graft bed preparation).

The commonest solution to the spine nonunion problem has been mechanical. However, controlling the local biomechanical environment at a fusion site by the use of internal fixation has not eliminated nonunions.[13, 117, 198, 203] Clearly, biologic factors must be implicated. Although many investigators have studied mechanical factors affecting spine fusion,[50, 111–113] a paucity of knowledge exists about the biology involved in achieving a successful fusion.

Advances in surgical techniques and in knowledge regarding gene-specific therapies, as well as the potential for biologic manipulation of bone formation, make it timely to reexamine the understanding of the biology of bone graft materials and the spine fusion process. This discussion reviews the multiplicity of local and systemic factors affecting spine fusion and discusses the properties and use of various graft materials. The results from studies using animal models to study fusion variables and the data from limited clinical studies are presented. Lastly, gaps in existing knowledge are identified, and future areas of research are discussed. An understanding of the biology of spine fusion will enable the clinician to apply sound principles in seeking solutions to the problems associated with achieving a successful spine fusion.

BIOLOGY OF SPINE FUSION

The outcome of a spine fusion depends on a complex process influenced primarily by the type of graft material used and the many local and systemic factors that affect the fusion healing response. These factors may have positive or negative effects on graft healing[20] (Table 1).

Local Factors

Soft Tissue Bed

The quality of the tissue bed into which the bone graft material is placed is paramount. The entire fusion process depends on the ingress of osteoprogenitor and inflammatory cells from the recipient bed as well as the few surviving bone cells transplanted when autogenous bone is used. The tissue bed must therefore be able to support all processes involved in bone graft healing. These processes are greatly affected by the adequacy of the local blood supply, the efficacy of the inflammatory response, and the availability of osteoprogenitor cells.

The adequacy of the blood supply in the fusion bed is a critical requisite for fusion healing. Host bed tissue must not be traumatized, and any avascular (nonviable) or traumatized tissue should be debrided. The fusion bed vasculature is a source of nutrients to the healing fusion, a vehicle for endocrine stimuli, and a pathway for the recruitment of inflammatory and osteoprogenitor cells, which are essential for the successful incorporation of graft material and the inhibition of infection.

Hurley and associates,[84] using a dog posterior spine fusion model, evaluated the role played by overlying soft tissues during fusion of the spine. Thirty-seven animals underwent one of the following procedures: (1) a modified Hibbs fusion as the control procedure, (2) a Hibbs fusion with nylon-reinforced sheets of Millipore (plastic membrane filter permeable to tissue fluids but impermeable to cells) interposed between the fusion site and overlying muscle mass, and (3) a Hibbs fusion with Silastic sheets (silicone rubber impermeable to both tissue fluids and cells). All 10 L5–L6 fusions with interposed Silastic sheets resulted in nonunion, whereas all 12 L5–L6 fusions with interposed Millipore filters resulted in a solid union. These results supported the role of the adjacent soft tissues in spine fusion in providing a source of nutrition for migrating osteoprogenitor cells and possibly a source of diffusible growth factors.

Table 1

Local and Systemic Factors Affecting Bone Healing

Local Factors		Systemic Factors	
Positive	Negative	Positive	Negative
Good vascular supply	Radiation	Growth hormone and somatomedins	Osteoporosis
Large surface area	Tumor		Corticosteroids
Mechanical stability	Local bone disease	Thyroid hormone	Vitamin D deficiency
Growth factors	Infection	Vitamin A	Methotrexate
Bone morphogenetic proteins	Mechanical instability	Vitamin D	Doxorubicin (Adriamycin)
Electrical stimulation	Bone wax	Insulin	NSAIDs
Mechanical loading	Denervation	Parathyroid hormone	Smoking
		Calcitonin	Anemia
		Anabolic steroids	Rheumatoid arthritis
			Sepsis
			Diabetes
			SIADH
			Malnutrition
			Sickle cell disease
			Thalassemia major

NSAIDs, nonsteroidal antiinflammatory drugs; SIADH, syndrome of inappropriate antidiuretic hormone secretion.

Graft Recipient Site Preparation

There are several methods of preparation of the bony surfaces onto which the graft material is placed; these include the use of a power bur, curets, rongeurs, and osteotomes. Regardless of the technique used, the goal is to maximize the area of exposed and viable vascular bone. Decortication by use of a power bur, as opposed to other methods, may induce thermal necrosis of the bone. This effect can be reduced by avoiding prolonged contact of the bur with the bone and by using continuous irrigation. Generally, the larger the surface area decorticated for fusion, the greater is the availability of potential osteogenic cells and the larger the contact area exposed to support a bony bridge large enough to carry a mechanical load. Decreased surface area may be responsible for the lower fusion rates seen in patients with myelomeningocele,[3] although other factors may also contribute (e.g., increased infection rate and difficulty of fixation).

Mechanical Stability

The mechanical stability of the spine segment or segments to be fused affects the rate of fusion.[64, 111–113, 126, 204] Several studies have shown higher union rates when internal fixation was used to decrease motion in the fusion segment,[13, 64, 111, 112, 203, 204] and when device loosening occurs, nonunion of the fusion mass is likelier to occur[7] (Fig. 1). Patients with muscular dystrophy or spinal muscular atrophy have higher-than-average fusion rates, which may be in part the result of decreased spine segment motion and improved mechanics from decreased voluntary motion.[5, 177] The level of fusion (L4–L5 versus L5–S1), the number of segments fused, the patient's weight and activity level, and the use of postoperative external mobilization (bracing)[167] are all important mechanical factors that may influence the rate of fusion.

In the study of the effects of spinal instrumentation and biomechanical stability on the spine, most research has focused on the acute or short-term in vitro biomechanical properties of the system under study.[62, 63, 87, 114, 197] Extrapolation of such laboratory findings to the clinical use of spinal instrumentation in spine fusions has been predicated on the information derived from this "bench-top" biomechanical testing rather than on results of studies on the long-term in vivo biologic effects on the fusion mass or vertebral bone. The common shortcoming of these bench-top studies is that the interaction between the biology of the fusion process and the instrumentation is not taken into account. Using in vivo animal models is therefore critical to study the relationship between spinal instrumentation and the long-term biologic effects on spine fusion.

Gurr and colleagues[64] and McAfee and colleagues[111–113] created a dog instability model to study the effect of spinal instrumentation on achieving a successful fusion and the radiographic incidence of spine fusion with respect to spine stability. Radiographic assessment of trabecular bridging 6 months after surgery revealed a greater probability of achieving a successful spine fusion if instrumentation was used. Nondestructive

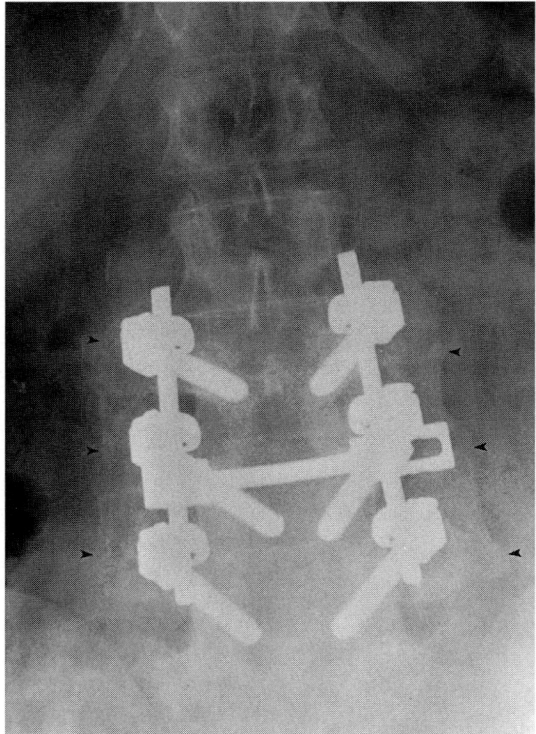

Figure 1. Radiograph taken 1 year after posterolateral intertransverse process fusion using autogenous iliac cancellous bone and internal fixation in a woman with spinal stenosis and degenerative spondylolisthesis. A well-corticalized margin *(arrowheads)* with continuous trabeculation suggests a mature fusion mass.

mechanical testing showed the instrumented fusions to be also significantly more rigid.[64, 111, 112] In 1991, Zdeblick and associates[204] reported on a model that used the coonhound to simulate an unstable L5 burst fracture. Use of anterior instrumentation resulted in an increased fusion rate radiographically and a more rigid fusion when the area was biomechanically tested. Using this model, Shirado and coworkers[121] replicated these results. Overall, the dog spine instability-corpectomy model has proved useful in studying the in vivo response to spinal instrumentation and stabilization.

Nagel and colleagues[126] developed an animal model of delayed union or nonunion following spine fusion in sheep. Posterior lumbar laminar and facet fusions achieved using iliac crest bone graft were performed in seven sheep. In six of seven sheep nonunions developed at the L6–S1 interspace, whereas all cephalad interlumbar spaces (21 of 21) fused solidly. In vivo flexion-extension radiographs were studied in an additional eight normal sheep, and spines from five normal sheep were studied ex vivo by use of displacement transducers to determine stiffness, linear displacement, and strain of the lumbar motion segments in flexion and extension. Notably increased motion occurred at the lumbosacral level compared with other lumbar levels. This paper established that motion was the major determinant of fusion outcome in the sheep model. Similar observations about nonunions at the more mobile lumbosacral junction have also been noted in dogs.[84]

The mechanical stresses (e.g., load and torque) experienced by the graft material itself also affect the fusion rate.[49] For example, 80% of the mechanical load of a motion segment is sustained by the intervertebral disc; thus, graft material placed into an intervertebral body location is subjected to compressive loading. These compressive forces act on the graft and promote fusion by stimulating the ingrowth of vascular buds and proliferating mesenchymal cells from the cancellous host bone into the donor graft. In contrast, graft placed posteriorly and, to a lesser extent, in the intertransverse process area experiences tensile forces, and healing is less favorable mechanically and is more dependent on biologic factors (e.g., osteogenic cells or osteoinductive factors).

Radiation

Irradiation to a healing spine fusion has an adverse effect on fusion rate and is especially detrimental within the first few weeks of fusion.[11] This effect may be caused by direct cytotoxic effects on the migrating, proliferating, and differentiating mesenchymal cells,[35] or it may be related to the alteration in vascularity from both the intense vasculitis induced by the radiation injury and the inhibition of angiogenesis. After the acute injury phase, radiation-induced osteonecrosis and dense hypovascular scar in the radiation bed make the fusion area a poor biologic environment for fusion; the use of vascularized grafts anastomosed to unirradiated vessels may increase the chance of successful fusion in this situation.

Tumor and Bone Disease

Local tumor or bone disease (e.g., that caused by fibrous dysplasia or Paget disease) may directly invade the fusion area and replace normal marrow, structurally weakening the recipient bone and fusion mass. These obstacles can be partly overcome by the use of specific fixation techniques[69, 96] and by the appropriate use of local irradiation and/or systemic chemotherapy. The use of autograft bone is desirable if the prognosis is favorable, but the harvest site must be maintained as a separate surgical field to prevent tumor seeding to the donor site.

Growth Factors

Several local growth factors are known to positively influence the migration, differentiation, and activity of potential bone-forming mesenchymal cells.[27-29] Bone morphogenetic proteins (BMPs) are the most widely investigated of these substances and were discussed in several reviews.[187, 200] In addition to BMPs, other local growth factors that influence these processes have been extracted from bone matrix and other tissues. Several of these proteins are already available through recombinant genetic technology. As the roles of these biologic mediators are elucidated, they will become an important clinical means of biologically manipulating the complex cascade of cellular events essential to the fusion process.

Electrical Stimulation

Several animal and clinical studies have documented the osteogenic effect of direct-current stimulation and pulsed electromagnetic fields on bone repair.[55, 70, 174, 201] Most studies have centered on long-bone delayed union or nonunion,[14, 71, 141, 142, 206] and on congenital pseudarthrosis of the tibia.[101, 143]

Electrical stimulation has been shown to enhance the rate of spine fusion in various animal studies[90–92, 129] and human clinical trials.[44, 45, 93, 121, 128, 173] Several mechanisms of action have been proposed; all appear to act directly or indirectly at the cellular level. Optimal biologic currents appear to be between 5 and 25 µA and can be delivered directly or via pulsed electromagnetic fields (PEMFs).

In an effort to study and evaluate the in vivo efficacy of both pulsed electromagnetic and direct constant current stimulation as an adjunct to improve the rate and quality of posterior spine fusions, four studies have been conducted employing the dog and pig as animal models.[90–92, 129] Kahanovitz and coworkers[91] investigated the ability of adjunctive noninvasive PEMFs to enhance spine fusions in dogs. Ten mongrel dogs underwent posterior three-level laminar and facet fusions with bilateral distraction instrumentation. Despite improved new bone formation and better organization of the fusion mass noted early in the stimulated specimens (by 12 and 15 weeks), no differences existed between the stimulated and control groups of dogs at the end point.

Two studies of direct constant current electrical stimulation on spine fusions in pig[129] and dog[90] spine fusion models have been conducted. Nerubay and associates[129] performed posterior L5–L6 laminar and facet fusions in 30 immature pigs by use of iliac graft with blinded implantation of an active versus an inactive bone growth stimulator. Results revealed a statistically significant increase in fusion score in the active bone growth stimulation group 2 months after surgery, as well as an increase in osteoblastic activity and bone formation. Kahanovitz and Arnoczky,[90] in a similar experiment using a dog model, performed facet fusions at L1–L2 and L4–L5 in 12 animals. An electrode pair was placed across each of the four facet joints, with only one pair at one level being functional and the other pair acting as a control. Although no differences were seen early, the stimulated specimens were radiographically and histologically more advanced at 12 weeks. No evidence of bony union was noted in the control group, whereas all facets demonstrated a complete bony fusion in the stimulated group. More recently, Kahanovitz and colleagues[92] evaluated the effect of the use of PEMFs on the healing of lumbar facet fusions in 24 dogs. No statistical difference in the radiographic or histologic appearance of the fusion mass could be detected between the stimulated and control groups at either 6 or 12 weeks.

Investigators who conducted clinical studies have reported results of electrical stimulation on spine fusion. In 1974, Dwyer and Wickham[45] first reported the clinical use of direct-current stimulation in spine fusions in 12 patients and concluded that it promoted earlier but more immature fusion. In a larger subsequent series, Dwyer[44] reported achieving radiographic fusion in 40 of 47 patients (85%). In 1984, Nerubay and Katznelson[128] observed that direct-current stimulation enhanced spine fusion in five patients with low-grade spondylolisthesis. At 10 weeks, clinical and radiographic assessment revealed that all patients had solid fusions. In 1988, Kane[93] reported the results of a randomized prospective study of direct-current stimulation in 59 patients considered to be at increased risk for nonunion. The fusion rate determined radiographically for the 28 control patients was 54%, whereas the rate of fusion in the 31 stimulated patients was 81%. In the same paper, Kane reported the results of a nonrandom multicenter study of 116 patients treated with electrical stimulation. Successful radiographic fusion was achieved in 108 of the 116 patients (93%).

The use of PEMFs to enhance the rate of spine fusion in high-risk patients has not gained as wide acceptance as the direct-current stimulation methods. Although PEMF stimulation is noninvasive, its success largely depends on patient acceptance and compliance. In 1985, Simmons[173] reported the use of PEMFs to treat failed posterior lumbar interbody fusions. An increase in bone formation was seen in 11 of 13 patients (85%), and solid radiographic fusion was achieved in 10 of 13 patients (77%) over a 4-month treatment period. In 1990, Mooney[121] reported the results of a randomized double-blind prospective study of the use of PEMFs to enhance the success rate of lumbar interbody fusions. In the group of 98 patients treated with an active stimulator, the radiographic fusion rate was 92%, whereas in the placebo group of 97 patients, the fusion rate was 65%.

Unfortunately, most of the clinical electrical stimulation studies were plagued with limitations, including mixed diagnoses, different fusion types, poor documentation of improved clinical outcomes, and randomization design errors. The authors believe that more data are needed before electrical stimulation can be recommended for routine posterolateral lumbar fusions.

Systemic Factors

Osteoporosis

Osteoporosis is the most prevalent metabolic bone disease, affecting 25 million Americans, and is commonly assumed to be a negative factor in bone healing. Although decreased bone mass is the hallmark of osteoporosis, alterations in bone marrow quality and the rate of bone turnover may also be present. The number of osteogenic stem cells may be deficient in the elderly patient and, in fact, may be more important than absolute bone mass. Additionally, osteoporotic vertebrae are weak and difficult to stabilize adequately with internal fixation, especially across the mobile lumbosacral junction. All of these factors may adversely affect the spine fusion rate.

Hormones

Over the past decade, a considerable amount of knowledge has been gained about the control of bone formation by hormones.[27] These chemical messengers have complex direct and indirect effects on bone formation and may influence spine fusion healing, both positively and negatively.

Growth hormone has no direct effects on cartilage or bone formation but exerts its stimulatory effects through somatomedins.[149, 150] Growth hormone stimulates bone healing in vivo by increasing intestinal absorption of calcium, bone formation, and bone mineralization.[120, 184]

Thyroid hormones are necessary for normal growth and development. They are required for the synthesis of somatomedins by the liver[164] and have a direct stimulatory effect on cartilage growth and maturation[21, 184] and thus have a positive effect on bone healing. Thyroid hormones act synergistically with growth hormone.[184]

In both experimental and clinical situations, corticosteroids have been shown to have deleterious effects on bone healing because they increase bone resorption and decrease bone formation.[65, 89] In cell culture experiments, corticosteroids have been shown both to inhibit and promote the differentiation of osteoblasts from mesenchymal cells[6, 172] and to decrease the synthesis rates of the major components of bone matrix that are necessary for bone healing.[36]

Estrogens and androgens (e.g., testosterone) are considered important in skeletal maturation of growing individuals and in the prevention of the bone loss associated with aging. The in vivo effects of these hormones on bone healing, however, are controversial. Although some studies indicate that they may stimulate bone formation,[8] most do not support this possibility.[97, 156] In vitro studies have shown that neither estrogens nor androgens affect bone collagen synthesis,[30] but estrogens may increase bone mineralization by increasing serum parathyroid hormone and 1,25-dihydroxycholecalciferol concentrations.[58]

Nutrition

Nutritional status has been shown to affect bone healing in the orthopedic patient.[46, 86] If suspected, nutritional deficiencies can be identified by use of serum albumin and transferrin levels, total lymphocyte count, skin antigen testing, anthropometric measurements, and nitrogen balance studies. These studies can be useful in assessing the nutritional status of selected patients to determine the need for nutritional support.

Hematologic disorders, such as sickle cell disease and thalassemia major, may also decrease the osteogenic potential of bone marrow by overgrowth of the hematopoietic elements at the expense of the osteoprogenitor cells. Iron deficiency anemia impairs fracture healing[161] and similarly may adversely affect fusion consolidation.

Drugs

Various drugs taken during the perioperative period can inhibit or delay bone formation. Chemotherapeutic agents, such as methotrexate and doxorubicin, inhibit bone formation and healing if they are administered early in the postoperative period.[23, 57, 134, 148] Nonsteroidal antiinflammatory drugs, such as ibuprofen, suppress the inflammatory response and may inhibit bone formation and spine fusion.[102]

Smoking

Cigarette smoking interferes with bone metabolism and revascularization and inhibits bone formation. Extracts from tobacco smoke have been reported to induce calcitonin resistance,[75] increase bone resorption at fracture ends,[99] and interfere with osteoblastic function.[39] The rate of nonunion in smokers who have undergone spine fusion has been shown to be higher than that in nonsmokers.[9, 15, 66, 117, 203]

PROPERTIES OF GRAFT MATERIALS

In addition to the local and systemic factors, the choice of graft material influences the outcome of a spine fusion. Graft materials placed into the spine fusion bed participate in the fusion process in several ways, depending on the properties they possess.[98, 152] These properties allow the grafts to (1) directly produce bone (osteogenic potential), (2) provide structural support conducive to bone formation (osteoconduction), and/or (3) stimulate osteoprogenitor cells to differentiate into osteogenic cells (osteoinduction). The ideal graft material possesses all these properties (Table 2).

Osteogenic Potential

The osteogenic potential of a graft is derived from its cellular content. Osteogenic graft materials contain viable cells that possess the ability to form bone (determined osteogenic precursor cells) or the potential to differentiate into bone-forming cells (inducible osteogenic precursor cells). These cells participate in the early stages of the healing process to unite the graft to the host bone and must be protected during the grafting procedure to ensure viability. This potential to produce bone is characteristic only of fresh autogenous bone and bone marrow cells.

Osteoconduction

Osteoconductivity is the physical property of a graft material that allows the ingrowth of neovasculature and the infiltration of osteogenic precursor cells during the process known as creeping substitution. A graft material that is only osteoconductive transfers neither osteogenic cells nor inductive stimuli but acts as a nonviable scaffold or trellis that supports the bone-healing response. Materials that are osteoconductive include autogenous and allograft bone, bone matrix, collagen, and calcium phosphate ceramics.

Osteoinduction

Bone induction is the process by which some factor or substance stimulates an undetermined osteoprogenitor stem cell to differentiate into an osteogenic cell type. This

Table 2

Properties of Graft Materials

Graft Material	Osteogenic Potential	Osteoinduction	Osteoconduction
Autogenous bone	X	X	X
Bone marrow cells	X	?	
Allograft bone		?	X
Xenograft bone			X
DBM		X	X
BMPs		X	
Ceramics			X

DBM, demineralized bone matrix; BMPs, bone morphogenetic proteins.

concept was introduced by Urist and associates[185, 191] in the 1960s after their initial studies on the osteoinductive properties of demineralized bone matrix (DBM) and BMPs. In addition to these materials, autogenous bone and allograft are known to possess osteoinductive properties.

GRAFT MATERIALS

Autograft

Autogenous bone is considered the most successful bone graft material and is presently the gold standard.* Complications with its use, however, may occur in as many as 25 to 30% of patients.[100, 202] Graft harvest complications include increased blood loss and risk of transfusion; increased surgical morbidity from an additional operative site for graft harvest, including chronic donor site pain[51]; increased operative time; and additional cost.[152] The quantity of bone available to harvest may be insufficient in patients requiring long, multisegment fusions or in those who have undergone previous graft harvests. These problems have motivated the investigation of growth factors DBM, BMPs, and bone graft substitutes (allograft bone, calcium phosphate ceramics) to achieve a spine fusion.

Autogenous cancellous bone is currently the most successful grafting material available for achieving a spine fusion (Fig. 2). Inherent to this material are all three of the ideal transplant properties: osteogenic potential, osteoconductivity, and osteoinductivity. These properties are present by virtue of the surviving bone cells, BMPs, bone mineral, and collagen. Additionally, a large trabecular surface area is available that can be incorporated through new bone formation, a property called connectivity.

Autogenous cortical bone is used as a graft material in situations in which structural support is needed at the graft site (Fig. 3). Except for the advantage of mechanical strength, cortical bone is less desirable than cancellous bone for many reasons. Fewer osteogenic cells are present in cortical bone because of the absence of marrow, and the cells that are present are less likely to survive because they are embedded in the more compact cortical matrix and are shielded

---

*References 48, 72, 82, 135, 152, 182, and 199.

from the diffusion of nutrients. Cortical bone has less surface area per unit weight than does cancellous bone, limiting the area onto which new bone can form and from which induction proteins can pass. Lastly, cortical bone is more resistant to vascular ingrowth and remodeling, both of which are necessary for bone healing and the development of mechanical strength. Whereas cancellous grafts tend to be completely repaired in time, cortical grafts remain as admixtures of viable and necrotic bone (Fig. 4).

Vascularized grafts of autogenous fibula, iliac crest, or rib have many advantages[12, 40, 115, 160, 168, 196] and are used in selected cases of anterior spinal fusion. The improved incorporation of these grafts makes their use desirable in cases in which avascular graft healing is poor, such as in areas of radiation-induced fibrosis or when radiation or chemotherapy is to be given in the perioperative period.

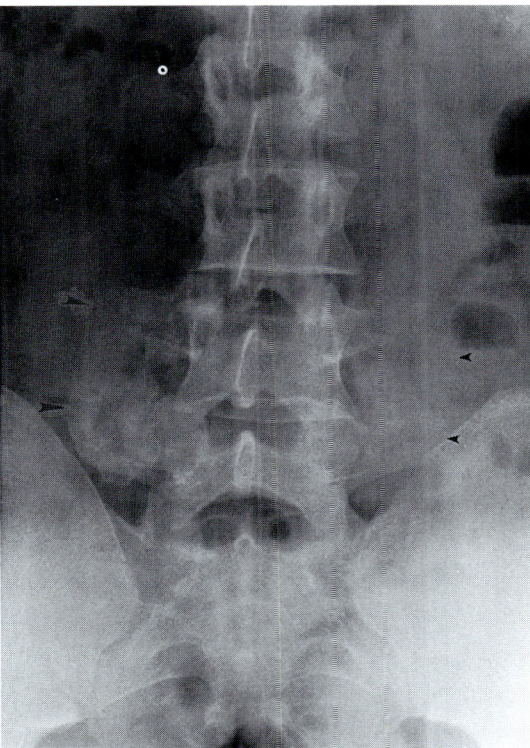

Figure 2. Radiograph taken 11 months after posterolateral intertransverse process fusion using autogenous iliac cancellous bone in a man with discogenic low back pain. Although one side has a robust fusion mass (arrowheads), the opposite side is not yet as well mineralized. This demonstrates the variability in healing that can be present even within the same patient.

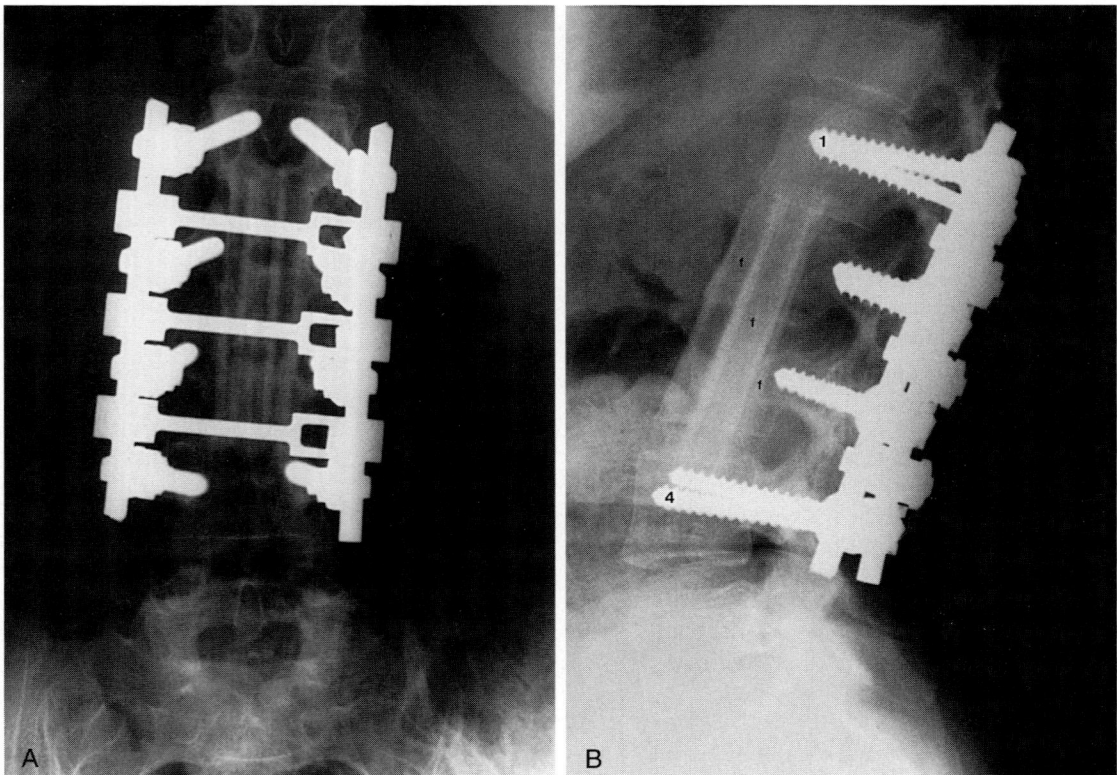

Figure 3. Anteroposterior *(A)* and lateral *(B)* radiographs taken 1 year after an anterior lumbar interbody fusion from L1 to L4 using three autogenous fibular strut grafts (f) in a woman with Pott disease at L2 and L3. A posterolateral fusion with internal fixation was also performed because of instability created by the two-level corpectomy.

Bone Marrow Cells

Bone marrow cells are osteogenic[24, 25, 29, 125, 136, 178] and have been used clinically as an adjunctive graft material for spine fusion. Osteogenic precursor cells exist in bone marrow and result in bone formation when they are transplanted to heterotopic sites (e.g., muscle or subcutaneous tissue). This bone-forming ability can be sustained or augmented in combination with bone[163] or with bone extracts containing BMPs.[178]

Allograft

The use of allograft bone as a graft material (an alloimplant) has been expanded as a result of improved methods of procurement, preparation, and storage; technical advances in surgical methods; and the desire to avoid the donor site complications associated with the use of autogenous bone. Although bone allografts are versatile and widely used in spine surgery, concerns exist regarding their ability to achieve a successful fusion consistently and the possibility of infectious disease transmission.[19, 31, 37, 116] Thus, knowledge regarding the methods of graft procurement, testing, processing, and storage is necessary for its efficient and safe use.[56] The ultimate decision to use allograft bone in a particular spine procedure depends on the underlying disease or pathologic process, the region of the spine where the graft is to be placed, the types of graft available, the surgical goals, and the preferences of the patient and the surgeon.

Obtaining allograft bone from living and cadaver donors is acceptable, but it requires meticulous attention to donor selection criteria. A comprehensive sociomedical history must be obtained, the cause of death determined, and serologic and other laboratory testing performed. If the results of screening are normal, the allograft bone is sterilely harvested within the first 12 to 24 hours of

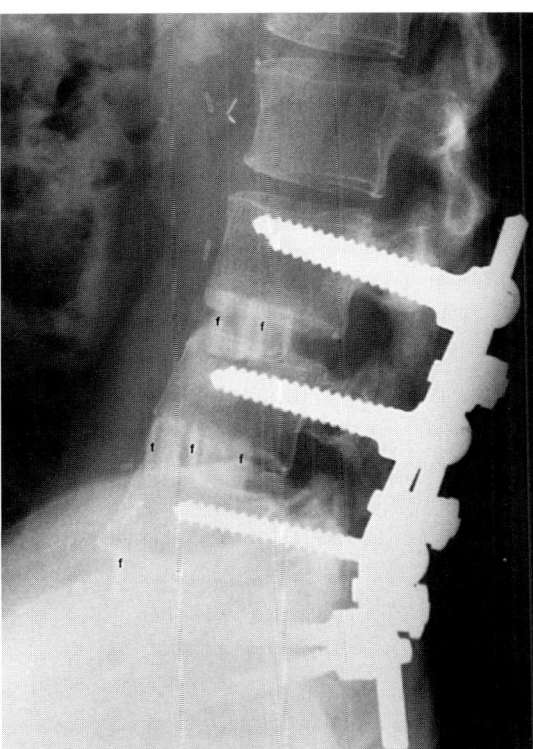

Figure 4. Radiograph of a three-level anterior lumbar interbody fusion using autogenous fibular grafts (f).

death, multiply cultured, and processed for preservation and storage.

Immunogenicity and maintenance of the osteoinductive and osteoconductive properties of the allograft bone are related to the method of graft processing and preservation. Preservation of allograft bone is generally accomplished by freezing or freeze-drying, carried out as soon after harvest as possible. These methods are effective in decreasing the immunogenicity of the graft and allow the graft to be stored for an extended period. Allograft bone that meets the criteria for use (i.e., negative results of screening) is processed by deep freezing at $-70°$ C or in liquid nitrogen at $-196°$ C.[37] Despite its being preserved in an inert, nonviable state, the mechanical properties of the bone are not affected.[145–147] The shelf life of frozen allograft bone stored at $-70°$ C is 5 years.[37] Alternatively, allograft bone may be processed by freeze-drying. This method is more effective in decreasing immunogenicity and inactivating viral agents but may result in a reduction in the mechanical strength of the graft.[145–147] Freeze-dried allograft bone must be dehydrated under vacuum and preserved in a sealed vacuum container, but it has the advantage of storage at room temperature and, as long as the vacuum is retained, an indefinite shelf life.

Sterilization of allograft bone is not a substitute for meticulous screening and sterile harvesting, but it can be an additional safety measure against infection. The most commonly used methods are gas sterilization with ethylene oxide (450 to 1500 mg/L at 30% to 60% humidity and 21° C) and high-dose gamma irradiation (1.5 to 2.5 megarads).[37] Although effective, these methods interfere with either the biologic properties (decreased osteoinduction) or the mechanical integrity of the allograft bone.[145] Other methods of graft sterilization, such as heating or autoclaving, are destructive to matrix proteins and are generally not used.

Xenograft

Xenogeneic graft materials have been used extensively in orthopedic surgery and have included ivory, cow horn, and bovine bone. Despite processing, xenografts evoke an immune response by the host and may become encapsulated, resulting in obstruction of microanastomoses between vessels of the recipient tissue and graft. Owing to their resistance to incorporation into host bone, ivory and cow horn are currently not used as graft materials. Freeze-dried[4, 68, 73, 151] and deproteinized (Kiel)[118, 162] bovine xenograft, which are both weakly antigenic, have been used in spine fusion surgery but have had mixed success in achieving a solid bony fusion and are not recommended alone as a graft material.

Demineralized Bone Matrix and Bone Morphogenetic Proteins

DBM is a less immunogenic form of allograft bone[61] and is prepared by decalcification of cortical bone. Since the initial studies performed by Urist and coworkers,[185, 191] the osteoinductive capacity of DBM has been well established.* The primary active components of DBM are a series of low-molecular-weight osteoinductive glycoproteins, including BMPs. These BMPs com-

---

*References 32, 38, 47, 59–61, 83, 106, 123, 138, 178, 183, 188, 193, and 194.

prise only 0.1% by weight of all bone protein and are most abundant in diaphyseal cortical bone. BMP exists in the extracellular matrix[190] and is not accessible until the bone matrix has been demineralized.[43, 191, 192] Once exposed, the active BMP induces the formation of cartilage and bone in vivo and stimulates a cascade of processes that are similar to fracture repair. Chemotaxis, proliferation, and differentiation of pluripotential mesenchymal cells result in the transient formation of cartilage and the production of mature bone with hematopoietic marrow.[200] Additionally, the demineralization of bone matrix destroys the highly antigenic cell membranes and the soluble hapten glycopeptides, thereby minimizing the host-versus-graft immune response.[61] Many variables are involved in the preparation of DBM and the purification of BMPs, and thus the osteoinductive activity of these substances may vary considerably.

Ceramics

Numerous biodegradable osteoconductive ceramic bone graft substitutes have received attention as alternatives to autogenous bone. The advantage of a biodegradable graft material is its compatibility with the new bone remodeling process required to attain optimum mechanical strength. A nonresorbable graft material may hinder remodeling and prolong the strength deficiency of new bone, as well as leave permanent stress risers in the fusion mass.[85] Calcium phosphate ceramics, which include hydroxyapatite and tricalcium phosphate (TCP), have been the most widely used in orthopedic surgery.[18]

For synthetic implants to be useful in vivo, they must have certain properties: (1) compatibility with surrounding tissues, (2) chemical stability in body fluids, (3) compatibility of mechanical and physical properties, (4) ability to be fabricated into functional shapes, (5) ability to withstand the sterilization process, (6) reasonable cost of manufacturing, and (7) reliable quality control. Calcium phosphate ceramics possess these properties[53, 85, 139] and have been used successfully as bone graft substitutes in dentistry and maxillofacial surgery,* in animal bone defect models,* and in humans, to a limited extent.[17, 18, 76, 140, 159, 169]

Hydroxyapatite and TCP ceramics are brittle materials with low fracture resistance and variability in their chemical and structural (crystalline) composition.[152] Different preparative methods lead to either a compact or a porous material with interconnective macropores that is the structural and spatial equivalent of cancellous bone. In a biologic system, greater crystalline formation and material density result in greater mechanical strength and resistance to dissolution, and they promote long-lasting stability. In contrast, an amorphous ultrastructure and greater porosity enhance interface activity and bone ingrowth, but they also enhance biodegradation of the implant.[85] Commercially available hydroxyapatite is resorbed slowly, if at all, under normal physiologic conditions,[79, 81, 85] whereas TCP is generally resorbed by 6 weeks after implantation.[52, 85]

ANIMAL STUDIES OF GROWTH FACTORS AND BONE GRAFT SUBSTITUTES

Because of the multiplicity of uncontrollable limitations in clinical spine fusion studies, animal investigations play a critical role in evaluating bone graft materials. Several animal models (dog, rabbit, and cat) have been established to study various growth factors (DBM, BMPs) (Table 3) and bone graft substitutes (allograft bone, hydroxyapatite, TCP) (Table 4) in spine fusion. Different types of spine fusions have been studied, including anterior or posterior interbody, spinous process, laminar, facet, and posterolateral intertransverse process fusion methods. Most experiments have compared quality and characteristics of fusion achieved through the use of these materials with the results obtained through the use of autograft bone or bone marrow cells in the same model.

To evaluate the ability of DBM to achieve or enhance spine fusion, many studies have used a rabbit posterior spine fusion model.[105, 106, 137, 154, 155] Most studies have shown that DBM combined with bone marrow cells, which are osteogenic them-

---

*References 34, 41, 85, 94, 103, 104, 119, 130–133, 158, 176, and 195.

*References 76–78, 80, 81, 122, 144, and 170.

Table 3

Animal Spine Fusion Models Using Growth Factors

Study	Year	Purpose	Animal	Number	Fusion Type	Graft Material	Histology	X-ray Study	Biomechanical Testing	Miscellaneous
Demineralized Bone Matrix										
Oikarinen[137]	1982	To compare DBM versus allograft versus autograft cancellous bone	Rabbit	29	Posterior spinous process L3–4	DBM Allograft Autograft (iliac)	H	R	—	DBM much better than allograft DBM and autograft had comparable results
Lindholm et al.[105]	1982	Pilot study using DBM and BM	Rabbit	12	Posterior spinous process and lamina T and L spine	Autograft BM DMB DBM + BM Iliac crest ± BM Tibial periosteum	H	—	—	DBM + BM better than BM. BM equal to iliac crest but worse than iliac crest + BM
Ragni et al.[154]	1987	To examine capability of DBM/BM to enhance T + L spine fusions	Rabbit	13	Posterior + intertransverse	DBM/BM	H	R	—	DBM/BM a sound alternative to using autograft bone
Lindholm et al.[106]	1988	To study BM +/− DBM as a graft material	Rabbit	23	Posterior T3–T4 and T7–T8	DBM BM DBM/BM	H	R	—	BM alone insignificant DBM/BM better than DBM alone
Ragni and Lindholm[155]	1989	To assess the healing time after spinal fusion with DBM and whether static changes develop after symmetric or asymmetric fusion	Rabbit	20	Posterior plus intertransverse T spine	DBM Autograft (iliac)	H	—	—	67% of fusion at 3 months, using DBM and 100% at 5 months
Guizzardi et al.[61]	1992	To test osteoinductive effect of DBM	Rat	20 / 12	Posterolateral Lumbar / Posterolateral T and L spine	Right side, DBM Left side, autograft / Local autograft in T spine DBM bilateral in L spine	H SEM	—	—	DBM had similar osteoinductive effect and callus development to autograft endochondral ossification
Frenkel et al.[54]	1993	To determine ability of DBM gel to act as an osteoconductive or inductive material	Dog	7	Posterolateral Thoracic	DBM gel Local autograft	HM	R	—	4 fusion procedures in each dog DBM gel may be a valuable means of enhancing spine fusion
Bone Morphogenetic Proteins										
Lovell et al.[107]	1989	To investigate action of BMP on local bone graft	Dog	13	Posterior laminar Thoracic	Local autograft ± BMP	H	R RM MR	—	4 fusion procedures in each dog with BMP, new bone and fusion ↑
Boden et al.[10a]	1995	To evaluate bovine BMP extract	Rabbit	48	Posterolateral lumbar	Autogenous iliac crest DBM	H	R	+	Autograft 62%, DBM 17%, DBM/BMP 100% fusion rate
Schimandle et al.[166a]	1995	To evaluate rhBMP-2	Rabbit	56	Posterolateral lumbar	DBM/bovine BMP iliac crest rhBMP-2/collagen; collagen alone	H	R	+	Autograft %: rhBMP-2, 100%; collagen, 0%

BM, autograft bone marrow cells; BMPs, bone morphogenetic proteins; DBM, demineralized bone matrix; H, routine histology; HM, histomorphometry; L, lumbar; MR, microradiography; R, plain radiography; RM, radiomorphometry; SEM, scanning electron microscopy; T, thoracic.

Table 4

Animal Spine Fusion Models Using Bone Graft Substitutes

Study	Year	Purpose	Animal	Number	Fusion Type	Graft Material	Histology	X-ray Study	Biomechanical Testing	Miscellaneous
Allograft										
Tsuang et al.[181]	1989	To compare allograft and autograft in anterior interbody and posterior spinal fusions	Dog	25	Anterior interbody Thoracic	Allograft Rib	H	R	—	Allograft nearly as effective as autograft in inducing bony anterior and posterior fusions. Allograft took longer to fuse and had ↑ infection rate
				31	Posterior L3–L4 with PMMA	Autograft Autograft (iliac)				
Ceramics										
Flatley et al.[53]	1983	To study the use of CaPO$_4$ ceramic as a bone graft substitute	Rabbit	26	Posterolateral vertebral body	CaPO$_4$ ceramic	H	R MR	—	Evaluated bony ingrowth into ceramic
Holmes et al.[76]	1984	To evaluate coralline HA as a bone graft substitute	Dog	16	Posterior L3–L6	Coralline HA on one side, local autograft on other	H	R	—	No solid fusions at 24 months. Bone incorporation similar on both sides
Ceramic Composites										
Ragni and Lindholm[153]	1991	To evaluate HA-DBM as a bone graft substitute	Rabbit	26	Anterior interbody L4–L5 and L5–L6	DBM HA-DBM HA Autograft	H HM	R DR	—	HA-DBM similar to autograft HA-DBM facilitates earlier stabilization of the fusion
Zerwekh et al.[205]	1992	To assess osteoconductive capacity of HA-TCP-collagen composite as a bone graft filler	Dog	12	Posterior L2–L4 with wire/pin	Composite/autograft Autograft (iliac)	H SEM	R	+	All fused with host bone Composite-autograft is a suitable alternative to autograft alone 2 experiments performed
Muschler et al.[124]	1993	To describe a canine segmental spinal fusion model for comparison of bone grafting materials	Dog	26	Posterior Lumbar with wire/PMMA	Autograft TCP-HA-collagen composite Composite/autograft Composite/matrix protein	H	—	+	Autograft best (12 of 13 fused) Composite was a good carrier and graft expander Composite alone not effective Cell count and viability measured

BM, autograft bone marrow cells; DBM, demineralized bone matrix; CaPO$_4$, calcium phosphate; DR, dynamic radiography; H, routine histology; HA, hydroxyapatite; HM, histomorphometry; MR, microradiography; PMMA, polymethyl methacrylate; R, plain radiography; SEM, scanning electron microscopy; TCP, tricalcium phosphate.

selves,[24, 25, 29, 125, 136, 178] was a more successful inducer of spine fusion than either DBM or marrow cells alone but was not as good as autograft bone with or without marrow cells.[105, 106, 137, 154] Oikarinen,[137] who performed posterior L3–L4 fusions in 29 rabbits, showed DBM to be a better autograft substitute than deep frozen allograft. In a posterior thoracic and lumbar spinal fusion model in rats, Guizzardi and coworkers[61] showed heterologous powdered DBM to have a comparable osteoinductive effect to that of autograft by virtue of similar fusion callus development seen on histologic sections. More recently, in a posterior thoracic dog spinal fusion model, Frenkel and colleagues[54] used DBM gel to enhance spinal fusion. DBM gel used in combination with autograft material produced the most vigorous osteoinductive response histologically, but the presence of fusion was not mechanically assessed.

To compare the action of bovine BMP with that of local bone graft in the spine, Lovell and associates[107] used a dog posterior spine fusion model. Four different fusion methods were used in the thoracic spine of each dog, including the use of BMP at one level. The fusions were examined by radiographs and histologic study and showed the BMP/autograft level to have two to three times more new bone than comparison levels and a 71% fusion rate, compared with 0%, 14%, and 29% in the three comparison levels. In a study using the rabbit posterolateral lumbar fusion model, Boden and colleagues demonstrated that a bovine BMP extract increased the fusion rate from 62% using autogenous iliac crest to 100% using the BMP extract.[10a] With the same model, a 100% fusion rate was achieved with recombinant human bone morphogenetic protein-2 (rhBMP-2) delivered in a collagen carrier.[166a] Further work is needed with growth factors such as BMP in both the naturally extracted form and with the various recombinant proteins, such as BMP-2 and OP-1 (BMP-7).

The use of allograft bone can minimize many of the limitations of autografts. Allograft bone, however, is less osteogenic, carries a small but finite risk of disease transmission[19, 31, 37, 116] and may elicit an immune response that can impair graft incorporation into the host.[22, 53] A study comparing autograft with allograft for anterior interbody and posterior fusions in a dog model showed a slower fusion rate a greater resorption of the graft material, and an increased infection rate in the dogs with allograft.[181] These problems have led many investigators to use allograft as a graft expander rather than as a graft substitute.

The ability of calcium phosphate ceramics to act as bone graft substitutes for spine fusion has been studied in dog and rabbit spine fusion models. Flatley and coworkers[53] used porous ceramic blocks of a 1:1 ratio of calcium hydroxyapatite and TCP to perform posterolateral vertebral body fusions across the intervertebral disc space in 21 rabbits. At 12 weeks, histologic sections showed bone ingrowth reaching the central portion of the ceramic block, and no fibrous tissue barrier was noted between the new bone and ceramic residue Holmes and colleagues,[76] using coralline hydroxyapatite in a canine posterior–facet spine fusion model, showed no solid fusions, even at 6 months, with the use of this ceramic but showed the distribution of new bone ingrowth to be similar in the ceramic and autograft fusion masses.

Ceramic composites consist of the osteoconductive ceramic combined with an osteoinductive agent, such as collagen, DBM, autograft bone, extracted BMP, and recombinant BMP,[122, 179, 189] and have also been investigated as bone graft substitutes in animal spine fusion models.[124, 153, 205] Ragni and Lindholm[153] used an experimental rabbit model of interbody fusion in which the incorporation of a porous hydroxyapatite block was enhanced by the addition of DBM. The animals implanted with the hydroxyapatite-DBM composite showed significantly earlier fusion consolidation than the animals implanted with DBM alone, hydroxyapatite alone, or autograft. By 6 months, however, the results were comparable with those attained with autograft bone. Zerwekh and associates[205] compared the efficacy of a collagen–ceramic (hydroxyapatite-TCP)–autograft composite with autograft bone alone in a dog L2–L4 posterior spine fusion model. At 12 months, histologic quantitation of bone ingrowth as well as results from biomechanical testing were similar in both groups.

Muschler and coworkers,[124] in two experiments using a dog segmental posterior spinal fusion model, compared posterior fusions attained using autograft, collagen-ceramic (hydroxyapatite-TCP) composite, collagen–ceramic (hydroxyapatite-TCP)–autograft composite, collagen–ceramic (hydroxyapatite-TCP)–bone matrix protein composite, and no graft material (control). Autograft bone was the most effective material tested and had a statistically superior union score. Results obtained with the ceramic composite alone were no better than those with no graft material. The addition of a BMP extract to the composite, however, significantly improved the union score, and the results were comparable with those obtained using composite plus autograft bone.

These animal studies have suggested that the use of ceramics and ceramic composites in spine fusion surgery holds promise as a viable alternative to autogenous bone grafting, either as a graft replacement or for graft augmentation.[18, 26, 85, 119] These findings will need to be confirmed in primate studies and ultimately in human clinical trials.

CLINICAL STUDIES USING BONE GRAFT SUBSTITUTES

The use of allograft bone as a graft material has expanded and appears to be a reasonable alternative to autogenous bone in meeting the need for supplemental or primary graft material for spine fusion. Although many animal studies have evaluated the use of allograft, few clinical studies of adequate design have been reported. Generally, the use of allograft has compared favorably with that of autogenous bone in interbody fusions (cervical, anterior, or posterior lumbar),* but the results have not been reliable when it has been used posteriorly in the lumbar spine.[88, 108] Thus, allograft seems to be more successful when it is placed in the anterior column under compression as opposed to posteriorly under tension (Fig. 5).

In 1981, Malinin and Brown[108] described the use of freeze-dried allograft bone in posterior lumbar spine fusions. They observed a high incidence of graft resorption leading to nonunion with the use of cortical strips of allograft wired to the facets, as well as with posterolateral intertransverse process fusions using corticocancellous matchsticks.

Urist and Dawson[186] used antigen-extracted allograft bone with local autogenous bone to perform posterior thoracolumbar and lumbosacral intertransverse process fusions for various diagnoses in 40 patients. Radiographic evidence of fusion was noted in 88% of patients. In 1987, Nasca and Whelchel[127] reported their series of consecutive spine fusions performed using a wide variety of anterior and posterior procedures. In posterior thoracolumbar and lumbosacral fusions using cryopreserved allograft, the fusion rate was 90% (65 of 72 patients), whereas in fusions using autogenous bone, the fusion rate was 86% (32 of 37 patients). Knapp and Jones,[95] in 1988, reported on the results of a retrospective review of 50 consecutive patients in whom allograft was used in instrumented posterior spinal fusions. Thirty-seven patients underwent fusion for spinal deformity and 13, for fractures. In procedures using freeze-dried corticocancellous allograft, the fusion rate was 98% (49 of 50 patients); the only nonunion occurred in the deformity group. These investigators believed that the graft material used was not as important as the fusion technique and that the use of allograft was justified.

Many published reports on allograft have addressed its use in fusions for spinal deformity. In 1967, May and Mauck[110] performed fusion mass explorations for nonunion in patients who underwent fusion for scoliosis. The nonunion rate at 6 months in patients who underwent fusion with autoclaved or frozen allograft was 66% (12 of 18 patients), whereas in fusions with autogenous bone, the nonunion rate was 36% (10 of 28 patients). Aurori and colleagues[7] reviewed the records of 208 patients with adolescent idiopathic scoliosis treated surgically with Harrington instrumentation and posterior fusion with autogenous bone or frozen allograft. In all patients with suspected nonunion, the fusion mass was explored. Nonunion was confirmed in 5.3% (five of 94 patients) when allograft was used and in 4.4% (five of 114 patients) when autogenous bone was used. The difference in nonunion rates was not statistically significant. In 1986, McCarthy and associates[116] used fresh frozen allograft exclusively in 32 patients undergoing instrumented posterior fusions for paralytic scoliosis. At 12 months, no nonunions had occurred, and all patients

---

*References 9, 16, 33, 67, 109, 115, and 157.

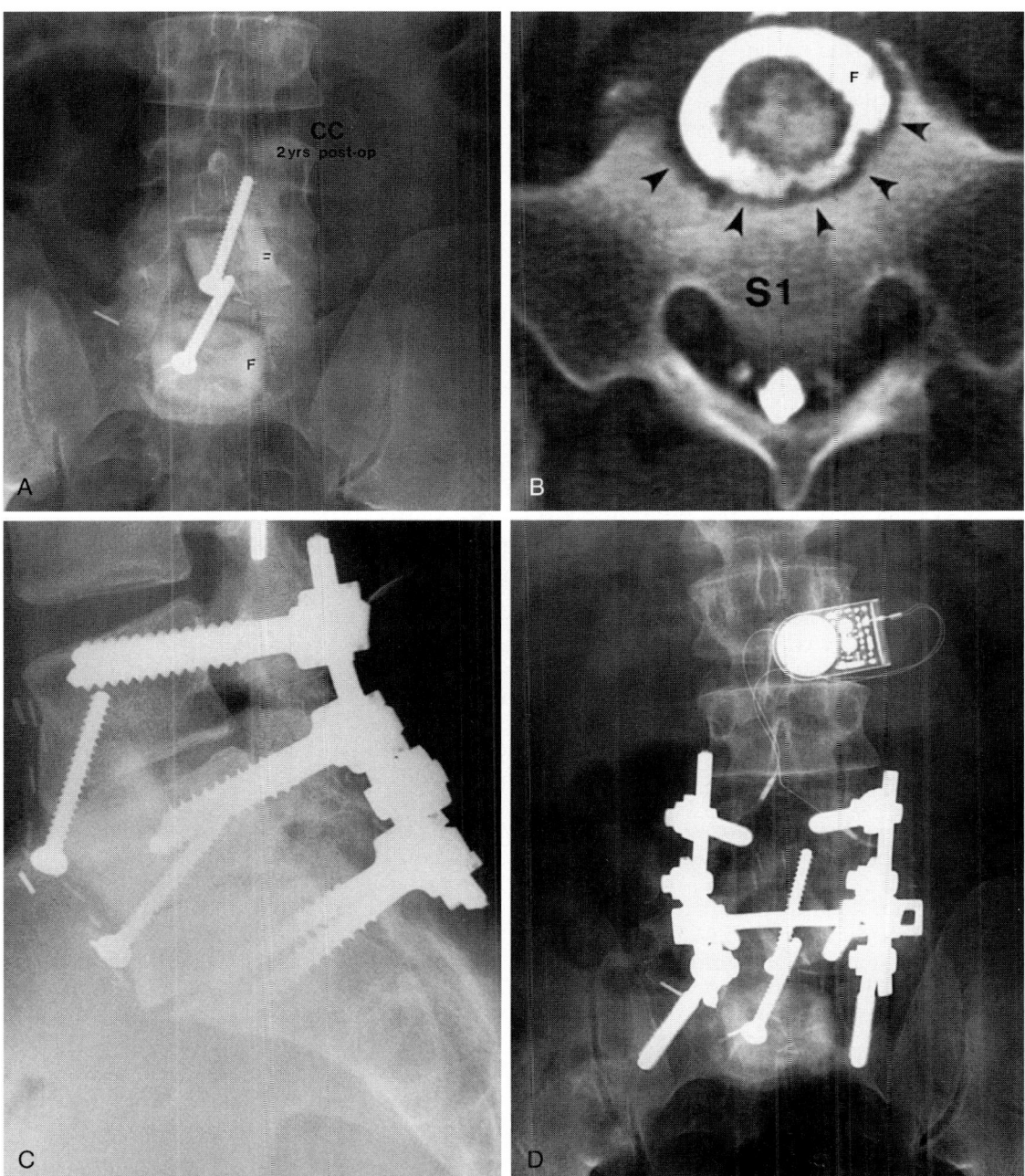

Figure 5. *A*, Radiograph taken 2 years after a failed anterior interbody fusion using femoral shaft allograft (F). *B*, Computed tomographic scan demonstrates lucency around the allograft (F), confirming the failure to incorporate. *C*, The patient was treated with a posterolateral fusion using autogenous iliac bone with internal fixation. *D*, The shotgun approach, evidenced by the use of electrical stimulation.

had well-marginated fusion masses with distinct trabecular markings radiographically.

The clinical efficacy of ceramics as a graft material or as a component in a composite graft for spinal fusion has not been clearly established. In a study of 12 patients with severe scoliosis, Passuti and colleagues[140] used internal fixation and blocks of hydroxyapatite-TCP (3:2) alone or mixed with autogenous cancellous bone to stabilize the spine and fuse the facet joints. Clinical and radiographic assessment of the fusions were performed, and in two cases, biopsies of the graft material were obtained. At an average follow-up of 15 months, all patients exhibited complete radiographic fusions. Histologic examinations of the biopsy specimens revealed the formation of new bone, which was directly bonded to the ceramic implant surface and inside the macropores. Although these results are favorable, they must be interpreted with consideration to the limitations of the study (i.e., the small number of patients, the mean age of 14 years, and the limited diagnoses).

KNOWLEDGE GAPS AND FUTURE RESEARCH DIRECTIONS

Despite the large amount of knowledge gleaned from previous studies on spine fusion, a large void exists in the basic understanding of this multifactorial process. As a result, several critical questions deserve consideration.

What type of healing occurs during fusion consolidation? Although much is known about the sequence of bone repair in fracture healing, little is known about spine fusion. Is fusion occurring through membranous bone formation, endochondral ossification, or both? Few previous studies have described the sequential histology during the spine fusion process, and reports have been conflicting and inconsistent.[154] Some studies reported cartilage as part of the early fusion mass,[76, 91, 137, 180] whereas others have suggested that endochondral ossification is not part of the healing process.[2, 84] Understanding this process at a histologic level can be the first step in preventing nonunions and predicting biologic interventions that enhance union.

What is the ideal rigidity required for the fastest healing and strongest fusion mass? Biomechanical studies have focused on the effects of rigid instrumentation and resultant osteopenia. No study has determined what degree of rigidity is sufficient and whether too much rigidity is detrimental.

The molecular biology of the spine fusion process is also a topic on which little knowledge exists. What triggers bone induction in this setting, and what is the sequence of gene expression occurring in the fusion healing process? Because the tissue and mechanical environment is different from that in fractures and long-bone defects, one cannot assume the biology is the same. Studies on gene expression in early fusion mass specimens allow the characterization on a molecular level of the temporal sequence of bone formation as well as the quantitation of specific osteoinductive proteins at various stages of fusion.

If an animal model is to be used to answer any question relevant to spine fusion, it must be carefully considered to be a good analog and to prevent the waste of excessive animal lives as well as the time, effort, and funding of the researcher.[166] The first requirement of any model used to study the spine fusion process should be the ability to replicate the surgical technique in the animal chosen. The second basic model requirement should be the replication of an outcome similar to that seen in humans —that is, a similar nonunion rate. Despite optimum planning, experimental design, and equipment, selection of an inappropriate animal model leads to useless, irrelevant, or, more seriously, misleading information. Determination of the appropriateness of an animal model, however, can in itself be the most difficult and time consuming aspect of the study design.[165]

The particular aspect of the fusion process to be studied must be carefully considered. Will the study focus on mechanical or biologic questions? If biomechanics or spinal instrumentation is of interest, larger, more expensive animals may be more suitable because they more closely approximate the size and bony anatomy of the human spine than do smaller animals. Although larger animals provide advantages for studies involving biomechanics, they offer little advantage for investigating biologic questions. Smaller, skeletally mature animals are useful in studying biologic questions, and by virtue of their lower cost and faster healing, they provide a larger data pool from which to base results.

Experimental design should follow valid scientific principles and replicate the specific clinical situation being modeled. Ideally, only one intervention should be studied in each animal, and only one level should be fused with the same technique on each side. For any valid fusion model, concurrent autograft controls should be established, optimum study lengths and observation intervals must be carefully determined, and evaluation or assessment techniques must be validated. The development and refinement of a valid animal model to investigate these growth factors would prove useful in realizing this potential and would allow the further study and characterization of the many factors affecting this complex process.[10]

The discovery, isolation, and availability of extractable and recombinant osteoinductive BMPs have introduced a new era of biologic manipulation of bone formation. Although previous bone graft substitutes have striven only to equal the results of autograft, the use of osteoinductive proteins may result in a more rapid, more reliable, and more biomechanically sound fusion than the autograft gold standard. After appropriate animal studies are performed, prospective, blinded, and randomized clinical trials must carefully validate any potential bone graft substitute in each spine application for which it will be used. The ultimate goal is that nonunion will no longer be of clinical concern.

REFERENCES

1. Albee, F. H.: Transplantation of a portion of the tibia into the spine for Pott's disease. JAMA 57:885–886, 1911.
2. Albee, F. H.: An experimental study of bone growth and the spinal bone transplant. JAMA 60:1044–1049, 1913.
3. Allen, B. L., and Ferguson, R. L.: The operative treatment of myelomeningocele spinal deformity—1979. Orthop. Clin. North Am. 10:845–862, 1979.
4. Anderson, K. J., LeCocq, J. F., and Mooney, J. G.: Clinical evaluation of processed heterologous bone transplants. Clin. Orthop. 29:248–263, 1963.
5. Aprin, H., Bowen, J. R., MacEwen, G. D., and Hall, J.: Spine fusion in patients with spinal muscular atrophy. J. Bone Joint Surg. 64:1179–1187, 1982.
6. Aronow, M. A., Gerstenfeld, L. C., Owen, T. A., et al.: Factors that promote progressive development of the osteoblast phenotype in cultured rat calvarial cells. J. Cell. Physiol. 143:213–221, 1990.
7. Aurori, B. F., Weierman, R. J., Lowell, H. A., et al.: Pseudarthrosis after spinal fusion for scoliosis: A comparison of autogeneic and allogeneic bone grafts. Clin. Orthop. 199:153–158, 1985.
8. Baran, D. T., Bergfeld, M. A., Teitelbaum, S. L., and Avioli, L. V.: Effect of testosterone therapy on bone formation in an osteoporotic hypogonadal male. Calcif. Tissue Int. 26:103–106, 1978.
9. Blumenthal, S. L., Baker, J., Dossett, A., and Selby, D. K.: The role of anterior lumbar fusion for internal disc disruption. Spine 13:566–569, 1988.
10. Boden, S. D., Schimandle, J. H., and Hutton, W. C.: An experimental lumbar intertransverse process spinal fusion model: Radiographic, histologic, and biomechanical healing characteristics. Spine 20:412–420, 1995.
10a. Boden, S. D., Schimandle, J. H., and Hutton, W. C.: Lumbar intertransverse process spinal arthrodesis with use of a bovine bone-derived osteoinductive protein: A preliminary report. J. Bone Joint Surg. 77A:1404–1417, 1995.
11. Bouchard, J. A., Koka, A., Bensusan, J. S., et al.: Effect of radiation on posterior spinal fusions: A rabbit model. Spine 19:1836–1841, 1994.
12. Bradford, D. S.: Anterior vascular pedicle bone grafting for the treatment of kyphosis. Spine 5:318–323, 1980.
13. Bridwell, K. H., Sedgewick, T. A., O'Brien, M. F., et al.: The role of fusion and instrumentation in the treatment of degenerative spondylolisthesis with spinal stenosis. J. Spinal Disord. 6:461–472, 1993.
14. Brighton, C. T.: The treatment of non-unions with electricity. J. Bone Joint Surg. 63A:847–851, 1981.
15. Brown, C. W., Orme, T. J., and Richardson, H. D.: The rate of pseudarthrosis (surgical nonunion) in patients who are smokers and patients who are nonsmokers: A comparison study. Spine 11:942–943, 1986.
16. Brown, M. D., Malinin, T. I., and Davis, P. B.: A roentgenographic evaluation of frozen allografts versus autografts in anterior cervical spine fusions. Clin. Orthop. 119:231–236, 1976.
17. Bucholz, R. W.: Clinical experience with bone graft substitutes. J. Orthop. Trauma 1:260–262, 1987.
18. Bucholz, R. W., Carlton, A., and Holmes, R. E.: Hydroxyapatite and tricalcium phosphate bone graft substitutes. Orthop. Clin. North Am. 18:323–334, 1987.
19. Buck, B. E., Malinin, T. I., and Brown, M. D.: Bone transplantation and human immunodeficiency virus. Clin. Orthop. 240:129–136, 1989.
20. Buckwalter, J. A., and Cruess, R. L.: Healing of the musculoskeletal tissues. In Rockwood, C. A., and Green, D. P. (eds.) Fractures in Adults, 3rd ed. Philadelphia, J. B. Lippincott, 1991, pp. 181–222.
21. Burch, W. M., and Lebovitz, H. E.: Triiodothyronine stimulation of in vitro growth and maturation of embryonic chick cartilage. Endocrinology 111:462–468, 1982.
22. Burchardt, H., and Enneking, W. F.: Transplantation of bone. Surg. Clin. North Am. 58:403–427, 1978.

23. Burchardt, H., Glowczewskie, F. P., and Enneking, W. F.: The effect of Adriamycin and methotrexate on the repair of segmental cortical autografts in dogs. J. Bone Joint Surg. 65A:103–108, 1983.
24. Burwell, R. G.: Studies in the transplantation of bone: VII. The fresh composite homograft-autograft of cancellous bone. An analysis of factors leading to osteogenesis in marrow transplants and in marrow-containing bone grafts. J. Bone Joint Surg. 46B:110–140, 1964.
25. Burwell, R. G.: The function of bone marrow in the incorporation of a bone graft. Clin. Orthop. 200:125–141, 1985.
26. Cameron, H. U., Macnab, I., and Pilliar, R. M.: Evaluation of a biodegradable ceramic. J. Biomed. Mater. Res. 11:179–186, 1977.
27. Canalis, E.: The hormonal and local regulation of bone formation. Endocr. Rev. 4:62–77, 1983.
28. Canalis, E.: Effect of growth factors on bone cell replication and differentiation. Clin. Orthop. 193:246–263, 1985.
29. Canalis, E., McCarthy, T., and Centrella, M.: Growth factors and the regulation of bone remodeling. J. Clin. Invest. 81:277–281, 1988.
30. Canalis, E., and Raisz, L. G.: Effect of sex steroids on bone collagen synthesis in vitro. Calcif. Tissue Int. 25:105–110, 1978.
31. Centers for Disease Control: Transmission of HIV through bone transplantation: Case report and public health recommendations. JAMA 260:2487–2488, 1988.
32. Chalmers, J., Gray, D. H., and Rush, J.: Observations on the induction of bone in soft tissues. J. Bone Joint Surg. 57B:36–45, 1975.
33. Cloward, R. B.: Gas-sterilized cadaver bone grafts for spinal fusion operations: A simplified bone bank. Spine 5:4–10, 1980.
34. Coviello, J., and Brilliant, J. D.: A preliminary clinical study on the use of tricalcium phosphate as an apical barrier. J. Endocrinol. 5:6–13, 1979.
35. Craven, P. L., and Urist, M. R.: Osteogenesis by radioisotope labelled cell populations in implants of bone matrix under the influence of ionizing radiation. Clin. Orthop. 76:231–243, 1971.
36. Cruess, R. L., and Sakai, T.: Effect of cortisone upon synthesis rates of some components of rat matrix. Clin. Orthop. 86:253–259, 1972.
37. Czitrom, A. A.: Principles and techniques of tissue banking. Instr. Course Lect. 42:359–362, 1993.
38. Dahners, L. E., and Jacobs, R. R.: Long bone defects treated with demineralized bone. South. Med. J. 78:933–934, 1985.
39. de Vernejoul, M. C., Bielakoff, J., and Herve, M., et al.: Evidence for defective osteoblastic function: A role for alcohol and tobacco consumption in osteoporosis in middle-aged men. Clin. Orthop. 179:107–115, 1983.
40. Dell, P. C., Burchardt, H., and Glowczewskie, F. P.: A roentgenographic, biomechanical, and histological evaluation of vascularized and non-vascularized segmental fibular canine autografts. J. Bone Joint Surg. 67A:105–112, 1985.
41. Denissen, H. W., and de Groot, K.: Immediate dental root implants from synthetic dense calcium hydroxyapatite. J. Prosthet. Dent. 42:551–556, 1979.
42. DePalma, A. F., and Rothman, R. H.: The nature of pseudarthrosis. Clin. Orthop. 59:113–118, 1968.
43. Dubuc, F. L., and Urist, M. R.: The accessibility of the bone induction principle in surface-decalcified bone implants. Clin. Orthop. 55:217–223, 1967.
44. Dwyer, A. F.: The use of electrical current stimulation in spinal fusion. Orthop. Clin. North Am. 6:265–279, 1975.
45. Dwyer, A. F., and Wickham, G. G.: Direct current stimulation in spinal fusion. Med. J. Aust. 1:73–75, 1974.
46. Einhorn, T. A., Bonnarens, F., and Burstein, A. H.: The contributions of dietary protein and mineral to the healing of experimental fractures: A biomechanical study. J. Bone Joint Surg. 68A:1389–1395, 1986.
47. Einhorn, T. A., Lane, J. M., Burstein, A. H., et al.: The healing of segmental bone defects induced by demineralized bone matrix: A radiographic and biomechanical study. J. Bone Joint Surg. 66A:274–279, 1984.
48. Enneking, W. F., Burchardt, H., Puhl, J. J., and Piotrowski, G.: Physical and biological aspects of repair in dog cortical bone transplants. J. Bone Joint Surg. 57A:237–252, 1975.
49. Evans, J. H.: Biomechanics of lumbar fusion. Clin. Orthop. 193:38–46, 1985.
50. Farey, I. D., McAfee, P. C., Gurr, K. R., and Randolph, M. A.: Quantitative histologic study of the influence of spinal instrumentation on lumbar fusions: A canine model. J. Orthop. Res. 7:709–722, 1989.
51. Fernyhough, J. C., Schimandle, J. H., Weigel, M. C., et al.: Chronic donor site pain complicating bone graft harvesting from the posterior iliac crest for spinal fusion. Spine 17:1474–1480, 1992.
52. Ferraro, J. W.: Experimental evaluation of ceramic calcium phosphate as a substitute for bone grafts. Plast. Reconstr. Surg. 63:634–640, 1979.
53. Flatley, T. J., Lynch, K. L., and Benson, M.: Tissue response to implants of calcium phosphate ceramic in the rabbit spine. Clin. Orthop. 179:246–252, 1983.
54. Frenkel, S. R., Moskovitch, R., Spivak, J., et al.: Demineralized bone matrix. Enhancement of spinal fusion. Spine 18:1634–1639, 1993.
55. Friedenberg, Z. B., and Brighton, C. T.: Bioelectric potentials in bone. J. Bone Joint Surg. 48A:915–923, 1966.
56. Friedlaender, G. E.: Current concepts review: Bone-banking. J. Bone Joint Surg. 64:307–311, 1982.
57. Friedlaender, G. E., Tross, R. B., Doganis, A. C., et al.: Effects of chemotherapeutic agents on bone: Short-term methotrexate and doxorubicin (Adriamycin) treatment in a rat model. J. Bone Joint Surg. 66:602–607, 1984.
58. Gallagher, J. C., Riggs, B. L., and DeLuca, H. F.: Effect of estrogen on calcium absorption and serum vitamin D metabolites in postmenopausal osteoporosis. J. Clin. Endocrinol. Metab. 51:1359–1364, 1980.
59. Gepstein, R., Weiss, R. E., Saba, K., and Hallel, T.: Bridging large defects in bone by demineralized bone matrix in the form of a powder. J. Bone Joint Surg. 69A:984–992, 1987.
60. Glowacki, J., Murray, J. E., Kaban, L. B., et al.: Application of the biological principle of induced osteogenesis for craniofacial defects. Lancet i:959–963, 1981.
61. Guizzardi, S., Di Silvestre, M., Scandroglio, R., et al.: Implants of heterologous demineralized bone

matrix for induction of posterior spinal fusion in rats. Spine 17:701–707, 1992.
62. Gurr, K. R., McAfee, P. C., and Shih, C.: Biomechanical analysis of anterior and posterior instrumentation systems after corpectomy. A calf spine model. J. Bone Joint Surg. 70A:1182–1191, 1988.
63. Gurr, K. R., McAfee, P. C., and Shih, C.: Biomechanical analysis of posterior instrumentation systems after decompressive laminectomy. J. Bone Joint Surg. 70A:680–691, 1988.
64. Gurr, K. R., McAfee, P. C., Warden, K. E., and Shih, C.: Roentgenographic and biomechanical analysis of lumbar fusions: A canine model. J. Orthop. Res. 7:838–843, 1989.
65. Hahn, T. J.: Corticosteroid-induced osteopenia. Arch. Intern. Med. 138:882–885, 1978.
66. Hanley, E. N., and Levy, J. A.: Surgical treatment of isthmic lumbosacral spondylolisthesis: Analysis of variables affecting results. Spine 14:48–50, 1989.
67. Hanley, E. N., Jr., Harvell, J. C., Shapiro, D. E., and Kraus, D. R.: Use of allograft bone in cervical spine surgery. Semin. Spine Surg. 1:262–270, 1989.
68. Harmon, P.: Processed heterologous bone implants (Boplant, Squibb) as grafts in spinal surgery. Acta Orthop. Scand. 35:98–116, 1964.
69. Harrington, K. D.: Metastatic tumors of the spine: Diagnosis and treatment. J. Am. Acad. Orthop. Surg. 1:76–86, 1993.
70. Hartshorne, E.: On the causes and treatment of pseudarthrosis, and especially of the form of it sometimes called supernumerary joint. Am. J. Med. Sci. 1:121–156, 1841.
71. Heckman, J. D., Ingram, A. J., Loyd, R. D., et al.: Nonunion treatment with pulsed electromagnetic fields. Clin. Orthop. 161:58–66, 1981.
72. Heiple, K. G., Chase, S. W., and Herndon, C. H.: A comparative study of the healing process following different types of bone transplantation. J. Bone Joint Surg. 45A:1593–1616, 1963.
73. Heiple, K. G., Kendrick, R. E., Herndon, C. H., and Chase, S. W.: A critical evaluation of processed calf bone. J. Bone Joint Surg. 49A:1119–1127, 1967.
74. Hibbs, R. A.: An operation for progressive spinal deformities. A preliminary report of three cases from the service of the Orthopaedic Hospital. N. Y. State J. Med. 93:1013–1016, 1911.
75. Hollo, I., Gergely, I., and Boross, M.: Smoking results in calcitonin resistance. JAMA 237:2470, 1977.
76. Holmes, R., Mooney, V., Bucholz, R., and Tencer, A.: A coralline hydroxyapatite bone graft substitute. Clin. Orthop. 188:252–262, 1984.
77. Holmes, R. E.: Bone regeneration within a coralline hydroxyapatite implant. Plast. Reconstr. Surg. 63:626–633, 1979.
78. Holmes, R. E., Bucholz, R. W., and Mooney, V.: Porous hydroxyapatite as a bone graft substitute in metaphyseal defects. J. Bone Joint Surg. 68A:904–911, 1986.
79. Holmes, R. E., Bucholz, R. W., and Mooney, V.: Porous hydroxyapatite as a bone graft substitute in diaphyseal defects: A histometric study. J. Orthop. Res. 5:114–121, 1987.
80. Holmes, R. E., and Salyer, K. E.: Bone regeneration in a coralline hydroxyapatite implant. Surg. Forum 29:611–612, 1978.
81. Hoogendoorn, H. A., Rencoij, W., Akkermans, L. M. A., et al.: Long-term study of large ceramic implants (porous hydroxyapatite) in dog femora. Clin. Orthop. 187:281–288, 1984.
82. Hopp, S. G., Dahners, L. E., and Gilbert, J. A.: A study of the mechanical strength of long bone defects treated with various bone autograft substitutes: An experimental investigation in the rabbit. J. Orthop. Res. 7:579–584, 1989
83. Hulth, A., Johnell, O., and Henricson, A.: The implantation of demineralized fracture matrix yields more new bone formation than does intact matrix. Clin. Orthop. 234:235–249, 1988.
84. Hurley, L. A., Stinchfield, F. E., Bassett, A. L., and Lyon, W. H.: The role of soft tissues in osteogenesis: An experimental study of canine spine fusions. J. Bone Joint Surg. 41A:1243–1254, 1959.
85. Jarcho, M.: Calcium phosphate ceramics as hard tissue prosthetics. Clin. Orthop. 157:259–278, 1981.
86. Jensen, J. E., Jensen, T. G., Smith, T. K., et al.: Nutrition in orthopaedic surgery. J. Bone Joint Surg. 64:1263–1272, 1982.
87. Johnston, C. E., Ashman, R. B., and Sherman, M. C., et al.: Mechanical consequences of rod contouring and residual scoliosis in sublaminar segmental instrumentation. J. Orthop. Res. 5:206–216, 1987.
88. Jorgenson, S. S., Lowe, T. G., France, J., and Sabin, J.: A prospective analysis of autograft versus allograft in posterolateral lumbar fusion in the same patient: A minimum of 1 year follow-up in 144 patients. Spine 19:2048–2053, 1994.
89. Jowsey, J., and Riggs, B. L.: Bone formation in hypercortisonism. Acta Endocrinol. (Copenh.) 63:21–28, 1970.
90. Kahanovitz, N., and Arnoczky, S. P.: The efficacy of direct current electrical stimulation to enhance canine spinal fusions. Clin. Orthop. 251:295–299, 1990.
91. Kahanovitz, N., Arnoczky, S. P. Hulse, D., and Shires, P. K.: The effect of postoperative electromagnetic pulsing on canine posterior spinal fusions. Spine 9:273–279, 1984.
92. Kahanovitz, N., Arnoczky, S. P., Nemzek, J., and Shores, A.: The effect of electromagnetic pulsing on posterior lumbar spinal fusions in dogs. Spine 19:705–709, 1994.
93. Kane, W. J.: Direct current electrical bone growth stimulation for spinal fusion. Spine 13:363–365, 1988.
94. Kent, J. K., Quinn, J. E., Zide, M. F., et al.: Alveolar ridge augmentation using nonresorbable hydroxyapatite with or without autogenous cancellous bone. J. Oral Maxillofac. Surg. 41:629–642, 1983.
95. Knapp, D. R., and Jones, E. T.: Use of cortical cancellous allograft for posterior spinal fusion. Clin. Orthop. 229:99–106, 1988.
96. Kostuik, J. P., Errico, T. J., Gleason, T. F., and Errico, C. C.: Spinal stabilization of vertebral column tumors. Spine 13 250–256, 1988.
97. Lafferty, F. W., Spencer, G. E., and Pearson, O. H.: Effects of androgens, estrogens, and high calcium intakes on bone formation and resorption in osteoporosis. Am. J. Med. 36:514–528, 1964.
98. Lane, J. M., and Sandhu, H. S.: Current approaches to experimental bone grafting. Orthop. Clin. North Am. 18:213–225, 1987.

99. Lau, G. C., Luck, J. V., Marshall, G. J., and Griffith, G.: The effect of cigarette smoking on fracture healing: An animal model. Clin. Res. 37:132A, 1989.
100. Laurie, S. W. S., Kaban, L. B., Mulliken, J. B., and Murray, J. E.: Donor-site morbidity after harvesting rib and iliac bone. Plast. Reconstr. Surg. 73:933–938, 1984.
101. Lavine, L. S., Lustrin, I., and Shamos, M. H.: Treatment of congenital pseudarthrosis of the tibia with direct current. Clin. Orthop. 124:69–74, 1977.
102. Lebwohl, N. H., Starr, J. K., Milne, E. L., et al.: Inhibitory effect of ibuprofen on spinal fusion in rabbits (abstract). Presented at the American Academy of Orthopaedic Surgeons Annual Meeting, 278, 1994.
103. Levin, M. P., Getter, L., Adrian, J., and Cutright, D. E.: Healing of periodontal defects with ceramic implants. J. Clin. Periodontol. 1:197–205, 1974.
104. Levin, M. P., Getter, L., and Cutright, D. E.: A comparison of iliac marrow and biodegradable ceramic in periodontal defects. J. Biomed. Mater. Res. 9:183–195, 1975.
105. Lindholm, T. S., Nilsson, O. S., and Lindholm, T. C.: Extraskeletal and intraskeletal new bone formation induced by demineralized bone matrix combined with bone marrow cells. Clin. Orthop. 171:251–255, 1982.
106. Lindholm, T. S., Ragni, P., and Lindholm, T. C.: Response of bone marrow stroma cells to demineralized cortical bone matrix in experimental spinal fusion in rabbits. Clin. Orthop. 230:296–302, 1988.
107. Lovell, T. P., Dawson, E. G., Nilsson, O. S., and Urist, M. R.: Augmentation of spinal fusion with bone morphogenetic protein in dogs. Clin. Orthop. 243:266–274, 1989.
108. Malinin, T. I., and Brown, M. D.: Bone allografts in spinal surgery. Clin. Orthop. 154:68–73, 1981.
109. Malinin, T. I., Rosomoff, H. L., and Sutton, C. H.: Human cadaver femoral head homografts for anterior cervical spine fusions. Surg. Neurol. 7:249–251, 1977.
110. May, V. R., and Mauck, W. R.: Exploration of the spine for pseudarthrosis following spinal fusion in the treatment of scoliosis. Clin. Orthop. 53:115–122, 1967.
111. McAfee, P. C., Farey, I. D., Sutterlin, C. E., et al.: Device-related osteoporosis with spinal instrumentation. Spine 14:919–926, 1989.
112. McAfee, P. C., Farey, I. D., Sutterlin, C. E., et al.: The effect of spinal implant rigidity on vertebral bone density: A canine model. Spine 16:S190–S197, 1991.
113. McAfee, P. C., Regan, J. J., and Farey, I. D., et al.: The biomechanical and histomorphometric properties of anterior lumbar fusions: A canine model. J. Spinal Disord. 1:101–110, 1988.
114. McAfee, P. C., Werner, F. W., and Glisson, R. R.: A biomechanical analysis of spinal instrumentation systems in thoracolumbar fractures. Comparison of Harrington distraction instrumentation with segmental spinal instrumentation. Spine 10:204–217, 1985.
115. McBride, G. G., and Bradford, D. S.: Vertebral body replacement with femoral neck allograft and vascularized rib strut graft: A technique for treating post-traumatic kyphosis with neurologic deficit. Spine 8:406–415, 1983.
116. McCarthy, R. E., Peek, R. D., Morrissy, R. T., and Hough, A. J.: Allograft bone in spinal fusion for paralytic scoliosis. J. Bone Joint Surg. 68A:370–375, 1986.
117. McGuire, R. A., and Amundson, G. M.: The use of primary internal fixation in spondylolisthesis. Spine 18:1662–1672, 1993.
118. McMurray, G. N.: The evaluation of Kiel bone in spinal fusions. J. Bone Joint Surg. 64B:101–104, 1982.
119. Metsger, D. S., Driskell, T. D., and Paulsrud, J. R.: Tricalcium phosphate ceramic—a resorbable bone implant: Review and current status. J. Am. Dent. Assoc. 105:1035–1038, 1982.
120. Misol, S., Samaan, N., and Ponseti, I. V.: Growth hormone in delayed fracture union. Clin. Orthop. 74:206–208, 1971.
121. Mooney, V.: A randomized double-blind prospective study of the efficacy of pulsed electromagnetic fields for interbody lumbar fusions. Spine 15:708–712, 1990.
122. Moore, D. C., Chapman, M. W., and Manske, D.: The evaluation of a biphasic calcium phosphate ceramic for use in grafting long-bone diaphyseal defects. J. Orthop. Res. 5:356–365, 1987.
123. Mulliken, J. B., Glowacki, J., Kaban, L. B., et al.: Use of demineralized allogeneic bone implants for the correction of maxillocraniofacial deformities. Ann. Surg. 194:366–372, 1981.
124. Muschler, G. F., Huber, B., and Ullman, T., et al.: Evaluation of bone grafting materials in a new canine segmental spinal fusion model. J. Orthop. Res. 11:514–524, 1993.
125. Nade, S., Armstrong, L., McCartney, E., and Baggaley, B.: Osteogenesis after bone and bone marrow transplantation. Clin. Orthop. 181:255–263, 1983.
126. Nagel, D. A., Kramers, P. C., Rahn, B. A., et al.: A paradigm of delayed union and nonunion in the lumbosacral joint: A study of motion and bone grafting of the lumbosacral spine in sheep. Spine 16:553–559, 1991.
127. Nasca, R. J., and Whelchel, J. D.: Use of cryopreserved bone in spinal surgery. Spine 12:222–227, 1987.
128. Nerubay, J., and Katznelson, A.: Clinical evaluation of an electrical current stimulator in spinal fusions. Int. Orthop. 7:239–242, 1984.
129. Nerubay, J., Margant, B., and Bubis, J. J., et al.: Stimulation of bone formation by electrical current on spinal fusion. Spine 11:167–169, 1986.
130. Nery, E. B., and Lynch, K. L.: Preliminary clinical studies of bioceramic in periodontal osseous defects. J. Periodontol. 49:523–527, 1978.
131. Nery, E. B., Lynch, K. L., Hirthe, W. M., and Mueller, K. H.: Bioceramic implants in surgically produced infrabony defects. J. Periodontol. 46:328–347, 1975.
132. Nery, E. B., Lynch, K. L., and Rooney, G. E.: Alveolar ridge augmentation with tricalcium phosphate ceramic. J. Prosth. Dent. 40:668–675, 1978.
133. Nery, E. B., Pflughoeft, F. A., Lynch, K. L., and Rooney, G. E.: Functional loading of bioceramic augmented alveolar ridge—a pilot study. J. Prosthet. Dent. 43:338–343, 1980.
134. Nilsson, O. S., Bauer, H. C. F., and Brostrom, L.:

Methotrexate effects on heterotopic bone in rats. Acta Orthop. Scand. 58:47–53, 1987.
135. Nisbet, N. W.: Antigenicity of bone. J. Bone Joint Surg. 59B:263–266, 1977.
136. Ohgushi, H., Goldberg, V. M., and Caplan, A. I.: Heterotopic osteogenesis in porous ceramics induced by marrow cells. J. Orthop. Res. 7:568–579, 1989.
137. Oikarinen, J.: Experimental spinal fusion with decalcified bone matrix and deep-frozen allogeneic bone in rabbits. Clin. Orthop. 162:210–218, 1982.
138. Oikarinen, J., and Korhonen, L. K.: The bone inductive capacity of various bone transplanting materials used for treatment of experimental bone defects. Clin. Orthop. 140:208–215, 1979.
139. Osborn, J. F., and Newesely, H.: The material science of calcium phosphate ceramics. Biomaterials 1:108–111, 1980.
140. Passuti, N., Daculsi, G., and Rogez, J. M., et al.: Macroporous calcium phosphate ceramic performance in human spine fusion. Clin. Orthop. 248:169–176, 1989.
141. Paterson, D. C., Carter, R. F., Maxwell, G. M., et al.: Electrical bone growth stimulation in an experimental model of delayed union. Lancet i:1278–1281, 1977.
142. Paterson, D. C., Lewis, G. N., and Cass, C. A.: Treatment of delayed union and nonunion with an implanted direct current stimulator. Clin. Orthop. 148:117–128, 1980.
143. Paterson, D. C., Lewis, G. N., and Cass, C. A.: Treatment of congenital pseudarthrosis of the tibia with direct current stimulation. Clin. Orthop. 148:129–135 1980.
144. Patka, P., den Otter, G., de Groot, K., and Driessen, A. A.: Reconstruction of large bone defects with calcium phosphate ceramics—an experimental study. Neth. J. Surg. 37:38–44, 1985.
145. Pelker, R. R., and Friedlaender, G. E.: Biomechanical aspects of bone autografts and allografts. Orthop. Clin. North Am. 18:235–239, 1987.
146. Pelker, R. R., Friedlaender, G. E., and Markham, T. C.: Biomechanical properties of bone allografts. Clin. Orthop. 174:54–57, 1983.
147. Pelker, R. R., Friedlaender, G. E., Markham, T. C., et al.: Effects of freezing and freeze-drying on the biomechanical properties of rat bone. J. Orthop. Res. 1:405–411, 1984.
148. Pelker, R. R., Friedlaender, G. E., Panjabi, M. M., et al.: Chemotherapy-induced alterations in the biomechanics of rat bone. J. Orthop. Res. 3:91–95, 1985.
149. Phillips, L. S., and Vassilopoulou-Sellin, R.: Somatomedins—part II. N. Engl. J. Med. 302:438–446, 1980.
150. Phillips, L. S., and Vassilopoulou-Sellin, R.: Somatomedins—part I. N. Engl. J. Med. 302:371–380, 1980.
151. Pieron, A. P., Bigelow, D., and Hamonic, M.: Bone grafting with Boplant: Results in thirty-three cases. J. Bone Joint Surg. 50B:364–368, 1968.
152. Prolo, D. J., and Rodrigo J. J.: Contemporary bone graft physiology and surgery. Clin. Orthop. 200:322–342, 1985.
153. Ragni, P., and Lindholm S.: Interaction of allogeneic demineralized bone matrix and porous hydroxyapatite bioceramics in lumbar interbody fusion in rabbits. Clin. Orthop. 272:292–299, 1991.
154. Ragni, P., Lindholm, S., and Lindholm, T. C.: Vertebral fusion dynamics in the thoracic and lumbar spine induced by allogenic demineralized bone matrix combined with autogenous bone marrow. An experimental study in rabbits. Ital. J. Orthop. Traumatol. 13:241–251, 1987.
155. Ragni, P. C., and Lindholm, T. S.: Bone formation and static changes in the thoracic spine at uni- or bilateral experimental spondylodesis with demineralized bone matrix (DBM). Ital. J. Orthop. Traumatol. 15:237–252, 1989.
156. Riggs, B. L., Jowsey J., Goldsmith, R. S., et al.: Short- and long-term effects of estrogen and synthetic anabolic hormone in postmenopausal osteoporosis. J. Clin. Invest. 51:1659–1663, 1972.
157. Rish, B. L., McFadden, J. T., and Penix, J. O.: Anterior cervical fusion using homologous bone grafts: A comparative study. Surg. Neurol. 5:119–121, 1976.
158. Roberts, S. C., and Brilliant, J. D.: Tricalcium phosphate as an adjunct to apical closure in pulpless permanent teeth. J. Endocrinol. 1:263–269, 1975.
159. Rokkanen, P., Vainionpaa, S., Tormala, P., et al.: Biodegradable implants in fracture fixation: Early results of treatment of fractures of the ankle. Lancet 1:1422–1424, 1985.
160. Rose, G. K., Owen, R., and Sanderson, J. M.: Transposition of rib with blood supply for the stabilisation of a spinal kyphos. J. Bone Joint Surg. 57B:112, 1975.
161. Rothman, R. H., Klemek, I. S., and Toton, J. J.: The effect of iron deficiency anemia on fracture healing. Clin. Orthop 77:276–283, 1971.
162. Salama, R.: Xenogeneic bone grafting in humans. Clin. Orthop. 174:113–121, 1983.
163. Salama, R., Burwell, R. G., and Dickson, I. R.: Recombined grafts of bone and marrow: The beneficial effect upon osteogenesis of impregnating xenograft (heterograft) bone with autologous red marrow. J. Bone Joint Surg. 55B:402–417, 1973.
164. Schalch, D. S., Heinrich, U. E., Draznin, B., et al.: Role of the liver in regulating somatomedin activity: Hormonal effects on the synthesis and release of insulin-like growth factor and its carrier protein by the isolated perfused rat liver. Endocrinology 104:1143–1151, 1979.
165. Schimandle, J. H., and Boden, S. D.: The use of animal models to study spinal fusion. Spine 19:1998–2006, 1994.
166. Schimandle, J. H., and Boden, S. D.: Animal use in spinal research. Spine 19:2474–2477, 1994.
166a. Schimandle, J. H., Boden, S. D. and Hutton, W. C.: Experimental spinal fusion with recombinant human bone morphogenetic protein-2 (rhBMP-2). Spine 20:1326–1337, 1995.
167. Schimandle, J. H., Weigel, M., and Edwards, C. C.: Indications for thigh cuff bracing following instrumented lumbosacral fusions (abstract). Presented at the North American Spine Society Annual Meeting, 1993.
168. Shaffer, J. W., Field, G. A., Goldberg, V. M., and Davy, D. T.: Fate of vascularized and nonvascularized autografts. Clin. Orthop. 197:32–43, 1985.
169. Shima, T., Keller, J., Alvira, M. M., et al.: Anterior cervical discectomy and interbody fusion. J. Neurosurg. 51:533–538, 1979.
170. Shimazaki, K., and Mooney, V.: Comparative

study of porous hydroxyapatite and tricalcium phosphate as bone substitute. J. Orthop. Res. 3:301–310, 1985.
171. Shirado, O., Zdeblick, T. A., McAfee, P. C., et al.: Quantitative histologic study of the influence of anterior spinal instrumentation and biodegradable polymer on lumbar interbody fusion after corpectomy. Spine 17:795–803, 1992.
172. Simmons, D. J., and Kunin, A. S.: Autoradiographic and biochemical investigations of the effect of cortisone on the bones of the rat. Clin. Orthop. 55:201–215, 1967.
173. Simmons, J. W.: Treatment of failed posterior lumbar interbody fusion (PLIF) of the spine with pulsing electromagnetic fields. Clin. Orthop. 193:127–132, 1985.
174. Spadaro, J. A.: Electrically stimulated bone growth in animals and man: Review of the literature. Clin. Orthop. 122:325–332, 1977.
175. Steinmann, J. C., and Herkowitz, H. N.: Pseudarthrosis of the spine. Clin. Orthop. 284:80–90, 1992.
176. Strub, J. R., Gaberthuel, T. W., and Firestone, A. R.: Comparison of tricalcium phosphate and frozen allogenic bone implants in man. J. Periodontol. 50:624–629, 1979.
177. Swank, S. M., Brown, J. C., and Perry, R. E.: Spinal fusion in Duchenne's muscular dystrophy. Spine 7:484–491, 1982.
178. Takagi, K., and Urist, M. R.: The role of bone marrow in bone morphogenetic protein induced repair of femoral massive diaphyseal defects. Clin. Orthop. 171:224–231, 1982.
179. Takaoka, K., Nakahara, H., and Yoshikawa, H., et al.: Ectopic bone induction on and in porous hydroxyapatite combined with collagen and bone morphogenetic protein. Clin. Orthop. 234:250–254, 1988.
180. Thomas, I., Kirkaldy-Willis, W. H., Singh, S., and Paine, K. W. E.: Experimental spinal fusion in guinea pigs and dogs: The effect of immobilization. Clin. Orthop. 112:363–375, 1975.
181. Tsuang, Y. H., Yang, R. S., Chen, P. Q., and Liu, T. K.: Experimental allograft in spinal fusion in dogs. J. Formos. Med. Assoc. 88:989–994, 1989.
182. Tuli, S. M.: Bridging of bone defects by massive bone grafts in tumorous conditions and in osteomyelitis. Clin. Orthop. 87:60–73, 1972.
183. Tuli, S. M., and Singh, A. D.: The osteoinductive property of decalcified bone matrix: An experimental study. J. Bone Joint Surg. 60B:116–123, 1978.
184. Udupa, K. N., and Gupta, L. P.: The effect of growth hormone and thyroxine in healing of fracture. Ind. J. Med. Res. 53:623–628, 1965.
185. Urist, M. R.: Bone: Formation by autoinduction. Science 150:893–899, 1965.
186. Urist, M. R., and Dawson, E.: Intertransverse process fusion with the aid of chemosterilized autolyzed antigen-extracted allogeneic (AAA) bone. Clin. Orthop. 154:97–113, 1981.
187. Urist, M. R., DeLange, R. J., and Finerman, G. A. M.: Bone cell differentiation and growth factors. Science 220:680–686, 1983.
188. Urist, M. R., Dowell, T. A., Hay, P. H., and Strates, B. S.: Inductive substrates for bone formation. Clin. Orthop. 59:59–96, 1968.
189. Urist, M. R., Lietze, A., and Dawson, E.: Beta-tricalcium phosphate delivery system for bone morphogenetic protein. Clin. Orthop. 187:277–280, 1984.
190. Urist, M. R., Lietze, A., Mizutani, H., et al.: A bovine low molecular weight bone morphogenetic protein (BMP) fraction. Clin. Orthop. 162:219–232, 1982.
191. Urist, M. R., Silverman, B. F., Buring, K., et al.: The bone induction principle. Clin. Orthop. 53:243–283, 1967.
192. Urist, M. R., and Strates, B. S.: Bone formation in implants of partially and wholly demineralized bone matrix. Including observations on acetone-fixed intra- and extracellular proteins. Clin. Orthop. 71:271–278, 1970.
193. Van de Putte, K. A., and Urist, M. R.: Osteogenesis of the interior of intramuscular implants of decalcified bone matrix. Clin. Orthop. 43:257–270, 1965.
194. Volpon, J. B., Xavier, C. A. M., and Concalves, R. P.: The use of decalcified granulated homologous cortical bone matrix in the correction of diaphyseal bone defect. An experimental study in rabbits. Arch. Orthop. Trauma. Surg. 99:199–207, 1982.
195. Walter, C., and Brunt, P. B.: Tricalcium phosphate as an implant material: Preliminary report. Br. J. Plast. Surg. 35:510–516, 1982.
196. Weiland, A. J., Phillips, T. W., and Randolph, M. A.: Bone grafts: A radiologic, histologic, and biomechanical model comparing aurografts, allografts, and free vascularized bone grafts. Plast. Reconstr. Surg. 74:368–379, 1984.
197. Wenger, D. R., Carollo, J. J., Wilkerson, J. A., et al.: Laboratory testing of segmental spinal instrumentation versus traditional Harrington instrumentation for scoliosis treatment. Spine 7:265–269, 1982.
198. West, J. L. III, Bradford, D. S., and Ogilvie, J. W.: Results of spinal arthrodesis with pedicle screw plate fixation. J. Bone Joint Surg. 73A:1179–1184, 1991.
199. Wilson, P. D., and Lance, E. M.: Surgical reconstruction of the skeleton following segmental resection for bone tumors. J. Bone Joint Surg. 47A:1629–1656, 1965.
200. Wozney, J. M.: Bone morphogenetic proteins. Prog. Growth Factor Res. 1:267–280, 1989.
201. Yasuda, I., Noguchi, K., and Sata, T.: Dynamic callus and electric callus. J. Bone Joint Surg. 37A:1292–1293, 1955.
202. Younger, E. M., and Chapman, M. W.: Morbidity at bone graft donor sites. J. Orthop. Trauma 3:192–195, 1989.
203. Zdeblick, T. A.: A prospective, randomized study of lumbar fusion: Preliminary results. Spine 18:983–991, 1993.
204. Zdeblick, T. A., Shirado, O., McAfee, P. C., et al.: Anterior spinal fixation after lumbar corpectomy. A study in dogs. J. Bone Joint Surg. 73A:527–534, 1991.
205. Zerwekh, J. E., Kourosh, S., Scheinberg, R., et al.: Fibrillar collagen-biphasic calcium phosphate composite as a bone graft substitute for spinal fusion. J. Orthop. Res. 10:562–572, 1992.
206. Zichner, L.: Repair of nonunions by electrically pulsed current stimulation. Clin. Orthop. 161:115–121, 1981.

Fusion: Its Current and Future Place in the Degenerative Lumbar Spine

Present Role of Lumbar Spine Fusion

HARRY N. HERKOWITZ

The role of spine fusion in the surgical management of scoliosis and traumatic conditions of the lumbar spine is well established. The indications for fusion in scoliosis include a progressive increase in the size of the curve and a loss of sagittal or coronal balance. For traumatic conditions, the indications include loss of structural stability and neurologic deficit with fracture fragments impinging on the nerve roots. These criteria are easily documented by the physical examination, plain radiography, and other appropriate imaging studies. In degenerative conditions of the lumbar spine, the indications for spine fusion are not nearly so clear-cut. Considerable controversy exists not only for when the fusion should be performed but also for whether it should be a posterolateral anterior interbody fusion, posterior interbody fusion, or a combination of these approaches. Increasing the confusion is the role of instrumentation as an adjunct to bony arthrodesis. If instrumentation is added, should it be posterior rods and hooks, pedicle fixation with plates or rods, or anterior fixation with plates or rods?

The picture is unclear for the following reasons. First, in degenerative disorders, no clear-cut definition of instability exists. Unless demonstrable translational movement on flexion or extension is greater than 4 mm or excessive angular end plate motion is present, as compared with the adjacent motion segments (greater than 10-degree change compared with the motion segment above and below), instability is a subjective concept. The degenerative conditions that can produce motion are isthmic or degenerative spondylolisthesis and prior surgery in which destabilization of the motion segment has occurred as a result of excessive removal of the facet joints.

Second, the term segmental instability has been used for low back pain occurring in conjunction with a degenerative lumbar disc. The theory is that the degenerative disc creates microinstability, which causes low back pain. If the micromotion is eliminated through spine fusion, clinical symptoms should be reduced or eliminated. The surgical results have been mixed, with success rates of 50% to 60%. The reason for the less than optimum outcome is the inability of clinicians to determine precisely the source of low back pain because disc degeneration occurs in patients with and those without low back pain and is part of the normal aging process. Interestingly, a multitude of operations have been performed for this condition through many approaches. The success rate, regardless of the approach selected, ranges from 50% to 75%, a number that approaches the natural history of improvement for low back pain when no active treatment is rendered.

Third, the literature is filled with retrospective and anecdotal articles on surgery for disc degeneration. The criteria for success differ from article to article. Until a prospective controlled study is undertaken that compares the results of surgery with those of nonoperative treatment, a definitive answer to the question of whether spine fusion is helpful for disc degeneration cannot be answered. Despite this lack of surety, the author believes that the indications for spine fusion in degenerative disorders of the lumbar spine can be broken down into the following categories:

I. Disc herniation
II. Disc degeneration
III. Spinal stenosis
   A. Stenosis associated with degenerative spondylolisthesis
   B. Scoliosis
      1. Flexible curve
      2. Progressive curve
      3. Coronal or sagittal imbalance
   C. Recurrent stenosis at same level
IV. Isthmic spondylolisthesis
V. Degenerative scoliosis
   A. Progressive curve
   B. Coronal or sagittal imbalance
   C. Painful scoliosis

DISC HERNIATION

Spine fusion may be considered in patients with a large central disc herniation at L4–L5 or above, where facet joint excision exceeds 50% or more bilaterally or complete excision of one facet is performed.

Patients who are undergoing a third surgery at the same disc segment that was operated on before are also candidates for a posterolateral fusion.

DISC DEGENERATION

Patients with mechanical low back pain with single-level disc degeneration who have positive results on provocative discography may be considered for surgery if they have failed to respond to nonoperative treatment. Whether the procedure is a posterolateral fusion, an anterior or posterior interbody fusion, or a circumferential arthrodesis depends on the surgeon's preference.

SPINAL STENOSIS

Stenosis Associated with Degenerative Spondylolisthesis

Posterolateral arthrodesis performed after decompressive laminectomy is indicated, except in cases in which the motion segment is essentially rigid from arthritis.

Scoliosis

If the lumbar curve is flexible or progressive or if coronal or sagittal imbalance is present, arthrodesis is indicated to stabilize the curve and to correct the imbalance. An osteotomy may also be necessary.

Recurrent Stenosis

When reoperation is necessary at the same level operated on before, an arthrodesis is indicated because a significant part of the facet joints may have to be excised to decompress the lateral recesses. If translational or angular instability of the motion segment is present after previous decompression, arthrodesis should be performed at the time of repeated surgery.

ISTHMIC SPONDYLOLISTHESIS

Isthmic spondylolisthesis, especially at L4–L5, with persistent or recurrent symptoms of low back pain and/or leg pain is an indication for arthrodesis. Concomitant nerve root decompression is recommended for clear-cut cases of radiculopathy in association with the spondylolisthesis.

DEGENERATIVE SCOLIOSIS

Surgery is indicated in patients with progressive lumbar scoliosis and low back pain with or without radiculopathy that is unresponsive to nonoperative treatment or a static lumbar curve that is out of balance in the coronal or sagittal plane.

SPINAL INSTRUMENTATION

The role of spinal instrumentation in degenerative disorders remains ill defined. Instrumentation is clearly indicated for correction of deformity and for stabilization when instability is present. Because the rate of pseudarthrosis increases with each additional level of fusion attempted, the addition of instrumentation may improve the rate of fusion when multilevel fusion is necessary.

Future of Spine Fusion

DIETER GROB

Surgical reconstruction of the anatomy of the spine after trauma or for congenital disorders is possible only in certain exceptional situations, such as reconstruction of the pars interarticularis in isthmic spondylolisthesis in young patients[8] or direct screw fixation of type II odontoid fractures (Bohler 81). Fusion will remain a therapeutic cornerstone for two specific purposes: (1) to correct deformities and (2) to reduce pain.

Measuring the success or failure in the first case is relatively easy through visual methods, including radiography and modern imaging techniques; therefore, fusion for the correction of deformities is generally accepted. However, the problem of pain measurement is still not solved. The visual analog pain scale is accepted as a common standard,[18] but it is far from a quantitative and qualitative indicator of such a subjective entity as pain. Little is known about the exact source of pain in a segment, but its mechanical origin has been confirmed in certain circumstances.[1, 5, 14]

The obvious goal of any fusion procedure is to achieve solid bony union. Unfortunately, no generally accepted method exists for confirming a solid fusion. Perhaps the commonest measure is the presence or absence of motion in flexion-extension radiographs in the fused segment, but even in these cases, no standard method exists to measure that range, and the error of measurement is considerable. Methods suggested include additional clinical evaluation with or without electronic assistance, manual or computer-assisted analysis of x-ray studies (digitization), and other imaging techniques.

A scientifically based comparison of different fusion techniques of the spine still lacks a safe, quick, simple-to-use, repeatable, clinically applicable method for the assessment of fusion, preferably consisting of a direct visualization technique or a mechanical test. In spite of this basic lack of knowledge, research should be directed to improve the present fusion techniques. A commonly accepted standard of instrumentation consists basically of two parallel rods that can be contoured to the desired shape.

The attachment of the rods to the spine is performed by hooks, wires, and/or screws. Whatever instrumentation is used, some form of fusion mass is needed. Autologous bone graft is the gold standard, but it has several inherent problems, especially at the donor site.

Fusion is equated with loss of both motion and function. Is it possible to entirely preserve function by replacing the altered part instead of performing fusion?

INSTRUMENTATION

Operative Techniques

Since their introduction 30 years ago, pedicle fixation systems have provided reliable stability. Their disadvantage is the increased risk of intraoperative complications[1] from nerve lesions that occur because of the technical difficulties of inserting the screws within the pedicles. This difficulty is increased by the considerable variation in the anatomy of the pedicles, especially in cases of scoliosis or congenital anomalies.[10, 22] Intraoperative screw placement may therefore be associated with perforation of the cortex of the pedicle[2] and damage to the neurologic structures. Most techniques of screw insertion rely on anatomic landmarks.[4, 14, 19] The use of fluoroscopy is generally recommended; however, it is cumbersome in the theater and provides only a two-dimensional view. The insertion of the screw relies heavily on the three-dimensional perception of the surgeon. Advanced technologies allow computer-assisted drilling of the pedicles[16] with real-time intraoperative imaging localization of surgical instruments. This goal is achieved by combining image-guided stereotaxis with advanced optoelectronic position-sensing techniques, and this technique allows a high degree of accuracy in the placement of pedicle screws. The practicability, however, is limited by the costs of the system.

Recommendations for minimizing the operative procedure are identical to those for reducing the chances for complications: successful unilateral instrumentations for fusions in the lumbar spine[7] may meet this need. Other attempts to reduce the operative trauma consist of the so-called minimally invasive procedures. Percutaneous techniques for disc removal and for segmental fusions have been developed. The present indications for these procedures seem to be restricted to a few pathologic situations; however, with improved technical facilities, a wider application might exist, such as for nucleotomy.[12]

Materials

Mechanical devices provide immediate stability but are not strong enough to withstand prolonged stress, and they eventually fail because of loosening or breakage. The material for such devices must be able to withstand continuous, cyclic stresses. A possible modification for the future might be the use of a biodegradable material, which would eliminate the necessity of reoperating for removal.

Titanium steel is the preferred material for implants for the spine because of its compatibility with modern imaging techniques. The mechanical properties of this alloy, however, require that a certain thickness be used to avoid failure. This may negatively interfere with the mass of bone graft for fusion in an anatomically limited place.

Design

The goal of instrumentation is to eliminate intersegmental motion. Virtually all currently available implants have the same structure: they consist of a combination of different multisegmental attachment systems (some combination of hooks, wires, and screws) with two longitudinal connection systems bilaterally. A problem that remains unsolved with the use of these implants is how much stiffness is necessary for fusion. Previous devices have sought to prevent intersegmental motion completely but that idea has been questioned, and some techniques have been proposed that restrict or alter the motion but do not completely eliminate it. One method is to reduce motion by changing from metallic rods or plates to ligamentous intersegmental connections.[3] Another possibility is the suppression of only part of the motion, such as elimination of painful flexion-extension (rotation in the sagittal plane) while allowing motion in the other planes. It is hoped that techniques such as these will allow the same benefits of fixation while decreasing the associated side effects.

Required properties of new, ideal spinal implants follow:

- Low profile
- Compatibility with modern imaging techniques
- Biodegradability
- Variable elasticity according to the bone quality
- Selective restriction of reducing motion
- Suitability for anterior and posterior use
- Ability to be used in both short and long fusions
- Possibility of reduction
- Low costs

BONE GRAFT

Enhancement

Enhancements to improve the success of bone grafts have included such exciting ideas as the use of carbon fiber cages to provide stable support with a potential for bony ingrowth if they are filled with autologous cancellous bone graft,[21] producing autologous bone graft by cancellous bone cell cultivation, and improving the vascularity and calcification of grafts with pulsed electromagnetic fields.[15]

Replacement

Some research has been published on the replacement of autogeneic bone grafts with other methods, but so far these methods have all had problems. The superiority of autogeneic bone graft to allogeneic material with lower fusion rates has been proved.[17] Synthetic substitutes based on polymethyl methacrylate tend to loosen at the bone-cement interface and provide stability only in compression.

Part of the problem in the development of new bone graft replacement techniques is the difficulty in testing new bone graft substitutes. A drawback is that of biocompatibility—animals have a different biologic potential than do humans. More accurate models are needed, possibly including the study of cultivated human tissue. Ways of testing new ideas include histomorphometry and microradiology.[20] Chemical bonding may be confirmed by efficient and sophisticated methods, such as scanning electron microscopy and energy-dispersive radiographic analysis.[9]

Tests with demineralized bovine bone matrix have been promising[6] to the extent that bone formation and ingrowth were stimulated (osteoinductivity) by this material.

Requirements of the future ideal bone graft follow:

- In vitro cultivation
- Mechanical stability
- Biocompatibility
- Osteoinductivity
- Variable shape (malleable mass, blocks of different shapes)
- Low costs

PRESERVATION OF FUNCTION

To return a patient to as normal a state as possible, operative techniques must target the problem accurately and cause minimum collateral damage. Important in this goal are techniques to improve biocompatibility and to reduce the negative effects of the surgery itself. Advances include the use of the omentum majus for reduced perineural scarring and improved vascularity of graft material.[13]

Disc replacement
    Artificial
    Transplant
Vertebral body
    Artificial
    Transplant

DOCUMENTATION

In spine fusion, as in all aspects of modern medicine, documentation and communication are paramount. To assess results and compare techniques, extensive collaboration among spine centers is needed. Modern computer techniques should be used to their full advantage in this communication.

REFERENCES

1. Esses, S. I., Sachs, B. L., and Dreyzin, V.: Complications associated with technique of pedicle screw fixation—a selected survey of ABS members. Spine 15:2231–2239, 1993.
2. Gertzbein, S. D., and Robbins, S. E.: Accuracy of pedicular screw placement in vivo. Spine 15:11–14, 1990.
3. Graf, H.: Instabilite vertebrale traitement a l'aide d'un systeme souple. (Lumbar instability surgical treatment without fusion: Soft system stabilization.) Rachis 4:123–137, 1992.
4. Grob, D., Magerl, F., and McGowan, D. P.: Spinal pedicle fixation: Reliability and validity of roentgenogram-based assessment and surgical factors on successful screw placement (letter). Spine 15:251, 1990.
5. Grob, D., Dvořák, J., Panjabi, M. M., and Antinnes, J. A.: Fixateur externe an der Halswirbelsäule—ein neue diagnostisches Mittel. (External fixation of the cervical spine, a new technique for diagnostics.) Unfallchirugie 96:416–421, 1993.
6. Guizzardi, S., DiSilvestre, M., Scandroglio, R., et al.: Implants of heterologous demineralized bone matrix for induction of posterior spinal fusion in rats. Spine 17:701–707, 1992.
7. Hambley, M. F., Wiltse, L. L., Peek, R. D., et al.: Unilateral lumbar fusion. Spine 16:S295–297, 1991.
8. Hefti, F., Seelig, W., and Morscher, E.: Repair of lumbar spondylolysis with a hook screw. Int. Orthop. 16:81–85, 1992.
9. Heikkila, J., Ahos, A. J., Yli-Urpo, A., et al.: Bioactive glass versus hydroxyapatite in reconstruction of osteochondral defects in the rabbit. Acta Orthop. Scand. 64:678–682, 1993.
10. Krag, M. H., Weaver, D. L., Beynnon, B. D., and Haugh, L. D.: Morphometry of the thoracic and the lumbar spine related to transpedicular screw placement for surgical spinal fixation. Spine 13:27–31, 1988.
11. Lenke, L. G., Bridwell, K. H., Bullis, D., Betz, R. R., et al.: Results of in situ fusion for isthmic spondylolisthesis. J Spinal Disord. 5:433–442, 1992.
12. Lozes, G., Fawaz, A., Mescola, P., et al.: Percutaneous interbody osteosynthesis in the treatment of thoracolumbar traumatic or tumoral lesions. A review of 51 cases. Acta Neurochir. (Wien) 102:42–53, 1990.
13. MacMillan, M., and Stauffer, E. S.: The effect of omental pedicle graft transfer on spinal microcirculation and laminectomy membrane formation. Spine 16:176–180, 1991.
14. Magerl, F.: External skeletal fixation of the lower thoracic and the lumbar spine. In Uthhoff H. (ed.): Current Concepts of External Fixation of Fractures. New York, Springer Verlag, 1982, pp. 353–366.
15. Mooney, V.: A randomized double-blind prospective study of the efficacy of pulsed electromagnetic fields for interbody lumbar fusions. Spine 15:708–712, 1990.
16. Nolte, L., Zamorano, L. J., Jiang, A., et al.: Image guided computer assisted spine surgery—a pilot study on spinal pedicle fixation. Submitted for Volvo award, 1994. Genau Lit bei Nolte, Bern erfragen.
17. Nugent, P. J., and Dawson, E. G.: Intertransverse

process lumbar arthrodesis with allogeneic fresh-frozen bone graft. Clin. Orthop. 287:107–111, 1993.
18. Reville, S., Robinson, J., Rosen, M., and Hogg, M.: The reliability of a linear analogue scale for evaluating pain. Anesthesia 31:1191–1194, 1976.
19. Roy-Camille, R., Saillant, G., Berteaux, D., et al.: Vertebral osteosynthesis using metal plates. Its different uses. Chirurgie 105:579–603, 1979.
20. Shirado, O., Zdeblick, T. A., McAfee, P. C., et al.: Quantitative histologic study of the influence of anterior spinal instrumentation and biodegradable polymer on lumbar interbody fusion after corpectomy. A canine model. Spine 17:795–803, 1992.
21. Shono, Y., McAfee, P. C., Cunningham, B. W., and Brantigan, J. W.: A biomechanical analysis of decompression and reconstruction methods in the cervical spine. Emphasis on a carbon fiber composite cage. J. Bone Joint Surg. 75A:1674–1684, 1993.
22. Zindrick, M. R., Wiltse, L. L., Doornik, A., et al.: Analysis of the morphometric characteristics of the thoracic and the lumbar pedicles. Spine 12:160–166, 1987.

25

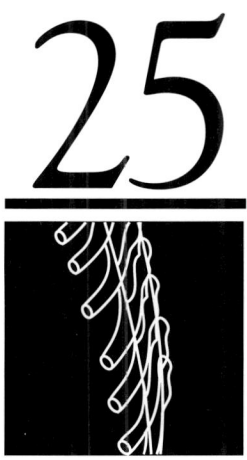

Measuring Clinical Outcomes

KEVIN F. SPRATT
JAMES N. WEINSTEIN

A fundamental axiom in virtually all learning theories is that feedback is a necessary condition for learning. Unfortunately, learning occurs regardless of feedback quality. In the clinical setting, if feedback indicates that a treatment is effective, clinicians are likely to learn that this treatment should be recommended. If this feedback is based on unreliable and invalid information (poor outcome measures), an ineffective treatment is being promoted. Similarly, if feedback indicates that a treatment is not effective, clinicians are likely to learn that this treatment should not be provided. If this feedback is based on poor outcome measures, an effective treatment is being abandoned. Thus, the importance of reliable and valid measures of outcome is clear: they provide the sources of the feedback. That is the basis from which clinicians and scientists make decisions about patient well-being and, therefore, treatment efficacy.

Measuring clinical outcomes and developing patient-based outcomes assessments are currently two of the most discussed topics in the medical community The increase in interest in this topic is clearly illustrated by comparing the number of citations found (commonly called hits) in MEDLINE (Medical Literature Analysis and Retrieval System on-line) searches across the years. A MEDLINE search for citations reporting on reliability or validity issues for questionnaires used in research involving human subjects obtained the hit rates summarized in Table 1.

Thus, the number of articles focusing on the psychometric properties of patient self-report data has nearly doubled in the past 5 years compared with the previous 5-year

Table 1

Summary of MEDLINE Citations Reporting on Reliability and Validity Issues

Years	Hits	Hits/100,000 Citations
1966–Mid-1976	50	2.11
Mid-1976–1984	272	11.85
1985–1989	420	24.87
1990–1994	719	46.64

This paper was supported, in part, by funding provided by the Iowa Measurement Research Foundation.

MEDLINE, Medical Literature Analysis and Retrieval System on-line.

period (46.64/24.87 ≅ 1.88:1), has nearly quadrupled in the past 5 years compared with the 1976–1984 period (46.64/11.85 ≅ 3.94:1), and has increased by more than 22-fold compared with the 1966–1976 period (46.64/2.11 ≅ 22.1:1). This increased interest undoubtedly has multiple causes but is fundamentally motivated by the need for a clear understanding of patients' conditions and progress and, by extension, treatment efficacy. Selected articles from these reviews that represent seminal work in the development of particular scales, that focus on establishing the psychometric properties of the scales, or that relate to populations of patients with low back trouble are provided in the reference section of this chapter.*

Of particular interest may be a book by McDowell and Newell,[125] which provides some basic structure for evaluating health outcome measures and then summarizes and reviews a large number of instruments used in the field. The Buros Institute of Mental Measurement is an independent entity now housed in the University of Nebraska–Lincoln with the mission of cataloguing and evaluating tests and instruments developed for use in education and psychology. Practitioners who build and develop instruments in these fields know that their efforts at establishing the reliability, validity, and general usefulness of the scales may be evaluated by the Buros Institute and that these results will appear in the *Mental Measurement Yearbook.* This publication is, in essence, the *Consumer Reports* of measurement instruments, and, just as in *Consumer Reports,* the nature of the reviews can affect the acceptance of the instruments. The interested reader might wish to examine the *Eleventh Mental Measurement Yearbook*[106] to appreciate the depth of information provided about each instrument and the quality of the reviews provided. Although the McDowell and Newell text is an impressive start in the direction of providing the health care community with desperately needed measurement resources, the ongoing effort needed to update and expand this work suggests that the health care community needs to establish an independent agency with a mission similar to that of the Buros Institute, focusing on health status outcome measures.

---

*References 1–19, 21–23, 25–34, 36, 38–60, 62–105, 107–130, 132–140, 142–187, and 189–197.

HARD VERSUS SOFT DATA

The intent of this chapter is to inform clinicians about numerous issues involved in the assessment of clinical outcomes. An assumption of this chapter is that patient self-report measures should form the basis of establishing the patient's health status. This notion is relatively new in clinical practice, in which for many years the hard data of the patient's biologic functioning and observable patient actions associated with a physical examination established the patient's health status. Thus, "hard" data are essentially representational in nature. That is, data that are associated with physical scales of measurement: counts of cells, millimeters of translation, or observed patient behaviors. Patient self-report, on the other hand, is designed to assess what has been called "soft" data, such as pain magnitude and psychologic factors such as depression, anxiety, and social support. These variables, typically called hypothetical constructs, are nonrepresentational in nature, meaning that they do not have analogs in physical measurement. Given all the technical issues and potential problems involved with patient self-report, many of which are addressed in this chapter, some might and have argued that these soft data elements have no place in clinical practice and that a return to the days when outcome was assessed using hard data only is clearly in order. Before making this decision, consider the following comparison of hard and soft data.

Clinical medicine has traditionally evaluated patient outcome in terms of hard data, meaning information derived from application of the biologic sciences, such as the results of blood tests and radiographic studies. However, the limitations of these hard data have become increasingly apparent to clinicians and the lay public.[188] The incidence of false-positive and false-negative results associated with drug testing and screening for the human immunodeficiency virus has major consequences for high-profile patients (e.g., professional and Olympic athletes) or for large segments of the total population, and erroneous testing results are common topics in both the local and national news, as well as in news magazine shows. Similarly, low reliabilities for evaluating plain roentgenograms for sagittal translation[164] and the general concern with low specificity (high false-positive rates) of magnetic resonance imaging and computed tomography has contributed to the increased practice of actually incorporating patients' perceptions and reports of their health status into the evaluation of treatment effectiveness.

In addition, the clinical community has become increasingly aware of the multifaceted nature of treatment, with an expanded emphasis on patient-centered factors associated with the home and work environment. Much of the work in this area was pioneered in the psychology, sociology, and education fields, in which self-report methods have been common practice. Perhaps because self-report data are considered soft data, a major area of study has developed to evaluate the psychometric properties of these data.

In direct comparisons of the psychometric properties (primarily reliability and validity, but also the related issues of false-positive and false-negative rates) of hard and soft data sources, the notion that hard data are superior to soft frequently does not hold. Reliability indices in the .8 to .9 range for self-report measures are often obtained. In addition, self-report scores have been demonstrated to be sensitive to patient improvement with sufficient accuracy and frequency to challenge the preeminence of hard data results in many clinical settings.

Perhaps the commonest criticism of self-report data is that the resultant score is arbitrary and is not clearly linked to the true nature of the underlying construct. The argumentative clinician might say: "When I evaluate a roentgenogram, I am looking at the anatomic structure and, with care, I can determine the percentage of slip (i.e., spondylolisthesis) or the status of the fusion, or the location of the break. But when I find that a patient has a pain rating of 6 on a 15-point visual analog scale, I do not really know what that means."

In response to these concerns about non-representational measurement, Dawes[37] identified five commonly used subjective rating scales (a six-point Likert scale, a seven-choice semantic differential, a four-option multiple-choice scale, a 100-point scale with five equally spaced anchor labels, and a 30-point scale with six equally spaced anchor labels) and modified the labeling on each so that subjects could rate the heights of coworkers. Correlations among the scales ranged from .72 to .92, correlations between each scale and height measured in inches ranged from .88 to .94, and a linear combination of the five scales (the first principal component from the five scales) had a correlation of .98 with the height of the subjects measured in inches.

Two fundamental points follow from the Dawes study. First, it is clear that in situations in which responders are reasonably aware and understanding of the underlying construct, in this case the height of well-known coworkers, rating scales commonly used in self-report questionnaires can accurately capture the essence of the underlying construct. In the clinical setting, the obvious question is whether patients are reasonably aware and have an understanding of the underlying constructs of interest when they evaluate outcomes such as symptoms and function. If patients are not aware of their own feelings and capabilities, who is? The goal when constructing self-report measures of patient status is to ask the necessary questions in a way that allows patients, who generally should be in the position to understand best what they are feeling and how they are functioning, to communicate their understandings accurately and completely.

A second point to consider from the Dawes study is that the cost of this equivalent accuracy when comparing hard with soft data is in the efficiency of the measurement. The subjects' height in inches was presumably obtained by a single reading from a standard ruler or tape measure. The equivalently accurate height ($r = .98$) from the rating scales required five assessments and a computer program to generate the composite score. Until the advent of virtually universal access to microcomputer technology, the inefficiency of the self-report approach was clearly too great to ignore. On the other hand, the computer dependency associated with many of the hard data measures, such as computed tomographic and magnetic resonance imaging findings, is rarely considered a limiting factor.

The inefficiency that remains concerns the relatively large number of data points (questions) that must be asked to maximize the chance of obtaining a reliable and valid score. On this front, computer technology may again provide part of the answer. Computer adaptive testing (CAT) uses the respondent's answers to each question to determine what next question should be asked and thereby substantially decreases the number of items needed to determine the respondent's score.[20] In CAT applications in standardized aptitude testing, reductions in the numbers of items needed to determine a respondent's score can average more than 50%.

At present, however, several concerns remain about attempts to implement CAT paradigms in clinical settings. First, relatively large samples, at least a few hundred in each population, are needed to accurately estimate the item parameters required in CAT applications. A second, related, problem concerns what might constitute a population in a clinical setting. In educational settings, populations are often obvious and simple to capture. For example, a population of interest may be all third graders. In clinical applications, however, populations might reasonably be based on diagnostic category, which may not be consistently classified across clinicians and, therefore, not obvious or simple to capture.

In some respects, the efficiency trade-off between hard and soft data in clinical settings is moot because many of the underlying constructions of interest, such as depression, hypochondriasis, ability to cope, job satisfaction, social functioning, health perceptions, and pain intensity, have no corresponding hard data methods available to capture the information. For factors that could be captured by hard data methods, such as activities of daily living, even in situations in which patients are confined to a limited environment, such as hospital wards or nursing homes, the resources necessary to track the patients' capabilities accurately are formidable.

In summary, when hard and soft data are examined under the same bright light provided by the measurement experts' psychometric tool kit, the higher reliability and validity assumed for hard data, because the measures essentially represent the underlying construct, is found to be myth. In general, the psychometric quality of hard and soft measures of patients' health status are comparable. In practice, however, hard data collection is well institutionalized in the clinical setting, where departments of radiology and histochemistry laboratories are part of the standard of care, but soft data collection is still often considered a side issue, useful only when clinical trials are conducted. This situation is slowly changing; some hospitals and clinical groups are establishing offices or departments whose primary goal is to evaluate clinical outcomes and patients' health status. The logical conclusion of this initiative would be to establish formal health status stations, laboratories, or clinics: just as clinicians order radiographic studies or blood work, they would also order a standard health status profile. Until measuring health outcomes from patient self-report attains the same status and institutional support that hard data sources of information enjoy, the battle to obtain and use patient self-report–based data to aid in the evaluation of the patient and the assessment of treatment efficacy and efficiency cannot be won.

TYPES OF PATIENT-BASED OUTCOME ASSESSMENT

During the past 30 years, a relatively large number of outcome instruments have been proposed, developed, and implemented that are applicable to populations of patients presenting with low back troubles. These instruments can broadly be classified into four basic types:

1. Pain measures, such as the McGill Pain Questionnaire, are those that quantify the magnitude of symptoms, predominately pain.
2. Function measures, such as the Sickness Impact Profile, are those that evaluate general health, typically in terms of the activities that patients can and cannot do as a function of their condition or conditions.
3. Psychosocial measures are those that measure psychosocial consequences such as depression, coping behaviors, illness behaviors, and fear avoidance, of illness.
4. Composite measures are instruments designed to measure a cross-section of all of these constructs.

Examples of each type of outcome instruments are listed in Table 2. More detailed information on selected instruments, including specific references, the populations studied, and how each instrument is administered, for general health and functional status, activities of daily living (ADL), and pain and psychosocial measures are provided in Tables 3, 4, and 5, respectively.

Some outcome measures, most notably the McGill Pain Questionnaire,[130, 131] have been conceptualized and constructed from a theoretic basis with scoring rules developed from psychometric methods in an attempt both to quantify and to explain the underlying construct (pain). The McGill Pain Questionnaire is made up of three basic sections: 20 groupings of pain adjectives, from which five pain rating indices are derived (sensory, affective, evaluative, miscellaneous, and total); a pain drawing to illustrate pain locations; and a six-point Likert scale (ranging from 0 [no pain] to 5 [excruciating]) measuring present pain intensity. All of this information can easily be formatted to fit on a single page.

Recognizing that quantifying pain level is one issue, and understanding it another, many researchers have designed surveys to complement the basic McGill Pain Questionnaire, including Melzack,[130] Duncan and associates,[54] Heaton and colleagues,[82] and Monks and Taenzer,[138] who developed the McGill Comprehensive Pain Questionnaire (MCPQ). The MCPQ assesses the patient's personal history (parents, siblings, childhood feelings, marriage, children, other dependents), past medical history, medications, and accompanying symptoms. It provides a multifaceted attempt to quantify the pain itself in terms of pain history, pain treatments, pain description (locations), pain patterns during the day, pain modifiers, and the effects of pain (on work, finances, legal proceedings, leisure, sleep, weight and diet, and habits).

The MCPQ, when administered in its entirety, undoubtedly provides the clinician with the most complete picture of the patient and his or her pain symptoms. However, at least four mitigating factors seem to argue against the implementation of this instrument as the gold standard of outcome measures. First, for many conditions, including low back trouble, pain is not always the symptom of greatest concern or importance. For some patients and clinicians, concern peaks when the pain subsides and is replaced by symptoms of numbness and weakness. Second, the relationship between pain and function is complex and nonmonotonic. Pain symptoms are directly and strongly related to level of dysfunction for some patients, but not for others. In fact, one of the strongest trends in rehabilitation therapy is to break or weaken links between pain symptoms and ability to function. Third, the amount of information provided by the MCPQ is overwhelming to many clinicians, who cannot adequately conceptualize all of the information provided. Fourth, the complexity and length of the instrument has led many patients not to provide complete information when the questionnaire is administered. These limitations may partly explain, why the MCPQ is typically not implemented in its entirety in many otherwise rigorous clinical trials.

Table 2

Examples of Health Outcome Instruments

Pain	Function	Psychosocial Measures	Composite
McGill Pain Inventory	Functional Status Index	Fear Avoidance	McGill Comprehensive Pain Questionnaire
Dallas Pain Inventory	Functional Rating Scale	Pain Beliefs Questionnaire	West Haven–Yale Multidimensional Pain Inventory
Pain Chart	Sickness Impact Profile	Pain Drawing	SF-36
Pain Rating Scale	Oswestry Disability Questionnaire	Illness Behavior Questionnaire	Health Status Index
Pain Interference Scale	Pain Disability	General Health Questionnaire	Duke–UNC Health Profile
Back Pain Classification Scale	Quality of Life Index	Beck Depression Inventory	McMaster Health Index Questionnaire
Pain Behavior Checklist	Disability and Impairment Interview Schedule	Minnesota Multiphasic Personality Inventory	Health Assessment Questionnaire

Table 3
General Health and Functional Status Outcome Measures

Measurement Tool	Population	Person Administering Measure	Study
Arthritis Impact Measurement Scale (influenced by QWB)	A, E	Self	Meenan et al.[129]
Comprehensive Assessment and Referral Evaluation	E	Other	Garland et al.[78]
Cornell Medical Index	A, E	Self	Brodman et al.[14, 15]
Duke–UNC Health Profile—	A	Self	Parkerson et al.[145]
Duke Health Profile	A, E	Self	Parkerson et al.[143, 144]
Functional Assessment Inventory	A	Other	Crewe et al.[34]
General Health Questionnaire	A	Self	Goldberg and Hillier[72]; Tarnopolsky et al.[175]
Health Assessment Questionnaire (HAQ) (same as Stanford HAQ)	A	Other	Fries et al.[69]; Wolfe et al.[192]
Modified Health Assessment Questionnaire (added to the HAQ)	A	Other	Wolfe and Pincus[193]
Health Status Index (Index of Well-Being)—Quality of Well-Being Scale	A, E	Other	Kaplan et al.[96]; Patrick et al.[146]
Illness Behavior Assessment Schedule	A, E	Other	Pilowsky et al.[151]
McMaster Health Index Questionnaire	A, E	Self, other	Chambers[28]
Medical Outcomes Study	A	Self	Anderson et al.[2]; McHorney et al.[128]; Parkersen et al.[144]
SF-36	A, C, E	Self, other	Riesenberg and Glass[158]; Stewart et al.[169]
SF-20	?	Self, other	McHorney et al.[127]; Ware and Sherbourne[186]
Health Status Questionnaire	A, C, E	Self, other	Kempen[103]; Schmid et al.[162]
Multilevel Assessment Instrument	E	Other	Lawton et al.[110]
Nottingham Health Profile	A, E	Self	Hunt et al.[85]
OARS Multidimensional Functional Assessment Questionnaire	A, E	Other	Fillenbaum and Smyer[66]
Oswestry Disability Index	A, E	Self	Baker et al.[4]; Co et al.[30]; Fairbank et al[59]; Haas and Nylendo[79]; Little and MacDonald[115]
Physical and Mental Impairment-of-Function Evaluation	E	Other	Gurel et al.[77]
Quality of Life Index	A	Self	Ferrans[64]; Ferrans and Powers[63, 65]
Sickness Impact Profile	A, C, E	Self, other	Bergner et al.[6, 7]; DeBruin et al.[38]; Deyo[46, 48]; Follick et al.[67]; Jensen et al.[89]; MacKenzie et al.[118]; Pincus et al.[153]; Pollard et al.[154]; Watt-Watson and Graydon[187]
Low Back Disability Questionnaire	A (ages 16–64 years)	Self	Roland and Morris[160]

A, adult; C, children; E, elderly; Other, administered by another in an interview; Self, self-administered; OARS, Older Americans' Resources and Services; QWB, quality of well-being; SF, short form.

Table 4

Activities of Daily Living Scales

Measurement Tool	Population	Person Administering Measure	Study
Barthel Index (formerly the Maryland Disability Index)	A, E	Other	Mahoney and Barthel[119]
Functional Rating Scale	A, C, E	Other	Evans and Kagan[58]
Functional Status Index	A, E	Other	Jette[93, 94]; Jette and Deniston[92]
Patient Assessment Form; Functioning Status Assessment Form	A, E	Other	Densen et al.[41]
PULHEMS Profile; PULSES Profile	E	Other	Granger et al.[74]
Index of ADL	A, C, E	Other	Brorsson and Asberg[15]; Katz[101]; Katz and Atdom[100]; Katz et al.[99]
Kenny Self-Care Evaluation	A, E	Other	Schoening[163]
Physical Self-Maintenance Scale	E (≥ 60 years)	Other	—
Functional Status Rating System	A	Other	—
Rapid Disability Rating Scale	E	Other	—
Patient Evaluation Conference System	A	Other	Harvey and Jellinek[80]
Functional Activities Questionnaire	A, E	Other	—
OECD Long-Term Disability Questionnaire	A	Self, other	—
Lambeth Health Survey; Lambeth Disability Screening Questionnaire	A	Self, other	Peach et al.[147]
Disability and Impairment Interview Schedule	A	Other	Garrad and Bennett[70]

A, adult; C, children; E, elderly; Other, administered by another in an interview; Self, self-administered; PULSES, Physical condition, Upper limb function, Lower limb function, Sensory components, Excretory functions, Support factors.

Problems one and two reflect content issues and probably explain the current thinking that patient function and dysfunction across multiple domains are more appropriate constructs on which to base patient health status and outcome than is the magnitude of a patient's pain. Problem three, that the information provided is too extensive and therefore overwhelming to clinicians who try to incorporate all of this information into their evaluation of the patient is essentially a problem of information management. The remarkable growth in the information systems field over the past decade suggests that an answer to this problem may lie in the application of information technologies now available to clinicians through the use of personal computers.

Problem four, that the MCPQ is too long and complicated to allow adequate patient completion, may be more a matter of style or construction than substance or content. In response to incomplete questionnaires, some investigators have suggested that a compromise between questionnaire length and completion rates be made.[48, 50, 160] The so-called length-completeness trade-off option, however, is illusory. With this option, short and simple questionnaires are developed in the belief that they will result in complete data bases with sufficient information. In practice, the experienced clinician comes to understand that virtually no useful questionnaire will be completed by all patients. Further, the short, easy-to-complete questionnaire that is designed to provide the minimally sufficient data set rarely succeeds at this goal unless the questions are simple. The consequence of not compromising length for compliance is apparently to develop long and complex questionnaires that result in incomplete data bases, which then also have insufficient information because of a lack of complete data. Thus, the length-completeness compromise is generally a lose-lose proposition. A better course of action is to develop questionnaires by use of carefully considered construction techniques that provide patients with the opportunity to describe their condition fully in a way that is not viewed by them as overly long or complex. The litmus test for this type of questionnaire is completion rate, not length. It matters not if the questionnaire is 100 pages and asks patients to consider complex issues regarding their physical and

Table 5

Pain and Selected Psychosocial Measurements

Measurement Tool	Population	Person Administering Measure	Study
Dallas Pain Questionnaire	A	Self	Lawlis et al.[109]
Fear Avoidance Beliefs Questionnaire	A	Self	Waddell et al.[182]
Illness Behavior Questionnaire	A, E	Self	Anderson et al.[2]; Callahan et al.[22]; Pilowsky et al.[151]; Pilowsky and Spenc[149, 150]
McGill Pain Questionnaire	A, E	Other	Haas and Nyiendo[79]; Holroyd et al.[83];
Low Back Pain Symptom Checklist	A, E	Self	Love et al.[116]; Lowe et al.[117]; Melzack[130, 133]; Wilkie et al.[190]
Back Pain Classification Scale	A, E	Self	Leavitt[111]; Sanders[161]
Pain Behavior Checklist	A, E	Other	Dirks et al.[51]; Kerns et al.[105]
Pain Beliefs Questionnaire	A, E	Self	Edwards et al.[55]
Pain Chart	A, C, E	Other	Margoles[121]
Pain Disability Index	A	Self	Jerome and Gross[91]; Tart et al.[172, 173]
Pain Drawing	A	Self	Love et al.[116]
Pain Perception Profile	A, E	Other	Tursky et al.[180]
Pain Rating Scale	A, E	Other	Dirks et al.[51]; Reading[157]
Self-Rating Pain and Distress Scale	A, E	Self	Zung[197]
Visual Analogue Scales	A	Self	Campbell and Lewis[25]; Langley and Sheppeard[108]; Leboeuf et al.[112]; Love et al.[116]
West Haven–Yale Multidimensional Pain Inventory	A, E	Self	Kerns et al.[105]
Minnesota Multiphasic Personality Inventory	A, C, E	Self	Adams et al.[1]; Armentrout et al[3]; Dennis et al.[40]; Dubro and Wetzler[53]; Hathaway and McKinley[81]; Hunsley et al.[84]; Sternbach et al.[168]

A, adult; C, children; E, elderly; Other, administered by another in an interview; Self, self-administered.

psychologic conditions if most patients can and do complete the questionnaire.

To summarize, clinical outcomes are used to assess patient wellness or health status. Health status is best determined when the assessment focuses on concrete aspects, such as patient functioning, which might include activities they can and cannot perform and their ability to function independently and to work. Unfortunately, although many outcome measures provide information about these abilities, in most situations, these instruments do not provide the additional information about the patient that is needed to interpret reasonably the meaning of the scores provided. Perhaps even worse, when an instrument has been developed that attempts to provide the contextual information necessary to interpret the meaning or meanings of the scores provided, the instrument is considered too complex, and the richness of the information provided is not used.

CONTEXT AS A NECESSARY COMPONENT OF OUTCOME ASSESSMENT

Context is the notion that information other than that directly associated with outcome must be known about the object of measurement (typically the patient) before meaning can be derived about the outcome measures. That some context is necessary for the evaluation of the meaning of outcome scores is evident. Even the most spartan outcome measures typically include patient age and gender as basic questions.

In clinical practice, patient context is typically implicit. The clinician generally sees the patient and, through an interview process and physical examination, comes to understand the general status of the patient. Thus, such basic information as patient age, gender, height, weight, address, phone number, type of work, place of work, education level, marital status, number of children, dependents, income, insurer, and general health history are all available or discovered by the clinician in the course of the patient examination. Unfortunately, much of this information available to the clinician is never explicitly coded as part of the patient's medical record. In dictated clinical notes, the aspects of the patient's situation (context) that made an impression on the clinician may be noted, but other aspects of the patient may be grouped together in a comment such as "no other remarkable conditions." This disparity between the vast amount of information available to the clinician as a result of direct contact and questioning of the patient during a clinic visit and the relative paucity of information typically available to the clinician from the clinic notes or the patient questionnaires may explain why some clinicians feel that clinic notes and patient questionnaires are of limited value in helping them to treat and evaluate a patient's progress.

A further illustration of the necessity of contextual patient information in the evaluation of patient health status or outcome is a mythical 20-item ADL scale in which the outcome measure of interest is the percentage of activities the patient reports that he or she can do. Suppose patient A (Bill) indicated that he could do 16 activities. His score would be 80% (16/20 × 100). Similarly, if patient B (Hill) indicated that she could do 12 activities, her score would be 60% (12/20 × 100). Now, which patient is less ill or more well or is enjoying a better health status? Without some patient context, this question cannot be satisfactorily answered.

Now suppose that the following information is made available to help fill in some patient context. What if Bill is an 18-year-old male college athlete who 1 week ago could do all 20 activities with no problem. Suppose further that the only reason he can do 80% of the activities now is because he uses crutches. Also suppose that Hill is a 65-year-old female who 1 week ago could only do 25% of the activities (5/20 × 100)? Suppose that for our 18-year-old male, an 80% ADL score is better than the scores of only 5% of typical 18-year-old men (i.e., a score of 80% indicates a percentile rank of 5 in his cohort). Suppose that for our 65-year-old female, a 60% ADL corresponds to percentile rank of 90 (i.e., her performance is better than that of 90% of her cohort). Now which patient is enjoying a better health status? Within the context provided, comparing Hill to her cohort and Bill to his cohort, clearly Hill is doing better than Bill.

Some might argue that this example is overly contrived, that it is not reasonable to directly compare an 18-year-old male athlete with a 65-year-old woman. In response, typical descriptions of patient populations reported in the literature on low back trouble should be considered. Patient information from five journal articles from a randomly selected issue of *Spine* are summarized in Table 6. Clearly, the age range of patients tends to be large, and, when patient sex was reported, the groups evaluated consisted of both male and female patients. Thus, it appears to be standard practice to evaluate the effects of treatment for mixed gender and age groups, at least when treatment efficacy was reported for patients presenting with low back trouble in 1985.

The approach used earlier to evaluate the outcome of Bill and Hill in terms of their outcome measure scores based on some context is fundamentally the approach that is used in many measurement situations: triangulation. An example of the use of triangulation is the measurement techniques used to determine location at sea by using a sextant. In navigation, triangulation allows sailors to determine their position by jointly consider-

Table 6

Summary of Patient Samples Used in Studies Evaluating Treatment Efficacy

Number of Patients	Male/Female Ratio	Age Range of Patients (years)	Journal	Vol	Pages	Year
34	—	15–70	*Spine*	10	307–312	1985
20	10:10	28–62	*Spine*	10	338–344	1985
200	96:104	17–74	*Spine*	10	345–349	1985
40	—	22–74	*Spine*	10	363–367	1985
77	55:22	7–32	*Spine*	10	937–943	1985

ing the angles between their location and two different objects, typically the horizon and the sun or another star of known latitude. The obtained angle distance is then compared with star charts that allow the navigator to fix the position.

In determining the nature of patient outcome, triangulation allows the clinician to determine patient outcome by jointly considering how well a patient was doing before compared with now (a horizon, or within-patient comparison), and how well a patient is doing now compared with how well a reasonable cohort does (a star of known properties, or an across-patient comparison). The major differences between navigating and assessing patient outcome by triangulation is that navigators have reliable sextants and a clear notion of where the horizon is, and they well understand what stars are in the sky. Clinicians, on the other hand, also have relatively reliable instruments (patient self-reports), but little or no knowledge about how to triangulate (level these sextants at the horizon and find an appropriate star in the sky). Finally, clinicians have little or no corresponding normative data (star charts) to allow them to convert the raw information they obtain into meaningful units that clearly indicate the patient's health status. In other words, the current state of the art in clinical outcomes assessment is not very helpful in accurately placing or ranking patients' outcome in their cohorts. To complete the metaphor, clinical outcome measures or instruments developed to study patients presenting with low back trouble are of limited value because our ship is in a fog bank. We can see neither the horizon nor the stars. In their medical training, many clinicians have never been provided with the basic information necessary to even attempt to look. Worse yet, if the fog were to lift and we knew enough to try to fix our bearings, we have no star charts (normative data) by which to convert our readings into meaningful interpretations.

GUIDELINES IN DEVELOPING SELF-REPORT MEASURES

The measurement literature and theory provides guidelines and suggestions that are helpful in developing questionnaires that simultaneously query complex topics and maximize completion rates. In the development of an outcome instrument, it must be remembered that the goals are relatively simple: to allow patients to describe their status accurately and completely. In many cases, when outcome assessments are developed, an additional implicit goal is also considered important: to gather additional information that will be useful in understanding, explaining, or predicting patient status. The following four general concepts should guide the construction of self-report measures.

Guideline 1. Patients should be allowed to describe their status, feelings, or situation rather than being forced to fit into some set of predetermined problems. For example, in many outcome instruments, the primary focus is on pain. Although pain is undoubtedly the commonest chief complaint, it is certainly not the only symptom that prompts patients to seek medical attention. Symptoms of numbness and weakness are also relatively common chief complaints in patients with low back trouble. If patients present with a chief complaint of numbness and weakness in the leg, how are they to respond to the following questions common in most outcome assessment instruments?

1. During the past week, how often have you taken medication for your back or leg pain?
2. During the past week, how often have you stayed home from work because of your pain?

If patients are literal minded, and the problem is not pain, patients who are taking medication and missing work because of their symptoms of numbness and weakness are likely to indicate that they took no medication or missed no work because of pain symptoms. Alternatively, pragmatic-minded patients, reasoning that the point of the question is what they are doing, not why they are doing it, may indicate that they are taking medications and are missing work because of their pain, even though the cause for their actions is not pain but their symptoms of numbness and weakness. In both cases, the goals of accurate and complete information are not achieved. A solution to this potential problem is to ask patients to describe their symptoms clearly and then to

How much of the time during the LAST WEEK	All of the time	Most of the time	A good bit of the time	Some of the time	Little of the time	None of the time
Have you been a very nervous person?						
Have you been a happy person?						

Figure 1. A typical presentation of a frequency Likert-type scale.

phrase all subsequent questions relative to their symptoms rather than assuming the symptom or cause of the various actions of interest is pain. Thus, once the nature of the patient's symptoms and chief complaint are ascertained, the two questions listed earlier could be rephrased as:

1. During the past week, how often have you taken medication because of your symptoms?
2. During the past week, how often have you stayed home from work because of your symptoms?

Guideline 2. When self-report assessments are developed, the underlying dimensions of a construct should be clearly delineated, and patients should be allowed to respond to each aspect of the situation separately. For example, when patients are asked to describe their pain, numerous underlying dimensions are involved: pain magnitude or intensity, pain duration, and pain pattern across time. For many patients, pain is not at a constant level all the time. Thus, if the goal is to obtain an accurate and complete indication of patients' pain, an approach might be to ask them to chart their pain intensity over a typical 24-hour period. In this way, patients are provided a concrete situation in which to evaluate their typical experience. In addition, this scenario might be expanded to allow patients to chart their usual activity levels over a typical 24-hour period. The advantage of providing the patient with a concrete situation in which to consider their status is more fully exploited by simultaneously allowing patients to consider and report about a second clinically important outcome. If the assessment simply asks patients to indicate their pain level on a typical day, patients must implicitly combine their experiences of pain intensity over the course of the day and mentally average their experiences to derive a single score. Individual differences in mental arithmetic virtually ensure that patients who might respond similarly in describing their pattern of pain across a typical 24-hour period would arrive at different overall pain intensity ratings.

Guideline 3. Ambiguous response scales should be avoided. A typical frequency Likert-type scale is illustrated in Figure 1, which shows an outcome measure currently in common use for the assessment of the frequency of patient behaviors or feelings. In this case, the problem is that discriminating among some of the categories is difficult, and little basis exists for assuming, for example, that any two patients would necessarily agree about what is meant by general time descriptors (e.g., "most of the time" versus "a good bit of the time"). In this instance, the adjustment to the scale is straightforward and, perhaps, once seen, is painfully obvious (Fig. 2).

Guideline 4. The content of the questions should be tailored to the underlying purpose for the questions. A classic example of this problem is the often-included question in many health status surveys of whether a patient smokes. Although the question may provide some useful information, in most instances, the underlying purpose of the question is not to establish the patient's smoking status, but to identify potential

Figure 2. Modification of the presentation and nature of a frequency Likert-type scale.

How many days in the LAST WEEK:	Number of Days 0 1 2 3 4 5 6 7
Have you been a very nervous person?	⓪ ① ② ③ ④ ⑤ ⑥ ⑦
Have you been a happy person?	⓪ ① ② ③ ④ ⑤ ⑥ ⑦

health and treatment risk factors. For example, the clinician may be considering using a spinal fusion with instrumentation in the hope of increasing the likelihood of solid fusion for a patient with a history of smoking. Of course, if the issue of smoking and the ability to achieve solid fusion is crucial, the clinician is not likely to rely solely on a single patient-reported piece of information regarding smoking status. However, in this instance, the single smoking status question may not be useful even as an initial screen. For most purposes, smoking status is reliably or accurately depicted by the simple yes or no question "do you smoke?" But if the purpose of asking the question is to establish risk factors, this purpose is not well served by this single question. What if the patient's history is one of smoking two packs a day for 30 years, but he or she quit 2 weeks ago. In this situation, the patient could legitimately respond that he or she does not smoke. At the relatively low cost of a few additional self-report questions aimed at detailing the patient's smoking history, the clinician would be provided with information useful for establishing risk factors in general, or the risks of fusion with or without adjunctive instrumentation.

These four guidelines are considerations in the development of an assessment instrument. For example, ADL scales are typically designed to assess patient function and are considered an important generic tool in the evaluation of patient health status. Instructions vary from scale to scale, but they are generally simple and ask patients to indicate which of the listed activities they can do. An excerpt from a typical ADL scale is provided in Figure 3.

Interviews of patients who have completed such ADL scales have suggested that numerous problems exist with the format. First, regardless of the instructions, patients tend to respond to each activity according to whether they do the activity, not whether they can do the activity. Thus, many patients incorrectly mark gender-stereotypic behaviors. For example, male patients tend to mark "wash dishes," with a "no," and female patients tend to mark "mow the lawn" with a "no." Second, some patients mark the activity as "no" when they can do the activity but require some assistance. Finally, even if patients' response is an accurate reflection of what they can do, the total score is more an estimate of their perceived efficacy rather than an indication of function because the score is not necessarily sensitive to the actual amount of the patients' activity.

The adjustments made to this ADL scale incorporate elements of all four basic guidelines summarized earlier and are illustrated in Figure 4. With this ADL scale restructured into this format, the result offers the clinician a wide range of information that is useful for evaluating patients' functional status. As indicated previously, the "can do" type of question speaks to patients' perceived efficacy, or how competent they feel they are to act. By explicitly distinguishing between "can do" and "do," the format forces the responder to consider and understand this fundamental distinction. By explicitly asking if assistance is needed to perform the activity, the format allows the responder to understand the issue is doing the activity and that if assistance is needed, the activity is still being done. By explicitly asking how often in a typical week the patient does the activity, the questions obtain a more accurate index of actual patient activity level, and by explicitly asking how the activity affects patient symptoms, the question enhances sensitivity to the progress of patient rehabilitation.

PROPERTIES OF HEALTH STATUS OUTCOME MEASURES

The two primary goals of health status outcome measures are simultaneously to

Instructions: Indicate if you can do each of the activities listed below:

Activity	Can you do this activity?	
1. Walk up a flight of stairs	Yes	No
2. Drive a car	Yes	No
3. Mow the lawn	Yes	No
4. Wash dishes	Yes	No

Figure 25-3. An excerpt of a typical activities of daily living (ADL) instrument.

Activity	❶ CAN you DO this activity?		If Yes →	❷ Do you Need Assistance to do this activity?		❸ How many days in a Typical Week do you do this activity?	❹ How does this activity Affect your Symptoms?		
	No	Yes		No	Yes	0 1 2 3 4 5 6 7	Makes Worse	No Affect	Makes Better
Walk up a flight of stairs	Ⓝ	Ⓨ	→	Ⓝ	Ⓨ	⓪①②③④⑤⑥⑦	○	○	○
Drive a car	Ⓝ	Ⓨ	→	Ⓝ	Ⓨ	⓪①②③④⑤⑥⑦	○	○	○
Mow the lawn	Ⓝ	Ⓨ	→	Ⓝ	Ⓨ	⓪①②③④⑤⑥⑦	○	○	○
Wash dishes	Ⓝ	Ⓨ	→	Ⓝ	Ⓨ	⓪①②③④⑤⑥⑦	○	○	○

Instructions: For each of the following activities, first indicate: ❶ If you CAN DO this activity. Then, if you indicate that Yes you CAN DO the activity, go on for that activity to indicate: ❷ if you Need Assistance to do the activity; ❸ How many days in a Typical Week you do the activity, and ❹ How doing the activity Affects your Symptoms

Figure 25–4. An extensive modification and "evolution" of the traditional ADL scale that explicitly forces the respondent to distinguish between "can do" and "do," which allows assessment of patient efficacy, activity level, and symptom interference with daily living.

1. Evaluate the wellness of the patient at any given time
2. Be sensitive to changes in wellness across time

These two goals are challenging to implement; they demand that the magnitude of the scores be meaningful at any given point in time and that changes in health status, both improvement and worsening, can be detected. In measurement terms, these demands mean that outcome measures need to minimize or avoid ceiling and floor effects.

Ceiling and Floor Effects

A health status instrument is said to have a ceiling effect if patients can score very high or at the top of the scale, even when they are not completely well. The instrument is said to have a floor effect if patients score very low or at the bottom of the scale, even if they are not seriously ill. In general, the instrument itself does not have the ceiling or floor effect, but rather the population or sample. For example, a mathematics placement examination designed to identify college freshmen who are ready to take calculus would have a serious floor effect if given to fifth grade students to assess their mathematics achievement because virtually any correct answers would be the result of guessing. Similarly, an instrument designed to assess the ability of fifth grade students to add, subtract, multiply, and divide would have a serious ceiling effect if given to college freshmen in a calculus course because, in this population, any incorrect answers would be the result of bad luck or silly mistakes.

Multilevel Instruments

In clinical applications, defining the gold standard outcome measure has been like a search for the Holy Grail. Given the range of possible health status outcomes, from extreme wellness or fitness to extreme illness or incapacity, one might gain some perspective concerning the difficulty of the problem by returning to the mathematics ability examples used to help conceptualize the notions of ceiling and floor effects. Because a gold standard outcome measure should be able to capture both a patient's current health status and any future health status, the analogous situation in assessing mathematics achievement would be to build a single instrument that can assess one's ability throughout the course of the person's development, from preschool through advanced graduate school years. Given that tests of mathematic and arithmetic skills are available for each age and ability segment, one might suggest that such a single instrument could conceivably be developed by simply combining all of these instruments. Clearly, such a test would be extremely long and impractical.

Measurement professionals who construct achievement tests have solved this problem by providing multilevel instruments, essentially dividing a single long test into separate tests that are appropriate for the particular age group or population being assessed. The analogous situation in clinical settings would be to devise different levels of health status instruments. Simply put, instruments for the very ill, the moderately ill, the slightly ill, and the well are separated. However, whereas in educational settings preselecting the appropriate test for the student is trivial, in clinical settings a health status instrument must be administered to determine the patient's general level of health status before one could determine which health status instrument should be administered. A nontrivial secondary problem, even if a screening health status measure were devised to classify the patient so that the appropriately sensitive health status instruments could be provided, is that the current state of development of outcome measures of health status is not sufficiently mature to allow the development of a battery of health status instruments appropriate for the detection of severity of illness. The primary obstacle is not the inability to conceptualize the structure of such an instrument, but the lack of the infrastructure that can provide a delivery system. Such a system must be able to capture the patients as they enter, progress, and leave the health care system. Until the health care system appreciates the importance of institutionalizing outcomes assessment, until clinicians and administrators understand that these data are just as important, if not more important, than billing codes, and until patients understand that the questionnaires and surveys they fill out are an important aspect of their medical treatment, the successful implementation of health status instruments is in jeopardy.

Clarification of Outcome Measures

Sensitivity to levels of health status must be both forward and backward looking. Some instruments focus on the present and hope to be sensitive to changes in patients' futures. However, this focus can be a problem because, as the old adage reminds us, it is sometimes difficult to know where you are going if you do not know where you have been. This problem often occurs in outcome studies that focus on return to work as the outcome of interest. In some clinical trials, especially those focusing on rehabilitation, return to work has been operationalized by the patient's response to a straightforward yes or no question: "Have you returned to work?" Patients who respond "yes" are considered to have a good outcome, those who respond "no," a poor one. However, just as in the example of the ADL scale with Bill and Hill, additional contextual information is needed before such evaluations can be made. In this case, at least four aspects of the patient's situation must be considered:

1. Was the patient working before the treatment? If not, what does the question of return to work mean to that patient? Similarly, what if the patient was never out of work?
2. Did the person who returned to work stay on the job? If the person returned to work for a day or two and then found that he or she could not continue, should this be considered a good outcome?
3. Was the job returned to the same job or one with restricted duties? If the patient returned to a job that had little or no physical requirements, is this as impressive as if the patient returned to a job that does require physical effort?
4. Was the reason the patient did not return to work related to the patient's condition or to the economic or other status of the employer? If the patient is well but did not return to work because no jobs exist, should this be considered a poor treatment outcome?

Without these and some other aspects of the situation in hand, the apparently simple question of return to work cannot be well established as a reliable outcome measure that is valid for inferring relationships between patients' work and health status.

Baseline Data

Including items in a patient self-report questionnaire to establish baseline information is a significant problem on two distinct levels. First, the process begs the question of how far back into the past the questions should examine. In other words, what baseline should be used? Second, the question of the accuracy of patients' recall of their presymptomatic past is a concern. The vagaries of memory, especially when patients are asked to think back to the days when they were well, suggest that the accuracy of these recall data will be suspect, especially if patients are motivated to exaggerate their prior state of wellness.

Arguing that they must work with what they get, some clinicians use patients' pretreatment status, that is, their condition at their initial presentation, as their wellness baseline. This choice presents many problems. First, baseline evaluations depend on a patient's access to treatment and the type of facility entered as well as the severity of the problem. Patients with quick access to a family physician are likely to be symptomatic, and those who must wait several days or weeks to be seen may be almost symptom free by the time they can see a clinician and, if they become symptom-free before their visit, may cancel their visit. Because a patient at initial visit is typically not feeling well, data obtained at this initial visit as a baseline measurement virtually ensure that current patient wellness is relatively low. In essence, this practice enlists the regression toward the mean phenomenon. Regression toward the mean, in this instance, simply means that on average, patients who are assessed and found to be in an extreme condition (i.e., when they are below their normal level of wellness) are likely at repeated assessment to generate less extreme scores as a consequence of errors of measurement rather than any real change in status. Thus, in treatments whose efficacy is based on improvement from initial visit or pretreatment wellness, treatment effects may be confounded with simple regression toward the mean effects. Treatment efficacy is less ambiguously considered when patients' presymptomatic wellness, pretreatment wellness, and posttreatment wellness are compared. Unfortunately, such a comparison is not possible in most systems that collect patient information.

One logical baseline measure would be to compare patients' current status relative to their condition just before their current complaints. However, for some patients, these data may date back a week or two; for others, a month or two; for still others, a year or two; and for an unfortunate few, several years. The person performing the assessment must then determine how information provided about the patient's presymptomatic past can be compared when the length of time since that past may be so variable. The assessor's ability to solve this problem depends on the extent of the second problem, namely that patients recall of their presymptomatic condition may be poor or biased and that the amount of memory loss and biased recollection may be a function of both the severity of the current problems and the length of time the problems have been experienced.

An obvious answer to these problems is to have patients complete clinical outcome measures before their symptoms appear and have patients make these records available to their treating physicians when they present with a problem. A detailed discussion of mechanisms that might be established to gather clinical outcome measures on individuals before they become patients and keeping these outcome measures updated is beyond the scope of this paper, but such discussions are clearly worth developing. It is interesting to note that AT&T, as part of a national television and print advertisement campaign in January 1994, indicated that they planned to have people's medical histories coded onto a "smart card" that could be carried with them at all times, much like a credit card. Given the dawn of these technologies, it seems a relatively small additional step to ensure that part of each citizens' health history would be, for lack of a better label, a clinical outcome profile.

Normative Data Base

Establishing the ability to ascertain patients' wellness or illness, although a major accomplishment in its own right, serendipitously provides the raw data necessary to resolve the problem of establishing the normative data base used to place or rank patients in their appropriate cohort. For example, suppose that as a part of a national health care plan it is required that citizens complete a clinical outcome profile. For school-aged children, the profile could become a part of their school registration.

For adults, completing the profile could be a part of renewing their driver's license, obtaining a picture identification card (for those who do not drive), or obtaining a social security card. In this scenario, over 250 million clinical outcome profile forms would be available in the United States alone, from which age- and gender-adjusted normative scales of performance could be established. In other words, these data would make it possible to compute age- and gender-adjusted percentile ranks like those used to rate Bill and Hill in the ADL example provided earlier.

Although it is not the inherent duty of the outcome measure to provide a normative interpretation of the score generated, such as age and gender cohort percentile ranks, outcome measures must provide sufficient information to define the appropriate cohort. Without this ability to establish a normative interpretation of the scores derived from outcome measures, adequate evaluation of patients' health status is not possible. Establishing normative data for scores derived from outcome measures is the role of researchers who wish to evaluate the validity of the measures. Sadly, this role has, in clinical outcome measure evaluation, not yet been played.

ASSESSING THE PSYCHOMETRIC PROPERTIES OF HEALTH STATUS OUTCOME MEASURES

The measurement properties of any assessment tool are generally categorized into issues of reliability and validity. For clinical relevance, the reliability and validity properties of an instrument used to help the clinician make decisions are associated with false-positive, or specificity, and false-negative, or sensitivity, rates. In general, to the extent that instruments are reliable and valid for the purpose for which they are being used, specificity and sensitivity are enhanced. Although the goal is to develop reliable and valid instruments, the underlying structure and understandings necessary to attain these goals are complex and are typically seen as unnecessarily so by clinicians who simply want to use the scores.

One of the problems in clinical studies is that the jargon often used to describe the psychometric properties of instruments is simultaneously assuring, intuitively obvious, and imprecise, typically to the point of being wrong. For example, in clinical studies, a common phrase used is "well-accepted measure of patient outcome." Over the years, most careful researchers have discovered that a well-accepted measure is defined as one used by someone else that resulted in a significant finding that we would like to find too. Another phrase commonly read in studies extolling the psychometric properties of a measure is "the results have demonstrated the instrument to be reliable and valid." To the trained measurement professional, this statement has little meaning. A general overview of issues associated with reliability and validity follows in the hope that the reader will come to appreciate what additional information must be provided before statements regarding the reliability of an instrument and its validity for some particular use can be understood and rationally evaluated.

Reliability

Reliability refers to the degree to which scores are free from errors of measurement. Given this definition, the notion suggested by some investigators, that reliability is not relevant in clinical situations, is clearly misguided. What these critics may be alluding to is that some of the methods used to assess reliability are not sufficiently sensitive to the problems uniquely associated with the measurement of clinically relevant factors. More likely yet, concern that reliability is not relevant in clinical settings is probably in response to a disagreement with the value of an approach used to establish reliability in a given situation. Readers interested in reliability in a wider context are referred to Feldt and Brennan.[61]

Classic measurement theory recognizes three basic approaches for establishing the reliability of a single instrument:

1. Reliability based on estimating score stability, usually evaluated using test-retest methods
2. Reliability based on consistency of scores when the single instrument is divided into two half-length parallel forms, typically called split-half reliability

3. Internal consistency reliability estimates, quantified in terms of Cronbach's α, also called coefficient α.[35]

Although coefficient α has been demonstrated to be algebraically equivalent to the average of all possible split-half reliability estimates, conceptually split-half reliability and internal consistency reliability estimates are distinct. These two forms are only directly comparable to the extent that the instrument being evaluated has been designed to assess a single trait that is considered unidimensional. In most clinical settings, these circumstances probably do not hold. For example, if the underlying construct being evaluated is pain, split-half and internal consistency reliability estimates are probably not comparable because pain is thought to have a multidimensional structure.

Beyond the theoretic vagaries of reliability theory, from the clinical perspective, the important question should be: How should reliability be evaluated for health status outcome measures? Unfortunately, as with most important questions, the answer is not straightforward. Because reliability is an estimate of the amount of error in the measurement, the answer depends on what sources of error are of greatest interest to the clinician to capture and, through instrument modification, to minimize.

Test-Retest Reliability

The notion of a stable, dependable score is probably the most comforting and most traditional view of reliability. Those who must make clinical decisions based on patient self-report scores would probably be happiest if score reliability based on stability estimates were maximized. Unfortunately, this type of reliability is also the most expensive and difficult to obtain, requiring that the respondent complete the instrument twice. The expense issue is obvious. The accompanying difficulties have also been well chronicled. The most fundamental concern is that the original assessment may change the respondents (patients) in some way that would affect their responses on a second administration. In other words, lack of consistency across time might be expected and not reflective of error but of real change. This problem is well understood in the clinical community with respect to physical capacity testing and with patients' responses during a physical examination, in which fatigue and wariness of the consequences of certain actions can affect subsequent performance.[167] Conversely, if the administration does not have any affect on respondents' subsequent performance, and if the scores across the two administrations are not similar, then either the underlying construct or the measurement procedure is unstable. Theoretically, it can be difficult to discriminate between these two possible sources of variation.

Split-Half Reliability

Techniques associated with split-half reliability can and have been used as a means for attempting to identify reasons or causes for low-stability reliability estimates. If the underlying construct is so unstable that true differences can be detected in short-interval test-retest situations, perhaps this same instability can be detected within the single administration of the instrument. Thus, constructing an instrument such that splitting it into two halves results in reasonably parallel or equivalent forms, and then assessing this split-half reliability, viewing it as a quasi test-retest reliability, is an approach for distinguishing between construct instability and error of measurement, or unreliability.

The major drawback with split-half reliability is the potential difficulty of forming reasonable splits, defined as two half-length instruments made up from the original, that can reasonably be considered as parallel or equivalent forms. This is an especially difficult problem in the area of health status assessment, in which the trend is to develop as short an instrument as possible. For example, consider the task of dividing the Health Status Questionnaire 2.0[155] into two parallel or equivalent halves. The Health Status Questionnaire 2.0, a variation or derivation from the Medical Outcomes Study 36-Item Short Form Health Survey (SF-36), has eight scales, which are constructed from 35 items. The various scales, the number of items on each, and a suggested split of items are presented in Table 7. Given that the total number of items used in the eight scales is an odd number (35), the two parallel or equivalent forms are not of equal length.

Table 7

Summary of the Scales and Item Counts for the Health Status Questionnaire

Scale	Total	First Half	Second Half
Health perception	5	3	2
Physical functioning	10	5	5
Role limitation			
Physical	4	2	2
Emotional	3	1	2
Social functioning	2	1	1
Mental health	5	2	3
Bodily pain	2	1	1
Energy/fatigue	4	2	2

Although this problem is not difficult to resolve when estimating split-half reliability, the number of scales with only one or two items in each of the splits is not encouraging, especially if the split-half reliabilities for each subscale are of interest.

Internal Consistency Reliability

Internal consistency reliability, most typically evaluated by coefficient α, is probably the single commonest form of reliability assessed, undoubtedly because of the ease with which the estimate can be obtained: no retesting is required, and the researcher need not split up the instrument into parts. With current statistical software, a simple request to compute coefficient α requires just a few keystrokes. As suggested earlier, however, the interpretation of the coefficient α reliability index is rarely consistent with the stability concept or the split-half formulation of reliability. In fact, this form of reliability finds its primary use in conjunction with instrument construction, where it is typically used to confirm that a set of items are behaving as they should if they are all functioning to measure the underlying construct of interest. Although this consideration is almost always important when an instrument is developed, it does not necessarily speak to score stability, and more important, scale modifications in pursuit of maximizing internal consistency estimates of reliability can have serious consequences for the validity of the score, especially when a major purpose of the score is to be sensitive to change.

Because it might be argued that the single most important use of a health status outcome score is to provide clinicians with the ability to reliably and accurately track real changes in patients' health status over time, the use of coefficient α to maximize internal consistency of items at any given time could result in a severe loss of sensitivity for the instrument. This point is especially important because the prevalence of coefficient α's use in the construction of self-report instruments is often based on the almost universally accepted, but wrong-minded, notion that maximizing reliability necessarily improves validity.

Most students with training in the sciences have heard the phrase "valid measures must be reliable." Unfortunately, many take this basic truism and turn it around, thinking that reliable measures must be valid, and then go on to infer that increasing the reliability of a measure must make it more valid. This relationship between reliability and validity does not hold, and two practices common in clinical research are clearly motivated by these false assumptions: (1) the tendency to maximize interrater reliability by minimizing the number of choices the clinician can choose and (2) the use of coefficient α to maximize internal consistency reliability of instruments designed to allow clinicians to track patients' health status across time.

The following example illustrates the way in which inappropriate use of coefficient α in instrument construction can simultaneously reduce the effective reliability of the instrument and decrease the validity of the instrument when the purpose is to be sensitive to change across time. Suppose that a 20-item ADL instrument were developed, and suppose further that the instrument were given to 100 patients. The resultant scores have a mean of 12 and a standard deviation of 4, they range from 3 to 17, and they have a coefficient α of .80. To further evaluate the psychometric properties of the instrument, the researcher numbers activities from easiest to hardest on the basis of this sample. The ambitious instrument builder notices that activities 1 and 2 (the two easiest) and activity 20 (the hardest) have no variance. In other words, all 100 patients said that they could do activities 1 and 2 and none of the 100 patients said they could do activity 20. When these activities are removed from the scale, coefficient α increases from .80 to .90.

The ambitious, but naive, researcher decides

that he or she is in a win-win situation: he or she can increase reliability and shorten the instrument. But at what cost? The researcher has now created an instrument with both a ceiling and a floor effect. Thus, this instrument, although maximally reliable now, has attained that status at the expense of disallowing some of these patients the ability to indicate accurately that over time, they can do more or less than they could before. Reliability has been temporarily served, the sensitivity of the instrument has been reduced, and given the imposed ceiling and floor effects on the revised instrument, the internal consistency of the instrument assessed at some future time will, in all likelihood, decrease.

In summary, for most clinical applications, test-retest reliability estimates of health status outcomes are the most preferable. Bearing in mind that this type of reliability estimate is the most expensive to obtain and can involve inherent difficulties that can affect the accuracy of the reliability estimate, split-half reliability estimates are typically acceptable substitutes if the nature of the instrument reasonably allows for split halves to be developed. Internal consistency estimates of reliability are probably the single most used index for evaluating the reliability of self-report measures, undoubtedly because they are the easiest to obtain. Unfortunately, the way in which these indices are occasionally used, especially when they are incorporated into the decision-making process for construction or refinement of new instruments, is inappropriate, resulting in instruments that are not more but less valid for their intended purpose. The notion that all reliability is the same is simple minded and untrue. The various forms of reliability are based on different underlying assumptions about the nature of the instrument being evaluated and are differentially sensitive to the types of error that are contributing to the unreliability or inaccuracy of a measure. In patient self-report instruments focusing on health status, stability estimates of reliability over relatively short intervals, with same-day assessments most preferable, should usually be considered the gold standard of reliability estimation.

Validity

Validity is the most important consideration in the evaluation of a measure. The concept refers to the appropriateness, meaningfulness, and usefulness of the inferences made from the scores.[141 (p9)] Thus, the outcome measures or the instruments themselves have no validity, and validity as a concept is not an attribute of a measure. Validity is completely associated with the way in which the information provided from the measure is used and interpreted. Thus, to say that a measure is valid is an incomplete sentence. To say that a measure has validity for the purpose of assessing the health status of a person is a complete sentence and more accurately describes the relationship of the instrument, the resulting score, and the use of the score. Validity has meaning only in reference to a measure's purpose.

Traditionally, the various means of accumulating validity evidence have been grouped into categories called content-related, criterion-related, and construct-related evidence of validity. These categories are convenient, as are other more refined categorizations (e.g., the division of the criterion-related category into predictive and concurrent evidence of validity), but the use of the category labels does not imply that distinct types of validity exist or that a specific validation strategy is best for each specific inference or test use.[141 (p9)]

Construct-related validity evidence focuses primarily on the measure as an accurate indicator of the underlying concept or variable of interest (e.g., health status). In clinical applications, pain, function, depression, coping, and activity level are all outcomes of interest in terms of health status. *Content-related validity* evidence attempts to demonstrate the degree to which the content (i.e., questions or tasks) making up the instrument are representative of the specified domain. If the scale is ADL, patients' blood type would be difficult to justify as being representative of that content domain. Walking up a flight of stairs, on the other hand, would be more representative of the domain. *Criterion-related evidence* demonstrates that the measures are systematically related to other, independent outcome measures. A popular and perhaps the preeminent methodology for developing criterion-related evidence is the use of the so-called multitrait-multimethod[24] protocols. In this methodology, different constructs (multitrait), some expected to be strongly related and others less strongly associated with each other, are measured by different approaches (multimethod), and the nature of these interrelationships is evaluated to determine if patterns of similarities and differences in traits are maintained under different measurement conditions.

In most validation schemes, multiple sources of evidence are required before the user should feel comfortable that the measures being used provide scores that are useful for the purposes that the measures were administered to provide. Two basic components are involved in the validation of an instrument. First, the user should feel comfortable that the magnitude of the score provided by the measures is related to the underlying construct that the instrument purports to measure. If the instrument is an ADL scale, the hope is that score magnitudes are related to the ability of the person responding to the scale to perform the ADL. If the scores are scaled so that higher scores indicate that a greater number of activities can be performed, the ADL score is showing validity evidence as a measure of health status if people in better health score higher than those in worse health. This aspect of validity could be assessed at a single point in time by gathering health-related information (e.g., age, gender, height, weight, blood pressure, pulmonary function, health history, range of motion, strength, flexibility, and endurance) about a group of persons and relating their ADL scores to these measures.

The second basic component involved is the ability of the score to function or behave in a manner consistent with the intended use of the score. Again, if the instrument is an ADL scale and the purpose is to use this scale to assess the effectiveness of a treatment in terms of improvement or worsening in health status, the ability of the ADL scale to be sensitive to changes in the person's health status must be assessed. This aspect of validity might be assessed by following various cohorts of patients longitudinally across time, with some cohorts being chosen on the basis of a general expectation that health status will improve over time and others being chosen on the basis of a general expectation that health status will worsen over time. Alternatively, cohorts might be identified that are known to be at different points on the health status continuum, and the ADL instrument may be administered to see if score magnitudes in these groups are distinct. Given that the stated purpose was to evaluate the ability of the instrument to be sensitive to changes in the treatments of various patient populations, better validity evidence would probably be gained from a longitudinal study that follows the progress of patients through treatment regimens. In general, the closer the validity evidence is to the intended purpose of the instrument, the more powerful the evidence should be considered.

CONCLUSIONS

This chapter has spanned a wide range of issues associated with assessing patient outcome in clinical settings. The focus has been on issues associated with patient self-report because this method is viewed as the way that health status is and will be assessed, and it is the area of patient assessment with which clinicians are least comfortable and familiar. In this chapter, an attempt has been made to

- Present reasons that patient self-report measures of health status are important
- Examine the fundamental differences and similarities in the so-called hard and soft data collected to document patient outcomes
- Identify the relatively large number of instruments available in the field
- Provide some basic guidelines for developing and, by extension, evaluating the quality of the instruments used to assess health care
- Identify some new approaches to more completely and accurately capture a patient's health status
- Promote an understanding of the need for context in the assessment of health status
- Stress the need to establish normative information as a way of more accurately communicating a patient's health status
- Identify the need to establish an infrastructure in medicine that will promote the collection, use, and maturation of health status information systems
- Define and describe some of the basic aspects of reliability and validity and provide some examples of these concepts in clinical applications

- Expose the reliability-validity myth, namely that increasing reliability must increase validity

The goals of this chapter were to spur clinicians' interest in these topics and to sensitize clinicians to some of the factors they should keep in mind when using outcome measures to aid in clinical decision-making. If after reading this chapter you have the feeling that the road to successful implementation of patient self-report measures of health status may be fraught with many pitfalls and potholes, then the intended message was received.

REFERENCES

1. Adams, K. M., Heolgronn, M., and Blumer, D. P.: A multimethod evaluation of the MMPI in a chronic pain patient sample. J. Counsel. Psychol. 42:878–886, 1986.
2. Anderson, J. St. C., Sullivan, F., and Underwood, T. P.: The Medical Outcomes Study Instrument (MOSI)—use of a new health status measure in Britain. Fam. Pract. 7:205–218, 1990.
3. Armentrout, D. P., Moore, J. E., Parker, J. C., et al.: Pain-patient MMPI subgroups: The psychological dimensions of pain. J Behav. Med. 5:201–211, 1982.
4. Baker, D. J., Pynsent, P B., and Fairbank, J. C. T.: The Oswestry Disability Index revisited: Its reliability, repeatability, and validity and a comparison with the St. Thomas's disability index. In Roland M. and Jenner J. (eds.): Back Pain: New Approaches to Rehabilitation and Education. Manchester, UK, Manchester University Press, 1989, pp. 174–186.
5. Bennett, A. E., and Ritchie, K.: Questionnaires in Medicine: A Guide to their Design and Use. London, Oxford University Press, 1975.
6. Bergner, M., Bobbitt, R. A., Pollard, W. E., et al.: The Sickness Impact Profile: Validation of a health status measure. Med. Care 14:57–67, 1976.
7. Bergner, M., Bobbitt, S. K., Pollard, W. E., et al.: The Sickness Impact Profile: Conceptual formulation and methodology for the development of a health status measure. Int. J. Health Serv. 6:393–415, 1976.
8. Bergner, M., Bobbitt, R. A., Carter, W. B., and Gilson, B. S.: The Sickness Impact Profile: Development and final revision of a health status measure. Med. Care 19:787–805, 1981.
9. Bergner, M.: Measurement of health status. Med. Care 23:696–704, 1985.
10. Bergner, M., and Rothman, M. L.: Health status measures: An overview and guide for selection. Annu. Rev. Public Health 8:191–210, 1987.
11. Bindman, A. B., Keane, D., and Lurie, N.: Measuring health changes among severely ill patients. Med. Care 28:1142–1152 1990.
12. Binkley, J., Finch, E., Hall, J., et al.: Diagnostic classification of patients with low back pain: Report on a survey of physical therapy experts. Phys. Ther. 73:138–155, 1993.
13. Boston, J. R., Rudy, T. E., and Kubinski, J. A.: Multiple statistical comparisons: Fishing with the right bait. J. Crit. Care 6:211–220, 1991.
14. Brodman, K., Erdmann, A. J., Lorge, I., and Wolff, H. G.: The Cornell Medical Index: An adjunct to medical interview. JAMA 140:530–534, 1949.
15. Brodman, K., Erdmann, A. J., Lorge, I., and Wolff, H. G.: The Cornell Medical Index–Health Questionnaire. JAMA 145:152–157, 1951.
16. Brook, R. H., Davies-Avery, A., Greenfield, S., et al.: Assessing the quality of medical care using outcome measures: An overview of the method. Med. Care 15:1–155, 1977.
17. Brorsson, B., and Asberg, K. H.: Katz Index of Independence in ADL: Reliability and validity in short-term care. Scand. J. Rehabil. Med. 16:125–132, 1984.
18. Brown, J. H., Kazis, L. E., Spitz, P. W., et al.: The dimensions of health outcomes: A cross-validated examination of health status measurement. Am. J. Public Health 74:159–161, 1984.
19. Budiman-Mak, E., Conrad, K. J., and Roach, K. E.: The foot function index: A measure of foot pain and disability. J. Clin. Epidemid. 44:561–570, 1991.
20. Bunderson, C. V., Inouye, D. K., Olsen, J. B.: The four generations of computerized educational measurement. In Linn, R. L. (ed.): Educational Measurement, 3rd ed. New York; Macmillan, 1989, pp. 367–408.
21. Burns, R. B., Moskowitz, M. A., Ash, A., et al.: Self-report versus medical record functional status. Med. Care 30:MS85–95, 1992.
22. Callahan, L. F., Smith, W. J. and Pincus, T.: Self-report questionnaire in five rheumatic diseases. Arthritis Care Res. 33:122–131, 1989.
23. Callahan, L. F., and Pincus, T.: A clue from a self-report questionnaire to distinguish rheumatoid arthritis from noninflammatory diffuse musculoskeletal pain. Arthritis Rheum. 33:1317–1322, 1990.
24. Campbell, D. T., and Fiske, D. W.: Convergent and divergent validity by the multitrait-multimethod matrix. Psychol. Bull. 56:81–105, 1959.
25. Campbell, W. I., and Lewis S.: Visual analogue measurement of pain. Ulster Med. J. 59:149–154, 1990.
26. Chalmers, T. C., Celan, P., Sacks, E. S., and Smith, H. J.: Bias in treatment assignment in controlled clinical trials. N. Engl. J. Med. 309:1358–1361, 1983.
27. Chambers, L. W., Haight, M., Norman, G., and MacDonald, L.: Sensitivity to change and the effect of mode of administration on health status measurement. Med. Care 25:470–479, 1987.
28. Chambers, L. W.: The McMaster Health Index Questionnaire: An update. In Walker, S. R., and Rosser, R. M. (eds.): Quality of Life: Assessment and Application. Boston, MTP Press, 1988, pp. 113–131.
29. Cleary, P. D., Goldberg, J. D. Kessler, L. G., and Nycz, G. R.: Screening for mental disorder among primary care patients. Arch. Gen. Psychiatry 39:837–840, 1982.
30. Co, Y. Y., Eaton, S., and Maxwell, M. W.: The relationship between the St. Thomas and Oswes-

try disability scores and the severity of low back pain. J. Manipulative Physiol. Ther. 16:14–18, 1993.
31. Colditz, G. A., Miller, J. N., and Mosteller, F.: How study design affects outcomes in comparisons of therapy: I. Medical. Stat. Med. 8:441–445, 1989.
32. Collen, M. F., Cutler, J. L., Siegelaub, A. B., and Cella, R. L.: Reliability of a self administered medical questionnaire. Arch. Intern. Med. 123:664–671, 1969.
33. Coons, S. J., Kaplan, R. M.: Quality of life assessment: Understanding its use as an outcome measure. Hosp. Formul. 28:486–498, 1993.
34. Crewe, N. M., Athelstan, G. T., and Meadows, G. K.: Vocational diagnosis through assessment of functional limitations. Arch. Phys. Med. Rehabil. 56:513–516, 1975.
35. Cronbach, L. J.: Coefficient alpha and the internal structure of tests. Psychometrika 16:297–334, 1951.
36. Cunny, K. A., and Perri, M.: Single-item vs multiple-item measures of health-related quality of life. Psychol. Rep. 69:127–130, 1991.
37. Dawes, R. M.: Suppose we measured height with rating scales instead of rulers. Appl. Psychol. Meas. 41:687–699, 1977.
38. DeBruin, A. F., DeWitte, L. P., Stevens, F., and Diederiks, J. P. M.: Sickness Impact Profile: The state of the art of a generic functional status measure. Soc. Sci. Med. 35:1003–1014, 1992.
39. Demjen, S., and Bakal, D.: Illness behavior and chronic headache. Pain 10:221–229, 1981.
40. Dennis, M. D., Greene, R. L., Farr, S. P., and Hartman, J. T.: The Minnesota Multiphasic Personality Inventory: General guidelines to its use and interpretation in orthopaedics. Clin. Orthop. 150:125–130, 1980.
41. Densen, P. M., Danehy, L., Flagle, C. D., and Katz, S.: Functioning status assessment form. *In* Ward, M. J. and Lindeman, C. A. (eds.): Instruments for Measuring Nursing Practice and Other Health Care Variables. Washington, DC, U.S. Government Printing Office, 1979, pp. 419–421.
42. Deyo, R. A., Inui, T. S., Leininger, J., and Overman, S.: Physical and psychosocial function in rheumatoid arthritis: Clinical use of a self-administered health status instrument. Arch. Intern. Med. 142:879–882, 1982.
43. Deyo, R. A., and Diehl, A. K.: Measuring physical and psychosocial function in patients with low-back pain. Spine 8:635–642, 1983.
44. Deyo, R. A., Inui, T. S., Leininger, J. D., and Overman, S. S.: Measuring functional outcomes in chronic disease: A comparison of traditional scales and a self-administered health status questionnaire in patients with rheumatoid arthritis. Med. Care 21:180–192, 1983.
45. Deyo, R. A.: Measuring functional outcomes in therapeutic trials for chronic disease. Controlled Clin. Trials 5:223–240, 1984.
46. Deyo, R. A.: Pitfalls in measuring the health status of Mexican Americans: Comparative validity of the English and Spanish Sickness Impact Profile. Am. J. Public Health 74:569–573, 1984.
47. Deyo, R. A., and Inui, T. S.: Toward clinical applications of health status measures: Sensitivity of scales to clinically important changes. Health Serv. Res. 19:275–289, 1984.
48. Deyo, R. A.: Comparative validity of the Sickness Impact Profile and shorter scales for functional assessment in low-back pain. Spine 11:951–954, 1986.
49. Deyo, R. A., and Centor, R. M.: Assessing the responsiveness of functional scales to clinical change: An analogy to diagnostic test performance. J. Chronic Dis. 39:897–906, 1986.
50. Deyo, R. A., and Patrick, D. L.: Barriers to the use of health status measures in clinical investigation, patient care, and policy research. Med. Care 27:S254–S268, 1989.
51. Dirks, J. F., Wunder, J., Kinsman, R., et al.: A Pain Rating Scale and a Pain Behavior Checklist for clinical use: Development, norms, and the consistency score. Psychother. Psychosom. 59:41–49, 1993.
52. Donaldson, S. W., Wagner, C. C., and Gresham, G. E.: A unified ADL evaluation form. Arch. Phys. Med. Rehabil. 54:175–179, 1973.
53. Dubro, A. F., and Wetzler, S.: An external validity study of the MMPI personality disorder scales. J. Counsel. Psychol. 45:570–575, 1989.
54. Duncan, G. H., Gregg, J. M., and Ghia, J. N.: The pain profile: A computerized system of assessment of chronic pain. Pain 5:275–284, 1978.
55. Edwards, L. C., Pearce, S. A., Turner-Stokes, L., and Jones, A.: The Pain Beliefs Questionnaire: An investigation of beliefs in the causes and consequences of pain. Pain 51:267–272, 1992.
56. Ellermeier, W., Westphal, W., and Heidenfelder, M.: On the "absoluteness" of category and magnitude scales of pain. Percept. Psychophys. 49:159–166, 1991.
57. Emerson, J. D., Burdick, E., and Hoaglin, D. C., et al.: An empirical study of the possible relations of treatment differences to quality, scores in controlled randomized clinical trials. Controlled Clin. Trials 11:339–352, 1990.
58. Evans, J. H., and Kagan, A. II: The development of a functional rating scale to measure the treatment outcome of chronic spinal patients. Spine 11:277–281, 1986.
59. Fairbank, J. C. T., Mboat, J. C., Davies, J. B., O'Brien, J. P.: The Oswestry Low Back Pain Disability Questionnaire. Physiotherapy 66:271–273, 1980.
60. Feldstein, A., Valanis, B., and Vollmer, W., et al.: The back injury prevention project pilot study: Assessing the effectiveness of back attack, an injury prevention program among nurses, aides, and orderlies. J. Occup. Med. 35:114–120, 1993.
61. Feldt, L. S., and Brennan, R. L.: Reliability. *In* Linn, R. L. (ed): Educational Measurement, 3rd ed. New York, Macmillan, 1989, pp. 105–146.
62. Fernandez, E., Nygren, T. E., and Thorn, B. E.: An "open-transformed scale" for correcting ceiling effects and enhancing retest reliability: The example of pain. Percept. Psychophys. 49:572–578, 1991.
63. Ferrans, C. E., and Powers, M. J.: Quality of Life Index: Development and psychometric properties. Adv. Nurs. Sci. 8:15–24, 1985.
64. Ferrans, C. E.: Development of a Quality of Life Index for patients with cancer. Oncol. Nurs. Forum 17(suppl.):15–21, 1990.
65. Ferrans, C. E., and Powers, M. J.: Psychometric assessment of the Quality of Life Index. Res. Nurs. Health 15:29–38, 1992.

66. Fillenbaum, G. G., and Smyer, M. A.: The development, validity, and reliability of the OARS Multidimensional Functional Assessment Questionnaire. J. Gerontol. 36:428–434, 1981.
67. Follick, M. J., Smith, T. W., and Ahern, D. K.: The Sickness Impact Profile: A global measure of disability in chronic low back pain. Pain 21:67–76, 1985.
68. Fries, J. F., Spitz, P., Kraines, R. G., and Holman, H. R.: Measurement of patient outcome in arthritis. Arthritis Rheum. 23:137–145, 1980.
69. Fries, J. F., Spitz, P. W., and Young, D. Y.: The dimensions of health outcomes: The Health Assessment Questionnaire, disability and pain scales. J. Rheumatol. 9:789–793, 1982.
70. Garrad, J., and Bennett A. E.: A validated interview schedule for use in population surveys of chronic disease and disability. Br. J. Prev. Soc. Med. 25:97–104, 1971.
71. Goldberg, D. P., Rickels, K., Downing, R., and Hesbacher, P.: A comparison of two psychiatric screening tests. Br. J. Psychiatry 129:61–67, 1976.
72. Goldberg, D. P., and Hillier, V. F.: A scaled version of the General Health Questionnaire. Psychol. Med. 9:139–145, 1979.
73. Gracely, R. H.: Evaluation of multi-dimensional pain scales. Pain 48:297–300, 1992.
74. Granger, C. V., Albrecht, G. L., and Hamilton, B. B.: Outcome of comprehensive medical rehabilitation: Measurement by PULSES Profile and the Barthel Index. Arch. Phys. Med. Rehabil. 60:5–154, 1979.
75. Greenwald, H. P.: The specificity of quality-of-life measures among the seriously ill. Med. Care 25:642–651, 1987.
76. Gronblad, M., Lukinmaa, A., and Konttinen, Y. T.: Chronic low-back pain: Intercorrelation of repeated measures for pain and disability. Scand. J. Rehabil. Med. 22:73–77, 1990.
77. Gurel, L., Linn, M. W., and Linn, B. S.: Physical and mental impairment-of-function evaluation in the aged: The PAMIE scale. J. Gerontol. 27:83–90, 1972.
78. Gurland, B., Kuriansky, J., Sharpe, L., et al.: The Comprehensive Assessment and Referral Evaluation (CARE)—rationale, development, and reliability. Int. J. Aging Hum. Dev. 8:9–42, 1977–78.
79. Haas, M., and Nyiendo, J.: Diagnostic utility of the McGill Pain Questionnaire and the Oswestry Disability Questionnaire for classification of low back pain syndromes. J. Manipulative Physiol. Ther. 15:90–98, 1992.
80. Harvey, R. F., and Jellinek, H. M.: Functional performance assessment: A program approach. Arch. Phys. Med. Rehabil. 62:456–461, 1981.
81. Hathaway, S. R., and McKinley, J. C.: A multiphasic personality schedule (Minnesota): I. Construction of the schedule. J. Psychol. 10:249–254, 1940.
82. Heaton, R. K., Getto, C. J., Lehman, R. A. W., et al.: A standardized evaluation of psychosocial factors in chronic pain. Pain 12(suppl.):165–174, 1982.
83. Holroyd, K. A., Holm, J. E., Keefe, F. J., et al.: A multi-center evaluation of the McGill Pain Questionnaire: Results from more than 1700 chronic pain patients. Pain 48:301–311, 1992.
84. Hunsley, J., Hanson, R. K., and Parker, K. C. H.: A summary of the reliability and stability of the MMPI scales. J. Counsel. Psychol. 44:44–46, 1988.
85. Hunt, S. M., McKenna, S. P., and McEwen, J., et al.: The Nottingham Health Profile: Subjective health status and medical consultations. Soc. Sci. Med. 15A:221–229, 1981.
86. Jacobson, N. S., Follette, W. C., and Revenstorf, D.: Psychotherapy outcome research: Methods for reporting variability and evaluating clinical significance. Behav. Ther. 15:336–352, 1984.
87. Jaeschke, R., Singer, J., and Guyatt, G. H.: Measurement of health status ascertaining the minimally clinically important difference. Med. Care 10:407–415, 1989.
88. Jensen, M. P., Karoly, P., and Braver, S.: The measurement of clinical pain intensity: A comparison of six methods. Pain 27:117–126, 1986.
89. Jensen, M. P., Strom, S. E., Turner, J. A., and Romano, J. M.: Validity of the Sickness Impact Profile Roland Scale as a measure of dysfunction in chronic pain patients. Pain 50:157–162, 1992.
90. Jensen, M. P., and McFarland, C. A.: Increasing the reliability and validity of pain intensity measurement in chronic pain patients. Pain 55:195–203, 1993.
91. Jerome, A., and Gross, R. T.: Pain Disability Index: Construct and discriminant validity. Arch. Phys. Med. Rehabil. 72:920–922, 1991.
92. Jette, A. M., and Deniston, O. L.: Inter-observer reliability of a functional status assessment instrument. J. Chronic Dis. 31:573–580, 1978.
93. Jette, A. M.: Functional Status Index: Reliability of a chronic disease evaluation instrument. Arch. Phys. Med. Rehabil. 61:395–401, 1980.
94. Jette, A. M.: The Functional Status Index: Reliability and validity of a self-report functional disability measure. J. Rheumatol. 14(suppl. 15):15–19, 1987.
95. Johnson, E. J.: Outcome measures . . . A chimera? Am. J. Phys. Med. Rehabil. 71:201, 1992.
96. Kaplan, R. M., Bush, J. W., and Berry, C. C.: Health status: Types of validity and the Index of Well-Being. Health Serv. Res. 11:478–507, 1976.
97. Kaplan, R. M., Coons, S. J., and Anderson, J. P.: Quality of life and policy analysis in arthritis. Arthritis Care Res. 5:173–183, 1992.
98. Kaplan, R. M., Anderson, J. P., and Ganiats, T. G.: The quality of well-being scale: Rationale for a single quality of life index. In Walker, S. R., and Rosser, R. M., (eds.): Quality of Life Assessment: Key Issues in the 1990s. Norwell, MA, Kluwer Academic Publishers, 1993, pp. 65–93.
99. Katz, S., Ford, A. B., Moskowitz, R. W., et al.: Studies of illness in the aged: The Index of ADL: A standardized measure of biological and psychosocial function. JAMA 185:914–919, 1963.
100. Katz, S., and Akpom, C. A.: Index of ADL. Med. Care 14:116–118, 1976.
101. Katz, S.: Index of Independence in Activities of Daily Living (Index of ADL). In Ward, M. J., and Lindeman, C. A. (eds.): Instruments for Measuring Nursing Practice and other Health Care Variables. Washington, DC, U.S. Government Printing Office, 1979, pp. 275–280.
102. Keller, C.: Psychological and physical variables as predictors of coping strategies. Percept. Mot. Skills 67:95–100, 1988.
103. Kempen, G. I. J. M.: The MOS short-form general health survey: Single item vs multiple measures of health-related quality of life: Some nuances. Psychol. Rep. 70:608–610, 1992.

104. Kerns, R. D., Turk, D. C., and Rudy, T. E.: The West Haven–Yale Multidimensional Pain Inventory (WHYMPI). Pain 23:345–356, 1985.
105. Kerns, R. D., Haythornthwaite, J., Rosenberg, R., et. al.: The Pain Behavior Check List (PBCL): Factor structure and psychometric properties. J. Behav. Med. 14:155–167, 1991.
106. Kramer, J. J., and Conoley, J. C. (eds.): The Eleventh Mental Measurement Yearbook. Lincoln, NE, University of Nebraska Press, 1992.
107. Kubinski, J. A., Rudy, T. E., and Boston, J. R.: Research design and analysis: The many faces of validity. J. Crit. Care 6:143–151, 1991.
108. Langley, G. B., and Sheppeard, H.: The Visual Analogue Scale: Its use in pain measurement. Rheumatol. Int. 5:145–148, 1985.
109. Lawlis, G. F., Cuencas, R., Selby, D., and McCoy, C. E.: The development of the Dallas Pain Questionnaire: An assessment of the impact of spinal pain on behavior. Spine 14:511–516, 1989.
110. Lawton, M. P., Moss, M., Fulcomer, M., and Kleban, M. H.: A research and service oriented multilevel assessment instrument. J. Gerontol. 37:91–99, 1982.
111. Leavitt, F.: Predicting disability time using formal low back pain measurement: The low back pain simulation scale. J. Psychosom. Res. 35:599–607, 1991.
112. Leboeuf, C., Love, A., and Crisp, T. C.: Chiropractic chronic low back pain sufferers and self-report assessment methods: Part II. A reliability study of the Middlesex Hospital Questionnaire and the VAS Disability Scales Questionnaire. J. Manipulative Physiol. Ther. 12:109–112, 1989.
113. Liang, M. H., Fossel, A. H., and Larson, M. G.: Comparisons of five health status instruments for orthopaedic evaluation. Med. Care 28:632–642, 1990.
114. Liang, M. H., Larson, M. G., Cullen, K. E., and Schwartz, J. A.: Comparative measurement efficiency and sensitivity of five health status instruments for arthritis research. Arthritis Rheum. 28:542–547, 1985.
115. Little, D. G., and MacDonald, D.: The Oswestry Disability Index in lumbar spinal surgery: Improvement in index versus subjective improvement. Read at the Annual Meeting of The Spine Society of Australia, 1992.
116. Love, A., Leboeuf, C., Crisp, T. C.: Chiropractic chronic low back pain sufferers and self-report assessment methods: Part I. A reliability study of the Visual Analogue Scale, the Pain Drawing and the McGill Pain Questionnaire. J. Manipulative Physiol. Ther. 12:21–25, 1989.
117. Lowe, N. K., Noble Walker, S., and MacCallum, R. C.: Confirming the theoretical structure of the McGill Pain Questionnaire in acute clinical pain. Pain 46:53–60, 1991.
118. MacKenzie, C. R., Charlson, M. E., DiGioia, D., and Kelley, K.: Can the Sickness Impact Profile measure change: An example of scale assessment. J. Chronic Dis. 39:429–438, 1986.
119. Mahoney, F. I., and Barthel, D. W.: Functional evaluation: The Barthel Index. M. Med. J. 14:61–65, 1965.
120. Main, C. J., Wood, P. L. R., Hollis, S., et al.: The distress and risk assessment method: A simple patient classification to identify distress and evaluate the risk of poor outcome. Spine 17:42–52, 1992.
121. Margoles, M.: The Pain Chart: Spatial properties of pain. In Melzack, R. (ed.): Pain Measurement and Assessment. New York, Raven Press, 1983, pp. 215–225.
122. Martin, M. J., Mayne, J. G., Taylor, W. F., and Swenson, M. N.: A health questionnaire based on paper-and-pencil medium, individualized and produced by computer: II. Testing and evaluation. JAMA 208:2064–2068, 1969.
123. Mayne, J. G., Martin, M. J., and Morrow, G. W., et al.: A health questionnaire based on paper-and-pencil medium, individualized and produced by computer. JAMA 208:2060–2063, 1969.
124. McCombre, P. F., Fairbank, J. C. T., Cockersole, B. C., and Pynsent, P. B.: Reproducibility of physical signs in low-back pain. Spine 14:908–918, 1989.
125. McDowell, I., and Newell, C.: Measuring Health: A Guide to Rating Scales and Questionnaires. New York, Oxford University Press, 1987.
126. McGuire, D. B.: Measuring pain. In Frank-Stromborg, M. (ed.): Instruments for Clinical Nursing Research. Norwalk, CT, Appleton & Lange, 1988, pp. 333–356.
127. McHorney, C. A., Ware, J. E., Jr., and Raczek, A. E.: The MOS 36-item short-form health survey (SF-36): II. Psychometric and clinical tests of validity in measuring physical and mental health constructs. Med. Care 31:247–263, 1993.
128. McHorney, C. A., Ware, J. E. Jr, and Rogers, W., et al.: The validity and relative precision of MOS short- and long-form health status scales and Dartmouth coop charts. Med. Care 30:MS253–265, 1992.
129. Meenan, R. F., Gertman, P. M., and Mason, J. H.: Measuring health status in arthritis. Arthritis Rheum. 23:146–152, 1980.
130. Melzack, R.: The McGill Pain Questionnaire: Major properties and scoring methods. Pain 1:277–299, 1975.
131. Melzack, R., and Torgerson, W. S.: On the language of pain. Anesthesiology 34:50–59, 1971.
132. Melzack, R.: Pain Measurement and Assessment. New York, Raven Press, 1983.
133. Melzack, R.: The short-form McGill Pain Questionnaire. Pain 30:191–197, 1987.
134. Metzner, H., and Mann, F.: A limited comparison of two methods of data collection: The fixed alternative questionnaire and the open-ended interview. Am. Soc. Rev. 17:486–491, 1952.
135. Millard, R. W., and Jones, R. H.: Construct validity of practical questionnaires for assessing disability of low-back pain. Spine 16:835–838, 1991.
136. Miller, J. E.: Guidelines for selecting a health status index: Suggested criteria. In Berg, R. L. (ed.): Health Status Indexes. Chicago, IL, Hospital Research and Education Trust, 1973, pp. 243–251.
137. Million, R., Hall, W., and Haavik Nilsen, K., et al.: Assessment of the progress of the back-pain patient. Spine 7:204–212, 1982.
138. Monks, R., and Taenzer, P.: A comprehensive pain questionnaire. In Melzack, R. (ed.): Pain Measurement and Assessment. New York, Raven Press, 1983, pp. 233–237.
139. Myers, A. M.: The clinical Swiss army knife: Empirical evidence on the validity of IADL functional status measures. Med. Care 30:MS96–MS111, 1992.

140. Nelson, E. C., and Berwick, D. M.: The measurement of health status in clinical practice. Med. Care 27:S77–90, 1989.
141. Novick, M. R. (ed.): Standards for Educational and Psychological Testing. Washington, DC, American Psychological Association, 1985.
142. Oxman, A. D., and Guyatt, G. H.: A consumer's guide to subgroup analysis. Ann. Intern. Med. 116:78–84, 1992.
143. Parkerson, G. R., Broadhead, W. E., and Tse, C. K.: The Duke Health Profile: A 17-item measure of health and dysfunction. Med. Care 28:1056–1069, 1990.
144. Parkerson, G. R., Broadhead, W. E., and Tse, C. K.: Comparison of the Duke Health Profile and the MOS short form in health young adults. Med. Care 29:679–683, 1991.
145. Parkerson, G. R., Gehlbach, S. H., and Wagner, E. H., et al.: The Duke-UNC Health Profile: An adult health status instrument for primary care. Med. Care 19:806–828, 1981
146. Patrick, D. L., Bush, J. W., and Chen, M. M.: Methods for measuring levels of well-being for a health status index. Health Serv. Res. 8:228–245, 1973.
147. Peach, H., Green, S., and Locker, D., et al.: Evaluation of a postal screening questionnaire to identify the physically disabled. Int. Rehab. Med. 2:189–193, 1980.
148. Pilowsky, I., and Spence, N. D.: Is illness behaviour related to chronicity in patients with intractable pain? Pain 2:167–173, 1976.
149. Pilowsky, I., and Spence, N. D.: Pain and illness behaviour: A comparative study. J. Psychosom. Res. 20:131–134, 1976.
150. Pilowsky, I., and Spence, N. D.: Pain, anger and illness behaviour. J. Psychosom. Res. 20:411–416, 1976.
151. Pilowsky, I., Bassett, D., Barrett, R., et al.: The Illness Behavior Assessment Schedule: Reliability and validity. Int. J. Psychiatry Med. 13:11–28, 1983.
152. Pincus, T., Callahan, L. F., and Vaughn, W. K.: Questionnaire, walking time and button test measures of functional capacity as predictive markers for mortality in rheumatoid arthritis. J. Rheumatol. 14:240–251, 1987.
153. Pincus, T., Callahan, L. F., Brooks, R. H., et al.: Self-report questionnaire scores in rheumatoid arthritis compared with traditional physical radiographic, and laboratory measures. Ann. Intern. Med. 10:259–266, 1989.
154. Pollard, W. E., Bobbitt, R. A., Bergner, M., et al.: The Sickness Impact Profile: Reliability of a health status measure. Med. Care 14:146–155, 1976.
155. Radosevich, D. M., Wetzler, H., and Wilson, S. M.: Health Status Questionnaire (HSQ) 2.0: Scoring comparisons and reference data. Bloomington, MN, Health Outcomes Institute, 1994.
156. Read, J. L., Quinn, R. J., and Hoefer, M. A.: Measuring overall health: An evaluation of three important approaches. J. Chronic Dis. 40(suppl. 1):7S–21S, 1987.
157. Reading, A. E.: A comparison of pain rating scales. J. Psychosom. Res. 24:119–124, 1980.
158. Riesenberg, D., and Glass, R. M.: The medical outcomes study. JAMA 262:943, 1989.
159. Robinson, J. P., Shaver, P. R., and Wrightsman, L. S. (eds.): Measures of Personality and Social Psychological Attitudes. San Diego, CA, Academic Press, 1991.
160. Roland, M., and Morris, R.: A study of the natural history of back pain: Part I: Development of a reliable and sensitive measure of disability in low-back pain. Spine 8:141–144, 1983.
161. Sanders, S. H.: Cross-validation of the Back Pain Classification Scale with chronic, intractable pain patients. Pain 22:271–277, 1985.
162. Schmid, A. A., Kiene, W., and Updegraff, G.: Health Status Questionnaire. In Ward, M. J., and Lindeman, C. A. (eds.): Instruments for Measuring Nursing Practice and other Health Care Variables. Washington, DC, U.S. Government Printing Office, 1979, pp. 397–404.
163. Schoening, H. A., Anderegg, L., Bergstrom, D., et al.: Numerical scoring of self-care status of patients. Arch. Phys. Med. Rehabil. 46:689–697, 1965.
164. Shaffer, W. O., Spratt, K. F., Weinstein, J. N., et al.: The reliability and validity of roentgenograms for measuring sagittal translation in the lumbar vertebral motion segment. Spine 15:741–750, 1990.
165. Sherbourne, C. D., and Stewart, A. L.: The MOS social support survey. Soc. Sci. Med. 32:705–714, 1991.
166. Spector, W. D., Katz, S., Murphy, J. B., and Fulton, J. P.: The hierarchical relationship between Activities of Daily Living and Instrumental Activities of Daily Living. J. Chronic Dis. 40:481–489, 1987.
167. Spratt, K. F., Lehmann, T. R., Weinstein, J. N., and Sayre, H. A.: A new approach to the low-back physical examination: Behavioral assessment of mechanical signs. Spine 15:96–102, 1990.
168. Sternbach, R. A., Wolf, S. R., Murphy, R. W., and Akeson, W. H.: Traits of pain patients: The low-back "loser." Psychosomatics 14:226–229, 1973.
169. Stewart, A. L., Hays, R. D., and Ware, J. E. Jr.: The MOS short-form general health survey: Reliability and validity in a patient population. Med. Care 26:724–735, 1988.
170. Stewart, A. L., Greenfield, S., Hays, R. D., et al.: Functional status and well-being of patients with chronic conditions. JAMA 262:907–913, 1989.
171. Streiner, D. L., and Norman, G. R.: Health measure scales: A practice guide to their development and use. Oxford, UK, Oxford Press, 1989.
172. Tait, R. C., Pollard, C. A., Margolis, R. B., et al.: The Pain Disability Index: Psychometric and validity data. Arch. Phys. Med. Rehabil. 68:925–930, 1987.
173. Tait, R. C., Chibnall, J. T., and Krause, S.: The Pain Disability Index: Psychometric properties. Pain 40:171–182, 1990.
174. Tarlov, A. R., Ware, J. E., Jr., and Greenfield, S., et al.: The medical outcomes study: An application of methods for monitoring the results of medical care. JAMA 262:925–930, 1989.
175. Tarnopolsky, A., Hand, D. J., McLean, E. K., et al.: Validity and uses of a screening questionnaire (GHQ) in the community. Br. J. Psychiatry 134:508–515, 1979.
176. Triano, J. J., McGregor, M., Cramer, G. D., and Emde, D. L.: A comparison of outcome measures for use with back pain patients: Results of a feasibility study. J. Manipulative Physiol. Ther. 16:67–73, 1993.

177. Turk, D. C., and Rudy, T. E.: Neglected factors in chronic pain treatment outcome studies—referral patterns, failure to enter treatment, and attrition. Pain 43:7–25, 1990.
178. Turk, D. C., and Rudy, T. E.: Neglected topics in the treatment of chronic pain patients—relapse, noncompliance, and adherence enhancement. Pain 44:5–28, 1991.
179. Turk, D. C., Rudy, T. E., and Sorkin, B. A.: Neglected topics in chronic pain treatment outcome studies: Determination of success. Pain 53:3–16, 1993.
180. Tursky, B., Jamner, L. D., and Friedman, R.: The Pain Perception Profile: A psychophysical approach to the assessment of pain report. Behav. Ther. 13:376–394, 1982.
181. Waddell, G., and Richardson, J.: Observation of overt pain behaviour by physicians during routine clinical examination of patients with low back pain. J. Psychosom. Res. 36:77–87, 1992.
182. Waddell, G., Newton, M., and Henderson, I., et al.: A Fear Avoidance Beliefs Questionnaire (FABQ) and the role of fear-avoidance beliefs in chronic low back pain and disability. Pain 52:157–168, 1993.
183. Ware, J. E., Jr., Davies-Avery, A., and Brook, R. H.: Conceptualization and Measurement of Health for Adults in the Health Insurance Study: Vol VI. Analysis of Relationships Amoung Health Status Measures. Santa Monica, CA, Rand Corporation, 1980.
184. Ware, J. E., Jr.: General health rating index. In Wenger, N. K., Mattson, M., Furburg, C. D., and Elinson, J. (eds.): Assessment of Quality of Life in Clinical Trials of Cardiovascular Disease. New York, LeJacq Publishing, 1984, pp. 184–188.
185. Ware, J. E., Jr.: Standards for validating health measures: Definition and content. J. Chronic Dis. 40:473–480, 1987.
186. Ware, J. E., Jr., and Sherbourne, C. D.: The MOS 36-item short-form health survey (SF-36): I. Conceptual framework and item selection. Med. Care 30:473–483, 1992.
187. Watt-Watson, J. H., and Graydon, J. E.: Sickness Impact Profile: A measure of dysfunction with chronic pain patients. J. Pain Symptom Manage. 4:152–156, 1989.
188. Wennberg, J.: Small area variations in health care delivery. Science 182:1102–1108, 1973.
189. Wesley, L., Gatchel, R. J., and Polatin, P. B., et al.: Differentiation between somatic and cognitive/affective components in commonly used measurements of depression in patients with chronic low-back pain: Let's not mix apples and oranges. Spine 16:S213–215, 1991.
190. Wilkie, D. J., Savedra, M. C., and Holzemer, W. L., et al.: Use of the McGill Pain Questionnaire to measure pain: A meta-analysis. Nurs. Res. 39:36–41, 1990.
191. Williams, A. C. de C., and Richardson, P. H.: What does the BDI measure in chronic pain? Pain 55:259–266, 1993.
192. Wolfe, F., Kleinheksel, S. M., Cathey, M. A., et al.: The clinical value of the Stanford Health Assessment Questionnaire Functional Disability Index in patients with rheumatoid arthritis. J. Rheumatol. 15:1480–1488, 1988.
193. Wolfe, F., and Pincus, T.: Standard self-report questionnaires in routine clinical and research practice—an opportunity for patients and rheumatologists. J. Rheumatol. 18:643–645, 1991.
194. Wu, A. W., Rubin, H. R., and Matthews, W. C., et al.: A health status questionnaire using 30 items from the medical outcomes study: Preliminary validation in persons with early HIV infection. Med. Care 29:786–798, 1991.
195. Young, D. W.: Comparison of information collected by a questionary with that in the patient's hospital record. Methods Inf. Med. 11:20–22, 1972.
196. Zung, W. W. K.: A self-rating depression scale. Arch. Gen. Psychiatry 12:63–70, 1965.
197. Zung, W. W. K.: A self-rating pain and distress scale. Psychosomatics 24:887–894, 1983.

26

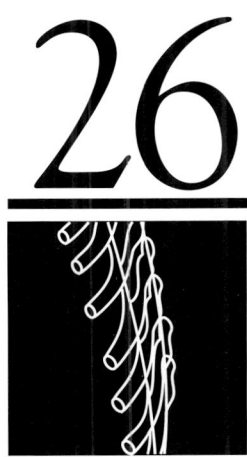

The Ethics of Spine Care

CHARLES V. BURTON

In today's world, the ethics of medical care are more often determined by sociologic and governmental, rather than medical, influences. External effects on medical practice are typically more visible in socialist than in free-enterprise systems, but this analysis may be deceptive because free-enterprise systems can become so controlled and regulated that freedom of medical practice may not be possible. The truly important issue, however, from the patient's standpoint, is not related to the nature of the system; it is a relatively simple and straightforward question, Is the health care provided really reflecting the patient's best interest?

It is increasingly evident that many of the socialized health care systems in the western world have engendered overwhelming and unsustainable economic burdens, long patient waits for service, increased patient dissatisfaction, inefficient delivery of modern health care technology, and poor incentives for health care providers to remain productive. These systems, however, have also provided uniform and consistent basic care for their populations, who have tended to believe that their system was primarily directed to their personal benefit. This perception is now undergoing significant change.

Is there really a health care crisis in the United States? Some investigators have suggested that, although there are significant problems that need attention, an actual crisis does not exist.[33] Is the expenditure of 14% of the gross domestic product for health care unreasonable if the public receives value? The basic problems with health care in the United States today really appear to reflect the following needs:

- To decrease the overall cost of health care
- To guarantee universal basic medical care for infants and children
- To provide the means by which adults can spend their own money for health care
- To provide catastrophic health insurance coverage for all
- To continue high-quality specialty care with associated patient freedom of choice
- To continue technologic leadership while also limiting the abuse of new technology
- To maintain ethical medical practices based on truth and integrity
- To maintain the patient's best interest over that of the physician, payer, or government
- To strive continually to maintain a high level of patient satisfaction regarding health care
- To develop practical means of outcome measurement
- To focus on medical management designed to make the patient independent of the health care system

CONFLICTS OF INTEREST IN DECISION-MAKING

Few medical environments have, in the past, better reflected the hippocratic ethic of "physicians practicing medicine primarily for their patient's benefit" than the state of Minnesota. Unfortunately for the patient, adversarial political influences have been at work to change this situation. With the advent of Health Maintenance Organizations (HMOs) and managed care systems, deviations from the hippocratic ethic of medical care have been increasingly evident. This insidious phenomenon has been described as the "veterinarian ethic."[31] Veterinarians do not owe their primary obligation to the animal but to the owner, who pays the bill. Increasingly, in the United States, patients are being directed into new types of health delivery systems in which the primary interest of the physicians is different from that of the patient, thus creating a conflict of interest related to health care delivery. Some physician "gatekeepers" are now being paid on the basis of how much care they deny rather than how much they provide. A similarly disturbing example is the fact that in many HMOs, a physician who refers a patient to an out-of-network specialist may have his or her personal compensation reduced by the cost difference between that specialist and an in-network specialist.

When this situation is considered on a global basis, participants in the socialist medical systems, in which all employed in health care work for the government, believe that their system eliminates the possibility of conflict of physician interest. It is their belief that the fee for service capitalist medical systems have the potentially adverse influence of personal financial gain, which is likely to place the physicians' financial interest ahead of care of the patient. In fact, however, if the litmus test of the hippocratic versus veterinary care ethic is applied, no current health care system can guarantee an absence of potential conflict in regard to the patient's best interest. Conflicts of interest in health care seem to more often reflect the professional ethics of the community and the prevailing social and medical educational systems than adherence to generally accepted standards.

The ethical dilemmas inherent in veterinary rather than hippocratic care become even more complex when the physician recommends treatment in the best interest of the patient only to have a third-party payer reject or modify this recommendation. This phenomenon, which is becoming more common, creates serious ethical dilemmas. Sometimes only a portion of a therapy or surgical procedure may be approved. What legal liability do treating physicians incur if they prescribe a course of therapy directed by another party rather than by themselves? In addition, who is then responsible for treatment decisions that go wrong? If a third-party payer denies payment or reimbursement to a patient who cannot otherwise afford treatment, is the payer determining care and thus assuming legal responsibility for the consequences? Third-party payers are saying they are not. They state that they are simply making decisions on benefit eligibility. On the basis of ERISA (Employee Retirement Income Security Act), United States federal legislation passed in 1974 to regulate pension and welfare benefits, some courts in the United States have swept away state laws that ordinarily provide a remedy for wrongful conduct and have sided with the third-party payers in this regard.[25]

When medically prescribed treatment is denied or modified by a health insurance system or a third-party payer, the physician's responsibility to the patient remains unchanged, but the physician may also be precluded from providing the appropriate care. If what is permitted by the payer represents a significant departure from what is the accepted standard of medical care, what recourse does the patient or physician have? Under a circumstance such as this, it is most prudent for the physician to document carefully these facts on the patient's medical record. The present legal influence on the health care delivery system in the United States today is most profound. It is also quite disturbing, because most physicians believe that they must practice "defensive medicine" in order to protect themselves from malpractice suits. One United States legal case held that a physician may have a duty to care for a patient, regardless of whether the course of recommended treatment would be paid for by another party. There is no means of predicting where this sort of thinking may ultimately lead.

There is little doubt that the future of health care will involve greater physician participation in generally agreed-to practice guidelines monitored by the accumulation of associated outcomes data. The benefits of this conformity should be better patient care. The danger of such conformity is the possibility of re-creating another Galenic (Cladius Galen, AD 130 to 200) era in medicine characterized by the exclusion of new thought and creativity (as occurred for more than 13 centuries after Galen's death). Our present challenge is to ensure that the care being provided not only reflects the best interests of the patient but also reflects a decrease in the overall cost of such care. It seems to this writer that the only way this could be achieved in the field of spine care would be the implementation of potent disease prevention programs with safe and effective disease treatment and valid post-treatment health maintenance programs designed to allow the patient to become *independent* of the health care system. To achieve this type of balance would clearly require a dramatic paradigm shift in our present philosophy of health care.

EXPERT CONFLICT OF INTEREST

Conflict of interest has been defined as "any situation where an individual with responsibility to others (which includes professional responsibilities) might be influenced, consciously or unconsciously, by financial or personal factors which involve self interest."[21, 27–29] The veterinary health care ethic[31] represents only a single example of a spectrum of potential conflicts of interest in health care delivery.

When a physician provides expert information, the ethical practices playing field becomes even more challenging. Usually, individuals who are truly experts (possessing the greatest knowledge and understanding of a specific subject) are those who do indeed have a potential conflict of interest. Their interest and expertise in the particular subject are generally a direct result of past effort directed to personal gain. Clearly, one way to preserve this important expertise for the benefit of society is to limit the effect of such bias by publicly identifying this potential bias or conflict of interest. Through consistent use of the so-called sunshine rules (public disclosure of all potential conflicts of interest), these liabilities can be greatly moderated while never being completely eliminated. The sunshine laws approach is an important means of avoiding one of the great pitfalls of the free enterprise system while maintaining competition in the health care system as a means of improving patient consideration, satisfaction, and treatment. It should be an inherent ethical responsibility of the professional caregiver to disclose, routinely and publicly, potential conflicts of interest. In fact, many organizations that sponsor medical seminars and medical journals require the advance submission of conflict of interest data sheets that identify any remuneration or associations that might influence the presentation.

INFORMED CONSENT

Informed consent is an interesting conceptual entity that has gradually evolved over time. What is considered adequate informed consent varies significantly throughout the world. The informed portion relates to the transfer of information to the patient, and the consent portion implies that this information has been effectively communicated and that the party being treated understands this information and, on the basis of this understanding, agrees to accept the risks of the proposed treatment.

As with many other endeavors in the modern world, informed consent has also been connected with the issue of patient rights. In the real "world of nature," there is no evidence that any animal has "rights." In early human history, only the monarchs of the world possessed rights. In today's world, rights extend to many topics and issues. Thomas Paine and James Madison divided rights into natural rights (e.g., freedom of thought and speech) and civil rights (e.g., the right to trial by jury). Informed consent is a civil right. Informed consent also strongly reflects the culture in which it resides.

In most western countries today, informed consent is expected to contain a comprehensive review of the most dangerous elements of the proposed treatment. In the case of proposed surgery, such as laminectomy, this process is straightforward and involves telling the patient that he or she may die, be paralyzed, have a nerve injured, experience a wound infection, medical problem, and so on. For diagnostic studies, such as myelography, informed consent has been much less clear in regard to true patient risk, and for some possible outcomes, such as arachnoiditis and myelopathy, has never really reflected the true potentially serious complications.

In the 1930s and 1940s, thorium dioxide (Thorotrast) was used as a myelographic contrast agent. The fact that thorium dioxide was radioactive (an α emitter with a half-life of 1.4×10^{10} years) and that significant numbers of patients exposed to it developed myelopathy and malignant lesions of the neuraxis years later was not well appreciated by the medical profession at that time.[8, 23] In the search for safer myelographic materials, iodinated sesame oil (Lipiodol) and then iophendylate (Pantopaque) were introduced in the 1940s. That these substances are potentially toxic and are capable of producing painful lifetime incapacitation secondary to adhesive arachnoiditis is still not well known by the medical community, despite extensive documentation.[7-9, 11] In the United States, England, and Australia, this situation led to the creation of lay self-help groups. It has been further reflected by the initiation of class-action legal suits in these countries based on informed consent issues. In these situations what would have constituted adequate patient information? A physician has the responsibility to inform a patient adequately regarding the nature of, and risks inherent in, any treatment or procedure. At what point should the physician be expected to know this information? At what point should a specialist be expected to know it?

USE OF INFORMATION

Experimental Versus Investigational

The appropriate use of information is the key not only to informed consent but also to the ethical practice of medicine. How information is used is often more important than the information itself. At present, significant difference of opinion exists as to what treatment constitutes standard practice, what is proved to be effective, and what is experimental or investigational. Although some variance will always exist in how these terms are defined, their legitimate definition is based on a consensus on safety and efficacy issues.

The terms experiment and investigational have been subject to particular abuse. The term experimental is commonly substituted for the more appropriate term investigational, often with the sole purpose of giving the communication a greater emotional impact because most individuals associate the term experimental with the concept of being a "guinea pig." The generally accepted definitions of these terms follow:

- Experimental: Experimental therapies and procedures are those for which basic safety and efficacy have not yet been determined (e.g., by cell culture or animal studies).
- Investigational: When basic safety and efficacy have been demonstrated by the scientific process, the investigational stage is reached. This typically represents the clinical phase of the scientific study, involving well-controlled patient groups as a prelude to the therapy's or the procedure's becoming standard.

Poor Medical Testimony

In addition to providing information regarding standard or accepted forms of therapy, physicians are often called on to provide expert testimony in the courtroom. A legitimate concern exists that sometimes the information presented is not of good quality and may be biased. In an adversarial system of law, each side produces its own witnesses and information, and the court must judge, and rule on, the legitimacy of this information. More frequently, the courts are becoming involved in issues relating to technology assessment. Specific examples of this trend are decisions made in regard to patient eligibility for such technologies, as well as court-ordered reimbursement for expensive treatment modalities.[3, 17, 18] Typically, many sources of information are invoked and range from the scientific to the anecdotal.

Randomized, double-blind, controlled and prospective studies provide the highest order of scientific information. The problem is that, at present, there is a paucity of such well-defined data. Despite their great value, these data provide only a small part of the information on which decisions regarding therapies, procedures, and legal matters are now being made and will continue to be made in the foreseeable future. We are therefore obliged to continue to use the best information available to us. In addition to the need to create legitimate information, there is also an ethical responsibility on the part of the medical profession, industry, and payers to disseminate such information openly. In Minnesota, a study on the cost-effectiveness of HMOs commissioned by the state human services department was found to have been suppressed. The reason given was that the study contained "flawed data," but internal department documents suggested that the report's release would have proved embarrassing for the politically powerful HMOs[14] (more than 34% of the population in Minnesota are now HMO members).

Studies pertaining to the spine are particularly hindered by the difficulties inherent in objectively measuring the anatomic, pathologic, and physiologic aspects of the normal as well as the diseased spine and its associated neurologic structures. This challenge to collecting scientifically meaningful data becomes even more evident when the study of the spine is compared with that of the heart or the eye, in which the difference between normal and abnormal can be accurately determined by many objective measurements.

Surprisingly, a 1993 survey stated that the judicial system seldom uses and may actually avoid published medical science because informal tradition and formal statutes dictate that the system use live witnesses.[16] This phenomenon may relate directly to the fact that contemporary medical practice, as we know it, really is not based on well-documented scientific information.[15, 26] When a physician is called on to provide information for patient care (or for the courtroom), the legacy of having a basically poor data base for reference invariably makes the endeavor a more challenging one. By defining the nature of the information (including its reliability), referencing its source, and disclosing any relevant personal conflicts of interest or bias, the value of this exchange is invariably enhanced.

In spine care, there exists a most particular and unique circumstance. Nowhere else in medicine are there so many differing treatments for the same condition. The multifocal nature of these therapies makes objective documentation difficult. The end result has been an area of medicine in which treatment has been, and continues to be, cost-ineffective. Despite the difficulties discussed, it appears that the meaningful documentation of outcomes data has the potential greatly to improve our ability to support health care decisions in the future. There are also those (this writer included) who believe that a paradigm shift from *treating disease* to *preventing disease* might be a productive endeavor for the future.

Second Opinion

In 1987 and 1988, the Health Program at RAND Corporation of Santa Monica, California, published a series of articles on the appropriateness of numerous medical procedures performed between 1979 and 1982.[12, 13, 34] These data suggested that a significant percentage of such procedures were unnecessary. Even though further clinical investigation of this methodology did not substantiate the RAND observations,[4, 20, 30] the effort was pounced on by many to justify stringent utilization and peer review and to continue to expend substantial resources in this type of effort. By 1992, 350 review firms existed in the United States to perform utilization review on about 80% of Americans receiving medical care. The concern with replacing medical care costs with administrative costs was reflected in a 1990 survey performed by the Inspector General of the United States Health and Human Services Department. This department reviewed 500,000 cataract operations funded by Medicare. In this study, the investigators demonstrated that the United States paid $13.3 million to utilization reviewers to save $1.4 million in possibly unnecessary surgery.[11]

Despite the well-documented high administrative cost of utilization review and second opinions, these services continue to flourish in the United States.[1] Concern exists that the reason for their continuance is more related to a desire by third-party payers to justify denial of medical coverage and care rather than truly to examine the merits of the therapy being recommended. For this reason, some medical organizations are now engaged in creating ethical guidelines to help to direct such peer review (Table 1).

PATIENT CARE AND THE POLITICAL PROCESS

As previously noted, the political environment has an important effect on how medicine is practiced. This influence varies, but it often involves how information is used and the nature of informed consent. In the United States, the Food and Drug Administration was empowered in 1976 through the medical device amendments to regulate medical devices. The specific purpose of this legislation was to protect the public from unsafe medical devices. The enabling legislation made clear that it was not intended to impede the development of new medical devices nor to empower the government to control the practice of medicine.[10] Unfortunately, the continuing interpretation of this legislation and the subsequent issuance of rules and regulations over the years have significantly limited the development and introduction of new medical devices in the United States. This legislation is now also being used by the United States federal government to control medical practice. In the field of spine care, the controversy surrounding the surgical use of pedicle screws is an example of this phenomenon.

Pedicle screw support systems are standard devices in spine practice and have been in use since the 1960s. Although these devices are in reality Class II (non–life-supporting devices for which standards can be written) under the United States medical device legislation they have been placed by the Food and Drug Administration in the Class III category of life-sustaining or supporting devices (e.g., heart valves). Essentially all of the approximately 20 pedicle screw systems used in the United States are referred to by the Food and Drug Administration as either experimental or investigational. This situation has created a dilemma for spine surgeons. Many surgeons have believed, with good reason, that the devices they have been recommending to their patients in the past were standard or approved devices. This controversy has created an unfortunate plethora of medical malpractice suits in the United States based on informed consent issues. In major United States cities, public advertisements are commonly placed by lawyers in newspapers directed to patients who have experienced "failed back fusion," indicating that such patients should "know their rights" and that they may be entitled to compensation for pain and suffering.

With the complexity in society today, more adversity is not needed in the health care system. All participating parties have some shared responsibility for this distressing situation, but government often creates the potential for adversarial relationships by not acting definitively in the public interest and, when it does, by not appropriately resolving the problem. The recognized role of government is to protect the public interest. The balance between regulation and freedom can become, if not carefully monitored, precarious.[6]

ACADEMIC INSTITUTIONS

These days, being a university is not easy. Universities have performed their job only

Table 1
■

Role of Peer Review in Treatment Authorization*

1. That those providing peer review be required to identify themselves, the organization they represent, and the party requesting the peer review.
2. That those providing peer review use standards consistent with the norms for the community.
3. If peer review is being performed by other than an M.D., D.O., or D.C., that their qualifications to conduct this review be stated.
4. Acceptable peer review requires that the professional training and expertise of the reviewer be similar to that of the original treatment provider being reviewed.
5. That peer review be performed within a reasonable period of time. If a second opinion is being given, this should ideally include an appropriate patient examination but must include a review of the actual diagnostic studies and not just the medical records and reports.
6. That if treatment is denied or significantly modified, the basis for this decision be clearly defined.

*These guidelines for peer review in the community were created by the Twin Cities Spine Society of Minneapolis/St. Paul, Minnesota as a means of attempting an ethical approach to addressing frequent abuses in the peer review process and delivery of second opinions.
From Peer Review: Leading to Authorization for Treatment. Adopted by the Twin Cities Spine Society, February 19, 1994.

too well; they have trained legions of highly qualified medical professionals, some of whom have established clinics and other organizations whose innovation, research, and clinical care have rivaled those of the source from which they have sprung. Burdened with unyielding academic traditions and tenure (which was intended to protect academic freedom), sometimes creating oppressive dynasties, inflexibilities, and sloth. Universities now appear to have lost their previous monopoly on excellence in intellectual pursuits.[5] In addition to this problem, the economic pressure on universities simply to survive has markedly increased.

As an important means of obtaining new funding, many universities have turned to collaborating with for-profit companies or even to initiating nonprofit commercial enterprises. Despite concerns relating to this "close encounter," the potential benefits of biomedical technology transfer to the United States economy and world competitiveness have led the American Congress to make bringing academia and industry together a national priority.[1,2] These industry-academia liaisons, however, have also created new potential conflicts of interest regarding the objectivity of scientific studies, the integrity of scientists (and institutions), and the safety of medical products. The board of regents of a prestigious Minnesota university closed down its $12.5 million manufacturing facility for antilymphocyte globulin (which is used for immunosuppressive purposes) 18 months after the federal government halted sales of the drug because of illegal sales and cover-up activities. Over a 22-year period, $80 million worth of antilymphocyte globulin had been sold in violation of federal laws.[24]

The industry-academia connection is a important area of ethical concern. In spine care, significant industrial pressures exist to bring new devices (e.g., those used in fusion) to market as soon as possible. This pressure creates conflicts between the researcher's academic and financial interests and promotes a greater industrial influence on the medical professionals. New societal concerns regarding questions of undue influence are evident in legislation. In Minnesota, a bill that would no longer allow elected officials to accept meals or gifts of even modest value from lobbyists and "interested persons" with business pending before those officials was passed.[32] It seems valid to wonder whether similar limitations would be appropriate in the relationship of industry to physicians and scientists involved in research studies.

There is reason to believe that the commercialization of biomedical research is a worthy public interest goal and that public and private research collaborations help to achieve this goal.[35] The challenge is to protect the public interest by creating consistent governmental and professional standards and rules that require public disclosure of such conflicts.

CONCLUSIONS

The ethics of spine health care, similar to the ethics of medical practice, are basically clear and are based on Hippocratic principles. The test for ethical decision-making lies in the answer to this question; Is what is being proposed primarily in the patient's or the public's best interest? Appropriately addressing the other potential ethical issues will certainly require great dedication and exceptional wisdom.

Acknowledgment

The author would like to express his particular appreciation to Drs. William Kirkaldy-Willis and Leon Wiltse for setting the example for an ethical basis in spine care and to Ronald Vantine, Esq., and William Leary, Esq., for editorial review.

REFERENCES

1. 35 USC 200 et seq.
2. 15 USC 3701 et seq.
3. Banta, H. D., and Thacker, S. B.: The case for reassessment of health care technology. Once is not enough. JAMA 264:235–240, 1990.
4. Bernstein, S. J., Hilborne, L. H., Leape, L. L., et al.: The appropriateness of use of coronary angiography in New York State JAMA. 269:766–769, 1993.
5. Brimelow, P.: Are universities really necessary? Forbes April:170–171, 1993.
6. Burton, C. V.: The balance between regulation and freedom. Neurosurgery 1:322–323, 1977.
7. Burton, C. V.: Adhesive arachnoiditis. *In* Youmans, J. R. (ed.): Neurological Surgery, 3rd ed. Philadelphia, W. B. Saunders, 1990.
8. Burton, C. V., and Wiltse, L. L.: Symposium: Lumbar arachnoiditis: Nomenclature, etiology, and pathology (editorial). Spine 3:23, 1978.

9. Burton, C. V.: Lumbosacral arachnoiditis. Spine 3:24–30, 1978.
10. Burton, C. V.: The medical device amendments of 1976. Neurosurgery 2:74–75, 1978.
11. Burton, T. M.: Firms that promise lower medical bills may increase them. *Wall Street Journal* July 28, 1992.
12. Chassin, M. R., Kosecoff, J., Park, R. E., et al.: Does inappropriate use explain geographic variations in the use of health care services? A study of three procedures. JAMA 258:2533–2537, 1987.
13. Chassin, M. R., Kosecoff, J., Solomon, D. H., and Brook, R. H.: How coronary angiography is used: Clinical determinants of appropriateness. JAMA 258:2543–2547, 1987.
14. Editorial. Secret study. *Minneapolis Star Tribune* March 19, 1994.
15. Evidence-Based Medicine Working Group: Evidence-based medicine: A new approach to teaching the practice of medicine. JAMA 268:2420–2425, 1992.
16. Ferguson, J. H., Dubinsky, M., and Kirsch, P. J.: Court-ordered reimbursement for unproven medical technology. Circumventing technology assessment. JAMA 269:2116–2121, 1993.
17. Fuchs, V. R., and Garber, A. M.: The new technology assessment. N. Engl. J. Med. 323:673–677, 1990.
18. Grimes, D. A.: Technology follies: The uncritical acceptance of medical innovation. JAMA 269:3030–3033, 1993.
19. Guyer, D. W., Wiltse, L. L., Eskay, M. L., and Guyer, B. H.: The long-range prognosis of arachnoiditis. Spine 14:1332–1340, 1989.
20. Hilborne, L. H., Leape, L. L., Bernstein, S. J., et al.: The appropriateness of use of percutaneous transluminal coronary angioplasty in New York State. JAMA 269:761–765, 1993.
21. Koshland, D. E. Jr.: Conflict of interest policy (editorial). Science 257:595, 1992.
22. Leape, L. L., Hilborne, L. H., Park, R. E., et al.: The appropriateness of use of coronary artery bypass graft surgery in New York State. JAMA 269:755–760, 1993.
23. Maltby, G.: Progressive thorium dioxide myelopathy. N. Engl. J. Med. 270:490–496, 1964.
24. Pinney, G. W.: "U" to shut down ALG program. *Minneapolis Star Tribune* March 11, 1994.
25. Platt, J. B.: Physician malpractice and managed care plans. New liability questions. Minnesota Physician, January 1994, pp. 1, 17, 18.
26. Relman, A. S.: On controversy in medicine. Pharos January: 18–22, 1978.
27. Relman, A. S.: Dealing with conflicts of interest. N. Engl. J. Med 316:1182–1183, 1984.
28. Rennie, D., Flanagin, A., Glass, R. M.: Conflict of interest in the publication of science. JAMA 266:266–267, 1991.
29. Rothman, K. J.: Conflict of interest. The new McCarthyism in science. JAMA 269:2782–2784, 1993.
30. Schoenbaum, S. C.: Toward fewer procedures and better outcomes. JAMA 269:794–796, 1993.
31. Schwartz, H.: Sad symptoms of changing American medicine. The veterinarian ethic. *Wall Street Journal* July 9, 1986.
32. Smith, D.: Strict ethics bill sent to Carlson. *Minneapolis Star Tribune* March 18, 1994.
33. Stelzer, I. M.: There is no health care crisis. *Wall Street Journal* January 25, 1994.
34. Winslow, C. M., Kosecoff, J. B., Chassin, M., et al.: The appropriateness of performing coronary artery bypass surgery. JAMA 260:505–509, 1988.
35. Witt, M. D., Gostin, L. O.: Conflict of interest dilemmas in biomedical research. JAMA 271:547–551, 1994.

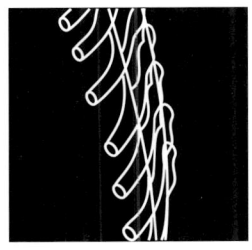

Index

Note: Page numbers in *italics* refer to illustrations; page numbers followed by (t) refer to tables.

A

Abdominal aneurysm, leaking, magnetic resonance imaging of, 372, *373*
Abdominal cavity, pressurization of, in lumbar spine loading, 169
Abdominal wall, anatomy of, 508, *510*
Abductor hallucis, segmental innervation of, 1233(t)
Abductors, hip, evaluation of, in low back pain, 94, 97
Abscess(es), epidural. See *Epidural abscess*.
  in spinal tuberculosis, 878, *881*
  paraspinal, after spinal stenosis surgery, 749
Acceleration transmissibility, 194
Accessory tubercle, 49, *50*
Acetaminophen, for low back pain, in pregnancy, 1062
Acetylsalicylic acid, for disc herniation, 484
Achilles reflex, in disc herniation, 480
Achondroplasia, developmental spinal stenosis in, 728
Achondroplastic stenosis, surgical treatment of, results of, 768
Acne, in SAPHO syndrome, 808
Acromed VSP plate fixation, 603
Actinobacillus actinomycetemcomitans, and vertebral osteomyelitis, 897
Action potential, 126
Activation program, for low back pain, 35–36
Activities of Daily Living (ADL) Scale, 1319(t)
  for outcome self-reporting, 1324, *1324*, *1325*
Acupuncture, for disc herniation, 485
  for spondylolisthesis, 666
Acute radicular syndrome, in disc herniation, diagnosis of, 494, 494(t)
Adaptation, in learning, definition of, 990
Addiction, to pain relief medication, 455
ADL (Activities of Daily Living) Scale, 1319(t)

ADL (Activities of Daily Living) Scale *(Continued)*
  for outcome self-reporting, 1324, *1324*, *1325*
Aerobic training, 1047
  for spondylolisthesis, 664
Aggrecan, 271–272
  concentration of, in pore size distribution, 275
  in intervertebral discs, 274
  solutions of, osmotic pressure of, 274–275
Aging, in low back pain, 88–89
  in osteophyte formation, 541
  in spinal stenosis surgery outcome, 772
  mechanism of, 459
  of facet joints, 540–541, *541*, *542*
  of intervertebral discs, 301–305
  primary vs. secondary, 459
AIF. See *Anterior interbody fusion (AIF)*.
Albers-Schönberg disease, pathologic spondylolisthesis in, 635, *636*
Albumin, measurement of, before spinal fusion, 595
Alexithymia, in low back pain, 1024
Allodynia, in nerve root compression, 131
Allograft(s), autograft vs., for spinal fusion, 591–592
  donor selection for, 1292
  in spinal deformity fusion, results of, 1298
  materials for, 1292–1293
  preservation of, 1293
  processing of, 1293
  sources of, 592
  sterilization of, 1293
  studies of, animal, 1294–1298, 1296(t)
    clinical, 1298–1300, *1299*
Amitriptyline, for chronic low back pain, 1030–1031, 1031(t)
Amphiarthrosis, definition of, 49
Amyloidosis, in ankylosing spondylitis, 801
Amyloids, in aging intervertebral disc, 302
Anal reflex, evaluation of, in low back pain, 98

Anal sphincter, reflex response of, to urethral stimulation, 151, *154*
Analgesics, for low back pain, 453
Anaphylaxis, chemonucleolysis and, 531, 960
Androgen, in fusion outcome, 1289
Anemia, iron deficiency, in fusion outcome, 1289
Anesthesia, for lumbar spine surgery, complications of, 946
　hypotensive, for hemostasis, in spinal fusion, 596
　saddle, in low back pain, 98
　spinal, in posterior lumbar spine surgery, advantages of, 946–947
Aneurysm, abdominal, leaking, magnetic resonance imaging of, 372, *373*
Aneurysmal bone cyst, of spine, 922, *926*
　plain film radiography of, 338, *339*
Aneurysmal syndrome, in spinal tuberculosis, 877, *877*
Angiography, of spinal tumors, 921
Ankle jerk, absence of, 1233–1234
　evaluation of, in disc herniation, 480
　in low back pain, 94
Ankylosing spondylitis (AS), 797–803
　amyloidosis in, 801
　cardiovascular system in, 801
　diagnosis of, criteria for, 798–799, 798(t), 799(t)
　　New York, 798, 798(t)
　　Rome, 798, 798(t)
　enthesopathies in, 800
　epidemiology of, 802
　etiology of, 802
　fractures in, 800
　in reactive arthritis, 805
　in women, 801
　kidney disorders in, 801
　neurologic manifestations of, 801
　pathology of, 798
　peripheral joints in, 800
　prognosis in, 802
　pulmonary disease in, 801
　radiography of, 799–801
　　plain film, 338–341, *340*
　treatment of, 802–803
　ulcerative colitis in, 808
　uveitis in, 800
Annulus fibrosus, age-related structural changes in, 302
　anatomy of, 51
　bulging of, computed tomography of, 390, *391*
　　in degenerative spondylolisthesis, 412
　　magnetic resonance imaging of, 356, *356*
　cells of, types of, 291, *292*
　collagen in, organization of, 273, 289, *289*
　　types of, 290, 312
　composition of, 271–272, 272(t)
　fissuring of, in disc degeneration, 311
　functions of, 286, *286*
　imaging of, in axial plane, 318, *319, 320, 322*
　in discogenic back pain, 463
　in lumbar spine loading, 172
　　in degeneration, 54
　　in health, 53
　partial injury of, animal model of, 314
　rupture/tear of, animal models of, 283–284
　　epidural hematoma with, computed tomography of, 380, *385*
　　magnetic resonance imaging of, 364–365, *365*

Annulus fibrosus *(Continued)*
　surgical defect of, creation of, in animal models, 282
Anterior interbody fusion (AIF), bone grafting in, 604–606, *605, 606*
　for degenerative spondylolisthesis, *706*, 706–707
　　results of, 769
　for disc degeneration, 465–466
　　results of, 466
　iatrogenic discitis after, 909–912, *912, 913*
　indications for, 604
　technique of, 604–606, *605, 606*
Anterior radicular artery, *62*
Anterior ramus, of spinal nerve, 51
Anterior spinal artery syndrome, 574
Anterior wedge fractures, 826, *826, 827*
Antibiotics, for iatrogenic discitis, 912–913
　for reactive arthritis, 805
Antidepressants, for chronic low back pain, 1029–1032, 1031(t)
　for disc herniation, 484
　tricyclic, for chronic low back pain, 1030–1032, 1031(t)
　in spondylolisthesis, 659
AO device, in vitro evaluation of, 216
Aorta, bifurcation of, location of, 508, *510*
　hemostasis of, in spinal fusion, 597
　incompetence of, in ankylosing spondylitis, 801
APLD (automated percutaneous suction lumbar discectomy), 516–517, *518*
　chemonucleolysis vs., 533
Apophyseal joints, in back pain, 87
Aprotinin, use of, history of, 3
Arachnoiditis, after lumbar spine surgery, 947–948
　after spinal stenosis surgery, 749
　evaluation of, postoperative, 420
　in multiply operated lumbar spine, 1109(t), 1112–1113
　　magnetic resonance imaging of, 371
　　treatment of, 1113
　myelography of, 417
Armstrong plate, for anterior fusion, *607*
Arteriovenous fistula, after lumbar spine surgery, 956
　dural, magnetic resonance imaging of, 573–574
　treatment of, 574
Arteriovenous malformations (AVMs), dural, 573
　diagnosis of, 573
　intradural, subarachnoid hemorrhage with, 573
　types of, 573
Artery(ies). See also names of specific arteries.
　injury to, during transpedicle fixation, 1205–1206
　vasodilation of, in neurogenic claudication, 720–721
Arthrectomy, for spinal stenosis, central, results of, 771
　technique of, 779
Arthritis, degenerative, of facet joints, 543
　postenteric, treatment of, 805
　postvenereal, 804
　　treatment of, 805
　reactive. See *Reactive arthritis.*
　rheumatoid, low back pain with, in pregnancy, 1059–1060, *1060*
Arthritis Impact Measurement Scale, 1318(t)
Arthritis mutilans, 806
Arthrodesis. See *Fusion.*
Arthrography, of facet joints, 109–112
　corticosteroid injection in, 109–110

Arthrography *(Continued)*
  diagnostic value of, 110–111
  indications for, 111–112, *112*
  recommendations for, 112
  technique of, 110, *111*
Arthrogryposis, pathologic spondylolisthesis in, 635, 637
Arthrology, of lumbar spine, 47–51, *50*
Arthroscopic discectomy, percutaneous, 519
AS. See *Ankylosing spondylitis (AS).*
Aspirin, for low back pain, 453
Asthma, Millar, 875
Astrocytoma, of spinal cord, 573
Atelectasis, after scoliosis surgery, 1127
Athlete, young, pars interarticularis stress fracture in, 633
  treatment of, 646–647, *648*
Athletic training, repetitive lumbar spine loading in, in vivo observation of, 187–188
  risk factors for, 184–185
Atrioventricular block, in ankylosing spondylitis, 801
Attention diversion, for chronic low back pain, 1033
Autograft(s), allograft vs., for spinal fusion, 591–592
  cancellous, properties of, 1291, *1291*
  cortical, properties of, 1291, *1292, 1293*
  harvesting of, complications of, 1291
  materials for, 1291, *1291–1293*
  sources of, 592, *593*
  vascularized, advantages of, 1291
Automanipulation, of lumbar spine, 1014, *1014*
Automated percutaneous suction lumbar discectomy (APLD), 516–517, *518*
  chemonucleolysis vs., 533
Autonomic nervous system, anatomy of, 570
Autotraction, for low back pain, 1008
AVMs. See *Arteriovenous malformations (AVMs).*
Axonal transport, 126–127
  antegrade, 126–127
  functions of, 127
  retrograde, 126–127
Azathioprine, for psoriatic spondyloarthropathy, 807

B

Back, flat, iatrogenic, in adult scoliosis, 1157–1164, *1160*
  etiology of, 1157
  lordosis restoration in, 1162–1164, *1163, 1164*
  prevention of, 1157–1162, *1159–1162*
  multiply operated. See *Lumbar spine, multiply operated.*
Back incident reports, industrial, predictors of, 1068–1070, 1069(t), *1070, 1071*
Back pain, low. See *Low back pain.*
Back Pain Classification Scale, 1317(t)
  in chronic low back pain, 1028
Back school, 994–995
  after spinal fusion, 610–611
  efficacy of, 994
  for low back pain, 35, 455
    in pregnancy, 1063
    industrial, follow-up of, 1090
  in combined rehabilitation program, 995
Back strain, differential diagnosis of, 449(t)
  etiology of, 452
  treatment of, local injection in, 455

Backrest, of chair, in lumbar support, 239–241, *240, 241*
BAK fixation system, for degenerative disease, 1220, *1220*
Balance point, 783, *785, 786*
Bamboo spine, 800
Barthel Index, 1319(t)
Basic multicellular units (BMUs), 971
Baston venous plexus, in neurogenic claudication, 722
Battered root, 955
Bayonet deformity, in spinal tuberculosis, 878, *879*
Beck Depression Inventory, 1317(t)
  in low back pain, 1048–1049
Becs de perroquet, in spinal tuberculosis, 878
Bed rest, for low back pain, 992–993
Belt, lifting, for manual materials handling, 249
  lumbar, for industrial low back pain, follow-up of, 1090
Bending, backward, in spinal manipulation, 1015, *1015*
Benzodiazepines, for chronic low back pain, 1030
Biceps femoris, in sacroiliac joint stability, 560, *560*
Biofeedback, for chronic low back pain, 1033–1034
Biomechanics, 163–269
Biopsy, in postoperative discitis, 951
  open, after discography, case histories of, 909, *909,* 910(t), 911, *911–914*
  percutaneous, of osteoblastoma, *920*
Bladder, decentralization of, 572
  dysfunction of, clinical neurophysiology in, 154–156, *156*
    in cauda equina syndrome, 577
    in disc herniation, 480
  function of, recovery of, in cauda equina syndrome, 579–580, 586–587
    secondary to disc herniation, 586–587
  paralysis of, in disc herniation, as surgical indication, 497
Blood, autologous donation of, before spinal fusion, 596
  flow of, in cauda equina, in neurogenic claudication, 720–721
  loss of, after scoliosis surgery, 1128
    during microdiscectomy, 960
  salvage of, during spinal fusion, 597
  supply of, to fusion bed, in surgical outcome, 1285
    to lumbar spine, 61, *62, 63,* 596–597, *597*
Blood transfusion, after scoliosis surgery, 1128
Blood vessels, injury to, during lumbar spine surgery, anterior, 961–962
  posterior, 956–957, *959*
  during spinal stenosis surgery, 750
  during transpedicle fixation, 1205–1206
  in mechanical back pain, 812–820
    pathogenesis of, 814–820, *815–820*
      biopsy studies of, 818–819, *819, 820*
      cadaveric studies of, 814–818, *815–818*
  of end plate, arrangement of, 296–297
  of nerve roots, *125,* 125–126
Blood-nerve barrier, 126
BMP (bone morphogenetic protein), in bone grafting, 1293–1294
  animal studies of, 1294–1298, 1295(t)
  in fusion outcome, 1287
BMUs (basic multicellular units), 971
Bohlman technique, 689
Bone(s), cancellous, characteristics of, 971

Bone(s) *(Continued)*
  cortical, aging, bone loss in, 975–976
    characteristics of, 971
  density of, compressive strength in, 973–974
  disease of, in fusion outcome, 1287
  loss of. See *Osteoporosis*.
  mass of, increase in, exercise for, 177
  mineral content of, estimation of, 974–975
  modeling of, 971–972
  new, formation of, in pyogenic spondylitis, 885, *890*
  physiology of, 970–972
  proliferation of, in psoriatic spondyloarthropathy, 807
  regrowth of, postoperative, and recurrent spinal stenosis, 748–749
  remodeling of, 971–972
    adaptive, in lumbar spine, 229–230, *230*
    lumbar spine loading and, 176–178
  resorption of, in psoriatic spondyloarthropathy, 806
  trabecular, aging, bone loss in, 975–976
    characteristics of, 971
    structural indices of, 977–978
      mechanical properties in, 978
Bone graft(s), biology of, 1284–1301
  for pyogenic spondylitis, 894–896, *895*
  future of, 1300–1301
  harvesting of, complications of, 963–965, *964*
  healing of, factors in, 1285(t)
  in spinal fusion. See *Fusion, bone graft in*.
  materials for, *1291–1293*, 1291–1294
    properties of, 1290–1291, 1290(t)
  osteoconductivity of, 1290
  osteogenic potential of, 1290
  osteoinductivity of, 1290–1291
  recipient site for, preparation of, in fusion outcome, 1286
  substitutes for, animal studies of, 1294–1298, 1296(t)
    clinical studies of, 1298–1300, *1299*
Bone marrow cells, in bone grafting, 1292
Bone morphogenetic protein (BMP), in bone grafting, 1293–1294
  animal studies of, 1294–1298, 1295(t)
  in fusion outcome, 1287
Bone scan, in adult scoliosis, 1136
  in discitis, iatrogenic, 908
    intervertebral, septic, 892
  in low back pain, 455
  in metastatic disease, accuracy of, 443
  in pyogenic spondylitis, 887–889
  in spinal tumors, 920
  in spondylolisthesis, degenerative, 672–673
  technetium 99m-labeled medronate disodium, in metastatic disease, 338, *339*
    in osteoid osteoma, 338, *339*
    in pyogenic spondylitis, 887–889
    in septic intervertebral discitis, 892
  in spinal infection, 338
Bowel(s), dysfunction of, clinical neurophysiology in, 154–156
  in cauda equina syndrome, 577
  neurogenic, evaluation of, 155–156, *156*
  paralysis of, in disc herniation, as surgical indication, 497
  perforation of, during transpedicle fixation, 1206
Bowstring test, in disc herniation, 479
Brace(s), for iatrogenic discitis, 913–914

Brace(s) *(Continued)*
  for low back pain, 454
  for spinal fractures, effectiveness of, 867
  for spinal tumors, 932–933
  for spondylolisthesis, 659
Brucellosis vertebral osteomyelitis, 897
Bulbocavernosus reflex, in sacral nerve root evaluation, 150
  in spinal cord lesion, 151, *152*
  testing of, utilization of, 142(t)
Bupivacaine, lidocaine injection with, for facet syndrome, 556
Buros Institute of Mental Measurement, 1314
Burst fractures, 827–828, *828*, 838(t), *839*, 839–840, *841*, *842*
  management of, 850–856, *854–857*
  plain film radiography of, 335–336, *337*
  with neurologic deficit, management of, 853, 855–856, *855–857*
Burst-split fractures, 840, *841*
Butterfly sign, 889

C

C fibers, in nerve root compression, 131, 133
C rods, in vitro evaluation of, 216
Cable tensiometer, in trunk muscle strength evaluation, 1077
Calcitonin, for neurogenic claudication, results of, 767
Calcium, concentration of, in intervertebral disc, 275
Calcium phosphate ceramics, in bone grafting, 1294
  animal studies of, 1297–1298
Cammed exercise equipment, for spondylolisthesis, 662
Campylobacter jejuni, and reactive arthritis, 804
CAP (computer adaptive testing), in clinical outcome measurement, 1315–1316
Cardiovascular fitness, in low back pain, 34
Cardiovascular system, disease of, in ankylosing spondylitis, 801
Carisoprodol, for muscle spasm, 453
Carrageenan, in low back pain, 80–81, *82*
Cartilage, rehabilitation of, in chronic low back pain, 1043–1045
CASP (contoured anterior spinal plate), in vitro evaluation of, 218
Cast, extension, for spondylolisthesis, in children and adolescents, 677–678
Cations, transport of, into intervertebral disc, 294
Cauda equina, anatomy of, 569–572
  blood flow in, in neurogenic claudication, 720–721
  entrapment of, evaluation of, clinical neurophysiology in, 150, *151*
  injury to, during anterior lumbar spine surgery, 962–963
  nerve conduction in, in neurogenic claudication, 157
  nerve roots of, imaging of, in axial plane, *320–323*, 324
    in sagittal plane, *328*
  spinal, vascular supply of, 126
  physiology of, 569–572, 572(t)
Cauda equina compression (CEC), animal models of, 577–578, 584–585
  diagnosis of, 452
    differential, 452
  in metastatic spinal tumor, posterior decompression for, neurologic deficit after, 934–935

Cauda equina compression (CEC) *(Continued)*
  in spinal stenosis, 128
  prolonged, *128,* 129, *129*
  symptoms of, 452
Cauda equina syndrome (CES), 569–581
  acute, 575
  after spondylolisthesis surgery, 643–644, *644*
  causes of, 575
  chemonucleolysis and, 532
  chronic, 575–576
    prognosis in, 580
  classification of, 575–576
  definition of, 582–583
  diagnosis of, 584–585
  disc herniation and, 576–578
    controversies in, 582–587
    prognosis in, 586–587
    treatment of, 585
      timing of, 585–586
  iatrogenic, 576
  in ankylosing spondylitis, 801
  incidence of, 576
  pathophysiology of, 576–577, 583–584
    animal models of, 576, 583
  physical findings in, 575
  prevention of, 577, 584
  prognosis in, 578–580
  treatment of, 578
    decompression for, 578
      timing of, 578–579
        animal models of, 579
CBC (complete blood count), before spinal fusion, 595
CEC. See *Cauda equina compression (CEC).*
Cells, osteoprogenitor, 1285
Central nervous system, developmental deficiencies of, malnutrition in, 715–716
Centralization, in low back pain, 97
Centrum, formation of, 45, *47,* 48
Cephazolin, in discography, discitis after, 900–901
  in iatrogenic discitis prevention, 912
Ceramic composites, in bone grafting, animal studies of, 1294–1298, 1296(t)
Ceramics, in bone grafting, 1294
  animal studies of, 1294–1298, 1296(t)
  clinical studies of, 1300
Cerebrospinal fluid (CSF), examination of, in disc herniation, 480
  in neurogenic claudication, 722
  flow of, disturbance in, in sciatica, 134–135
Cerebrospinal fluid (CSF) fistula, dural tear and, in multiply operated lumbar spine, 1116
  during laminectomy, treatment of, 739
  during spinal stenosis surgery, 747–748
  recurrent, treatment of, 741
Cervical spine, in psoriatic spondyloarthropathy, 806
CES. See *Cauda equina syndrome (CES).*
c-fos gene, expression of, in nerve root compression, 134
Chair, backrest of, in lumbar support, 239–241, *240, 241*
Chairback orthosis, 254, *254*
Chance fracture, 829
Chemonucleolysis, 524–534
  alternatives to, comparison of, 533–534
  chymopapain, 528–534
  complications of, 960–961
  contraindications to, 529

Chemonucleolysis *(Continued)*
  discitis after, 899
  discography before, 528
  economic consequences of, 534
  efficacy of, 529–530
  for disc prolapse, 1241–1242
  history of, 3
  imaging variables in, 530
  indications for, 529
  morbidity of, 531–532
  results of, long-term, 530–531
  surgery after, 532
  technique of, 528–529
Chemotherapy, for spinal tuberculosis, 880–882
  in fusion outcome, 1290
Chest, excursion of, evaluation of, in low back pain, 94
Chlamydia trachomatis, and reactive arthritis, 803(t), 804–805
Chloride, concentration of, in intervertebral disc, 275
Cholecystitis, after scoliosis surgery, 1128
Chondrification, of lumbar spine, 46
Chondrocytes, in disc degeneration, 461
Chondroitin 4-sulfate, biochemistry of, 313
  concentration of, in fused spine, 314
Chondroitin sulfate (CS), biochemistry of, 313
  changes in, in disc degeneration, 461
  in fixed charge density, 288
  in intervertebral discs, 274, *287, 287*
Chondroitinase ABC, injection of, studies of, 533
Chondroma, synovial cyst vs., 384, *387*
Chondromalacia facetae, 542
Chondrosarcoma, of spine, 927
  survival in, 928(t)
Chordoma, of spine, 927
  survival in, 928(t)
Chromatolytic reaction, 127
Chronic intractable benign pain, 1023
Chyloperitoneum, after scoliosis surgery, 1127
Chylothorax, after scoliosis surgery, 1127
Chymopapain, complications of, 960
  in chemonucleolysis. See *Chemonucleolysis.*
  intrathecal injection of, complications of, 531
  use of, history of, 3
Circulation, to nerve roots, *125,* 125–126
Claudication, neurogenic. See *Neurogenic claudication.*
Clomipramine, for chronic low back pain, 1030, 1031(t)
Cobb angle, in adult scoliosis, 1128, 1131
Cognitive programs, for chronic low back pain, 1034–1035
Colitis, ulcerative, inflammatory spondyloarthropathy in, 807–808
Collagen, *289,* 289–290
  biochemistry of, 312–313
  changes in, in disc degeneration, 461
  content of, in disc degeneration, 304
  cross-linking of, 273, 290
    aging in, 312
    defective, 290
  functions of, 286–287, *287*
  laxity of, in pregnancy, and low back pain, 1060
  molecular structure of, 272–273
  organization of, 273–274, 289, *289*
    in annulus fibrosus, 289, *289*
    in end plate, 273–274

Collagen *(Continued)*
 in nucleus pulposus, 289, *289*
 synthesis of, after outer annular tear, in animal models, 284
  in cartilage, in low back pain, 1044
  loading in, 279
  types of, 290
Collagenase, injection of, studies of, 533
 use of, history of, 3
Colon, injury to, during transpedicle fixation, 1206
Colonic compliance, measurement of, in neurogenic bowel dysfunction, 155
Colonic motility, testing of, utilization of, 142(t)
Colonometry, in neurogenic bowel dysfunction, 155–156
 normal, *156*
 utilization of, 142(t)
Complete blood count (CBC), before spinal fusion, 595
Comprehensive Assessment and Referral Evaluation, 1318(t)
Compression fractures, *826,* 826–827, *827*
 anterior, subtypes of, 826–827
 lateral, management of, 860
 management of, 849–850, *851, 852*
Compression rods, development of, 1178
Compression test, in sacroiliac joint dysfunction, 562
Computed tomography (CT), 376–424
 before laminectomy, 1235–1236
  retrospective analysis of, 415–418, *417*
 for corticosteroid injection, in facet syndrome, 551
 high resolution, in up-down stenosis, with lytic spondylolisthesis, 404, 406–408
  indications for, 423–424
 in diagnostic anatomy, 59–60
 magnetic resonance imaging vs., 317
 of anatomic variations, 379–380, *381, 382*
 of degenerative disc disease, 384–409, *388–392*
 of disc abnormality, myelography vs., *417,* 417–418
 of disc herniation, accuracy of, 442, 442(t)
  blinded prospective analysis of, 414, 414(t)
  myelography vs., 413–418, 413(t), 414(t), *417*
  recurrent, *521,* 522
  retrospective analysis of, 413–414
 of discitis, 420, *421, 422*
 of epidural hematoma, 380–384, *383, 385, 386*
 of lumbar spine fracture, 336, 846
 of multiply operated lumbar spine, 1108
 of neoplasms, 420, *423*
 of osteoid osteoma, 338, *339*
 of osteomyelitis, 420, *421, 422*
 of osteoporosis, 983
 of postoperative spine, 418–420, *419*
 of sacroiliac joint dysfunction, 563, *563*
 of scoliosis, with spinal stenosis, *754, 755*
  myelography with, *754*
 of segmental instability, *791*
 of spinal stenosis, accuracy of, 442–443, 443(t)
  blinded prospective analysis of, 414–415, 414(t)
  "burned-out," 408–409
  degenerative, 734–735
   advantages of, 734
   disadvantages of, 734–735
  dynamic, 409, *410*
  far-lateral, 404–408, *407*
  front-back, with pinhole stenosis, 408
  lateral, 392–397, *395–397*
  myelography vs., 413–418, 414(t)

Computed tomography (CT) *(Continued)*
  recurrent, myelography with, *751, 752*
  subarticular, 390, *391*
  up-down, 398–402, *399, 401–403*
   with lytic spondylolisthesis, 403–404, *405, 406*
 of spinal tumors, 920, *920*
 of spondylitis, ankylosing, 799
  pyogenic, 887
 of spondylolisthesis, 686
  degenerative, 409–413, *411*
 of spondylosis, 392–397
 of synovial cyst, 384, *387*
 of trauma, to lumbar spine, 423
  to thoracolumbar junction, 420–423
 radiation exposure during, 369–379
 results of, in normal subjects, 436, 436(t)
 technique of, *378,* 378–379
 three-dimensional, 379
  of spinal stenosis, 394, *396*
 uses of, 377
 with multiplanar reformations, *378,* 378–379
  in postoperative spine evaluation, 418
  in traumatic injury, 420, 423
Computer adaptive testing (CAP), in clinical outcome measurement, 1315–1316
Concentric exercise, for spondylolisthesis, 661
Conduction velocity, of nerve endings, in lumbar facet capsule, 79, 79(t)
Conjunctivitis, in reactive arthritis, 804
Connectivity, of autograft, 1291
Conray 60, injection of, into facet joint, results of, 544–545
Consent, informed, in spine care, 1341–1342
Construct-related validity, of health status outcome measure, 1331
Content-related validity, of health status outcome measure, 1331
Contoured anterior spinal plate (CASP), in vitro evaluation of, 218
Contraction, isometric, of multifidus, in spinal manipulation, 1015, *1015*
Contrast medium, injection of, into sacroiliac joint, method of, 563–564, *564*
Conus medullaris, anatomy of, 569–570
 imaging of, in coronal plane, *331*
 in sagittal plane, 325, *327*
Conus medullaris syndrome, 572–574
Cornell Medical Index, 1318(t)
Corset(s), for low back pain, 454
 in pregnancy, 1062–1063
 for lumbosacral strain, 256
 for spondylolisthesis, 659
 lumbosacral, 254, *254*
 use of, after spinal fusion, 610–611
Cortical evoked potential, utilization of, 142(t)
Corticosteroids, in fusion outcome, 1289
 injection of, facet arthrography with, 109–110
  for back strain, 455
  for disc herniation, 484
  for facet syndrome, prospective studies of, 556
   results of, 550–551
   technique of, 551–555, *553, 554*
  for iatrogenic discitis, 914
  for low back pain, neurophysiology of, 81, *83*
  for psoriatic spondyloarthropathy, 807
  for reactive arthritis, 805
  for sacroiliac joint dysfunction, 566

Corticosteroids *(Continued)*
   for sciatica, 486
   for spondylolisthesis, 665–666
Cortisone, injection of, facet arthrography with, 109–110
Cosmesis, in adult scoliosis, surgery for, 1138–1139
Costal cartilage, splitting of, in tenth rib approach, to anterior spine surgery, 1256, *1256, 1257*
Costal process, formation of, 45, *48*
Costotransversectomy, for metastatic spinal tumors, 934
   in anterior spine surgery, 1254
Cotrel-Dubousset instrumentation, 746
   evaluation of, in vitro, 218
   fatigue strength of, 1193
   for adult scoliosis, 1139, *1140, 1141*, 1143–1149, *1146–1148*
      complications of, 1149, *1150, 1151*
         in elderly, 1155
      with extended fusion, 1156, *1159*
      with iatrogenic flat back deformity, *1159*, 1159–1160, *1162*, 1163, *1164*
      with severe rigid deformity, 1152
   for sacral fusion, results of, 1161
   for spinal stenosis, with degenerative spondylolisthesis, 777, 778
Coupled motion coefficient, in spinal stability evaluation, 209
Cranial shear test, in sacroiliac joint dysfunction, 562
Creep effect, 286
Creeping substitution, 1290
Criterion-related evidence, in health status outcome measurement, 1331
Crock device, in vitro evaluation of, 213–215, *215*
Crohn disease, inflammatory spondyloarthropathy in, 808
Crossed straight leg raising test, in disc herniation, 479
Crossover pain, well leg lifting vs., 96
Crosstalk, in sciatica, 134–135
Cryomicrotomy, in disc disease evaluation, 18, *18*
Cryptococcal vertebral osteomyelitis, 897
CS. See *Chondroitin sulfate (CS)*.
CSF. See *Cerebrospinal fluid (CSF)*.
CT. See *Computed tomography (CT)*.
CT-discography, in chemonucleolysis, 530
   indications for, 429
CT/MPR (computed tomography with multiplanar reformations), *378*, 378–379
   in postoperative spine evaluation, 418
   in traumatic injury, 420, 423
CT-myelography, before laminectomy, 1236–1237
   in postoperative spine evaluation, 418, 420
   in traumatic injury, 423
Cyclic adenosine monophosphate, measurement of, before spinal fusion, 595
Cyclooxygenase, inhibition of, nonsteroidal antiinflammatory drugs in, 134
Cyst(s), bone, aneurysmal, of spine, 922, *926*
   plain film radiography of, 338, *339*
   synovial. See *Synovial cyst(s)*.
Cystometry, in bladder function assessment, 155, *156*
   in spinal cord lesion, *152*
   utilization of, 142(t)
Cytokines, in compressed nerve root pain, 131–132, *132*
   synovial, leakage of, in sciatica, 134

D

Daily adjustable progressive resistive exercise (DAPRE), for spondylolisthesis, 661
Dallas Pain Inventory, 1317(t), 1320(t)
d'Anquin syndrome, congenital spinal stenosis in, 727–728
DAPRE (daily adjustable progressive resistive exercise), for spondylolisthesis, 661
DBM (demineralized bone matrix), in bone grafting, 1293–1294
   animal studies of, 1294–1298, 1295(t)
DDS device, in vitro evaluation of, 219, *220*
Deceleration injuries, 832
Decompression, anterior, for spinal fracture, 863, *868, 869*
   for spinal tumor, 934
   for cauda equina syndrome, 578
      timing of, 578–579
   for fractures, burst, with neurologic deficit, 856
      techniques of, 863–865, *870*
   for lateral recess stenosis, results of, 1244
   for nerve root entrapment, 1249
   for spinal stenosis, 1245–1246
      degenerative adult scoliosis after, 1170
      extent of, 770–772
      fusion with, in degenerative spondylolisthesis, 775–776, *776*
      method of, *770*, 770–772, *771*
         selection of, 775, *775*
      prophylactic, indications for, 778, *779*
      technique of, 779
   for spondylolisthesis, 687
      congenital, 643
      degenerative, fusion with, 957
         results of, 769
         types of, 649, *650*
      in children and adolescents, 677(t), 678
      isthmic, 746
      for tumors, 933
   isthmic spondylolisthesis after, 957
   of lumbosacral nerve roots, indications for, 1241, 1241(t)
   orthosis use after, 257
   posterior, for cauda equina compression, in metastatic spinal tumor, neurologic deficit after, 934–935
      for degenerative spondylolisthesis, 704–705
      for spinal cord compression, in metastatic spinal tumor, neurologic deficit after, 934–935
      for spinal tumor, 934
   posterolateral, transpedicle, for spinal fracture, 863–865, *870*
   repeated, of lumbar nerve roots, results of, 1247
   of multiply operated lumbar spine, 1113–1114
Deep venous thrombosis (DVT), after lumbar spine surgery, 947–949
   prophylaxis for, 948–949
Defecation, neurologic control of, 570–571, 572(t)
Degenerative cascade, 177
Degenerative lumbar stenosis (DLS), diagnosis of, 731–736
   computed tomography in, 734–735
   differential, 732
   electrodiagnostic, 735–736
   electromyography in, 735–736
   history of present illness in, 731–732
   magnetic resonance imaging in, 735

Degenerative lumbar stenosis (DLS) *(Continued)*
  myelography in, 734
  nerve conduction studies in, 736
  past history in, 732–733
  physical examination in, 733
  plain radiography in, 733–734
  somatosensory evoked potentials in, 736
Demineralization, in osteoporosis, 970
Demineralized bone matrix (DBM), in bone grafting, 1293–1294
  animal studies of, 1294–1298, 1295(t)
Denervation, in facet syndrome, results of, 549–550
  of facet joints, difficulty in, 544
Depression, in low back pain, 1018–1020
  pharmacologic treatment of, 1030–1031, 1031(t)
  rating of, 1048–1049
Derangement syndrome, in low back pain, 1004–1005
  treatment of, mechanical, 1009
Dermatan sulfate, in intervertebral disc, 288
Dermatomal somatosensory evoked potentials, eliciting of, before laminectomy, 1237
  methods of, 146–147
  in radiculopathy localization, 149
  surgical monitoring of, 153–154
  utilization of, 142(t)
Dermatomes, formation of, 44–45, *46*
  in low back pain, *108*, 108–109, *109*
  in disc herniation, 478
Dermomyotome, formation of, 44, *45, 46*
Desipramine, for chronic low back pain, 1030, 1031(t)
Determinant system, of lumbar load calculation, 165
Dexamethasone suppression test, in low back pain, with depression, 1019
Diabetes, disc degeneration in, 305
  spinal stenosis with, surgical treatment of, indications for, 775
    results of, 773
Diagnostic tests, accuracy of, 441–444
  comparison of, bias in, reduction of, 437–438, 437(t), 438(t)
  efficacy of, levels of, 435–436
  evaluation of, population choice for, 438–439
    receiver operating characteristic curves in, 439–440
    strategies for, 434–440
    termination in, 434–440
  "gold standard" for, establishment of, 436–437, 436(t)
  predictive value of, disease prevalence in, 438, 439(t)
Diaphragm, anatomy of, 1254–1255
  crus of, removal of, in eleventh rib approach, to anterior spine surgery, 1260, *1261*
  resection of, in tenth rib approach, to anterior spine surgery, 1258
Diarthrosis, definition of, 49
Diatrizoate, in discography, 464
Diazepam, addiction to, 455
  for muscle spasm, in low back pain, 453
Diffuse idiopathic spinal hyperostosis (DISH), and neurogenic claudication, 717
  plain film radiography of, 344, *345*
Diffusion coefficient, 294, *295*
1,25-dihydroxyvitamin D_3, measurement of, before spinal fusion, 595
Direct dynamics, in trunk muscle strength testing, 1084–1087, *1085, 1086*

Disability, low back pain and, 92
Disability and Impairment Interview Schedule, 1317(t), 1319(t)
Disc, intervertebral. See *Intervertebral disc(s)*.
Disc space, infection of, after posterior microdiscectomy, 506–507
Discectomy, alternatives to, complications of, 958–961
  complications of, 953–958
  definition of, 1231
  economic consequences of, 534
  endoscopic, 1231
  extraperitoneal, anterior, sympathetic ganglionectomy with, 1281
    without fusion, 1271–1283
      case study of, 1275, *1275–1279*
      complications of, 1278, 1281
      patient selection for, 1275, *1275–1279*, 1275(t)
      results of, 1278, *1279, 1280*, 1281, *1281*, 1281(t), *1282*
      technique of, *1272–1274*, 1272–1275
  for cauda equina syndrome, 585
  for nerve root entrapment, 1249
  for spinal stenosis, fusion after, 762
    technique of, 779–780
  laser, 1231
  limited, posterior, technique of, 500–502, *500–503*
  microlumbar, for disc herniation, 1242
  percutaneous, 524–534
    arthroscopic, 519
    automated, 1231
    complications of, 526, 961
    laser, 517–518, 525
    lumbar, 515–519, *518*
      automated, chemonucleolysis vs., 533
      suction, 516–517, *518*
    history of, 3
    mechanisms of, *527*, 527–528
    patient selection for, 525
    results of, 526–527
    technique of, 525–526
  segmental instability after, 792
  surgical, chemonucleolysis vs., 533
Discitis, after chemonucleolysis, 532, 899–900, 961
  after discography, 899–900
    pathology of, 901, *906, 907*
  after lumbar spine surgery, 950–951, *952*
    diagnosis of, 950–951, *952*
    treatment of, 951
  after percutaneous discectomy, 961
  after spinal stenosis surgery, 749–750
  computed tomography of, 420, *421, 422*
  iatrogenic, 899–915
    case histories of, 909–912, 910(t), *911–914*
    clinical course of, 907
    diagnosis of, 907–909, *908, 909*
    etiology of, 900–901
    incidence of, 899–900
    nomenclature of, 914–915
    pathology of, 901, 902(t), *903–906*, 907
    presentation of, 907
    prevention of, 912
    prognosis in, 907
    treatment of, 912–914
  in children, 914–915
  in multiply operated lumbar spine, 1109(t), 1113
    treatment of, 1113
  intervertebral, septic, 889–892

Discitis *(Continued)*
   and paraplegia, 896
   bone scan of, 892
   laboratory tests in, 892
   magnetic resonance imaging of, 892
   radiography of, *891,* 891–892
   treatment of, conservative, 893–894
      surgical, 896
   magnetic resonance imaging of, 420, *421, 422*
Discography, 428–432
   accuracy of, 444
   advantages of, 429, 429(t)
   and pain provocation, 431
   before chemonucleolysis, 528
   complications of, 432
   discitis after, 899–900
      cephazolin administration in, 900–901
      pathology of, 901, *906, 907*
   history of, 429
   in adult scoliosis, 1121, 1136, *1137*
      degenerative, 1168
   in chemonucleolysis, 530
   in disc degeneration, 464–465
      magnetic resonance imaging with, 465
   in discogenic pain, 429–431
   in low back pain, 31
      in pain localization, 946
   indications for, after magnetic resonance imaging, 431
      historical, 428–429
      current, 432
   magnetic resonance imaging vs., 366–367
   open biopsy after, case histories of, 909, *909,* 910(t), 911, *911–914*
   technique of, 432
DISH (diffuse idiopathic spinal hyperostosis), and neurogenic claudication, 717
   plain film radiography of, 344, *345*
Disseminated intravascular coagulation, after scoliosis surgery, 1128
Distraction, for adult scoliosis, 1125
   for chronic low back pain, 1033
   in lumbar spine manipulation, 1013(t)
   positional, 1016, *1016*
Distraction injury, plain film radiography of, 336
Distraction test, in sacroiliac joint dysfunction, 562
DLS. See *Degenerative lumbar stenosis (DLS).*
Dorsal horn, changes in, in nerve root compression, 132–133
Dorsal ramus syndrome, in spondylolisthesis, 658
Dorsal root ganglion (DRG), anatomy of, 124, *124, 125*
   compression of, and vascular injury, 136
      in spondylolisthesis, and back pain, 657–658
   electrophysiology of, 127
   imaging of, in axial plane, 318, *323, 324*
      in coronal plane, *331*
      in sagittal plane, *329*
   in neuropeptide synthesis, 127
Dorsiflexion, of great toe, evaluation of, 94
Double-crush phenomenon, 953
Doxepin, for chronic low back pain, 1030
DRG. See *Dorsal root ganglion (DRG).*
Drill, Midas Rex, for laminectomy, in spinal stenosis, 738
Driving point impedance, 194
Drugs. See also named drug or drug group.
   in fusion outcome, 1290

Duke–UNC Health Profile, 1317(t), 1318(t)
Dunn's anterior fixation device, in vitro evaluation of, 216
Dura mater, anatomy of, 124
   compression of, in spinal stenosis, magnetic resonance imaging of, 360
   imaging of, in axial plane, 318, *319, 320*
   tear of, during posterior microdiscectomy, 505–506
      during transpedicle fixation, 1204
      repair of, during laminectomy, for spinal stenosis, 739
      in multiply operated lumbar spine, 1114–1116, *1115*
Durotomy, after posterior lumbar spine surgery, 954–955
DVT (deep venous thrombosis), after lumbar spine surgery, 947–949
   prophylaxis for, 948–949
Dwyer screws, in iatrogenic flat back deformity correction, in adult scoliosis 1163, *1163*
Dynamic stenosis, computed tomography of, 409, *410*
Dynamic testing, direct, of trunk muscle strength, 1084–1087, *1085, 1086*
   inverse, of trunk muscle strength, 1084–1087, *1085, 1086*
Dynamometer, in strength testing, 1073
   of trunk muscles, 1077–1078
      follow-up of, 1090–1091
   triaxial, in strength testing, of trunk muscles, 1078
Dysfunction syndrome, in low back pain, 1004
   treatment of, mechanical, 1009
Dysraphism, spinal, in congenital spinal stenosis, 727

E

Eccentric exercise, for spondylolisthesis, 661
Edema, of spinal nerve roots, in nerve root compression, 130
Edge effect, 129
Education, clinician-patient interaction in, 990–994
   expectation setting in, 991–992
   explanation of condition in, 990–991
   health care consumerism information in, 993
   symptom control advice in, 992–993
   work/leisure activity recommendations in, 993
   written material in, 993–994
   in rehabilitation, 989–996
   in workplace, 995–996
   learning process in, 990
Edwards rods, 692, *694,* 1191
   for spinal fracture, *863, 864*
Effort assessment, in spinal function testing, 1048
Ejaculation, retrograde, after anterior retroperitoneal transverse spine surgery, 1269–1270
   after scoliosis surgery, 1128
Elastic bands, in strength training, in spondylolisthesis, 662
Electrical stimulation, for disc herniation, 485
   of fusion mass. See *Fusion, electrical stimulation of.*
Electromyography (EMG), before laminectomy, 1237
   in abdominal muscle testing, 1081–1082
   in degenerative lumbar stenosis, 735–736
      disadvantages of, 736
   in lumbar load evaluation, 169–170
   in muscle dysfunction, 157–158
   in trunk muscle strength testing, 1079
   in vibrational studies, 196

Electromyography (EMG) *(Continued)*
  needle, in entrapment neuropathy localization, 150
    in neurologic deficit evaluation, 148
    in radiculopathy localization, 149
  sensitivity/specificity of, 144
  utilization of, 142(t)
Electron microscopy, of disc degeneration, 311–312
Electrophoresis, protein, serum, measurement of, before spinal fusion, 595
Electrotherapy, for disc herniation, 484–485
Elemental resource model, of industrial low back pain, 1087–1088
EMG. See *Electromyography (EMG)*.
Empyema, after spinal stenosis surgery, 749
End plate, age-related structural changes in, 303
  blood vessels of, arrangement of, 296–297
  cells of, types of, 291
  changes in, plain film radiography of, 343, *344*
  collagen network of, organization of, 273–274
  composition of, 271–272, 272(t)
  fractures of, in osteoporosis, 981, *982*
    types of, 827
  herniation in, magnetic resonance imaging of, 366
  imaging of, in axial plane, *324*
    in coronal plane, *332*
  in cation transport, into intervertebral disc, 294
  in spinal infection, plain film radiography of, 337, *338*
  response of, to lumbar loading, 172
  sclerosis of, plain film radiography of, 349, *350*
Endothoracic fascia, of diaphragm, 1255
End-range motion, repeated, in low back pain diagnosis, 979–980, *1003*
Endurance training, for spondylolisthesis, 663
Enterobacteriaceae, and reactive arthritis, 804
Enthesopathy, 236
  in ankylosing spondylitis, 800
  in psoriatic spondyloarthropathy, 807
Entrapment neuropathy, evaluation of, clinical neurophysiology in, 150
Environment, in inflammatory spondyloarthropathies, 809
Eosinophilic granuloma, of spine, 922, *927*
  plain film radiography of, 338
Ependymoma, in children/adolescents, magnetic resonance imaging of, 368
  of spinal cord, 573
  treatment of, case history of, 938, *940*
Epidural abscess, after lumbar spine surgery, 952–953, *953*
  diagnosis of, 952–953
  treatment of, 953
  magnetic resonance imaging of, 372
  spinal, 892
    clinical features of, 892
    diagnosis of, 892, *893*
    treatment of, conservative, 894
      surgical, 896
Epidural fibrosis, after lumbar spine surgery, 947–948
  in multiply operated lumbar spine, magnetic resonance imaging of, 371, *371*
Epidural hematoma, after posterior lumbar spine surgery, 955–956
  annular tear with, 380, *385*
  computed tomography of, 380–384, *383, 385, 386*
  degenerative disc disease with, *383, 385*
  magnetic resonance imaging of, *383,* 384

Epidural space, anatomy of, 61–62
Erector spinae, in spinal stability, 207
  in trunk movement, 1080, *1081, 1082*
Ergonomics, goal of, 1087
Erythrocyte sedimentation rate (ESR), in iatrogenic discitis, 907–908
  in infection, after spinal stenosis surgery, 749–750
Estrogen, in fusion outcome, 1289
Ethambutol, for spinal tuberculosis, 880–882
Euler buckling, 978
Ewing sarcoma, of spine, 927
  survival in, 928(t)
Exercise(s), and increased bone mass, 177
  for disc herniation, 483, 485
  for low back pain, 33–34, 34(t), 454, 1008–1009
    industrial, follow-up of, 1090–1091
  for sacroiliac joint dysfunction, *565,* 565–566
  for spondylolisthesis, concentric, 661
    eccentric, 661
    isometric, 662
    isotonic, 662
    manual resistance, 662
    program of, prescription of, 664–665
    progressive resistance, 661
    water-based, 662
  in intervertebral disc nutrition, 297–299, *298*
  in lactate concentration, in intervertebral disc, 298, *298*
  in lactate production, 295
  in proteoglycan synthesis, 298–299
  in sulfate concentration, in intervertebral disc, 298, *298*
  oxygen consumption during, in intervertebral disc, 295
Exostosis, multiple, hereditary, and developmental spinal stenosis, 728
Extension, repetitive, of motion segments, mechanical effects of, 189–190
Extension casting, for spondylolisthesis, in children and adolescents, 677–678
Extension fractures, 832, *833*
  management of, 860–862
Extensor digitorum brevis, segmental innervation of, 1233(t)
Extensor hallucis longus, segmental innervation of, 1233(t)
External fixator, in segmental instability testing, 788
External oblique muscles, in trunk movement, 1080, *1081,* 1082, *1082*
Extremity(ies), lower, in neurogenic claudication, 722
  strength training of, in spondylolisthesis, 660–661

F

F responses, abnormal, *145*
  disadvantages of, 145
  in neurogenic claudication, 157
  in neurologic deficit evaluation, 148
  in radiculopathy localization, 149
  normal, *146*
  testing of, utilization of, 142(t)
FABER test, in low back pain, 96
Facet blocks, in adult scoliosis, 1136
Facet joint(s), aging of, 540–541, *541, 542*
  anatomy of, 49, *50,* 68
  arthrography of. See *Arthrography, of facet joints.*
  asymmetry of, plain film radiography of, 351

Facet joint(s) *(Continued)*
  capacity of, 543
  capsule of, in low back pain, 75–76
    neurophysiology of, 78, 78–79, 79
    nerve endings of, conduction velocity of, 79, 79(t)
  degeneration of, arthritis in, 543
    clinical implications of, 56
  denervation of, difficulty in, 544
  fracture of, after spinal stenosis surgery, 749
  functions of, 540–541, 541
  hypertrophy of, in degenerative spondylolisthesis, computed tomography of, 409, 411
    in front-back stenosis, 408
  in degenerative spondylolisthesis, 700–701
  in facet syndrome, evaluation of, criteria for, 544–548
    treatment of, criteria for, 544–548
  in load bearing, 53
  in low back pain, 31, 543
    historical aspects of, 87
  in spinal stability, 203–204
  innervation of, 435, 544, 545
  loading of, 542–543
    in low back pain, 75–76
    response to, 173–174, 174–176
  meniscus of, 541–542, 542
  osteoarthritis of, plain film radiography of, 345, 346, 349, 350
  pain in, diagnosis of, 90
  pressure measurements across, cadaveric studies of, 462
  removal of, excessive, in spinal stenosis surgery, fusion for, 762
  rotation of, in spondylolisthesis, 633
    congenital, 626, 627, 629
    degenerative, 634
  symptomatic, pathologic changes in, 542
Facet screws, for internal fixation, in degenerative disease, 1220, 1221
Facet syndrome, 538–557
  anatomy of, 540–544, 541, 542, 544–546
  evaluation of, criteria for, 544–548
  future studies of, 555
  historical background of, 538–540
  orthoses for, 257
  symptoms of, 547
  treatment of, corticosteroid injection in, prospective studies of, 556
    results of, 550–551
    technique of, 551–555, 553, 554
  criteria for, 544–548
  denervation in, results of, 549–550
  options for, 548
  results of, 548–551
Facetectomy, for degenerative spondylolisthesis, 704–705
  for nerve root entrapment, 1244, 1244
  for spinal stenosis, laminectomy with, 739
    technique of, 779
  oblique, for central spinal stenosis, results of, 772
  partial, 1231
    for nerve root entrapment, 1249–1250
  spinal stability after, 204, 204
Failed back surgery syndrome, 5
Far-lateral stenosis, 741–742
  computed tomography of, 397, 404–408, 407
Far-out stenosis, 397
Fascia, lumbar, anatomy of, 62
Fat graft, nerve compression by, after posterior lumbar spine surgery, 956, 957
Fatigue fracture, 971–972
  definition of, 182
FCaE (fractional calcium excretion), measurement of, before spinal fusion, 595
Fear Avoidance, 1317(t)
Fear Avoidance Beliefs Questionnaire 1320(t)
Femoral nerve, injury to, during bone grafting, 965
Femoral stretch test, 1232
  in disc herniation, 479–480
  in low back pain, 97–98
Fenestration, definition of, 1231
  for central canal stenosis, 740
  for degenerative spondylolisthesis, 744–745
  for lateral recess stenosis, 740
  wide, for central spinal stenosis, results of, 771
Fenfluramine, for chronic low back pain, 1030
Fetus, development of, stages of, 43
Fibrinolysis, defective, back pain with, 813–814
  mechanical, stanozolol for, 814
  in disc herniation, 483
  in sciatica, 134–135
Fibromyalgia syndrome, 29
Fibrosis, epidural, after lumbar spine surgery, 947–948
  in multiply operated lumbar spine, magnetic resonance imaging of, 371, 371
  in mechanical back pain, 812–820
Fibrous dysplasia, in fusion outcome, 1287
Fibula, bone grafting from, for spinal fusion, 592
Figure 4 test, in low back pain, 96
Finite element method, of lumbar loading analysis, 170–172
Fistula, cerebrospinal fluid. See *Cerebrospinal fluid (CSF) fistula.*
Fitts' law, 1092
Fixation. See also *Instrumentation.*
  devices for, in vitro studies of, 213–221, 214, 215, 220, 220(t)
Fixed charge density, 274
  chondroitin sulfate/keratan sulfate ratio in, 288
Flat back, iatrogenic, in adult scoliosis, 1157–1164, 1160
  etiology of, 1157
  lordosis restoration in, 1162–1164, 1163, 1164
  prevention of, 1157–1162, 1159–1162
Flaval ligaments, anatomy of, 49
Flexibility training, for spondylolisthesis, 663–664
Flexion, repetitive, of motion segments, mechanical effects of, 189–190
Flexion-distraction injuries, 828–832, 829–832
  burst, 833, 836
  classification of, 829, 829, 830
  management of, 857–860, 858, 859, 861, 862
Flexion-extension injury, plain film radiography of, 335–336
Flexion-rotation injuries, 832–833, 833
Flexors, hip, evaluation of, in low back pain, 95
Fluoroscopy, for contrast medium injection, in sacroiliac joint dysfunction, 563–564, 564
  in facet joint evaluation, in facet syndrome, 544–545
Fluoxetine, for chronic low back pain, 1030, 1031(t)
Foot, weakness of, in disc herniation, 480
Foramen, intervertebral. See *Intervertebral foramen.*
Foraminotomy, laminectomy with, for spinal stenosis, 739

Fractional calcium excretion (FCaE), measurement of, before spinal fusion, 595
Fracture(s), 822–871. See also specific sites of fracture.
  anatomy of, 822–824
  biomechanics of, 822–824, *824*
  burst. See *Burst fractures.*
  burst-split, 840, *841*
  Chance, 829
  classification of, 822–871
    comprehensive, 836–845, 838(t)
    conventional, 825–836
    sequence of, 840, 844
  compression. See *Compression fractures.*
  decompression for, techniques of, 863–865, *870*
  evaluation of, 822–871
    clinical, 845–846
    diagnostic, 846–848, *847, 848*
  extension, 832, *833*
    management of, 860–862
  fatigue, 971–972
    definition of, 182
  flexion-distraction, 828–832, *829–832*
    classification of, 829, *829, 830*
    management of, 857–860, *858, 859, 861, 862*
  impaction, 838(t), 839, *839*
  in ankylosing spondylitis, 800
  management of, 822–871
    goals of, 848–849
    surgical vs. nonsurgical, 849
  mechanisms of, 825–836
  minor, management of, 849
  orthoses for, 256, 865–871
  plain film radiography of, 335–336, *336, 337*
  posterior arch, 833, 836
  primary, types of, *837*, 837–839
  slice, 840, *844*
  spinal instability in, 824–825, *825*, 825(t)
  split, 838(t), 839, *839*
  stable, orthoses for, 867
  stress, of ilium, after bone grafting, 963, *964*
    of pars interarticularis, in young athlete, 633
      treatment of, 646–647, *648*
  surgical stabilization of, considerations in, 862–865, *863–869*
  thoracic, classification of, 838(t)
  Type A, *839*, 839–840, *841, 842*
    management of, 849–856, *851, 852, 854–857*
  Type B, 840, *843*
    management of, 857–860, *858, 859, 861, 862*
  Type C, 840, *843–845*
  types of, identification of, algorithm for, 844–845, *845*
  wedge, anterior, 826, *826, 827*
Fracture-dislocation injuries, 832–833, *833–836*
  burst, flexion-distraction, 833, *836*
  flexion-rotation, 832–833, *833*
  management of, 860
  shear, 833, *834, 835*
Free nerve endings, 76, *77*
Freezing, in nerve destruction, in facet syndrome, 550
Frequency, natural, definition of, 182
  in vibration studies, 194–195
Frequency Likert-type scale, 1323, *1323*
Front-back stenosis, *395, 396*
  pinhole stenosis with, computed tomography of, 408
Frost's criteria of everyday trauma, 970

FSU (functional spinal unit), mechanical properties of, during lumbar spine loading, 170, 171(t)
Functional Activities Questionnaire, 1319(t)
Functional Assessment Inventory, 1318(t)
Functional Rating Scale, 1317(t), 1319(t)
Functional spinal unit (FSU), mechanical properties of, during lumbar spine loading, 170, 171(t)
Functional Status Index, 1317(t), 1319(t)
Functional Status Rating System, 1319(t)
Functioning Status Assessment Form, 1319(t)
Fusion, 588–611, 1284–1311
  and disc nutrition, 299, *299*
  anterior, 604–606
    for spinal tuberculosis, 882–883, 883(t), *884, 887*
    history of, 590–591
    indications for, 604
    instrumentation for, 606, *607*
    internal fixation with, 606
      indications for, 606, *607*
    technique of, 604–606, *605, 607*
  assessment of, 1309
  biology of, 1284–1301, 1285(t)
  bone graft in, allograft, sources of, 592
    augmentation of, 593
    autograft, allograft vs., 591–592
      sources of, 592, *593*
    future of, 1310–1311
    harvesting of, complications of, 963–965, *964*
      from iliac crest, 598–599, *599*
        anterior, 598–599
        posterior, 598, *599*
    sources of, 591–593, *593*
    supplementation of, 593
    technique of, 591–593, *593*
  combined anterior-posterior, 606–607
    indications for, 606–607
  decompression with, for burst fracture, with neurologic deficit, 856
    for spinal stenosis, with degenerative spondylolisthesis, 775–776, *776*
  electrical stimulation of, 608–610
    external, 610
    history of, 608
    implantable, 608–610
      external stimulation vs., 610
    indications for, 610
    outcome of, 1288–1289
  exposure for, 596
  for disc degeneration, 1308
  for disc herniation, 1308
    laminectomy with, 1243
  for discogenic pain, 1220, *1221*
  for pyogenic spondylitis, 894–896, *895*
  for sacroiliac joint dysfunction, 566–567
  for scoliosis, 1308
    adult, extension of, 1155–1157, *1157–1159*
      operative approach to, 1157
      results of, 1156–1157, *1157–1159*
    indications for, 1138–1139
    prognosis in, 1134
  degenerative, 1308
  history of, 589
  for segmental instability, after discectomy, 792
  for spinal stenosis, 757–764, 1308
    indications for, structural alterations in, intraoperative, 762
      preoperative, 757–762, *758–763*

Fusion (Continued)
  instrumentation for, 762–764, 764
  recurrent, 1303
  with degenerative spondylolisthesis, 1308
  for spondylolisthesis, 687
    cauda equina syndrome after, 643–644, 644
    congenital, 643
    degenerative, decompression with, 957
      results of, 769
      types of, 649, 650
    in children and adolescents, anterior, 672
      anterior/posterior, 674
      laminectomy with, 671–672
      one level, 671, 676, 677(t)
      posterolateral, technique of, 679–680, 680
      two level, 671, 677–678, 677(t), 678
    isthmic, 640, 642, 643, 1308
  function preservation in, 1311
  future of, 1309–1311
  global, for disc degeneration, 466
  hemostasis in, 596–597, 597
  history of, 3–5, 588–591
  in situ, anterior, for spondylolisthesis, 689–691, 691
    posterior, for spondylolisthesis, 687–689, 690
  indications for, 593–594
  instrumentation with, 1308
    future of, 1309–1310
  interbody, anterior. See *Anterior interbody fusion (AIF)*.
    for iatrogenic discitis, 914
    for spondylolisthesis, transpedicle fixation with, 644, 646
    history of, 4
    in disc oxygen consumption, 295
    in lactate production, 295
    posterior. See *Posterior lumbar interbody fusion (PLIF)*.
    postsurgical evaluation of, plain film radiography in, 348
  lateral, bilateral, for disc degeneration, 465
    advantages of, 465
    results of, 465
  long-term follow-up of, 611
  nonunion of, 1284
    animal studies of, 1287
  of degenerative lumbar spine, 1307–1311
  of multiply operated lumbar spine, indications for, 1114
  of pars interarticularis fracture, indications for, 647–649
  of sacrum, Cotrel-Dubousset instrumentation for, results of, 1162
  outcome of, drugs in, 1290
    electrical stimulation in, 1288–1289
    graft recipient site preparation in, 1286
    growth factors in, 1287
    hormones in, 1289
    mechanical stability in, 1286, 1286–1287
    nutrition in, 1289
    osteoporosis in, 1289
    radiation in, 1287
    smoking in, 1290
    soft tissue bed in, 1285
    tumor/bone disease in, 1287
  posterior, history of, 3–4, 588–589
    indications for, 599
    internal fixation with, 600–604

Fusion (Continued)
    devices for, 601–604, 602, 603
    indications for, 600–601
    patient position for, 596
    postsurgical evaluation of, plain film radiography in, 348
    technique of, 599–600, 600
  posterolateral, for disc degeneration, 465
    advantages of, 465
    results of, 465
    for spondylolisthesis, with lysis, 745–746
    history of, 4
    pseudarthrosis after, 764
  postoperative care in, 610–611
  preoperative care/planning in, 594–596
    autologous blood donation in, 596
    metabolic work-up in, 594–596
    patient preparation in, 594
  procedure for, 596–608
  proteoglycan concentration in, animal model of, 314
  results of, documentation of, 1311
  role of, 1307–1308
  segmental instability after, 793–794
  somatosensory evoked potential monitoring during, 597
  spine evaluation after, computed tomography in, 418, 419

G

Gadolinium-labeled diethylenetriamine pentacetate (Gd-DTPA), in magnetic resonance imaging, in annular rupture/tear, 365, 365
  in infection, 372
  in metastatic disease, 373–374
  in multiply operated lumbar spine, 371, 371, 1108
  in root entrapment syndrome, 355–359, 358
GAG (glycosaminoglycan), in intervertebral discs, 274
Gallium 67 imaging, in pyogenic spondylitis, 889
  in septic intervertebral discitis, 892
Ganglion, dorsal root. See *Dorsal root ganglion (DRG)*.
Ganglionectomy, sympathetic, anterior peritoneal discectomy with, 1281
Gastrocnemius, segmental innervation of, 1233(t)
Gauvain test, 91
Gd-DTPA. See *Gadolinium-labeled diethylenetriamine pentacetate (Gd-DTPA)*.
Gender, in low back pain, 89
Gene, *c-fos*, expression of, in nerve root compression, 134
General Health Questionnaire, 1317(t), 1318(t)
Genetics, in inflammatory spondyloarthropathies, 809
Giant cell tumor, of spine, 922, 926
Gibbs-Donnan equilibrium, 275, 288
Gill procedure, for spondylolisthesis, with lysis, 745
  pedicle screws in, 644
Glioma, intramedullary, in children/adolescents, magnetic resonance imaging of, 368
Gluteus maximus, evaluation of, in low back pain, 98
  in sacroiliac joint stability, 560, 560
Glycoproteins, in intervertebral discs, 291
Glycosaminoglycan (GAG), in intervertebral discs, 274
Gold, for psoriatic spondyloarthropathy, 807
Goniometer, in range-of-motion measurement, 1046–1047
Graft(s), bone, in spinal fusion. See *Fusion, bone graft in*.

Graft(s) *(Continued)*
  fat, nerve compression by, after posterior lumbar spine surgery, 956, *957*
Granuloma, eosinophilic, of spine, 922, *927*
  plain film radiography of, 338
Gravity, effect of, on locomotion, 266–268, *267, 268*
Great toe, dorsiflexion of, evaluation of, 94
Group programs, for chronic low back pain, 1035–1036
Growth factors, in bone grafting, animal studies of, 1294–1298, 1295(t)
  in fusion outcome, 1287
Growth hormone, in fusion outcome, 1289

H

H reflexes, abnormal, *145*
  disadvantages of, 145
  in neurologic deficit evaluation, 148
  in radiculopathy localization, 149
  normal, *146*
  testing of, magnetic stimulator in, 145, *147*
  utilization of, 142(t)
Halo vest, for metastatic spinal tumor, 932–933
Hamilton Depression Rating Scale, 1049
Hamstring reflexes, evaluation of, in low back pain, 98
Hamstrings, tightness of, in spondylolisthesis, causes of, 646, *647, 648*
  surgery for, 643
HAQ (Health Assessment Questionnaire), 1317(t), 1318(t)
Harrington rods, complications of, 1219
  evaluation of, in vitro, 216
  fatigue strength of, 1193
  for adult scoliosis, and iatrogenic flat back deformity, 1157, *1160*
    complications of, 1155
    in elderly, 1155
    prognosis in, 1134
    with extended fusion, 1156, *1159*
    with severe rigid deformity, 1152
  for spondylolisthesis, in children and adolescents, 678, 681
  history of, 589
  modifications to, 1178
HCAs (heterocyclic antidepressants), for chronic low back pain, 1030
Head, derotation of, during locomotion, 264–266, *265*
Headache, spinal, after lumbar spine surgery, 954–955
Health Assessment Questionnaire (HAQ), 1317(t), 1318(t)
Health Maintenance Organizations (HMOs), in spine care, 1340
Health status, measures of, ceiling/floor effects of, 1325
  clarification of, 1326
  data in, baseline, 1326–1327
    normative, 1327–1328
  multilevel, 1325–1326
  properties of, 1324–1328
    psychometric, 1328–1332, 1330(t)
Health Status Index, 1317(t)
Health Status Index–Quality of Well-Being Scale, 1318(t)
Health Status Questionnaire, 1318(t)
Heart block, in ankylosing spondylitis, 801
Hemangioma, of spine, 922, *923*

Hematoma, epidural. See *Epidural hematoma*.
  paraspinal, plain film radiography of, 336
Hemilaminectomy, definition of, 1231
  for cauda equina syndrome, 578, 585
  for degenerative spondylolisthesis, 744–745
Hemivertebra, spinal tuberculosis vs., 878, *878*
Hemorrhage, meningeal, chemonucleolysis and, 531
  subarachnoid, arteriovenous malformation with, 573
Hemostasis, in spinal fusion, 596–597, *597*
Hensen node, 44, *44*
Hereditary multiple exostosis, and developmental spinal stenosis, 728
Hernia(tion), and anterior thigh pain, 457
  of end plate, magnetic resonance imaging of, 366
  of intervertebral discs. See *Intervertebral disc(s), herniation of*.
Heterocyclic antidepressants (HCAs), for chronic low back pain, 1030
High-resolution computed tomography (HRCT), in up-down stenosis, with lytic spondylolisthesis, 404, 406–408
  indications for, 423–424
Hip(s), abductors of, evaluation of, in low back pain, 94, 97
  flexors of, evaluation of, in low back pain, 95
  fractures of, osteoporosis in, 969–970
  in anterior thigh pain, 457
  pain in, low back pain vs., 95–96
    determination of, lumbar nerve root sheath infiltration in, *119*, 119–120
  pattern of, 91
Hip spica, 255, *255*
HLA-B27, in ankylosing spondylitis, 798
  frequency of, 802
  with Crohn disease, 808
  with ulcerative colitis, 808
  in Reiter syndrome, 803–804
  in spondyloarthropathy, inflammatory, 809
    psoriatic, 807
HLA-B38, in psoriatic spondyloarthropathy, 807
HMOs (Health Maintenance Organizations), in spine care, 1340
Hoffmann-Slatis frame, for sacroiliac joint dysfunction, 566
Hook fixation, for adult scoliosis, 1125
  for spinal fracture, 863, *863, 864*
  segmental, for spinal fracture, 863, *865*
Hormones, in fusion outcome, 1289
HRCT (high-resolution computed tomography), in up-down stenosis, with lytic spondylolisthesis, 404, 406–408
  indications for, 423–424
Human leukocyte antigens. See *HLA* enteries.
Hyaluranon, in intervertebral discs, 274
Hyaluronic acid–binding region, of intervertebral disc, *287*, 287–288
Hybridization, in situ, in mechanical back pain evaluation, 818
Hydration, of intervertebral discs. See *Intervertebral disc(s), hydration of*.
Hydraulic permeability coefficient, 294, *295*
Hydrocortisone, for low back pain, neurophysiology of, 81, *83*
Hydroxyapatite ceramics, in bone grafting, 1294
  animal studies of, 1297–1298
Hydroxypyridinium, 290, 312
Hypaque, in discography, 464

Hyperalgesia, in nerve root compression, 131
Hyperbaric oxygenation, for spinal epidural abscess, 896
Hypercalciuria, measurement of, before spinal fusion, 595
Hyperextension, and pars interarticularis fracture, 191
　for low back pain, 454
Hyperlordosis, in spondylolisthesis, 685
Hypermobility, vertebral, after spinal stenosis surgery, 770
Hyperostosis, in SAPHO syndrome, 808
　spinal, idiopathic, diffuse, and neurogenic claudication, 717
　　plain film radiography of, 344, *345*
Hypnosis, for chronic low back pain, 1035
Hypochondriasis, in low back pain, 1023
Hypogastric plexus, superior, injury to, during anterior lumbar spine surgery, 962
　location of, 508, 511, *511*
Hyponatremia, after adult scoliosis surgery, 1171–1172
Hysteria, in low back pain, 1023

I

Ibuprofen, for low back pain, 453
Ileus, after lumbar spine surgery, 947
　after scoliosis surgery, 1127–1128
Iliac arteries, hemostasis of, in spinal fusion, 597
Iliac crest, bone graft harvesting from, in spinal fusion, 598–599, *599*
Iliac vein, left, protection of, in anterior retroperitoneal transverse spine surgery, 1270
Iliac veins, hemostasis of, in spinal fusion, 597
Iliohypogastric nerve, injury to, during bone grafting, 965
Ilioinguinal nerve, injury to, during bone grafting, 965
Iliolumbar ligament, anatomy of, 67, *68*
Iliolumbar vein, injury to, during anterior lumbar spine surgery, 961
　ligation of, in twelfth rib approach, to anterior spine surgery, 1266, *1267*
Ilium, bone grafting from, for spinal fusion, 592, *593*
　stress fracture of, after bone grafting, 963, *964*
Illness Behavior Assessment Schedule, 1318(t)
Illness Behavior Questionnaire, 1317(t)
　in pain measurement, 1320(t)
Imagery, for chronic low back pain, 1033
Imaging. See also *Computed tomography (CT); Magnetic resonance imaging (MRI); Radiography.*
　interpretation of, variability in, 440–441, 440(t)
　of disc degeneration, 463–464
　of lumbar spine, in axial plane, 318, *319–326*, 324–325
　　in coronal plane, 327, *331, 332*, 332
　　in sagittal plane, 325–327, *327–330*
　overuse of, 440–441
　quality of, variability in, 440–441
　results of, irrelevant, 441
Imipramine, for chronic low back pain, 1031(t)
Immobilization, in segmental instability testing, 788
Immune system, in vertebral canal development, 715–716
Immunohistochemistry, in mechanical back pain evaluation, 818–819, *819, 820*
Immunophoresis, serum, measurement of, before spinal fusion, 595
Impaction fractures, 838(t), 839, *839*

Impedance, driving point, 194
　mechanical, definition of, 182
Implant, intolerance of, in transpedicle fixation, 1214
Impotence, after anterior lumbar spine surgery, 962
　measurement of, 155
Impulse propagation, nerves in, 126–127
In situ hybridization, in mechanical back pain evaluation, 818
Inclinometer, in range-of-motion measurement, 1046–1047
Index of ADL, 1319(t)
Indomethacin, for ankylosing spondylitis, 803
　for low back pain, 453
　injection of, for outer annular tear, in animal models, 284
Infection(s), after adult scoliosis surgery, 1172
　after anterior extraperitoneal discectomy, without fusion, 1278
　after microdiscectomy, 960
　after spinal stenosis surgery, 749–750
　after transpedicle fixation, 1211–1212
　diagnosis of, differential, 449(t)
　　tests for, accuracy of, 443
　in low back pain algorithm, 452
　of bone graft site, 963
　of disc space, after posterior microdiscectomy, 506–507
　of intervertebral disc, magnetic resonance imaging of, 371–372, *372, 373*
　of lumbar spine, plain film radiography of, 336–338, *338*
　pyogenic, 874–897
　　treatment of, conservative, 892–894
　　　surgical, 894–896, *895*
　spinal, 874–915
　tuberculous. See *Tuberculosis, of spine.*
　urinary tract, after scoliosis surgery, 1128
　wound. See *Wound infection.*
Inflammation, and nerve root irritation, historical aspects of, 87
　chronic, in mechanical back pain, 812–820
　of lumbar spine, plain film radiography of, 338–341, *340*
Inflammatory bowel disease, inflammatory spondyloarthropathy in, 807–808
Informed consent, in spine care, 1341–1342
Injury. See *Trauma.*
Insertion disorder, 236
Instrumentation, 1177–1227
　anterior, for adult scoliosis, 1140–1143, *1142, 1143*
　　complications of, 1142–1143
　　indications for, 1140–1141
　　limitations of, 1141
　　postoperative care in, 1141
　　results of, 1142
　for compression fractures, 850, *851, 852*
　history of, 591
　in vitro evaluation of, 213
　Cotrel-Dubousset. See *Cotrel-Dubousset instrumentation.*
　disadvantages of, 601
　external, for sacroiliac joint dysfunction, 566
　fixation, in vitro studies of, 213–221, *214, 215, 220*, 220(t)
　for spinal tumors, failure of, 940–941
　for spondylolisthesis surgery, 689
　for thoracolumbar stabilization, evaluation of, artificial spine models in, 221–225, *222–224*, 222(t)

Instrumentation *(Continued)*
    canine models in, 225–231, *226–228, 230*
    in vitro, 213–225
  fusion with, 1308
    anterior, 606, *607*
    for spinal stenosis, 762–764, *764*
      indications for, 764
    future of, 1309–1310
  in fusion outcome, *1286,* 1286–1287
  internal, 1216–1227
    biomechanics of, 1219
    definition of, 1218–1219
    disadvantages of, 601
    for degenerative disease, 1220, *1220, 1221*
    for metastatic disease, 1222, *1225*
    for scoliosis, 1222, 1226, *1227*
    for spondylolisthesis, 1222, *1226*
    for trauma, 1220–1222, *1222–1224*
    fusion with, anterior, 606
      indications for, 606, *607*
      posterior, 600–604
        devices for, 601–604, *602, 603*
        indications for, 590–591
    goals of, 1218–1219
    history of, 4–5, 1217–1218
    indications for, 1216–1227
    posterior, history of, 589–590
    results of, 1216–1227
    technique of, 1216–1227
  Jackson, for adult scoliosis, with iatrogenic flat back deformity, 1160, *1162*
  Jacobs, in vitro evaluation of, 216
  Kostuik-Harrington, for adult scoliosis, with iatrogenic flat back deformity, *1163, 1164*
    in vitro evaluation of, 218
  Luque. See *Luque instrumentation.*
  posterior, for adult scoliosis, 1125–1127, *1126*
    complications of, 1149, *1150, 1151*
    results of, 1149
    for burst fractures, 853, *854, 855*
      with neurologic deficit, 855
    for flexion-distraction injuries, 857
    indications for, 862
  Roy-Camille, 1179–1181
    history of, 590
    in vitro evaluation of, 216
  segmental, posterior, for adult scoliosis, 1143–1149, *1144–1148, 1150, 1151*
    complications of, 1149, *1150, 1151*
  spine evaluation after, computed tomography in, 418, *419*
  transpedicle. See *Transpedicle fixation.*
Interbody spacers, in vitro evaluation of, 218
Intercostal arteries, ligation of, in tenth rib approach, to anterior spine surgery, 1258, *1258*
Intercostal muscles, 52
Interference patterns, measurement of, needle electromyography in, 148
Interleukin–1, in mechanical back pain evaluation, 819, *820*
Intermediate mesoderm columns, 44
Internal consistency reliability, in health status outcome measurement, 1330–1331
Internal disc disruption, definition of, 17–18
Internal fixation systems, history of, 4–5
Internal vertebral venous plexus, *63*
Interspinal muscles, 52

Interspinous ligaments, anatomy of, 51
Intertransverse ligaments, anatomy of, 51, 67, *68*
Intertransverse muscles, 52
Intervertebral disc(s), abnormality of, diagnosis of, computed tomography vs. myelography in, *417,* 417–418
  aging of, biochemistry of, 301–304, *302*
    degeneration vs., 310–314
  anatomy of, 63
  biochemistry of, 271–314
    in animal models, 283, 313–314
  bulging of, trunk muscle testing in, 1093–1095, *1094*
  cells of, *291,* 291–292, *292*
    biology of, 310–314
    density of, 291, *291*
    types of, 291, *292*
  collagen of, organization of, 273–274
  components of, 271–272, 272(t)
    biochemical, 286–291, *287–289*
      changes in, aging in, 272
      degeneration/disease in, 272
    structural, 285–286, *286*
      biochemistry of, 312–314
  decompression of, chemonucleolysis in, 524–534
    percutaneous discectomy in, 524–534
  degeneration of, 17–18, *18*
    aging vs., 310–314
    and low back pain, 459–460
      mechanical, 816, *816*
    animal models of, 281–284
    autopsy studies of, *20,* 20–21
    biochemistry of, 301–304
    clinical implications of, 55–56
    computed tomography of, 384–409, *388–392*
    electron microscopy of, 311–312
    epidural hematoma with, *383, 385*
    etiology of, 304–305, 458–467
    factors in, 54
    fusion for, 1308
      results of, 1307
    histologic, 311–312
    in spondylolisthesis, and back pain, 657
    macroscopic, 311
    magnetic resonance imaging of, 22–24, *23,* 362–364, *363–365,* 391–392
    pathoanatomy of, 460–465
      biochemical changes in, 460–462
      discographic changes in, 464–465
      studies of, 462–463
      imaging, 463–464
    pathogenesis of, 304–305
    radiographic studies of, 21–22
      in sagittal plane, 327, *330, 331*
      plain film, 343–344, *344, 345*
    treatment of, surgical, methods of, 465–467
      results of, 465–467
  disease of, clinical behavior of, 475–476
    definition of, 16–18, *17*
    epidemiology of, 16–25
    evaluation of, *18,* 18–19
    occurrence rate of, 19–25
    orthoses for, 256
    risk factors for, 19–25, 19(t), *20*
    spinal stenosis with, 741
  displacement of, 792
    in degenerative lumbar stenosis, 732

Intervertebral disc(s) *(Continued)*
  disruption of, definition of, 17–18
  distortion of, terminology for, *493,* 493–494, *494*
  excision of. See *Discectomy.*
  fissures of, in mechanical back pain, 816, *816, 817*
  function of, 285–286
  herniation of, 477
    after spinal stenosis surgery, case report of, 750, *751*
      magnetic resonance imaging of, 753, *753*
    and cauda equina syndrome. See *Cauda equina syndrome (CES), disc herniation and.*
    central, 354
    classification of, 477
    clinical implications of, 473–487
    combined spinal loading with, 175
    computed tomography of, 386–392, *388*
      blinded prospective analysis of, 414, 414(t)
      myelography vs., 413–418, 413(t), 414(t), *417*
      retrospective analysis of, 413–414
    conjoined nerve roots with, 380, *382*
    contained vs. noncontained, computed tomography of, 390, *391*
      magnetic resonance imaging of, 356–358, *357, 358, 392*
    diagnosis of, 476–481
      clinical, 478–481
        cerebrospinal fluid examination in, 480
        mobility in, 478
        motor deficits in, 480
        pain/suffering in, 481
        posture in, 478
        present pain in, 478
        radiographic examination in, 480–481
        reflex changes in, 480
        sensory disturbances in, 480
        tension sign in, 478–480
      differential, 477–478
      pathoanatomy in, 476–477
      physical examination in, 441–442, 442(t)
      tests for, accuracy of, 442
    factors in, 475
    foraminal, surgical treatment of, *519,* 519–520, *520*
    fusion for, 1308
    impact of, 474–475
    in adolescents, magnetic resonance imaging of, 369
    in mechanical back pain, *815,* 815–816
    in multiply operated lumbar spine, 1109(t), 1111
    in pregnancy 1058
    in spinal stenosis, surgical treatment of, 520
    in spondylolisthesis, and back pain, 658
      degenerative, 412
      surgical treatment of 520
    in up-down stenosis, with lytic spondylolisthesis, 404, *405, 406*
    incidence of, 24–25
    lateral, 354–355
      computed tomography of, 386, *389*
    lateral stenosis with, nerve root entrapment in, *494,* 494, 494(t)
    location of, 477
    magnetic resonance imaging of, 358–359, *359*
    midline, computed tomography of, 388–390, *390*
    myelography of, blinded prospective analysis of, 414, 414(t)

Intervertebral disc(s) *(Continued)*
      retrospective analysis of 413–414
    natural history of, 473–487
    nerve root compression in, biomechanics of, 128
    nerve root displacement in, computed tomography of, 384, *388*
    nonorganic disability in, signs/symptoms of, 522, 522(t)
    ontogenetics of, 473–474
    pain mechanisms in, 481–482
    pattern of, 476–477
    phylogenetics of, 473–474
    plain film radiography of, 348
    posterolateral, 354
    recurrent, after lumbar spine surgery, posterior, 954
      scar formation vs., 954
    chemonucleolysis in, 529
    imaging of, *521,* 522
      magnetic resonance imaging of, 369–370
    sciatica with, magnetic resonance imaging of, 358–359
    size of, 476
    speed of, 476–477
    staging of, 494–495, *494–497*
    surgical anatomy of, 60
    surgical treatment of, anterior approaches to, 507–515
      advantages of, 508
      disadvantages of, 508
      extraperitoneal, 514–515, *515–517*
      indications for, 507–508, *508, 509*
      postoperative care in, 515
      surgical anatomy for, 508–511, *510, 511*
      transperitoneal, 511–514, *511–514*
    contraindications to, 498 498(t)
    diagnostic testing before, 498
    indications for, 456, 483, 492–522
    options for, 498–519
    patient selection for, 483
    percutaneous lumbar discectomy in, 515–519, *518*
    posterior approaches to, *499,* 499–507, 499(t)
      limited discectomy in, 500–502, *500–503*
      microdiscectomy in, 502–505, *504–506.* See also *Microdiscectomy.*
    results of, 483
    techniques for, 492–522
  surgically induced, animal model of, 313–314
  treatment of, 482–486
    agenda for, 486
    bed rest in, 484
    causal, 483
    coping in, 485–486
    current approach to, 520–522, *521,* 522(t)
    effectiveness of, 33(t)
    exercise in, 485
    future of, 486–487
    manipulation in, 1016–1017
    medication in, 484
    microsurgical, complications of, 505–507
    operative vs. nonoperative, 1238
    physical therapy in, 484–485
    results of, 497, 497(t)
    symptomatic, 483–486
  histology of, 281–284
  hydration of, aging in, 461

Intervertebral disc(s) *(Continued)*
   factors in, 287, *287*
   in loading, 277
      disc composition in, 277, *278*
      proteoglycans in, 288, *288*
   proteoglycans in, 276–277
   swelling/leaching in, 286–287, *287*
  imaging of, in axial plane, 318, *319*, *320*
  in low back pain, 30, 999
   historical aspects of, 87
  in water/solute transport, 294–297, *295*, *296*
  infection of, magnetic resonance imaging of, 371–372, *372*, *373*
  lesions of, anterior, magnetic resonance imaging of, 366
  loading of, 53
   repetitive, mechanical effects of, 190
   response to, 172–173
  matrix of, 292–293, *293*
   components of, 272–274
     metabolism of, 277–279
  mechanical properties of, during lumbar spine loading, 171(t)
  metabolism of, 294–297, *295*, *296*
  narrowing of, after anterior extraperitoneal discectomy, without fusion, 1278, *1279*
  in spinal tuberculosis, *876*, 877
  neural elements of, 293–294
  nutrition of, 285–305
   factors in, 297–301, *297*–*301*
  pain in, diagnosis of, 90
  pathophysiology of, 285–305
  prolapse of, clinical presentation of, 1234, 1234(t)
   treatment of, 1241–1243
  proteoglycans of, 274
  resorption of, spontaneous, magnetic resonance imaging of, 365–366
  sequestered, 477
  surgery of, development of, history of, 492, 493(t)
   open, history of, 1–2
Intervertebral foramen, imaging of, in axial plane, 318, *323*
  in coronal plane, *331*, *332*
  in sagittal plane, *329*
  stenosis of, in spinal stenosis, magnetic resonance imaging of, 361–362, *362*
   surgical treatment of, indications for, 774–775
     results of, 769
Intervertebral motion device, in spinal stability evaluation, 209
Intervertebral nerve, root canal stenosis of, in spondylolisthesis, and back pain, 658
Intestines, injury to, during transpedicle fixation, 1206
Intradiscal procedures, percutaneous, history of, 3
Inverse dynamics, in trunk muscle strength testing, 1084–1087, *1085*, *1086*
Ionic solutes, concentration of, factors in, 275, *276*
Iophendylate, injection of, in myelography, sequelae of, 417
Iothalamate meglumine, injection of, into facet joint, results of, 544–545
Iritis, in ankylosing spondylitis, 800
ISOLA system, in vitro evaluation of, 218
  of transpedicle fixation, *866*
Isometric exercise, for disc herniation, 485
  for low back pain, 454
  for spondylolisthesis, 662

Isometric testing, dynamic lifting tests with, 1083–1084
Isoniazid, for spinal tuberculosis, 880–882
Isostation B200, in trunk muscle strength testing, 1077–1078, *1078*, 1080, *1082*, 1099
Isotonic exercise, for spondylolisthesis, 662
Isthmic defect repair, for spondylolisthesis, in children and adolescents, 674

J

Jackson instrumentation, for adult scoliosis, with iatrogenic flat back deformity, 1160, *1162*
Jacobs instrumentation, in vitro evaluation of, 216
Jewett hyperextension orthosis, 252, *253*
Job satisfaction, as low back injury predictor, 1070, *1070*
Joint(s). See also named joint, e.g., *Hip(s)*.
  apophyseal, in back pain, 87
  facet. See *Facet joint(s)*.
  in reactive arthritis, 804
  manipulation of, definition of, 1012–1013
  peripheral, disease of, in ankylosing spondylitis, 800
   in psoriatic spondyloarthropathy, 806–807
  sacroiliac. See *Sacroiliac joint*.
  zygapophyseal. See *Zygapophyseal joint*.
Jugular vein, compression of, in low back pain, 94

K

Kaneda device, evaluation of, artificial spine models in, 221
  in vitro, 218
  for anterior decompression, in spinal fracture, *869*
  for anterior fusion, *607*
  for compression fractures, *851*
Kenny Self-Care Evaluation, 1319(t)
Keratan sulfate (KS), biochemistry of, 313
  changes in, in disc degeneration, 461
  in fixed charge density, 288
  in intervertebral discs, 274, 287, *287*
Keratoderma blennorrhagicum, in reactive arthritis, 804
Kerrison rongeur, for laminectomy, in spinal stenosis, 738–739
Kidney, disorders of, in ankylosing spondylitis, 801
Kidney rest, use of, in anterior interbody fusion, 606
Klebsiella pneumoniae, and reactive arthritis, 803(t)
  in ankylosing spondylitis, 802
Kluger fixateur interne, in vitro evaluation of, 216
Knee jerk, evaluation of, in disc herniation, 480
  in low back pain, 95
Kneeling position, for posterior lumbar surgery, 499, *499*
  precautions with, 499, 499(t)
Knodt rods, complications of, 1219
  for internal fixation, in posterior fusion, 601, *602*
Knuttson sign, 792
Kostuik-Harrington device, for adult scoliosis, with iatrogenic flat back deformity, *1163*, *1164*
  in vitro evaluation of, 218
KS. See *Keratan sulfate (KS)*.
KTP laser, in percutaneous discectomy, 517–518
Kuskokwim disease, pathologic spondylolisthesis in, 637
Kyphoscoliosis, adult, posterior instrumentation for, 1146, *1147*

Kyphosis, angle of, after spinal tuberculosis treatment, 882, 883(t)
  congenital spondylolisthesis with, 628–630
  in osteoporosis, 983–984
  in pregnancy, 1060
  lumbosacral, in spondylolisthesis, 685
  spinal stenosis with, fusion for, 759–761, *760, 761*
  spinal tuberculosis and, 875

L

L5 vertebra, deep-seated, lumbar nerve root sheath infiltration with, *120,* 120–121
Labor, low back pain during, 1059
Lactate, concentration of, in intervertebral disc, after exercise, 298, *298*
  after fusion, 299
Lactic acid, production of, in intervertebral disc, in animal model, 295
Lambeth Disability Screening Questionnaire, 1319(t)
Lambeth Health Survey, 1319(t)
Lamella(e), collagen network of, organization of, 273
  functions of, 286, *286*
  imaging of, in axial plane 318, *319, 320, 325*
    in sagittal plane, *329*
  in disc degeneration, 311
Laminar hooks, for internal fixation, history of, 589
Laminectomy, 1230–1250
  approach to, 1247–1250, 1247(t), *1248*
  complications of, 953–953
  computed tomography before, retrospective analysis of, 415–418, *417*
  decompressive, for spinal stenosis, 1245–1246
    segmental instability after, 792–793, *793*
  definition of, 1230–1231
  diagnostic criteria for, 1232–1238, 1232(t), *1233,* 1233(t), 1234(t), 1235(t), *1236*
  for cauda equina syndrome, 578, 585
  for disc herniation, fusion with, 1243
  for isolated root canal stenosis, results of, 768–769
  for nerve root compromise 1234–1235, 1234(t), 1235(t)
  for spinal cord compression, in metastatic spinal tumor, neurologic outcome in, 935
  for spinal epidural abscess 896
  for spinal stenosis, 737–740
    central, results of, 770–771, *771*
    expansive laminoplasty vs., 740
  for spinal tumors, indications for, 933
  for spondylolisthesis, 687
    degenerative, 704–705, 744–745
    results of, 769
    in children and adolescents, 676, 678, *679*
  history of, 1–2
  posterior, for neurologic deficit, in metastatic spinal tumor, 934–935
  for spinal tumor, 934–935
  repeated, for multiply operated lumbar spine, technique of, 1114
  retrospective analysis of, myelography in, 415–418, *417*
  revision, 1246–1247
  techniques of, 1232–1238, 1232(t), *1233,* 1233(t), 1234(t), 1235(t), *1236*
  total, for spinal stenosis, selection of, 775, *775*
  instability after 769–770
Laminoplasty, expansive, laminectomy vs., for spinal stenosis, 740

Laminotomy, definition of, 1231
  for isolated root canal stenosis, results of, 768–769
  multiple, for spinal stenosis, central, results of, *770,* 771
    selection of, 775
    technique of, 778–779
Laminotomy fenestration, definition of, 1231
Laminotomy-discectomy, limited, technique of, 500–502, *500–503*
Laser, low-energy, for industrial low back pain, follow-up of, 1090
Laser discectomy, 1231
  percutaneous, 517–518, 525
Lateral femoral cutaneous nerve, injury to, during bone grafting, 965
Lateral lumbar circumferential wedge osteotomy, for imbalanced adult scoliosis, 1164–1167, *1165, 1166*
Lateral mesoderm plate, 44
Lateral recess stenosis (LRS), decompression for, results of, 1244
  pain in, 732
Lateral stenosis, 360
  causes of, 394, 398
  chemonucleolysis in, 529
  clinical presentation of, 729–730
  computed tomography of, 392–397 *395–397*
  disc herniation with, nerve root entrapment in, 494, *494,* 494(t)
  fenestration procedures for, 740
  imaging of, 394, *395*
  in degenerative spondylolisthesis, computed tomography of, *411,* 412
  in spondylosis, 393–394
  terminology in, 728–729, 728(t)
  types of, 396
Lateral wedge injuries, management of, 860
Left iliac artery, injury to, during anterior lumbar spine surgery, 962
Left iliac vein, protection of, in anterior retroperitoneal transverse spine surgery, 1270
Leg(s), affected vs. healthy, strength of, in disc herniation, 480
  pain in, low back pain vs., 454–457
Leg lifting, in low back pain evaluation, 96
  well, crossover pain vs., 96
Leg referral zone pain, back pain with, in spondylolisthesis, 658
  causes of, 658
Leksell rongeur, for laminectomy in spinal stenosis, 738
Lesion maker, for facet syndrome, historical background of, 540
Levator muscles, 52
Lido Active Back System, 1083
Lido Lift Rehabilitation System, 1083, 1084, *1085*
Lidocaine, for back strain, 455
  for facet syndrome, bupivacaine injection with, 556
  for low back pain, neurophysiology of, 81, *83*
Lift testing, 1047
  dynamic, 1083–1084
  isoinertial, 1047, 1083–1084
  isokinetic, 1047, 1083–1084
  isometric, 1047, 1083–1084
  preemployment, 1096
Lifting, biomechanics of, *242–247* 242–248
  guidelines for, 244–246, *246*

Lifting (Continued)
    lumbar motion during, 248, 249
    weight restrictions for, 246–248, 247
Lifting strength, as low back injury claims predictor, 1068
Ligament(s). See also names of specific ligaments.
    in chronic low back pain, rehabilitation of, 1045
    in spinal stability, 204, 204
    spinal, anatomy of, 67–68, 68
        loading of, response to, 173, 173(t)
Ligamentum flavum, hypertrophy of, in spinal stenosis, magnetic resonance imaging of, 360, 361
    imaging of, in axial plane, 318, 319, 320, 323
        in sagittal plane, 325, 328, 329
            in degenerative disc disease, 330, 331
        in degenerative spondylolisthesis, 701
        computed tomography of, 409, 411
    preservation of, in posterior microdiscectomy, 503
Likert-type scale, frequency, 1323, 1323
Limbus vertebral fractures, in spinal stenosis, 742, 742–744, 743
Link proteins, in aging intervertebral disc, 313
Lipofuscin, in aging intervertebral disc, 302
Lipoma, in children/adolescents, magnetic resonance imaging of, 368
Liquid crystal tomography, before laminectomy, 1237
Locomotion, gravity in, 266–268, 267, 268
    spine in, 262, 262–263, 263
    trunk in, 264–268
Longissimus muscle, 52
Longitudinal ligament(s), failure of, 823–824
    ossification of, in ankylosing spondylitis, plain film radiography of, 340, 340
    posterior. See Posterior longitudinal ligament.
Longitudinal vein, imaging of, in axial plane, 318, 319, 320
Lopamidol, in discography, 464
Lordosis, in pregnancy, 1060
    restoration of, in iatrogenic flat back deformity, in adult scoliosis, 1162–1164, 1163, 1164
Louis plate fixation system, 746
Loupes, in spinal fragment excision, 500–502, 500–503
Low Back Disability Questionnaire, 1318(t)
Low back pain, activity-related, magnetic resonance imaging of, 362
    in older patient, 367
    in young adult, 367
    acute, progression of, 1026
    after anterior extraperitoneal discectomy, without fusion, 1281, 1281(t)
    after chemonucleolysis, 532, 961
    algorithm for, 447–457, 448(t), 449(t)
        back vs. leg pain in, 454–457
        cauda equina compression in, 452
        concepts of, 450–451
        goals of, 447–450
        guidelines in, 451
        medical conditions in, 452–454
            acute, 452
            braces/corsets for, 454
            drug therapy for, 453
            exercise for, 454
            rest for, 453
        patient evaluation in, 450
        sciatica in, 456–457
            spinal stenosis in, 456–457

Low back pain (Continued)
    standards in, 451
    thigh pain in, anterior, 457
        posterior, 457
    and disability, 11–12, 12–14
    biochemical factors in, 80–82, 82, 83
    biomechanics of, 75–76, 76(t)
    causes of, extraspinal, 455
        identification of, 74–75
    chronic, biopsychosocial factors in, 1026
        definition of, 1018
        functional restoration in, 1042–1053
            need for, 1042
            outcomes of, 1051–1052
            policies for, 1052–1053
            politics in, 1052–1053
            program for, 1049–1051, 1050(t)
            variations of, 1051–1052
        organic vs. functional, 1026–1029
        progression of, to acute pain, 1026
        psychiatric assessment in, indications for, 1022–1026, 1029
        psychosocial factors in, 1018–1022
        treatment of, behavioral intervention procedures in, 1032–1034
            cognitive approaches in, 1034–1035
            group treatment in, 1035–1036
            hypnosis in, 1035
            operant behavioral programs in, 1032–1033
            pharmacologic, 1029–1032, 1031(t)
            psychodynamic psychotherapy in, 1035
            psychologic, 1018–1036
            respondent treatment approaches in, 1033–1034
    classification of, 98–101, 99(t), 100(t)
    derangement syndrome in, 1004–1005
        treatment of, mechanical, 1009
    dermatomes in, 108, 108–109, 109
    diagnosis of, 31, 74–158
        differential, 449(t)
        electrodiagnostic testing in, 141–158
        facet joints in, 543
        historical aspects of, 86–88
        history taking in, 85–101
            age in, 88–89
            disability in, 92
            diurnal pattern in, 90–91
            exacerbating/relieving factors in, 90
            family history in, 92
            occupation in, 89–90
            pain description in, 91–92
            pain pattern in, 91
            pain periodicity in, 90
            psychologic factors in, 92
            reliability of, 88
            sex in, 89
            smoking in, 92
        mechanical, 998–1010, 1000–1006
            history in, 1000–1001
            pain patterns in, 1001–1006, 1003, 1004
            palpation in, 1000–1001
        medical, 1000
        physical examination in, 85–101
            of musculoskeletal system, while bending over examining table, 95
                while lying prone, 97
                while lying supine, 95–96
                while side-lying, 97

Low back pain *(Continued)*
  while standing, 93–94
  of nervous system, while kneeling on chair, 94
    while lying prone, 97–98
    while lying supine, 96–97
    while side-lying, 97
    while sitting on chair/feet on floor, 94–95
    while sitting on examining table/legs hanging free, 95
    while standing, 93–94
  disc degeneration and, 30, 459–460
  discography in, 431–432
  during labor, 1059
  dysfunction syndrome in, 1004
    treatment of, mechanical, 1009
  economic consequences of, 12–14, 15(t)
  facet joints in, arthrography of. See *Arthrography, of facet joints.*
  fitness in, 33–34, 34(t)
  frequency of, 8–9
  future of, 28–37
  health care service utilization for, 10–11, 10–12, 11(t)
  hip pain vs., 95–96
    determination of, lumbar nerve root sheath infiltration in, 119, 119–120
  idiopathic, orthoses for, 256
    psychosocial factors in, 32–33
  impact of, 10–12
  impairment in, evaluation of, 1074
  in adult scoliosis, 1134
  in children/adolescents, magnetic resonance imaging of, 367–369
    posture in, 368–369
  in degenerative lumbar stenosis, 731
  in discitis, 907
  in osteoporosis, 983
  in pregnancy. See *Pregnancy, low back pain in.*
  in scoliosis, adult, history of, 1119–1120
    incidence of, 1119
    treatment of, 1121–1122
  in spinal tumors, 918, 918(t)
  in spondylolisthesis, 656–658
    causes of, 657
    degenerative, 701
    leg referral zone pain with, 658
      causes of, 658
    pathophysiology of, 657
  industrial. See *Occupations, industrial, low back pain from.*
  intensity of, 1001–1002
  loading and, 163–164
  location of, 1001–1002, 1003, 1004
  lumbar nerve root sheath infiltration in. See *Lumbar nerve(s), root sheath infiltration of.*
  mechanical, clinical features of, 812–814
    defective fibrinolysis with, 813–814
      stanozolol for, 814
    fibrosis in, 812–820
    inflammation in, chronic, 812–820
    nerve root compression in, 814
    smoking in, 814
    vascular damage in, 812–820
      pathogenesis of, 814–820, 815–820
        biopsy studies of, 818–819, 819, 820
        cadaveric studies of, 814–818, 815–818
  motion segment mechanics in, 30–31

Low back pain *(Continued)*
  muscles in, 29–30
  nervous system in, 28–29
  neuromechanisms of, 74–153
  neurophysiology of, 76–80, 77–81, 77(t), 79(t)
  nonspecific, classification of, 1002–1005
    identification of, 1005–1006
    treatment of, mechanical, 1009
  occupational, mechanisms of, 235, 235–236
  pathology of, 819–820, 999–1000
  patterns of, 105–121
  plain film radiography of, 335
  postpartum, 1062
  postural syndrome in, 1002–1003
    treatment of, mechanical, 1009
  prevention of, 36
  problem of, magnitude of, 8–15
  psychosocial assessment in, 1048–1049
  radicular, nonradicular vs., 105–108, 106, 107(t)
  radiologic abnormalities in, 436(t)
  recovery from, natural history of, 9, 9
  repetitive tasks and, 182–192
  rheumatoid arthritis with, in pregnancy, 1059–1060, 1060
  sacroiliac joint dysfunction in, incidence of, 561
  sciatica vs., 492
  sclerotomes in, 108, 108–109, 109
  signs of, nonorganic, 1234, 1235(t)
  sources of, 59
  transitory, 476
  treatment of, 31–32, 32(t), 33(t), 998–1010
    activation program in, 35–36
    autotraction in, 1008
    bed rest in, 992–993
    chemonucleolysis in, 529
    diagnostic blocks in, 105–121
    exercise in, 33–34, 34(t), 1008–1009
    massage in, 1008
    mechanical, 1006–1009
      methods of, 1006–1009
    psychosocial evaluation in, 455
    self-treatment in, 1006–1008
    spinal manipulative therapy in, 1006–1008
    surgical, indications for, 492–522
      techniques for, 492–522
    traction in, 1008
  workers' compensation for, 12–14, 13(t), 14
Lower extremity(ies), in neurogenic claudication, 722
  muscles of, segmental innervation of, 1233, 1233(t)
  neurologic deficit of, diagnostic testing of, 143–144, 144
LRS (lateral recess stenosis), decompression for, results of, 1244
  pain in, 732
Lumbago, etiology of, 452
  facet syndrome in, historical background of, 538
Lumbar artery, anatomy of, 62
  shunting of, during walking, in neurogenic claudication, 722
Lumbar disc surgery, development of, history of, 492, 493(t)
Lumbar discectomy, percutaneous, history of, 3
Lumbar nerve(s), anatomy of, 569–570
  root sheath infiltration of, 112–121
    diagnostic value of, 115–117
    indications for, 118–120, 119
    pitfalls in, 115, 116, 121

Lumbar nerve(s) *(Continued)*
  predictive value of, 117–118
  recommendations for, *120,* 120–121
  replicability of, 116–117
  sensitivity of, 117
  specificity of, 117
  technique of, 113–115, *113–116*
  validity of, 117
Lumbar spine, algorithm for, 447–457, 448(t), 449(t)
  anatomy of, 43–69, 379–384
    applied, 47–52
    clinical, *58,* 58–59, *59*
    developmental, 43–47, *44–48*
    diagnostic, 59–60
    imaging, 317–332
    pathologic, 60
    regional, 61–68, *62–68*
    surgical, 60–61
    theoretical, 58
    variations in, computed tomography of, 379–380, *381, 382*
  arthrology of, 47–51, *50*
  automanipulation of, 1014, *1014*
  care of, academic institutions in, 1344–1345
    conflicts of interest in, 1340–1341
      among experts, 1341
    ethics of, 1339–1345
    experimental vs. investigational, 1342
    information use in, 1342–1344
    informed consent in, 1341–1342
    politics in, 1344
    poor medical testimony in, 1342–1343
    second opinion in, 1343–1344, 1344(t)
  curvature of, in adult scoliosis, types of, 1145–1146, *1146–1148*
  disorders of, epidemiology of, 1–15
    treatment of, vs. spontaneous resolution, 1238–1246, 1239(t), *1240,* 1241(t), *1244*
  embryology of, 43–47, *44–48*
  evaluation of, postsurgical, plain film radiography in, 348, *349*
  fracture of, internal fixation for, 1220–1222
  hypokyphotic, posterior instrumentation for, 1148
  imaging of, accuracy of, 434–445
    in axial plane, 318, *319–326,* 324–325
    in coronal plane, 327, *331,* 332, *332*
    in sagittal plane, 325–327, *327–330*
    plain film, 333–351
      views in, *334,* 334–335
    reproducibility of, 434–445
  infection of, plain film radiography of, 336–338, *338*
  inflammation of, plain film radiography of, 338–341, *340*
  injury to, plain film radiography of, 335–336, *336, 337*
  loading of, and bone remodeling, 176–178
    biomechanical analyses of, 163–179, 171(t), 173(t), *174–176*
    combined, 174–175
    evaluation of, 164–170, *165,* 165(t), *167*
      electromyographic models in, 169–170
      optimization models in, 166–169, *167*
    facet joints in, 173–174, *174–176*
    intervertebral disc in, 172–173
    multisegment studies of, 175–176
    neurophysiologic studies of, 79–80, *80, 81*
    repeated, and spondylolysis, 185–186

Lumbar spine *(Continued)*
    effects of, 181–197
      in vitro investigations of, 188–192
      frequency/endurance of, 186–187
      in vivo observation of, in exposed cohorts, 187–188
      risk factors for, in athletic training, 184–185
        in industrial labor environments, 183–184
    spinal ligaments in, 173, 173(t)
  magnetic resonance imaging of, 353–375
  manipulation of. See *Manipulation, of lumbar spine.*
  multiply operated, algorithmic approach to, 1106–1116
    differential diagnosis in, 1108–1113, 1109(t), *1110*
      of extraspinal problems, 1108–1111
      of mechanical lesions, 1109(t), 1111–1112
      of nonmechanical entities, 1109(t), 1112–1113
    magnetic resonance imaging of, 370–371, *371*
    patient evaluation in, 1107–1108
      history in, 1107
      imaging in, 1108
      physical examination in, 1107
    surgery of, techniques of, 1113–1116, *1115*
  myology of, 51–52
  neoplasm of, plain film radiography of, 338, *339, 340*
  neurology of, 51–52
  osteology of, 47–51, *50*
  surgery of, anterior, 1252–1271
    complications of, 961–963
    eleventh rib approach to, 1258–1260, *1259, 1261*
      closure in, 1260
    incisions for, 1253
    patient positioning for, 1253
    retroperitoneal, 1254
    tenth rib approach to, 1255–1258, *1255–1258*
      closure in, 1258
    transperitoneal, 1254
    twelfth rib approach to, 1262–1269, *1263–1265, 1267, 1268*
      closure in, 1266–1269, *1267, 1268*
  approaches to, 1230–1283
  complications of, 945–965
    intraoperative, 946–947
    preoperative, 945–946
  failed, causes of, 418
    lumbar nerve root sheath infiltration for, 120
  frequency of, 10–11, *11,* 11(t), *12*
  history of, 1–15
  outlook for, 5–6
  posterior, complications of, 953–961
    prone positioning for, complications of, 946
  postoperative, 947–953
  vibration of, effects of, 181–197
    studies of, 195–196
  vulnerable, plain film radiography of, 348–351, *350*
Lumbar sympathetic chain, injury to, during anterior lumbar spine surgery, 962
Lumbosacral junction, degenerative disease of, internal instrumentation for, 1220, *1220, 1221*
Lumbosacral plexus, injury to, during anterior lumbar spine surgery, 963
  during transpedicle fixation, 1204
Lumbosacral spine, imaging of, in axial plane, 318, *324*

Lumbosacral spine *(Continued)*
  surgery of, anterior, 1252–1271
    eleventh rib approach to, 1258–1260, *1259, 1261*
      closure in, 1260
    incisions for, 1253
    patient positioning for, 1253
    retroperitoneal, 1254
    transverse, *1268, 1269–1271, 1270*
    tenth rib approach to, 1255–1258, *1255–1258*
      closure in, 1258
    transperitoneal, 1254
    twelfth rib approach to, 1262–1269, *1263–1265, 1267, 1268*
      closure in, 1266–1269, *1267, 1268*
Lumbosacral strain, orthoses for, 256
Lung, disease of, in ankylosing spondylitis, 801
Luque instrumentation, development of, 1178
  fatigue strength of, 1193
  for adult scoliosis, 1143, *1144*
  for internal fixation, in posterior fusion, 601, *602*
  in vitro evaluation of, 215–217
Lymphoma, of spine, 927
  survival in, 928(t)

M

Macromolecular solutes, distribution of, factors in, 277–278
Magnesium, concentration of, in intervertebral disc, 275
Magnetic resonance imaging (MRI), 353–375
  before laminectomy, 1235–1236
  discography after, indications for, 431
  in diagnostic anatomy, 59–60
  in low back pain activity-related, 362
    in older patient, 367
    in young adult, 367
  in children/adolescents, 367–369
  in trunk muscle evaluation, in industrial low back pain, 1098
  indications for, 423–424
  of adult scoliosis, 1121, 1136
  of annular bulging, 356, *356*
  of annulus rupture/tear, 364–365, *365*
    Gd-DTPA in, 365, *365*
  of deep wound infection, 950
  of disc degeneration, 362–364, *363–365*, 391–392, 464
    discography with, 465
    studies of, 22–24, *23*
  of disc disease, 18
    anterior, 366
  of disc herniation, 358–359, *359*
    accuracy of, 442, 442(t)
    after spinal stenosis surgery, 753
    contained vs. noncontained, 356–358, *357, 358, 392*
    in adolescents, 369
    recurrent, 369–370, *521,* 522
    with sciatica, 358–359
  of discitis, 371–372, *372, 373,* 420, *421, 422*
    accuracy of, 443
    Gd-DTPA in, 372
    intervertebral, septic, 892
    postoperative, 951, *952*
  of dural arteriovenous fistula, 573–574

Magnetic resonance imaging (MRI) *(Continued)*
  of epidural hematoma, *383* 384
  of leaking abdominal aneurysm, 372, *373*
  of metastatic disease, accuracy of, 443
  of multiply operated lumbar spine, 370–371, *371,* 1108
    Gd-DTPA in, 371, *371*
  of neoplasms, 420, *423*
  of osteomyelitis, 420, *421, 422*
  of root entrapment syndrome, 355–359, *355–359*
    Gd-DTPA in, 355–359, *358*
  of spinal epidural abscess, 892, *893*
  of spinal fractures, 846
  of spinal stenosis, 360–362, *361, 362,* 409, *410,* 752
    accuracy of, 442–443, 443(t)
    degenerative, advantages of, 735
      disadvantages of, 735
    up-down, with lytic spondylolisthesis, 404, *406,* 408
  of spinal tuberculosis, 878, *881*
  of spondylitis, pyogenic, 889, *891*
    tuberculous, 878, *881*
  of spondylolisthesis, 367, 686 *686*
    degenerative, 672
  of spondylolysis, 367, *367*
  of spontaneous disc resorption, 365–366
  of synovial cysts, 384, *388*
  of trauma, 374–375
  of tumors, 372–374, 920–921
    intraspinal, 374
    metastatic, 373–374, *374*
      Gd-DTPA in, 373
    primary, 372–373
  results of, in normal subjects, 436, 436(t)
  uses of, 377
  vs. computed tomography, 317
  vs. discography, 366–367
Magnetic stimulator, for low back pain, 141–142
  in H reflex testing, 145, *147*
  in paraspinal muscle stimulation, *157,* 157–158
  in somatosensory evoked potential testing, 147
Malignancy, lumbar nerve root entrapment in, lumbar nerve root sheath infiltration for, 120, *120*
Malnutrition, in neuroosseous development, 715–716
Mamillary process, 49, *50*
Mamilloaccessory ligament, anatomy of, 67
Manipulation, for disc herniation, 485
  for sacroiliac joint dysfunction, 566
  for spondylolisthesis, 659
    lytic, 659
  of joint, definition of, 1012–1013
  of lumbar spine, 1012–1017
    contraindications to, 1016
    effects of, 1014
    history of, 1013–1014
    indications for, 1014–1016, *1015*
    limitations of, *1016,* 1016–1017
    purpose of, 1014, *1014*
    techniques of, classification of, 1013, 1013(t)
Manual materials handling, biomechanics of, 241–249, *242–249*
  lifting belts for, 249
  pushing/pulling in, 249
  static strength models of, 248, *248*
  unexpected loading during, 248–249
Manual resistance exercise, for spondylolisthesis, 662
Manual therapy, for disc herniation, 485

Maprotiline, for chronic low back pain, 1031(t)
Massage, for disc herniation, 484
  for low back pain, 1008
Maximum voluntary exertion (MVE), in trunk muscle strength testing, 1079
McGill Comprehensive Pain Questionnaire (MCPQ), 1317, 1317(t)
  limitations of, 1317
McGill Pain Inventory, in chronic low back pain, 1028, 1320(t)
  in patient-based outcome assessment, 1316–1317, 1317(t)
McMaster Health Index Questionnaire, 1317(t), 1318(t)
MCPQ (McGill Comprehensive Pain Questionnaire), 1317, 1317(t)
  limitations of, 1317
Mechanoreceptors, discharge of, during spinal loading, 80, *81*
  in low back pain, 76–77, *77*
Medical Outcomes Study, 1318(t)
Medullary arteries, anatomy of, *125,* 125–126
MedX Lumbar Extension Machine, 1078–1079
Meningeal hemorrhage, after chemonucleolysis, 531
Meningioma, of spinal cord, 573
Meningitis, after spinal stenosis surgery, 749
Meniscus, of facet joints, 541–542, *542*
Mensana Clinic Back Pain Test, 1028
Meralgia paresthetica, bone grafting and, 965
Mesoderm, formation of, 44
  paraxial, 44
Metabolic work-up, before spinal fusion, 594–596
Metastatic disease, bone scan of, 338, *339*
  diagnostic tests of, accuracy of, 443, 443(t)
  internal instrumentation for, 1222, *1225*
  magnetic resonance imaging of, 373–374, *374*
  plain film radiography of, 338, *339*
Methocarbamol, for muscle spasm, in low back pain, 453
Methotrexate, for psoriatic spondyloarthropathy, 807
Mianserin, for chronic low back pain, 1031(t)
Microdiscectomy, complications of, 959–960
  posterior, 502–505, *504–506*
    advantages of, 502
    complications of, 504–507
    disadvantages of, 503
    follow-up after, long-term, 507
    indications for, 503
    results of, 504–505
Microfracture, 971–972
Microscopy, electron, of disc degeneration, 311–312
Midas Rex drill, for laminectomy, in spinal stenosis, 738
Middle sacral artery, hemostasis of, in spinal fusion, 597, *597*
  injury to, during anterior lumbar spine surgery, 962
Millar asthma, 875
Million Visual Analog Scale, 1048
Minerals, bone content of, estimation of, 974–975
Min/max contraction intensity, 166
Minnesota Multiphasic Personality Inventory (MMPI), 1317(t)
  correlation of, with pain drawing, 1026–1027
  in low back pain, 1049, 1320(t)
    chronic, 1023
    in organic vs. psychogenic cause determination, 1027–1028
Mixed nerve somatosensory evoked potentials, testing of, 142(t)

MMPI. See *Minnesota Multiphasic Personality Inventory (MMPI).*
Mobility, evaluation of, in disc herniation, 478
Mobilization, for sacroiliac joint dysfunction, 566
Modeling, of bone, 971–972
Modified Health Assessment Questionnaire, 1318(t)
Modified Steffee (MVSP) system, evaluation of, canine models in, *228,* 228–229
Morning stiffness, 90–91
Morquio disease, and developmental spinal stenosis, 728
Motion, end-range, repeated, in low back pain diagnosis, 979–980, *1003*
Motion radiography, of segmental instability, 787–788, *789*
Motion segment, adjacent, spinal fusion effect on, 1213
  collapse of, imaging of, in sagittal plane, 327, *330, 331*
  degeneration of, after scoliosis surgery, 1155–1157, *1157–1159*
    evaluation of, 1156
    operative approach to, 1156
    treatment of, results of, 1156–1157, *1157–1159*
  disorders of, mechanical, plain film radiography of, 341
  evaluation of, postsurgical, plain film radiography of, 348
  instability of, clinical implications of, 56
  mechanics of, in degenerative disc disease, 54, *55*
    in low back pain, 30–31
  neuroanatomy of, 544, *545, 546*
  repetitive loading of, in vitro investigations of, 189–190
    mechanical effects of, 189–190
  response of, biomechanical, to lumbar spine loading, 170–172
    to external forces, 174, *175, 176*
Motor deficit, in disc herniation, as surgical indication, 497
  evaluation of, 480
Motor function, in cauda equina syndrome, recovery of, 580, 587
  secondary to disc herniation, 587
Motor nerve conduction, testing of, in radiculopathy localization, 149–150
  utilization of, 142(t)
Movement, sagittal, in industrial low back pain, evaluation of, 1091–1096, *1092–1095*
  patterns of, 1091, *1092*
MRI. See *Magnetic resonance imaging (MRI).*
MTS system, in vitro evaluation of, 218
  studies of, in artificial spine, 221, *222*
Multifidus, 52
  isometric contraction of, in spinal manipulation, 1015, *1015*
Multifidus triangle syndrome, 91
Multilevel Assessment Instrument, 1318(t)
Muscle(s). See also names of specific muscles.
  action of, 1075–1077
    isoinertial, 1075
    isokinetic, 1075
    isometric, 1075
    isotonic, 1075
  dysfunction of, evaluation of, clinical neurophysiology in, *157,* 157–158
  endurance of, definition of, 1076–1077

Muscle(s) *(Continued)*
   in low back pain, 29–30
      rehabilitation of, 1045
   in spinal instability, 206–207
   mechanics of, during lifting, 243–244, *244–246*
   of lumbar spine, anatomy of, 62
   strength of, definition of, 1076–1077
Muscle relaxants, for low back pain, 453
Muscle spasm, treatment of, 453
Muscle training, 29
Musculoskeletal system, in low back pain, physical examination of, while bending over examining table, 95
      while lying prone, 97
      while lying supine, 95–96
      while side-lying, 97
      while standing, 93–94
MVE (maximum voluntary exertion), in trunk muscle strength testing, 1079
MVSP (Modified Steffee) system, evaluation of, canine models in, *228*, 228–229
Myelography, 376–424
   before laminectomy, 1235
      retrospective analysis of, 416
   computed tomography with, before laminectomy, 1236–1237
   in postoperative spine evaluation, 418, 420
   in traumatic injury, 423
   in laminectomy retrospective analysis, 415–418, *417*
   iophendylate injection in, sequelae of, 417
   limitations of, 376–377
   of arachnoiditis, 417
   of disc abnormality, computed tomography vs., *417*, 417–418
   of disc herniation, accuracy of, 442, 442(t)
      blinded prospective analysis of, 414, 414(t)
      computed tomography vs., 413–418, 413(t), 414(t), *417*
      retrospective analysis of, 413–414
   of multiply operated lumbar spine, 1108
   of postoperative spine, 418–420, *419*
   of scoliosis, adult, 1136
      degenerative, 1168
   of segmental instability, *791*
   of spinal fractures, 846
   of spinal stenosis, accuracy of, 442–443, 443(t)
      blinded prospective analysis of, 414–415, 414(t)
      computed tomography vs., 413–418, 414(t)
      degenerative, 734
         advantages of, 734
         disadvantages of, 734
      recurrent, *751*
   of spinal tumors, 920
   of spondylolisthesis, degenerative, after spinal stenosis surgery, *753*
   radiation exposure during, 379
   uses of, 377
Myeloma, of spine, 927
Myelopathy, thoracic, 572–574
      causes of, 573
Myocoele, formation of, 44
Myofascial pain syndrome, in low back pain, 1023
   pain patterns in, 91
Myofasciitis, 548
Myology, of lumbar spine, 51–52
Myotome, formation of, 45, *46*

N

Naproxen, for low back pain, 453
Narcotic analgesics, for chronic low back pain, 1029
National Institute for Occupational Safety and Health (NIOSH), weight lifting guidelines of, 247, *247*
Needle electromyography, in entrapment neuropathy localization, 150
   in neurologic deficit evaluation, 148
   in radiculopathy localization, 149
Nefazodone, for chronic low back pain, 1031(t)
Neisseria gonorrhoeae, and reactive arthritis, 803(t)
Neoplasms, computed tomography of, 420, *423*
   plain film radiography of, 338, *339*, *340*
Nerve(s). See also names of specific nerves.
   decompression of, inadequate, after posterior lumbar spine surgery, 953–954
   disease of, in ankylosing spondylitis, 801
   dysfunction of, and neurogenic claudication, 718
   in impulse propagation, 126–127
   injury to, during anterior lumbar spine surgery, 962–963
      during transpedicle fixation, 1203–1205
   of lumbar spine, anatomy of, 62–63, *64*
   sensory, classification of, 76, 77(t)
   supply of, to intervertebral discs, 293–294
Nerve block, for disc herniation, 484
   for sciatica, 136
Nerve conduction, in cauda equina, in neurogenic claudication, 157
   studies of, disadvantages of, 144–145
      in degenerative lumbar stenosis, 736
      in entrapment neuropathy localization, 150
      in radiculopathy localization, 149–150
Nerve endings, free, 76, *77*
   in low back pain, neurophysiologic studies of, *78*, 78–79, *79*, 79(t)
   in lumbar facet capsule, conduction velocity of, 79, 79(t)
Nerve root(s), anatomy of, 63, *65*, 123–126, *124*, *125*
   asymmetry of, causes of, 379–380, *381*
   blood supply to, *125*, 125–126
      watershed area in, 135–136
   compression of, and edema, 130
      and nerve conduction changes, 130
      and pain, 462–463
         low back, in disc herniation, 481–482
         mechanical, 814, 820
      and vascular injury, 136
      animal models of, 129–131
      biology of, 129–134, *132*
   biomechanics of, 127–129, *128*, *129*
      in disc herniation, 128
      in spinal stenosis, 128
   clinical syndromes of, 1234–1235, 1234(t), 1235(t)
   cytokines in, 131–132, *132*
   definition of, 725
   dorsal horn changes in, 132–133
   electrophysiologic abnormalities in, 134–135, *135*
   gene expression in, 134
   in degenerative disc disease, *392*
   in spinal stenosis, magnetic resonance imaging of, 361–362
   in subarticular recess stenosis, 390, *391*
   in subarticular stenosis, 393
   mechanisms of, 123–136
   N-methyl-D-aspartic acid in, 133–134
   physiologic changes in, pressure limits for, 130

Nerve root(s) *(Continued)*
  spontaneous afferent activity in, 131
  tachykinins in, 123
 conjoined, 379–380, *381, 382*
  disc herniation with, 380, *382*
 displacement of, in disc herniation, computed tomography of, 384, *388*
 dorsal, anatomy of, 123, *124*
 electrophysiology of, 127
 entrapment of. See *Root entrapment syndrome.*
 imaging of, in coronal plane, *331*
  in sagittal plane, 327, *329*
 in up-down stenosis, 398, 400
 injection studies of, before laminectomy, 1237
 injury to, during posterior lumbar spine surgery, 955
  during transpedicle fixation, 1204
  in mechanical back pain, 813
 irritation of, inflammatory, historical aspects of, 87
 lumbar, lateral border of, location of, pitfalls in, 500
  sheath of, infiltration of. See *Lumbar nerve(s), root sheath infiltration of.*
 lumbosacral, decompression of, indications for, 1241, 1241(t)
  dysfunction of, nonsurgical treatment of, 1247, 1247(t)
   surgical treatment of, positioning for, *1248,* 1248–1249
 nutrition to, *125,* 125–126
  impairment of, in disc herniation, 482
 of cauda equina, imaging of, in axial plane, 320–323, *324*
  in sagittal plane, *328*
  spinal, vascular supply of, 126
 pathway of, zones of, 728–729, 728(t)
 physiology of, *126,* 126–127
 sacral, electrodiagnostic evaluation of, 150
 sciatic, irritation of, evaluation of, 96–97
 ventral, anatomy of, 123, *124*
Nerve root canal, anatomy of, 66, *66*
 compression of, in up-down stenosis, 398, *399*
 stenosis of. See *Root canal stenosis.*
Nerve root evoked potential, utilization of, 142(t)
Nerve root foramen, anatomy of, 66, *67*
Nerve root ganglion, compression of, and low back pain, in disc herniation, 482
 in up-down stenosis, 398, 400
Nervous system, disorders of, after chemonucleolysis, 531
 in low back pain, 28–29
  physical examination of, while kneeling on chair, 94
   while lying prone, 97–98
   while lying supine, 96–97
   while side-lying, 97
   while sitting in chair/feet on floor, 94–95
   while sitting on examining table/legs hanging free, 95
   while standing, 94
 sympathetic, anatomy of, 570
Net reaction, in lumbar spine loading, 165, *165,* 165(t)
Neural arch, closure of, failure of, 714–715
 formation of, 45
 intact, degenerative spondylolisthesis with, spinal stenosis in, 744–745
 repetitive loading of, in vitro investigations of, 190–191

Neural tube, defects of, 714–715
 formation of, 44, *45*
Neurocentral synchondrosis, 47
Neurogenic claudication, atypical, lumbar nerve root sheath infiltration for, 118–119
 calcitonin for, results of, 767
 clinical neurophysiology in, 156–157
 definition of, 725
 diagnosis of, difficulties in, 113
 in back pain evaluation, 85–86
 in degenerative adult scoliosis, 1124
 in degenerative spondylolisthesis, 701
 lower extremities in, 722
 pathophysiology of, 717–722
  abnormal nerve function in, 718
  cerebrospinal fluid in, 722
  root canal stenosis in, 718–719, *720, 721*
  spinal stenosis in, central, 718–719, *719–721*
   degenerative, 717
   developmental, 717
   two level, 719–720, *720, 721*
  vertebral displacement in, 717–718, *718*
  walking in, 720–722
 vascular claudication vs., 90, 1232
Neurokinins, in compressed nerve root pain, 133
Neuroleptanalgesia, for chemonucleolysis, 528
Neurologic deficit, burst fracture with, management of, 853, 855–856, *855–857*
 documentation of, clinical neurophysiology in, 143–147, *144–148*
 in adult scoliosis, surgery for, 1138, *1139*
 in disc herniation, as surgical indication, 497
 in sciatica, evaluation for, 456
 in spinal tumors, 918, 918(t)
  metastatic, 930–931
   after posterior decompression, of cauda equina, 934–935
   of spinal cord, 934–935
   posterior laminectomy for, 934–935
 localization of, clinical neurophysiology in, 149–151, *151–154*
 of lower extremity, diagnostic testing of, 143–144, *144*
 severity of, rating of, clinical neurophysiology in, 148–149
Neurology, of lumbar spine, 51–52
Neuromuscular efficiency ratio (NMER), in trunk muscle strength testing, 1079
Neuropathy, entrapment, evaluation of, clinical neurophysiology in, 150
 peripheral. See *Peripheral neuropathy.*
Neuropeptides, changes in, in nerve root compression, 131
 in low back pain, 81
 synthesis of, disturbance in, in sciatica, 135
  dorsal root ganglion in, 127
Neurophysiology, clinical, in bladder dysfunction, 154–156, *156*
 in bowel dysfunction, 154–156
 in cauda equina entrapment, 150, *151*
 in entrapment neuropathy, 150
 in low back pain, 141–158
  questions answered by, 143, 143(t)
 in muscle dysfunction, *157,* 157–158
 in neurogenic claudication, 156–157
 in neurologic deficits, in deficit localization, 149–151, *151–154*

Neurophysiology (Continued)
  in documentation, 143–147, 144–148
    in severity rating, 148–149
  in peripheral neuropathy, 149–150
  in radiculopathy, 149
  in reflex sympathetic dystrophy, 156
  in sacral nerve entrapment, 150
  in sexual dysfunction, 154–156
  in spinal cord lesions, 150–151, 152–154
  in surgical monitoring, 153–154, 155
  tests in, 142(t)
Neutral zone, in spinal stability evaluation, 209
Night pain, 90
NIOSH (National Institute for Occupational Safety and Health), weight lifting guidelines of, 247, 247
Nitric oxide (NO), in compressed nerve root pain, 133–134
NMDA (N-methyl-D-aspartatic acid), in compressed nerve root pain, 133–134
NMER (neuromuscular efficiency ratio), in trunk muscle strength testing, 1079
N-Methyl-D-aspartatic acid (NMDA), in compressed nerve root pain, 133–134
NO (nitric oxide), in compressed nerve root pain, 133–134
Nocardial vertebral osteomyelitis, 897
Nociception, mechanism of, 127
Nociceptors, in low back pain, 76
Nonsteroidal antiinflammatory drugs (NSAIDs), for ankylosing spondylitis, 803
  for compressed nerve root pain, 134
  for disc herniation, 484
  for low back pain, 453
    in pregnancy, 1062
    industrial, follow-up of, 1090
  for outer annular tear, in animal models, 284
  for psoriatic spondyloarthropathy, 807
  for reactive arthritis, 805
  for sciatica, 456, 1240–1241
  for spondylolisthesis, 658–659
  in fusion outcome, 1290
Nortriptyline, for chronic low back pain, 1031(t)
Notochord, formation of, 44, 44
Nottingham Health Profile, 1318(t)
Novocain, for sciatica, 456
NSAIDs. See Nonsteroidal antiinflammatory drugs (NSAIDs).
Nucleography, in nucleus pulposus shape delineation, 430
Nucleotomy, percutaneous, for disc herniation, 1242
Nucleus pulposus, age-related structural changes in, 302
  anatomy of, 51
  cells of, types of, 291, 292
  collagen in, organization of, 273, 289, 289
    types of, 290, 312
  components of, 271–272, 272(t)
    leakage of, in sciatica, 134–135
  displacement of, in animal models, 282–283
  functions of, 286, 286
  herniation of, differential diagnosis of, 449(t)
  imaging of, in axial plane, 318, 319, 320, 323
  in load bearing, 172
    in degeneration, 54
    in health, 53
  loss of, in disc degeneration, 311
  shape of, delineation of, nucleography in, 430

Nutrients, concentration of, in intervertebral disc matrix, factors in, 296
Nutrition, in fusion outcome, 1289
  of intervertebral discs, 285–305
    factors in, 297–301, 297–301
    insufficient, and disc degeneration, 304
  of nerve roots, 125, 125–126
    impairment of, in disc herniation, 482
  spinal, changes in, in nerve root compression, 130

O

OARS (Older Americans' Resources and Services) Multidimensional Functional Assessment Questionnaire, 1318(t)
Oblique muscles, exercise of, for sacroiliac joint dysfunction, 565, 565–566
Obstacle course, in spinal function testing, 1048
Occupational biomechanics, 235–250
Occupations, in low back pain, 89
  mechanisms of, 235, 235–236
  industrial, low back pain from, 1055–1100
    at-risk patient identification in, 1088–1089, 1089
    claims reporting in, 1066–1067
      impact of, 1067
      predictors of, 1068–1070, 1069(t), 1070, 1071
      safety concerns in, 1066–1067
      symptoms in, 1066
    elemental resource model of, 1087–1088
    etiology of, 1066
    prevention of, 1065, 1091–1096, 1092–1095
    resource economics paradigm in, 1087–1088
    risk factors for, 1065–1072
      prospective studies of, 1067–1068
      retrospective studies of, 1067
    treatment of, follow-up of, 1089–1091
    trunk muscle strength testing in, 1074–1100
      applications of, 1096–1097
  repetitive lumbar spine loading in, risk factors for, 183–184
  with vibration exposure, 192–194
OECD Long-Term Disability Questionnaire, 1319(t)
Older Americans' Resources and Services (OARS) Multidimensional Functional Assessment Questionnaire, 1318(t)
Ölerud rod, fatigue strength of, 1193
Oligoarthritis, in reactive arthritis, 804
Open disc surgery, history of, 1–2
Operant behavioral programs, for chronic low back pain, 1032–1033
Optimization models, of lumbar load evaluation, 166–169, 167
Orthosis(es), 251–257
  biomechanics of, 252–255, 253–255
  clinical applications of, 255–257
  for adult scoliosis, 1122, 1136–1138
  for fractures, 865–871
    stable, 867
  for sacroiliac joint dysfunction, 566
  for spinal instability, minimal, 867, 870–871
    postsurgical, 871
  future studies of, 257
  history of, 251–252
  negative effects of, 257
  thoracolumbosacral. See Thoracolumbosacral orthosis (TLSO).

Oscillations, in lumbar spine manipulation, 1013(t)
Ossification, of longitudinal ligament, in ankylosing spondylitis, plain film radiography of, 340, *340*
  of lumbar spine, 46–47
Osteitis, in SAPHO syndrome, 808
Osteoarthritis, of facet joints, plain film radiography of, 345, *346*, 349, *350*
Osteoblastoma, in children/adolescents, magnetic resonance imaging of, 369
  of spine, 922, *924*
    percutaneous biopsy of, *920*
Osteochondroma, of spine, 922, *925*
Osteoconductivity, of bone graft, 1290
Osteogenic sarcoma, of spine, survival in, 928(t)
Osteoid osteoma, bone scan of, 338, *339*
  computed tomography of, 338, *339*
  of spine, 922, *923*
Osteoinductivity, of bone graft, 1290–1291
Osteology, of lumbar spine, 47–51, *50*
Osteoma, osteoid, bone scan of, 338, *339*
  computed tomography of, 338, *339*
  of spine, 922, *923*
Osteomyelitis, after spinal stenosis surgery, 749–750
  computed tomography of, 420, *421*, *422*
  magnetic resonance imaging of, 420, *421*, *422*
  plain film radiography of, 336–338, *338*
  vertebral, *Actinobacillus actinomycetemcomitans*, 897
    brucellosis, 897
    cryptococcal, 897
    nocardial, 897
    pyogenic, after lumbar spine surgery, 951–952
      diagnosis of, 952
      treatment of, 952
Osteophyte(s), formation of, after outer annular tear, in animal models, 284
  aging in, 303, 541
  plain film radiography of, 344, *344*
Osteophytic spurs, in lateral stenosis, 402, *403*
Osteoporosis, 969–984
  clinical aspects of, 983–984
  demineralization in, 970
  epidemiology of, 969–970
  failure patterns in, 981, *982*
  in fusion outcome, 1289
  in hip fractures, 969–970
  in vertebral fractures, 969–970
  radiography of, 981–983
    plain film, 341, *341*
  rate of, in aging trabecular/cortical bone, 975–976
  simulations of, 978–979, *979, 980*
  transpedicle fixation in, 1213–1214
Osteoprogenitor cells, 1285
Osteosarcoma, of spine, 927
Osteotomy, for adult scoliosis, with iatrogenic flat back deformity, *1163*, 1163–1164, *1164*
  wedge, for imbalanced adult scoliosis, 1164–1167, *1165, 1166*
  vertebral, for ankylosing spondylitis, 803
Oswestry Disability Questionnaire, 1317(t), 1318(t)
Outcome, clinical, assessment of, context in, 1320–1322, 1321(t)
  measurement of, 1313–1333, 1313(t)
    hard vs. soft data in, 1314–1316
    patient self-reporting of, 1314–1316
      guidelines for, 1322–1324, *1323–1325*
  functional status, measures of, 1318(t)

Outcome *(Continued)*
  health status, measures of, properties of, 1324–1328
    psychometric, 1328–1332, 1330(t)
  patient-based, assessment of, instruments for, 1316–1320, 1317(t), 1318(t), 1319(t), 1320(t)
Overexertion, and spine injuries, 236
Oxycodone, addiction to, 455
Oxygen, concentration of, in intervertebral disc, after fusion, 299
  consumption of, in intervertebral disc, in animal model, 295
Oxygenation, hyperbaric, for spinal epidural abscess, 896

P

Pacinian corpuscles, 76, *77*
Paget disease, in fusion outcome, 1287
Pain, after bone grafting, 963
  back. See *Low back pain.*
  crossover, well leg lifting vs., 96
  discogenic, diagnosis of, 90
    discography in, 429–431
    internal instrumentation for, 1220, *1220, 1221*
    pathoanatomic studies of, 463
  during discography, 431
  evaluation of, clinical neurophysiology in, 158
    in disc herniation, 478, 481
  extraspinal, Pynsent-Fairbank-Hall classification of, 99(t), 100–101
  in adult scoliosis, factors in, 1131–1132
    history of, 1135
  in disc herniation, mechanism of, 481–482
  in lateral recess stenosis, 732
  intraspinal, Pynsent-Fairbank-Hall classification of, 100–101, 100(t)
  lumbar spine, origins of, *58*, 58–59, *59*
  measurements of, 1320(t)
  myofascial, 548
  night, 90
  nonradicular, definition of, 105
    pattern of, 105, *106*
    radicular pain vs., 105–108, *106*, 107(t)
    synonyms for, 107(t)
  radicular, chemonucleolysis for, 529
    definition of, 105
    in adult scoliosis, 1120
    in degenerative lumbar stenosis, 731–732
    in disc herniation, 479
    in spinal tumors, 918, 918(t)
    inadequate relief of, after chemonucleolysis, 961
      postoperative, 953–954
    nonradicular pain vs., 105–108, *106*, 107(t)
    pathomechanism of, 135, *135*
    pattern of, 105, *106*
    referred pain vs., 1232, 1232(t)
    synonyms for, 107(t)
  referred, assessment of, 87
    facet syndrome in, historical background of, 539
    in posterior thigh, 457
    pattern of, 91
    radicular pain vs., 1232, 1232(t)
  sacroiliac joint dysfunction and, 562, *562*
  sclerodermal, historical aspects of, 87
  thigh, in low back pain algorithm, 457
Pain and Impairment Relationship Scale (PAIRS), 1028–1029

Pain Behavior Checklist, 1317(t), 1320(t)
Pain Beliefs Questionnaire, 1317(t), 1320(t)
Pain Chart, 1317(t), 1320(t)
Pain control class, for chronic low back pain, 1035–1036
Pain Disability Index, 1317(t), 1320(t)
Pain Drawing, 1317(t), 1320(t)
  correlation of, with Minnesota Multiphasic Personality Inventory, 1026–1027
  in chronic low back pain, 1028, 1048
  quantified, 1048
Pain Interference Scale, 1317(t)
Pain Perception Profile, 1320(t)
Pain Rating Scale, 1317(t), 1320(t)
PAIRS (Pain and Impairment Relationship Scale), 1028–1029
Palpation, in low back pain diagnosis, 1000–1001
Paracetamol, for disc herniation, 484
Paraplegia, chemonucleolysis and, 531
  Pott, 876–877
  pyogenic spondylitis and, 894
  septic intervertebral discitis and, 896
Paraspinal abscess, after spinal stenosis surgery, 749
Parasympathetic nerves, anatomy of, 570
  injury to, during anterior lumbar spine surgery, 962
Parathyroid hormone, measurement of, before spinal fusion, 595
Paravertebral fascia, of diaphragm, 1255
Paravertebral pressure test, 478
Paraxial mesoderm, 44
Paresthesia syndrome, in spondylolisthesis, 658
Parietal pleura, dissection of, in eleventh rib approach, to anterior spine surgery, 1259, 1259–1260
Paroxetine, for chronic low back pain, 1031(t)
Pars artery, hemostasis of, in spinal fusion, 597, 597
Pars interarticularis, defect of, plain film radiography of, 341–342, 342
  repetitive lumbar spine loading in, 185–186
  fracture of, 631
    during laminotomy, for spinal stenosis, 779
    fusion of, indications for, 647–649
    hyperextension and, 191
    in spondylolisthesis, 632, 633, 684–685
      congenital, 626, 628
      isthmic, 630–631, 632
      pathologic, 635, 636
    plain film radiography of, 341–342, 343
    stress, in young athlete, 633
      treatment of, 646–647, 648
Partition coefficient, 275
  in solute concentration, 294
  physiologic importance of, 275
Patient Assessment Form, 1319(t)
Patient Evaluation Conference System, 1319(t)
Pedicle screws, for internal fixation, in posterior fusion, 601, 603, 604
Pedicles, anatomy of, 66–67
  surgical, 60–61
  cortex of, penetration of, during transpedicle fixation, 1204
  fixation of. See Transpedicle fixation.
Peer review, in spine care, 1343–1344, 1344(t)
Pelvic tilt, in pregnancy, 1060
Pelvic torsion–left posterior rotation test, in sacroiliac joint dysfunction, 562
Pelvic torsion–right posterior rotation test, in sacroiliac joint dysfunction, 562

Pelvic visceral dysfunction, 569–531. See also *Cauda equina syndrome (CES)*.
Pelvis, rotation of, during locomotion, spine in, 262–263, 263, 264
PEMFs (pulsed electromagnetic fields), in fusion outcome, 1288–1289
D-Penicillamine, for psoriatic spondyloarthropathy, 807
Penile tumescence, nocturnal, studies of, in impotence measurement, 155
  testing of, utilization of, 142(t)
Percodan, addiction to, 455
Percutaneous intradiscal procedures, history of, 3
Pericarditis, in ankylosing spondylitis, 801
Periostitis, in psoriatic spondyloarthropathy, 806
Peripheral neuropathy, and anterior thigh pain, 457
  degenerative lumbar stenosis vs., 732
  evaluation of, clinical neurophysiology in, 149–150
  production of, experimental, 131
Peripheral vascular disease, degenerative lumbar stenosis vs., 732
Peritoneum, perforation of, during anterior lumbar spine surgery, 963
  protection of, in tenth rib approach, to anterior spine surgery, 1256, 1257
  removal of, in twelfth rib approach, to anterior spine surgery, 1263, 1265
  retraction of, in anterior extraperitoneal discectomy, 1272, 1274
Personality, in low back pain, 1024–1025
Phenobarbital, in low back pain, 453
Phenol, injection of, for facet syndrome, 550
Phenothiazines, for chronic low back pain, 1031–1032
Phenylbutazone, for ankylosing spondylitis, 803
Phospholipase A_2, leakage of, in sciatica, 134
Physical and Mental Impairment-of-Function Evaluation, 1318(t)
Physical fitness, as low back injury claims predictor, 1068–1069
Physical Self-Maintenance Scale, 1319(t)
Physical therapy, for adult scoliosis, 1121
  for disc herniation, 484–485
Physiotherapy, for sciatica, frequency of, 10, 10
PILE (progressive isoinertial lifting evaluation), 1047
Pinhole stenosis, 395, 396
  front-back stenosis with, computed tomography of, 408
Piriformis muscle, in sacroiliac joint stability, 560, 560
Plantar flexion, evaluation of, in low back pain, 94–95
Plasmacytoma, of spine, 927
  survival in, 928(t)
Pleura, parietal, dissection of, in eleventh rib approach, to anterior spine surgery, 1259, 1259–1260
  protection of, in twelfth rib approach, to anterior spine surgery, 1262
PLIF. See *Posterior lumbar interbody fusion (PLIF)*.
PMMA (polymethyl methacrylate), for fusion, in vitro evaluation of, 217
  in transpedicle fixation, 1189–1191
Pneumonia, after scoliosis surgery, 1127
Pneumothorax, after scoliosis surgery, 1127
Polymethyl methacrylate (PMMA), for fusion, in vitro evaluation of, 217
  in transpedicle fixation, 1189–1191
Positive predictive value, of lumbar nerve root sheath infiltration, 117–118

Positive stress sign, in spinal stenosis, 1112
Posterior arch fractures, 833, 836
Posterior internal venous plexus, imaging of, in axial plane, *321, 322,* 324, *324*
Posterior longitudinal ligament, anatomy of, 49–51
 imaging of, in axial plane, 318, *319, 320, 322, 323*
 in sagittal plane, *328*
 in discogenic back pain, 463
Posterior lumbar interbody fusion (PLIF), 607–608
 advantages of, 466
 for degenerative spondylolisthesis, 705, 707
 for disc degeneration, 466–467
 for disc herniation, 1243
 history of, 590
 indications for, 607
 technique of, 607–608, *609*
Posterior radicular artery, *62*
Posterior ramus, of spinal nerve, 51
Posterior shear test, in sacroiliac joint dysfunction, 562
Posttraumatic stress disorder, low back pain in, 1019–1020
Postural syndrome, in low back pain, 1002–1003
 treatment of, mechanical, 1009
Posture, biomechanics of, 236–241, *238–241*
 erect, effects of, 474
 evaluation of, in disc herniation, 478
 in low back pain, in children/adolescents, 368–369
 sitting, biomechanics of, 237–241, *239–241*
 standing, biomechanics of, 237, *238*
Pott paraplegia, 876–877
Pregnancy, ankylosing spondylitis in, 801
 disc herniation in, 1058
 low back pain in, 1057–1063
  clinical presentation of, 1058–1060, *1059, 1060*
  diagnosis of, 1061
  epidemiology of, 1057–1058
  pathogenesis of, 1060–1061
  prevention of, 1062–1063
  rheumatoid arthritis with, 1059–1060, *1060*
  sacroiliac joint in, 564–565
  treatment of, 1061–1062
 symphysiolysis in, 1061
PRIDE (Progressive Rehabilitation Institute of Dallas for Ergonomics) program, 1049–1050
 functional restoration outcome in, 1051
Procaine, for sciatica, 456
Progressive isoinertial lifting evaluation (PILE), 1047
Progressive Rehabilitation Institute of Dallas for Ergonomics (PRIDE) program, 1049–1050
 functional restoration outcomes in, 1051
Progressive resistance exercise, for spondylolisthesis, 661
Protein(s), link, in aging intervertebral disc, 313
 morphogenetic, bone, in bone grafting, 1293–1294
  animal studies of, 1294–1298, 1295(t)
  in fusion outcome, 1287
 noncollagenous, in intervertebral disc, 291
 serum, in intervertebral disc, 292
Protein electrophoresis, serum, measurement of, before spinal fusion, 595
Proteoglycans, 274, 287–289, *287–289*
 biochemistry of, 313
 concentration of, after fusion, animal model of, 314
 in pore size, 275, 292
 functions of, 274–277, *276,* 286–287, *287*
 in disc degeneration, 312, 461

Proteoglycans *(Continued)*
 in disc hydration, during loading, 288, *288*
 osmotic pressure of, factors in, 288–289, *289*
 synthesis of, 277–279
  exercise in, 298–299
  in aging intervertebral disc, 303–304
  in cartilage, in low back pain, 1044
  loading in, 279
Pseudarthrosis, after adult scoliosis surgery, 1172
 in elderly, 1155
 with extended fusion, 1156
 with iatrogenic flat back deformity, 1161
 after fusion, for segmental instability, 794
 posterolateral, 465, 764
 after transpedicle fixation, 1212
 repair of, in spondylolisthesis, in children and adolescents, 675
Pseudomeningocele, after lumbar spine surgery, 954–955
 after spinal stenosis surgery, 747–748
 evaluation of, postoperative, 420
Psoas muscle, 52
 identification of, in twelfth rib approach, to anterior spine surgery, 1263, *1265*
Psoriasis, in reactive arthritis, 804
 spondylitis with, 806
Psoriatic spondyloarthropathy, 805–807
 classification of, 806, 806(t)
 laboratory findings in, 807
 prognosis in, 807
 symptoms of, extraarticular, 807
  peripheral, 806–807
  sacroiliac, 806
  spinal, 806
 therapy for, 807
Psychologic factors, in low back pain, 92
Psychomotor therapy, for disc herniation, 486
Psychosocial function, measurements of, 1320(t)
Psychotherapy, psychodynamic, for chronic low back pain, 1035
Pudendal nerve, organs innervated by, *151*
Pudendal somatosensory evoked potentials, in sacral nerve root evaluation, 150
PULHEMS Profile, 1319(t)
Pulmonary embolism, after lumbar spine surgery, 947–949
 after scoliosis surgery, 1127
Pulmonary function, in adult scoliosis, 1120, 1135
Pulsed electromagnetic fields (PEMFs), in fusion outcome, 1288–1289
PULSES profile, 1319(t)
Pustulosis, in SAPHO syndrome, 808
Pynsent-Fairbank-Hall Classification, of pain, extraspinal, 99(t), 100–101
 intraspinal, 100–101, 100(t)
Pyrazinamide, for spinal tuberculosis, 880–882

Q

Quadratus lumborum, 52
Quality of Life Index, 1317(t), 1318(t)

R

Radiation, exposure to, during computed tomography, 369–379
 during myelography, 379

Radiation *(Continued)*
   during plain film radiography, 379
   in fusion outcome, 1287
Radicular syndrome, acute, disc herniation and, diagnosis of, 494, 494(t)
Radicular veins, 63
Radiculitis, chemical, in disc degeneration, 460–461
   in sciatica, 134–135
Radiculopathy, definition of, 725
   evaluation of, clinical neurophysiology in, 149
Radiography, 317–334
   of adult scoliosis, 1121, 1135–1136
   of ankylosing spondylitis, 799–800
   of disc degeneration, 463–464
     studies of, 21–22
   of disc herniation, 480–481
   of discitis, iatrogenic, 908, 908
     intervertebral, septic, 891, 891–892
   of osteoporosis, 981–983
   of sacroiliac joint dysfunction, 563, 563–564, 564
   of segmental instability, 737, 787, 788
     motion studies in, 787–788, 789
   of spinal fractures, 846
   of spinal instability, motion studies in, 207–208
   of spinal tuberculosis, 876–880, 877–878
   of spinal tumors, 919, 919–921, 920
   of spondylolisthesis, 685–686
     degenerative, 672–703
   plain film, 333–351
     before laminectomy, 1235
     of degenerative lumbar stenosis, 733–734
     of multiply operated lumbar spine, 1108
     of pyogenic spondylitis, 885–887, 889, 890
     radiation exposure during, 379
     views in, 334, 334–335
   weight-bearing, of segmental instability, 1111
Radiotherapy, for spinal tumors, 932
   complications of, 941
   metastatic, 929
Raney jacket, 252, 253
Range of motion, measurement of, in chronic low back pain, 1046–1047
Rapid Disability Rating Scale, 1319(t)
Reactive arthritis, 803–805
   ankylosing spondylitis in, 805
   bacteria in, 803(t), 804
   diagnosis of, 805
   evolution of, 805
   symptoms of, articular, 804
     extraarticular, 804
   treatment of, 805
Recalibrage, of spinal canal, for spinal stenosis, 770–771
Receiver operating characteristic (ROC) curves, in diagnostic test evaluation, 439–440
Recruitment, measurement of, needle electromyography in, 148
Rectal examination, in low back pain, 98
Rectus abdominis, in trunk movement, evaluation of, 1082
   retraction of, in anterior extraperitoneal discectomy, 1272, 1273
Reduction, of spondylolisthesis, 691–692
   anterior/posterior, 693–694, 696
     in children and adolescents, 674–675, 678–679, 679, 680–681
     indications for, 691

Reduction *(Continued)*
   posterior, 692–693, 694, 695
     vertebral body resection in, 694–698, 697
   of spondyloptosis, vertebral body resection in, 694–698, 697
Reflex(es), anal, in low back pain, 98
   ankle, absence of, 1233–1234
     in disc herniation, 480
     in low back pain, 94
   bulbocavernosus, in sacral nerve root evaluation, 150
     in spinal cord lesion, 151, 152
     testing of, utilization of, 142(t)
   evaluation of, in disc herniation, 480
   H. See *H reflexes.*
   hamstring, in low back pain, 98
   knee, in low back pain, 95
Reflex sympathetic dystrophy, clinical neurophysiology in, 156
Rehabilitation, 989–1053
   education in, 989–996
     clinician-patient interaction in, 990–994
   for industrial low back pain, follow-up of, 1090
   functional restoration in, 1042–1053
   learning process in, 990
   lumbar spine manipulation in, 1012–1017
   principles of, 655–656, 655(t), 656(t), 657(t)
   psychologic approaches to, 1018–1036
   training in, 989–996
Reiter syndrome, 803
   evolution of, 805
   extraarticular symptoms of, 804
   pathogenesis of, 809
Relaxation, for chronic low back pain, 1033
Relaxin, in low back pain, in pregnancy, 1060
Reliability, of health status outcome measure, 1328–1331, 1330(t)
Remodeling, adaptive, of lumbar spine, 229–230, 230
   of bone, 971–972
     lumbar spine loading and, 176–178
Resource economics paradigm, in industrial low back pain, 1087–1088
Respondent treatment programs, for chronic low back pain, 1033–1034
Retrodisplacement, 649
Retrograde ejaculation, after anterior retroperitoneal transverse spine surgery, 1269–1270
   after scoliosis surgery, 1128
Retrolisthesis, 649
Retroperitoneal tumor, and anterior thigh pain, 457
Retrospondylolisthesis, treatment of, 745
Rhizotomy, for facet syndrome, results of, 549–550
Ribs, bone grafting from, for spinal fusion, 592
Rifampin, for spinal tuberculosis, 830–832
ROC (receiver operating characteristic) curves, in diagnostic test evaluation, 439–440
Rod–transpedicle screw system (RTS), in vitro evaluation of, 213–215, 215
Rongeur, Kerrison, for laminectomy, in spinal stenosis, 738–739
   Leksell, for laminectomy, in spinal stenosis, 738
Root canal stenosis, 31
   and neurogenic claudication, 718–719, 720, 721
   isolated, surgical treatment of, indications for, 774
     results of, 768–769
   of intervertebral nerve, in spondylolisthesis, 658
   treatment of, effectiveness of, 33(t)

Root entrapment syndrome, 354–359
  causes of, 393
  clinical presentation of, 1234, 1234(t)
  disc protrusion in, central, 354
    lateral, 354–355
    posterolateral, 354
  in disc herniation, with lateral recess stenosis, 494, *494,* 494(t)
  in malignancy, lumbar nerve root sheath infiltration for, 120, *120*
  localization of, for lumbar nerve root sheath infiltration, 115, *116*
  lumbosacral, decompression for, 1249
    discectomy for, 1249
    preoperative planning in, 1249
  natural history of, 1239, 1239(t)
  radiographic assessment of, 355–359, *355–359*
    magnetic resonance imaging in, 355–359, *355–359*
    with Gd-DTPA, 355–359, *358*
  treatment of, 1243–1245, *1244*
Root sheath, imaging of, in axial plane, *325*
Root sleeve, anatomy of, 123–124
Rotator muscles, 52
Roy-Camille instrumentation, 1179–1181
  history of, 590
  in vitro evaluation of, 216
RTS (rod–transpedicle screw system), in vitro evaluation of, 213–215, *215*
Ruffini end organs, 76, *77*

S

Sacral arteries, hemostasis of, in spinal fusion, 597, *597*
  protection of, in anterior retroperitoneal transverse spine surgery, 1270
Sacral nerves, anatomy of, 569–570
  entrapment of, evaluation of, clinical neurophysiology in, 150
Sacral thrust, in sacroiliac joint dysfunction, 562
Sacral veins, protection of, in anterior retroperitoneal transverse spine surgery, 1270
Sacroiliac joint, anatomy of, *559,* 559–561, *560*
  dysfunction of, clinical significance of, 561–563
    diagnosis of, 561–563, *562*
    evaluation of, 559–568
      radiographic, *563,* 563–564, *564*
    in low back pain, incidence of, 561
    treatment of, 559–568, *565, 567*
  evaluation of, in low back pain, 96
  imaging of, in axial plane, *325, 326*
  in pregnancy, 564–565
    pain in, 1058, *1059,* 1061
  motion of, 561
  stability of, 559–560, *560*
Sacroiliitis, in ankylosing spondylitis, 798
  radiography of, 799, 799(t)
  in Crohn disease, 808
  in psoriatic spondyloarthropathy, 806
  in Reiter syndrome, 805
  in SAPHO syndrome, 809
Sacrospinal muscle, 52
Sacrotuberous ligament, in sacroiliac joint stability, 560, *560*
Sacrum, anatomy of, 67
  surgical, 60–61
  fusion of, Cotrel-Dubousset instrumentation for, 1161

Sacrum *(Continued)*
  imaging of, in axial plane, 324, *325, 326*
  nerve roots of, electrodiagnostic evaluation of, 150
  opening of, in congenital spondylolisthesis, 626, *628*
  transpedicle fixation of, screw placement in, 1185, 1185(t)
Saddle anesthesia, in low back pain, 98
Salicylates, for low back pain, in pregnancy, 1062
Saline, injection of, in chemonucleolysis trials, 529
  into facet joint, results of, 545–546
SAPHO syndrome, 808–809
Sarcoma, Ewing, of spine, 927
  survival in, 928(t)
  osteogenic, of spine, survival in, 928(t)
Scalp, evoked potentials at, recording of, *157,* 157–158
Scarring, after lumbar spine surgery, 947–948
  recurrent disc herniation vs., 954
  epidural, in multiply operated lumbar spine, 1109(t), 1113
    treatment of, 1113
Scheuermann disease, 343
  magnetic resonance imaging of, 366
  in children/adolescents, 369
Schmorl nodes, formation of, aging in, 303
  fracture of, in osteoporosis, 981, *982*
  magnetic resonance imaging of, 366
  plain film radiography of, 343
Schwannoma, of spinal cord, 573
Sciatic nerve, injury to, during bone grafting, 965
  irritation of, evaluation of, 96
Sciatica, definition of, 725
  diagnosis of, 31
    differential, 499(t)
  disc herniation with, magnetic resonance imaging of, 358–359
    recurrent, magnetic resonance imaging of, 369–370
  etiology of, *59,* 123–136
  facet syndrome in, historical background of, 538
  in adult scoliosis, surgery for, 1125
  in cauda equina syndrome, 577
  in low back pain algorithm, 456–457
  incidence of, 9–10, 24–25
  low back pain vs., 492
  natural history of, 492
  nerve block for, 136, 456
  pain mechanisms in, 134–135, *135*
  physiotherapy for, frequency of, 10, *10*
  recovery from, 9–10, *10*
  recurrent, characteristics of, 498(t)
    surgical treatment of, indications for, 498(t)
  treatment of, 31–32, 32(t), 33(t)
    conservative, 1240–1241
    surgical, 1241, 1241(t)
Sclerodermal pain, historical aspects of, 87
Sclerosants, for sacroiliac joint dysfunction, 567, *567*
Sclerotomes, formation of, 44–45, *45, 46*
  in low back pain, *108,* 108–109, *109*
Scoliosis, adult, 1118–1173
  characteristics of, 1131
  decision-making in, 1118–1128
  definition of, 1130
  degenerative, 1122–1124, 1167–1170
    after spinal stenosis decompression, 1170
    curve magnitude in, 1167

Scoliosis *(Continued)*
  curve progression in, risk factors for, 1124
  demographics of, 1167
  discography in, 1168
  idiopathic scoliosis vs., 1167–1168
  myelography in, 1168
  pain in, 1167
  prevalence of, 1167
  surgery of, 1168–1170, *1169, 1170*
    indications for, 1168, *1169*
    preoperative evaluation before, 1168–1169
  treatment of, 1124, 1168
  epidemiology of, 1118–1119
  evaluation of, 1118–1128, 1130–1173
    discography in, 1136, *1137*
    facet blocks in, 1136
    history in, 1119–1120, 1134–1135
    imaging studies in, 1121, 1135–1136
    physical examination in, 1120–1121, 1135
  fusion for, extension of, 1155–1157, *1157–1159*
    operative approach to, 1157
    results of, 1156–1157, *1157–1159*
    previous, motion segment disorder after, 1155–1157, *1157–1159*
  iatrogenic flat back deformity in, 1157–1164, *1160*
    lordosis restoration in, 1162–1164, *1163, 1164*
    prevention of, 1157–1162, *1159–1162*
  imbalanced, lateral lumbar circumferential wedge osteotomy for, 1164–1167, *1165, 1166*
  in elderly, 1152–1155, *1154*
    treatment results in, 1153, 1155
  low back pain in, history of, 1119–1120
    incidence of, 1119
  natural history of, 1118–1119
  onset of, before skeletal maturity, 1130–1167
  paralytic curve in, 1152, *1153*
  posterior instrumentation for, 1125–1127, *1126*
  prevalence of, 1130–1131
  problem of, magnitude of, 1130–1134, *1132, 1133*
  prognosis in, 1131
    after surgery, 1132–1134
  progression of, factors in, 1131
  severe rigid deformity in, 1152
    treatment of, 1152
    results of, 1152
  special problems in, 1149–1155, *1153, 1154*
  surgery of, anterior, 1140–1143, *1142, 1143*
    complications of, 1127–1128, 1170–1172, 1171(t)
    considerations in, 1124–1125
    indications for, 1122, *1123*, 1138–1139, *1139*
      cosmesis as, 1138–1139
      deformity progression as, 1138
      neurologic deficit as, 1138, *1139*
      pain as, 1138
    posterior, 1143–1149, *1144–1148, 1150, 1151*
    staging of, 1172–1173
  treatment of, 1130–1173
    nonoperative, 1121–1122, 1136–1138
  types of, 1130
degenerative, fusion for, 1308
  progressing, 792
  spinal stenosis with, 746
fusion for, 1308
  history of, 589
  indications for, 1307
idiopathic, in children/adolescents, magnetic resonance imaging of, 369

Scoliosis *(Continued)*
  internal instrumentation for, 1222, 1226, *1227*
  intervertebral disc composition in, 272
  plain film radiography of, 349
  spinal stenosis with, case report of, 753–756, *754, 755*
    fusion for, 759–761, *760, 761*
    surgical treatment of, planning of, 777–778
  spondylolisthesis with, in children and adolescents, 676
    treatment of, 687, *688*
  transpedicle fixation in, neurologic complications of, 1205
Seat belt injuries. See *Flexion-distraction injuries.*
Segmental arteries, anatomy of, 125, *125*
Segmental instability, 782–794. See also *Spinal instability.*
  after decompressive laminectomy, 792–793, *793*
  after disc excision, 792
  after posterior lumbar spine surgery, 957–958
  after spinal fusion, 793–794
  axial rotational, 790–791, *791*
  biomechanics of, 783, *784–786*, 787
  classification of, 790–794, 790(t), *791, 793*
  definition of, 782, *783*
  degenerative, 788–790
    classification of, 790(t)
  differential diagnosis of, 449(t)
  fusion for, results of, 1307
  in multiply operated lumbar spine, 1109(t), 1111–1112
  in spondylolisthesis, and back pain, 657
    leg referral zone pain with, 658
  pathology of, 782
  radiography of, motion studies in, 787–788, *789*
    plain film, 347–348
  retrospondylolisthetic, 792
  signs/symptoms of, clinical, 787
    radiographic, 787, *787, 788*
  translational, 791
Segmental nerve, formation of, 45, *48*
Segmental rotation, in walking, in neurogenic claudication, 721–722
Segmental vessels, hemostasis of, in spinal fusion, 597
Selby II instrumentation, *603*
Self-Rating Pain and Distress Scale, 1320(t)
Selvik method, 30–31
Semispinal muscles, 52
Sensation, evaluation of, in disc herniation, 480
  recovery of, after cauda equina syndrome, 580, 587
    secondary to disc herniation, 587
Sensory nerve conduction, testing of, in radiculopathy localization, 149–150
  utilization of, 142(t)
Sensory nerves, classification of, 76, 77(t)
SEPs. See *Somatosensory evoked potentials (SEPs).*
Sequestration, chemonucleolysis in, 529
Serotonin, depletion of, in chronic low back pain, 1030
Sexual function, after lumbar sympathectomy, 571–572
  evaluation of, clinical neurophysiology in, 154–156
  neurologic control of, 571, 572(t)
  recovery of, after cauda equina syndrome, 580, 587
    secondary to disc herniation, 587
SF–20, 1318(t)
SF–36, 1317(t), 1318(t)

Sharpey fibers, 51
Shear injuries, 833, *834, 835*
Shigella flexneri, and reactive arthritis, 803(t), 804
Shiny corner sign, 339
SIADH (syndrome of inappropriate antidiuretic hormone secretion), after lumbar spine surgery, 947
    after scoliosis surgery, 1128
    in adults, 1171–1172
Sickle cell disease, in fusion outcome, 1289
Sickness Impact Profile, 1317(t), 1318(t)
Single-photon emission computed tomography (SPECT), of spondylolisthesis, 686
Sinuvertebral nerves, *64*
    anatomy of, 51
    in discogenic back pain, 463
Sitting, biomechanics of, 237–241, *239–241*
Sit-ups, in low back pain evaluation, 96
Skeleton, adaptation of, stimulus for, 972
    strength of, estimation of, 974–975
        experimental assessment of, 973–975
Slice fractures, 840, *844*
Slump test, in disc herniation, 479
Small sensory nerve evoked responses, in radiculopathy localization, 149
    testing of, methods of, 146–147
    utilization of, 142(t)
Smoking, in fusion outcome, 594, 1290
    in intervertebral disc nutrition, 300–301, *301*
    in low back pain, 92
    mechanical, 814
SMT (spinal manipulative therapy), for low back pain, 998–999, 1006–1008
Sodium, concentration of, in intervertebral disc, 275
Soft tissue, adjacent, in fusion outcome, 1285
Soleus, segmental innervation of, 1233(t)
Solute(s), concentration of, in intervertebral disc matrix, 296
    ionic, concentration of, 275, *276*
    macromolecular, distribution of, 277–278
    transport of, into intervertebral disc, 294–297, *295, 296*
        smoking in, 300, *301, 302*
Somatosensory evoked potentials (SEPs), dermatomal. See *Dermatomal somatosensory evoked potentials.*
    disadvantages of, 144–145
    eliciting of, magnetic stimulator in, 147
        methods of, 146–147, *148*
    in degenerative lumbar stenosis, 736
    in spinal cord lesions, 150–151, *152*
    in spinal stenosis, 156
    intraoperative monitoring of, 153–154, *155*
        during spinal fusion, 597
    mixed nerve, utilization of, 142(t)
    pudendal, in sacral nerve root evaluation, 150
Somites, formation of, 44, *45, 46*
Spasm, muscle, in low back pain, treatment of, 453
SPECT (single-photon emission computed tomography), of spondylolisthesis, 686
Spica, hip, 255, *255*
Spina bifida, spondylolisthesis with, 632
    congenital, 626–627, *628*
    spondylolysis with, 714–715, *715*
Spina bifida occulta, plain film radiography of, 349
Spinal anesthesia, in posterior lumbar spine surgery, advantages of, 946–947

Spinal canal, patency of, intraoperative ultrasonographic assessment of, 847, *847, 848*
    recalibrage of, for spinal stenosis, 770–771
    shape of, in disc herniation, 475
    ultrasonographic measurement of, in low back injury prediction, 1069
Spinal cord, arterial supply of, 574
    compression of, in ankylosing spondylitis, 801
        in spinal tumor, metastatic, laminectomy for, 935
            posterior decompression for, 934–935
            neurologic function in, 930–931, 932(t)
    infarction of, 573
        causes of, 574
    lesions of, evaluation of, clinical neurophysiology in, 150–151, *152–154*
    tumors of, 573
        extramedullary, 573
        intramedullary, 573
        treatment of, 574
    vasocorona of, vascular branches of, 125–126
Spinal dysraphism, in congenital spinal stenosis, 727
Spinal headache, after lumbar spine surgery, 954–955
Spinal instability, 203–210. See also *Segmental instability.*
    causes of, 203–207, *204, 205*
    degeneration and, *205,* 205–206
    diagnosis of, 207–209, *209*
        radiographic motion studies in, 207–208
    injury and, 203–205, *204, 205*
    lumbar fractures and, 824–825, *825,* 825(t)
    minimal/moderate, orthoses for, 867, 870–871
    postsurgical, orthoses for, 871
    spinal muscles in, 206–207
    three-column model of, 824–825, *825,* 825(t)
    treatment of, 209
        future of, 210
    two-column model of, 824
Spinal manipulative therapy (SMT), for low back pain, 998–999, 1006–1008
Spinal nerves, anatomy of, 51
    in up-down stenosis, 398, 400
Spinal rhythm, evaluation of, in low back pain, 93
Spinal rotation, evaluation of, in low back pain, 94
Spinal sclerosis, in pyogenic spondylitis, 885, *890*
Spinal stenosis, 359–362, 711–780
    absolute vs. relative, 726
    acquired, 726
        spondylolisthesis in, lysis with, 745–746
    "burned-out," computed tomography of, 408–409
    canal, classification of, 726–727
        surgical treatment of, results of, 767–768
        taxonomy of, 727
    central, 359–360
        and neurogenic claudication, 718–719, *719–721*
        chemonucleolysis in, 529
        fenestration procedures for, 740
        in degenerative spondylolisthesis, computed tomography of, 409, *411*
        in spondylosis, 394
        natural history of, 766–767
        postoperative, evaluation of, 418
        surgical treatment of, indications for, 773–774
    classification of, 724–764
    clinical presentation of, 359–360, 1234, 1234(t)
    combined, 726–727
    computed tomography of, blinded prospective analysis of, 414–415, 414(t)

Spinal stenosis *(Continued)*
    myelography vs., 413–418, 414(t)
    congenital, classification of, 727–728
    decompression for, degenerative adult scoliosis after, 1170
        extent of, 770–772
        method of, 770, 770–772, *771*
        prophylactic, indications for, 778, *779*
    definition of, 724–725
    degenerative. See *Degenerative lumbar stenosis (DLS)*.
    developmental, classification of, 728
    diagnosis of, 456–457
        differential, 449(t)
        tests for, accuracy of, 442–443, 443(t)
    disc disease with, 741
    disc herniation with, surgical treatment of, 520
    dynamic, computed tomography of, 409, *410*
    far-lateral, 741–742
        computed tomography of, *397*, 404–408, *407*
    far-out, 397
    front-back, *395*, *396*
        with pinhole stenosis, computed tomography of, 408
    fusion for, 757–764, 1308
        indications for, structural alterations in, intraoperative, 762
            preoperative, 757–762, *758–763*
        instrumentation for, 762–764, *764*
    history of, 724
    in low back pain algorithm, 456–457
    in multiply operated lumbar spine, 1109(t), 1112
    in spondylolisthesis, degenerative, fusion for, 1308
        intact neural arch with, 744–745
        surgical treatment of, 775–777, *776–778*
    laminectomy for, 737–740
        expansive laminoplasty vs., 740
    lateral. See *Lateral stenosis*.
    limbus vertebral fractures with, *742*, 742–744, *743*
    magnetic resonance imaging of, 360–362, *361*, *362*, 409, *410*
    movement analysis in, trunk muscle testing in, 1093–1094, *1095*
    myelography of, blinded prospective analysis of, 414–415, 414(t)
    natural history of, 725–726, 766–767, 1239–1240, *1240*
    nerve root compression in, biomechanics of, 128
    orthoses for, 257
    pathogenesis of, 393
    pinhole, *395*, *396*
    posttraumatic, 746–747
    primary vs. secondary, 727
    radiography of, 360–362, *361*, *362*
        plain film, 346–347, *347*
    recurrent, at same segment, fusion for, 761–762, *763*
        case report of, 750, *751*
        computed tomography of, myelography with, *751*, *752*
        fusion for, 1308
        postoperative bone regrowth and, 748–749
        secondary surgery for, 740–741
    scoliosis with, case report of, 753–756, *754*, *755*
        degenerative, 746
        surgical treatment of, planning of, 777–778
    somatosensory evoked potentials in, 156
    subarticular, computed tomography of, 390, *391*, *397*

Spinal stenosis *(Continued)*
    in degenerative spondylolisthesis, computed tomography of, 409, *411*
    surgical anatomy of, 60
    taxonomy of, 726–730
    treatment of, 724–764, 1245–1246, 1250
        conservative, results of, 767
        effectiveness of, 33(t)
        surgical, 737–756
            and cerebrospinal fluid fistula, 747–748
            and facet fracture, 749
            and infection, 749–750
            and pseudomeningocele, 747–748
            and vascular injury, 750
            complications of, 747–756
                age-related, 747
                case reports of, 750, *751–755*, 753, 755–756
                psychosocial, 747
            guidelines for, 773–780
            indications for, 773–775
            instability after, 769–770
            planning of, 775–778, *775–779*
            results of, 767–773
                age at operation in, 772
                comorbidity in, 773
                follow-up duration in, 772–773
                long-term, 766–780
                previous surgery in, 773
                recurrence in, 773, *774*
                stenosis type/severity in, 772
            technique of, 778–780
    two level, and neurogenic claudication, 719–720, *720*, *721*
    up-down. See *Up-down stenosis*.
Spinalis muscle, 52
Spine, bamboo, 800
    biomechanical adaptation of, 979–981, *981*
    curvature of, acquisition of, 265–266, *266*
        need for, 263–264, *265*
    degeneration of, stages of, 205
    disability of, evaluation of, guidelines for, 1075
    disorders of, direct costs of, 13, 15(t)
    evaluation of, postoperative, computed tomography in, 418–420, *419*
        myelography in, 418–420, *419*
    function of, evolutionary perspective of, 259–269
        fundamentals of, 1042–1045
        measurement of, 1045–1048
            functional capacity testing in, 1047–1048
                aerobic capacity testing in, 1047–1048
                effort assessment in, 1048
                lift testing in, 1047
                obstacle course in, 1048
            physical capacity testing in, 1046–1047
                range-of-motion measurements in, 1047–1048
                trunk strength measurement in, 1048
    healthy, 20–21, *21*
    in psoriatic spondyloarthropathy, 806
    lumbar. See *Lumbar spine*.
    mobility of, loss of, in dysfunction syndrome, 1004
    stiffness of, measurement of, 783, 787
    thoracic, hypokyphotic, posterior instrumentation for, 1148
    thoracolumbar. See *Thoracolumbar spine*.
SPINE Institute of New England program, functional restoration outcomes in, 1051
Spitalfield study, 713

Split fractures, 838(t), 839, *839*
Split-half reliability, in health status outcome measurement, 1329–1330, 1329(t)
Spondylitis, ankylosing. See *Ankylosing spondylitis (AS).*
  in Reiter syndrome, 805
  orthoses for, 257
  psoriasis with, 806
  pyogenic, 885–889
    and paraplegia, 894
    bone scan of, 887–889
    computed tomography of, 887
    diagnosis of, 885
    magnetic resonance imaging of, 889, *891*
    radiography of, 885–887, *889, 890*
    treatment of, conservative, 892–893
      surgical, 894–896, *895*
  tuberculous, magnetic resonance imaging of, 878, *881*
Spondylitis deformans, occurrence rate of, 20, *20*
Spondyloarthropathy(ies), classification of, European criteria for, 798, 799(t)
  differential diagnosis of, 449(t)
  inflammatory, 797–810
    definition of, 797
    etiology of, 809–810
    historical review of, 797
    pathogenesis of, 809–810
  psoriatic. See *Psoriatic spondyloarthropathy.*
Spondylolisthesis, 621–708
  acquired, after spinal fusion, for segmental instability, 794
  back pain in, 656–658
    causes of, 657–658
    leg referral zone pain with, 658
      causes of, 658
  classification of, 621–637
    anatomic, *622–625,* 623–626, 623(t)
  clinical subtypes of, 656–658
  congenital, 626–630, *627–629*
    etiology of, 631–633
    inheritance of, 626–627, 633
    isthmic vs., 649
    kyphosis with, 628–630
    natural history of, 638
    spina bifida with, 626–627, *628*
    surgery for, 643
    types of, *622,* 623
  controversy in, 644–649
  definition of, 621
  degenerative, 623, *634,* 634–635
    after spinal stenosis surgery, *752,* 753, *753*
    and neurogenic claudication, 717–718, *718*
    anterior surgery for, 508, *509*
    computed tomography of, 409–413, *411*
    decompression for, fusion with, 957
      types of, 649, *650*
    definition of, 700–701
    disc herniation in, 412
    etiology of, 701
    fusion for, types of, 649, *650*
    in adults, differential diagnosis of, 703
      epidemiology of, 701
      physical examination of, 701–702
      radiologic evaluation of, 702–703
      symptoms of, 701–702
      treatment of, 703–708

Spondylolisthesis *(Continued)*
      conservative, 703–704
      surgical, 700–708, 704–708, *706, 708*
    natural history of, 639
    pathoanatomy of, 700–701
    pathophysiology of, 701
    plain film radiography of, 345, *346*
    spinal stenosis with, computed tomography of, 409, *411*
      fusion for, 757–759, *758, 759,* 1308
      intact neural arch in, 744–745
      surgical treatment of, planning of, 775–777, *776–778*
    surgical treatment of, instability after, 770
      results of, 769
    synovial cyst in, imaging of, 384, *387*
  diagnosis of, 623–637
    differential, 449(t)
  disc herniation with, surgical treatment of, 520
  dysplastic, surgery for, 684–698
  etiology of, 684–685
  evaluation of, 685–686, *686*
  hamstring tightness in, causes of, 646, *647, 648*
    surgery for, 643
  in children and adolescents, above previously fused level, 676
    fusion for, anterior, 672
      anterior/posterior, 674
      in situ, 671
      laminectomy with, 671–672
      posterolateral, 679–680, *680*
    iatrogenic, 676
    isthmic defect repair for, 674
    laminectomy for, 671–672
    pseudarthrosis repair in, 675
    reduction of, 674–675, 680–681
    scoliosis with, 676
    surgery for, 669–681
      care after, 675
      considerations in, 669–670
      indications for, 671, *672, 673,* 676–679, 677(t), *678, 679*
      methods of, 671–675
      risk factors in, clinical, 670
        radiographic, 670
      selection of, 676, 677(t)
  inheritance of, 631(t)
  intervertebral disc composition in, 272
  isthmic, *630,* 630–631, 631(t)
    after decompression, 957
    congenital vs., 649
    etiology of, 631–633
    fusion for, 1308
    inheritance of, 633
    natural history of, 638–639
    surgery for, 640, *640–643,* 684–698
    types of, 623, *623, 624*
    vertebral canal in, *714,* 715, *715*
  localized, 637
  lytic, 630, *630*
    and acquired spinal stenosis, 745–746
    treatment of, nonoperative, 654–667
      corticosteroid injections in, 665–666
      exercise training in, 659–665
      goal setting in, 654–655
      lumbar braces/corsets in, 659
      manipulation/traction in, 659

Spondylolisthesis *(Continued)*
  medications in, 658–659
  rehabilitation in, 655–656, 655(t), 656(t), 657(t)
  surgical, referral for, 666–667
  up-down stenosis with, computed tomography of, 403–404, 405, 406
    magnetic resonance imaging of, 404, 406, 408
    mechanism of, 404
  magnetic resonance imaging of, 367
  natural history of, 637–639
  orthoses for, 256
  paresthesia syndrome in, 658
  pars interarticularis defect with, plain film radiography of, 341–342, 343
  pathogenesis of, 684–685
  pathologic, 635–637, 636
    types of, 623, 626
  postsurgical, 635
    types of, 623
  posttraumatic, 623, 625, 635
  progression of, 684
  reduction of, 691–692
    anterior/posterior, 693–694, 696
    indications for, 691
    posterior, 692–693, 694, 695
    vertebral body resection in, 694–698, 697
  research on, 644–649
  reversed, in spinal tuberculosis, 878, 880
  scoliosis with, treatment of, 687, 688
  spondylolytic, anterior surgery in, 508, 509
  transpedicle fixation in, neurologic complications of, 1205
  treatment of, 686–698
    conservative, 686
    decompression in, 687
    fusion in, 687
      in situ, anterior, 689–691, 691
        posterior, 687–689, 690
      instrumentation for, 689
      internal, 1222, 1226
    spondylolysis repair in, 687
    surgical, 640–644, 640–646
      cauda equina syndrome after, 643–644, 644
      pedicle screws in, 644, 645, 646
  types of, 626–637, 627–630, 631(t), 632, 634, 636
Spondylolysis, classification of, 623–626
  healed, diagnosis of, 631
  in low back pain, 454–455
  inheritance of, 631(t)
  magnetic resonance imaging of, 367, 367
  natural history of, 637–639
  orthoses for, 256
  plain film radiography of, 341–342, 342, 343
  repair of, 687
  repetitive lumbar spine loading and, 185–186
  spina bifida with, 714–715, 715
Spondyloptosis, reduction of, vertebral body resection in, 694–698, 697
Spondylosis, computed tomography of, 392–397
  pathogenesis of, 393
  spinal stenosis in, 393–394
Spondylosis deformans, in miners, 183
Spur, traction, in segmental instability, 787, 787
Stabilization, of thoracolumbar spine, biomechanics of, 212–231
Standing, biomechanics of, 237, 238

Standing *(Continued)*
  vibration effects on, 196
Stanozolol, for mechanical back pain, 814
Steel, titanium, for spinal implants, 1310
Steffee screws, 1183
Steffee (VSP) system, 1191–1192
  complications of, 1206–1207
  evaluation of, canine models in, 229
    in vitro, 213–215, 215, 217, 218
  fatigue strength of, 1193
  screw-plate fixation in, 1210
Steinmann pins, in twelfth rib approach, to anterior spine surgery, 1269
Stenosis, achondroplastic, surgical treatment of, results of, 768
  "burned-out," computed tomography of, 408–409
  of intervertebral foramen, in spinal stenosis, magnetic resonance imaging of, 361–362, 362
  surgical treatment of, indications for, 774–775
    results of, 769
  spinal. See *Spinal stenosis*.
  subarticular, computed tomography of, 390, 391, 397
    pathogenesis of, 393
Steroids. See *Corticosteroids*.
Stiffness, morning, 90–91
Straight leg raising test, after anterior extraperitoneal discectomy, without fusion 1275, 1278
  before anterior extraperitoneal discectomy, without fusion, 1275, 1275
  components of, 1232, 1233
  crossed, in disc herniation, 479
  in disc herniation, 479
  passive, in low back pain, 96
  positive, as low back injury predictor, 1070
Strain, back, differential diagnosis of, 449(t)
  etiology of, 452
  treatment of, local injection in, 455
  lumbosacral, and low back disorders, 236
  orthoses for, 256
Strength, lifting, as low back injury claims predictor, 1068
  testing of, 1079–1080
    isometric testing with, 1083–1084
  submaximum testing of, preemployment, 1096
  ultimate, definition of, 182
Strength training, for spondylolisthesis, 661–663
  of extremities, for spondylolisthesis, 660–661
Streptomycin, for spinal tuberculosis, 880–882
Stress fracture, of ilium, after bone grafting, 963, 964
  of pars interarticularis, in young athlete, 633
    treatment of, 646–647, 648
Stressors, interpersonal, in low back pain, 1025–1026
Stretching, in lumbar spine manipulation, 1013, 1013(t)
Stromer's law, 43
Subarachnoid hemorrhage, arteriovenous malformation with, 573
Subarticular entrapment, 115, 116
Subarticular stenosis, computed tomography of, 390, 391, 397
  pathogenesis of, 393
Sublaminar plexus, imaging of, in axial plane, 321, 322, 324, 324
Sublaminar wires, for adult scoliosis, 1143, 1144
  for internal fixation, history of, 589–590
Subluxation, in pyogenic spondylitis, 885, 890

Subluxation *(Continued)*
　in spinal tuberculosis, 878, *879*
Submaximum strength testing, preemployment, 1096
Substance P, changes in, in nerve root compression, 131, 133
　in low back pain, 81–82
Sulfasalazine, for ankylosing spondylitis, 803
Sulfate, concentration of, in intervertebral disc, 275
　after exercise, 298, *298*
Sunshine laws, 1341
Superior cluneal nerves, injury to, during bone grafting, 965
Superior gluteal artery, hemostasis of, in spinal fusion, 597, *597*
　injury to, during bone grafting, 964, 965
Superior gluteal nerve, injury to, during bone grafting, 965
Superior hypogastric plexus, location of, 508, 511, *511*
　protection of, in anterior retroperitoneal transverse spine surgery, 1269–1270, *1270*
Superior mesenteric artery syndrome, after scoliosis surgery, 1128
Supraspinous ligament, anatomy of, 51
Sympathectomy, lumbar, sexual functioning after, 571–572
Sympathetic nervous system, anatomy of, 570
Sympathetic plexus, injury to, during anterior lumbar spine surgery, 962
Symphysiolysis, in pregnancy, 1061
Symphysis, definition of, 49
Synarthrosis, definition of, 47, 49
Synchondrosis, neurocentral, 47
Syndesmophyte(s), in ankylosing spondylitis, 798
　radiography of, 800
　　plain film, 340, *340*
　in psoriatic spondyloarthropathy, 806
Syndesmosis, definition of, 49
Syndrome of inappropriate antidiuretic hormone secretion (SIADH), after lumbar spine surgery, 947
　after scoliosis surgery, 1128
　in adults, 1171–1172
Synovial cyst(s), chondroma vs., 384, *387*
　computed tomography of, 384, *387*
　in degenerative spondylolisthesis, imaging of, 384, *387*
　magnetic resonance imaging of, 384, *387*
Synovitis, in SAPHO syndrome, 808

T

T_4, measurement of, before spinal fusion, 595
Tachykinins, in compressed nerve root pain, 133
TCAs (tricyclic antidepressants), for chronic low back pain, 1030–1032, 1031(t)
　in spondylolisthesis, 659
TCP (tricalcium phosphate) ceramics, in bone grafting, 1294
　animal studies of, 1297–1298
Technetium 99m-labeled medronate disodium bone scan. See *Bone scan, technetium 99m-labeled medronate disodium.*
Tendons, in chronic low back pain, rehabilitation of, 1045
Tensiometer, cable, in trunk muscle strength evaluation, 1077
Tension sign, in disc herniation, 478–480
　in multiply operated lumbar spine, 1107

Tension sign *(Continued)*
　in sciatica, 456
Testosterone, measurement of, before spinal fusion, 595
Test-retest reliability, in health status outcome measurement, 1329
Tetracycline, for reactive arthritis, 805
Texas Scottish Rite Hospital (TSRH) system, 746
　for adult scoliosis, 1141–1142
　in vitro evaluation of, 218
Thalassemia major, in fusion outcome, 1289
Thecal sac, imaging of, in axial plane, 318, *319, 320, 322, 324, 325*
　in coronal plane, *331*
　in sagittal plane, *328*
Thermography, in disc herniation, accuracy of, 442, 442(t)
　in reflex sympathetic dystrophy, 156
　utilization of, 142(t)
Thermotherapy, for disc herniation, 484
Thigh, pain in, in low back pain algorithm, 457
Thigh thrust test, in sacroiliac joint dysfunction, 562
Third-party payers, in spine care, 1340
Thoracic myelopathy, 572–574
　causes of, 573
Thoracic spine, hypokyphotic, posterior instrumentation for, 1148
Thoracolumbar junction, imaging of, in coronal plane, *331*
　surgery of, anterior approach to, ninth rib resection in, 1254
　trauma to, imaging of, 420, 423
Thoracolumbar spine, curvature of, in adult scoliosis, 1145–1146, *1146–1148*
　stabilization of, biomechanics of, 212–231
　surgery of, anterior, 1252–1271
　　eleventh rib approach to, 1258–1260, *1259, 1261*
　　　closure in, 1260
　　incisions for, 1253
　　patient positioning for, 1253
　　retroperitoneal, 1254
　　tenth rib approach to, 1255–1258, *1255–1258*
　　　closure in, 1258
　　transperitoneal, 1254
　　twelfth rib approach to, 1262–1269, *1263–1265, 1267, 1268*
　　　closure in, 1266–1269, *1267, 1268*
Thoracolumbosacral orthosis (TLSO), 253, 253–254
　for burst fractures, 850, 853
　for compression fractures, 850
　for lateral wedge injuries, 860
　for spinal instability, minimal to moderate, 867, 870–871
　　postoperative, 871
　for spinal tumor, 933
Thoracoplasty, for adult scoliosis, 1139
Three-joint complex, 52–57
　degeneration of, clinical implications of, 54–56, *55*
　　end stage of, 56
　　natural history of, 54, *55*
　　surgical intervention for, 56–57
　healthy, 53–54
Thrombus, formation of, in mechanical back pain, 817, *817, 818*
Thrust techniques, of lumbar spine manipulation, 1013, 1013(t)

Thymosin α_1, in vertebral canal size, 715
Thyroid hormones, in fusion outcome, 1289
Tiaprofenic acid, injection of, for outer annular tear, in animal models, 284
Tibia, bone grafting from, for spinal fusion, 592
Tibialis anterior, segmental innervation of, 1233(t)
Titanium steel, for spinal implants, 1310
TLSO. See *Thoracolumbosacral orthosis (TLSO).*
Toe, great, dorsiflexion of, evaluation of, 94
Tomography, computed. See *Computed tomography (CT).*
  liquid crystal, before laminectomy, 1237
Torsion, repetitive, of motion segments, mechanical effects of, 189–190
Traction, for disc herniation, 484
  for low back pain, 1008
  for spondylolisthesis, 659
Traction spur, 51
  in segmental instability, 787, *787*
Training, aerobic, 664
  athletic, repetitive lumbar spine loading in, in vivo observation of, 187–188
    risk factors for, 184–185
  endurance, 663
  exercise, 659–666
  flexibility, 663–664
  in workplace, 995–996
  muscle, for low back pain, 29
  strength, 661–663
  weight, 660–661
Tranquilizers, for chronic low back pain, 1029–1030
Transcutaneous electrical nerve stimulation, for disc herniation, 484
Transforaminal ligament, anatomy of, 67
Transfusion, blood, after scoliosis surgery, 1128
Transpedicle fixation, biomechanical testing of, 1194–1196, 1195(t)
  biomechanics of, 1177–1197
  complications of, 1203–1214, 1309
    intraoperative, 1203–1206
      neurologic, 1203–1205
      vascular, 1205–1206
      visceral, 1206
    postoperative, 1211–1213
      infection in, 1211–1212
      juxtafusion deterioration in, 1213
      pseudarthrosis in, 1212
    technical, 1206–1211, *1207–1212*
  development of, 1177–1181, *1179*
  distraction rods in, 1180
  fixators in, 1180–1181
  for adult scoliosis, 1125, *1126*
  for burst fractures, 853, *856*
  for flexion-distraction injuries, *858*, 860, *861, 862*
  for osteoporosis, 1213–1214
  for posterior fusion, devices for, 601, *603*, 604
    for disc degeneration, 466–467
  for posterolateral fusion, for disc degeneration, 465
  for spinal fracture, 863, *866*
  for spinal stenosis, 763–764, *764*
    advantages of, 763
    disadvantages of, 763–764
    with degenerative spondylolisthesis, 776–777, *777, 778*
  for spinal tumors, 941
  for spondylolisthesis, 644, *645, 646*, 689
    degenerative, 707, *708*

Transpedicle fixation *(Continued)*
    results of, 769
  in children and adolescents, 680
  history of, 5, 590
  implant intolerance after, 1214
  implant removal in, 1197
  morphometry in, 1181, *1182*, 1182(t)
  of sacrum, screw placement in, 1185, 1185(t)
  postoperative management in, 1196–1197, 1196(t)
  risk-benefit ratio in, 862
  screw design in, 1181–1183
  screw placement in, 1183–1191, *1184–1186*, 1185(t), *1188, 1189*, 1190(t)
    depth of, 1187–1188, *1188, 1189*
    entry site/orientation in, 1183–1187, *1184–1186*, 1185(t)
    hole preparation for, 1188–1189, 1190(t)
    longitudinal linkage between, 1191–1194
      fatigue strength in, 1193
      implant stiffness in, 1192
      positional control in, 1191–1192
      reduction in, 1193
    polymethyl methacrylate in, 1189–1191
  systems for, evaluation of, artificial spine models in, 221
    in vitro, 217–218
  transverse connectors in, 1194
Transversalis fascia, of diaphragm, 1255
  opening of, in twelfth rib approach to anterior spine surgery, 1262, *1264*
Transverse process, anatomy of, 49, *50*
Transverse process artery, hemostasis of, in spinal fusion, 596–597, *597*
Transversus abdominis, opening of, in twelfth rib approach, to anterior spine surgery, 1262, *1264*
Trauma, and disc degeneration, 305
  and low back pain, 89
  computed tomography of, 423
  fusion for, indications for, 1307
  internal instrumentation for, 1220–1222, *1222–1224*
  magnetic resonance imaging of, 374–375
  to thoracolumbar junction, computed tomography of, 420–423
Trazodone, for chronic low back pain, 1031(t)
Trendelenburg test, in low back pain, 94
Tricalcium phosphate (TCP) ceramics, in bone grafting, 1294
  animal studies of, 1297–1298
Tricyclic antidepressants (TCAs), for chronic low back pain, 1030–1032, 1031(t)
  in spondylolisthesis, 659
Trunk, in locomotion, 264–268
  motion of, during lifting, 248, *249*
Trunk muscles, activity of, during lumbar spine loading, 169
  endurance of, 1080–1083, *1081, 1082*
    in healthy subjects, 1097–1098
    testing of, applications of, 1097–1100, *1099*
  evaluation of, in industrial low back pain, 1074–1100
  fatigue of, in industrial low back pain, 1097–1100, *1099*
  movement of, dynamic, 1080–1083, *1081, 1082*
  performance of, quantification of, 1075–1077
  strength of, measurement of, 1047
    dynamic, 1077–1079, *1079*
    isokinetic, 1047

Trunk muscles *(Continued)*
    isometric, 1047
    static, 1077–1079, *1079*
    testing of, clinical applications of, 1088–1096, *1089, 1092–1095*
        functional capacity in, 1087
        inverse/direct dynamics in, 1084–1087, *1085, 1086*
        occupational applications of, 1096–1097
        preemployment, 1096–1097
        task demands in, 1087
TSRH (Texas Scottish Rite Hospital) system, 746
    for adult scoliosis, 1141–1142
    in vitro evaluation of, 218
Tuberculosis, of spine, 874–897
    diagnosis of, *876–881*, 877–878
        magnetic resonance imaging in, 878, *881*
        radiography in, *876–880*, 877–878
    distribution of, 874–875, *875*
    Pott paraplegia in, 876–877
    presentation of, patterns of, 875–876
    reactivation of, 875
    treatment of, 880–885
        conservative, 880–882
        preferred, 883–885, *884, 886–888*
        surgical, 882–883, 883(t)
Tumor(s), of spine, 917–942
    anatomic extent of, 935, *936*
    angiography of, 921
    benign, 921–922, *923–927*
    bone scan of, 920
    clinical presentation of, 918–919, 918(t)
    computed tomography of, 920, *920*
    differential diagnosis of, 449(t)
    in fusion outcome, 1287
    in low back pain algorithm, 452
    magnetic resonance imaging of, 372–374, *374*, 920–921
        in children/adolescents, 368
    malignant, 922, 927–928, 928(t), 929(t)
        survival in, 929(t)
    metastatic, 928–931
        distribution of, 929–930
        magnetic resonance imaging of, 373–374, *374*
        neurologic status in, 930–931, 932(t)
        origins of, 928
        pathogenesis of, 930, *931*
        pathophysiology of, 929–930
        prognosis in, 928–929
        treatment of, 929
    myelography of, 920
    primary, 921, *921, 922*
        magnetic resonance imaging of, 372–373
    radiography of, *919*, 919–921, *920*
    surgical stabilization of, 935–941, *936, 937, 939–941*
        case history of, 938, *940, 941*
        complications of, 938–941
        resection zones for, 935–938, *937, 939*
    treatment of, 931–933
        algorithm for, 919, *919*
        braces in, 932–933
        goals of, 917
        radiotherapy in, 932
        surgery in, 931–932
            approaches to, 933–935, 933(t)
            indications for, 933

Tumor(s) *(Continued)*
    margin extent in, 936

U

Ulcerative colitis, inflammatory spondyloarthropathy in, 807–808
Ultrasonography, during laminectomy, for spinal stenosis, 739
    in spinal canal measurement, in low back injury prediction, 1069
    intraoperative, 847, *847, 848*
    of spinal fractures, 847
Uncinate spur, 394–396, *395, 397*
    in up-down stenosis, 398, *399*, 400, *401*, 402, *403*
Up-down stenosis, 394, *395*
    computed tomography of, 398–402, *399, 401–403*
    etiology of, 398
    lytic spondylolisthesis with, computed tomography of, 403–404, *405, 406*
        magnetic resonance imaging of, 404, *406*, 408
        mechanism of, 404
    uncinate spurring in, 398, *399*, 400, *401*, 402, *403*
Ureaplasma urealyticum, and reactive arthritis, 803(t)
Ureter, injury to, bone grafting and, 965
    during anterior lumbar spine surgery, 963
Urethra, stimulation of, anal sphincter reflex in, 151, *154*
Urethritis, in reactive arthritis, 804
Urinary retention, after lumbar spine surgery, 947
    after scoliosis surgery, 1128
Urinary tract, disorder of, and anterior thigh pain, 457
    infection of, after scoliosis surgery, 1128
Urination, neurologic control of, 570–571, 572(t)
Uveitis, in ankylosing spondylitis, 800
    in psoriatic spondyloarthropathy, 807
    in reactive arthritis, 804

V

Vacuum sign, 341, *341, 344*
Validity, in health status outcome measurement, 1331–1332
Valvulitis, in reactive arthritis, 804
Variable screw placement (VSP) system. See *Steffee (VSP) system.*
Vasocorona, of spinal cord, vascular branches of, 125–126
Vasodilation, arterial, in neurogenic claudication, 720–721
VDS (ventral derotation system), 1222, 1226
Vein(s). See also names of specific veins.
    injury to, transpedicle fixation and, 1205–1206
Velocity, conduction, of nerve endings, in lumbar facet capsule, 79, 79(t)
Vena cava, inferior, hemostasis of, in spinal fusion, 597
    protection of, in anterior retroperitoneal transverse spine surgery, 1271
Ventral derotation system (VDS), 1222, 1226
Ventral ramus syndrome, in spondylolisthesis, 658
Vermont fixator, 1183
    in vitro evaluation of, 216
Vertebra(e), concertina collapse of, in spinal tuberculosis, 877, *877*
    destruction of, symmetric, in pyogenic spondylitis, 885, *889*

Vertebra(e) *(Continued)*
  displacement of, and neurogenic claudication, 717–718, *718*
  failure of, loading in, 823
  fracture of, limbus, spinal stenosis with, *742*, 742–744, *743*
    osteoporosis in, 969–970
    risk of, estimation of, 974–975
      experimental assessment of, 973–975
    threshold for, 973
  hypermobility of, after spinal stenosis surgery, 770
  level of, in mechanical/physical properties, 975
  loading of, aging in, 823
  lumbar, formation of, 45, *48*
    repetitive loading of, in vitro investigations of, 188–189
  morphology of, *976*, 976–979, *979*, *980*
  segmentation of, failure of, in congenital spinal stenosis, 727
  slipping of, after spinal stenosis surgery, 770
  strength of, 972–976
  transitional, plain film radiography of, 349, *350*
Vertebral body(ies), anatomy of, 49, *50*
  changes in, aging in, 400–402
  elements of, posterior, *494*, 495, *495*
    superior, 495, *495*
  fracture of, orthoses for, 256
  imaging of, in axial plane, 318, *321*
    in sagittal plane, 325, *327*, *328*
  resection of, for spondylolisthesis, 694–698, *697*
    for spondyloptosis, 694–698, *697*
  zones of, for surgical resection, 935–938, *937*
Vertebral canal, bony component of, importance of, 711–712
  maturation of, *712*, 712–713
  clinical relevance of, 711, *712*
  development of, 711–716
    factors in, 713–714, *714*
    immune system in, 715–716
  imaging of, in axial plane, 318, *322*
    in sagittal plane, 327, *328*
  in isthmic spondylolisthesis, *714*, 715, *715*
  size of, 713–714, *714*
  soft tissue component of, importance of, 711–712
  trefoil-shaped, development of, 713
  in subarticular stenosis, *390*, *391*
Vertebral wedge osteotomy, for ankylosing spondylitis, 803
Vertebrectomy, for spondyloptosis, 694–698, *697*
"Veterinarian ethic," 1340
Vibration, electromyographic studies of, 196
  human response to, 194–196
  in intervertebral disc nutrition, 299–300, *300*
  natural frequency of, studies of, 194
  occupational exposure to, 192–194
    in aircraft, 193–194
    in automobiles, 192–193
    in earth-moving equipment, 194
  of lumbar spine, effects of, 181–197
  studies of, 195–196
  transmissibility of, studies of, 194–195
Visual Analogue Scales, in pain measurement, 1320(t)
Vitamin D, measurement of, before spinal fusion, 595
von Willebrand factor (vWf), in mechanical back pain evaluation, 818–819, *819*
VSP (variable screw placement) system. See *Steffee (VSP) system.*

vWf (von Willebrand factor), in mechanical back pain evaluation, 818–819, *819*

W

Waddell score, in chronic low back pain, 1027
Waddell's nonorganic physical signs, in chronic low back pain, 1028
WAIS-R (Wechsler Adult Intelligence Scale), in low back pain, 1049
Walking. See also *Locomotion.*
  in neurogenic claudication, Baston venous plexus in, 722
    dynamics of, 720–722
    failed arterial response in, 720–721
    lumbar artery shunt during, 722
    segmental rotation in, 721–722
Water, in intervertebral discs, 290–291
  biochemistry of, 312
Water-acceptance test, in chemonucleolysis, 528
Water-based exercise, for spondylolisthesis, 662
WBC (white blood cell) count, in infection, after spinal stenosis surgery, 749–750
Wechsler Adult Intelligence Scale (WAIS-R), in low back pain, 1049
Weight, reduction of, for adult scoliosis, 1121
  restriction of, for lifting, 246–248, *247*
Weight training, for spondylolisthesis, 660–661
  repetitive lumbar spine loading in, 184
Well leg lifting, crossover pain vs., 96
West Haven–Yale Multidimensional Pain Inventory, 1317(t), 1320(t)
Whipple disease, inflammatory spondyloarthropathy in, 808
White blood cell (WBC) count, in infection, after spinal stenosis surgery, 749–750
Wiltse instrumentation, *603*
Wolff's law, 976, 980
Women, ankylosing spondylitis in, 801
Workers' compensation, for low back pain, 12–14, 13(t), *14*
Workplace, education in, 995–996
Wound infection, after lumbar spine surgery, 949–950
  deep, 949–950
    treatment of, 950
  superficial, 949
    treatment of, 949

X

Xenograft, materials for, 1293

Y

Yersinia enterocolitica, and reactive arthritis, 803(t), 804
Yersinia pseudotuberculosis, and reactive arthritis, 803(t), 804
Yuan I-beam plates, for adult scoliosis, 1156, *1158*
Yuan Syracuse plate, for anterior fusion, 607

Z

Zielke device, 746
  for adult scoliosis, 1141
  in elderly, complications of, 1153, 1155
  results with, 1142–1143

Zielke device *(Continued)*
   with paralytic curves, *1153*
Zygapophyseal joint, anatomy of, 68
   fracture of, 556

Zygapophyseal joint *(Continued)*
   in low back pain, 999
   pain from, etiology of, 556–557
   pathology of, disc degeneration with, 393

ISBN 0-7216-6943-3

90038